Quick Reference to Occupational Therapy
Second Edition

Kathlyn L. Reed, PhD, OTR, FAOTA, MLIS, AHIP
Visiting Professor
School of Occupational Therapy
Texas Woman's University–Houston Center
Houston, Texas

Rhona Reiss Zukas, Consulting Editor

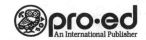
pro·ed
An International Publisher
8700 Shoal Creek Boulevard
Austin, Texas 78757-6897
800/897-3202   Fax 800/397-7633
www.proedinc.com

Library of Congress Cataloging-in-Publication Data

Reed, Kathlyn L.
Quick reference to occupational therapy / Kathlyn L. Reed; Rhonda Reiss
Zukas, consulting editor,—2nd ed.
   p. ; cm.
Originally published: Gaithersberg, Md. : Aspen Publishers, 2001
   Includes bibliographical references and index.
   ISBN-13: 978-094448080-9
   ISBN-10: 0-944480-80-2
1. Occupational Therapy-Handbooks, manuals, etc.   I. Tilte
(DNLM: 1. Occupational therapy-Handbooks. WB 39R324q 2001a]
RM735.3.R42 2002
615.8'515—DC21

2003043186

6   7   8   9   10   11   12   13   17   16   15   14   13   12   11

Table of Contents

Introduction

The purpose of this handbook is to provide students, practitioners, and researchers with a ready source of information about disorders or conditions seen in occupational therapy practice, as documented in published literature. Each disorder or condition is summarized using the same outline and headings. This consistency allows for quick review and for comparison between topics. The summary may be useful in conferring with a team of professionals regarding aspects of intervention and approaches used in practice or research, as documented in the occupational therapy literature. The references can be consulted to seek additional information, to write a literature review, or to summarize findings for a research project. References for this edition were restricted to 1993 forward, except for the occasional citation to a classic article.

The organization of each disease or disorder is designed to reflect the "top-down" approach to assessment and intervention. That is, occupations or performance areas are discussed before components of function. In other words, self-care, productivity, and leisure are discussed before sensorimotor, cognitive, and psychosocial issues. Although the profession has made an effort to talk about occupational performance areas before performance components, the literature remains heavily dominated by the "bottom-up" approach. Nearly all of the literature reviewed discusses sensorimotor, cognitive, and psychosocial issues before discussing self-care or activities of daily living, work or homemaking tasks, and leisure activities. The "bottom-up" approach is apparent even in textbooks with the most current copyright dates. If the profession is going to talk "top-down," there needs to be a concerted effort to walk (and write) top-down.

Because the profession continues to write "bottom-up," many of the presentations for self-care, productivity, and leisure occupations appear lean and anemic. Lack of content is to blame. More assessment and intervention needs to address the occupation or performance areas before the outline for each disease or disorder will begin to look more balanced.

This handbook is based solely on published literature on the application of occupational therapy to service delivery and research. The author has made a conscious effort to record the printed or published information while avoiding personal interpretation to the extent that is possible. No unpublished or personal knowledge has been deliberately included. Where information seems scant or lacking, that information has not been published in a format identifiable to the author. If oversights have occurred, the author would be pleased to know about them. All references used in the preparation of the handbook have been listed in the References section following each topic. Usually, a particular reference is used once, but a few cover more than one topic in some detail and, thus, were used twice or, rarely, three times.

The person who is the focus of assessment, intervention, or research is usually referred to as *the person*. In context where the person is not appropriate, the word *individual* or *client* is used. If the person is a child, the term *the child* has been used. Because individuals can interact with occupational therapy personnel in many roles and titles, the most generic term has been used. Humans are persons first—an important consideration in all intervention and research. Professional and technical-level persons educated in occupational therapy are referred to as *occupational therapy personnel*. No attempt has been made to separate roles and functions of different levels of occupational therapy personnel because management and legal issues are not the focus of the handbook. The author assumes that occupational therapy personnel know what education and skills have been attained and how to apply that knowledge to occupational therapy assessment, intervention, and research. Occasionally, a note has been added regarding special requirements that all or most occupational therapy personnel would need to use specific physical agent modalities or techniques not routinely taught to occupational therapy personnel at any level. An example is the treatment of hand injuries, in which numerous physical modalities are used by some occupational therapy personnel but for which specialized training or continuing education is usually attained.

More named assessment instruments were noted in this revision than in the first edition, especially in regard to conditions seen in children. To help occupational therapy personnel sort which assessments were developed within the profession versus those developed by other professionals, the assessment instruments have been divided into two subsections. The major concern is that assessments developed by other professionals may not actually measure what occupational therapy personnel want to measure, and the results may not be consistent with the philosophy and/or frame of reference inherent in the domain of occupational therapy. When assessment instruments have been developed for other purposes in other professions, occupational therapy personnel need to determine whether the assessment can be used successfully within the context of occupational therapy theory and practice.

Of concern are the many errors noted in citations to assessment instruments. To the extent possible, corrections regarding spelling of names, correct and full titles, and correct primary sources of assessments have been made. Also, the most current edition of the assessment instrument available at the time of publication has been cited in this handbook, although an older version was frequently cited in the original reference. Use of the most current edition of an assessment instrument would seen to be appropriate for all occupational therapy service delivery programs. In research studies, use of an older edition might be justified to replicate a previous study. Otherwise, updating assessment instruments used in service delivery programs should be considered an important administrative function by service managers.

Some specific subjects covered in the 1991 edition were not included in this edition because insufficient new information was located with a publication dated 1993 or later.

Sufficient literature usually means three or more references, unless one reference is a review of current practice. The topics eliminated include kidney disease, polymyositis, and dermatomyositis. Several topics have been added. Also, some terminology has changed, such as the subtopics under sensory integration disorders. The reader is reminded that the changes reflect analysis of published literature and not surveys of actual practice. The actual number and type of named disorders or conditions seen in occupational therapy practice may be quite different than the published literature suggests. For example, intervention strategies not identified in the published literature may be successful but the results remain unpublished, even though several conference presentations may have been made. Presentation at a conference is not defined as publication. Gaps in published knowledge do exist and are fertile ground for the attention and writing of an enterprising practitioner, educator, or researcher.

Occupational therapy personnel have used a number of words to describe the intervention process. For the purpose of this handbook, the following terms are used and defined:

Prevention—Intervention designed to decrease the known risk of developing a specific deficit, dysfunction, disorder, problem, or undesirable condition, such as preventing contractures, which might limit the person's ability to perform self-care occupations by using range of motion exercises, positioning techniques, or applying a splint. Prevention is based on the idea that avoiding the deficit, dysfunction, disorder, problem, or undesirable condition is more cost-effective in terms of time, money, and energy than incurring and dealing with those same situations.

Development/Acquisitional— Intervention designed to facilitate the attainment or learning of sequentially or chronologically appropriate functional skills and task performance. The developmental/acquisitional approach may be used with persons of any age who, for whatever reason, have never attained or failed to learn certain functional skills or to perform certain tasks. The term *development* tends to be used with children and adolescents, whereas the term *acquisitional* may be applied to any age.

Learning, Educating, Training—Intervention designed to increase the person's knowledge, comprehension, and understanding of task performance. Opportunity for practice is often—but not always—included, depending on the situation and context. Examples might include advice or recommendations on selecting furniture or clothing techniques for developing better coping strategies, such as time and stress management; better problem-solving or reasoning approaches, such as organizing frequently used utensils or tools within easy arm's reach; or goal-setting techniques of prioritizing what is most important to do today and what can be done next week.

Remedial, Remediation—Intervention designed to help a person to learn certain functional skills and to perform certain tasks that may have been incompletely or inaccurately learned or performed, thus contributing to deficits, dysfunction, or disorder. The remedial approach may be used with persons of any age who want or need to learn information, a skill, or how to perform certain tasks and routines. Remedial techniques are sometimes applied to learning tasks after the chronologic age in which most people learned specific information, skill, or task performance. Such application of the term may be confusing and may require clarification in individual situations.

Restorative, Cure—Intervention designed to cure or correct function so that little or no evidence exists that deficit, dysfunction, or disorder has occurred, such as using intervention strategies to enable a person to regain the ability to eat independently with standard (nonadapted) eating utensils or to return to productive living tasks without restrictions, special needs for accommodation, or specialized equipment.

Adaptive, Substitute, Augmentative, or Supportive—Intervention that focuses on using substitute actions of the body or modified equipment to optimize functional skills and task performance, thus reducing the evidence or appearance of deficit, dysfunction, or disorder, such as using the left hand instead of the right hand to sign a signature, using a built-up handle on a spoon to assist weak grasp, or using makeup to camouflage surgical scars or uneven pigmentation of the skin.

Compensatory, Environmental Adaptation—Intervention that uses alternative strategies to accomplish a specific task or function when the person is unable to perform a task or needs to conserve energy by not performing the task in the standard way. Most frequently, the alternative strategies involve assistive technology, such as use of a feeder system that eliminates hand grasp, a wheelchair to compensate for lack of walking skills, or electronic activities of daily living (EADLs) to facilitate answering the doorbell and turning the lights on/off. Modifications of the physical environment, such as building a ramp or widening a doorway, may also be included.

Humanistic, Phenomenologic, Client-Centered—Intervention that focuses on the person's point of view or perspective about intervention, rather than the medical or therapy point of view. Emphasis is placed on respecting and incorporating directly into the intervention process the individual's needs, wishes, interests, values, or wants. Goals are determined by the individual, not by therapy personnel or team members. The intervention program centers around the person, not around a preset or preestablished therapy program in which the person participates but does not control. Examples include helping a person to determine how to fix his or her hair without assistance because that's the most important task that the individual wants to achieve, or helping a person to develop self-confidence in selecting groceries or clothes because the person indicates that shopping is a problem.

Maintain, Sustain—Intervention designed to keep or sustain the current level of function and to avoid further loss of functional skills (deficit, dysfunction, or disorder) and task performance for as long as possible. Maintenance approaches are used primarily with persons who have degenerative disorders or with persons who want to counteract the effects of aging on the body.

Palliative—Intervention that provides physical comfort or peace of mind by empowering the person to focus on goals of his or her choosing that may have little or nothing to do with changing or maintaining functional skills or task performance. Used primarily with persons who have terminal illnesses.

Advocate, Advocacy—Intervention designed to help the person "cut through the red tape" to secure services from public or private agencies. Actions for specific individuals may include providing correct information, calling ahead to clear the communication channel, writing a letter of introduction or summary of facts about the person, and/or physically accompanying the person to the office or facility in question. Therapy personnel can also participate in community planning, lobbying for passage of certain legislation, or file complaints about quality of services provided, but such actions are not the focus of this book.

There are other services and roles that occupational therapy personnel can provide that are not part this project, such as participating in research, writing, and publishing; instructing future professionals; providing continuing education; or designing environments that are universally accessible.

Finally, the author wishes to acknowledge the assistance of Allison Toncrey, a graduate from the School of Occupational Therapy, Texas Woman's University-Houston Center, who did the preliminary literature search for and organization of published literature on occupational therapy as her professional project in the Master's of Occupational Therapy program. Journals, textbooks, newsletters, and trade newspapers were the principal sources, although a few video- and audiotapes were also identified.

Part I

Developmental Disorders

Arthrogryposis Multiplex Congenita

DESCRIPTION

Arthrogryposis multiplex congenita (AMC), called also multiple congenital contractures or arthrogryposis, is characterized by multiple joint contractures (especially of the upper limbs and neck) without other serious congenital abnormalities and with relatively normal intelligence. Arthrogryposis is prenatal fixation (partial or complete) of joints in a flexed (contracted) position. When there is generalized fixation or ankylosis of joints at birth, the condition is termed arthrogryposis multiplex congenita (AMC), but it can also occur as an isolated finding (Merck 1999, 2221). AMC is nonprogressive. Types of AMC include neuropathic, myopathic, and mixed. AMC may also be classified according to the type of limb involvement: (1) primarily limb involvement, (2) limb involvement plus abnormalities in other areas of the body, and (3) limb involvement plus dysfunction of the central nervous system (Sala, Rosenthal, and Grant 1996).

CAUSE

AMC can result from neurogenic, myopathic, or connective tissue disorders. Congenital myopathies, anterior horn cell disease, and maternal myasthenia gravis have been proposed as causes of the associated amyoplasia. AMC is not genetic, although genetic disorders (e.g., trisomy 18, spina bifida) have an increased incidence of arthrogryposis. Joint development occurs in the second month of gestation, and disorders that impair in utero movement (uterine malformation, multiple gestations, oligohydramnios) can result in arthrogryposis (Merck 1999, 2221). In addition to the joint and connective tissue disorders, other abnormalities may include cardiac, respiratory, or urinary tract anomalies, cryptorchidism or undescended testes, hypoplasia of labia or scrotum, facial hemangioma, mild micrognathia, short anteverted nostrils, facial asymmetry, and hernia. Complications include breech presentation, Caesarean section, and fractures. Muscle imbalance, in which the muscle on one side of the joint is more active than its antagonist, is responsible for the appearance of the deformity (Sala, Rosenthal, and Grant 1996, 74).

ASSESSMENT

Areas

- passive range of motion
- active motion
- postural alignment of head, neck, trunk, and extremities
- joint mobility and/or contractures
- hand functions
- sensory modulation and self-regulation
- level of alertness

Instruments

Instruments Developed by Occupational Therapy Personnel
- *Movement Assessment of Infants* (MAI) by L.S. Chandler, M.S. Andrews, and M.W. Swanson, Rolling Bay, WA: Infant Movement Research, 1980.
- *Toddler and Infant Motor Evaluation (TIME)* by L.J. Miller and G.H. Roid, San Antonio, TX: Therapy Skill Builders, 1994.

Instruments Developed by Other Professionals and Used by Occupational Therapy Personnel
- *Battelle Developmental Inventory* (BDI) by J. Newborg, J.R. Stock, and L. Wnek, Itasca, NY: Riverside Publishing Co., 1984.
- *Developmental Profile II* (DPII) by G.D. Alpren, T.J. Boll, and M.S. Shearer, Los Angeles: Western Psychological Services, 1984.
- *Vineland Adaptive Behavior Scales—Revised* (VABS-R) by S.S. Sparrow, D.A. Balla, and D.V. Cicchetti, Circle Pines, MN: American Guidance Services, 1984.

PROBLEMS

Sensorimotor
- Postural problems in neck may occur due to contracture of the sternocleidomastoid muscle and hyperextension of neck.
- Postural problems in trunk may occur due to thoraco-lumbar scoliosis, hyperextension of the spine, and tight trunk musculature.
- Scapulae may be abducted and tipped forward with inferior angle winging.
- Shoulder may be adducted, internally rotated, and extended.
- Elbows may be extended or hyperextended with forearm pronation.
- Wrist flexion contracture may be present.
- Thumb-in-palm deformities may be present.
- Fingers and thumb may not align in coronal plane.
- Fingers may be extended at the metacarpophalangeal joint and partially flexed at the proximal interphalangeal joint.
- Passive flexion of the digits may not be possible.
- Fingers may be deviated toward the ulna.
- Normal palmar creases may be absent, exaggerated, and partially misplaced.
- Passive movement of hip joints may be limited to a few degrees.
- Bilateral equinovarus deformities may be observed.
- Active motion may be very limited and restricted by joint contractures and resulting deformities.
- Atrophy of musculature may be evident in all extremities.
- Infantile reflexes may be difficult to evaluate because of joint contractures.
- Gross motor skills may be limited by joint contractures.
- Attainment of neutral position of the body may be impossible due to joint contractures.
- Difficulty with swallowing may occur due to head and neck alignment problems.

- Regulatory functions such as calming to gentle rocking or comforting by mother are not usually involved.
- Sensory systems are usually normal.

Cognitive
- Intelligence is usually normal or above normal.
- Child is usually able to demonstrate alert behavior by smiling and looking at caregiver within limits of active movement.

Psychosocial
- Child or adult is able to interact socially within limits of movement and mobility.

TREATMENT/INTERVENTION

Self-Care
- Facilitate positioning that will increase potential for independent feeding, dressing, performing personal hygiene, and mobility.

Productivity and Leisure
- Facilitate positioning that will promote play activities.
- Teach caregivers simple games to play with child.

Sensorimotor
- Improve passive range of motion to facilitate:
  1. shoulder external rotation, abduction, and flexion
  2. elbow flexion
  3. forearm supination
  4. wrist extension and radial/ulnar deviation
  5. thumb extension and abduction
  6. flexion and extension of all finger joints
  7. hip flexion/extension, adduction, and internal rotation
  8. knee flexion and extension
  9. ankle dorsiflexion
  10. eversion and abduction of the foot
- Increase active movement:
  1. Increase joint mobility.
  2. Improve positioning and alignment (see next objective).
  3. Determine need for compensatory techniques when more normal mobility and alignment are not possible due to paralysis or paresis.
- Improve joint alignment to attain more functional positions:
  1. Promote neutral alignment and midline orientation of the head, trunk, and extremities by fabrication of positioning equipment such as side-lying or supine board and by gentle stretching exercises, joint manipulation, and serial casting or splinting. Splints might include resting splints, flexion splints.
  2. Improve axial alignment to prevent structural spinal deformities.

3. Increase potential for sitting by promoting better body alignment of head, trunk, and hips.
4. Promote hand-to-hand activity through positioning such as side-lying or supine position.
5. Promote eye-hand coordination through positioning such as side-lying or supine position.
6. Promote hip abduction through positioning of hips.
7. Gradually increase the amount of time the person is held in positioning board.

- Encourage the achievement of developmental milestones by providing developmentally appropriate activities.
- Promote proper swallowing.
- Provide for sensory stimulation through visual, auditory, tactile, proprioceptive, and vestibular input.

Cognitive
- Educate the parents about the disorder and therapy techniques.
- Teach parents proper positioning to improve alignment while carrying, holding, and feeding. Infant should be supported with the head in the cubital fossa of the parent's arm with the parent's forearm encircling the infant's head to facilitate head and trunk flexion and normal neck rotation.
- Teach caregivers to check skin carefully for signs of pressure sores.
- Provide visual and auditory stimulation through toys and interaction with adults to counteract the limited ability to explore the environment independently.
- Promote localization of sights and sounds through visual gaze and then neck turning.
- As active movement is available, follow localization with swiping, touching, reaching, assisted grasp, and active grasp.

Psychosocial
- Encourage interaction between child, caregivers, and other adults.
- Encourage child to recognize familiar and unfamiliar people.

PRECAUTIONS
- Always be aware of respiratory function and do not position person in any manner that will compromise respiration.
- Always be aware of skin condition to avoid pressure sores, especially when using positioning equipment.

PROGNOSIS AND OUTCOME
Prognosis and outcome are varied and depend on the level and number of joints involved. Those with fewer joints involved and joints that respond to treatment may be able to live independently and productively, although vocational barriers are likely to persist. Those with more joint involvement and increased severity will need assistive living arrangements.
- The person has maximum range of motion possible given structural and physiologic limitations.

- The person achieves gross and fine motor skills, although the development of skills does not progress normally.
- The person has functional hand skills, although the use of the hands may be unorthodox.
- The person has independent mobility with or without powered mobility. Two-thirds can become ambulatory (Merck 1999).
- The person achieves independence in self-care and daily living skills.
- The person develops and applies productive skills.

REFERENCES

Beers, M.H., and R. Berkow, eds. 1999. *The Merck Manual of Diagnosis and Therapy*, 17th ed. Whitehouse Station, NJ: Merck Research Laboratories.
Sala, D.A. et al. 1996. Clinical concerns: Early treatment of an infant with severe arthrogryposis. *Physical and Occupational Therapy in Pediatrics* 16, no. 3: 73–89. (case report)

BIBLIOGRAPHY

Gordon, C.Y. et al. 1996. Diagnostic problems in pediatrics—arthrogryposis multiplex congenita. In *Occupational therapy for children*. 3rd ed., eds. J. Case-Smith et al., 121–122. St. Louis, MO: Mosby.
Joe, B.E. 1995. Prepared for anything. *OT Week* 9, no. 49: 12.
Tomcheck, S.D. 1999. The musculoskeletal system—arthrogryposis multiplex. In *Pediatric therapy: A systems approach*, eds. S.M. Poor and E.B. Rainville, 217–219. Philadelphia: F.A. Davis.

Attention Deficit/Hyperactivity Disorder

DESCRIPTION

Attention deficit/hyperactivity disorder involves a persistent and frequent pattern of developmentally inappropriate inattention and impulsivity, with or without hyperactivity (DSM-IV). A child without hyperactivity has attention deficit disorder (ADD); a child with hyperactivity has attention deficit/hyperactivity disorder (ADHD). Both are implicated in learning disorders and can influence the behavior of a child at any cognitive level, except for moderate to profound mental retardation. Boys are more commonly affected than girls in a ratio of 10:1. Estimates are that 5 percent to 10 percent of school-aged children are affected. Other terms associated with this disorder are minimal brain dysfunction (MBD), hyperkinesis, hyperkinetic impulse disorder, and hyperactive child syndrome (Merck 1999, 2255–2256).

CAUSE

The cause is unknown. Several theories advocating biochemical, sensorimotor, physiologic, and behavioral correlates and manifestations have been proposed. The disorder tends to occur in families and is common in first-degree biological relatives. Many now believe that

Criteria for Attention Deficit/Hyperactivity Disorder

A. Either (1) or (2)

  (1) Six (or more) of the following symptoms of **inattention** have persisted for at least six months to a degree that is maladaptive and inconsistent with developmental level.

    (a) Often fails to give close attention to details or makes careless mistakes in schoolwork, work, or other activities.

    (b) Often has difficulty sustaining attention in tasks or play activities.

    (c) Often does not seem to listen when spoken to directly.

    (d) Often does not follow through on instructions and fails to finish schoolwork, chores, or duties in the workplace.

    (e) Often has difficulty organizing tasks and activities.

    (f) Often avoids, dislikes, or is reluctant to engage in tasks that require sustained mental effort.

    (g) Often loses things necessary for tasks or activities (e.g., toys, school assignments, pencils, books, or tools).

    (h) Is often easily distracted by extraneous stimuli.

    (i) Is often forgetful in daily activities.

  (2) Six (or more) of the following symptoms of **hyperactivity-impulsivity** have persisted for at least six months to a degree that is maladaptive and inconsistent with developmental level.

Hyperactivity

    (a) Often fidgets with hands or feet or squirms in seat.

    (b) Often leaves seat in classroom or in other situations in which remaining seated is expected.

    (c) Often runs about or climbs excessively in situations in which it is inappropriate (in adolescents or adults, may be limited to subjective feelings of restlessness).

    (d) Often has difficulty playing or engaging in leisure activities quietly.

    (e) Is often "on the go" or often acts as if "driven by a motor."

    (f) Often talks excessively.

Impulsivity

    (g) Often blurts out answers before questions have been completed.

    (h) Often has difficulty awaiting turn.

    (i) Often interrupts or intrudes on others (e.g., butts into conversations or games).

B. Some hyperactivity-impulsivity or inattention systems that cause impairments were present before age 7 years.

continues

continued

> C. Some impairment from the symptoms is present in two or more settings (e.g., at school [or work] and at home).
> D. There must be clear evidence of clinically significant impairments in social, academic, or occupational functioning.
> E. The symptoms do not occur exclusively during the course of a pervasive developmental disorder, schizophrenia, or other psychotic disorder and are not better accounted for by another mental disorder (e.g., mood disorder, anxiety disorder, dissociative disorder, or a personality disorder).
>
> *Source:* Reprinted with permission from the *Diagnostic and Statistical Manual of Mental Disorders, Fourth Edition.* Copyright 1994, American Psychiatric Association.

the disorder is a difference in brain chemistry rather than a deficit or impairment that results in a difference in the person's approach to learning. The leading hypothesis suggests neurotransmitter abnormalities in dopaminergic and noradrenergic systems with decreased activity or stimulation in upper brain stem and frontal-midbrain tracts. Other hypotheses include effects of toxins, neurologic immaturity, infections, drug exposure in utero, head injuries, and environmental factors (Merck 1999, 2256).

ASSESSMENT

Areas

- gross motor skills and coordination
- fine motor skills, manipulation, dexterity, and bilateral coordination
- balance and postural control
- motor planning or praxis
- regulatory and sensory modulation skills
- sensory discrimination and perception
- level of arousal and alertness: attention span or sustained attention
- memory skills
- impulsivity and impulse control
- amount or level of impersistence
- awareness and judgment regarding safety of self and others
- socialization and communication skills
- daily living skills and performance (personal and instrumental activities of daily living)
- play development and skills
- productive skills
- leisure skills
- time management

Instruments

There is no single comprehensive assessment instrument for this disorder. Several assessments will be needed to complete the evaluation for any given individual. Also, the therapist should be sure to note which, if any, medication the person is taking, since the medication may alter the testing results. Common medications are methylphenidate (Ritalin), dextroamphetamine (Dexedrine or DextroStat), and pemoline (Cylert).

Instruments Developed by Occupational Therapy Personnel
- *Sensorimotor History* by P. Montgomery and E. Richter, in *Sensorimotor integration for developmentally disabled children*, Los Angeles: Western Psychological Services, 1977.
- *Sensory Integration and Praxis Tests* by A.J. Ayres, Los Angeles: Western Psychological Services, 1989.
- *Touch Inventory for Elementary-School-Aged* by C.B. Royeen, *American Journal of Occupational Therapy* 44, no. 2 (1990): 155–159.

Instruments Developed by Other Professionals and Used by Occupational Therapy Personnel
- *Aggregate Neurobehavioral Student Health and Educational Review* by M.D. Levine, Cambridge, MA: Educators Publishing Services, 1989.
- *Attention Deficit Disorder Evaluation Scale–Revised* by S.B. McCarney, Columbia, MO: Hawthorne Educational Services, 1995.
- *The Beery-Buktenica Developmental Test of Visual-Motor Integration* (VMI-4), 4th ed. by K.E. Beery and N.A. Buktenica, Parsippany, NJ: Modern Curriculum Press, 1997.
- *Bruininks-Oseretsky Test of Motor Proficiency* (BOTMP) by R. Buininks, Circle Pines, MN: American Guidance Services, 1978.
- *Child Behavior Checklist* by T.M. Achenbach and C. Edelbrock, Burlington, VT: University of Vermont, Department of Psychology, 1983.
- *Conners Parent and Teacher Rating Scales* by C.H. Goyette, C.K. Conners, and R.F. Ulrich, in Normative data on revised Conners Parent and Teacher Rating Scales, *Journal of Abnormal Child Psychology* 6 (1978): 221–236.
- *Louisville Behavior Checklist* by L.C. Miller, Los Angeles: Western Psychological Services, 1981.
- *Motor-Free Visual Perception Test–Revised* (MVPT-R) by R. Colarusso and D.D. Hamill, Novato, CA: Academic Therapy Press, 1996.
- *Peabody Development Motor Scales* by M.R. Folio and R.R. Fewell, Austin, TX: Pro-ed, 1983.
- *Pediatric Early Elementary Examination–Revised* by M.D. Levine, Cambridge, MA: Educators Publishing Services, 1995.
- *Pediatric Examination of Educational Readiness* by M.D. Levine, Cambridge, MA: Educators Publishing Services, 1982.
- *Pediatric Examination of Educational Readiness at Middle School–Revised*, Cambridge, MA: Educators Publishing Services, 1995.
- *Pediatric Extended Examination at Three* by M.D. Levine, Cambridge, MA: Educators Publishing Services, 1982.
- *Quick Neurological Screening Test-II* by M. Mutti, H.M. Sterling, and N.V. Spalding, Novato, CA: Academic Therapy Publications, 1998.
- *Tinkertoy Test* by M.D. Lezak, in *Neuropsychological Assessment*, 3rd ed., New York: Oxford University Press, 1995.

PROBLEMS

Self-Care
- The person is often forgetful in daily activities (DSM-IV).

Productivity
- The person often fails to give close attention to details or makes careless mistakes in schoolwork, work, or other activities (DSM-IV).
- The person often has difficulty playing quietly (DSM-IV).
- The person may have poor writing skills and illegible printing or handwriting. Common problems reported are inability to stay on baseline, crossovers and markovers, poor stroke quality, confusing upper- and lower-case letters, disproportionate letter size, a mixture of upper- and lower-case letters within a single word, and inappropriate spacing within and between words (Marmer 1995).

Leisure
- The person often has difficulty engaging in leisure activities quietly (DSM-IV).

Sensorimotor
- The person often fidgets with hands or feet or squirms in seat (DSM-IV).
- The person often leaves seat in classroom or in other situations in which remaining seated is expected (DSM-IV).
- The person often runs about or climbs excessively in situation in which it is inappropriate (DSM-IV).
- The person is often "on the go" or often acts as if "driven by a motor" (DSM-IV).
- The person often talks excessively (DSM-IV).
- The person may have poor perceptual motor skills.
- The person may have poor fine motor skills. (Note: Poor performance in fine motor skills may be related to impulsivity and short attention span rather than inability to perform the task [Doyle et al. 1995].)

Cognitive
- The person often has difficulty sustaining attention in tasks or play activities (DSM-IV).
- The person often does not seem to listen when spoken to directly (DSM-IV).
- The person often does not follow through on instructions and fails to finish schoolwork, chores, or duties in the workplace (DSM-IV).
- The person often has difficulty organizing tasks and activities (DSM-IV).
- The person often avoids, dislikes, or is reluctant to engage in tasks that require sustained mental effort (DSM-IV).
- The person often loses things necessary for tasks or activities (DSM-IV).
- The person is often easily distracted by extraneous stimuli (DSM-IV).
- The person may have poor processing skills.

Psychosocial
- The person often blurts out answers before questions have been completed (DSM-IV).
- The person often has difficulty awaiting his or her turn (DSM-IV).

- The person often interrupts or intrudes on others (DSM-IV).
- The person may have limited tolerance for frustration and may lose his or her temper with little provocation or justification.
- The person may have a high level of anxiety when experiencing stress.
- The person may have perfectionist standards but poor level of performance.
- The person may have poor communication and interaction skills.
- The person may feel dissatisfied and have difficulty experiencing contentment or satisfaction in life.
- The person may approach tasks with a "get it over with" attitude rather than trying to do the task correctly the first time.
- The person may ignore or be inattentive to social feedback cues, facial expression, or verbal comments.

Environment
- Teachers may view person as lazy or careless.
- The person's behavior may be viewed by others as aggressive or disruptive.

TREATMENT/INTERVENTION
Treatment should be within an interdisciplinary team approach that focuses on cognitive, behavior, emotional, and sensorimotor outcomes. Within occupational therapy the primary approaches have been regulatory functioning (Williams and Shellenberger 1996), sensory integration and the model of human occupation. The model of human occupation considers intake, feedback, and the three subsystems of throughput-performance, habituation, and volition. Emphasis is on performance and habituation rather than volition, which is assumed to follow when performance and habituation improve. Models of practice developed by other professionals include: psychostimulant medication trials, cognitive training, development of coping behavior, developmental therapy, and neurobehavioral control.

Self-Care
- Improve ability to follow routines required in performance of self-care skills by using charts, checklists, and/or audiotapes to provide structure and organization.

Productivity
- Reduce "out of seat" behavior at school by setting boundaries using carpet squares or taped areas on the floor.
- Learning keyboard skills for use in word-processing programs can provide an alternate written communication skill. Student might use oral communication for short assignments if handwriting (motor coordination) is a problem.
- Consider whether engaging in volunteer work may help the person develop skills in areas that do not require skills in which the person is deficient.

Leisure
- Facilitate selection and performance of leisure skills such as constructing shapes with plastic building toys.
- Help the person explore leisure activities that can be successful and rewarding to the person and do not require the skills with which the person has difficulty.

Sensorimotor
- Improve regulatory functioning and sensory modulation by teaching the person ways to calm down.
- Improve fine motor skills such as manual dexterity.
- Improve visual perception and visual-motor skills.

Cognitive
- Break tasks into short segments to compensate for impulsivity. Example: Listen for instructions (intake), accomplish task (performance), or complete one page of an assignment and turn it into the teacher. Then go to the next page.
- Provide structure and cues in organization and planning skills to increase independence in accomplishing self-care tasks and homework assignments.
- Provide memory and organizational aids such as day planners, schedules, and assignments written on the chalkboard, or a beeper to remind the person what needs to be done and when.
- Increase concentration through play activities such as hiding pennies in Theraplast.
- Increase judgment of safety by using verbal reminders such as Stop, Look, Listen, or making a contract with the person to hold an adult's hand while crossing the street.

Psychosocial
- Role playing may be helpful in improving social interaction behaviors such as correct behavior in a competitive game whether winning or losing.
- Reduce impulsive and distractive behavior by structuring tasks with "to do" lists and setting an alarm clock for completion of task.
- Increase self-esteem through selection of a hobby or activity within the person's strengths.

Environment
- Explain to caregivers and teachers which behaviors the person can control and which he or she cannot control.
- Teach caregivers and teachers techniques for calming the person when hyperactivity becomes a problem.
- Recommend to the classroom teacher that the student's desk be moved to the least distracting area of the classroom.
- Consider whether giving the student extra time to complete assignments might be helpful.
- Suggest that the teacher (and caregivers) write assignments, along with materials needed, on the blackboard for easy review.
- Suggest that the teacher find tasks the student can do that permit getting out of the seat at specified times, such as taking a note to the principal's office.
- Consider whether it might be useful for the child to sit on a small inflatable ring to provide sensory feedback.
- Consider the usefulness of assistive technology such as slant board for writing activities, modified pencil grips and scissors, adaptations to computers, specialized computer software to practice eye-hand coordination, or adaptations to computers.

PRECAUTIONS
- A person with ADD or ADHD may have more than one diagnosis. Tourette's syndrome, obsessive-compulsive disorder, and learning disability are common additional diagnoses. In assessment and intervention these additional diagnoses must be considered.

• Avoid concentrating only on the negative situations in the person's life. Focus on increasing opportunities for positive feedback for actions, activities, and occupations that are performed well.

PROGNOSIS AND OUTCOME

Attention deficit disorder is a lifelong condition. A child with ADD or ADHD becomes an adult with ADD or ADHD. Compensatory techniques will be required for a lifetime, although the specific techniques may need to be modified.

• The person demonstrates improved ability to regulate his or her own responses to sensory modulation and is less dependent on the external environment.
• The person is able to attend to a task selectively without responding to distractions.
• The person is able to sustain attention to a task until it is completed.
• The person is able to attend to and follow verbal commands.
• The person is able to describe alternate approaches to solving a problem.
• The person is able to play and work quietly with self-control.
• The person is able to play and work in a group and observe the rules.

REFERENCES

American Psychiatric Association. 1994. *Diagnostic and Statistical Manual of Mental Disorders: DSM-IV*, 4th ed. Washington, DC: American Psychiatric Assocation. Task Force on DSM-IV.
Beers, M.H., and R. Berkow, eds. 1999. *The Merck Manual of Diagnosis and Therapy*, 17th ed. Whitehouse Station, NJ: Merck Research Laboratories.
Doyle, S. et al. 1995. Motor skills in Australian children with attention deficit hyperactivity disorder. *Occupational Therapy International* 2, no. 4: 229–240.
Marmer, L. 1995. ADHD: Handwriting on the wall. *Advance for Occupational Therapists* 11, no. 31: 12.
Williams, M.S., and S. Shellenberger. 1996. *How does your engine run? A leader's guide to the alert program for self-regulation*. Albuquerque, NM: Therapy Works.

BIBLIOGRAPHY

Campbell, M.B. 1994. The fizzle effect. *OT Week* 8, no. 42: 20–22. (Discusses adult ADD.)
Florey, L. 1998. Attention deficit hyperactivity disorder. In *Willard and Spackman's occupational therapy*. 9th ed., eds. M.E. Neistadt and E.B. Crepeau, 630–631. Philadelphia: Lippincott-Raven Publishers.
Hanft, B.E. 1997. *Occupational therapy practice guidelines for attention-deficit/hyperactivity disorders*. Bethesda, MD: The American Occupational Therapy Association.
Klein, M.D., and T.A. Delaney. 1994. Conditions affecting feeding and nutrition—attention deficit hyperactive disorder. In *Feeding and nutrition for the child with special needs: Handouts for parents*, eds. M.D. Klein and T.A. Delaney, 345–347. Tucson, AZ: Therapy Skill Builders.
Mulligan, S. 1996. An analysis of score patterns of children with attention disorders on the Sensory Integration and Praxis Tests. *American Journal of Occupational Therapy* 50, no. 8: 647–654.
Peterson, C.Q. 1993. Attention deficit hyperactivity disorder: Evaluation and treatment. *Developmental Disabilities Special Interest Section Newsletter* 16, no. 1: 2–4.
Porr, S.M. 1999. The psychological system—attention deficit disorder. In *Pediatric therapy: A systems approach,* eds. S.M. Poor and E.B. Rainville, 289–294. Philadelphia: F.A. Davis.

Segal, R. 1998. The construction of family occupations: a study of families with children who have attention deficit/hyperactivity disorder. *Canadian Journal of Occupational Therapy* 65, no. 5: 286–292.

Stahl, C. 1995. Using computers to aid visual-motor processing. *Advance for Occupational Therapists* 11, no. 2: 17.

Stancliff, B.L. 1998. Understanding the "whoops" children. *OT Practice* 3, no. 11: 18–25.

Woodrum, S.C. 1993. A treatment approach for attention deficit hyperactivity disorder: Using the model of human occupation. *Developmental Disabilities Special Interest Section Newsletter* 16, no. 1: 1–2.

Autism or Autistic Disorder

DESCRIPTION

The essential features of autism or autistic disorder are the presence of markedly abnormal or impaired development of social interaction and communication and a markedly restricted repertoire of activities of interest. Manifestations of the disorder vary greatly depending on the developmental level and chronologic age of the individual. Usually the disorder is apparent between birth and age 3 (American Psychiatric Association, 66).

The disorder was originally described in 1943 by Leo Kanner, a psychiatrist at Johns Hopkins University, who thought it was due to psychogenic factors related to cold and unloving parents. Other names for the disorder include early infantile autism, childhood autism, Kanner's autism or Kanner's syndrome, and pervasive developmental disorder.

Autism is often described as having two types of clinical onset. In the first type, the child exhibits signs of autism shortly after birth (early onset). Symptoms may include lack of anticipatory response to being picked up, absent or delayed smiling, and poor eye contact. In the second type, the child is usually described as developing normally until 12 to 24 months of age and then regressing, losing previously acquired skills and exhibiting symptoms of autism (late onset). Symptoms may have been present earlier but were not identified clearly enough to be diagnostic.

CAUSE

The exact cause is unknown. Current theory classifies autism as a neurobiological disorder, and the focus is on changes in the neuroanatomy and neurochemistry of the brain. Computed tomographic scans have isolated a subgroup of autistic children with enlarged ventricles , and magnetic resonance imaging (MRI) has identified a subgroup of autistic adults with hypoplasia of the cerebellar vermis. Individual cases of autism have been associated with the congenital rubella syndrome, cytomegalic inclusion disorder, phenylketonuria, and the fragile X syndrome (Merck 1999, 2420). The ratio of male to female cases is 4:1. The incidence is four to five per 10,000 births. All races and ethnic groups seem to be similarly affected. Family income, lifestyle, and educational level do not determine frequency.

ASSESSMENT

Areas

- daily living skills and performance
- play skills
- preacademic or readiness skills
- regulatory and sensory processing skills: sleeping patterns, response to food, activity level (hyperactivity)
- motor skills: developmental milestones, gross motor skills, bilateral coordination
- fine motor skills: manipulation, dexterity, and eye-hand coordination
- postural control and balance: muscle tone, reflex development, and maturation
- stereotypical patterns (unusual use of the hands, feet, or body)
- sensory modulation: sensory sensitivity (hypo- or hyperresponsiveness)
- adaptive movement: praxis or motor planning
- sensory discrimination and perceptual skills
- attending and arousal behavior: orienting behavior, concentration, or attention span
- anticipatory response to being picked up
- learning skills, such as imitation
- object relations, human and nonhuman
- social and communication skills: smiling, eye contact, degree of vocalization, and use of language
- coping skills

Instruments

Instruments Developed by Occupational Therapy Personnel

- *Preschool Play Scale* by S. Knox, in A play scale, *Play as exploratory learning*, ed. M. Reilly, 247–266, Beverly Hills, CA: Sage, 1974. *Revised Knox Preschool Play Scale* by S. Knox, in *Play in occupational therapy for children,* eds. L.D. Parham and L.S. Fazio, 35–51, St. Louis, MO: Mosby, 1997.
- *Sensory Integration and Praxis Tests* (SIPT) by A.J. Ayres, Los Angeles: Western Psychological Services, 1989. (Note: Not appropriate for some autistic children. Check criteria before administering.)
- *Sensory Profile* by W. Dunn, San Antonio, TX: Therapy Skill Builders, 1999.

Instruments Developed by Other Professionals and Used by Occupational Therapy Personnel

- *Bayley Scales of Infant Development-II* (BSID-II) by N. Bayley, San Antonio, TX: The Psychological Corporation, 1993.
- *Motivation Assessment Scale* (MAS) by V.M. Duran and D.B. Crimmins, in Identifying the variables maintaining self-injuries behavior, *Journal of Autism and Developmental Disorders* 18, no. 1 (1988): 99–117.
- *Vineland Adaptive Behavior Scales–Revised* (VABS-R) by S.S. Sparrow, D.A. Balla, and D.V. Cicchetti, Circle Pines, MN: American Guidance Services, 1984.

PROBLEMS

Self-Care
- The person may have difficulty transferring from bottle to textured food or from baby food to table food.
- The person may refuse to chew or swallow and present intense gagging.
- The person does not attain normal self-care milestones such as assisting with dressing and feeding.

Productivity
- The person may not demonstrate varied, spontaneous make-believe or pretend play and show no imagination in play activities.
- The person may not demonstrate socially imitative play appropriate to developmental level.
- The person may have no or impaired social play skills and prefer to play alone.
- The person may have difficulty learning to consistently perform job tasks as required.

Leisure
- The person may have difficulty developing interests beyond those involved in ritual or perseverate behaviors.

Sensorimotor
- The person may demonstrate stereotyped and repetitive motor mannerisms such as hand or finger flapping or twisting, head banging, or complex whole-body movements such as body spinning, rocking, and twirling. These behaviors are classified as self-stimulating or self-abusive behaviors.
- The person may repeat or perseverate a certain motor mannerism such as twirling or spinning a variety of objects in the environment.
- The person may refuse to hold objects, which suggests difficulty with grasp, but may readily hold a favorite object such as a piece of string.
- The person often has inconsistent patterns of attaining motor developmental milestones.
- The person may exhibit decreased muscle tone, inadequate postural control, poor co-contraction, inadequate joint stability in the neck muscles, and poor gross motor coordination.
- The person may have delayed response to reflex stimulation.
- The person may tend to avoid activities that require physical exertion.
- The person may have sensory modulation disorders (faculty sensory modulation) even though there is no damage to the sensory systems themselves. Examples include the following:
  1. The person may stiffen the body when being picked up, which may be related to tactile defensiveness.
  2. The person may respond as if deaf, cover ears, or run away from sound (auditory defensiveness).
  3. The person may seek large amounts of vestibular input such as by spinning or turning.
  4. The person may seek large amounts of proprioceptive input such as by pulling, pushing, or jumping.

5. The person may have shortened postrotary nystagmus.
6. The person may not respond to pain.

- The person may have poor spatial relationships (insist on maintaining the same organization or relation of objects in the environment).
- The person may demonstrate a paradoxical response to stimuli. For example, the person may not respond to touch or may have an aversion to touch (tactile defensiveness) but seek certain tactile input. The person may not respond to certain visual or auditory stimuli but overrespond to other visual or auditory stimuli.
- The person may have a sensory processing disorder in which the nervous system is easily put into a high state of arousal so that the person is overwhelmed and shuts down. However, the next day the opposite pattern may occur in which the person actively seeks more sensory input.
- When presented with a multisensory experience, the person may appear to overfocus in one sensory modality to the exclusion of other sensory input. In other words, there appears to be a failure of the nervous system to manage multisensory input.
- The person usually avoids eye gaze or seems to stare through a person rather than at the person, behavior which may be related to regulatory dysfunction.
- The person may have poor motor planning skills such as how to get a swing and make the swing move.
- The person is often assessed for apparent deafness because the person does not respond or delays response to the human voice.

Cognitive

- The person demonstrates preoccupation with one or more stereotyped and restricted patterns of interest that is abnormal either in intensity or focus.
- The person may be persistently preoccupied with parts of an object to the exclusion of the whole.
- The person may have a learning disorder such as dyslexia, possibly related to poor registration and modulation of sensory input. The person does not correctly register information, filter extraneous input, and select an optimal state of arousal to attend to tasks.
- The person may have poor attending or orienting behavior and poor eye contact (poor orienting reflex, which may be related to a sensory modulation disorder).
- The person may have short attention span and poor concentration skills.
- The person may have poor ideation and organization of behavior response.
- The person may be unable to form novel concepts or imitate and purposefully interact with the environment.
- The person may demonstrate good rote memory and special skills such as superior musical ability, spatial skills (doing difficult puzzles easily), or skills for memorization skills of details.
- The person may have difficulty making a transition from one activity to another.

Psychosocial

- The person shows marked impairment in the use of nonverbal communication, such as aversion of eye gaze, flat facial expression, failure to face the person speaking, performance of avoidance gestures, or failure to perform social gestures.

- The person does not relate to others or relates only briefly. For example, the person may show no interest in siblings.
- The person does not show, bring, or point out objects of interest to people.
- The person does not demonstrate social or emotional reciprocity.
- The person has delayed or totally lacks spoken language and does not compensate by using alternative modes of communication such as gesture or mime.
- The person may be mute or have idiosyncratic speech, such as echolalia, and may reverse pronouns, saying "you" when meaning "I."
- The person usually does not imitate or maintain a conversation with others even though the person is capable of speaking.
- The person may not demonstrate goal-directed behavior.
- The person may have marked lack of awareness of the existence or feelings of others and a lack of attachment to caregivers.
- The person usually fails to cuddle when held and does not seek comfort at times of distress.
- The person may have strong attachment to objects and relate well to objects but not to humans.
- The person may show no signs of distress when separated from parent or caregiver.
- The person does not imitate social behaviors, such as waving good-bye or copying parent's activities around the house.
- As a teenager, the person may become aware of poor social skills and become depressed and suicidal.

Environment

- The person may demonstrate strong resistance to change in the environment and respond to change with crying or screaming.
- The person demonstrates apparently inflexible adherence to specific nonfunctional routines and rituals.
- The person may demonstrate extreme stress if routine or ritual is not followed or is interrupted.
- The person may insist on following routines in precise detail.

TREATMENT/INTERVENTION

Treatment is based on the models of sensory integration, occupational role and functioning, neurodevelopmental therapy, sensory diet approach, social communications approach, behavior modification, auditory integrative training, and play therapy. Often treatment uses a team approach, especially in the school. Sensory integration seems to work best for individuals who are sensitive to input. The goal of this therapy is to encourage adaptive responses such as postural reactions, purposeful activities, self-direction, imitation, and social interaction. Neurodevelopmental therapy appears to work best for individuals with postural, tonal, and movement deficits, such as unusual weight-bearing patterns, low tone, inadequate postural control, reduced movement, and clumsiness. The sensory diet approach is used for individuals who need assistance in meeting arousal needs. A sensory diet provides a variety of activities and adaptations based on the person's sensory needs that assists the individual in maintaining an appropriate level of arousal and performance.

Self-Care

• Increase independence in performance of activities of daily living.
• In adolescence, increase independence in daily living skills to permit living in a group home.

Productivity

• Increase play skills by beginning play within a familiar environment such as the person's home, with an active play partner, few cognitive and communication demands, and involvement of parents. Use modeling and reinforcement techniques.
• Increase the level of play skills from solitary to parallel and cooperative play. Computer games may be useful.
• Increase symbolic play skills.
• Reinforce schoolwork whenever possible. Examples might include having the student read simple directions for baking cookies or figure the costs of items in a grocery list.
• In adolescence, promote vocational readiness skills.
• Increase home-management skills, including meal preparation, shopping, budgeting, and housecleaning.

Leisure

• Explore interests that could be developed into leisure activities.

Sensorimotor

• Improve gross motor skills through directed practice in a variety of play activities.
• Increase muscle tone and co-contraction to promote stability, especially in the midline trunk muscles and shoulder and hip joints, using linear vestibular input (in a hammock or on a large ball), proprioception (all-fours position), prone extension position during play activities (scooter board), and sucking.
• Improve muscle tone by facilitating coactivation during activities that provide vestibular input while stopping and holding.
• Improve balance reactions by challenging the equilibrium reactions during function activities that provide vestibular input, which is altered by slowing down, stopping, and holding.
• Increase motor planning skills using mazes or obstacle courses.
• Decrease self-abusive or self-stimulating behaviors, which are assumed to be related to stress and therefore are treated by reducing stress, such as by reducing the noise level, reducing the number of people in the environment, or reducing the complexity of the environment. The behaviors may also indicate what sensory information is lacking or is not registering, and is needed to increase sensitivity and discrimination.
• For hyperresponsiveness and hyperactivity, reduce environmental visual and auditory stimuli while providing vestibular, proprioceptive, and tactile input.
• Provide vestibular stimulation, such as swinging, riding, or rocking. For hyperresponsiveness, use slow, regular input; for hyporesponsiveness, use rapid, irregular input.
• Increase body awareness (proprioceptive and kinesthetic) through the use of obstacle courses or resistive activities and joint compression and traction, beginning with symmetrical flexion patterns organized at the midline, such as holding onto a bolster swing.
• Decrease tactile defensiveness, if present, and increase tactile discrimination through activities and games that use deep pressure (rolling in a blanket, sandwiching between mats,

or swaddling) and provide the opportunity to experience a variety of tactile sensations (feeling a variety of textured cloths, locating articles buried in sand, pulling objects out of a "feely" bag). See also section on tactile defensiveness.
- Increase skills in spatial relations and ability to negotiate space by creating mazes for the scooter board or a navigation pathway around the room; then use fine motor mazes and finally paper and pencil mazes.

Cognitive
- Provide directive commands and repeat them frequently to assist the person in focusing attention on the activity or listening to directions, for example, "Look at me," or "Look at the picture."
- Increase attending behavior and attention span by decreasing extraneous visual and auditory stimuli. Computer programs such as games and drawing programs may be useful.

Psychosocial
- Teach rules for social interaction with others and provide opportunity to practice in a small-group situation first. The group may form a club in which participants set the rules and work on any of the following objectives:
  1. Increase comfort level in maintenance of proximity to others.
  2. Increase imitation and social responsiveness through use of behavior modification and modeling of peer group.
  3. Increase ability to share activities and cooperation.
  4. Increase adaptive and coping skills.
  5. Increase ability to take turns and wait for a turn.
  6. Increase ability to take initiative in social interaction.
- Improve ability to ask for help and information by teaching the person to use gestures, point to objects, or use words to demonstrate that the person needs help.
- Increase understanding of social contexts and use of appropriate behaviors for those contexts.
- Increase understanding and appropriate expression of affect.
- Decrease dependence on routines or repetitive behaviors by encouraging the person to engage in novel behavior.
- Teach relaxation techniques and other stress-reduction behaviors.
- Encourage development of social skills through games and sports.
- Assist in the promotion of language. Sign language is frequently used. Music may be useful. Vestibular stimulation has been correlated with increased verbalization.

Environment
- If team members are not all working at the same site, consider using a communication book that parents take to each session so the team members can share what they are doing, what responses or gains the person is making, and any questions that may occur regarding how to proceed.
- Help parents learn about autism and its effects on their child.
- Provide parents with social support so they can learn how to deal with, understand, and help their child at home.

- Facilitate parental involvement in the home program for their child. Use of videotape on sensory integrative therapy may help parents understand better than explanation or printed materials. Also find out what the parents are already doing that may be useful in the occupational therapy program.
- Suggest to teachers and parents that they create a quiet space in the classroom and at home where the child can move away from others or activity when overloaded to calm down and collect himself or herself.
- Suggest therapy equipment and activity materials that the parents can make or purchase easily (within a limited budget) to use at home.

PRECAUTIONS
- Monitor the person for signs of overload. Each person may react differently, so careful attention to individual variations is important.
- Keep rooms where children play or perform large movements free of sharp corners and unsafe objects.
- Use protective gear such as helmets or joint guards (wrist, knee, and elbow) if skating activity is used.
- Keep jumping surfaces low to the ground and provide padding such as a springy mat or mattress on the floor.
- If swings and hammocks are used, be sure they have soft surfaces underneath and are properly fastened into ceilings or walls.
- Use only objects designed to be put into the mouth or oral motor and chewy toys.
- Substitute food such as cereal pieces in fine motor tasks if there is a concern about the child's putting objects in the mouth.

PROGNOSIS AND OUTCOME
The prognosis is guarded because autism can be a chronic disorder. Response to treatment varies. Some individuals may be able to function in a semi-independent environment, such as a group home. Others will need a highly structured environment, such as a nursing home or state hospital. Children with higher intelligence, early language development, hyperresponsiveness, and good play skills seem to do better.
- The person is able to perform daily living skills without assistance.
- The person is able to play with other children in parallel or engage in cooperative play with children at or near his or her own age level.
- The person is progressing in academic skills.
- The person demonstrates increased muscle tone, co-contraction, and joint stability.
- The person demonstrates increased discriminative skills to sensory stimuli.
- The person demonstrates increased ability to orient or attend to stimuli.
- The person demonstrates increased attention span or concentration.
- The person spends less time in ritual and repetitive behavior and more in purposeful activities.
- The person is more able to adapt to or cope with changes in the environment.
- The person demonstrates improved social skills.

REFERENCES

American Psychiatric Association. 1994. *Diagnostic and Statistical Manual of Mental Disorders: DSM-IV*, 4th ed. Washington, DC: American Psychiatric Assocation. Task Force on DSM-IV.
Beers, M.H., and R. Berkow, eds. 1999. *The Merck Manual of Diagnosis and Therapy*, 17th ed. Whitehouse Station, NJ: Merck Research Laboratories.

BIBLIOGRAPHY

Anderson, J.M. 1998. *Sensory motor issues in autism*. San Antonio, TX: Therapy Skill Builders.
Another OT approach to treating autism. 1996. *OT Practice* 1, no. 7: 26.
Blanche, E.I. et al. 1995. The use of neuro-developmental treatment and sensory integration in the assessment and treatment of children with developmental disorders—Autism. In *Combing neuro-developmental treatment and sensory integration principles: An approach to pediatric therapy*, eds. E.I. Blanche et al., 103–114. Tucson, AZ: Therapy Skill Builders.
Cammisa, K.M., and S.G. Hobbs. 1993. Etiology of autism: A review of recent biogenic theories and research. *Occupational Therapy in Mental Health* 12, no. 2: 39–67.
Christie, A., and S. Robertson. 1993. Katie, a child with autism: An occupational therapy case history. *New Zealand Journal of Occupational Therapy* 44, no. 2: 3–10.
Cook, D. 1996. The impact of having a child with autism. *Developmental Disabilities Special Interest Section Newsletter* 19, no. 2: 1–4. (case reports)
Gorman, P.A. 1997. Sensory dysfunction in dual diagnosis: Mental retardation/mental illness and autism. *Occupational Therapy in Mental Health* 13, no. 1: 3–22.
Greene, S. 1995. Social skills in context: Group intervention for children with autism. *School System Special Interest Section Newsletter* 2, no. 4: 3–5.
Joe, B.E. 1995. Confronting autism: Parents learn to cherish small gains. *OT Week* 9, no. 24: 16–17.
Kientz, M.A. 1996. Sensory-based needs in children with autism: Motivation for behavior and suggestions for intervention. *Developmental Disabilities Special Interest Section Newsletter* 19, no. 3: 1–3.
Kientz, M.A., and W. Dunn. 1997. A comparison of the performance of children with and without autism on the Sensory Profile. *American Journal of Occupational Therapy* 51, no. 7: 530–537.
Miller, H. 1996. Eye contact and gaze aversion: Implications for persons with autism. *Sensory Integration Special Interest Section Newsletter* 19, no. 2: 1–3.
Mora J., and N. Kashman. 1998. "Teaming" model provides holistic approach to autism treatment. *Advance for Occupational Therapists* 14, no. 17: 27–29.
Restall, G., and J. Magill-Evans. 1994. Play and preschool children with autism. *American Journal of Occupational Therapy* 48, no. 2: 113–120.
Stahl, C. 1995. Treating autism throughout the life span. *Advance for Occupational Therapists* 11, no. 13: 17, 62.
Stancliff, B.L. 1996. Autism: Defining the OT's role in treating this confusing disorder. *OT Practice* 1, no. 7: 18–21, 23–29.
Tapper, B.E. 1994. Linking social functioning and the brain. *OT Week* 8, no. 24: 18–19.
Zarella, S. 1996. Sound therapy helps children focus. *Advance for Occupational Therapists* 12, no. 3: 19.

Cerebral Palsy Syndromes

DESCRIPTION

The term cerebral palsy syndromes is used broadly to describe a number of motor disorders characterized by impaired voluntary movement resulting from prenatal developmental abnormalities or perinatal or postnatal central nervous system (CNS) damage occurring before age 5 years. The term cerebral palsy is not a diagnosis but identifies children with nonprogressive spasticity, ataxia, or involuntary movements (Merck 1999, 2416).

Four major groups of syndrome are recognized: spastic, athetoid or dyskinetic, ataxic, and mixed forms.

Spastic syndromes occur in about 70 percent of cases. The spasticity, which is an upper motor neuron symptom, may range from mild to severe. The spastic syndromes may be categorized by the part of the body affected such as hemiplegia, paraplegia, quadriplegia (tetraplegia), or diplegia.

Athetoid or dyskinetic syndromes occur in about 20 percent of cases and result from basal ganglia dysfunction. Slow, writhing involuntary movements may affect the extremities (athetoid form) or the proximal parts of the limbs and the trunk (dystonic form); abrupt, jerky, distal movement (choreiform form) may also occur. The movements increase with emotional tension and disappear during sleep.

Ataxic syndromes occur in about 10 percent of cases and result from dysfunction of the cerebellum or its pathways. Weakness, incoordination, and intention tremor produce an unsteady, wide-based gait and difficulty with rapid or fine movements.

Mixed forms are common, especially spasticity and athetosis. Less often, ataxia and athetosis occur together.

CAUSE

The cause is often hard to establish, but prematurity, in utero disorders, neonatal jaundice, birth trauma, and perinatal asphyxia are implicated. Birth trauma and perinatal asphyxia appear to cause about 15 percent of cases. Spastic paraplegia is especially common after premature birth, spastic quadriparesis after perinatal asphyxia, and athetoid and dystonic forms after perinatal asphyxia or kernicterus. CNS trauma or severe systemic disease during early childhood (e.g., meningitis, sepsis, dehydration) may also cause a cerebral syndrome (Merck 1999, 2416).

Causes can be divided into prenatal, perinatal, and postnatal. Prenatal causes included chromosomal abnormalities or genetic syndromes, congenital brain malformation, problems with fetal or placental functioning, radiation exposure, teratogen exposure relating to material use, twin or multiple pregnancies, and viral infections. Perinatal causes include asphyxia or anoxia, intraventricular hemorrhage, perinatal trauma, preeclampsia, respiratory disorders of prematurity, or sepsis or CNS infection. Postnatal causes include anoxia, toxin exposure, traumatic head injury, and viral or bacterial meningitis.

ASSESSMENT

Subtypes Classified by Part of Body Involved (Topographical)

- Spastic hemiplegia: involvement of the arm and leg on one side of the body.
- Spastic diplegia: involvement of all four extremities, but the lower extremities are more involved than the upper extremities.
- Spastic monoplegia: involvement primarily of one extremity (rare).
- Spastic triplegia: involvement of three extremities.
- Spastic quadriplegia, spastic tetraplegia, or bilateral hemiplegia: involvement of all four extremities.

Subtypes Classified by Characteristics of Movement Disorder

- Athetosis/athetoid: characterized by alternating, writhing, or rotary movements that affect primarily the distal portions of the extremities and tend to increase in response to emotional tension and decrease as the person relaxes.
- Dystonic: characterized by slow, writhing involuntary movements that affect primarily the proximal parts of the limbs and trunk.
- Choreiform: characterized by abrupt, jerky, distal movements.
- Ataxic: characterized by uncoordinated movements that adversely affect the performance of fine and gross motor skills, posture, and balance.
- Flaccid: characterized by fluctuating, markedly low muscle tone in infants, which later changes to spastic, athetoid or ataxic form.
- Rigid: characterized by high muscle tone that continuously resists slow passive movement; sometimes called lead pipe rigidity (rare).
- Tremor: characterized by a rhythmic, alternating muscle contraction and relaxation that is involuntary (rare).
- Atonic: characterized by a lack of muscle tone, leading to the use of the term floppy infant (rare).

Subtypes Classified by Physiologic Characteristics

- Pyramidal: indicates damage to the motor cortex or to the pyramidal tracts of the brain and associated with spasticity, hyperreflexia, and hypertonia
- Extrapyramidal: indicates damage occurring outside the pyramidal tracts in areas such as the basal ganglia or cerebellum and associated with involuntary or incoordinated movements (athetosis) and rigid or floppy muscle tone.
- Mixed: indicates damage to both the pyramidal and extrapyramidal tracts.

Areas

- daily living skills
- play skills
- academic skills
- leisure skills
- reflex development and maturation (note all abnormal and obligatory reflex patterns)
- motor skills: functional range of motion; gross motor skills: rolling, sitting, standing, walking; functional mobility; ability to move self or use assistive technology
- fine motor skills: eye-hand coordination, manipulation, dexterity

---

Positive and Negative Symptoms of Upper Extremity Dysfunction

Positive symptoms (excess or exaggerated movements)
Hypertonicity
- Abnormal postures of the upper extremity that also affect total body posture
- Hyperreflexia, especially increased proprioceptive reflexes, resulting in spasticity and exaggerated cutaneous reflexes producing flexion withdrawal spasms
- Extensor spasms
- Clonus
- Synergistic movement patterns

Negative symptoms (deficits or losses in movement)
- Hypotonia
- Muscle weakness, resulting in loss of functional movement and power
- Muscle fatigability
- Loss of coordination in the hands and upper extremities
- Loss of dexterity in the hands

Source: From *Management of Upper Limb Hypertonicity.* Copyright 1998 by Therapy Skill Builders, a Harcourt Health Sciences Company. Reproduced by permission. All rights reserved.

- hand functions: grasp, pinch, release, opposition
- postural control: muscle tone: hyper- and hypotonia, balance and postural tone, midline stability, bilateral integration
- sensory processing and registration (note especially visual disorders, such as altered eye motility, strabismus, diplopia, amblyopia, cranial nerve paralysis, retrolental fibroplasia, hemianopia)
- sensory modulation and adaptive movement skills
- sensory discrimination and perception skills (note especially visual perceptual skills)
- praxis skills (motor planning) and ideation
- cognitive skills: attention span, concentration, memory, problem solving
- psychosocial skills: self-perception, coping skills, social skills
- language/communication skills
- self-help skills, especially feeding (oral motor skill), dressing, and grooming
- architectural and environmental barriers

Instruments

Instruments Developed by Occupational Therapy Personnel

- *Hawaii Early Learning Profile–Revised* by S. Furuno et al., Palo Alto, CA: VORT Corporation, 1997.
- *Observation List: Sensory Processing in Children with Cerebral Palsy* by E.I. Blanche, T.M Botticelli, and M.K. Hallway, eds., in *Combining neuro-developmental treatment and*

sensory integration principles: An approach to pediatric therapy, 45, San Antonio, TX: Therapy Skill Builders, 1995.

- *Pediatric Evaluation of Disability Inventory* (PEDE) by S. Haley et al., San Antonio, TX: Psychological Corporation–Therapy Skill Builders, 1992.
- *Quality of Upper Extremities Skills Test* (QUEST) reviewed by M. Law, D. Cadman, P. Rosenbaum, S. Walter, D. Russell, C. DeMatteo, in Neuro-developmental therapy and upper-extremity inhibitive casting for children with cerebral palsy, *Developmental Medicine and Child Neurology*, 33 (1991): 379–387.
- *Rehabilitation Institute of Chicago Functional Assessment Scale* by S. Intagliata and B.E. Sullivan, in Development and implementation of the Rehabilitation Institute of Chicago Functional Assessment Scale, *Occupational Therapy Practice* 2, no. 2 (1991): 26–37. Current manual: K. Cichowski, eds., *Rehabilitation Institute of Chicago Functional Assessment Scale manual*, version IV, Chicago IL: Rehabilitation Institute of Chicago, 1996.
- *Sensory Integration and Praxis Tests* (SIPT) by A.J. Ayres, Los Angeles: Western Psychological Services, 1989.
- *Sitting Assessment for Children with Neuromotor Dysfunction* (SACND) by D. Reid, San Antonio, TX: Therapy Skill Builders, 1997.
- *Toddler and Infant Motor Evaluation* (TIME) by L.J. Miller and G.H. Roid, San Antonio, TX: The Psychological Corporation, 1994.
- *Wee Functional Independence Measure* (WeeFIM) by Uniform Data Systems, Buffalo, NY: Uniform Data Systems, 1993.

Instruments Developed by Other Professionals and Used by Occupational Therapy Personnel

- *Battelle Developmental Inventory* (BDI) by J. Newborg, J.R. Stock, and J. Wnek, Itasca, NY: Riverside Publishing Company, 1984.
- *Bayley Infant Neurodevelopmental Screen* (BINS) by G.P. Aylward, San Antonio, TX: The Psychological Corporation, 1995.
- *The Beery-Buktenica Developmental Test of Visual-Motor Integration* (VMI-4), 4th ed. by K.E. Beery and N.A. Buktenica, Parsippany, NJ: Modern Curriculum Press, 1997.
- *Developmental Profile II* (DPII) by G.D. Alpern, T.J. Boll, and M.S. Shearer, Los Angeles: Western Psychological Services, 1984.
- *Goodenough-Harris Drawing Test* by F.L. Goodenough and D. Harris, San Antonio, TX: The Psychological Corporation, 1963.
- *Infant Motor Screen* by R.E. Nickel, C.A. Renken, and J.S. Gallenstein, in The infant motor screen, *Developmental Medicine and Child Neurology* 31, no. 1 (1989): 35–42.
- *Milani-Camparetti Motor Development Screening Test*, 3rd ed rev. by W. Stuberg, Omaha, NE: Meyer Rehabilitation Institute, 1992.
- *Peabody Developmental Motor Scales* by M.R. Folio and R.R. Fewell, Austin, TX: Pro-ed, 1983.
- *Vineland Adaptive Behavior Scales–Revised* by S.S. Sparrow, D.A. Balla, and D.V. Cichetti, Circle Pines, MN: American Guidance Services, 1984.

PROBLEMS

Self-Care

- The person usually has difficulty performing basic activities of daily living, such as eating independently, dressing, toileting, grooming, and hygiene, and lacks the ability to be mobile.
- The person usually needs assistance to develop and achieve independent living status.

Productivity

- The child's play skills may be delayed due to lack of exploratory play behavior.
- The person may need assistance in adapting the working environment to his or her own abilities.
- The person may need assistance in determining how to assume responsibilities at home.
- The person may have difficulty with schoolwork such as learning how to read and how to write.
- In adolescence, the person may need assistance in exploring career options.

Leisure

- The person may need assistance in exploring leisure options.
- The person may need assistance in adapting the leisure environment to his or her own abilities.

Sensorimotor

Spastic Subtype

Muscle Tone

- The person may have hypertonicity in certain muscles, while hypotonicity appears in the opposing muscle groups. In the upper extremities, hypertonicity is most common in the flexors, adductors, pronators, and internal rotators. In the lower extremities, hypertonicity is most common in the extensors, adductors, invertors, and internal rotators. High tone appears in extremities, while low tone appears in trunk musculature. Around a specific joint, the tone may fluctuate, making movement unreliable. Tone may vary from the right to the left side of the body, which makes coordinate movements and bilateral integration difficult.
- The neonate or infant may initially appear normal or hypotonic, but gradually the tone increases or begins to fluctuate, with hypertonicity in extremities and hypotonicity in the trunk and neck.
- The person with hypertonicity in the upper extremity may have any or all of the following characteristics (Copley and Kuipers 1999):
  1. increased resistance to passive movement of the limb
  2. posturing of the limb in positions of deformity at rest
  3. posturing of the limb in positions of deformity during active movement of the affected limb, of the opposing limb, or of other body parts
  4. weakness or paralysis of specific hypertonic and/or nonhypertonic muscle groups, which contributes to a lack of specific movements or movement patterns

5. reduced muscle balance between hypertonic and nonhypertonic muscle groups
6. compensatory or synergistic movement patterns in place of controlled and coordinated voluntary movement
7. functional, organic, or fixed contractures or deformities of the limb resulting from posturing, immobilization, and changes to the structure of joints, muscles, and soft tissue
8. reduced stability and integrity of specific joints
9. limitations to bone growth and density in the affected upper limbs
10. lack of preservation of the architecture of the hand, including the three arches
11. limitations to upper limb function ranging from reduced dexterity or speed during the performance of fine motor tasks to complete absence of active movement
12. sensory deficits ranging from specific loss of discriminative sensation to total neglect of the limb

Reflexes and Reactions
- The person may have primitive reflexes that persist, such as the asymmetrical tonic neck reflex, symmetrical tonic neck reflex, tonic labyrinthine reflex, Moro's reflex, and positive supporting reflex. Nonintegrated primitive reflexes cause muscle tone and movement changes in the extremities.
- The person may engage in toe walking as a result of the positive support reflex.
- The person may have incomplete or abnormal development of the postural (righting, protective, and equilibrium) reactions.

Postural Control, Static and Dynamic
- The person may have delayed, incomplete, and abnormal motor development and decreased voluntary motor control, including lack of stability or base of support, mobility or point of movement, weight shift or change of body position, and reaction weight shift or postural adjustment.
- The person may dislike the prone position because of difficulty with antigravity muscle control. The neck may be hyperextended and the scapula retracted (lack of scapular stability), with inability or difficulty in bearing weight on the forearms.
- The person may have difficulty with flexion against gravity in the supine position, such as inability to flex the trunk against gravity and tendency to maintain upper extremities at the side of the body.
- The person may have a scissor gait as a result of the extension, adduction, and internal rotation of the hip muscles.
- The person may exhibit stereotypical (patterned) movements that include compensatory movements.
- In a sitting position, the person falls into flexion, cannot reach with ease, and maintains the pelvis in posterior tilt with a kyphotic trunk.
- The person has no rotation of the trunk and may use hyperextension as a compensatory movement.

Synergistic Patterns
- Associated reactions (overflow) may be present.
- The person may tend to exhibit the same stereotypic synergy in all positions.

Motor Development and Movement
- The person may have developmental delays (development blocks) that stop the developmental process or result in atypical development. Both delayed and atypical development may lead to compensatory movements or patterns of movement. The more common blocks are neck hyperextension, neck asymmetry, scapulohumeral tightness and scapular adduction, anterior pelvic tilt (lordosis), posterior pelvic tilt, pelvic femoral tightness, and hip extension adduction.
- The person may have difficulty moving in and out of different positions.
- The person may stiffen in anticipation of movement or completely lack any anticipation of movement.
- The person may react to movement after the action has occurred.
- The person may tend to maintain asymmetric position after 6 months of age.
- The person may show delays in hand reach, grasp, release, and bilateral coordination.

Range of Motion
- The person may have contractures and joint tightness, which tend to lead to orthopedic deformities.
- The person may have extremities that are maintained in midrange of motion.

Other Central Nervous System Dysfunctions
- The person may have seizures.

Sensory Functions
- The person may have eye motility problems, including diplopia, strabismus, amblyopia, lack of upward gaze, and hemianopia.
- The person may have visual perception problems, such as impaired visual discrimination or impaired space and form perception.
- In cases of hemiplegic palsy, the person may neglect or ignore one side of the body.
- The person may have vestibular responses that are hyper- or hyporeactive, including gravitational insecurity.
- The person may have tactile responses that are hyper- or hyporesponsive, including tactile defensiveness.
- The person may have diminished awareness of pain.
- The person may have auditory hypersensitivity.
- The person may exhibit fluctuation of muscle tone from low to normal, accompanied by hyperextensor tone.

Athetoid Subtype

Muscle tone
- The person may have writhing and involuntary movements, which are usually seen in distal joints. Spasticity may be present in proximal joints.
- The person may have muscle spasms.

Postural Control, Static and Dynamic
- The person has difficulty stabilizing joints.
- The person may have difficulty performing gross motor activities.
- The person may have difficulty performing fine motor activities.

- The person may have transient subluxation or dislocation of joints.
- The person may have a lack of co-contraction of muscles.
- The person may have a lack of muscle grading.
- The person may be unable to hold a segment of the body, such as a forearm, at various points within the range of motion.
- The person may have asymmetry in both posture and movement.

Synergistic Patterns
- Moving the head affects trunk and limbs.

Reflexes and Reactions
- The person has incomplete righting reflexes, equilibrium reactions, and protective responses that lead to problems in balance and equilibrium.
- The person may have primitive reflexes, such as an inability to hold the head in midline because of the asymmetrical tonic neck reflex, that dominate motor activity.

Sensory Functions
- The person may have hearing loss or other auditory disorder.
- The person may have hyper- or hyporesponsiveness to vestibular stimulation.
- The person may have hyper- or hyporesponsiveness to tactile stimulation.
- The person may have eye motility problems.
- The person may have visual perceptual disorders.

Choreathetotic Subtype

Muscle Tone
- The person usually has constant fluctuations from low to high with no co-contraction.
- The person has low tone (weakness) in hands and fingers.

Movement
- The person has jerky, involuntary movements, more proximal than distal.
- The person has no gradation of movement or ability to select movement.
- The person has difficulty with stabilization or fixation of movement.

Range of Motion
- The person has many involuntary movements with extreme ranges but no control at midrange.
- The person may have subluxation in the shoulder and fingers.

Reflexes and Reactions
- The person may have an intermittent tonic neck reflex.
- The person may not have upper extremity protective extension or performance may be abnormal.
- The person may have equilibrium reactions but these may be ineffective.

Ataxic Subtype

Muscle Tone
- The person has near-normal to normal tone in upper extremities but may have hypertonicity in flexion of the lower extremities.

Range of Motion
- The person's range of motion is usually adequate but may be decreased in flexion.

Movement
- The person may lack a point of stability, so activation is difficult.
- The person may use primitive patterns of movement that are gross, total patterns.
- The person may be incoordinated (dysmetria disdiadochokinesia).
- The person may have tremors at rest.
- The person may show asymmetries.

Cognitive
- The person may have learning disabilities related to perceptual disorders.
- The person may have difficulty learning due to mental retardation.

Psychosocial
- The person may become depressed and express feelings of hopelessness and helplessness.
- The person may have a poor self-image and low self-esteem.
- The person may have inadequate coping skills and become easily frustrated.
- The person may have limited opportunities for self-expression.
- The person may have dysarthric speech and delayed language development.
- The person may have difficulty making friends and developing social skills.
- The person may be emotionally labile.
- The person may have low frustration tolerance and poor coping skills.
- The person may have difficulty developing social relations.

TREATMENT/INTERVENTION

Treatment and management of cerebral palsy usually require an interdisciplinary team approach. Treatment models in occupational therapy are based on neurodevelopmental therapy, sensorimotor therapy, sensory integration, occupational behavior, and model of human occupation. Although these models do not reflect the alteration of neuromotor functioning, there is a change of emphasis in treatment from the neuromaturational and reflex-hierarchical models to systems and motor learning principles and from measurement in a neurodevelopmental framework to measurement in a disablement framework (McEwen and Shelden 1995).

Self-Care
- Promote oral motor skills to facilitate feeding.
- Suggest clothing adaptations that may facilitate independent dressing.
- Suggest various positions that promote stability during dressing.
- Suggest adaptive equipment that may facilitate activities of daily living, such as bolsters, wedges, aids for standing and side lying, adapted chairs, and mobility aids.
- Promote development and independence in performing activities of daily living.

Productivity
- Increase opportunities for play development. Adapted toys and computer-aided games and toys may expand the child's play environment.

Principles of Positioning for Activities of Daily Living

Functional area	Principle	Technique/equipment
Feeding	Provide stability through the trunk to enable a child to have optimal use of a stable base on which to maintain the head in proper alignment for proper oral-motor function and digestion of food.	Commercially available adapted chair, wheelchair, therapeutic holding to adapt a standard chair, or tray attached to chair or wheelchair
Bathing	Provide a safe environment while in a tub or shower for a child and/or a caregiver as well as provide appropriate stability to optimize function.	Tub/shower chair, reclined bath seat, commercially available baby bath rings, or bed bath
Grooming/hygiene	Provide adequate support through the trunk to encourage optimal hand skills.	Appropriate positioning (e.g., chair in front of sink) or appropriate placement and setup of supplies
Toileting	Provide appropriate postural support and stability to enable a child to perform toileting needs in a safe manner.	Adapted toilet seat, commode, or footstool to support feet
Dressing	Provide postural stability, inhibit the effect of abnormal tonal patterns, and eliminate the need to work against gravity.	Chair (regular or adapted) or positioning on floor or in corner
School/play	Provide postural stability to enable a child to engage in classroom or play activities.	Adapted seat or positioning on floor

Source: Reprinted with permission from Dormans, J.P., Pellegrino, L. (Eds.) (1998) *Caring for Children with Cerebral Palsy: A Team Approach* (p. 335). Baltimore. Paul H. Brookes.

- Encourage parents, caregivers, or teachers to assign responsibilities and duties for child to perform.
- Develop work habits and work tolerance.
- Explore vocational interests and career options.
- Promote development of work habits, work skills, and work tolerance.
- Provide opportunities for career exploration.
- Encourage development of independent living skills.

Leisure

- Explore leisure interests.
- Develop leisure skills by providing opportunities to participate in activities.

Sensorimotor

Spasticity

- Inhibit the person's abnormal reflex patterns and facilitate normal posture and movement patterns by handling (guiding) the head and trunk to help the person feel and learn normal sequences of movement in head control, trunk control, weight shifting, weight bearing, and mobility.
- Facilitate head control by improving the balance of neck flexion and extension, lateral flexion, midline control (co-contraction), midline orientation (alignment of head and body) against gravity, and neck mobility (elongation and chin tuck).
- Increase postural tone in trunk musculature and reduce postural tone throughout the extremities to increase postural stability in the trunk while promoting the opportunity for movement in the extremities.
- Balance postural tone (decrease hypertonicity) between opposing groups of muscles to increase co-contraction and alternate contraction and elongation.
- Increase functional range of motion in the extremities as hypertonicity is reduced.
- Promote postural reflex development and maturation (equilibrium and righting reactions) to permit balance (stability) and encourage voluntary movement (mobility).
- Encourage greater variety and differentiation of movement patterns, including varied positions (flexion, extension, rotation), speed, and direction by using key points of control (head, shoulder girdle, trunk, pelvis, calcaneus, knees, and the thenar eminence of the hand).
- Promote use of arms and hands to support, reach, grasp, and hold, and decrease dependence on arms for postural control and stability as trunk stability increases.
- Promote weight bearing with movement designed to increase postural control against gravity.
- Inhibit associated (overflow) reactions by anchoring the opposite limb through weight bearing and such actions as grasping a peg with the hand.
- Encourage the person to initiate movements and avoid remaining in static postures and positions for long periods.
- Work toward muscle elongation, joint mobility, proximal stabilization (co-contraction), and active function of muscles around the joint.
- Consider inhibitive casting of the ankle and foot or hand and wrist to reduce distal muscle tone.

- Consider using hand splints to promote thumb abduction, wrist extension, and functional positioning of the digits.
- Consider powered mobility for persons with poor motor control.
- Encourage movement against gravity to facilitate learning how to control movement.
- Facilitate experiencing the sensation of movement (with vestibular, proprioceptive, and kinesthetic input) to promote learning about movement.
- Use vestibular stimulation to promote equilibrium reactions.
- Provide tactile stimulation to promote oral motor and hand functions.
- For visual perceptual problems, developmental apraxia, gravitational insecurity, and tactile defensiveness, see sections on these specific problems.

Athetosis
- Normalize postural muscle tone by increasing low tone and decreasing high tone.
- Increase symmetric muscle activity.
- Focus activity toward the midline.
- Increase muscle control proximally, then work distally.
- Improve holding posture or motion at various points within the range of motion during active movement.
- Assist person to separate movements of the head from those of the trunk.
- Promote control of muscle spasms.
- Facilitate integration of righting reflexes and the development of equilibrium reactions and protective responses.
- Normalize response to sensory stimulation, if necessary.

Cognitive
- Instruct parents, caregivers, and teachers in seating and positioning techniques to (1) decrease abnormal tone, such as extensor tone, and (2) facilitate trunk and lower limb stability while promoting mobility in the upper extremities.
- Increase attending behavior and attention span.
- Instruct person to instruct others regarding need for assistance.
- Instruct person, family, or caregivers on the adapted equipment available and methods of adapting the home to increase mobility while maintaining safety.
- Use of computers may facilitate learning tasks and improve the person's ability to function in the classroom.

Psychosocial
- Provide a safe environment in which the person can experience movement without fear.
- Provide activities designed to improve self-image and increase self-esteem and a sense of mastery through the use of creative activities such as art, crafts, music, drama, dance, or creative writing. (Note: A computer may be useful for writing and art.)
- Provide opportunities for socialization.
- Assist in development of functional communication and language skills.
- Encourage person, parents, or caregivers to participate in self-help groups, if available.
- Encourage parents to assist the person in understanding role expectations in the home and community.
- Help the family identify community resources.

- Facilitate improvement of self-image.
- Encourage development of social skills.

Environment
- Provide inservice assistance to staff.
- Provide education to parents regarding techniques for managing at home and modifications to home to facilitate care.
- Assist parents in locating community resources.

PRECAUTIONS
- Be alert for signs of sensory overload when using sensory stimulation, especially vestibular stimulation.
- Be aware of any history of seizures and report all seizures to the physician.
- Be alert to signs of illness. The person's performance may deteriorate rapidly during minor illnesses such as the common cold.
- Be alert to any changes in medication and reactions to medications.
- Be sure any assistive technology that uses battery power does not overheat. If electronic power is used, be sure the system is grounded. If the item is constructed, it should be sturdy.

PROGNOSIS AND OUTCOME
The degree of disability from cerebral palsy varies from very mild to very severe. In addition, the level of cognitive function also varies from superior intelligence to severe mental retardation. Those with mild disability from cerebral palsy and average or above average intelligence are more likely to become independent.
- The person has increased self-care skills.
- The person has increased play skills.
- The person demonstrates productive skills.
- The person demonstrates leisure skills.
- The person demonstrates more normal movement patterns.
- The person shows improved postural tone, control, and balance.
- The person demonstrates improved gross motor skills.
- The person shows improved hand skill development and fine motor coordination, manipulation, and dexterity.
- The person demonstrates improved sensory processing skills.
- The person demonstrates improved perceptual skills.
- The person has increased attention span and concentration.
- The person has improved learning skills.
- The person demonstrates increased self-esteem.
- The person shows improved coping skills.

REFERENCES
Beers, M.H., and R. Berkow, eds. 1999. *The Merck Manual of Diagnosis and Therapy*, 17th ed. Whitehouse Station, NJ: Merck Research Laboratories.

Copley J, and K. Kuipers. 1999. *Management of Upper Limb Hypertonicity.* San Antonio, TX: Therapy Skill Builders.
McEwen, I.R., and M.L. Shelden. 1995. Pediatric therapy in the 1990s: The demise of the educational versus medical dichotomy. *Physical and Occupational Therapy in Pediatrics* 15, no. 2: 33–45.

BIBLIOGRAPHY

Anderson, S. 1998. Daily care. In *Children with cerebral palsy: A parents' guide.* 2nd ed., ed. E. Geralis, 101–145. Bethesda, MD: Woodbine House.
Beauregard, R. et al. 1998. Quality of reach during a game and during a rote movement in children with cerebral palsy. *Physical and Occupational Therapy in Pediatrics* 18, no. 3/4: 67–84.
Beck, A.J. et al. 1993. Improvement in upper extremity function and trunk control after selective posterior rhizotomy. *American Journal of Occupational Therapy* 47, no. 8: 704–707.
Black, T. 1993. The child with cerebral palsy. In *Practice issues in occupational therapy: Intraprofessional team building,* ed. S.E. Ryan, 45–56. Thorofare, NJ: Slack.
Blanche, E.I. 1997. Doing with—not doing to: Play and the child with cerebral palsy. In *Play in Occupational Therapy for Children,* eds. L.D. Parham and L.S. Fazio, 202–218. St. Louis, MO: CV Mosby.
Blanche, E.I. et al. 1995. Sensory processing problems in children with cerebral palsy. In *Combining neuro-developmental treatment and sensory integration principles: An approach to pediatric therapy,* eds. E.I. Blanche et al., 67–84. Tucson, AZ: Therapy Skill Builders.
Boulton, J.E. et al. 1995. Reliability of the Peabody Developmental Gross Motor Scale in children with cerebral palsy. *Physical and Occupational Therapy in Pediatrics* 15, no. 1: 35–51.
Buckon, C.E. et al. 1997. Developmental skills of children with spastic diplegia: functional and qualitative changes after selective dorsal rhizotomy. *Archives of Physical Medicine & Rehabilitation* 78, no. 9: 946–951.
Burstein, A.R. et al. 1998. Promoting function in daily living skills. In *Caring for children with cerebral palsy: A team approach,* eds. J.P. Dormans and L. Pellegrino, 371–389. Baltimore: Paul H. Brookes.
Case-Smith, J. 1996. Fine motor outcomes in preschool children who receive occupational therapy services. *American Journal of Occupational Therapy* 50, no. 1: 52–61.
Case-Smith J., and M.A. Nastro. 1993. The effect of occupational therapy intervention on mothers of children with cerebral palsy. *American Journal of Occupational Therapy* 47, no. 9: 811–817.
Colangelo, C. 1994. Powered mobility and the child with cerebral palsy. *Advance for Directors in Rehabilitation* 3, no. 7: 24–27.
Colangelo, C., and D. Gorga. 1996. *Occupational therapy practice guidelines for cerebral palsy.* Bethesda, MD: American Occupational Therapy Association.
Copley, J. et al. 1996. Upper limb casting for clients with cerebral palsy: A clinical report. *Australian Occupational Therapy Journal* 43, no. 2: 39–50.
DeGangi, G.A. 1994. Examining the efficacy of short-term NDT intervention using a case study design: Part 1. *Physical and Occupational Therapy in Pediatrics* 14, no. 1: 71–88.
DeGangi, G.A. 1994. Examining the efficacy of short-term NDT intervention using a case study design: Part 2. *Physical and Occupational Therapy in Pediatrics* 14, no. 2: 21–61.
Dorval, G. et al. 1996. Impact of aquatic programs on adolescents with cerebral palsy. *Occupational Therapy International* 3, no. 4: 241–261.
Dudgeon, B.J. et al. 1994. Prospective measurement of functional changes after selective dorsal rhizotomy. *Archives of Physical Medicine and Rehabilitation* 75, no. 1: 46–53.
Eliasson, A.C. et al. 1998. Hand function in children with cerebral palsy after upper-limb tendon transfer and muscle release. *Developmental Medicine & Child Neurology* 40: 612–621.
Erhardt, R.P., and S.C. Merrill. 1998. Neurological dysfunction in children—cerebral palsy. In *Willard and Spackman's occupational therapy,* eds. M.E. Neistadt and E.B. Crepeau, 589–598. Philadelphia: J.B. Lippincott Co.

Foltz, L.C. et al. 1998. Physical therapy, occupational, and speech and language therapy. In *Children with cerebral palsy: A parents' guide.* 2nd ed., ed. E. Geralis, 231–290. Bethesda, MD: Woodbine House.

Freeman, J.E. 1995. Treatment of hand dysfunction in the child with cerebral palsy. In *Hand function in the child: Foundations for remediation*, eds. A. Henderson and C. Pehoski, 282–298. St. Louis, MO: Mosby.

Geyer, L.A. et al. 1998. Promoting function in daily living skills. In *Caring for children with cerebral palsy: A team approach*, eds. J.P. Dormans and L. Pellegrino, 323–346. Baltimore: Paul H. Brookes.

Gisel, E.G. 1996. Effect of oral sensorimotor treatment on measures of growth and efficiency of eating in the moderately eating-impaired child with cerebral palsy. *Dysphagia* 11, no. 1: 48–56.

Greiner, B.M. et al. 1993. Gait parameters of children with spastic diplegia: A comparison of effects of posterior and anterior walkers. *Archives of Physical Medicine and Rehabilitation* 74, no. 4: 381–385.

Grimby, G. et al. 1996. Structure of a combination of Functional Independence Measure and instrumental activity measure items in community-living persons: A study of individuals with cerebral palsy and spina bifida. *Archives of Physical Medicine and Rehabilitation* 77, no. 11: 1109–1114.

Hagesstedt, J.L. 1993. Splint adaptation encourages functional activity. *OT Week* 7, no. 20: 20–21.

Harburn, K.L., and P.J. Potter. 1993. Spasticity and contractures. *Physical Medicine and Rehabilitation: State of the Art Reviews* 7, no. 1: 113–132.

Hickey, A., and J. Ziviani. 1998. A review of the Quality of Upper Extremities Skills Test (QUEST) for children with cerebral palsy. *Physical and Occupational Therapy* 18, no. 3/4: 123–135.

Klein, M.D., and T.A. Delaney. 1994. Conditions affecting feeding and nutrition—cerebral palsy. In *Feeding and nutrition for the child with special needs: Handouts for parents*, eds. M.D. Klein and T.A. Delaney, 363–379. Tucson, AZ: Therapy Skill Builders.

Klinghorn, J., and G. Roberts. 1996. The effect of an inhibitive weight-bearing splint on tone and function: A single case study. *American Journal of Occupational Therapy* 50, no. 10: 807–815.

Lange, M.L. 1995. Aiming high. *TeamRehab Report* 6, no. 9: 26–30.

Lange, M.L. et al. 1995. A custom fit. *TeamRehab Report* 6, no. 1: 22–26.

Law, M. et al. 1997. A comparison of intensive neurodevelopmental therapy plus casting and a regular occupational therapy program for children with cerebral palsy. *Developmental Medicine and Child Neurology* 39, no. 10: 664–670.

Leonard, J.F. et al. 1997. *Keys to parenting a child with cerebral palsy.* Hauppauge, NY: Barron's Education Services.

Lewin, J.E. et al. 1993. Self-help and upper extremity changes in 36 children with cerebral palsy subsequent to selective posterior rhizotomy and intensive occupational and physical therapy. *Physical and Occupational Therapy in Pediatrics* 13, no. 3: 25–42.

MacKinnon, J.R. et al. 1995. A study of therapeutic effects of horseback riding for children with cerebral palsy. *Physical and Occupational Therapy in Pediatrics* 15, no. 1: 17–34.

Majnemer, A. 1999. Occupational therapy. *Exceptional Parent* 29, no. 6: 51–52.

Muraki, T. et al. 1993. Effect of respiratory and cardiometabolic responses to tub bathing on elderly with cerebral palsy: A preliminary investigation. *Physical and Occupational Therapy in Geriatrics* 11, no. 2: 39–56.

Nelson, CA. 1995. Cerebral palsy. In *Neurological Rehabilitation.* 3rd ed., ed. D.A. Umphred, 263–286. St. Louis, MO: Mosby.

Pimm, P.L. 1996. Some of the implications of caring for a child or adult with cerebral palsy. *British Journal of Occupational Therapy* 59, no. 7: 335–341.

Reid, D.T. 1995. Development of preliminary validation of an instrument to assess quality of sitting of children with neuromotor dysfunction. *Physical and Occupational Therapy in Pediatrics* 15, no. 1: 53–81.

Reid, D.T. 1995. The effects of the saddle seat on seated postural control and upper extremity movement in children with cerebral palsy. *Developmental Medicine and Child Neurology* 38, no. 9: 805–815.

Reid, D.T., and P. Rigby. 1996. Research in progress: Development of improved anterior pelvic stabilization devices for children with cerebral palsy. *Physical and Occupational Therapy in Pediatrics* 16, no. 3: 91–96.

Shamberg, S., and A. Shamberg. 1996. Building an accessible home from the ground up. *TeamRehab Reports* 7 no. 4: 16–17, 20–22.

Tcheremenska, A.R., and E.G. Gisel. 1994. Use of substitute food textures for standard eating assessment in children with cerebral palsy and children without disabilities. *American Journal of Occupational Therapy* 48, no. 7: 626–632.

Tomcheck, S.D. 1999. The nervous system—cerebral palsy. In *Pediatric therapy: A systems approach*, eds. S.M. Poor and E.B. Rainville, 161–174. Philadelphia: F.A. Davis.

Tona, J.L., and C.M. Schneck. 1993. The efficacy of upper extremity serial inhibitive casting: A single-subject pilot study. *American Journal of Occupational Therapy* 47, no. 10: 901–910.

Trefler, E., and J. Angeo. 1997. Comparison of anterior trunk supports for children with cerebral palsy. *Assistive Technology* 9, no. 1: 15–21.

Vogle, L.K. et al. 1998. An aquatic program for adults with cerebral palsy living in group homes. *Physical Therapy Case Reports* 1, no. 5: 250–259.

Wilsdon, J. 1996. Cerebral palsy. In *Occupational therapy and physical dysfunction: Principles, skills, and practice*, eds. A. Turner et al., 395–432. New York: Churchill Livingstone.

Wright, F.V. et al. 1998. Evaluation of effective dorsal rhizotomy for the reduction of spasticity in cerebral palsy: A randomized controlled trial. *Developmental Medicine and Child Neurology* 40, no. 4: 239–247.

Child Abuse and Neglect

DESCRIPTION

Child abuse and neglect is defined as physical or mental (emotional) injury, sexual abuse, negligent treatment, or maltreatment of a child under the age of 18. **Physical abuse** involves the physical battery of a child. **Emotional abuse** involves the emotional or mental battery of a child, which often damages the child's emotional growth and self-esteem. **Sexual abuse** or molestation involves exposure, genital manipulation, sodomy, fellatio, and coitus. **Neglect** includes failure to meet a child's basic physical and medical needs, emotional deprivation, and desertion (Merck 1999, 2300).

The Child Abuse Prevention and Treatment Act (Public Law 95-266) defines child abuse as "the physical or mental injury, sexual abuse or exploitation, negligent treatment or maltreatment of a child under the age of eighteen or the Child Protective Law of the State in question, by a person who is responsible for the child's welfare under circumstances which would indicate that the child's health or welfare is harmed or threatened therapy" (*U.S. Code Annotated* 1978, 228). Note that most states have a mandatory notification system if child abuse or neglect is known to or suspected by another person. The occupational therapy practitioner should know these requirements and follow the procedures for fulfilling them.

Other relevant terms include battered child syndrome and maltreated children.

CAUSE

- **Abuse** is the breakdown of impulse control in the parent, guardian, or other caregiver. There are four factors involved:
  1. **Personality features**. The caregiver experienced lack of affection and support as a child and thus does not know how to provide these for his or her child, or the caregiver is out of control due to substance abuse or psychotic illness.

2. **The "difficult" child**. Examples include hyperactive, handicapped, premature, or sickly children or stepchildren.
3. **Inadequate support**. The caregiver feels isolated or abandoned by relatives or friends who could provide guidance and assistance.
4. **Crisis situation**. Stress overcomes the caregiver's ability to function.
- **Neglect** is observed in families with multiple problems and disorganized lifestyles. Depression, desertion, drug or alcohol abuse, and chronic medical conditions may be seen in one or more caregivers (Merck 1999, 2301).

ASSESSMENT

Areas
- daily living skills
- academic readiness or academic skills
- play skills
- motor skills: muscle strength, gross motor development, and coordination skills
- fine motor skills, manipulation, dexterity, and bilateral coordination
- reflex development and maturation
- postural control: muscle tone, joint stability, and mobility
- sensory modulation
- sensory discrimination and perceptual skills
- attending behavior and concentration
- ability to follow directions/sequencing
- motivation or self-initiation of activity
- mood or affect
- self-control
- coping skills
- social conduct skills
- parenting skills and practices
- stress within the family unit

Instruments
Instruments Developed by Occupational Therapy Personnel
- *A Play Scale* (also called *Preschool Play Scale*) by S. Knox, in *Play as Exploratory Learning*, ed. M. Reilly, 247–266, Beverly Hills, CA: Sage, 1974. *Revised Knox Preschool Play Scale* by S. Knox in *Play in occupational therapy for children,* eds. L.D. Parham and L.S. Fazio, 35–51, St. Louis, MO: Mosby, 1997.
- *Miller Assessment for Preschoolers* (MAP) by L.J. Miller, San Antonio, TX: Therapy Skill Builders, 1988.

Instruments Developed by Other Professionals and Used by Occupational Therapy Personnel
- *Battelle Developmental Inventory* (BDI) by J. Newborg, J.R. Stock, and J. Wnek, Itasca, IL: Riverside Publishing Company, 1984.

- *Bruininks-Oseretsky Test of Motor Proficiency* (BOTMP) by R. Bruininks, Circle Pines, MN: American Guidance Services, 1978.
- *Denver Developmental Screening Test, Revised* (Denver-II) by W.K. Frankenburg et al., Denver, CO: Denver Developmental Materials, 1990.

PROBLEMS

The problems associated with child abuse can be varied and many. The list of problems should be considered as examples and not as a comprehensive list.

Self-Care
- The person may be delayed in developing activities of daily living, such as dressing, tying shoes, or eating with a fork.
- The person may be unable to perform certain activities of daily living if motor skills are involved.

Productivity
- The person may have developmental delays in acquiring play skills.
- The person may use less imagination in play.
- The person may be unable to organize play activities.
- The person may show little exploratory behavior in play.

Leisure
- The person may have few leisure interests beyond watching television or video.

Sensorimotor
- The person's developmental milestones may be delayed, especially gross and fine motor skills.
- The person may have muscle weakness or paralysis if nerve or brain damage has occurred.
- Contractures may be present if the condition has existed for some time.
- The person may have decreased of range of motion, depending on the type of injury.
- The person may have incomplete reflex maturation: primitive reflexes may still be present.
- The person may have sensory loss in vision, hearing, touch, proprioception, or kinesthesia, or less commonly in taste or smell.
- The person may have a poor body image or an impaired body image may develop.
- The person may have sensory integrative dysfunction: sensory modulation may be hypo- or hyperreactive.

Cognitive
- The person may have learning disabilities, including dyslexia, short attention span, and hyperkinetic behavior.
- The person may have poor problem-solving skills.

Psychosocial
- The person may have a poor self-image and lack self-confidence.

- The person may feel guilty for "causing so much trouble." (Note: The child is not the cause but may be made to feel so by repeated statements from one or more adults.)
- The person may have a blunted or flat affect.
- The person may lack self-control; for example, the person may be negative and aggressive or have a low tolerance for frustration.
- The person may act helpless or be overly compliant or withdrawn.
- Role identity within the family unit may be ill-defined or fluctuating.
- Parent(s) and child may lack coping skills.
- The person may have delayed development of social interaction and conduct skills.
- The person may be delayed in acquiring speech or vocabulary.
- Bonding between parent and child may be inadequate or lacking.
- The person may lack group interaction skills.

Environment
- Caregiver may not have appropriate parenting skills.
- Caregiver may lack knowledge about normal growth and development of children.
- Caregiver may be under stress with insufficient coping skills.

TREATMENT/INTERVENTION

Intervention requires an interdisciplinary team approach that addresses the needs of the family and child. Usually occupational therapists will be part of a team of professionals. Models of treatment include sensory integration and neurodevelopmental therapy.

Self-Care
- Promote self-feeding skills.
- Decrease oral motor sensitivity, if needed.
- Increase skills in dressing and other tasks of daily living.

Productivity
- Teach parents or caregivers the child's level of play skills and how to participate in play activities with the child.
- Promote development of play skills.
- Assist in promoting academic readiness skills.

Leisure
- Encourage exploration of interests and development of leisure skills.

Sensorimotor
- Promote development of gross and fine motor skills according to developmental level.
- Increase muscle strength through progressive resistive exercises, if needed.
- Maintain or increase joint range of motion through passive exercises and active involvement in activities.
- Facilitate integration of primitive reflexes.
- If sensory loss has occurred, facilitate development of remaining senses.
- Increase body awareness and position in space.

- If sensory integrative dysfunction is noted, see section on the specific disorder for treatment suggestions.

Cognitive
- Improve attending behavior and attention span.
- Improve the child's ability to follow directions and sequences.
- Improve problem-solving skills by assisting the child to think through a situation, by asking questions, and by prompting responses.

Psychosocial
- Facilitate bonding between caregiver and child by encouraging holding and cuddling, feeding, and grooming, and by teaching developmentally appropriate skills.
- Increase interaction between caregiver and child by grading the amount of interaction and adult-imposed structure required based on developmental level of caregiver and child.
- Select or help caregiver select activities that are mutually enjoyable; provide opportunity for gentle physical contact and pleasant interactive communication.
- Improve self-image and sense of mastery through use of creative activities such as crafts, games, music, dance, or drama.
- Increase self-control by assisting the child to think of alternative approaches to situations and tasks.
- Provide an opportunity for the child to practice social conduct in a group situation.

Environment
- Provide caregiver with a social support system that is available to help, not criticize, while focusing on ways to reduce caregiver stress and sense of frustration, especially in single-parent homes.
- Assist caregiver in understanding the importance of reliability, gentleness, and communication of caring to the child.
- Educate caregiver about normal child development, such as how and when a child learns to perform daily living and social skills, to reduce unrealistic expectations of caregiver regarding child's behavior.
- Educate caregiver about parenting skills, especially appropriate discipline through nonpunitive behavior-management techniques such as praising approximations of desired behavior, using sticker charts or other reward systems, and instituting time out.
- Facilitate development and continuation of a parent group for mutual support.
- Help caregiver learn to plan ahead and seek assistance from various sources such as friends, other family members, or community resources as needed.
- Practitioner should be prepared to demonstrate and teach some of the activities during initial sessions. Role-playing techniques may be useful.
- Practitioner should consider whether assertiveness training may be helpful in teaching caregiver to manage child, improve communication skills, and increase self-esteem.

PRECAUTIONS
- Observe child for signs of any additional abuse or neglect.

- Observe caregiver for signs of increased stress and frustration, which may result in abuse or neglect of the child.
- Be prepared to take action, if necessary, according to team protocol, to prevent abuse or neglect.
- Be aware that a child with a disability, behavioral disorder, and/or chronic condition is more likely to be abused and/or neglected.

PROGNOSIS AND OUTCOME

- The primary goal is to prevent further incidents of child abuse or neglect.
- Parent or caregiver is able to interact with the child without violent, abusive, or neglectful behavior.
- Parent or caregiver demonstrates knowledge of the child's level of development and adjusts expectations to the child's level of development and performance.
- Parent or caregiver is able to manage his or her own life situation and stresses without taking out anger or frustrations on the child.
- The child demonstrates improved developmental profile in sensorimotor, cognitive, psychosocial, self-care, and play skills.

REFERENCES

Beers, M.H., and R. Berkow, eds. 1999. *The Merck Manual of Diagnosis and Therapy*, 17th ed. Whitehouse Station, NJ: Merck Research Laboratories.
The Public Health and Welfare, Section 4541–6500. 1978. *U.S. Code Annotated*. St. Paul, MN: West Publishing Company.

BIBLIOGRAPHY

Abromovich, T. 1995. Adult survivors of sexual abuse in childhood: One case study. *Israel Journal of Occupational Therapy* 4, no. 3: 78–84.
Davidson, D.A. 1995. Physical abuse of preschoolers: Identification and intervention through occupational therapy (review). *American Journal of Occupational Therapy* 49, no. 3: 235–243.
Davidson, D.A. 1998. Child abuse and neglect. In *Willard and Spackman's occupational therapy*. 9th ed., eds. H.L. Hopkins and H.D. Smith, 636–639. Philadelphia: Lippincott-Raven Publishers.
Forrest, K., and S. Wright. 1994. Letter to the editor. Physical and emotional abuse: Comment and reply to "Physical and emotional abuse and neglect of preschool children: A literature review." *Australian Occupational Therapy Journal* 41, no. 4: 184–185.
Joe, B.E. 1996. Expressive therapy helps adults cope with past abuse. *OT Week* 10, no. 30: 17. (adults)
Joe, B.E. 1996. Overcoming childhood trauma. *OT Week* 10, no. 23: 18–19.
O'Neill, D., and L. Bradley. 1993. Developmental approach to victimized youth: Integrating occupational therapy into current service delivery. *Occupational Therapy Forum* 8, no. 14: 4–5, 8.
Wright, S.A. 1994. Physical and emotional abuse and neglect of preschool children: A literature review. *Australian Occupational Therapy Journal* 41, no. 2: 55–63.

Developmental Coordination Disorder

DESCRIPTION

According to the DSM-IV, developmental coordination disorder should be considered when "performance in daily activities that require motor coordination is substantially below that expected given the person's chronologic age and measured intelligence." The manifestations include marked delays in achieving motor milestones such as walking, crawling, and sitting, dropping things, clumsiness, poor performance in sports, and poor handwriting. These manifestations should be severe enough to interfere with academic achievement or activities of daily living. However, neither medical conditions such as cerebral palsy, hemiplegia, or muscular dystrophy, nor any type of pervasive developmental disorder such as autism, should be present. Mental retardation may be present, but the motor difficulties must exceed those usually associated with the degree of mental retardation.

A number of terms have been used in the past to describe motor incoordination. According to Willoughby and Polatajko (1995), Ayres used the term developmental dyspraxia (see section on sensory integration—developmental dyspraxia or apraxia). Other terms considered to be similar or equivalent are clumsy child syndrome, physical awkwardness, poor coordination, incoordination, mild motor problems, perceptual motor dysfunction, motor delay, developmental agnosia, and minimal brain dysfunction. The condition is often associated with learning disability, communication disorders, disruptive behavior, and attention deficit/hyperactivity disorder.

CAUSE

There is general agreement that developmental coordination disorder is the result of problems in sensory processing. The disputes begin with the exact nature of the sensory processing problem. Explanations include the presence of unisensory, intersensory, and multisensory problems. Furthermore, there is no agreement as to which sensory systems are involved or which is(are) the primary cause(s). Candidates for primary causation include the vestibular, proprioceptive, kinesthetic, and visual systems. In addition, the role of sensory processing deficits is not clearly understood. Thus, it is unclear whether remediation should stress unimodal intervention (within one sensory system such as vision) or cross-modal intervention (involving two sensory systems such as touch to vision). Finally, one view suggests that the problem is simply one of maturational lag and that, with time, the problem will resolve itself. The latter view has been shown to be shortsighted. Children with developmental coordination disorder do not outgrow the problems, which remain throughout adulthood, although compensatory techniques may mask some symptoms. McConnell (1995) has reviewed the four primary perspectives underlying the developmental coordination disorder, which are the neuropathologic, visual perceptual, kinesthetic processing, and motor programming perspectives.

Criteria for Developmental Coordination Disorder

- Performance in daily activities that require motor coordination is substantially below that expected given the person's chronologic age and measured intelligence. This deficit may be manifested by marked delays in achieving motor milestones (e.g., walking, crawling, sitting), tendency to drop things, "clumsiness," poor performance in sports, or poor handwriting.
- The disturbance in the above criterion significantly interferes with academic achievement or activities of daily living.
- The disturbance is not due to a general medical condition (e.g., cerebral palsy, hemiplegia, or muscular dystrophy) and does not meet criteria for pervasive developmental disorder.
- If mental retardation is present, the motor difficulties are in excess of those usually associated with it.

Source: Reprinted with permission from *Diagnostic and Statistical Manual of Mental Disorders*, 4th ed., pp. 54–55, © 1994, American Psychiatric Association.

ASSESSMENT

Areas
- fine and gross motor patterns of development, such as catching a ball
- performance of motor tasks appropriate for current age
- quality of movement, such as difficulty drawing
- kinesthetic awareness
- functional performance at home, play, and school
- performance of novel motor-based tasks
- self-esteem
- social acceptance
- coping strategies
- life experience, temperament, environment, and genetic endowment

Instruments
Instruments Developed by Occupational Therapy Personnel
- *About Me* by C. Missiuna, in Development of "All About Me," a scale that measures children's perceived motor competence, *Occupational Therapy Journal of Research* 18, no. 2 (1998): 85–108.
- *Canadian Occupational Performance Measure* (COPM), 2nd ed. by M. Law et al., Toronto, Canada: CAOT/L'ACE Publications, 1994.
- *Sensory Integration and Praxis Tests* by A.J. Ayres, Los Angeles: Western Psychological Services, 1989. (Replaces the Southern California Sensory Integration Tests.)

Instruments Developed by Other Professionals and Used by Occupational Therapy Personnel

- *The Beery-Buktenica Developmental Test of Visual-Motor Integration* (VMI-4), 4th ed. by K.E. Beery and N.A. Buktenica, Parsippany, NJ: Modern Curriculum Press, 1997.
- *Bruininks-Oseretsky Test of Motor Proficiency* (BOTMP) by R.H. Bruininks, Circle Pines, MN: American Guidance Services, 1978.
- *Developmental Test of Visual Perception-2* (DTVP-2) by D.D. Hammill, N.A. Pearson, and J.F. Voress, Austin, TX: Pro-ed, 1993. (Replaces the Marianne Frostig Developmental Test of Visual Perception.)
- *Goodenough Draw-a-Man Test* by F.L. Goodenough and D.B. Harris, San Antonio, TX: The Psychological Corporation, 1963.
- *Gubbay's Screening Test* by S. Gubbay, in Clumsy children in normal schools, *Medical Journal of Australia* 1 (1975): 233–236.
- *Kinaesthetic Sensitivity Test* by J.I. Laszlo and P.J. Bairstow, in The measurement of kinaesthetic sensitivity in children and adults, *Developmental Medicine and Child Neurology* 22 (1985): 454–464. (Test is published by Senkit, Ltd., in Perth, Australia.)
- *McCarron Assessment of Neuromuscular Development* by L.T. McCarron, Dallas, TX: Common Market Press, 1982.
- *Movement Assessment Battery for Children* (Movement ABC, formerly the Test of Motor Impairment) by S.E. Henderson and D.A. Sugden, San Antonio, TX: The Psychological Corporation, 1992.
- *Perceptual-Motor Abilities Test* by J. Laszio and P. Bairstow, in *Perceptual-motor behaviour: Developmental assessment therapy*, London: Holt, Rhinehart and Winston, 1985.
- *The Pictorial Scale of Perceived Competence and Social Acceptance for Young Children* by S. Harter and R. Pike, *Child Development* 55, no. 6 (1984): 1969–1982.
- *Test of Visual-Perceptual Skills (non-motor), Revised* by M.F. Gardner, Hydesville, CA: Psychological and Educational Publications, 1996.

PROBLEMS

Self-Care
- The person may have difficulty performing activities of daily living such as self-feeding.

Productivity
- The person may have poor handwriting.

Leisure
- The person often performs poorly in sports activities.

Sensorimotor
Overall
- The person may be able to perform an action or movement if prompted but does not initiate or use the action or movement spontaneously in coping with the environment during exploratory play or completion of a specific task. Therapist must differentiate between

actions or movements that cannot be performed and those that can be performed but are not routinely used.

Motor Development
- The person may have developmental delay in the achievement of milestones in severe cases.
- The person may register in the low-normal range of achievement of developmental milestones in mild cases.

Muscle and Postural Tone
- The person may have decreased postural tone as evidenced by stiffening in the shoulder girdle area to gain stability.
- The person may have decreased stability in neck and shoulder girdle musculature apparent in prone and supine positions.
- The person may avoid challenging postural control.
- The person may have deficits in anticipatory postural control.
- The person may have a tendency to maintain the pelvis in anterior pelvic tilt to gain stability.
- The person may tend to use a wide base of support in sitting and standing.

Movement Synergies
- The person may have a variety of movement synergies but has a reduced repertoire of movement strategies to meet the demands of the task.
- The person may have poor flexion in antigravity positions, especially in the abdominal area.
- The person may have ability to rotate the trunk but does not use rotation spontaneously.

Weight Bearing and Shifting
- The person may have difficulty shifting weight from side to side.
- The person may have a tendency to elevate the shoulder and decrease degrees of freedom by fixing and locking the elbows.

Movement
- The person may have difficulty with transitions: may maintain higher, more demanding postures against gravity but may not sequence lower-level transition.
- The person may have poor anticipatory control: may react after the action has occurred.

Upper Extremity Control
- The person may have poor scapular stability as evidenced by winging of the scapulae.
- The person may have a tendency to fist the hands during weight bearing, although no difficulty is seen in opening the hands in other situations.
- The person may tend to stabilize the upper extremities by adducting the humerus against the trunk.

Perceptual Motor
- The person may have difficulty with spatial organization.
- The person may be clumsy or may be considered to be clumsy by others.
- The person may be incoordinated.

- The person may have motor dyspraxia and poor motor planning skills as evidenced in the performance of closed and open tasks.
- The person may have mixed hand dominance.
- The person may have difficulty with eye-hand coordination tasks such as stacking blocks.

Cognitive

- The person may have limited concentration span.
- The person may have poor information-processing skills.
- The person may have difficulty with sequencing tasks and activities.
- The person may have difficulty acting on feedback.

Psychosocial

- The person may be socially isolated.
- The person may perceive himself or herself as having lower levels of physical competence than peers.
- The person may not believe he or she has the ability to perform tasks requiring motor planning and coordination.

TREATMENT/INTERVENTION

Since no clear explanation exists as to cause, there are many differing approaches to treatment and intervention. Which approach is best cannot be ascertained unless the fundamental problem can be clearly defined, explained, and assessed. In educational environments, the perceptual motor approach has been popular. Within occupational therapy, the most popular approach has been sensory integrative therapy. However, the practitioner should consider the response of the person. If the response to multisensory input is poor, perhaps a unisensory approach should be tried.

Other treatment approaches that have been tried include process-oriented treatment using kinesthetic training (Polatajko et al. 1995) and the verbal self-guidance approach (Martini and Polatajko 1998).

Sensorimotor

- Facilitate use of those actions or movements that are not routinely used by the person through application of cueing or reminders.
- Facilitate development of gross and fine motor activities that have not been learned within a developmental continuum.
- Provide sensory integrative activities such as those using scooter boards and bolster swings.
- Provide perceptual motor activities such as those involving pegboards, balance beams, and painting materials.
- Improve kinesthetic skills.
- Assist the person in attaining specific motor planning and coordination skills.
- Provide multisensory stimulation, as by rolling a large ball back and forth with the person, with each calling out the name of the other before rolling the ball; making a group collage using beans, pasta, and lentils; going through an obstacle course; identifying colors; playing Simon Says; using a life-size body picture for identifying body parts; making a chart to

record achievement; playing sleeping lions; playing charades; making a dragon out of paper and cardboard; telling a story about the dragon; playing matchsticks or pick-up sticks; using a tactile box; folding paper; making cards; copying gestures; videotaping a variety of fine and gross motor activities; playing memory games; drawing around the hand to make reindeer antlers; cutting out forms; icing biscuits and decorating with small sweets; playing crab football.

- Provide information relating object to object (mainly visual), self to earth (mainly vestibular), self to self (mainly proprioceptive/kinesthetic), and self to object (mainly somatosensory) to promote dynamic integration.

Cognitive

- Consider use of the kinesthetic learning approach: Child is taught to say to himself or herself (self-instruction or verbal self-guidance) the words *Goal, Plan, Do,* and *Check* (GPDC strategy) during the performance of an occupational task. **Goal** is what the child wants to do; **Plan** is how the child will do it; **Do** is carrying out the plan; and **Check** is seeing if the plan worked and, if not, where it went wrong.

Psychosocial

- Improve self-esteem and self-confidence through participation and skill building, reward for effort, social feedback, and peer comparison.
- Provide alternate strategies that can lead to success if direct intervention in motor planning and coordination does not yield positive results.

Environment

- Help caregivers and teachers understand that behavioral problems will probably decrease as sensorimotor abilities increase.

PRECAUTIONS

- Be aware that children with developmental coordination disorder should be assessed and treated for both motor and sensory development and integration. Working only to overcome developmental delays in reaching milestones will leave motor planning skills untouched.
- Be aware that children with developmental coordination disorder may appear to have an uneven level of development that allows the performance of some items higher in the developmental continuum while lower-level tasks are not performed.

PROGNOSIS AND OUTCOME

- The child will be able to perform self-care activities appropriate to normal age range.
- The child's play skills will be age appropriate.
- Individuals with developmental coordination disorder do respond to intervention and can improve their ability to perform sensorimotor activities and tasks.
- The person's sensorimotor performance will improve toward the normal for his or her chronologic age.
- The person's disruptive behavior will decrease and cooperative behavior will improve.

REFERENCES

American Psychiatric Association. 1994. *Diagnostic and Statistical Manual of Mental Disroders: DSM-IV*, 4th ed. Washington, DC: American Psychiatric Assocation. Task Fource on DSM-IV.

Martini, R., and H.J. Polatajko. 1998. Verbal self-guidance as a treatment approach for children with developmental coordination disorder: A systematic replication study. *Occupational Therapy Journal of Research* 18, no. 4: 157–181.

McConnell, D. 1995. Processes underlying clumsiness: a review of perspectives. *Physical and Occupational Therapy in Pediatrics* 15, no. 3: 33–52.

Polatajko, H.J. et al. 1995. A clinical trial of the process-oriented treatment approach for children with developmental co-ordination disorder. *Developmental Medicine and Child Neurology* 37: 310–319.

Willoughby, C., and H.J. Polatajko. 1995. Motor problems of children with developmental coordination disorder: Review of the literature. *American Journal of Occupational Therapy* 49, no. 8: 787–794.

BIBLIOGRAPHY

Blanche, E.I. 1998. Intervention for motor control and movement organization disorders. In *Pediatric occupational therapy and early intervention.* 2nd ed., ed. J. Case-Smith, 268–269. Boston: Butterworth-Heinemann.

Howard, L. 1997. Developmental coordination disorder: Can we measure our intervention? *British Journal of Occupational Therapy* 60, no. 5: 219–220.

Klein, S., and J. Magill-Evans. 1998. Perceptions of competence and peer acceptance in young children with motor and learning difficulties. *Physical and Occupational Therapy in Pediatrics* 18, no. 3/4: 39–52.

Lockhart, J., and M. Law. 1994. The effectiveness of a multisensory writing programme for improving cursive writing ability in children with sensorimotor difficulties. *Canadian Journal of Occupational Therapy* 61, no. 4: 206–214.

Malloy-Miller, T. et al. 1995. Handwriting error patterns of children with mild motor difficulties. *Canadian Journal of Occupational Therapy* 62, no. 5: 258–267.

Missiuna, C. 1998. Development of "All About Me," a scale that measures children's perceived motor competence. *Occupational Therapy Journal of Research* 18, no. 2: 85–108.

Missiuna, C., and H. Polatajko. 1995. Developmental dyspraxia by any other name: Are they all just clumsy children. *American Journal of Occupational Therapy* 49, no. 7: 619–627.

Polatajko, H.J. et al. 1995. National perspective: An international consensus on children with developmental coordination disorder. *Canadian Journal of Occupational Therapy* 62, no. 1: 3–6.

Sellers, J.S. 1995. Clumsiness: Review of causes, treatments, and outlook. *Physical and Occupational Therapy in Pediatrics* 15, no. 4: 39–55.

Wilson, B. et al. 1992. Reliability and construct validity of the clinical observation of motor and postural skills. *American Journal of Occupational Therapy* 46, no. 9: 775–783.

Developmental Delay—Child

DESCRIPTION

As defined in the criteria for eligibility in the Individuals with Disabilities Education Act of 1990 (Public Law 101-476), developmental delay indicates delay in one or more of the following developmental areas: cognitive, physical (including vision and hearing), communication, social or emotional, and adaptive, as measured by an appropriate diagnostic instrument or procedure. States differ in the criteria for determining an "appropriate" instrument or procedure. Within the law, the age range is limited to 5 years or younger. Two programs are covered. The first is early intervention, which encompasses children 0 to 2 years of age and is based on the medical model. The second is a special education program for children 3 to 5 years of age.

Developmental delay is a catch-all term used for government funding programs. The term is not specific enough for this handbook. Please refer to sections dealing with a more specific diagnosis for the child, such as attention deficit/hyperactivity disorder, autism, Rett's disorder, developmental coordination disorder, mental retardation, etc.

REFERENCE

Public Law 101–476. Disabilities Education Act of 1990, 1990.

BIBLIOGRAPHY

Hanft, B.E. 1997. *Occupational therapy practice guidelines for young children with delayed development.* Bethesda, MD: American Occupational Therapy Association.

Developmental Disabilities—Adult

DESCRIPTION

As described in the Developmental Disabilities laws (Public Law 88-162, Public Law 100-146), persons with developmental disabilities are those with severe and chronic disabilities that are attributable to a mental or physical impairment or a combination of mental or physical impairments. The disability must have manifested itself before age 22 and must be likely to continue indefinitely. The results of disability must be evident in three or more of the following areas of major life activities: self-care, receptive and expressive language, learning, mobility, self-direction, capacity for independent living, and economic sufficiency.

Persons with adult developmental disabilities may have diagnoses such as mental retardation, autism, sensory and/or neurologic impairments, epilepsy, and other lifelong disabilities.

CAUSE

The causes for developmental disabilities are varied and include all causes discussed in this section of the handbook as well as those that are unknown. Examples include genetic disorders, hereditary causes, infectious diseases, birth trauma, in utero growth retardation, accidents, substance abuse and addictions, and other factors that are known to slow or delay growth and development.

ASSESSMENT

Areas
- self-care components: feeding and swallowing, performance of daily living skills, home-making skills
- productivity: functional capacity evaluation, also called physical or work capacity evaluation; work performance skills; job analysis
- leisure skills and interests
- sensorimotor components: developmental profile, gross motor skills and coordination, fine motor skills, manipulation, dexterity, and bilateral coordination
- sensory integrative components: sensory responsiveness (hypo- or hyperresponsiveness); perceptual skills, including matching and discrimination; motor planning/praxis skills
- cognitive components: attention span, short-term and long-term memory for general knowledge, learning style
- psychosocial components: social interaction skills, community skills
- temporal contexts
- environmental contexts

Instruments

Instruments Developed by Occupational Therapy Personnel
- *Let's Do Lunch: A Comprehensive Nonstandardized Assessment Tool* by S. Bachner, in *Adults with developmental disabilities: Current approaches in occupational therapy*, eds. M. Ross and S. Bachner, 263–306, Bethesda, MD: American Occupational Therapy Association, 1998.
- *Sensory Integration Inventory for Individuals Who Have Developmental Disabilities (Revised)* by J. Reisman and B. Hanschu, San Antonio, TX: Therapy Skill Builders, 1996.

PROBLEMS

Self-Care
- The person may have poor grooming and hygiene skills.
- The person may not have learned to perform self-care or homemaking tasks such as eating, grooming and hygiene, dressing, and health maintenance.
- The person may have specific deficits in the performance of certain self-care or homemaking tasks.
- The person may be unable to live independently in the community due to one or more deficits in the performance of occupational roles or components.
- The person may have dysphagia and loss of interest in food due to decreased taste buds.

- The person may be disinterested in food and liquids, which could result in renal insufficiency.
- The person may have inadequate food intake, which could place the person at risk for bedsores as well as poor skin and soft-tissue healing.
- The person may be unable to perform activities of daily living without supervision.

Productivity
- The person may not have developed work skills suitable for employment.
- The person may have a deficit in work skills.
- The person may not have mastered basic educational tasks such as reading, writing, and math.
- The person may have poor or no work habits and skills.

Leisure
- The person may not have leisure skills.
- The person may have a deficit in chosen leisure skills.

Sensorimotor
- The person may have low muscle tone.
- The person may have deficits in gross and fine motor skills.
- The person may have poorly developed gross motor skills and difficulty executing purposeful movements.
- The person may have decreased eye-hand coordination and dexterity.
- The person may have disordered sensory registration and modulation such as sensory defensiveness.
- The person may have a specific sensory integration dysfunction disorder or characteristics such as difficulty crossing the midline of the body.
- The person may have poor or decreased discrimination skills in vestibular, tactile, proprioceptive, and visual systems.
- The person may exhibit stereotypical behaviors (head banging, rocking, face or eye rubbing) related to poor integration of sensory input, especially tactile, vestibular, and proprioceptive input.
- The person may be decreasing in mobility and increasing in sedentary lifestyle. Note: The risk is thus increased for constipation, osteoporosis, skeletal deformities, circulatory problems, decreased endurance, decreased muscle tone, decreased muscle strength, and loss of functional skills.

Cognitive
- The person usually does not learn from incidental experiences and generally requires structured learning situations.
- The person may have an acquired cognitive disability in addition to mental retardation.
- The person may have poor eye contact.
- The person may have poor attending behavior and short attention span.
- The person may not exhibit goal-directed and task-oriented behavior.

Psychosocial

- The person may have poor imitation skills.
- The person may not have learned basic social skills such as social interaction and behavior control.
- The person may have a deficit in social skills.
- The person may exhibit unacceptable behaviors such as hitting, slapping, pushing, throwing objects, destroying property, and injuring the self.
- The person may have poor self-perception.
- The person may have poor impulse control.
- The person may have poor coping skills, especially in handling stress.
- The person may frequently withdraw from social situations.
- The person may have difficulty in relating to authority figures.
- The person may have difficulty relating to peers and peer group.

Environment

- The person may be unable to manage time without guidance from others.
- The person may have declining functions, especially in mobility and transfers, which may put increasing stress on family and institutional caregivers.
- Caregivers may lack social resources or knowledge about such resources.

TREATMENT/INTERVENTION

Intervention depends on the overall level of function the individual has achieved. Some persons with adult developmental disabilities will need sensory integrative activities for continuing problems in sensory modulation and discrimination. Others may need biomechanical and manual therapy approaches to increase physical and structural efficiency. Still others may be ready to learn more independent living tasks and participate in employment and community-based programs with specific assistive technology to compensate for limited ability to perform some tasks.

Self-Care

- Improve eating habits and mealtime behavior.
- Promote good positioning for safe chewing and swallowing.
- Reinforce hand washing after toileting or before a meal or snack.
- Improve willingness and ability to get dressed and/or stay dressed.
- Assist the person in learning to shop for groceries from a list.
- Assist the person in learning to plan and prepare meals, starting with simple meals such as a sandwich and drink.
- Assist the person in learning to use the telephone.
- Increase the person's ability to function as independently as possible in all areas of daily living through structured learning situations. Note: Consider cultural aspects. Some cultures provide a role for a young person to care for an older disabled person.
- Provide adaptive equipment and teach the person to use the equipment if it is needed to help the person perform daily living tasks.

Productivity

- Develop prevocational skills such as following directions, working with others, performing self-correction, seeking directions, being punctual.

- Provide practice filling out application forms.
- Assist person in learning to read a bus schedule, catch a bus, and pay bus fare.
- Encourage use of assistive technology provided to improve performance.
- Increase the person's home management skills, including meal planning, cooking, house-work, clothes washing, home safety skills, budgeting, shopping, and performance of simple maintenance tasks.

Leisure
- Encourage the person to attend recreational activities or events.
- Encourage the person to explore and develop leisure activities.

Sensorimotor
- Improve hand use and function. For a person with palmar grasp only, use handles from laundry and dishwasher bottles to attach to other objects. Dropping objects into containers provides grasp-release patterns. Attaching items by use of Velcro also provides opportunity for practice in grasp and release.
- Provide an enriched sensory diet to enhance brain efficiency for persons with hyporesponsiveness.
- Use hands-on techniques, such as pressure and touch to body surfaces, or compression or stretch to joints.
- Use activities with natural or built-in opportunities to move, exert, or make physical contact, such as performing heavy work.
- Set up or structure activities that incorporate strong brain-stem sensation, such as going through an obstacle course.
- Use visually stimulating materials with bright colors, color contrast, and movement, such as a clear plastic bottle filled with water and tiny plastic pieces, which invites shaking and visual attention.
- Reduce tactile sensory defensiveness (hyperresponsiveness) while increasing tactile explo-ration through use of brushing, vibration, and touching of materials covered with interesting textures such as fur, terry cloth, or felt.
- Increase eye-hand coordination using games such as ring stack and ring toss.
- Promote motor planning skills through performance of functional activities and tasks.
- Increase ability to regulate alertness and arousal.
- Promote sleep-related behavior.
- Increase motor development through involvement in gross motor activities and repetitive actions, such as locomotion, ball playing, and balancing.
- Increase vestibular, tactile, proprioceptive, and visual input to facilitate motor performance and decrease stereotypical behaviors.
- Improve discrimination skills by using various movements, various textures, and various positions, and by having the person match various sizes, colors, and shapes.

Cognitive
- Increase interest, attention, and motivation to learn and perform activities and tasks. An example is to use a weight-sensitive switch that will activate music or radio after a certain number of rings are stacked.
- Provide opportunity to learn about health promotion.
- Provide information to aid learning about nutrition in foods.

- Provide sex education, including information about sexually transmitted diseases and birth control.
- Provide information for learning about first aid.
- Provide information for learning about crime prevention and personal safety.
- If possible provide teaching experience within the context of a real situation, such as teaching cooking skills during meal preparation or practicing safety skills while getting into a van or while crossing a street.
- Increase the person's ability to manage and organize time into cycles of self-care, productivity, leisure, rest, and sleep.
- Increase the person's attention span (amount of time spent working on a task).
- Improve the person's ability to follow directions in completing a task.

Psychosocial
- Increase initiation of interaction with others.
- Develop social skills.
- Practice communication skills.
- Decrease undesirable behaviors such as self-stimulation and avoidance of social contact.
- Help person overcome fear of failure by providing tasks of appropriate ability level and providing supervision as needed to complete the tasks successfully.
- Provide opportunities for increasing self-esteem and sense of mastery through successful completion of projects with simple, short-term activities.
- Encourage self-confidence and pride in appearance.
- Provide instruction in stress management to increase the person's coping skills.
- Provide group experiences through group activities.
- Promote and develop the person's language and communication skills.
- Increase the person's social skills, including concepts of socially acceptable behavior, tolerance, and respect for others.

Environment
- Develop community skills such as getting a library card or completing a medical form.
- Provide practice in time management, such as by using a time card from an actual job environment or using a calendar to organize weekly activities.
- Provide extra time to learn and practice new skills.
- Provide a variety of settings and environments in which the person can try out new skills to facilitate generalization.

PRECAUTIONS
- Many persons with adult developmental disabilities have multiple diagnoses and/or multiple areas of dysfunction. Comprehensive assessment and analysis may be necessary to document and address the multiple problems.
- Frequent illness or need for medical interventions may slow progress of the intervention program.
- Avoid overstimulation. Be sure activity can be stopped quickly by dropping or turning off the item used, such as a vibrator or bright light.
- Watch for signs of dysphagia during mealtimes.

PROGNOSIS AND OUTCOME

- The person is able to perform self-care and mobility tasks independently, such as eating, grooming, hygiene tasks, and dressing.
- The person is able to perform independent living tasks, including home management, meal planning and preparation, budgeting, and shopping, either alone or in a group living arrangement.
- The person is able to apply and interview for a job and demonstrates skills needed to keep a job, such as coming to work on time, performing assigned duties, and interacting with peers.
- The person is able to perform vocational tasks.
- The person is able to participate in community activities using public transportation safely.
- The person demonstrates knowledge of how to use adaptive equipment, when to use it, and how to maintain it.
- The person is able to perform avocational tasks.
- The person demonstrates leisure interests and skills.
- The person is able to function and move about the community as needed with adequate concern for safety.
- The person is able to demonstrate social interaction skills and behavior control.
- The person has mastered socially acceptable behaviors, including awareness of self, basic conversation skills, and cooperative behavior.
- The person demonstrates knowledge of community agencies that can assist in promoting individual rights, providing government services, and providing personal services.

REFERENCES

Public Law 88–162. Mental Retardation Facilities and Community Health Act, 1963.
Public Law 100–146. Developmental Disabilities Assistance and Bill of Rights Amendments, 1987. 42 U.S.C. § 6000 (1989).

BIBLIOGRAPHY

Ashby, M. et al. 1995. Snoezelen: Its effects on concentration and responsiveness in people with profound multiple handicaps. *British Journal of Occupational Therapy* 58, no. 7: 303–307.
Burnett, S., and J. Weinstein. 1998. Developing occupational skills with adults who have developmental disabilities and are slow learners. *Developmental Disabilities Special Interest Section Quarterly* 21, no. 4: 3.
De Mello, M.A.F., and W.C. Mann. 1995. The use of mobility related devices by older individuals with developmental disabilities living in community residences. *Technology and Disability* 4, no. 4: 275–285.
Hanschu, B. 1998. Using a sensory approach to serve adults who have developmental disabilities. In *Adults with developmental disabilities: Current approaches in occupational therapy,* eds. M. Ross and S. Bachner, 165–212. Bethesda, MD: American Occupational Therapy Association.
Herge, E.A., and J.E. Campbell. 1998. The role of the occupational and physical therapist in the rehabilitation of the older adult with mental retardation. *Topics in Geriatric Rehabilitation* 13, no. 4: 12–21.
Kluver, J. et al. 1998. A community program for adults with developmental disabilities. *OT Practice* 3, no. 8: 31–36. (case reports)

Mann, W.C. et al. 1995. Custom device development and professional training in developmental disabilities. *Technology and Disability* 4, no. 4: 295–329.

Pedersen, J.P. 1995. Wheelchair seating intervention for person with developmental disabilities living in a skilled nursing facility: The "Bogard" consent decree. *Technology and Disability* 4, no. 3,4: 269–273.

Renwick, R. 1998. Quality of life: a guiding framework for practice with adults who have developmental disabilities. In *Adults with developmental disabilities: Current approaches in occupational therapy*, eds. M. Ross and S. Bachner, 23–41. Bethesda, MD: American Occupational Therapy Association.

Reisman, J. 1993. Using a sensory integrative approach to treat self-injurious behavior in an adult with profound mental retardation (review). *American Journal of Occupational Therapy* 47, no. 5: 403–411.

Ross, M. 1998. A five-stage model for adults with developmental disabilities. In *Adults with developmental disabilities: Current approaches in occupational therapy*, eds. M. Ross and S. Bachner, 329–348. Bethesda, MD: American Occupational Therapy Association.

Ross, M., and S. Bachner. 1998. *Adults with developmental disabilities: Current approaches in occupational therapy*. Bethesda, MD: American Occupational Therapy Association.

Simpson, D. 1996. Seeing the forest for the trees: Treating adults with mental retardation through structurally based manual therapy. *OT Practice* 1, no. 11: 40–45.

Smith, B. 1997. Creating functional activities for the DD population. *Advance for Occupational Therapists* 13, no. 48: 8–10.

Stahl, C. 1995. The success of deinstitutionalization in DD: People with mental retardation do live safely in the community. *Advance for Occupational Therapists* 11, no. 21: 12, 16.

Willems, B., and D. Loebl. 1995. Care study—adapting a TV/VCR control for a person with severe developmental disability. *Technology and Disability* 4, no. 3,4: 287–294.

Wysocki, D.J., and A.T. Neulicht. 1998. Adults with developmental disabilities and work: What can I do as an occupational therapy practitioner? In *Adults with developmental disabilities: Current approaches in occupational therapy*, eds. M. Ross and S. Bachner, 45–88. Bethesda, MD: American Occupational Therapy Association.

Down Syndrome

DESCRIPTION

Down syndrome, also called trisomy 21, trisomy G, or mongolism, is a chromosomal disorder usually resulting in mental retardation, a characteristic facies, and other features such as microcephaly and short stature. There are three types of Down syndrome: trisomy, translocation, and mosaicism. In about 95 percent of cases, there is an extra or third whole chromosome 21 (trisomy), which is usually derived from the mother. Some persons with Down syndrome have the translocation type in which the additional chromosome 21 has been translocated or attached to another chromosome, such as number 14 or 22. The third type, mosaicism, occurs when two different cell lines or types are present in one person. One cell line is normal, with 46 chromosomes, and the other cell line has 47 chromosomes. Down syndrome mosaicism presumably results from an error in chromosomal separation during cell division (nondisjunction) in the growing embryo (Merck 1999, 2233–2234).

CAUSE

The exact cause of Down syndrome is not completely understood. In the typical trisomy type, the extra chromosome is usually from the mother but occurs spontaneously. In some types of translocation (21;22) a parent, usually the mother, is a carrier. In other types of translocation (14;21) the parents' karyotypes are normal, thus the occurrence is de novo. The incidence is about 1 in 800 live births. A marked variability is seen, however, depending on maternal age: for mothers younger than 20 years, the incidence is about 1 in 2,000; for mothers older than 40 years, it rises to about 1 in 40 overall.

ASSESSMENT

Areas

- daily living skills
- productivity history, skills, interests, values
- leisure interests
- motor skills: developmental milestones, gross motor skills and coordination, range of motion, hand functions
- postural control and balance: muscle tone, reflex development, maturation, and integration
- fine motor skills, manipulation, dexterity
- oral motor skills
- sensory modulation
- sensory discrimination and perceptual skills
- attending behavior: span of attention, concentration
- problem solving and decision making
- learning and memory skills
- self-perception
- coping skills
- social interaction skills
- communication skills

Instruments

Instruments Developed by Occupational Therapy Personnel

- *Erhardt Developmental Prehension Assessment* rev. by R.P. Erhardt, San Antonio, TX: Therapy Skill Builders, 1994.
- *Movement Assessment of Infants* (MAI) by L.S. Chandler, M.S. Andrews, and M.W. Swanson, Rolling Bay, WA: Infant Movement Research, 1980.
- *Sensory Integration and Praxis Test*s by A.J. Ayres, Los Angeles: Western Psychological Services, 1989. (Caution: Consider possible effects of hypotonicity or gravitational insecurity.)

Instruments Developed by Other Professionals and Used by Occupational Therapy Personnel

- *Bayley Scales of Infant Development-II* (BSID-II) by N. Bayley, San Antonio, TX: The Psychological Corporation, 1993.
- *Bruininks-Oseretsky Test of Motor Proficiency* (BOTMP) by R.H. Bruininks, Circle Pines, MN: American Guidance Services, 1978.
- *Gesell Developmental Schedules—Revised*, in *Developmental Diagnosis*, 3rd ed., eds. H. Knoblock and B. Pasamanick, Hagerstown, MD: Harper & Row, 1974.

- *Neonatal Behavioral Assessment Scale (Brazelton)*, 3rd ed. by T.B. Brazelton and J.K. Nugent, in *Clinics in Developmental Medicine* no. 137, London: Mac Keith Press, 1995.
- *Peabody Developmental Motor Scales* by M.R. Folio and R.R. Fewell, Austin, TX: Pro-ed, 1983.

PROBLEMS

Self-Care
- The person usually needs assistance to learn activities of daily living.
- Skills for independent living may not be learned.
- The person's tongue tends to be forward in the mouth, which presents as a slight tongue thrust, and development of tongue movements is delayed. The tongue may appear large due to a small oral cavity secondary to midfacial hypoplasia.
- The person's palate may be short and narrow. Underdevelopment of the maxilla may alter the position of the muscles used for chewing.
- Duration of the chewing cycle is longer than normal and chewing is less vigorous. The person may tend to hold food in the mouth without chewing and demonstrate difficulty in moving food from side to side with the tongue.
- The person may be a mouth breather due to decreased size of the nasal passages, which interferes with chewing and swallowing.
- The person may have generalized facial and oral hypotonia, which contributes to poor lip closure, poor sucking, poor tongue control, and jaw instability.
- The person may experience difficulty drinking from a glass or cup because of problems in sucking and swallowing.

Productivity
- The person is usually most successful at jobs that require repetitive, easy-to-master tasks.

Leisure
- The person may have difficulty developing leisure skills.
- The person may not use leisure skills already developed without assistance.

Sensorimotor
- The person usually has hypotonicity in muscle tone (floppy infant) and hypermobility of the joints due to laxness of joint ligaments.
- The person usually has delayed milestones in physical development.
- The person may have missed milestones, such as creeping on hands and knees.
- The person may use alternate forms of locomotion, such as scooting on buttocks or creeping on feet (with extended knees) and hands.
- The person's hands tend to be short and broad, and interfere with coordination and dexterity.
- Congenital heart disease may limit the person's physical capacity and lower endurance.
- The person may have malalignment of the neck vertebrae (atlantoaxial joint instability at C1 and C2) that exposes the spinal cord to injury.
- The person usually has shortened bones, especially in the arms and legs, which increases the difficulty in performing tasks such as climbing stairs and propping on elbows.

- The person may have muscle weakness, especially in the trunk and flexor muscle groups. Grip strength is reduced.
- The person may have poor bilateral motor coordination and poor midline stability.
- The person may have poor motor planning skills or dyspraxia.
- The person may have delayed reflex development and maturation.
- The person may underrespond to sensory input and exhibit
  1. decreased awareness and attention to tactile stimulation that leads to lack of discrimination and stereognosis through tactile senses and failure to manipulate objects
  2. decreased awareness of the position of the body, which is related to decreased kinesthetic feedback
  3. failure to alter force of movements to accomplish different tasks or results, which is related to decreased kinesthetic feedback
  4. decreased sense of balance and equilibrium responses
  5. decreased duration of postrotary nystagmus
- The person may overrespond to sensory input and exhibit
  1. resistance to handling, including touching and being touched (tactile defensiveness)
  2. avoidance of weight bearing on the arms, legs, hands, and knees (proprioceptive hyperresponsiveness)
  3. fear of heights and unstable or moving surfaces (gravitational insecurity), such as ramps, swings, slides, ladders, or stairs

Cognitive

- The person usually has subnormal intelligence.
- The person's mental development may be delayed.
- The person may have poor attending behavior.
- The person may have poor concentration and be easily distracted.
- The person's ability to plan ahead may be limited.
- The person's ability to solve problems may be delayed.

Psychosocial

- The person tends to be passive and appears to lack motivation.
- The person may have low self-esteem.
- The person's affective behavior may be delayed.
- Quality of speech production may be affected by the person's thick, broad tongue.
- Lack of physical skills may interfere with the person's ability to develop sports skills and engage in other group activities.
- The person may not initiate social contacts for fear of being laughed at or rejected.
- Social development may be delayed.

TREATMENT/INTERVENTION

Self-Care

- Encourage oral motor development toward self-feeding. Decrease the person's sensitivity and increase tongue control and chewing movement.
- Encourage self-dressing and self-grooming.

Productivity

Encourage exploratory and symbolic play activities.

Sensorimotor

- For an infant, concentrate on handling (holding, lifting, carrying) and positioning (on stomach, back, side, sitting):
  1. Hold and carry the child with his or her head slightly flexed and arms and legs close together; avoid carrying straddling the hips.
  2. Support the infant's head when lifting to avoid hyperextension of the neck.
  3. Position the infant so he or she can see and reach for toys or objects.
  4. Position the legs in knee flexion; avoid "frog leg" position of hip abduction.
  5. Always turn the infant to your stomach and push into sitting position; never "pull to sit" because of neck instability.
- Increase the person's muscle strength, especially in the neck, shoulder, trunk, and pelvis, to provide stability by pushing away from surfaces and working against gravity.
- Increase range of motion with activities while supporting the person's major joints and working with gravity.
- Encourage gross motor skills (rolling, propping on elbows, crawling, creeping, sitting, knee standing, pulling to stand) by incorporating skill practice with visual and auditory stimulation, reaching for toys, and simple games.
- Increase movement patterns and improve ability to grade movement by increasing active production of postural responses, especially abdominal muscle activity and controlled movement patterns.
- Encourage reflex maturation through tilting and bouncing in the air.
- Improve tone by facilitating coactivation during functional activities that provide vestibular sensory experiences.
- Decrease hypermobility and improve body alignment by inhibiting abnormal movement patterns and using postural control.
- Improve motor planning by encouraging imitation and gestures.
- Improve bilateral integration by placing objects and requiring the person to pick up the object using the opposite hand (across the body midline).
- Provide tactile activities, including differentiation of textures, shapes, and surfaces, and experience in sand and water, with tactile boxes and "feely" bags, and with art materials.
- Provide proprioceptive input through playing games of localization and identification of body parts, wearing a weighted vest or ankle or wrist weights, and bouncing on an inner tube or in a hammock.
- Provide vestibular input by encouraging climbing, riding, sliding, swinging, spinning, and hanging upside down.
- Provide auditory input through activities such as differentiating sounds, playing rhythm instruments, and moving to different rhythms.
- Provide practice in balance and equilibrium by having the person use balance beams and step through the rungs of a ladder, over low hurdles, and in and out of hoops placed on the floor.
- Decrease tactile sensitivity and defensiveness through application of firm tactile stimulation to the body. (See section on tactile defensiveness.)

- Decrease proprioceptive hyporesponsiveness by encouraging the person to bear weight on his or her bare feet.
- Decrease gravitational insecurity by encouraging vestibular activities in linear and circular form. (See section on gravitational insecurity.)

Cognitive

- Instruct the person's parents in a home program to increase mobility and hand skills or other developmental skills depending on the child's developmental level.
- Encourage attending behavior and concentration, especially in visual and auditory activities.
- Increase ability to initiate activities and tolerate novel activities by providing a variety of activities to increase repertoire of interactions.

Psychosocial

- Encourage parental involvement in a therapy program that carries over into the home.

PRECAUTIONS

- Be aware of possible instability or subluxation at the occipitoatlantal or atlantoaxial (C1, C2) joints. There may be laxity of ligaments, malformations, or absence of the odontoid process. Spinning may be contraindicated. Physical contact sports may be contraindicated, including participation in Special Olympics (Committee on Sports Medicine 1984).
- Be aware of possible cardiac pathology, such as congenital heart disease, which may reduce physical endurance.
- Be aware of possible seizure disorders.
- Be aware of possible allergies to food, chemicals, or fabrics. Asthma may be present also.
- Be aware of difficulties with ears (wax buildup, ear infection, blocked tubes) that may affect balance and hearing.
- Be aware of possible visual disorders related to strabismus, astigmatism, or optic nerve hypoplasia.

PROGNOSIS AND OUTCOME

- The person achieves independent mobility.
- The person achieves oral control and self-feeding skills.
- The person is independent in self-care activities.
- The person demonstrates marketable productive skills.
- The person demonstrates homemaking skills needed for independent living.
- The person demonstrates leisure skills and interests.

REFERENCES

Beers, M.H., and R. Berkow, eds. 1999. *The Merck Manual of Diagnosis and Therapy*, 17th ed. Whitehouse Station, NJ: Merck Research Laboratories.
Committee on Sports Medicine. 1984. Atlantoaxial instability in Down syndrome. *Pediatrics* 74: 152–154.

BIBLIOGRAPHY

Adams, R.C. 1996. Treating kids with hypotonia: Patience is more than a virtue. *Advance for Occupational Therapists* 12, no. 7: 18.

Blanche, E.I. et al. 1995. The use of neuro-developmental treatment and sensory integration in the assessment and treatment of children with developmental disorders—Down syndrome. In *Combining neuro-developmental treatment and sensory integration principles: An approach to pediatric therapy*, eds. E.I. Blanche et al., 86–103. Tucson, AZ: Therapy Skill Builders.

Breske, S. 1995. Mom and Dad join rehab team: Treating children with developmental disabilities. *Advance for Directors in Rehabilitation* 4, no. 7: 59–63.

Bruni, M. 1998. *Fine motor skills in children with Down syndrome: A guide for parents and professionals.* Bethesda, MD: Woodbine House.

Crowe, T.K. et al. 1996. The impact of child characteristics on mothers' sleep patterns. *Occupational Therapy Journal of Research* 16, no. 1: 3–22.

Earith, K. 1995. The Down syndrome project: Quilting on the Internet. *Advance for Occupational Therapists* 11, no. 49: 18.

Edwards, S. 1998. Hand function of children with Down's syndrome. *Developmental Disabilities Special Interest Section Quarterly* 21, no. 1: 1–3.

Edwards, S.J., and M.K. Lafreniere. 1995. Hand function in the Down syndrome population. In *Hand function in the child: Foundations for remediation*, eds. A. Henderson and C. Pehoski, 299–326. St. Louis, MO: CV Mosby.

Edwards, S.J., and H.K. Yuen. 1996. Heart rate response to vestibular stimulation in two children with Down's syndrome: A pilot study. *Australian Occupational Therapy Journal* 43, no. 3/4: 167–171.

Kellegrew, D.H., and D. Allen. 1996. Occupational therapy in full-inclusion classrooms: A case study from the Moorpark model. *American Journal of Occupational Therapy* 50, no. 9: 718–724.

Klein, M.D., and T.A. Delaney. 1994. Conditions affecting feeding and nutrition—Down syndrome. In *Feeding and nutrition for children with special needs: Handouts for parents,* eds. M.D. Klein and T.A. Delaney, 395–412. San Antonio, TX: Therapy Skill Builders.

Nommensen, A., and F. Maas. 1993. Sensory integration and Down's syndrome. *British Journal of Occupational Therapy* 56, no. 12: 451–454.

Failure To Thrive

DESCRIPTION

The term failure to thrive (FTT) is applied to infants whose weight consistently is below the third percentile for chronologic age; who show progressive decrease in weight to below the third percentile; who weigh less than 80 percent of the ideal weight for height and age; or who show a decrease in expected rate of growth based on the child's previously defined growth curve, irrespective of whether the weight falls below the third percentile.

Subtypes include organic FTT, nonorganic FTT, and mixed FTT. **Organic FTT** refers to growth failure due to an acute or chronic disorder known to interfere with normal nutrient intake, absorption, metabolism, or excretion or to result in increased energy requirements to sustain or promote growth. **Nonorganic FTT** refers most commonly to growth failure due to environmental neglect (e.g., lack of food) or stimulus deprivation in the absence of a physiologic disorder that accounts for the growth failure. In **mixed FTT**, organic and nonorganic causes overlap. The diagnosis of FTT should be based on information from a growth chart, the dietary history of the child, and assessment of the child's elimination pattern, medical history, family, and social history (Merck 1999, 2241–2243).

CAUSE

Causes of organic FTT may include cleft lip or palate, gastroesophageal reflux, rumination, celiac disease, cystic fibrosis, disaccharidase (e.g., lactase) deficiency, fructose intolerance, transferase deficiency, diabetes mellitus, proteinuria, bronchopulmonary dysphasia, and hyperthyroidism. The mechanisms are decreased nutrient intake, malabsorption, impaired metabolism, increased excretion, and increased energy requirements. Causes of nonorganic FTT may be lack of food as a result of impoverishment, poor understanding of feeding techniques, improperly prepared formula (e.g., overdilution of formula to stretch it because of financial difficulties), or an inadequate supply of breast milk (e.g., because the mother is under stress, exhausted, or poorly nourished). Psychological causes include depression secondary to stimulus deprivation, which may lead to apathy and ultimately anorexia. Lack of stimulation may occur because the caregiver is depressed or apathetic, has poor parenting skills, is anxious about or unfulfilled by the caregiving role, feels hostile toward the child, or is responding to real or received external stresses (Merck 1999, 2242).

ASSESSMENT

Areas
- developmental profile
- reflex maturation and development (especially poor sucking reflex in infants)
- posture (note atypical postures)
- oral motor functions (note also such behaviors as perseveration of sucking, turning head away from food, pushing food away, crying, refusing the nipple, falling asleep during feedings, vomiting, fighting with caregiver, and refusing solid foods)
- gross motor skills and coordination
- fine motor skills, manipulation, dexterity, and bilateral coordination
- sensory modulation (especially oral motor sensory defensiveness)
- sensory discrimination (especially gustatory discrimination)
- arousal and attending behaviors (note avoidance behaviors)
- auditory and communication skills
- mood or affect (note level of irritability, listlessness, or apathy)
- infant-caretaker interaction (note lack of cuddling behavior, inability to be soothed)
- social interaction skills (note interaction with persons other than primary caretaker)
- daily living skills

Instruments
- *Occupational Therapy Protocol for Infants Who Fail to Thrive* by R. Denton, *American Journal of Occupational Therapy* 40, no. 5 (1986): 354, 356.

- *Vulpe Assessment Battery—Revised* by S.G. Vulpe, East Aurora, NY: Slosson Educational Publications, 1994.

PROBLEMS

The list of problems can vary from child to child because FTT is not a single disorder.

Self-Care

- The person may be anorexic or have a voracious appetite.
- The person may have developmental delay in attaining independence in activities of daily living.

Productivity

- The person may have poorly developed or absent play skills.

Leisure

- The person may have little, if any, interest in toys, games, or group activities.

Sensorimotor

- The person may have low muscle tone (hypotonicity).
- The person may have developmental delay in attaining motor milestones.
- The person may have decreased motor activity (hypoactivity) and lack of purposeful movements.
- The person may have infantile posture (note flexed hips and knees, arms flexed 90 degrees or more at the elbow, or forearms held above the head).
- The person may have increased hand and finger activity.
- The person may have muscle weakness.
- The person may have primitive reflexes that are not integrated.
- The person may under- or overreact to stimuli (hypo- or hypersensitivity).
- The person may have developmental delay in sensory modulation and discrimination.

Cognitive

- The person may have poor attending behavior.
- The person may have short attention span.
- The person may have poor or impaired memory.

Psychosocial

- The person may be hyperalert or disinterested.
- The person may have no facial expression and lack of affect.
- The person may be withdrawn.
- The person may be listless or apathetic.
- The person may be irritable.
- The person may ruminate.
- The person may lack vocalization or have developmental delays in communication skills, including a decrease or absence of cooing, squealing, babbling, laughing, vocalizing syllables, or saying words.

- The person may cry when approached.
- The person may avoid eye contact, stare, or look disinterested.
- The person may not smile in social situations.

TREATMENT/INTERVENTION

Treatment models are the neurodevelopmental model and the sensory integration model. Treatment should be aimed at decreasing the impact of the root cause. A multidisciplinary approach is frequently used.

Self-Care
- Develop or improve feeding skills, integrate oral reflexes, reduce oral-tactile hypersensitivity, and promote swallowing pattern.
- Increase independence through improvement of skills in daily living tasks.

Productivity and Leisure
- Develop or improve play skills.

Sensorimotor
- Increase/improve gross and fine motor skills to range of normal development.
- Increase or decrease response to stimuli to range of normal. (See sections on sensory integration for specific examples.)

Cognitive
- Increase or improve attention span.
- Increase or improve memory and retention skills.
- Instruct caregiver regarding normal growth and development, selection of toys and games, play activities with infants and young children, and adequate nutrition.

Psychosocial
- Decrease signs of apathy, withdrawal, and irritability by engaging the child in play activities that require physical motor skills that are within the child's developmental level and are fun for the child to do.
- Encourage and promote interaction and communication between child and caregivers by establishing eye contact; talking, singing, or gesturing to the child; and touching or holding the child within the level of the child's tolerance. Avoid overfatigue and overstimulation.

PRECAUTIONS
- Observe the child carefully for any signs of organic pathology that might contribute to the problem of FTT.
- Make sure the child is not overstimulated or fatigued.

PROGNOSIS AND OUTCOME
- The person has improved skills in daily living.

- The person has improved play skills.
- The person demonstrates improved reflex maturation such as integration of primitive reflexes.
- The person demonstrates improved postural reflexes.
- The person demonstrates improved oral motor development.
- The person has progressed developmentally in the areas of gross and fine motor skills.
- The person demonstrates improved orienting to sensory stimuli.
- The person demonstrates normalized response to stimuli and less hyper- or hyporesponsiveness.
- The person is able to attend to tasks and activities for a longer time.
- The person is able to smile, coo, or laugh when enjoying an activity.
- The person interacts with caregiver by cuddling or reaching to be picked up.
- Parents or caregivers demonstrate improved skills in interacting with the child.

REFERENCE

Beers, M.H., and R. Berkow, eds. 1999. *The Merck Manual of Diagnosis and Therapy*, 17th ed. Whitehouse Station, NJ: Merck Research Laboratories.

BIBLIOGRAPHY

Abarbanel-Can'ani, L. 1995. Developmental feeding disorders and chronic illness: A case study. *Israel Journal of Occupational Therapy* 4, no. 1: E9-E20.

Foy, T. et al. 1997. Treatment of severe feeding refusal in infants and toddlers. *Infants and Young Children* 9, no. 3: 26–35.

Joe, B.E. 1996. Little miracles. *OT Week* 10, no. 49: 12–13.

Ramsey, M. et al. 1993. Non-organic failure to thrive: Growth failure secondary to feeding-skills disorder. *Developmental Medicine and Child Neurology* 35, no. 4: 285–297.

Wavrek, B.B. 1996. Hospital services—failure to thrive. In *Occupational therapy for children*. 3rd ed., eds. J. Case-Smith et al., 753–755. St. Louis, MO: Mosby.

Yossem, F. 1998. The case of many challenges: Severe brain damage, neuromuscular disorders, and failure to thrive. In *Clinical management of feeding disorders: Case studies,* ed. F. Yossem, 91–111. Boston: Butterworth-Heinemann.

Fetal Alcohol Syndrome

DESCRIPTION

Fetal alcohol syndrome (FAS) is due to maternal alcohol abuse during pregnancy. FAS is the most common type of drug-induced teratogenesis. The most serious consequence is severe mental retardation due to impaired brain development. Severely affected newborns have growth retardation and are microcephalic. Malformations may include microphthalmia, short palpebral fissures, midfacial hypoplasia, abnormal palmar creases, cardiac defects, and joint contractures (Merck 1999, 2158). FAS and its effects were first formally labeled in 1973, although the concerns regarding FAS had been reported for many years.

CAUSE

FAS has been diagnosed in neonates born to chronic alcoholics who drank heavily throughout pregnancy. Lesser degrees of alcohol abuse result in a less severe manifestation of FAS termed alcohol-related birth defects. Maternal alcohol abuse during pregnancy is considered to be the most common cause of drug-induced teratogenesis. The associated mental retardation is thought to be due to the ethanol in alcohol. Rates of FAS are higher in North America than in other countries. The incidence of FAS is highest among American Indians, blacks, and those of low socioeconomic status.

ASSESSMENT

Areas

- postural mechanisms: balance, joint mobility, muscle tone, muscle strength, neurodevelopmental level
- praxis; gross and fine motor skills, sensorimotor skills, developmental milestones
- perceptual and sensory integration
- cognitive mechanisms: attending behavior, orientation, recognition, sequencing, categorization, concept formation, intellectual operations in space, learning, memory and retention, problem solving and processing skills, generalization of learning, integration and synthesis of learning
- psychosocial mechanisms: motivation, initiation and termination of activities, cooperative behavior, roles and role behavior, values, interests, self-concept, social conduct, self-expression, self-management, coping skills, self-control
- environmental mechanisms: time management

Instruments

Instruments Developed by Occupational Therapy Personnel

- *Ayres Clinical Observation of Sensory Integration* by A.A. Poulson and K.E. Peachey, in Ayres' clinical observations: Performance of four and five year old children, *American Journal of Occupational Therapy* 30, no. 1 (1976): 15–22.
- *DeGangi-Berk Test of Sensory Integration* (DBTSI) by R.A Berk and G.A. DeGangi, Los Angeles: Western Psychological Services, 1983.
- *Test of Sensory Functions in Infants* (TSFI) by G. DeGangi and S.I. Greenspan, Los Angeles: Western Psychological Services, 1989.
- *Sensory Integration and Praxis Tests* by A.J. Ayres, Los Angeles: Western Psychological Services, 1989.

Instruments Developed by Other Professionals and Used by Occupational Therapy Personnel

- *Bayley Scales of Infant Development-II* (BSID-II) by N. Bayley, San Antonio, TX: The Psychological Corporation, 1993.
- *The Beery-Buktenica Developmental Test of Visual-Motor Integration* (VMI-4), 4th ed. by K.E. Beery and N.A. Buktenica, Parsippany, NJ: Modern Curriculum Press, 1997.

- *Bruininks-Oseretsky Test of Motor Proficiency* (BOTMP) by R.H. Bruininks, Circle Pines, MN: American Guidance Services, 1978.
- *Carolina Record of Individual Behavior* by R.J. Simeonsson et al., in The Carolina record of individual achievement: Characteristics of handicapped infants and children, *Topics in Early Childhood Special Education* 1 (1982): 43–55.
- *Infant Motor Screen* by R.E. Nickel, C.A. Renken, and J.S. Gallenstein, in The infant motor screen, *Developmental Medicine and Child Neurology* 31, no. 1 (1989): 35–42.
- *Peabody Developmental Motor Scale*s by M.R. Folio and R.R. Fewell, Austin, TX: Pro-ed, 1983.
- *Tennessee Self Concept Scale* rev. by W.H. Fitts and W.L. Warren, Los Angeles: Western Psychological Services, 1988.
- *Test of Visual-Motor Skills—Revised* (TVMS-R) by M.F. Gardner, Hydesville, CA: Psychological and Educational Publications, 1995.
- *Test of Visual-Perceptual Skills (Non-motor)—Revised* by M.F. Gardner, Hydesville, CA: Psychological and Educational Publications, 1996.

PROBLEMS

Self-Care
- The person may have difficulty learning routines in activities of daily living.

Productivity
- The person usually will fall behind peers in academic performance in later elementary grades.

Sensorimotor
- The person usually has pre- and postnatal growth deficiencies, especially in weight and head circumference.
- The person usually was born with a low birth weight.
- The person usually experiences developmental delays (see section on developmental delays in children).
- The person may have symptoms of failure to thrive (see section on failure to thrive).
- The person usually has central nervous system dysfunctions, including
  1. microcephaly
  2. hypotonia
  3. irritability and restlessness in infancy
  4. hyperactivity in childhood
- The person usually has facial anomalies, including maxillary hypoplasia, small palpebral fissures (eye openings in skull), cleft palate, flat maxillary, poorly developed philtrum, and thin upper lip.
- The person usually has musculoskeletal problems, including
  1. congenital dislocations
  2. foot positional defects
  3. cervical spine abnormalities, including short neck and spina bifida

4. specific joint alterations
5. flexion contractures in the elbows
6. tapering of the terminal phalanges

- The person may have cerebellar disorders, including axial ataxia and kinetic tremors.
- The person may have fine motor dysfunction demonstrated by weak grasp and poor eye-hand coordination.
- The person may have a weak suck as an infant.
- The person may having hearing loss and auditory perceptual problems due to otitis media.
- The person may have sensorimotor deficits, including deficits in vision, hearing, vestibular sense, and motor coordination.
- The person may have sensory integrative dysfunction—sensory modulation (see section on sensory integrative dysfunction and sensory modulation disorders).
- The person may have difficulty habituating to ordinary stimuli such as clothing (tactile defensiveness).
- The person may have symptoms of regulatory disorder, including sleep problems and difficulty in adapting to change and transition (see section on regulatory disorders).
- The person may have cardiac murmurs and septal defects.
- The person may have renogenital anomalies.
- The person may have seizures.

Cognitive

- The person usually is mentally retarded.
- The person usually has difficulty with cause-and-effect relations.
- The person may have a short attention span.
- The person usually has speech problems.
- The person may have learning disabilities, especially poor retention.
- The person usually has more difficulty with sequential processing than with simultaneous processing.
- The person may be impulsive and not use good judgment.
- The person may have difficulty following directions.

Psychosocial

- The person may have an unstable home environment because of mother's drinking.
- The person may have no permanent home.
- The person may have a history of abuse and neglect (see section on child abuse and neglect).
- The person may have a low tolerance for frustration and have temper tantrums.
- The person may have difficulty accepting adult direction or authority but have difficulty with self-initiated behaviors.
- The person may exhibit disobedient behavior.
- The person usually has difficulty understanding social roles and expectations.
- The person may be easily influenced by peer behavior without understanding the consequences of his or her actions.
- In adolescence, the person's behavior may become more aggressive and unpredictable. Problem behaviors may include lying, stealing, and vandalism.
- The person may become depressed, which increases risk for substance abuse and suicide.

TREATMENT/INTERVENTION

Treatment may begin in infancy but will need to continue into adulthood. Levels of intervention may include prevention, skill development, remediation, and compensatory techniques. Techniques in neurodevelopment, sensory integration, perceptual motor training, and functional skill training may be used. Interdisciplinary approach to identification of problems and supportive planning is important.

Self-Care
• Assist in teaching activities of daily living.

Productivity
• In adolescence focus on vocational training, functional skills, and independent living skills.

Leisure
• Assist in teaching leisure skills.

Sensorimotor
• Address issues of regulatory dysfunction.
• Address issues of sensory integrative dysfunction.
• Address issues of neurosensorimotor delay.
• Address issues of visual-perceptual delay.

Cognitive
• Teach compensatory techniques such as new problem-solving techniques, establishment of repetitive tasks, use of lists (or other cuing devices) for tracking of routine responsibilities, or use of adaptive equipment.
• Focus on strategies to facilitate appropriate behavior that will carry over into the real world.

Psychosocial
• Address issues in social skills.

Environment
• Direct, individual therapy session in a distraction-free environment may be useful, rather than therapy in a small-group setting or a session in a room with many distractions.
• Organizing the therapy session into a constant temporal routine can help clarify tasks and set boundaries. Change should be introduced in small increments.
• Consider what services the caregivers may need to reduce stress, such as education in techniques to calm and regulate an irritable, crying infant.
• For infants consider massage, swaddling with a blanket, provision of vestibular input, use of soothing music, and slow introduction to new tactile stimuli.
• For toddlers and children consider creation of a predictable, positive routine.

PRECAUTIONS
• Initiation of a task without prompting is often a major problem for persons with FAS. Do not assume person is able to perform independently in any situation where safety may be an

issue unless the person has performed satisfactorily on several occasions in the immediate past.
• Be aware of the potential for seizures. Plan activities accordingly.

PROGNOSIS AND OUTCOME
• A person with FAS may always need a guardian, coach, or house parent to live independently. Those with lesser symptoms are more likely to be able to live independently.
• The person is able to perform self-care skills with or without cues.
• The person is able to use public transportation as needed.
• The person is able to perform work tasks.
• The person is able to perform leisure activities.

REFERENCE
Beers, M.H., and R. Berkow, eds. 1999. *The Merck Manual of Diagnosis and Therapy*, 17th ed. Whitehouse Station, NJ: Merck Research Laboratories.

BIBLIOGRAPHY
Gordon, C.Y. et al. 1996. Diagnostic problems in pediatrics—fetal alcohol syndrome. In *Occupational therapy for children*. 3rd ed., eds. J. Case-Smith et al., 148–149. St. Louis, MO: CV Mosby.
Kerr, T. 1998. The ravages of FAS. *Advance for Occupational Therapy Practitioners* 14, no. 38: 24–26.
Rotert, D.A., and L. Svien. 1993. Fetal alcohol syndrome: Implications for practice. *Occupational Therapy Practice* 4, no. 2: 24–32.

Fragile X Syndrome

DESCRIPTION
Fragile X syndrome was first identified as an X-linked anomaly in 1969 (Friefeld and MacGregor 1994). The X chromosome has a constriction near the end of the long arm, so that a section is separated from the main portion of the chromosome by a thin stalk. The stalk is referred to as a fragile site, thus the name fragile X syndrome. Males are usually affected more than females. Most, but not all, males with the syndrome are mentally retarded and have a long face, prominent ears, macroorchidism (enlarged testes), strabismus, larger than normal head, and puffiness around the eyes (Blanche et al. 1995). Learning disabilities, attentional problems, motor coordination deficits, and sensory integrative dysfunction are common in both males and females. Females may have prominent jaw, prominent ears, a long face, and overgrowth syndrome present from birth. Cognitive abilities begin to decrease in childhood and continue to decline through adolescence, but the decrease tapers off in adulthood. Next to Down syndrome, fragile X syndrome is the most common cause of mental retardation that can be specifically diagnosed.

Some children with fragile X syndrome have been diagnosed as autistic because of extreme gaze aversion and lack of visible social connectedness.

CAUSE

The cause is a mutant gene, but what causes the gene to mutate is unclear. Females may be carriers but usually are not affected, presumably because their second X chromosome is normal. The gene sequence was described in 1991. The sequence (FMR-1) is repeated more than 200 times, and as a result, the FMR-1 protein is not produced. The lack of the protein causes fragile X syndrome. Also, the posterior cerebellar vermis is smaller than normal, which may contribute to the lack of inhibition, attentional problems, and sensory integration dysfunction seen in fragile X syndrome (Hagerman 1994).

ASSESSMENT

Areas
- sensory defensiveness: tactile, oral, auditory, visual, and olfactory defensiveness; gaze aversion, movement or gravitational insecurities
- poor self-regulation: modulation problems, arousal difficulties, attention deficits; disordered sleep cycles, respiration
- postural mechanisms: muscle tone, joint laxity, joint hypermobility, body segment alignment problems, especially pronation of the feet, problems with equilibrium and balance, ataxic gait, body/movement dissociation
- praxis: initiation and ideation difficulties; poor sensory discrimination and information gathering; generalized planning/organizing and sequencing problems; lack of self-monitoring; gross, fine, and oral motor dyspraxia; visual and somato-based dyspraxias; pragmatic difficulties (Note: Optical spatial praxis necessary in imitation may be a strength.)
- visual-perception: space and form perception, visual-somatic perception, closure
- fine motor skills: hand development, distal-to-proximal relations, sensorimotor functions, handwriting (Note: Fine motor skills may be better than gross motor skills. Bimanual dexterity may be good in children but may decrease in adolescence [Friefeld and MacGregor 1994].)
- stereotypical behaviors: hand flapping, biting, rocking, poor eye contact, aggressive outbursts
- life role development: parent/child relations; functioning in home, school, work, play, community, occupational options

Instruments
Persons with fragile X syndrome are reported to be difficult to assess using standard techniques. Modifications include working in a small or overly large space depending on the person's reaction; letting the child hold a vibrator, sit on the floor, or work inside a barrel during testing; testing while sitting on a swing, inverted on a ball, or sitting on a parent's lap; allowing child to put gum, candy, or fruit in the mouth, or suck on a milk shake or water bottle during testing. Testing may need to be done in small segments. Clinical observation and

information obtained from parents or other caregivers using questionnaires and interviews may need to replace standardized direct testing techniques.

Note also that paradoxical responses are common in persons with fragile X syndrome. A person with auditory defensiveness may make loud sounds; an orally defensive child may chew on anything available as a means of gaining some control over the environment. Understanding paradoxical responses may facilitate interpretation of seemingly conflicting data from direct testing, questionnaires, or interviews.

A sensory history questionnaire and interview that carefully review each sensory system and reactions or behaviors associated with each sensory modality can be very useful in determining the need for intervention with therapy or change in routines at home and school. (Wilbarger 1995).

Instruments Developed by Occupational Therapy Personnel

* *Praxis Test for Children* by K.E. Conrad, S.A. Cermak, and C. Drade, in Differentiation of praxis among children, *American Journal of Occupational Therapy* 37 (1983): 466–473.

Instruments Developed by Other Professionals and Used by Occupational Therapy Personnel

* *The Beery-Buktenica Developmental Test of Visual-Motor Integration* (VMI-4), 4th ed. by K.E. Beery and N.A. Buktenica, Parsippany, NJ: Modern Curriculum Press, 1997.
* *McCarron Assessment of Neuromuscular Development: Fine and Gross Motor Abilities*, rev. ed. by L.T. McCarron, Dallas, TX: Common Market Press, 1982.
* *Motor-Free Visual Perception Test* (MVPT) by R.P. Colarusso and D.D. Hammill, Novato, CA: Academic Therapy Publications, 1972.

PROBLEMS

Self-Care

* The person may have feed/eating problems due to oral motor sensitivity.

Productivity

* The person may have difficulty learning academic subjects, especially difficulty with reading and math skills.

Leisure

* The person may have difficulty with sequencing, processing, pacing, social interaction, and problem solving required in team sports. May be able to participate in solo sports.

Sensorimotor

* The person has sensory defensiveness/hypersensitivity to visual, auditory, olfactory, and tactile stimuli, and gaze aversion. Tactile defensiveness is reported to occur in 90 percent of cases (Stackhouse 1994).
* The person has poor self-regulation, which may be observed as hyperactivity.
* Postural mechanisms are poorly developed, which results in rigid "fixing" patterns of movement to counteract postural instability.

- The person may have low muscle tone, loose connective tissues, and ligament laxity.
- The person has difficulty isolating body parts for specific functions.
- The person has difficulty with praxis, motor planning, and sequencing.
- The person has diminished smooth and accurate movement patterns.
- The person may develop splinter skills, such as the ability to memorize entire movie dialogues, but show an inability to communicate with imitating.
- The person has difficulty making physical transitions.
- The person has disorganized or diminished processing of sensory input.
- The person has poor visual-perceptual, visual-motor, and fine motor skills.
- The person may have strabismus or turning of the eyes from center.
- The person has difficulty with visual space perception, body space perception, and judgment of visual information.

Cognitive

- The person may have difficulty maintaining arousal and attention.
- The person may have communication difficulties, including phrase, sentence, and topical perseveration.
- The person may have cognitive deficits ranging from learning disabilities to severe retardation.

Psychosocial

- The person may demonstrate impulsive behavior.
- The person may have emotional lability.
- The person may have reactionary aggressiveness that does not have a clear antecedent.
- The person, when excited or overwrought, may demonstrate hand flapping, hand biting, or chewing on clothes (considered signs that proprioceptive input is needed).
- Perseverative or tangential behavior may occur.
- The person may have difficulties with social interaction and may show alternating periods of avoidance and seeking behavior.

TREATMENT/INTERVENTION

The treatment model of choice in occupational therapy is sensory integrative therapy (see section on sensory modulation disorders—sensory defensiveness), which may be combined with neurodevelopmental treatment for postural and movement objectives. Behavior modification is often recommended but is usually ineffective.

Self-Care

- Increase independent toileting.

Productivity

- Increase play skill competencies.

Leisure

- Help child participate in leisure activities that can meet sensory needs.

Sensorimotor
- Decrease sensory defensiveness and hypersensitivity to tactile, visual, olfactory, gustatory, and auditory stimuli.

Visual
- Simplify visually presented materials to eliminate clutter or excessively stimulating format.
- Provide visual cues such as color coding, numbering, and arrows to organize written tasks.

Auditory
- Give specific concrete cues when giving oral directions.
- Give instructions in a slow, simple, and concrete manner.
- When giving instructions, be in close proximity to the person.
- Structure the environment to avoid auditory distraction: use earphones or carrels, or seat person away from air conditioner or heater noise.
- Use sensory diet approach developed by Wilbarger (Wilbarger 1995; Wilbarger and Wilbarger 1991), which incorporates various sensory input throughout the day, such as deep tactile pressure, proprioceptive input, heavy work or co-contraction, movement, oral-respiratory activity, and other sensorimotor-based activities.
- Improve tactile defensiveness and poor discrimination of tactile input with activities that provide inhibitory input, such as deep pressure, and opportunities to experience a variety of self-imposed tactile inputs, including tactile discrimination.
- Improve modulation of vestibular input by providing opportunities to engage in purposeful activities that incorporate vestibular and proprioceptive input.
- Improve postural adjustments by facilitating postural adjustments during functional activities such as swinging.
- Improve quality of movement by facilitating coactivation during functional activities and coordinating the use of a variety of movement patterns through handling.
- Improve motor planning skills and body awareness in relationship to the environment by providing a variety of sensory inputs, beginning with activities that require simple adaptive responses and moving to more complex activities.
- Improve the person's ability to make adaptive responses in a developmentally appropriate sequence by facilitating use of gross and fine motor skills.

Cognitive
- Increase attending behaviors in all situations by encouraging active initiation and self-direction.
- Increase compliance to direct cues.
- Increase problem-solving skills by providing a choice of a variety of activities.
- Suggest to caregivers that clothing be made of natural fibers to decrease irritation.
- Suggest to caregivers that careful recording of foods eaten along with observations of behaviors may reveal a link between consumption of certain foods and a worsening of behavior problems such as hyperactivity.
- Suggest to caregivers that color and olfactory stimuli can alter emotional state.
- Teach caregivers ways to calm the person, such as by initiating quieting sounds, having the person chew crushed ice, applying firm pressure, wedging or squeezing, having the person wear headphones, using vibrating objects or massage, or having the person pet animals.

Psychosocial
- Decrease mouthing, hand biting, and chewing on clothing by sensory modulation techniques.
- Decrease ritualistic behaviors.
- Decrease the occurrence of tantrums by increasing coping strategies.
- Help the person explore life roles and role functioning as a family member, peer, friend, student, worker, and player.

Environment
- Increase tolerance of changes in routine and environment.
- Decrease person- and environment-specific behaviors.
- Consider using natural lighting whenever possible.

PRECAUTIONS
- In using the sensory diet approach, never brush the stomach and generally avoid the head, neck, and chest. The stomach area tends to show a delayed reaction of discomfort and/or irritation from brushing.
- Never using brushing techniques with children under 2 months of age. The nervous system is considered too immature in these children.
- Avoid light touch stimuli. Aggressive behaviors may occur in response to fight or flight response.
- Seizures may occur in about 20 percent of persons.
- The person may be taking several drugs to improve attention and concentration, to decrease impulsivity and aggression, to improve coordination, and to prevent seizures. Both individual responses and possible synergistic effects should be considered. Negative symptoms should be reported to the physician.
- The use of folic acid is a controversial therapy.

PROGNOSIS AND OUTCOME
- The person's sensory processing has been normalized.
- The person is able to perform self-care tasks and activities.
- The person may be able to live independently, especially in a group situation.
- The person is able to initiate functional daily activities.

REFERENCES

Blanche, E.I. et al. 1995. The use of neuro-developmental treatment and sensory integration in the assessment and treatment of children with developmental disorders—Fragile X syndrome. In *Combining neuro-developmental treatment and sensory integration principles: An approach to pediatric therapy*, eds. E.I. Blanche et al., 114–123. Tucson, AZ: Therapy Skill Builders.
Friefeld, S.J., and D. MacGregor. 1994. Sensorimotor coordination in boys with fragile X syndrome. *Occupational Therapy International* 1, no. 3: 174–183.
Hagerman, R. 1994. Medical aspects of fragile X syndrome. *Sensory Integration Special Interest Section Newsletter* 17, no. 1: 7–8.

Stackhouse, T.M. 1994. Sensory integration concepts and fragile X syndrome. *Sensory Integration Special Interest Section Newsletter* 17, no. 1: 2–6.

Wilbarger, P. 1995. The sensory diet: Activity programs based on sensory processing theory. *Sensory Integration Special Interest Section Newsletter* 18, no. 2: 1–4.

Wilbarger, P., and J.L. Wilbarger. 1991. *Sensory defensiveness in children aged 2–12: An intervention guide for parents and other caretakers.* Santa Barbara, CA: Avanti Educational Programs.

BIBLIOGRAPHY

Roley, S.S. 1994. From the chair. *Sensory Integration Special Interest Section Newsletter* 17, no. 1: 1.

Scharfenaker, S.K. 1994. Speech and language skills in males with fragile X syndrome. *Sensory Integration Special Interest Section Newsletter* 17, no. 1: 6.

Scharfenaker, S. et al. 1991. An integrated approach to intervention. In *Fragile X syndrome: Diagnosis, treatment and research*, eds. R.J. Hagerman and A.C. Silverman, 327–372. Baltimore: Johns Hopkins University Press.

Wilbarger, J. 1994. From the editor. *Sensory Integration Special Interest Section Newsletter* 17, no. 1: 8.

High Risk or At Risk Infants

DESCRIPTION

Risk factors are those elements that suggest that a child has a greater than normal probability of developing a disabling condition, although at present no evidence of a disability is manifest. Risk factors can be divided into three categories: established risk, biological risk, and environmental risk. **Established risk** applies to those infants with known chromosomal, structural, or metabolic defects classified as having an established risk. Prenatal diagnostic tests such as amniocentesis, chorionic villus biopsy, and restriction enzyme analysis can determine if a child has an established risk. **Biological risk** applies to infants and children with a potential for exhibiting neurodevelopmentally or educationally identifiable disorders secondary to a history of prenatal, perinatal, or neonatal insult, such as apnea, asphyxia, hypoxic-ischemic encephalopathy, intraventricular hemorrhage, respiratory distress syndrome, bronchopulmonary dysplasia, meconium aspiration, necrotizing entero- colitis, retinopathy of prematurity, brachial plexus injury, congenital dislocation of the hip, talipes equinovarus (clubfoot), metatarsus varus, tibial torsion, and patent ductus arteriosus. **Environmental risk** applies to infants and children with potential for delayed development secondary to family and social stressors such as adolescent parenting, low socioeconomic status, history of drug abuse, child abuse or neglect, problems in the parents' mental health, lack of family support, and poor parent-child interaction (Cook 1993, 62–64).

CAUSE

Causes may be related to hereditary factors, maternal history, labor and delivery problems, gestational weight and age, prematurity, postmaturity, and social or psychological factors.

ASSESSMENT

Areas
- regulatory management skills: ability to calm oneself after stimulation
- self-care skills: oral motor skills
- motor skills: range of motion (note discrepancies between the two sides of the body), gross motor skills and coordination, hand functions
- fine motor skills: eye-hand coordination, dexterity
- postural control: muscle tone (hyper- or hypotonicity), reflex development and maturation, bilateral integration
- praxis, motor planning
- sensory registration and processing
- sensory modulation, hyper- or hyporesponsiveness
- sensory discrimination and perception: visual perception, visual motor integration
- attending behavior: alerting, arousal
- cognition: focus of attention, attention span, concentration
- response to being picked up or handled
- communication: vocalization and crying
- psychosocial skills

Instruments
Instruments Developed by Occupational Therapy Personnel
- *Hawaii Early Learning Profile–Revised* by S. Furuno et al., Palo Alto, CA: VORT Corporation, 1997.
- *Miller Assessment for Preschoolers* (MAP) by L.J. Miller, San Antonio, TX: The Psychological Corporation, 1988.
- *Movement Assessment of Infants* (MAI) by L.S. Chandler, M.S. Andrews, and M.W. Swanson, Rolling Bay, WA: Infant Movement Research, 1980.
- *Test of Sensory Functions in Infants* (TSFI) by B.A. DeGangi and S.I. Greenspan, Los Angeles: Western Psychological Services, 1988.

Instruments Developed by Other Professionals and Used by Occupational Therapy Personnel
- *Assessment of Preterm Infant's Behavior* (APIB) by H. Als et al., in *Theory and research in behavioral pediatrics*, vol. 1, ed. H. Fitzgerald, 65–132, New York: Plenum Publishing, 1982.
- *Chandler Movement Assessment of Infants Screening Test* by L. Chandler, Rolling Bay, WA: Infant Movement Research, 1997.
- *Clinical Assessment of Gestational Age of the Newborn Infant* by L.M.S. Dubowitz, V. Dubowitz, and C. Goldberg, *Journal of Pediatrics* 77, no. 1 (1970): 1–10.
- *Denver Developmental Screening Test* (Denver II) by W.K. Frankenberg et al., Denver, CO: Denver Developmental Materials, 1990.
- *Developmental Profile II* (DPII) by G. Alpern, T. Boll, and M. Shearer, Los Angeles: Western Psychological Services, 1984.

- *Einstein Neonatal Neurobehavioral Assessment Scale* (ENNAS) by C. Daum, B. Grellong, D. Kurtzberg et al. in C. Limperopoulos et al., Agreement between the neonatal neurologic examination and a standardized assessment of neurobehavioural performance in a group of high-risk newborns, *Pediatric Rehabilitation* 1, no. 1 (1997): 9–14; and A. Majnemer et al., Predicting outcome in high-risk newborns with a neonatal neurobehavioral assessment, *American Journal of Occupational Therapy* 48, no. 8 (1994): 723–732.
- *Home Observation for Measurement of the Environment* by B. Caldwell and R. Bradley, Little Rock, AR: University of Arkansas, 1984.
- *Milani-Comparetti Developmental Examination,* 3rd ed. by W. Stuberg, Omaha, NE: Meyer Rehabilitation Institute, University of Nebraska Medical Center, 1993.
- *Morgan Neonatal Neurobehavioral Examination* in M.S. Sheahan and N.F. Brockway, The high-risk infant, *Pediatric physical therapy*, ed. J.S. Tecklin, 56–88, Philadelphia: J.B. Lippincott Co., 1994.
- *Neonatal Behavioral Assessment Scale (Brazelton)*, 3rd ed. by T.B. Brazelton and J.K. Nugent, in *Clinics in Developmental Medicine* no. 137, London: MacKeith Press, 1995; distributed by Cambridge University Press, Cambridge, MA.
- *Neurological Assessment of the Preterm and Full-term Newborn Infant* (NAPFI) by L. Dubowitz and V. Dubowitz, in *Clinics in Developmental Medicine* no. 79, Philadelphia: J.B. Lippincott Co., 1981.
- *Neurological Examination of the Full-term Newborn Infant*, 2nd ed. by H. Prechtl, in *Clinics in Developmental Medicine* no. 63, Philadelphia: J.B. Lippincott Co., 1977.
- *Peabody Developmental Motor Scales* by M.R. Folio and R.R. Fewell, Austin, TX: Pro-ed, 1983.

PROBLEMS

Self-Care
- The person may have poor oral motor skills and difficulty with feeding.
- The person may have delays in learning self-care skills.

Productivity and Leisure
- The person may have delays in play skills.

Sensorimotor
- The person may have a regulatory disorder such as difficulty with sleeping and eating.
- The person may show signs of physiologic stress, including color changes, cyanosis around the mouth (circumoral), skin mottling, changes in respiratory rate or rhythm, change in heart rate, coughing, sneezing, yawning, vomiting, bowel movement, or hiccups (Sheahan and Brockway 1994, 60).
- The person may show signs of stress in motor actions, such as sudden change in muscle tone; flaccidity in the trunk extremities or face; stiffness, including leg bracing, opisthotonos, finger splaying, facial grimacing, tongue extension, or hyperflexion; or alterations in the quality of movement, such as disorganized movement, jitteriness, or squirminess (Sheahan and Brockway 1994, 60).
- The person may have delayed motor milestones.

- The person may have abnormal muscle tone (hypo- or hypertonicity).
- The person may have an obligatory response to reflex stimuli, such as asymmetrical tonic neck reflex.
- The person may have decreased range of motion.
- The person may have atypical movement patterns—asymmetries, constant jerkiness.
- The person may have poor coordination between the two sides of the body.
- The person may have a sensory processing disorder such as hyporesponsiveness to sensory input—visual, aural, tactile, touch, temperature, proprioceptive, and/or kinesthetic.
- The person may have hypersensitivity to sensory input, such as tactile defensiveness.

Cognitive
- The person may be unable to remain alert even for brief periods of time.

Psychosocial
- The person may show signs of stress with behavioral indicators such as irritability (crying, inconsolability), staring, gaze aversion, hyperalertness, roving eye movements, glassy-eyed appearance, sleeplessness, and restlessness (Sheahan and Brockway, 1994, 60).
- The person may have poor eye contact.
- The person may show no change in facial expression when approached.
- The person may cry all the time and be unable to be consoled.
- The person may not respond to human contact or may stiffen or arch the back when picked up.
- The person does not make sounds or makes sounds outside of the human speech range (unusual sounds).
- The person may have poor impulse control.

Environment
- Parents may have their occupational roles as nurturers and caregivers preempted by the staff in the neonatal intensive care unit. They may have limited opportunity to touch, feed, change, or protect the infant. They cannot use their own creativity and problem solving in caring for the infant.
- Parents' expectations of having a healthy baby may have been jarred.
- Parents may feel denial and guilt, as well as anger at their small, fragile, unattractive infant.
- Parents may have to become technicians first to learn to monitor data.

TREATMENT/INTERVENTION
Models of treatment include neurodevelopmental therapy and sensory integration.

Self-Care
- Encourage oral motor skills, including the suck-swallow reflex to permit feeding with a nipple, by using tactile stimulation of the mouth and gums, pressure on the cheeks, and nonnutritive sucking.

Productivity
- Help the person develop play skills to entertain himself or herself.

Leisure
• Help the person discover preferred activities.

Sensorimotor
• Enhance self-regulatory behavior through environmental modification such as assisting the child to calm herself or himself through relaxation techniques designed to reduce stress, including slow, rhythmical rocking, deep proprioceptive input, and tight swaddling.
• Improve muscle tone in trunk, shoulder girdle, and hip girdle (axial skeleton) to increase stability, and in arms and legs (appendicular skeleton) to increase movement.
• Increase flexor patterns in premature infants; increase extension patterns in full-term infants.
• Promote more normal patterns of movement by decreasing hyperextension of the neck and trunk, reducing elevation of the shoulder, decreasing retraction of the scapula, and reducing extension of the lower extremities. At the same time, promote activation of the primary flexor muscle groups through planned positioning and therapeutic handling, such as gently flexing the hips and knees to reduce hyperextension and bringing the hands toward the buttocks to reduce shoulder elevation. Side-lying position is useful in reducing scapula retraction and lower extremity extension.
• Promote postural alignment including increased orientation to midline through planned positioning, such as placement in a hammock-like sling (Sheahan and Brockway 1994, 74–76).
• Improve visual reactions and responses by putting faces or mobiles in the child's line of vision.
• Improve auditory reactions and responses by talking, singing, or exposing the child to sounds and music.
• Improve tactile reactions and responses by stroking, rubbing with lotions or oils, or allowing the child to touch various textures.
• Improve vestibular reactions and responses by gentle rocking or swinging the child in a hammock.
• Improve proprioceptive reactions and responses by placing weight and deep pressure on the soles of the child's feet.
• Facilitate the development of the child's reflex patterns, beginning with head righting on through primitive reactions to equilibrium reactions.
• Decrease tactile defensiveness, if present, through the use of deep, rhythmical tactile input.

Cognitive
• Encourage child to attend by using a hammock-like sling made with a doubled blanket with sides rolled toward the infant for stability (Sheahan and Brockway 1994, 74–76).

Psychosocial
• Encourage responses to handling, talking, and seeing human faces.
• Promote appropriate parent-infant or parent-child interaction.

Environment
• Provide consultation to team members, including the nursing staff and parents, regarding developmental intervention.

- Participate in interagency collaboration designed to facilitate transition to the home environment.
- Provide appropriate remediation of orthopedic complications, such as with splints or serial casting.
- Instruct parents about normal growth and developmental patterns.
- Instruct parents or caregivers about positioning and handling techniques.
- Instruct parents about methods of increasing alert state through the use of arrhythmic vestibular stimuli, such as bouncing and upright position, or tactile stimuli, such as a light touch to the face and body.

PRECAUTIONS

- Watch for signs of physiologic stress and sensory overload, including gaze aversion, staring, facial hypotonia, alterations in respiration or heart rate, jerkiness, hiccups, spitting, changes in the color of skin to dark or light tones, and mottling. (See "Problems" section above.)
- Watch for iatrogenic musculoskeletal abnormalities caused by failure to maintain best positioning.
- When flexing the neck, avoid hyperflexion, which may cause airway obstruction and pulmonary compromise.
- Avoid the use of lotions and oils during tactile awareness activities because they may irritate the skin.

PROGNOSIS AND OUTCOME

- Infant has better oral motor skills.
- Infant's quality of muscle tone has improved, as evidenced by such actions as less extensor thrust.
- Infant's rate of gaining developmental milestones and reflex maturation has increased.
- Infant's response to sensory input has improved, as evidenced by tactile awareness.
- Infant has increased attending behavior (eye contact).
- Infant has increased attention span.
- Infant responds to being picked up by flexing (cuddling) or changing facial expression (smiling).
- Infant is able to calm himself or herself.

REFERENCES

Cook, D.G. 1993. Screening and identification in early prevention. In *Pediatric occupational therapy and early intervention*, ed. J. Case-Smith, 62–80. Boston: Andover Medical Publishers.
Sheahan, M.S., and N.F. Brockway. 1994. The high-risk infant. In *Pediatric physical therapy*, ed. J.S. Tecklin, 56–88. Philadelphia: J.B. Lippincott Co.

BIBLIOGRAPHY

Churcher, E. et al. 1993. Fine motor development of high-risk infants at 3, 6, 12, and 24 months. *Physical and Occupational Therapy in Pediatrics* 13, no. 1: 19–37.

Hunter, J.G. 1996. The neonatal intensive care unit. In *Occupational therapy for children.* 3rd ed., eds. J. Case-Smith et al., 583–631. St. Louis, MO: Mosby.

Joe, B.E. 1996. Little miracles. *OT Week* 10, no. 49: 12–13.

Lewerenz, T.L., and R.C. Schaaf. 1996. Sensory processing in at-risk infants. *Sensory Integration Special Interest Section Newsletter* 19, no. 1: 1–4.

Limperopoulos, C. et al. 1997. Agreement between the neonatal neurologic examination and a standardized assessment of neurobehavioural performance in a group of high-risk newborns. *Pediatric Rehabilitation* 1, no. 1: 9–14.

Majnemer, A. et al. 1994. Predicting outcome in high-risk newborns with a neonatal neurobehavioral assessment. *American Journal of Occupational Therapy* 48, no. 8: 723–732.

Mohr, N. 1993. Studying the effect of delayed oral feeding in severely ill infants. *OT Week* 7, no. 43: 62.

Olson, J.A., and K. Baltman. 1995. Infant mental health in occupational therapy practice in the neonatal intensive care unit. *Neonatal Intensive Care* 8, no. 2: 48–52, 54, 58.

Tomchek, S.D., and S.J. Lane. 1993. Full-term low birth weight infants: Etiology and developmental implications. *Physical and Occupational Therapy in Pediatrics* 13, no. 3: 43–65.

Vergara, E. 1993. Medical management of high-risk neonates. In *Foundations for practice in the neonatal intensive care unit and early intervention: A self-guided practice manual,* 77–85. Vol 1. Rockville, MD: American Occupational Therapy Association.

Warren, I. 1994. Getting started on the special care baby unit: Preparation and protocol. *British Journal of Occupational Therapy* 57, no. 12: 462–466.

Homelessness—Child and Adolescent

DESCRIPTION

Children and adolescents are considered to be homeless when they and/or their family have no permanent address. Generally the children and adolescents do not have any specific medical condition or diagnostic condition. Homeless families with children constitute about 40 percent of all homeless persons, according to estimates by the National Coalition for the Homeless. In urban areas, approximately 30 percent of the homeless population may be composed of children and unaccompanied minors, according to the U.S. Conference of Mayors. Once the children or adolescents become homeless, they may be forced to move frequently and their schooling may be interrupted (Kerr 1998).

CAUSE

The cause of homelessness appears to have little or nothing to do with children or adolescences themselves. Typically the child or youth is from a poor family and/or broken home, especially in the urban areas (Marmer 1997).

ASSESSMENT

Areas

- motor skills, including fine and gross motor skills

- cognitive and language skills
- adaptive and socioemotional skills
- school readiness
- job readiness

Instruments

Instruments Developed by Occupational Therapy Personnel

- *FirstSTEp: Screening Test for Evaluating Preschoolers* by L.A. Miller, San Antonio, TX: The Psychological Corporation, 1993.

PROBLEMS

Self-Care

- The person is dependent on others for instrumental activities of daily living.

Productivity

- Skills in school readiness for young children may be below the norm for age on screening test.
- Skill performance in academic subjects, especially reading and writing, may be several grade levels below expectation in school-age children and adolescents.
- The person usually has been in trouble with the school system for failure to perform, truancy, or breaking the rules.

Sensorimotor

- The person may be at risk for developmental delays but actual performance will vary from below the norm to above the norm.
- The person may have sensory deficits.
- The person may have fine motor deficits.
- The person may have poor perceptual motor skills.

Cognitive

- Skills in cognitive performance, including language skills, may be below the norm for age on screening test.
- The person may have deficits in problem-solving and organizational skills.
- The person may have difficulty following verbal and written directions.
- The person may have difficulty with memory skills.

Psychosocial

- Skills in adaptive and socioemotional areas may vary from below the norm to above the norm.
- The person may not trust or feel safe with anyone except an immediate circle of friends.
- The person may have history of physical and sexual abuse.

Environment
- The child may be used to "hanging out" on the streets with little structure to the day's activities unless the child attends school.
- The person may be familiar with drugs and violence.
- The person may have a history of having lived in several different foster homes.

TREATMENT/INTERVENTION

Self-Care
- Foster independence skills by teaching the person to use public transportation, employment and health care services, and other community resources.
- Provide instruction in parenting, cooking, and budgeting.

Productivity
- Help person focus skills and interests on potential careers that enhance personal meaning.
- Focus on employment readiness, job skills, resume building, interviewing, and job application processes.
- Discuss job opportunities through formalized training such as trade school, junior college, or the future job market.

Leisure
- Assist person in exploring the community and available resources through field trips, lectures, or discussion.

Cognitive
- Encourage individuals to think for themselves and trust their own thoughts.
- Use demonstration as well as verbal instructions for those who have poor perceptual skills and difficulty following directions.
- Break cognitive tasks into smaller units of learning.

Psychosocial
- Increase self-esteem.
- Focus on the student's interests and skills.
- Use group activities.
- Help the person explore values.
- Teach stress-management skills.
- Instruct the person in socially acceptable skills in dating and friendship.
- Make an educational videotape for others or videotape a talk show segment to get individuals to talk about their feelings and stories.

Environment
- Provide opportunity for novelty and variety as well as consistency and familiarity.
- Provide alternative lifestyle to living on the streets, such as a structured routine of daily activities.

- Help the person explore options in the community, especially the arts, recreation, and cultural activities.
- Arrange for the person to take trips into the community to try out newly acquired skills.

PRECAUTIONS
- Avoid stereotypes about homelessness, such as poor motivation on the part of certain ethnic groups, families who are poor, or people who live in certain areas of the community.

PROGNOSIS AND OUTCOME
- The person will continue normal development of skills and will not experience developmental delays.
- The person will continue to receive an education and continue to learn.

REFERENCES
Kerr, T. 1998. Getting homeless kids ready to become students: Their social development was higher than the norm. *Advance for Occupational Therapy Practitioners* 14, no. 39: 25, 28.
Marmer, L. 1997. Pilot program brings OT to "City of Angels" street kids. *Advance for Occupational Therapists* 13, no. 22: 11.

BIBLIOGRAPHY
Stahl, C. 1998. Social workers value occupational therapy at The Working Zone. *Advance for Occupational Therapy Practitioners* 14, no. 36: 7, 26.

Learning Disorders

DESCRIPTION

Learning disorders are characterized by an inability to acquire, retain, or generalize specific skills or sets of information because of deficiencies or defects in attention, memory, or reasoning, or deficiencies in producing responses associated with a desired and skilled behavior. Other related terms are learning disability, neurologic impairment, minimal brain dysfunction, perceptual motor dysfunction, perceptual deficit disorder, dyslexia, attention deficit disorder, and hyperkinesis. A learning disability is a specific disorder and assumes normal cognitive abilities. It refers to a problem in reading (dyslexia), arithmetic (dyscalculia), spelling, written expression, or handwriting (dysgraphia), and in the understanding and/or use of verbal communication (dysphasia, dysnomia, difficulties with expressive language) and nonverbal communication. Learning disorders encompass cognitive problems in acquiring daily living, social, language or communication, and academic skills (Merck 1999, 2251).

CAUSE

No single cause or set of symptoms has been identified. Genetic and neurologic causes may be involved. Theories about causation focus on ideas about brain dysfunction such as left-hemisphere maturation lag or damage, lack of hemispheric specialization, inadequate inter-hemispheric communication, and sensory integration dysfunction (Szklut et al. 1995, 315–318). The ratio of affected males to females is about 5:1. Between 3 percent and 15 percent of schoolchildren may be affected.

ASSESSMENT

Areas

- postural control and gross motor performance: muscle tone and strength; functional range of motion; integration of primitive postural reflexes; development of righting, equilibrium, and vestibular function; automatic postural reactions; gross motor skills development
- fine motor and visual motor performance: proximal and distal movement patterns, eye-hand coordination, handwriting and fine motor skill development
- motor planning abilities: ideation, planning, and execution
- sensory integration: sensory modulation, sensory discrimination, and perception
- physical fitness: muscle strength, endurance, and flexibility

Instruments

Instruments Developed by Occupational Therapy Personnel

- *DeGangi-Berk Test of Sensory Integration* (DBTSI) by G.A. DeGangi and R.A. Berk, Los Angeles: Western Psychological Services, 1983.
- *FirstSTEp: Screening Test for Evaluating Preschoolers* by L.A. Miller, San Antonio, TX: The Psychological Corporation, 1993.
- *Loewenstein Occupational Therapy Cognitive Assessment* by M. Itzkovich, E. Elazar, S. Averbueh and N. Katz, distributed by Pequanock, NJ: Maddak Inc., 1990.
- *Miller Assessment for Preschoolers* (MAP) by L.J. Miller, San Antonio, TX: The Psychological Corporation, 1988.
- *Sensory Integration and Praxis Tests* by A.J. Ayres, Los Angeles: Western Psychological Corporation, 1989. (Replaces the Southern California Sensory Integration Tests.)

Instruments Developed by Other Professionals and Used by Occupational Therapy Personnel

- *Basic Motor Ability Tests* by D.D. Arnheim and W.A. Sinclair, in *The Clumsy Child*, St. Louis, MO: Mosby, 1979.
- *The Beery-Buktenica Developmental Test of Visual-Motor Integration* (VMI-4), 4th ed. by K.E. Beery and N.A. Buktenica, Parsippany, NJ: Modern Curriculum Press, 1997.
- *Bender Gestalt Test for Young Children* by E.M. Koppitz, New York: Grune & Stratton, 1963.
- *Bruininks-Oseretsky Test of Motor Proficiency* (BOTMP) by R.H. Bruininks, Circle Pines, MN: American Guidance Services, 1978.

- *Developmental Test of Visual Perception-2* (DTVP-2) by D.D. Hammill, N.A. Pearson, and J.K. Voress, Austin, TX: Pro-ed, 1993. (Replaces the Marianne Frostig Developmental Test of Visual Perception.)
- *Motor-Free Visual Perceptual Test–Revised* by R.P. Colarusso and D.D. Hammill, Novato, CA: Academic Therapy Publications, 1996.
- *Movement Assessment Battery for Children* (Movement ABC) by S.E. Henderson and D.A. Sugden, San Antonio, TX: The Psychological Corporation, 1992. (Replaces Test of Motor Impairment.)
- *Peabody Developmental Motor Scales* (PDMS) by M.R. Folio and R.R. Fewell, Austin, TX: Pro-ed, 1983.
- *Pediatric Clinical Tests of Sensory Interaction for Balance* (B-CTSIB) by J.C. Deitz et al., in Performance of children with learning disabilities and motor delays on the Pediatric Clinical Test of Sensory Interaction for Balance (B-CTSIB), *Physical and Occupational Therapy in Pediatrics* 16, no. 3 (1996): 1–21.
- *Pediatric Examination of Educational Readiness* by M.D. Levine, Cambridge, MA: Educators Publishing Services, 1982.
- *Perceptual Motor Assessment for Children* (P-MAC) by J.G. Dial, L. McCarron, and G. Amann, Dallas, TX: McCarron-Dial Systems, 1988.
- *Purdue Pegboard Test* by J. Tiffin, Lafayette, IN: Lafayette Instrument Co., 1960.
- *Quick Neurological Screening Test-II* by M. Mutti, H.M. Sterling, and N.V. Spalding, Novato, CA: Academic Therapy Publications, 1998.
- *Soft Neurological Signs* by S.E. Szklut et al., in Learning disabilities, *Neurological rehabilitation*, ed. D.A. Umphred, 325, St. Louis, MO: Mosby, 1995.
- *Test of Visual-Motor Skills—Revised* (TVMS-R) by M.F. Gardner, Hydesville, CA: Psychological and Educational Publications, 1995.
- *Tests for Motor Proficiency* by S.S. Gubbay, in *The Clumsy Child*, Philadelphia: W.B. Saunders Co., 1975.
- *Wide Range Achievement Test—3* by G.S. Wilkinson, Wilmington, DE: Jastak Associates/ Wide Range, 1993.
- *Woodcock-Johnson Psycho-Educational Battery* by R.W. Woodcock and M.J. Johnson, Itasca, IL: Riverside Publishing Co., 1977.

Other Assessment Procedures
- *Minor neurologic indicators*: left-right discrimination, finger agnosia, visual tracking, extinction of simultaneous stimuli, choreiform movements, tremor, exaggerated associated movements, and reflex asymmetries.
- *Coordination indicators:* finger-to-nose touching, sequential thumb-finger touching, diadochokinesia, heel-to-shin movement, and slow controlled movements.
- *Postural and motor measures*: muscle tone and strength; arm extension at 90 degrees (Schilder's posture); standing with feet together, eyes closed (Romberg's position); standing with feet in tandem (heel to toe), eyes closed (Mann's position); standing on one leg, eyes closed; walking a line; tandem walking (heel to toe, forward and backward); hopping, jumping, or skipping; ball throwing and catching; imitation of tongue movements; paper and pencil tasks; and fine motor tasks.
- *Sensory indicators*: graphesthesia, stereognosis, and localization of touch input.

PROBLEMS

Self-Care

- The person may have difficulty performing some activities of daily living, such as tying shoelaces.

Productivity

- The person may have poorly developed play skills.
- The person does not want to participate in games and athletic activities due to poor motor functioning.
- The person is at least two years behind age level in one or more school areas, such as reading, spelling, or math.

Leisure

- The person may have few leisure activities.

Sensorimotor

Postural Control and Automatic Postural Reactions

- The person may have low muscle tone and poor joint stability. Observations of low tone are "floppy" positioning and open mouth, lordotic back and sagging belly, knees positioned close together. Signs include locking elbows, winging of the scapula, or lordosis of the trunk. Note: Increased tone is not common in learning disorders but may be a sign of mild cerebral palsy.
- The person's posture is poor with lordosis (curvature) of the upper trunk, kyphosis (pot belly) of the lower trunk, and recurvatum of the knees.
- The person may be unable to rotate upper and lower segments on the body's axis.
- The person may develop patterns of compensation for low tone called fixing patterns, which include elevated and internally rotated shoulders, internally rotated hips, and pronated feet.
- The person has difficulty moving against gravity in static holding (arms out like an airplane on stomach) and dynamic activities (throwing a ball, climbing a jungle gym). Note: Standard muscle testing and range of motion testing are usually not done. Assessment of strength and range is based on functional performance.

Reflex Maturation and Integration of Primitive Postural Reflexes

- The person may show signs of residual primitive postural reflexes in stressful motor performance, especially the asymmetrical and symmetrical tonic neck reflexes.
- The person may have difficulty sitting straight forward at the table for fine motor or writing tasks or with other midline-focused activities such as pulling or hanging on a rope with both hands.

Righting, Protective, and Equilibrium Reactions and Vestibular Function

- The person may have difficulty righting the head and neck in changing positions of the body to vertical position.
- The person may have difficulty using equilibrium reactions when balance is challenged and respond using protective (propping or parachute) reactions.

Gross Motor Skills

- The person may have delays in developing gross motor skills needed for such functions as smooth gait, running, skipping, jumping, or throwing and catching a ball.
- The person may have unusual movements, such as choreiform (jerky, rapid, irregular) movements of the face, arms, or legs, especially when performing a movement that is difficult for the person.

Fine Motor Skills, Eye-Hand Coordination, Dexterity, and Handwriting

- The person has difficulties in fine motor dexterity and manipulation that lead to problems such as poor control of a pencil and an inability to cut on a line or color within the lines.
- The person lacks skill in eye-motor coordination, including being labeled clumsy and performing poorly on eye-tracking tasks.
- The person may have ocular motor apraxia, such as an inability to track or scan smoothly due to strabismus (motor imbalance of the eye muscles), amblyopia, diplopia, nystagmus, or paralysis of gaze.

Adaptive Movement Responses, Motor Planing, and Ideation

- The person has difficulty in motor planning (dyspraxia), motor sequencing, and flexibility of motor responses.
- The person may have dysdiadochokinesia or an inability to rapidly and smoothly repeat alternating movements, such as supination and pronation of the forearm.

Sensory Modulation

- The person may show tactile defensiveness.
- The person may be hyper- or hyporesponsive to vestibular stimulation and may have gravitational insecurity or intolerance to movement.

Sensory Discrimination and Perception

- The person may have difficulties in visual perception, especially figure-ground, part-whole relationships, and position in space.
- The person may have poor proprioceptive skills and may be unaware of the position of body or body parts in space (laterality and directionality).
- The person may lack tactile discrimination and localization.
- The person may have difficulties in auditory perception, especially auditory discrimination.
- The person may have disturbances in body image, especially integration of the two sides of the body.

Cognitive

- The person may have a short attention span and be inattentive or overattentive (fixate on one aspect of a situation or object).
- The person may be easily distracted.
- The person may have short-term memory loss.
- The person may perseverate.
- The person may have difficulty orienting to time, space, or distance.
- The person may have difficulty understanding concepts of size, color, shape, sameness, and difference.

Psychosocial

• The person has poor self-perception.
• The person may show poor impulse control.
• The person has non–goal-directed behavior.
• The person may be withdrawn or act as the class clown.
• The person may have mild dysphasia or inability to process language.

TREATMENT/INTERVENTION

The major models for treatment in occupational therapy are sensory integration, vision therapy (Downing-Baum and Maino 1996; Scheiman 1997), and metacognition strategies with information-processing theory (Mason 1994). Occupational therapists should be aware that sensory integration techniques are controversial and that negative critiques on the effectiveness of sensory integration appear in the literature (Hoehn and Baumeister 1994; Kadrman 1993).

Self-Care

• Improve daily living skills. Use schedule boards to list daily tasks, provide checklists of activities to perform, and use timers to signal the end of an activity. Use picture sequences to help the person learn tasks such as tying shoelaces.

Productivity

• Improve level of play skills in exploration and imaginative activities.
• Improve level of academic skills by promoting better adaptive and organizational skills. For example, person may be considered lazy because adaptive strategies are difficult for the individual. Suggest that the teacher provide more structure to assignments. In handwriting, determine whether printing or cursive writing is easier or if keyboarding would be better. Recommend use of calendars for scheduling assignments and notebook binder organization for class notes. For math work, provide worksheets that reduce the number of problems to two per line and gradually increase in number as spatial orientation skills increase. If the person uses too much pressure in handwriting, have the individual practice with a watercolor brush.

Leisure

• Increase the person's exposure to leisure activities of possible interest.

Sensorimotor

• Promote effective total body management in a wide variety of activities that require dynamic balance and agility.
• Promote object management including manipulation, propulsion, and reception.
• Integrate primitive reflexes and improve muscle tone through positions and tasks designed to counter the effects of the reflex.
• Improve gross motor skills through active participation on the playground.
• Improve fine motor skills using construction toys.
• Improve ability to deal with daily schedule of activities by providing a flip picture schedule with one-step photos of each activity done during the day.

- Improve capacity to register, process, and integrate sensory information by direct intervention through active participation in activities that elicit an adaptive response. For example, to increase ability to deal with objects in the classroom, set up a kinesthetic "feely" box containing 10 common classroom objects to be identified.
- Increase the frequency, duration, or complexity of adaptive responses to sensory input.
- Improve motor planning skills.
- Increase visual tracking skills by having the person read the letters from left to right on a sheet of letters printed in random order. See how many letters can be read correctly in 30 seconds or 1 minute. Letters can be typed in a large font initially and gradually reduced in size. Have the person find the letters of the alphabet in sequence from a page of randomly ordered letters. Have the person find words that are embedded in a page with randomly ordered letters. Begin with left to right orientation only and increase difficulty by introducing words oriented up and down. For variety, change to numbers.

Cognitive

- Improve the person's ability to organize ideas, plan a sequence of actions (steps to take), and execute a plan. For example, to organize the morning routine and reduce dawdling time, suggest prompts to be given verbally and with visual cues, lay out clothes the night before, or use a checklist with a reward for timely completion of tasks.
- Increase attention span and concentration.
- Increase memory skills. For example, if visual memory is poor, have the person stand in a dark room, shine a flashlight on two objects selected by the therapist, switch off the light, and describe details of the objects. Later replace pictures for objects. Place the person prone in a net or platform swing and rotate it while the person looks for puzzle-piece letters on the floor, which must be placed in alphabetical sequence in a form board. To aid in remembering letter formation, have the person form the letters using a finger in a tactilely stimulating medium such as modeling clay, sand, or shaving cream. Begin with one letter and gradually increase the number of letters to be formed at one time.
- Teach the person compensatory techniques and metacognition strategies. Examples include counting the number of blocks or pegs in the original before beginning patterns, such as copying block designs or peg and parquetry patterns, marking off the corners of the design, and working in a particular orientation (e.g., top to bottom or left to right).
- Teach the person always to check the work that has been done to see if it is correct or is as the person intended.

Psychosocial

- Increase the person's self-esteem, positive self-concept, and self-confidence.
- Improve coping skills and emotional control.
- Improve social interaction skills.
- Increase communication skills.

Environment

- Adapt the environment to take advantage of the person's strengths and to compensate for the areas of deficit.
- Conduct sessions with teachers on ideas they can use in class to improve fine motor skills and visual perception skills.

- Provide information to teachers on sensory modulation disorders and the way in which sensory overload affects performance.
- Provide sessions with parents to explain management techniques and activities that can be used at home.

PRECAUTIONS

- Observe child for signs of sensory overload, such as flushing, blanching, or perspiring.
- Observe child for signs of overinhibition of brain-stem functions, such as depressed respiratory functions.
- Monitor child for potential accidents due to lack of skills or lack of judgment on the part of the child.

PROGNOSIS AND OUTCOME

- The person is able to perform activities of daily living appropriate to age level.
- The person demonstrates improvement in play and academic skills.
- The person demonstrates improvement in leisure skills.
- The person demonstrates integration of primitive reflexes and correct use of protective and equilibrium reflexes.
- The person demonstrates normal muscle tone.
- The person performs gross and fine motor skills appropriate to age level.
- The person demonstrates dexterity and coordination tasks appropriate to age level.
- The person demonstrates improvement in motor planning and praxis behavior.
- The person demonstrates improved attention span and concentration.
- The person shows improvement in coping skills.
- The person demonstrates improved social skills.

REFERENCES

Beers, M.H., and R. Berkow, eds. 1999. *The Merck Manual of Diagnosis and Therapy*, 17th ed. Whitehouse Station, NJ: Merck Research Laboratories.
Downing-Baum, S., and D. Maino. 1996. Case studies show success in OT-OD treatment plans. *Advance for Occupational Therapists* 12, no. 44: 18, 46. (case reports)
Hoehn, T.P., and A.A. Baumeister. 1994. A critique of the application of sensory integration therapy to children with learning disabilities. *Journal of Learning Disabilities* 27, no. 6: 338–350.
Kadrman, C.J. 1993. Is sensory integration therapy an effective treatment for children with learning disabilities. *Journal of Occupational Therapy Students* 7, no. 2: 15–22.
Mason, M. 1994. Utilizing metacognitive strategies with learning disabilities. *Occupational Therapy Forum* 9, no. 22: 4–5, 10.
Scheiman, M. 1997. Visual problems associated with learning disorders. In *Understanding and managing vision deficits: A guide for occupational therapists,* ed. M. Scheiman, 217–232. Bethesda, MD: American Occupational Therapy Association. (case reports)
Szklut, S.E. et al. 1995. Learning disabilities. In *Neurological rehabilitation*, ed. D.A. Umphred, 312–359. St. Louis, MO: Mosby.

BIBLIOGRAPHY

Deitz, J.C. et al. 1996. Performance of children with learning disabilities and motor delays on the Pediatric Clinical Test of Sensory Interaction for Balance (B-CTSIB). *Physical and Occupational Therapy in Pediatrics* 16, no. 3: 1–21.

Erhardt, R., and S.C. Merrill. 1998. Learning disabilities. In *Willard and Spackman's occupational therapy.* 9th ed., eds. M.E. Neistadt and E.B. Crepeau, 598–601. Philadelphia: J.B. Lippincott Co.

Fanchiang, S.P. 1996. The other side of the coin: Growing up with a learning disability. *American Journal of Occupational Therapy* 50, no. 4: 277–285. (case report)

Humphries, T. et al. 1996. Evidence of nonverbal learning disability among learning disabled boys with sensory integrative dysfunction. *Perceptual and Motor Skills* 82: 979–987.

Humphries, T.W. et al. 1993. Clinical evaluation of the effectiveness of sensory integrative and perceptual motor therapy in improving sensory integrative function in children with learning disabilities. *Occupational Therapy Journal of Research* 13, no. 3: 163–182.

Kemmis, B.L., and W. Dunn. 1996. Collaborative consultation: The efficacy of remedial and compensatory interventions in school contexts. *American Journal of Occupational Therapy* 50, no. 9: 709–717.

Klein, S., and J. Magill-Evans. 1998. Perceptions of competence and peer acceptance in young children with motor and learning difficulties. *Physical and Occupational Therapy in Pediatrics* 18, no. 3/4: 39–52.

McFall, S.A. et al. 1993. Test-retest reliability of visual perceptual skills with children with learning disabilities. *American Journal of Occupational Therapy* 47, no. 9: 819–824.

Moryosef-Ittah, S., and J. Hinojosa. 1996. Discriminant validity of the Development Test of Visual Perception-2 for children with learning disabilities. *Occupational Therapy International* 3, no. 3: 204–211.

North, K. et al. 1994. Specific learning disability in children with neurofibromatosis type 1: Significance of MRI abnormalities. *Neurology* 44: 878–883.

Parush, S., and J. Hahn-Markowitz. 1997. A comparison of two settings for group treatment in promoting perceptual-motor function of learning disabled children. *Physical and Occupational Therapy in Pediatrics* 17, no. 1: 45–57.

Porr, S.M. 1999. The cognitive system—learning disorders. In *Pediatric therapy: A systems approach*, eds. S.M. Porr and E.B. Rainville, 276–287. Philadelphia: F.A. Davis.

Spitzer, S. et al. 1998. Occupational therapy provision for children with learning disabilities (statement). In *Reference manual of the official documents of the American Occupational Therapy Association,* 357–370. 6th ed. Bethesda, MD: American Occupational Therapy Association.

Wilson, B.N., and J.B. Kaplan. 1994. Follow-up assessment of children receiving sensory integration treatment. *Occupational Therapy Journal of Research* 14, no. 4: 244–266.

Mental Retardation— Child and Adolescent

DESCRIPTION

Mental retardation in children (called learning disabilities in Great Britain and Australia) is characterized by significantly subaverage intellectual functioning (intelligence quotient [IQ] of less than 70 to 75), which exists concurrently with related limitations in two or more of the following applicable skill areas: communication, self-care, home living, social skills, community use, self-direction, health and safety, functional academics, leisure, and work (American Association on Mental Retardation [AAMR] 1992). The three major criteria are significantly subaverage intellectual functioning, limitations in adaptive skills, and onset prior to age 18 years. In 1992, the AAMR changed the definition of mental retardation from one that relied primarily on IQ to one that includes consideration of the environment and interaction with others, especially the amount of support needs. Thus, there are two classifications:

1. *Classification based on IQ*
   Mild: 52–68
   Moderate: 36–51
   Severe: 20–35
   Profound: <20
2. *Classification based on level of support*
   Intermittent: Does not require constant support.
   Limited: Requires ongoing support of varying intensity, for example, introduction to a sheltered workshop.
   Extensive: Requires daily and ongoing consistent levels of support.
   Pervasive: Requires an ongoing high level of support for all activities of daily living.

CAUSE

The *Merck Manual* (1999) lists three categories of cause:

1. Prenatal factors
   A. Chromosomal abnormalities (trisomies, partial deletions, translocations, abnormalities in sex chromosomes or various mosaicisms)
   B. Genetic metabolic and neurologic disorders (autosomal recessive disorders, peroxisomal disorders, lysosomal defects, X-linked recessive disorders)
   C. Congenital infections (rubella, cytomegalovirus, *Toxoplasma gondii*, *Treponema pallidum*)
   D. Prenatal drug exposure (alcohol, cocaine, heroin, methadone, hydantoin)
   E. Malnutrition
2. Perinatal factors: prematurity, central nervous system bleeding, periventricular leukomalacia, breech or high forceps delivery, multiple births, placenta previa, preeclampsia, and asphyxia neonatorum
3. Postnatal factors: viral and bacterial encephalitides, meningitides, poisoning, severe malnutrition, and accidents

Ten groups of etiologic factors are recognized by the American Association on Mental Deficiency: (1) infections and intoxications, (2) trauma or physical agents, (3) metabolism or nutrition, (4) gross brain disease (postnatal), (5) unknown prenatal influence, (6) chromosomal anomalies, (7) other conditions originating in the prenatal period, (8) following psychiatric disorder, (9) environmental influences, and (10) other conditions.

ASSESSMENT

Areas

- self-care skills

- play skills
- preacademic (readiness) and academic skills
- productivity history, skills, values, interests
- leisure skills and interests
- motor skills: range of motion, gross motor development and coordination, hand functions
- postural control: muscle tone, muscle strength in antigravity positions, reflex development and integration, bilateral integration
- fine motor skills: eye-hand coordination, manipulation, dexterity
- sensory awareness and processing
- sensory modulation and adaptive movements
- sensory discrimination and perception
- praxis or motor planning, ideation
- attention span
- ability to follow directions
- self-perception
- communication skills
- coping skills
- social skills
- social and life roles

Instruments

Instruments Developed by Occupational Therapy Personnel

- *Hawaii Early Learning Profile—Revised* by S. Furuno et al., Palo Alto, CA: VORT Corporation, 1997.
- *Miller Assessment for Preschoolers* (MAP) by L.J. Miller, San Antonio, TX: The Psychological Corporation, 1988.
- *Sensorimotor Performance Analysis* by E.W. Richter and P.C. Montgomery, Hugo, MN: PDP Press, 1989.
- *Vulpe Assessment Battery*, rev. ed. by S.G. Vulpe, East Aurora, NY: Slosson Educational Publications, 1987.

Instruments Developed by Other Professionals and Used by Occupational Therapy Personnel

- *Battelle Developmental Inventory* (BDI), by J. Newborg, J.R. Stock, and J. Wnek, Itasca, IL: Riverside Publishing Company, 1984.
- *Bayley Scales of Infant Development-II* (BSID-II) by N. Bayley, San Antonio, TX: The Psychological Corporation, 1993.
- *Denver Developmental Screening Test, Revised* (Denver-II) by W.K. Frankenburg et al., Denver, CO: Denver Developmental Materials, 1990.
- *Early Intervention Developmental Profile* by S.J. Rogers and D.B. D'Eugenio, Ann Arbor, MI: University of Michigan Press, 1981.
- *Milani-Comparetti Motor Developmental Screening Test,* 3rd ed. rev. by W. Stuberg, Omaha, NE: Meyer Rehabilitation Institute, 1992.
- *Peabody Developmental Motor Scales* by M.R. Folio and R.R. Fewell, Austin, TX: Pro-ed, 1983.

- *Tennessee Self Concept Scale*, rev. by W.H. Fitts and W.L. Warren, Los Angeles: Western Psychological Services, 1988.
- *Vineland Adaptive Behavior Scales–Revised* by S.S. Sparrow, D.A. Balla, and D.V. Cicchetti, Circle Pines, MN: American Guidance Services, 1984.

PROBLEMS

Self-Care
- The person may have regulatory disorders such as difficulty with sleeping.
- The person may have feeding problems such as mouth breathing; cleft lip or palate; enlarged, thick, or protruding tongue; dysphagia (see section on deglutition disorders); drooling; and diminished gag reflex.
- The person may have difficulty learning dressing skills.
- The person may have difficulty learning personal care and toileting skills.
- The person may have difficulty learning to get around in the community and use public transportation.

Productivity
- Play skills may be underdeveloped.
- The person usually has difficulty with readiness and academic skills.

Leisure
- The child may have few or no leisure skills or interests.

Sensorimotor
- The person may have difficulty gaining mobility skills.
- The person may have any of the following skeletal and joint problems: spinal deformities such as scoliosis, lordosis, or kyphosis; dislocated hips; ankylosing (fusing) of back, elbow, hips, and shoulders; stiff joints; hyperflexible or hyperextensible joints.
- The person may have any of the following hand deformities: syndactyly (fusion of fingers), brachydactyly (shortness of fingers), polydactyly (partial extra finger), oligodactyly (missing finger), clinodactyly (short, tapered fingers), or claw hand deformities.
- The person may have lymphedema (puffy swelling) on the dorsum of the hand.
- The person may have any of the following neuromuscular problems: atrophy of various tissues, athetosis or choreoathetosis, hypotonia or hypertonia, tetany, spastic paralysis of extremities.
- The person may be hypokinetic or hyperkinetic.
- The person may have ataxia.
- The person may have seizures.
- The person may have various visual disorders, such as homonymous hemianopsia, cataracts, strabismus, or nystagmus.
- The person may be hypo- or hyperresponsive to tactile, vestibular, proprioceptive, visual, auditory, taste, smell, and/or pain stimuli.
- The person may have an auditory disorder such as a hearing loss.

- The person may engage in self-stimulation behaviors, such as head banging, rocking, or head rolling (see section on self-injuries and stereotypical behavior).
- The person may have poor discrimination and perceptual skills in areas such as tactile discrimination and localization, visual perception, visual motor perception, and body scheme.

Cognitive
- The person may have poor attending behavior and lack concentration or have a short attention span.
- The person may have poor memory skills including, short-term, visual, and auditory memory skills.
- The person may lack good problem-solving skills.
- The person may have difficulty following directions.

Psychosocial
- The person may have a poor self-image.
- The person may engage in self-mutilation behavior.
- The person may have a poor sense of self-mastery or internal locus of control.
- The person may lack self-control.
- The person may lack communication skills.
- The person may lack interaction or social skills in one-on-one, small-group, or large-group situations.

TREATMENT/INTERVENTION

Treatment models include a neurodevelopmental approach, behavior modification, sensory integration, and human occupation. Treatment may occur over several years from infancy through adolescence as the nature of the problems changes with new role demands.

Self-Care
- Assist in development of self-care skills when special problems exist, such as the feeding problems listed above. Note: Occupational therapy is not needed for routine training but may be needed if there are problems with positioning or oral motor sensitivity.
- Promote independence in daily living tasks.

Productivity
- Develop play skills, especially exploration and manipulation.
- Explore vocational interests through stimulated work activities and career interest batteries.
- Develop work habits and skills through sheltered workshop programs.
- Develop home management skills through simulation techniques.

Leisure
- Explore and develop the person's leisure interests.

Sensorimotor

Occupational therapy is usually needed only in special cases in which multiple disabilities are present or a persistent developmental lag has occurred in spite of intervention by teachers and parents.

- Increase the child's reflex integration when primitive reflexes continue to present.
- Improve postural control and balance reactions, especially trunk stability, through increased proprioceptive input.
- Increase muscle strength, especially of trunk muscles.
- Increase range of motion and flexibility.
- Increase physical endurance.
- Promote hand skills, especially development of reach, grasp, and release.
- Increase gross motor skills and coordination.
- Increase fine motor skills, manipulation, and dexterity.
- Improve bilateral coordination and integration (see section on vestibular-bilateral disorder).
- Improve motor planning skills (see section on developmental dyspraxia).
- Decrease activity level if the person is overactive and increase activity level if the person is underresponsive.
- Decrease tactile defensiveness if present (see section on tactile defensiveness).
- Increase gravitational security if present (see section on gravitational insecurity).
- Decrease self-stimulating activities through use of sensory integrative techniques.
- Improve visual fixation, tracking, and scanning if needed (see section on visual perceptual disorders).

Cognitive

Usually occupational therapy services are requested for specific problems that have not been remediated by teachers and parents.

- Increase attending behaviors such as concentration and focus by decreasing distracting stimuli. Note: Which stimuli are distracting must be observed for each person because individuals react differently depending on their degree of hyper- or hyposensitivity.
- Improve ability to follow directions.

Psychosocial

- Improve self-image through the use of creative activities such as art, crafts, drama, dance, music, and games.
- Increase group interaction skills.
- In cooperation with a speech pathologist, consider if sign language skills might augment language skills. Determine if hand skills are sufficient to make hand signing possible or if a pictorial language system such as Bliss symbols would be better.

Environment

- Provide adaptive equipment or assistive technology as needed. Examples include adapting a chair to provide for support by adding a footrest or arm supports.
- Consult with parents regarding suitable community social activities such as scouting and recreational programs.

- Encourage parents to arrange play dates at home with a peer from the school or neighborhood.
- Consult with parents about appropriate toys to facilitate developmental skills at home.
- Consult with parents about concerns regarding sexuality and menstrual periods.
- Consult with school regarding safe transportation of students. For example, discuss creating a file that stays on the bus containing essential directory information on each student, providing identification tags for each student to wear, and equipping each bus with a mobile phone for bus driver to call for assistance.
- Hold education and training sessions for teachers and parents that provide basic information about types of mental retardation and specific management techniques such as wheelchair management and positioning for function.

PRECAUTIONS
- Avoid developing splinter skills (isolated skills) that will not generalize to other situations.
- Be aware of other medical conditions that are often associated with mental retardation, such as seizures, vision disorders, and anatomical variations in the face, hands, and spine.

PROGNOSIS AND OUTCOME
The prognosis varies depending on the severity of the mental retardation and response to intervention. The outcomes listed below are samples and do not necessarily apply to all persons since intervention frequently is highly specific.
- The person has improved self-care skills, such as feeding.
- The person demonstrates an ability to perform productive activities.
- The person demonstrates an ability to perform leisure activities.
- The person shows improvement in specific motor skills.
- The person has improved sensory integrative skills.
- The person has improved attending skills.
- The person is able to function in a group setting, performing an individual task or participating as a group member.

REFERENCES
American Association on Mental Retardation. 1992. Mental retardation: Definition, classification and systems of support. 9th ed. Washington, D.C.
Beers, M.H., and R. Berkow, eds. 1999. *The Merck Manual of Diagnosis and Therapy*, 17th ed. Whitehouse Station, NJ: Merck Research Laboratories.

BIBLIOGRAPHY
Allen, S., and M. Donald. 1995. The effect of occupational therapy on the motor proficiency of children with motor/learning difficulties: A pilot study.* *British Journal of Occupational Therapy* 58, no. 9: 285–291.

Balouff, O. 1998. Developmental delay and mental retardation. In *Willard and Spackman's occupational therapy*. 9th ed., eds. M.E. Neistadt and E.B. Crepeau, 576–581. Philadelphia: J.B. Lippincott Co.

Fleming, A. et al. 1997. Learning disabilities.* In *Occupational therapy and mental health*. 2nd ed., ed. J. Creek, 399–418. New York: Churchill Livingstone.

Joe, B.E. 1994. Williams syndrome. *OT Week* 8, no. 45: 18–19.

Jones, D. 1995. Learning disability: An alternative frame of reference.* *British Journal of Occupational Therapy* 58, no. 10: 423–426.

Lifshiz, N. 1994. Comparison between the classical approach and the dynamic approach in reference to cognitive modifiability and social adaptation of the retarded child. *Israel Journal of Occupational Therapy* 3, no. 1: E31.

Lissy, S.S. 1997. Sensory stimulation as treatment for self-injurious behavior in severe or profound mental retardation. *Developmental Disabilities Special Interest Section Quarterly* 20, no. 1: 1–4.

Marmer, L. 1995. Treating the baffling symptoms of Lesch-Nyhan disease. *Advance for Occupational Therapists* 11, no. 29: 16.

McFadden, S.M. 1993. The child with mental retardation. In *Practice issues in occupational therapy: Intraprofessional team building*, ed. S.E. Ryan, 35–44. Thorofare, NJ: Slack.

Miller, L.J., and G.H. Roid. 1993. Sequence comparison methodology for the analysis of movement patterns in infants and toddlers with and without developmental delays. *American Journal of Occupational Therapy* 47, no. 4: 339–347.

Molineux, M. 1993. Improving home programme compliance of children with learning disabilities. *Australian Occupational Therapy Journal* 40, no. 1: 23–32.

Nicol, M.M., and A. Anderson. 1997. Computer-assisted versus teacher-directed teaching of community living skills in people with mild learning disability.* *British Journal of Occupational Therapy* 60, no. 11: 498–502.

Pimentel S., and S. Ryan. 1996. Working with clients with learning disabilities and multiple handicaps: A comparison between hospital and community based therapists.* *British Journal of Occupational Therapy* 59, no. 7: 313–318.

Platts, L. 1993. Social role valorisation and the model of human occupation: A comparative analysis for work with people with a learning disability in the community. *British Journal of Occupational Therapy* 56, no. 8: 278–282.

Porr, S.M. 1999. The cognitive system—mental retardation. In *Pediatric therapy: A systems approach*, eds. S.M. Porr and E.B. Rainville, 268–276. Philadelphia: F.A. Davis.

Soper, G., and C.R. Thorley. 1996. Effectiveness of an occupational therapy programme based on sensory integration theory for adults with severe learning disabilities.* *British Journal of Occupational Therapy* 59, no. 10: 475–482.

Sutcliffe, P. 1995. Rehabilitation and special education: Measuring outcomes in mentally retarded children in India. *British Journal of Occupational Therapy* 58, no. 3: 107–110.

Thiers, N. 1993. AAMR's new mental retardation definition includes function. *OT Week* 7, no. 30: 10.

Thompson, S.B.N. 1994. Sexuality training in occupational therapy for people with a learning disability, four years on: Policy guidelines.* *British Journal of Occupational Therapy* 57, no. 7: 255–258.

Thompson, S.N., and S. Martin. 1994. Making sense of multisensory rooms for people with learning disabilities.* *British Journal of Occupational Therapy* 57, no. 9: 341–344.

---

*In Great Britain and Australia, the term learning disabilities is now used for mental retardation.

Prematurity

DESCRIPTION

A premature infant is any infant born before 37 weeks gestation. The premature infant is small, usually weighing less than 2.5 kg, and tends to have thin, shiny, pink skin through which the underlying veins are easily seen. Little subcutaneous fat, hair, or external ear cartilage exists. Spontaneous activity and tone are reduced, and extremities are not held in a flexed position (Merck 1999, 2127–2128).

CAUSE

The cause of premature labor, whether or not the labor is preceded by premature rupture of the membranes, is usually unknown. However, the histories of women having premature deliveries commonly show that the women are of low socioeconomic status, have had inadequate prenatal care, have poor nutritional habits, have little education, are not married, and have intercurrent, untreated illness or infection. Other risk factors include untreated material bacterial vaginosis and previous preterm birth (Merck 1999, 2128).

ASSESSMENT

Areas

- postural control: muscle tone, hyper- or hypotonic
- reflex development and maturation, especially primitive reflexes and oral motor skills
- motor skills: range of motion (note especially discrepancies between two sides of the body), gross motor skills and coordination, hand functions
- sensory processing and modulation: awareness and response to touch, movement, sound, and light; response to being picked up or handled, visual gaze and tracking
- attending behavior: alertness, arousal, ability to focus attention, attention span, concentration
- regulatory behavior: ability to calm self after stimuli
- socialization: eye contact, cuddling, vocalization, and crying behavior

Instruments

Instruments Developed by Occupational Therapy Personnel

- *DeGangi-Berk Test of Sensory Integration* (DBTSI) by G.A. DeGangi and R.A. Berk, Los Angeles: Western Psychological Services, 1983.
- *Hawaii Early Learning Profile* (HELP), rev. ed. by S. Furuno et al., Palo Alto, CA: VORT Corporation, 1985.
- *Movement Assessment of Infants* by L.S. Chandler, M.S. Andrew, and M.W. Swanson, Rolling Bay, WA: Infant Movement Research, 1980.

Development of the Fetus and Neonate from Conception

Week	Behavior
0–4	Twitching movements
4–8	Flexor posture
9–12	Isolated head and limb movements
13–16	Eye opening and eye movements
17–20	Coordinated hand-to-face movements
21–24	Rapid eye movements
25–27	Fetal respiratory movement
28–31	Complex movements and thumb sucking
32–36	Rapid eye movement and coordinated respiratory movement
37–41	Focused alertness (full-term birth)
42–46	Social reciprocation
47–52	Object play

Source: Adapted with permission from J. Hunter, The Neonatal Intensive Care Unit, in *Occupational Therapy for Children*, 3rd ed., J. Case-Smith, A.S. Allen, and P.N. Pratt, eds., p. 592, © 1996, Mosby-Year Book, Inc.

Instruments Developed by Other Professionals and Used by Occupational Therapy Personnel

- *Bayley Scales of Infant Development-II* (BSID-II) by N. Bayley, San Antonio, TX: The Psychological Corporation, 1993.
- *Milani-Comparetti Motor Development Screening Test,* 3rd ed. rev. by W. Stuberg, Omaha, NE: Meyer Rehabilitation Institute, 1993.
- *Neonatal Behavior Assessment Scale (Brazelton),* 3rd ed. by T. Brazelton, in *Clinics in Developmental Medicine* no. 137, Philadelphia: J.B. Lippincott, 1995.
- *Neonatal Neurobehavioral Evaluation* (NNE) by A.M. Morgan et al., in Neonatal neurobehavior examination: A new instrument for quantitative analysis of neonatal neurological status, *Physical Therapy* 68, no. 9 (1988): 1352–1358.
- *Neonatal Neurological Examination* (NEONEURO) by M. Sheridan Pereira, P.H. Ellison, and V. Helgeson, in The construction of a scored neonatal neurological examination for assessment of neurologic integrity in full-term neonates, *Journal of Developmental and Behavioral Pediatrics* 12, no. 1 (1991): 25–30.
- *Neonatal Oral Motor Assessment Scale* (NOMAS) by M.A. Braun and M. Palmer, in A pilot study of oral motor dysfunction in "at risk" infants, *Physical and Occupational Therapy in Pediatrics* 5, no. 4 (1986): 13–25.
- *Neurobehavioral Assessment for Preterm Infants* (NAPI) by A.F. Korner et al., in Establishing the reliability and developmental validity of a neurobehavioral assessment for preterm infants: A methodological process, *Child Development* 62, no. 5 (1991): 1200–1208.
- *Neurological Assessment of the Preterm and Full-Term Infant* (NAPFI) by L. Dubowitz and V. Dubowitz, *Clinics in Developmental Medicine* no. 79, Philadelphia: J.B. Lippincott, 1981.

PROBLEMS

Self-Care

- The infant may be unable to feed from the breast or bottle, necessitating nasogastric or gavage feeding.
- The infant may suck weakly and have poor rooting reflexes.

Productivity and Leisure

- The infant may be unable to engage in play behavior or have poorly developed play skills.

Sensorimotor

- The infant usually has low spontaneous activity.
- The infant usually has low muscle tone (hypotonicity).
- The infant's extremities usually are partially extended rather than flexed.
- The infant may have respiratory distress syndrome due to underproduction of surfactant needed to prevent alveolar collapse and atelectasis.
- The infant is prone to hemorrhage of the periventricular germinal matrix.
- The infant may have hypotension and inadequate brain perfusion, and peaks in blood pressure may cause cerebral injury.
- Infants born prior to 34 weeks gestation usually have inadequate sucking and swallowing reflexes.
- The infant's sensory modulation may be hyper- or hyporesponsive.
- The infant's temperature regulation may be poor.

Cognitive

- The infant may have difficulty maintaining an alert state for any length of time.

Psychosocial

- The infant may have difficulty calming him- or herself.
- The infant usually has some difficulty maintaining eye contact initially.
- The infant may not cuddle when held.

TREATMENT/INTERVENTION

Self-Care

- Improve oral motor skills, including sucking and swallowing.

Productivity and Leisure

- Promote play skills, especially exploration of body and manipulation of objects.

Sensorimotor

- When the infant is medically stable, begin promoting flexion of body and limbs to increase muscle tone.
- Promote development and integration of reflexes and reactions.

- Promote development of gross motor skills, including rolling, sitting, creeping, crawling, and standing.
- Promote sensory awareness and discrimination, including vestibular, tactile, proprioceptive, gustatory, olfactory, visual, and auditory.
- If hyper- or hyposensitivity is present, work toward normalizing response.

Cognitive
- Increase the length of time the infant can maintain an organized, alert state by encouraging sucking, maintaining eye contact, and swaddling or talking to the infant. Initially, the infant may be able to tolerate only one input at a time and then gradually tolerate two or more inputs.
- Instruct the parents on holding, moving, or feeding the infant through demonstration and coaching.

Psychosocial
- Help the infant learn calming behavior (coping skills).
- Promote bonding with the parents or caregivers through use of developmental age-appropriate toys, games, and activities.

Environment
- When handling the infant, observe his or her reaction and note physiologic changes.
- Hold the infant's limbs close to the body and in flexed position to keep the infant calm.
- Provide slow, gentle motions to help the infant maintain his or her state of control and stability.
- Apply normal sensory motor experiences during routine care.
- Provide support to trunk and control to distal segments.

PRECAUTION
- Do not overload the infant with stimuli. Watch for signs of overload such as gaze aversion, staring, facial hypotonia, alterations in respiration or heart rate, jerkiness in movements, hiccups, spitting, changes in color of skin to dark or light tones, and mottling.

PROGNOSIS AND OUTCOME
- The infant is able to calm him- or herself.
- The infant has improved oral motor skills.
- The infant's quality of muscle tone has improved, including increased flexion.
- The infant's rate and level of reflex maturation has increased.
- The infant's response to sensory input has improved.
- The infant has increased attending behavior (eye contact).
- The infant has increased attention span.
- The infant responds to being picked up by flexing (cuddling) or changing facial expression (smiling).

REFERENCE

Beers, M.H., and R. Berkow, eds. 1999. *The Merck Manual of Diagnosis and Therapy*, 17th ed. Whitehouse Station, NJ: Merck Research Laboratories.

BIBLIOGRAPHY

Case-Smith, J. 1993. Postural and fine motor control in preterm infants in the first six months. *Physical and Occupational Therapy in Pediatrics* 13, no. 1: 1–17.

DeMaio-Feldman, D. 1994. Somatosensory processing abilities of very low-birth weight infants at school age. *American Journal of Occupational Therapy* 48, no. 7: 639–645.

Einarsson-Backes, M. et al. 1994. The effect of oral support on sucking efficiency in preterm infants. *American Journal of Occupational Therapy* 48, no. 6: 490–498.

Gaebler, C.P., and J.R. Hanzlik. 1996. The effects of a prefeeding stimulation program on preterm infants. *American Journal of Occupational Therapy* 50, no. 3: 184–192.

Glass, R.P., and L.S. Wolf. 1994. A global perspective on feeding assessment in the neonatal intensive care unit (review). *American Journal of Occupational Therapy* 48, no. 6: 514–526.

Gorga, D. 1994. The evolution of occupational therapy practice for infants in the neonatal intensive care unit. *American Journal of Occupational Therapy* 48, no. 6: 487–489.

Holloway, E. 1994. Parent and occupational therapist collaboration in the neonatal intensive care unit. *American Journal of Occupational Therapy* 48, no. 6: 535–538.

Holloway, E. 1997. Fostering parent-infant playfulness in the neonatal intensive care unit. In *Play in occupational therapy for children,* eds. L.D. Parham and L.S. Fazio, 171–183. St. Louis, MO: Mosby.

Holloway, E. 1998. Relationship-based occupational therapy in the neonatal intensive care unit. In *Pediatric occupational therapy and early intervention*, 2nd ed., ed. J. Case-Smith, 111–126. Boston: Butterworth-Heinemann.

Huelshamp, S. 1998. Fragile babies: Rehab gives early babies a chance to thrive. *Advance for Occupational Therapy Practitioners* 14, no. 44: 36–38, 66.

Hunter, J. 1996. The neonatal intensive care unit. In *Occupational therapy for children*, 3rd ed., eds. J. Case-Smith et al., 583–631. St. Louis, MO: Mosby.

Hunter, J. et al. 1994. Medical considerations and practice guidelines for the neonatal occupational therapists (review). *American Journal of Occupational Therapy* 48, no. 6: 546–560.

Hyde, A.S., and B.W. Jonkey. 1994. Developing competency in the neonatal intensive care unit: A hospital training program. *American Journal of Occupational Therapy* 48, no. 6: 539–545.

Klein, M.D., and T.A. Delaney. 1994. Conditions affecting feeding and nutrition—prematurity. In *Feeding and nutrition for the child with special needs: Handouts for parents*, eds. M.D. Klein and T.A. Delaney, 427–442. Tucson, AZ: Therapy Skill Builders.

Klepitsch, L.W. 1995. Having a preemie changed my outlook as a therapist. *Occupational Therapy Forum* 10, no. 13: 4–6.

Lane, S.J. et al. 1994. Prediction of preschool sensory and motor performance by 18-month neurologic scores among children born prematurely. *American Journal of Occupational Therapy* 48, no. 5: 391–396.

Marmer, L. 1996. Quiet, please: Babies at work (growing). *Advance for Occupational Therapists* 12, no. 13: 14.

Matthews, C.L. 1994. Supporting suck-swallow-breath coordination during nipple feeding. *American Journal of Occupational Therapy* 48, no. 6: 561–562.

Miller, M.Q., and M. Quinn-Hurst. 1994. Neurobehavioral assessment of high-risk infants in the neonatal intensive care unit. *American Journal of Occupational Therapy* 48, no. 6: 506–513.

Mohr, N. 1993. Studying the effect of delayed oral feeding in severely ill infants. *OT Week* 7, no. 43: 62.

Monfort, K., and J. Case-Smith. 1997. The effects of a neonatal positioner on scapular rotation. *American Journal of Occupational Therapy* 51, no. 5: 378–384.

Monfort, K.B. 1995. A comparison of two methods of prone positioning of premature infants in the neonatal intensive care unit (thesis). *Physical and Occupational Therapy in Pediatrics* 14, no. 3/4: 134–135.

Mouradia, L.E., and H. Als. 1994. The influence of neonatal intensive care unit caregiving practice on motor functioning of preterm infants. *American Journal of Occupational Therapy* 48, no. 6: 527–533.

Olson, J.A., and K. Baltman. 1994. Infant mental health in occupational therapy practice in the neonatal intensive care unit. *American Journal of Occupational Therapy* 48, no. 6: 499–505.

Shepherd, J.T. et al. 1999. Working in the neonatal intensive care unit. In *Pediatric therapy: A systems approach,* eds. S.M. Poor and E.B. Rainville, 313–378. Philadelphia: F.A. Davis.

Vergara, E. 1992. Preterm infant development. In *Foundations for practice in the neonatal intensive care unit and early intervention: A self-guided practice manual,* ed. E. Vergara, 41–76. Rockville, MD: American Occupational Therapy Association.

Wiener, A.S. et al. 1996. Sensory processing of infants born prematurely or with regulatory disorders. *Physical and Occupational Therapy in Pediatrics* 16, no. 4: 1–17.

Yossem, F. 1998. The case of the finger in the mouth: Prematurity and developmental delay. In *Clinical management of feeding disorders: Case studies,* ed. F. Yossum, 113–130. Boston: Butterworth-Heinemann.

Prenatal Exposure to Cocaine

DESCRIPTION

Prenatal exposure to cocaine results from the maternal use of cocaine (powder) or crack cocaine (smokeable form) during pregnancy. Cocaine crosses the placenta, and the same physiologic effects that occur in the mother are believed to occur in the fetus. Cocaine inhibits reuptake of neurotransmitters such as norepinephrine and epinephrine (Merck 1999, 2158). Reuptake is a neural mechanism used to stop the action of a neurotransmitter by taking the excess transmitter out of the synaptic cleft and returning the excess to the neuron (Lane 1992, 1). Thus the cocaine produces a short euphoria or "high" and also mimics the adrenergic effects of the sympathetic nervous system, causing vasoconstriction and hypertension. Cocaine use may cause fetal death or neurologic damage due to the lack of blood supply and oxygen. Infants born to addicted mothers have low birth weight, reduced body length and head circumference, and lower Apgar scores. Anomalies associated with cocaine use are related to the vascular disruption and hypoxia secondary to the vasoconstriction. These anomalies include cardiac difficulties, short limbs, prune-belly syndrome (missing layers of abdominal musculature), and intestinal atresia or necrosis. Some infants with cerebral infarcts noted at birth may have the blood supply to the brain impaired secondary to cocaine effects in utero. At birth, the infants may show withdrawal symptoms if cocaine was used by the mother just prior to delivery. The long-term effects of cocaine on growth and development are not well understood because many mothers use several types of drugs and because other social factors such as crime, inadequate diet, and disruptive home life make the effects of cocaine on the infant difficult to isolate.

CAUSE

Cocaine is a central nervous system stimulant with both anesthetic and vasoconstrictive effects. In the placenta cocaine is assumed to cause intense vasoconstriction, which significantly decreases blood flow to the fetus, resulting in periods of hypoxia. The specific effects on the fetus probably relate to the time during fetal development in which cocaine was used by the mother and the amount absorbed by the fetus. Exact correlations have not been established. It has been suggested that exposure to cocaine by the fetus may lead to defective synaptic development (Lane 1992, 1).

Cocaine is also an appetite depressant. The mother may be malnourished, which often leads to low birth weight and small head circumferences.

ASSESSMENT

Areas

- neurodevelopmental status: quality of movement, muscle tone, reflexes, and reaction patterns
- physical development: fine and gross motor skills, grasp, hand functions, eye-hand coordination, manual dexterity, adaptive motor functions
- sensory processing: reaction to sound and light, tactile deep pressure, visuotactile integration, oculomotor control, reactivity to vestibular stimulation
- regulatory/neurobehavioral status
- social and physical environment

Instruments

Instruments Developed by Occupational Therapy Personnel

- *Miller Assessment for Preschoolers* (MAP) by L.J. Miller, San Antonio, TX: The Psychological Corporation, 1988.
- *Movement Assessment of Infants* (MAI) by L.S. Chandler, M.S. Andrews, and M.W. Swanson, Rolling Bay, WA: Infant Movement Research, 1980.
- *Test of Sensory Functions in Infants* (TSFI) by G.A. DeGangi and S.I. Greenspan, Los Angeles: Western Psychological Services, 1989.

Instruments Developed by Other Professionals and Used by Occupational Therapy Personnel

- *Bayley Scales of Infant Development-II* (BSID-II) by N. Bayley, San Antonio, TX: The Psychological Corporation, 1993.
- *The Beery-Buktenica Developmental Test of Visual-Motor Integration* (VMI-4), 4th ed. by K.E. Beery and N.A. Buktenica, Parsippany, NJ: Modern Curriculum Press, 1997.
- *Fagan Test of Infant Intelligence* (FTII) by J.F. Fagan and D.K. Detterman, in The Fagan Test of Infant Intelligence: A technical summary, *Journal of Applied Developmental Psychology* 13 (1992): 173–193.
- *Neurological Assessment of the Preterm and Full-Term Infant* (NAPFI) by L. Dubowitz and V. Dubowitz, *Clinics in Developmental Medicine* no. 79, Philadelphia: J.B. Lippincott, 1981.

- *Peabody Developmental Motor Scales* (PDMS) by M.R. Folio and R.R. Fewell, Austin, TX: Pro-ed, 1983.

PROBLEMS

Productivity
- The infant's development of play skills is at risk.

Sensorimotor
- The infant's regulatory/modulation disorders may include hyperirritability, hypersensitivity to stimuli, gastrointestinal dysfunction, respiratory distress, yawning, sneezing, mottling, low-grade fever, high-pitched crying, and seizures.
- The infant's musculoskeletal problems may include increased muscle tone, especially in the extensors, tremors and jitteriness, feeding difficulties, poor motor abilities, abnormal reflexes, and asymmetries.
- The infant's physical characteristics may include low birth weight or small size for gestational age and decreased head circumference.
- The infant's postural control issues may include poor head control, poor midline functions, poor rotation, and lack of placing reaction.

Cognitive
- The infant may have difficulty with arousal.
- The infant may have impaired orientation.
- The infant may have delayed language skills.

Psychosocial
- Parent-child relationships are at risk.

Environment
- The mother may have been abusing other substances such as tobacco, marijuana, alcohol, narcotics, and other drugs during pregnancy. Using multiple substances or drugs is common.
- The caregivers and the infant may be living in a high-stress environment.
- The caregivers and the infant may have a low socioeconomic status.
- The mother may have psychopathology or an identified mental disorder such as depression.
- The child may experience physical, sexual, or emotional abuse.
- The parents or other caregivers may not know good parenting techniques.
- The mother or other caregivers may have little social support.

TREATMENT/INTERVENTION

Sensorimotor
- Gradually increase the amount of time the infant spends in prone position as head control improves.

- Provide gentle range of motion, including gentle stretching.
- Increase tolerance to sensory stimulation and ability to self-regulate through use of deep pressure, slow and gentle linear motions, and slow rocking.
- Increase sensory responsiveness, one sensory modality at a time.
- Use pediatric massage to provide calming deep pressure and joint input, improve circulation, reduce sensory hypersensitivity and pain, and promote a normal touch experience.

Cognitive

- Instruct caregivers on methods of calming infant through use of environmental modification such as swaddling, positioning hands near the face for self-soothing, and reducing light and noise during sleep time in crib.
- Instruct caregivers on techniques of sensory modification to reduce sensory defensiveness.
- Increase caregivers' awareness that avoidance behaviors are an attempt to reduce sensory input, not rejection of the caregivers.
- Increase caregivers' awareness of signs of overstimulation, such as gaze aversion, yawns, hiccups, spitting up, changes in skin color, and changes in respiration.
- Instruct caregivers in pediatric massage.

Psychosocial

- Improve parent-child attachment through education of mother or primary caregiver, clinical intervention, and environmental modification of the infant responsiveness and cues.
- Provide a role model of how to interact with an infant and encourage him or her to maintain a calm, alert state while avoiding or reducing overstimulation.
- Use pediatric massage to promote interaction, enhance attachment, and reduce stress behavior.

Environment

- Encourage caregivers during feeding and dressing to provide deep touch, to swaddle the infant, to hold the infant snugly in either a vertical or horizontal position, and to use very slow movements.
- Encourage caregivers to use environmental modifications such as reductions in light and noise as techniques to modify infant behavior.
- Increase caregivers' self-confidence by giving them the opportunity to practice and discuss methods of modifying infant's responses.

PRECAUTIONS

- Be aware that few mothers have ingested only cocaine. Look for signs of use of other drugs, including alcohol. (See "Prenatal Exposure to Drugs" below and "Substance Abuse" in Mental Disorders in Part X.)
- Always watch for signs of distress and discontinue stimulation when noted.

PROGNOSIS AND OUTCOME

- There is an increased risk of sudden infant death syndrome in infants with prenatal exposure to cocaine (Miller 1997, 120).

- By 12 months, many problems related to prenatal exposure to cocaine are resolved (Tona and Adamitis 1992, 4).
- The person may retain primitive reflexes, have excessive extensor muscle tone, and be deficient in volitional movement patterns.

REFERENCES

Beers, M.H., and R. Berkow, eds. 1999. *The Merck Manual of Diagnosis and Therapy*, 17th ed. Whitehouse Station, NJ: Merck Research Laboratories.

Lane, S.J. 1992. Assessment of infants born after prenatal cocaine exposure. *Developmental Disabilities Special Interest Section Newsletter* 15, no. 3: 2–4.

Miller, H. 1997. Prenatal cocaine exposure and mother-infant interaction: Implications for occupational therapy intervention. *American Journal of Occupational Therapy* 51, no. 2: 119–131.

Tona, J., and A.M. Adamitis. 1992. Occupational therapy with an infant exposed to cocaine in utero. *Developmental Disabilities Special Interest Section Newsletter* 15, no. 2: 3–4.

BIBLIOGRAPHY

Bayer, D.J. et al. 1996. The relationship between the Movement Assessment of Infants and the Fagan Test of Infant Intelligence in infants with prenatal cocaine exposure. *Physical and Occupational Therapy in Pediatrics* 16: 145–153.

Benson, A.M., and S.J. Lane. 1994. Interrater reliability of the Test of Sensory Function with infants exposed to cocaine in utero. *Occupational Therapy Journal of Research* 14, no. 3: 170–177.

Drehobl, K.F., and M.G. Fuhr. 1991. *Pediatric Massage for the Child with Special Needs*. Tucson, AZ: Therapy Skill Builders.

Lane, S.J. 1996. Cocaine: An overview of use, actions, and effects. *Physical and Occupational Therapy in Pediatrics* 16: 15–33.

Parks, R.A. 1994. Understanding drug dependence. In *Working with substance-exposed children: Strategies for professionals,* ed. C.H. Puttkammer, 3–8. San Antonio, TX: Therapy Skill Builders.

Stallings-Sahler, S. 1993. Prenatal cocaine exposure and infant behavioral disorganization. *Sensory Integration Special Interest Section Newsletter* 16, no. 3: 1–4.

Prenatal Exposure to Drugs Other than Cocaine

DESCRIPTION

Withdrawal from opiates (heroin, morphine, methadone): The newborn should be observed for withdrawal symptoms, which usually occur with 72 hours after delivery. Characteristic signs of withdrawal include irritability, jitteriness, hypertonicity, vomiting, diarrhea, sweating, convulsions, and hyperventilation that produces respiratory alkalosis (Merck 1999, 2159).

Withdrawal from barbiturates: Prolonged maternal abuse may cause neonatal drug withdrawal with jitteriness, irritability, and fussiness that often does not develop until 7 to 10 days after birth, when the newborn has been discharged from the nursery (Merck 1999, 2159).

Other drugs mentioned are diazepam (Ritalin) and pentazocine (Talwin).

Because of the variety of drugs, amounts of drugs taken, and times taken during pregnancy, no general profile of drug-exposed infants is available. Observation of normal and abnormal behavioral responses and knowledge of possible problems is important with drug-exposed infants.

CAUSE

The general cause is assumed to be exposure to drugs in utero. However, other factors such as malnutrition, general health status of the mother, lower socioeconomic status, and lack of prenatal care must be considered. Present living status such as foster home or adoption may contribute positively or negatively to overall performance.

ASSESSMENT

Areas

- sensory processing of tactile, vestibular, and proprioceptive input
- behavioral response to sensory input
- eating habits
- sleep patterns
- state of alertness
- communication skills (verbal and nonverbal)
- emotional reactions and temperament
- medical problems, including seizures, reflux, bleeds in the brain, surgery for insertion of G-tube or shunt, and episodes of apnea

Instruments

Drug-exposed neonates and infants tend to have short attention spans. Assessments may have to be modified into short segments, or information may need to be obtained from caregivers. Videotaping may be useful to provide comparison between initial assessment and changes after therapy was instituted.

Instruments Developed by Occupational Therapy Personnel

- *DeGangi-Berk Test of Sensory Integration* (DBTSI) by G.A. DeGangi and R.A. Berk, Los Angeles: Western Psychological Services, 1983.
- *Developmental Hand Dysfunction: Theory Assessment and Treatment* by R. Erhardt, Tucson, AZ: Therapy Skill Builders, 1982.
- *Early Coping Inventory* (ECI) by S. Zeitlin, G.G. Williamson, and M. Scezpanski, Bensenville, IL: Scholastic Testing Services, Inc., 1990.
- Miller Assessment for Preschoolers (MAP) by L.J. Miller, San Antonio, TX: The Psychological Corporation, 1988.
- *Movement Assessment of Infants* (MAI) by L.S. Chandler, M.S. Andrews, and M.W. Swanson, Rolling Bay, WA: Infant Movement Research, 1980.

- *Movement Assessment of Infants—Screening Test* (MAIST) by L.S. Chandler, M.S. Andrews, and M.W. Swanson, Rolling Bay, WA: 1983.
- *Test of Sensory Functions in Infants* (TSFI) by G.A. DeGangi and S.I. Greenspan, Los Angeles: Western Psychological Services, 1989.

Instruments Developed by Other Professionals and Used by Occupational Therapy Personnel

- *Adult-Adolescent Parenting Inventory* (AAPI) by S.J. Bavolek, Eau Claire, WI: Family Development Resources, Inc., 1984.
- *Bayley Scales of Infant Development-II* (BSID-II) by N. Bayley, San Antonio, TX: The Psychological Corporation, 1993.
- *Child Abuse Potential Inventory* (CAPI), 2nd ed. by J.S. Milner, DeKalb, IL: Psytec Inc., 1986.
- *Child Behavior Checklist for Ages 2–3* by T. Achenbach, Burlington, VT: Center for Children, Young and Families, University of Vermont, 1988.
- *Neurological Assessment of the Preterm and Full-Term Infant* (NAPFI) by L. Dubowitz and V. Dubowitz, *Clinics in Developmental Medicine* no. 79, Philadelphia: J.B. Lippincott, 1981.
- *Nursing Child Assessment Satellite Training Teaching Scale* by K.E. Barnard, ed., Seattle, WA: Nursing Child Assessment Training Publications, 1980.
- *Observation Scale for Mother-Infant Interaction during Feeding* by I. Chatoor et al., Washington, DC: Children's Hospital Medical Center, 1988.
- *Parent/Caregiver Involvement Scale* by D. Farran et al., Chapel Hill, NC: The University of North Carolina at Chapel Hill, 1986.
- *Parenting Stress Index—Short Form* by R.R. Abidin, Charlottesville, VA: Pediatric Psychology Press, 1990.
- *Peabody Developmental Motor Scales* (PDMS) by M.R. Folio and R.R. Fewell, Austin, TX: Pro-ed, 1983.
- *Transdisciplinary Play-Based Assessment: A Functional Approach to Working with Young Children* by T.W. Linder, Baltimore: Paul H. Brooks, 1990.

PROBLEMS

Self-Care
- The infant may have poor feeding skills and problems with reflux or other gastrointestinal problems.

Productivity and Leisure
- The infant may have poor play skills, such as making little effort to explore the world around him- or herself.

Sensorimotor
- Problems with the infant's motor skills may include delayed motor milestones; poor quality of movement; weak abdominal muscles; little dissociation between the lower extremities (inability to place legs in different positions) or legs mirroring each other, making asym-

metrical movements difficult; little trunk rotation; inability to control and grade movements to slow down or speed up; avoidance of upper-extremity weight bearing; walking on toes; posturing with one or both arms; refusing to use both arms at the same time.
- The infant's motor learning problems may include difficulty rising to stand from a half-kneel position and difficulty imitating tongue movements.
- The infant's postural control problems may include difficulty with body position in space while stepping on marked spots on the floor, difficulty with dynamic balance while walking a straight line, abnormal muscle tone, and "fixing" of shoulders to maintain postural control.
- The person may have difficulty with accuracy of hand movement on paper such as vertical writing.
- The person may have difficulty identifying which finger was touched when vision is occluded (finger localization), may have trouble matching an object placed in the hand with vision occluded (stereognosis), or may have an over- or underactive sense of touch.
- Tremors may be present, especially in the upper extremities and jaw.
- The person may be self-stimulating and become self-abusive.

Cognitive
- The infant may have a short attention span.
- The infant may be easily distracted.
- The person may have poor generalization of learning.

Psychosocial
- The infant may have a low frustration level.
- The infant may have difficulty calming him- or herself.
- The infant may have poor social skills.

Environment
- The infant may be defensive in response to being handled, leading the caregiver to assume that the neonate or infant does not like the caregiver.

TREATMENT/INTERVENTION

Treatment approaches involving normal growth and development, neurodevelopment treatment and sensory integration are the most widely used. Cultural differences in infant care and child rearing should be considered when working with caregivers (Jackson 1994).

Self-Care
Feeding
- Helping the infant to gain weight is often a major goal. Drug-exposed neonates do not breastfeed well, and, depending on the mother's response to the infant, may not have the option.
- It is best to hold the infant at a 45-degree angle for feeding.
- Massaging the cheeks may increase lip closure and decrease loss of milk. Rub the soft part of the infant's cheeks in a circular pattern.

- For older infants, gently stroke the back of gums forward to the center seam to encourage a more normal and efficient suck.
- Use a hard preemie nipple with a small hole initially.
- Encourage the infant to hold onto the bottle. A cloth cover or tube sock on the bottle can increase tactile input.
- Hold the infant upright on your lap when burping him or her. Exert slight pressure on the abdomen and up the infant's back. Alternate position is prone on a 45-degree wedge. Do not do heavy pats on the back, which can lead to spitting up and vomiting.
- Feed the infant small amounts of food frequently on a demand schedule until desired weight is obtained, at which time a set schedule can be established.

Dressing
- Use all-cotton clothing. It absorbs perspiration well and allows the body to regulate its own temperature. Also, it can be bleached easily.
- Use cotton diapers because they "breathe" and are less likely to cause skin rashes, a frequent problem with drug-exposed infants.
- Use long gowns with drawstrings or booties to keep feet warm because temperature regulation is a common problem in drug-exposed infants.
- Use loose-fitting garments. Do not use tight-fitting garments because infants become frantic when anything restricts them.

Productivity and Leisure
- Play games with infants to improve their development. Simple games include touching and imitating games such as sticking out the tongue or opening the mouth wide, singing, or rhythmic touching. Avoid sudden movement or light touch.
- With older infants, play peek-a-boo, or hide a toy under a washcloth.

Sensorimotor
Sensory Stimulation
- Stimulate only one sensory system at a time. For instance, limit as much as possible motion, sound, or light touch while stimulating vision.
- Start with the tactile system because it is highly developed at birth and many drug-exposed infants are tactilely defensive.
- Stimulation to the vestibular system must be approached carefully because of the direct connections of the vestibular system to stomach innervation, which may cause stomach upsets and regurgitation. When using steady movement (vestibular input), monitor eyes for signs of nystagmus (rapid, rhythmical movements of the eyes, which show the infant is dizzy).

Sensory Dampening (Calming)
- Calming techniques should simulate the womb environment: dark, quiet, confining, with gentle movement.
- Consider effective methods for reducing noise and light whenever possible because of the high incidence of hypersensitivity in drug-exposed infants. A blanket placed over the incubator or crib can muffle sound and reduce the light in a nursery or at home.

- Provide a small pacifier that is soft and pliable and all one piece. Drug-exposed neonates tend to suck frantically and can quickly cause the rubber nipple to detach from the plastic mounting. The nipple may become lodged in the trachea, causing anoxia.
- Keep the neonate swaddled as much of the time as possible. Hold the hand near the face to encourage self-calming by hand sucking.
- Hold the infant firmly, putting deep pressure into the joints and muscles, with as much body contact as possible to facilitate calming.
  1. Football hold (anterior-posterior position). Hold the neonate or infant prone, with your hand and arm under the length of the stomach and chest. Spread your fingers to support the head, and hold the infant as close to your body as possible with the neonate's left or right side pressed against your stomach and chest. Your other hand can provide firm pressure to the infant's back.
  2. Vertical hold. For neonates who spit up, place the neonate against your chest with both hands, providing deep proprioceptive input all down the back and buttocks. Shifting your weight from side to side in a gentle rocking motion may be helpful.
- When the neonate or infant starts to cry, try to respond quickly. Drug-exposed neonates become inconsolable and frantic in a very short time and will continue to cry until they vomit or collapse into a deep sleep. They also start to cry if any other child is crying. Prompt soothing is important.
- A warm bath may be calming, but the dressing and undressing may negate the calming effects unless they are done slowly and deliberately.
- Oil massages may be helpful if done using deep proprioceptive input and constant contact with the skin. Avoid the palms or the soles of the feet. Keep the neonate warm by using a radiator, register, or other source of heat.
- Vocal or instrumental music from a tape recorder or CD player may be helpful if it is soft and repetitive.
- Mechanical simulators that provide vibration and sounds similar to those in the womb may have a calming effect.

Musculoskeletal

- Use normal patterns of movement to try to elicit normal responses.
- At 12 weeks, infants voluntarily feel one hand with the other. At 16 weeks, they touch their hands to their knees. At 19 weeks, they touch hands to feet. Then they bring their feet to their mouths. Facilitating these movement patterns can be a satisfying game to caregiver and infant.
- Work on weight shifting, trunk rotation, dissociation between lower extremities, transitional movements, and upper extremity weight bearing.

Visual Perception

- Visual stimulation is especially difficult for the neonate to handle. As a result, the neonate often keeps the eyes closed. Keep lights low.
- At the beginning, use high-contrast objects such as a white paper plate with black circles made with a magic marker. Hold the plate 7 to 8 inches from the neonate's face.
- Other large objects that reflect light, such as a foil balloon or foil-covered paper plate, are attractive to neonates.

- Start with peripheral vision, which is relatively well developed in neonates. Begin at about a 45-degree angle from the face with a moving stimulus. Move the item toward the midline, or from ear to nose. Sequence moving is slow movement from left to right, and back again, movement in an arc, movement in a circle, and finally movement on the diagonal.
- Use vision only at the beginning, then add touch or vestibular, which can help integrate vision.

Psychosocial
- The neonate needs to be in a quiet and alert state to begin seeing and interacting with others. Such a state is difficult to achieve for more than a short time but should be encouraged.

Environment
- Provide or participate in a program of caregiver education.
- Help all caregivers to use calming techniques to reduce and avoid frustration, hostility, and abuse toward the infant and feelings that the infant is rejecting the caregiver.
- Adapt high chairs, strollers, car seats, and tables and chairs so the infant can have appropriate seating for optimum functioning. In seating, hips and knees should be flexed at greater than 90 degrees.
- Increase caregivers' sense that they will be able to meet the infant's needs.

PRECAUTIONS
- Always watch for signs of neonate or infant distress from overstimulation such as yawns, hiccups, sneezes, grimaces, changes in skin color, changes in respiration, and eye aversion or tightly closed eyes. Discontinue stimulation techniques and begin using calming techniques.
- Always monitor the eyes for signs of nystagmus, which indicates dizziness when using vestibular input.
- Have changes of clothing available for both the neonate or infant and caregiver because of incidences of regurgitation, diarrhea, and perspiration.
- Try to avoid any treatment that upsets the neonate's or infant's stomach. Many infants need to gain weight, and an upset stomach often leads to regurgitation, causing loss of calories.
- Loud, stimulating music is contraindicated and should be avoided, if possible.
- When using oral stimulation, be aware that some neonates or infants may be HIV-positive. Use gloves.

PROGNOSIS AND OUTCOME
- With early intervention, the person may be able to function within normal range between ages 2 and 18 depending on severity of symptoms.

REFERENCES

Beers, M.H., and R. Berkow, eds. 1999. The Merck Manual of Diagnosis and Therapy, 17th ed. Whitehouse Station, NJ: Merck Research Laboratories.

Jackson, S.J. 1994. Theoretical approaches to treatment. In *Working with substance-exposed children: Strategies for professionals,* ed. C.H. Puttkammer, 57–61. Tucson, AZ: Therapy Skill Builders.

BIBLIOGRAPHY

Fulks, M.L. 1995. Children exposed to drugs in utero: Their scores on the Miller Assessment for Preschoolers. *Canadian Journal of Occupational Therapy* 62, no. 1: 7–15.
Lange, R.L. 1994. Occupational therapy with substance-exposed toddlers and preschool children. In *Working with substance-exposed children: Strategies for professionals,* ed. C.H. Puttkammer, 73–82. Tucson, AZ: Therapy Skill Builders.
Murphy, J. 1995. Infants who have been drug exposed aided with therapy. *Advance for Occupational Therapists* 11, no. 36: 11.
Puttkammer, C.H. 1994. Emotional concerns. In *Working with substance-exposed children: Strategies for professionals,* ed. C.H. Puttkammer, 19–24. Tucson, AZ: Therapy Skill Builders.
Puttkammer, C.H. 1994. Intervention techniques with substance-exposed infants. In *Working with substance-exposed children: Strategies for professionals,* ed. C.H. Puttkammer, 63–72. Tucson, AZ: Therapy Skill Builders.
Puttkammer, C.H. 1994. Toys for special infants. In *Working with substance-exposed children: Strategies for professionals,* ed. C.H. Puttkammer, 185–188. Tucson, AZ: Therapy Skill Builders.
Sherman, I. 1994. Early intervention and drug-exposed infants: A case study. In *Working with substance-exposed children: Strategies for professionals,* ed. C.H. Puttkammer, 175–178. Tucson, AZ: Therapy Skill Builders.
Stewart, K.B. et al. 1996. Clinical considerations in the assessment of infants and young children affected by parental substance abuse. *Physical and Occupational Therapy in Pediatrics* 16: 51–72.

Regulatory Disorders

DESCRIPTION

Regulatory disorders involve difficulties in regulating physiologic, sensory, attention, motor, or affective processes and in organizing a calm, alert, or affectively positive state. In addition to the behavior symptoms, there must be at least one sensory, sensory-motor, or processing difficulty that is observed. There are three major types of regulatory disorders: hypersensitive with either fearful and cautious or negative and defiant behavior; underreactive with either withdrawn and difficult to engage or self-absorbed behavior; and motorically disorganized with impulsive behavior. A fourth type involves children who have motor or sensory processing difficulty but do not appear to have a behavior symptom (Diagnostic Classification of Mental Health and Developmental Disorders in Infancy and Early Childhood 1994).

CAUSE

Evidence suggests that constitutional and early maturational patterns contribute to the difficulties in regulatory disorders, but it is also recognized that early caregiving patterns can

---

Characteristic Behavioral Patterns in Regulatory Disorders

- physiological or state repertoire (e.g., irritable, startles, hiccups, gags)
- gross motor activity (e.g., motor disorganization, jerky movements, constant movement)
- fine motor activity (e.g., poorly differentiated or sparse, jerky, or limp movements)
- attentional organization (e.g., "driven" behavior, inability to settle down, or, conversely, perseveration about a small detail)
- affective organization, including the predominant affective tone (e.g., sober, depressed, or happy); the range of affect (e.g., broad or constricted); and the degree of modulation expressed (e.g., infant shifts abruptly from being completely calm to screaming frantically) and the capacity to use and organize affect as a part of relationships and interaction with others (e.g., avoidant, negativistic, clinging and demanding behavior patterns)
- behavioral organization (e.g., aggressive or impulsive behavior)
- sleep, eating, or elimination patterns
- language (receptive and expressive) and cognitive difficulties

Source: Reprinted with permission from *Diagnostic Classification: 0–3: Diagnostic Classification of Mental Health and Developmental Disorders of Infancy and Early Childhood*, Copyright © 1994, Washington, DC. ZERO to THREE/National Center for Clinical Infant Programs.

---

influence how the constitutional and maturational patterns develop and become part of the person's evolving personality. Prematurity is a risk factor because it can contribute to problems in maturation. More males than females are affected.

ASSESSMENT

Areas
- productivity: response to play situations such as existence of stereotypical play behaviors, amount of reciprocal interaction, amount of symbolic play, amount of exploratory play
- self-regulation: level of irritability, ability to self-calm, activity level, sleep cycle, feeding and eating habits, temperament
- postural and motor maturity: muscle tone (hyper- or hypotonicity), gross and fine motor skills, motor planning and praxis skills, coordination, balance and postural control
- processing of sensory input
  1. auditory stimuli—hyper- or underresponsive
  2. visual stimuli—hyper- or underresponsive
  3. tactile or touch stimuli—hyper- or underresponsive
  4. pain stimuli—hyper- or underresponsive
  5. vestibular stimuli—hyper- or underresponsive

6. oral stimulation—hyperresponsive
7. oral-motor coordination
8. visual spatial processing skills
9. auditory and verbal processing skills

- sensory processing to movement: hypersensitive to or fear of movement in space, gravitational insecurity
- cognitive processing: attention span, concentration and focus skills, level of distractibility, termination or change of task
- psychosocial: level of frustration tolerance, ability to separate from caregivers, ability to tolerate limits set by adults, aggressive behavior, behavioral control
- environmental: tolerance to changes in the environment, level of adaptability

Instruments

Instruments Developed by Occupational Therapy Personnel

- *Erhardt Developmental Prehension Assessment,* rev. by R. Erhardt, San Antonio, TX: Therapy Skill Builders, 1994.
- *Infant-Toddler Symptom Checklist* by G.A. DeGangi et al., San Antonio, TX: Therapy Skill Builders, 1995.
- *Test of Attention in Infants* by G.A. DeGangi, Dayton, OH: Southpaw Enterprises, 1995.
- *Test of Sensory Functions in Infants* (TSFI) by G.A. DeGangi and S.I. Greenspan, Los Angeles: Western Psychological Services, 1989.

Assessments Developed by Other Professionals and Used by Occupational Therapy Personnel

- *Bates' Infant Characteristics Questionnaire* by J.E. Bates, San Antonio, TX: The Psychological Corporation, 1984.
- *Bayley Scales of Infant Development-II* (BSID-II) by N. Bayley, San Antonio, TX: The Psychological Corporation, 1993.
- *Child Behavior Checklist* by T.M. Achenbach, Burlington, VT: University of Vermont, 1989.
- *Dimensions of Temperament Scale, Revised* (DOTS-R) by M. Windle and R.M. Lerner, in Reassessing the dimensions of temperamental individuality across the life span: The revised dimensions of temperament survey (DOTS-R), *Journal of Adolescent Research* 1, no. 2 (1986): 213–230.
- *Parenting Stress Index* by R.R. Abidin, Charlottesville, VA: Pediatric Psychology Press, 1986.

PROBLEMS

Self-Care

- The child often has poor eating skills.

Productivity and Leisure

- The child may have poor play skills, including no reciprocal interactions during play, lack of symbolic play, lack of exploratory behavior during play.

**Signs of Defensive/Disorganized/Unstable and Approachable/
Organized/Stable Behavior in Infants**

System	Defensive	Approachable
Autonomic	Irregular respiration	Regular respiration
	Pauses or holds breath	Continuous breathing
	Tachypnea or gasping	Normal breathing rate
	Skin color changes: pale, mottled, flushed, grey, or cyanotic	Good, stable color
	Tremors, twitching	No or minimal tremulousness
	Seizures	No seizure activity
	Visceral signs: gagging, hiccupping, straining, spitting up, sneezing, and yawning	No or minimal visceral signs
Motor	Flaccidity	Well-regulated tone
	Hypotonicity in extension: fingers/toes splaying, saluting (arms extended), airplane position, high-guard with hands, sitting in air (legs extended), leg bracing, "scorpion" position, tongue protrusion, grimacing, squinting, "ape-like" face	Well-organized postures: hand clasp, hand to mouth, finger fold, grasping caregiver's finger, grasping pacifier, foot clasp, oral searching and sucking
	Hypotonicity in flexion:	
	Fetal tuck	Ability to assume flexion tuck
	Fisting of hands	Hands in midline
	Abrupt, jerky movements	Smooth movements
	General frantic activity and squirming movements	Organized movement
State organization	Diffuse sleep states	Robust sleep states
	Diffuse alert states:	Periods of quiet alertness:
	Gaze locking	Focused alertness
	Glassy "floating" eyes	Bright eyes
	Roving eye movements	
	Hyperalertness	
	Poor transitions or lability, abrupt state change	Smooth state transitions
	Cannot be consoled	Consolable by caregiver
Attention/ Interaction	Gaze aversion	Ability to attend visually and auditorily
	Visually staring	Prolonged attention

Source: Reprinted with permission from J. Case-Smith, *Pediatric Occupational Therapy and Early Intervention*, pp. 115 and 243, © 1993, Butterworth-Heineman.

Sensorimotor

• The child may have self-regulatory problems, including irritability, inability to calm self, frantic motor activity, disturbed sleep cycles, difficulty with feeding.

- The child may have sensory processing problems.
  1. The child may exhibit over- or underreactivity to loud or high- or low-pitched noises.
  2. The child may exhibit over- or underreactivity to bright lights or new and striking visual images.
  3. The child may exhibit tactile defensiveness.
  4. The child may exhibit oral hypersensitivity.
  5. The child may have oral-motor difficulties or incoordination influenced by poor muscle tone and oral tactile hypersensitivity.
  6. The child may exhibit underreactivity to touch or pain.
  7. The child may exhibit gravitational insecurity.
  8. The child may exhibit under- or overreactivity to odors.
  9. The child may exhibit under- or overreactivity to temperature.
- The child may have postural and motor control difficulties.
  1. The child may exhibit poor muscle tone and muscle stability.
  2. The child may have deficits in motor planning skills.
  3. The child may have deficits in the ability to modulate motor activity.
  4. The child may have deficits in fine motor skills.
  5. The child may have deficits in visual spatial processing capacities.

Cognitive

- The child often have deficits in the capacity to attend and focus.
- The child may have difficulty initiating a new activity or terminating an existing activity.
- The child may have deficits in auditory and verbal processing.
- The child may have deficits in articulation capacity—disarticulation.

Psychosocial

- The child may be fearful of new or strange situations.
- The child may be cautious in interactions with others.
- The child may be negativistic and/or defiant.
- The child may have tantrums.
- The child may be withdrawn and avoid some situations.
- The child may show signs of depression.
- The child may be self-absorbed.
- The child may be impulsive.
- The child may show affective lability.

Environment

- The child may be destructive of property.
- The child may have difficulty making transitions.
- Caregivers may view the child as demanding, moody, distractible, nonadaptable, and unresponsive.
- Caregivers may lack parenting and caregiving skills, have health problems such as malnutrition, be dependent on substances, lack social support, be depressed, have difficulties with being a single parent or caregiver, or be overcontrolling in interactions with the person.

TREATMENT/INTERVENTION

Sensory integration techniques and ego psychology based on Greenspan (1989) have been reported. For instructions to caregivers, behavioral management, supportive counseling, practical management techniques, and developmental therapy have been used.

Self-Care
- Help caregiver to establish a regular feeding schedule that is based on calming the hyperreactive child before feeding begins.
- Recommend all-cotton clothing if defensive behaviors occur during dressing.

Productivity and Leisure
- Use play activities to address irritability, sensory hypersensitivities, and inattention.
- Improve ability to experience the sense of touch and handle textured toys.
- Assist in development of symbolic and vestibular play activities using linear movement, bouncing, and swinging.

Sensorimotor
- Promote development of self-regulation.
  1. Teach techniques to modulate physiologic states, including sleep and waking cycles, hunger and satiety.
  2. Teach techniques to promote self-calming activities and modulation of arousal states through selected sensory input.
  3. Teach mastery of sensory functions through
     - reducing tactile defensive behaviors
     - providing and promoting vestibular activities to increase response to movement
     - increasing sense of gravitational security during movements off the ground
     - increasing motor planning skills
     - improving bilateral interaction of two sides of body
     - improving postural control
- Facilitate attainment of developmental milestones.
- Facilitate development of perceptual motor skills.

Cognitive
- Increase attention span through organized, purposeful activity.
- Increase skills in self-directed activities.

Psychosocial
- Increase opportunities for engagement with objects and persons.
- Provide consistent communication and signaling in verbal and gestural interactions.

Environment
- Instruct caregivers in play activities designed to address specific problems of the person.
- Provide a role model to caregivers for methods of handling and playing with the person.
- Help caregivers to interpret the person's communication—verbal and behavioral.

• Instruct caregivers on methods to improve interaction between caregiver and child by focusing on synchrony, pace, and time of interactions.

PRECAUTIONS
• The response of the person to intervention should be monitored closely. An infant or child with a regulatory disorder is easily overstimulated and may be very difficult to calm down after such stimulation.
• Watch for signs of hyperarousal: behaving in a disorganized manner, averting the gaze, being easily distracted, being wide-eyed, being emotionally labile.
• Be aware that the caregiver may also be overwhelmed and need as much therapy as the person.
• Be sure that medical problems such as allergies or food intolerances have been identified.

PROGNOSIS AND OUTCOME
Regulatory disorders involve a complex of diagnostic problems. Prognosis and outcome depend on the number and type of problems and the response to intervention.
• The person is able to calm him- or herself to go to sleep.
• The person is able to self-console after experiencing an emotionally difficult situation.
• The person is able to perform daily living tasks independently at developmental age.
• The person is able to play with objects and peers using skills appropriate for developmental age.
• The person is able to attend preschool or elementary school in regular classroom.
• The person demonstrates less hyper- or hyposensitivity to sensory input.
• The person is attaining developmental milestones at appropriate ages.
• The person is able to use cognitive skills to learn new skills.
• The person is able to interact with others using age-appropriate skills.
• Parents or caregivers are able to manage the person's behavioral problems to their satisfaction.
• Parents or caregivers demonstrate reduced stress in parenting or caregiving tasks.

REFERENCES
Diagnostic Classification of Mental Health and Developmental Disorders in Infancy and Early Childhood. 1994. Washington, DC: Zero to Three.
Greenspan, S.I. 1989. *Development of the Ego.* New York: International University Press.

BIBLIOGRAPHY
DeGangi, G.A. 1991. Assessment of sensory, emotional, and attentional problems in regulatory disordered infants. *Infants and Young Children* 3, no. 3: 1–8.
DeGangi, G.A. et al. 1991. Psychophysiological characteristics of the regulatory disordered infant. *Infant Behavior and Development* 14: 37–50.
DeGangi, G.A. et al. 1991. Treatment of sensory, emotional, and attentional problems in regulatory disordered infants. *Infants and Young Children* 3, no. 3: 9–19.

DeGangi, G.A. et al. 1993. Four-year follow-up of a sample of regulatory disordered infants. *Infant Mental Health Journal* 14, no. 4: 330–343.

DeGangi, G.A. et al. 1996. Fussy babies: To treat or not to treat. *British Journal of Occupational Therapy* 59, no. 10: 457–464.

DeGangi, G.A. et al. 1997. Mother-infant interactions in infants with disorders of self-regulation. *Physical and Occupational Therapy in Pediatrics* 17, no. 1: 17–44.

Wiener, A.S. et al. 1996. Sensory processing of infants born prematurely or with regulatory disorders. *Physical and Occupational Therapy in Pediatrics* 16, no. 4: 1–17.

Williamson, G.G., and G. White-Tennant. 1997. Regulatory disorders: Type I: Hypersensitive. In *DC:0–3 Casebook: A guide to the use of Zero to Three's "Diagnostic classification of mental health and developmental disorders of infancy and early childhood" in assessment and treatment planning*, eds. A. Lieberman et al., 219–232. Washington, DC: Zero to Three: National Center for Infants, Toddlers, and Families.

Rett's Disorder

DESCRIPTION

Rett's disorder, also called Rett syndrome or Rett's syndrome, is a neurodegenerative disorder characterized by progressive loss of intellectual function, loss of fine and gross motor skills, and development of stereotypic hand movement. The disorder was named for Dr. Andreas Rett, who reported the syndrome in 1966 in Austria. It was recognized in the United States in 1983 when the research was reported in English. Rett's disorder is sometimes confused with autism.

According to the DSM-IV, Rett's disorder is classified as a pervasive developmental disorder. The essential feature of Rett's disorder is the development of multiple specific deficits following a period of normal functioning after birth. Individuals appear to have a normal prenatal period with normal psychomotor development through the first five months of life. Head circumference at birth is within normal limits, but between ages 5 months and 48 months, head growth decelerates. There is a loss of previously acquired purposeful hand skills between ages 5 months and 30 months, with subsequent development of characteristic stereotyped hand movements resembling hand-wringing or hand washing. Interest in the social environment diminishes during the first few years after onset but may develop later. Problems in coordination of gait or trunk movements are noted. There is also severe impairment of expressive and receptive language development, with severe psychomotor retardation (American Psychiatric Association, 71).

CAUSE

While the exact cause of Rett's disorder is unknown, the disorder may be a hereditary X-linked disorder of females caused by an inborn error in metabolism. Onset usually occurs between 6 months and 18 months. The course of the disorder alternates between periods of progression and periods of rapid decline. Death occurs usually between ages 20 and 30.

ASSESSMENT

Areas
- daily living skills
- play skills
- hand functions
- fine motor skills: manipulative, dexterity, and bilateral coordination
- praxis and motor planning
- stereotypic movement or motions
- reflex maturation and development
- attending behavior and concentration
- mood and affect
- communication skills

Instruments
No instruments were identified as developed by occupational therapy personnel in the literature. However, some other instruments may be useful:
- *Peabody Developmental Motor Scales* (PDMS) by M.R. Folio and R.R. Fewell, Austin, TX: Pro-ed, 1983.
- reflex development test
- activities of daily living scale
- play history

PROBLEMS

Self-Care
- The person may have progressive loss of the ability to perform activities of daily living that depend on fine motor hand skills, such as feeding and dressing.

Productivity
- The person usually loses play skills due to loss of hand skills, trunk balance, and gait skills.

Leisure
- The person may be unable to continue leisure interests that depend on mobility, cognitive functioning, or fine motor skills.

Sensorimotor
- The person usually has spasticity present in respiratory muscles, in swallowing, and in the leg flexors, which leads to toe walking.
- The person usually has a progressive loss of purposeful, fine motor hand skills.
- The person may have gait ataxia, which may result in loss of ambulation skills. Early signs include wide-based gait and locking of joints, such as knees in hyperextension and ankles in pronation.

- The person may have ataxia and apraxia of the trunk muscles, which may lead to loss of gross motor skills.
- The person may have a spinal deformity, and scoliosis may be present.
- The person may hyperventilate and hold breath.
- The person usually has stereotypical hand-wringing, hand washing, hand biting, hand sucking or licking, and stretching and flexing the middle finger joints.
- The person may exhibit bruxism, or grinding of the teeth.
- The person may have seizures.
- The person may have contractures that are related to spasticity, especially in distal joints.
- The person may have loss of balance and equilibrium reactions.

Cognitive
- The person usually has progressive loss of intellectual functions.
- The person may have decreased awareness of the environment.

Psychosocial
- The person may be irritable.
- The person may lose contact with the environment, similar to autistic withdrawal.
- The person may have impaired expressive and receptive language.

TREATMENT/INTERVENTION
Treatment approaches are not well identified.

Self-Care
- Increase purposeful hand-to-mouth activities to help the person feed him- or herself. Behavior modification techniques may be useful to facilitate achieving this objective.
- Promote better swallowing by decreasing tone and improving positioning.
- Increase ability to perform other self-care activities, such as dressing, brushing teeth and hair, and bathing.

Productivity
- Promote play skills to support hand skills and encourage interpersonal relationships.

Leisure
- Develop the person's leisure interests.

Sensorimotor
- Assist the person in developing and maintaining ambulation skills by encouraging weight-bearing activities in the upper extremities.
- Consider splinting joints to maintain functional position, such as knee splints to reduce hyperextension and hand splints to decrease wrist flexion and hand-to-mouth stereotypical movements. (Note: Stereotypical hand movements are not learned behavior and do not respond to behavior therapy; the problem is neurologic.)
- Normalize or decrease hypertonicity (spasticity) through positioning, aquatic therapy, and vibration.

- Promote good positioning in seating (strollers, wheelchairs, regular chairs) to decrease tendency toward scoliosis.
- Increase or maintain the person's equilibrium and protective reactions through activities that require changing body position, such as the use of vestibular boards.

Cognitive
- Increase the level of awareness through use of visual and auditory stimulation, such as brightly colored or battery-operated musical toys.

Psychosocial
- Relaxation techniques and sensory desensitization may be helpful in reducing irritability.
- Promote verbal communication.
- Encourage socialization and interaction. (Note: Lack of eye gaze is not intentional aversion but part of the basic neurologic disorder.)
- Act as an empathic listener, source of information, and referral source for the family.

PRECAUTION
- Do not promise more than can be delivered. Be realistic about the outcome.

PROGNOSIS AND OUTCOME
The prognosis is generally poor, and the outcome is death. Therapy is focused on slowing the decline, maintaining function as long as possible, and enhancing the quality of life.
- The person demonstrates increased hand function.
- The person demonstrates decreased stereotypical hand movements or motions.
- The person increases self-care skills, such as feeding.

REFERENCE
American Psychiatric Association. 1994. *Diagnostic and Statistical Manual of Mental Disroders: DSM-IV*, 4th ed. Washington, DC: American Psychiatric Assocation. Task Force on DSM-IV.

BIBLIOGRAPHY
Bat-Haee, M.A. 1994. Behavioral training of a young woman with Rett syndrome. *Perceptual and Motor Skills* 78, no. 1: 314.
Diffendal, J. 1998. Women with Rett syndrome: Don't discount them. *Advance for Occupational Therapy Practitioners* 14, no. 32: 36, 66.
Klein, M.D., and T.A. Delaney. 1994. Conditions affecting feeding and nutrition—Rett syndrome. In *Feeding and nutrition for children with special needs: Handouts for parents*, eds. M.D. Klein and T.A. Delaney, 443–444. Tucson, AZ: Therapy Skill Builders.
Kosnosky, G. 1995. A case report on Rett's syndrome. *Advance for Occupational Therapists* 11, no. 14: 16.
Porr, S.M. 1999. The psychological system—Rett's syndrome: The clinical picture. In *Pediatric therapy: A systems approach*, eds. S.M. Porr and E.B. Rainsville, 296–297. Philadelphia: F.A. Davis.

Tomcheck, S.D. 1999. The nervous system—Rett's syndrome. In *Pediatric therapy: A systems approach*, eds. S.M. Porr and E.B. Rainsville, 197–199. Philadelphia: F.A. Davis.

Spina Bifida

DESCRIPTION

Spina bifida is defective closure of the vertebral column. It is one of the most serious neural tube defects compatible with prolonged life. Varieties range from the occult (closed) type with no neurologic findings to a completely open spine (rachischisis) with severe neurologic disabilities. Problems with closed defects include compression of the spinal cord and stretched spinal cord (ethered cord). In spina bifida cystica or operata (open), the protruding sac can contain meninges (meningocele), spinal cord (myelocele), or both (myelomeningocele).

When the spinal cord or lumbosacral nerve roots are involved, varying degrees of paralysis occur below the involved level. Since the paralysis occurs in the fetus, orthopaedic problems can present at birth, such as hydrocephalus, clubfoot, arthrogryposis, or dislocated hip. The paralysis usually affects bladder and renal functions (Merck 1999, 2224; Tomchek 1999, 184–185).

CAUSE

What causes the neural tube to not close properly during fetal development is unknown, although lack of folic acid is suspected in about 50 percent of cases. Environmental and genetic influences may also be involved. Spina bifida occurs during the first month of embryonic life, when the central nervous system is forming. At the end of the first month, the embryo becomes a flat layer of cells or plate. The plate then begins to roll up and form a tube. One end of the tube becomes the brain and the other the spinal cord. The tube should close up completely. If the tube fails to close, an opening occurs called a neural tube defect. Usually the defect occurs in the lumbar, low thoracic, or sacral region of the spine and extends three to six vertebral segments.

The incidence of spina bifida is about 1 in 1,000 in the United States but is greater in Ireland. Boys are more frequently affected than girls. A shunt (plastic tube) may be inserted in the ventricle(s) of the brain to drain excess fluid to the kidneys, thereby reducing hydrocephalus.

ASSESSMENT

Areas

- daily living skills
- academic skills, handwriting
- play and work skills

- leisure skills
- level of lesion or sac
- physical abnormalities: head size, brainstem, chest, and hips
- motor skills: muscle strength, especially antigravity postures and movements; active and passive range of motion; gross motor development and skills; mobility (with and without aids and equipment)
- reflex maturation development—presence of primitive reflexes or abnormal movements
- postural control: proximal and distal muscle tone, protective and equilibrium reactions, midline stability and orientation, and symmetrical and asymmetrical movement
- coordination: visual motor, bilateral, and reciprocal
- fine motor hand skills: grasp and release, dexterity, and manipulation
- ocular motor control, including tracking and scanning
- physical endurance and work tolerance
- motor planning (praxis)
- sensory processing (awareness and orientating behavior)
- sensory sensitivity and modulation
  1. tactile: level of sensation, light touch, pressure, temperature, vibration, and two-point discrimination
  2. vestibular: linear (vertical and horizontal) and angular
  3. proprioceptive
  4. visual: acuity, peripheral vision, color vision
  5. auditory: localization, discrimination, identification
- sensory discrimination and perceptual skills
  1. visual: form constancy, position in space, visual closure, figure-ground, depth perception, part-whole discrimination, object permanence
  2. auditory
  3. tactile: stereognosis, graphesthesia
  4. kinesthesia
  5. body scheme: laterality, directionality, right-left discrimination
- attending behavior: attention span or concentration
- memory skills
- self-perception
- social conduct skills

Instruments

Instruments Developed by Occupational Therapy Personnel

- *Miller Assessment for Preschoolers* (MAP) by L.J. Miller, San Antonio, TX: The Psychological Corporation, 1988. (Motor skills, 2.9 years to 5.8 years)
- *Movement Assessment of Infants* (MAI) by L.S. Chandler, M.S. Andrews, and M.W. Swanson, Rolling Bay, WA: Infant Movement Research, 1980.
- *School Assessment of Motor and Process Skills* (SAMPS) by A. Fisher, K. Bryze, and L. Magalhaes, Fort Collins, CO: Occupational Therapy Department, Colorado State University, 1998.
- *Toddler and Infant Motor Evaluation* (TIME) by L.J. Miller and G.H. Roid, San Antonio, TX: Therapy Skill Builders, 1994. (Motor skills, birth to 3.5 years)

Instruments Developed by Other Professionals and Used by Occupational Therapy Personnel

- *Battelle Developmental Inventory* by J. Newborg et al., Itasca, IL: Riverside Publishing Co., 1984.
- *The Beery-Buktenica Developmental Test of Visual-Motor Integration* (VMI-4), 4th ed. by K.E. Beery and N.A. Buktenica, Parsippany, NJ: Modern Curriculum Press, 1997. (Visual-motor integration, 3 years to 18 years)
- *Bruininks-Oseretsky Test of Motor Proficiency* (BOTMP) by R. Bruininks, Circle Pines, MN: American Guidance Services, 1978. (Motor skills, 4.5 years to 14.5 years)
- *Developmental Profile II* (DPII) by G.D. Alpren, T.J. Boll, and M.S. Shearer, Los Angeles: Western Psychological Services, 1984. (Self-care, independent living skills)
- *Motor-Free Visual Perception Test—Revised* (MVPT-R) by R. Colarusso and D.D. Hamill, Novato, CA: Academic Therapy Publications, 1995. (Visual perception, 4 years to 11 years)
- *Peabody Developmental Motor Scales* (PDMS) by M.R. Folio and R.R. Fewell, Austin, TX: Pro-ed, 1983. (Motor skills)
- *Test of Visual-Motor Skills—Revised* (TVMS-R) by M.F. Gardner, Hydesville, CA: Psychological and Educational Publications, 1995. (Visual-motor integration, 3 years to 3 years, 11 months.)
- *Test of Visual-Perceptual Skills—Revised* (TVPS-R) by M.F. Gardner, Hydesville, CA: Psychological and Educational Publications, 1996. (Visual perception, 4 years to 12 years, 11 months.)
- *Vineland Behavioral Scales* (VBS) by S.S. Sparrow, D.A. Balla, and D.V. Cicchetti, Circle Pines, MN: American Guidance Services, 1982. (Self-care, independent living skills)
- *Wee Functional Independence Measure* (WeeFIM) by Uniform Data Systems, Buffalo, NY: Uniform Data Systems, 1993. (Self-care, independent living skills)

PROBLEMS

Self-Care

- The person may have incomplete bowel and bladder control.
- The person's performance in some activities of daily living may be limited due to limited range of motion, instability of the trunk, difficulty learning how to do the task, difficulty with visual perception, or difficulty with fine motor skills.
- The person may have difficulty performing self-care skills independently.

Productivity

- The person may have poorly developed play skills.
- The person may be behind in academic skills, including handwriting, spelling, arithmetic, and reading. Timed tests are often difficult because of sensorimotor impairments.
- The person may not contribute to independent living and home management within the family or living unit.
- As an adolescent or adult, the person may have few, if any, work skills or identified vocational interests.

Leisure
- The person may have few leisure interests or skills.

Sensorimotor
- At or above the lesion, muscle weakness may be present. The person may have paralysis below the involved level when spinal cord or lumbosacral nerve roots are involved.
- The person may have various physical abnormalities.
  1. The person may have hydrocephalus, which, if unarrested, increases the size of the head and may create problems in milestone development because the person cannot raise his or her head.
  2. The person may have Arnold-Chiari malformation, a defect in the formation of the brainstem.
  3. The person may have kyphosis, or posterior rounding of the thorax region.
  4. The person may have a dislocated hip or hips.
- The person may have low or abnormal muscle tone and muscle imbalance, which can lead to other deformities, including scoliosis, kyphosis, or both (kyphoscoliosis).
- The person may have a limited range of motion in the upper extremities. Limitations in the lower extremities may result from a dislocated hip.
- The person may have delays in attainment of obtainable gross motor skills, such as sitting.
- The person may have primitive reflexes that have not integrated and/or abnormal reflexes.
- The person may have poor postural control in the trunk with poor midline stability.
- The person may have poor coordination of the two sides of the body or of sensorimotor tasks, such as eye-hand coordination.
- The person may have delays in development of fine motor and hand skills, such as primitive grasp patterns and failure to develop hand dominance.
- The person may have low endurance and low physical tolerance.
- Mobility will be limited, although level of lesion is important in determining problems in mobility.
- The person may have poor ocular motor control due to strabismus or paralysis of gaze or fixation. Tracking (following a moving object), scanning (locating objects in the environment), and fixating may be performed poorly, especially at the midline.
- The person may have dyspraxia and poor motor planning skills.
- Sensations of touch, pressure, kinesthesia and temperature, and proprioception may be lost or impaired below the level of spinal cord or nerve root involvement.
- Perceptual problems may occur, especially in persons with unarrested or poorly arrested hydrocephalus.
  1. visual: visual discrimination (color, size, shape, position, sameness and difference), visual closure (part-whole), figure-ground, form constancy, depth perception, visual orientation in space
  2. auditory: localization, discrimination, identification
  3. proprioceptive: body scheme, right-left discrimination, spatial relationships
  4. tactile: stereognosis
  5. kinesthetic: position in space

- The person may be hyper- or hyporesponsive to stimuli, with such reactions as tactile defensiveness, auditory defensiveness, intolerance of movement, gravitational or postural insecurity, and inadequate bilateral integration.

Cognitive

- If hydrocephalus is arrested early, there are no complications from shunts, no seizures, no anoxia, and no central nervous system infections, then intelligence and cognitive functions may be normal. But if hydrocephalus is not arrested, or any of the other conditions have occurred, mental retardation and other cognitive disorders usually are present. (Note discrepancies between verbal and motor performance.)
- The person may have poor attending behavior.
- The person may have a short attention span and be easily distracted.
- The person may have deficits in short- and long-term memory.
- The person may have learning disabilities.

Psychosocial

- The person may have a poorly developed self-concept, including poor self-mastery.
- The person may have poor social control, including a poor sense of responsibility for actions.
- The person may have poor coping skills.
- The person may have poor dyadic skills.
- The person may have poor group interaction skills.
- The person may have limited responsibilities in the family or support group.
- The person may be hyperverbal (continuous talking; also called chatterbox personality or cocktail personality). He or she may use words fluently but have a limited fund of knowledge on subject matters. The level of conversation is shallow or superficial. The person changes topics if pressed for details. This may lead some team members to think the person is brighter than the level of measured intelligence indicates. Hyperverbal behavior may be related to auditory defensiveness (i.e., talking to avoid listening to unwanted sounds).

TREATMENT/INTERVENTION

Treatment is usually provided by a team of professionals and is habilitative, stressing the development of childhood and adolescent occupations. Treatment models in occupational therapy are based on developmental stages, sensory integration, and rehabilitation (compensation techniques).

Self-Care

- Alleviate or compensate for missing self-care skills due to paralysis and weakness.
- Provide step-by-step instruction to assist in the development of self-care skills. Use reminder charts and other multisensory learning aids to assist learning and memory.
- Provide adaptive devices to assist with bowel and bladder care.

- Provide adaptive methods and devices to perform other self-care tasks and activities of daily living that the person may be unable to perform without specific aids. Example: To compensate for lower extremity weakness, have the person use adaptive equipment for dressing such as reachers and long-handled shoehorns, adapt clothing by adding Velcro, and use elastic shoelaces. To compensate for bladder incontinence, have the person wear diapers to school or teach the person to self-catheter.

Productivity
- Provide a play situation designed to increase play skills for children.
- Facilitate motor development skills within limits of lesion through selected play activities.
- If sitting on the floor during play or group activities is a problem for the person, try using an air cushion or beanbag chair.
- Use computers and structured, repetitive learning. Step-by-step instruction may be helpful, and because the person does not have to write, he or she may respond more quickly to academic instruction.
- To compensate for decreased fine and visual-motor control, consider allowing more time for written work in school, de-emphasizing written work, and relying more on oral reports or computer keyboards.
- If walking is functional but slow, consider giving the person more time to move from class to class. Leaving a class early or arriving late may help, as might using a wheelchair when time is critical.
- Provide practice situations designed to increase skills in independent living and home management.
- Provide opportunities to develop work skills, work tolerance, work habits, and good attitudes in vocational activities.
- Alleviate or compensate for missing skills in home life, school, or work.

Leisure
- Help the person to explore and develop leisure interests. For instance, the person might enjoy belonging to a recreational club (e.g., Scouts, Camp Fire, 4-H).
- Help the person to participate in noncompetitive activities where decreased physical abilities will be less of a factor.

Sensorimotor
- Maintain or increase muscle strength in the person's weak or underused muscles, especially in the trunk and shoulder girdle, to increase stability and facilitate transfers.
- Maintain or improve positioning to prevent deformities and reduce incidence of decubiti.
- Promote integration of primitive reflexes and reduce the influence of abnormal reaction patterns.
- Promote development of gross motor skills through opportunities for frequent (high-dose) practice.
- Improve postural control and proximal stability to facilitate seating and positioning.
- Increase fine motor and perceptual motor skills in dexterity, manipulation, and coordination.

- Encourage development of hand skills through structured, repetitive practice using such activities as putting small objects in containers, stringing beads, pinching clothespins, buttoning, or using zipper boards.
- Maintain or improve endurance and physical tolerance through graded activities.
- Assist in increasing mobility through selective use of walkers, wheelchairs, or powered mobility equipment.
- Improve ocular motor skills through the use of toys with bright colors or auditory output in a light-controlled environment.
    1. Fixation of visual gaze: Place any of the following about 10 to 12 inches in front of the eyes: human face, pinwheels, spinning toys, finger puppets with penlight.
    2. Shifting of gaze: Use two toys or two penlights placed to the left and right, up and down, or in a diagonal.
    3. Tracking: Start at midline, moving to the left or right, up or down, or diagonally using battery-operated toys, hand or finger puppets, or a small ball in a clear plastic tube.
    4. Scanning: Try games of "find it" or 20 Questions for older children, pointing to items in a row, uncovering items in a sequence, sequence cards, or duplicating a colored bead or block pattern.
- Improve motor planning skills.
- Promote increased vestibular processing through tactile and proprioceptive inputs to the trunk and hips.
- Consider sensory integration techniques to improve interaction of sensory systems.
- Provide sensory stimulation to increase sensory awareness and discrimination within each sensory modality.

Cognitive
- Use visual memory devices, such as wall charts or posters, to outline steps of important tasks that need to be performed.
- Use multisensory instruction combining visual, tactile, and auditory elements for reinforcement. Structured learning using cuing and fading of instruction and reinforcement of successive approximations of desired performance may also be useful.
- Instruct the person in concepts of energy conservation and work simplification.
- Instruct the person in time management.

Psychosocial
- Provide therapeutic activities designed to increase self-confidence and mastery of the environment.
- Provide opportunities to increase the person's coping skills.
- Encourage development of dyadic skills.
- Provide opportunities to develop group interaction skills.
- Help the family or support group expand the individual's role in the family or group structure.
- Decrease feelings of depression and withdrawal by encouraging the person and family to participate in a spina bifida support group or recommend professional counseling.

Environment
- Assist caregivers in learning how to manage the shunt, use urinary catheter, clean scar area, and put on brace, splints, or casts correctly.
- Assist in teaching caregivers how to manage the person at home, including how to spot problems with shunts and skin tissue, check urinary catheter, check for infections at the site of the scar, and check splints for pressure areas.
- Provide information to classmates about the person's disability to decrease teasing.
- Provide assistive technology and adapted techniques that facilitate care of the person and teach caregivers how to use and maintain the technology.

PRECAUTIONS
- Watch for signs of a malfunctioning shunt, such as increased head size, or behavioral changes, such as increased irritability or fussiness, increased sleepiness or drowsiness, seizures, vomiting, headaches, or "setting sun" eyes (partially visible iris).
- Always maintain good skin care techniques. Check skin for pressure sores from sitting or from wearing a splint. Change the person's position frequently. Avoid tight-fitting clothing and shoes. Consider which seating devices serve the person best.
- If hip dislocation is present, use proper joint alignment techniques at all times.

PROGNOSIS AND OUTCOME
Prognosis and outcome depend in part on the level of lesion. A person with a sacral or low lumbar defect can walk with support (bracing) or an adaptive device such as a walker frame. A person with midlumbar or high-lumbar lesions may walk with braces or adaptive equipment. Another important factor is mental functioning. A person with normal intelligence is usually able to achieve a better outcome than one with mental retardation.
- The person is performing at his or her maximum level of independence in self-care and daily living management skills.
- When indicated, the person has developed work skills, work habits, and attitudes related to possible vocational choices.
- The person demonstrates sufficient strength and endurance to perform functional activities.
- The person demonstrates basic sensory-motor skills to facilitate perception and learning.
- The person demonstrates socially acceptable behavior patterns and participates in age-appropriate activities.
- The person demonstrates emotional and psychological skills necessary to cope with his or her living situation.

REFERENCES
Beers, M.H., and R. Berkow, eds. 1999. *The Merck Manual of Diagnosis and Therapy*, 17th ed. Whitehouse Station, NJ: Merck Research Laboratories.
Tomchek, S.D. 1999. The nervous system: Neural tube defects. In *Pediatric therapy: A systems approach*, eds. S.M. Porr and E.B. Rainville, 184–192. Philadelphia: F.A. Davis.

BIBLIOGRAPHY

Erhardt, R.P., and S.C. Merrill. 1998. Neurological dysfunction in children: Neural tube defects. In *Willard and Spackman's occupational therapy,* 9th ed., eds. M.E. Neistadt and E.B. Crepeau, 601–604. Philadelphia: J.B. Lippincott.

Grimby, G. et al. 1996. Structure of a combination of Functional Independence Measure and instrumental activity measure items in community-living persons: A study of individuals with cerebral palsy and spina bifida. *Archives of Physical Medicine and Rehabilitation* 77, no. 11: 1109–1114.

Latcha, C.M. et al. 1993. A comparison of the grip strength of children with myelomeningocele to that of children without disability. *American Journal of Occupational Therapy* 47, no. 6: 498–503.

Scoggin, A.E., and K.M. Parks. 1997. Latex sensitivity in children with spina bifida: Implications for occupational therapy practitioners (review). *American Journal of Occupational Therapy* 51, no. 7: 608–611.

Unruh, A.M. et al. 1993. Parents' and therapists' ratings of self-care skills in children with spina bifida. *Canadian Journal of Occupational Therapy* 60, no. 3: 145–148.

Sensory Integrative Dysfunction—General

DESCRIPTION

Sensory integration is the ability to synthesize, organize, and process sensory information received from the body and the environment to produce purposeful goal-directed responses (Arkwright 1998, 1). Sensory integrative dysfunction is a developmental disorder in which the person has difficulty with the processing of sensory input. There are several types of sensory integrative dysfunction problems, and there are several systems used to classify those problems. For the purposes of this handbook, the various types of sensory integrative dysfunction will be organized as follows:

- sensory modulation disorders
  1. sensory defensiveness (hyperresponsivity, overreactivity)
     - tactile defensiveness
     - gravitational insecurity
  2. sensory dormancy/sensory registration problems (hyporesponsivity, underreactivity)
- adaptive movement response disorders
  1. vestibular processing disorder
  2. developmental dyspraxia
- sensory discrimination and perceptual disorders
  1. tactile discrimination
  2. proprioceptive perception
  3. visual perceptual
  4. other senses

CAUSE

The origin of sensory integrative dysfunction is assumed to be within the processing centers of the central nervous system, although the exact cause is unknown.

PROBLEMS

The following list of problems is based on Arkwright (1998, 2–3).

* sensory processing: hypersensitive to sensory stimuli such as touch or noise, touches everything or nothing, hates being hugged or craves physical contact, afraid of movement or loves movement, lethargic or unusually active
* postural control: slouches, props head when sitting, uses support when standing
* fine motor: difficulty manipulating objects such as scissors, blocks, beads; awkward grasp on objects such as pencils (too tight or too weak); difficulty tying shoes, buttoning skirt
* gross motor: skipping, hopping, running awkward or impossible; stumbles; bumps into things; clumsy
* perceptual skills: difficulty matching objects, loses place when copying or reading, difficulty putting puzzles together
* cognitive skills: distractible, unable to transfer or generalize skills, of average or above average intelligence
* psychosocial skills: poor self-esteem, throws tantrums, gets frustrated easily

TREATMENT/INTERVENTION

The following discussion of intervention strategies and treatment is based on Kimball (1993).

* Intervention techniques should address the specific underlying sensory system deficit, not the observable behavior. Direct intervention regarding a specific skill may improve that skill but will not improve the ability to generalize from one situation to the next.
* Intervention should begin with sensory system modulation problems first. If the person is responding with sympathetic arousal, the adaptive response will reflect survival needs, not integration within the nervous system.
* Begin the therapy session with sensory modulation activities. Functional support capabilities should follow sensory modulation, and finally, end-product abilities should be included. Do not start with a complex motor planning activity.
* Get the person actively involved in the activities and help the person succeed. Work *with* the person, not *on* the person (except for brushing to treat tactile defensiveness). Facilitate, do not control, the person's interaction with therapy activities.
* Strive for a balance in treatment sessions between structured, therapist-directed and -selected activities and unstructured, free-choice activities. The approach will depend on the nature of the person's problems. Persons with learning disabilities tend to need less help with structure than those with autism. The therapy session should begin with structure and progress to free choice.
* Therapy should be fun, not hard work. The challenge to the therapist is to select activities that are within the person's ability to achieve. Activities that are too easy organize nothing and those that are too difficult disorganize.

Categories of Sensory Integrative Functions

Sensory System Modulation
- tactile response
- auditory response
- vestibular response—relationship to gravity
- postrotary nystagmus response
- movement level—self-initiated movement
- attention level
- emotional level
- oral arousal
- olfactory arousal
- visual arousal
- sensitivity to movement—initiated by others
- proprioceptive sensitivity

Functional Support Capabilities
- suck-swallow-breathe
- tactile discrimination
- other sensory modalities and discriminative abilities
- muscle concontraction
- muscle tone
- proprioception
- balance and equipment reactions
- developmental reflexes
- lateralization
- bilateral integration

End-Product Abilities
- praxis
- form and space perception
- behavior
- academics
- language and articulation
- emotional tone
- activity level
- environmental mastery

Source: Data from J.G. Kimbell, Sensory Integrative Frame of Reference, in *Frames of Reference for Pediatric Occupational Therapy*, pp. 87–175, J.P. Kramer and J. Hinjosa, © 1993, Williams and Wilkins.

- The therapist must be able to adapt and modify the day's activities at any time because the person's sensory system modulation may change from day to day. Activities may need to be made easier or more difficult during a therapy session.

PRECAUTIONS

- Be sure there is sufficient space to allow swinging movements, running and jumping activities, and a scooter board ramp.
- Be sure there is sufficient padding on the floors. Mats must provide sufficient padding to cushion a fall of 4 feet. Mats should be constructed with dense foam of 2 to 4 inches. If the floor is cement, additional mats will be needed.
- Floor space that is not padded should have a nondistracting color and pattern to reduce optokinetic nystagmus.
- Overhead suspension systems should be able to hold at least 500 pounds and withstand swinging motions.
- Always observe the person in therapy at all times for signs of overarousal to avoid shutdown of the nervous system or shock.
- Monitor the person in therapy to make sure that equipment is used safely and activities will not cause injury.

REFERENCES

Arkwright, N. 1998. *An Introduction to Sensory Integration.* San Antonio, TX: Therapy Skill Builders.
Kimball, J.G. 1993. Sensory integrative frame of reference. In *Frames of reference for pediatric occupational therapy,* eds. P. Kramer and J. Hinojosa, 87–167. Baltimore: Williams & Wilkins.

BIBLIOGRAPHY

Ayres, A.J. 1979. *Sensory Integration and the Child.* Los Angeles: Western Psychological Services. (Classic reference)
Baloueff, O. 1998. Sensory integration. In *Willard and Spackman's occupational therapy,* 9th ed., eds. M.E. Neistadt and E.B. Crepeau, 546–550. Philadelphia: J.B. Lippincott.
Blanche, E.I. et al. 1995. *Combining Neuro-Developmental Treatment and Sensory Integration Principles: An Approach to Pediatric Therapy.* San Antonio, TX: Therapy Skill Builders.
Cermak, S.A., and L.A. Daunhauer. 1997. Sensory processing in the postinstitutionalized child. *American Journal of Occupational Therapy* 51, no. 7: 500–507.
DeGangi, G.A. 1997. Sensory patterns in infants and young children: introduction and infancy; sensory patterns in infants and young children: the toddler; sensory patterns in infants and young children: the preschool child. In *Handbook of child and adolescent psychiatry,* ed. J.D. Noshpitz, 43–55, 83–88, 144–149. New York: Wiley & Sons.
Frick, S.M., and N. Lawton-Shirley. 1994. Auditory integrative training from a sensory integrative perspective. *Sensory Integration Special Interest Section Newsletter* 17, no. 4: 1–3.
Haack, L., and M. Haldy. 1998. Adaptations and accommodations for sensory processing problems, no. 4. In *Occupational therapy: Making a difference in school system practice,* ed. J. Case-Smith, 1–39. Bethesda, MD: American Occupational Therapy Association.
Hickman, L. 1995. Two clinical stories of sensory integration. *Sensory Integration Special Interest Section Newsletter* 18, no. 1: 1–3. (Case reports)
Mailloux, Z. 1997. Sensory integration and role performance in students. *Sensory Integration Special Interest Section Newsletter* 20, no. 3: 3–4.
Miller, H., and T. Heaphy. 1998. Sensory processing in preschool children, no. 3. In *Occupational therapy: Making a difference in school system practice,* ed. J. Case-Smith, 1–49. Bethesda, MD: American Occupational Therapy Association.

Oetter, P. et al. 1995. *MORE: Integrating the Mouth with Sensory and Postural Functions*, rev. ed. Hugo, NH: PDP Press.

Orr, C. 1998. *Mouth Madness: Oral Motor Activities for Children*. San Antonio, TX: Therapy Skill Builders.

Parham, L.D., and Z. Mailloux. 1996. Sensory integration. In *Occupational therapy for children*, 3rd ed., eds. J. Case-Smith et al., 307–356. St. Louis, MO: Mosby.

Sarracino, T. 1997. Sensory integration in the schools. Part I: Applying a sensory integrative frame of reference in school practice. *Sensory Integration Special Interest Section Quarterly* 20, no. 3: 1–2.

Sheda, C.H., and P.R. Ralston. 1997. *Sensorimotor Processing Activity Plans*. San Antonio, TX: Therapy Skill Builders.

Stallings-Sahler, S. 1998. Sensory integration: Assessment and intervention with infants and young children. In *Pediatric occupational therapy and early intervention*, 2nd ed., ed. J. Case-Smith, 223–254. Boston: Butterworth-Heinemann.

Stephens, L.C. 1997. Sensory integrative dysfunction in young children. *AAHBEI (American Association for Home-Based Early Interventions) News Exchange* 2, no. 1.

Tryon, P.N. 1997. Sensory integration in the schools. Part II: Communication and collaboration with parents and between school- and clinic-based therapists. *Sensory Integration Special Interest Section Quarterly* 20, no. 4: 1–2.

Sensory Integrative Dysfunction— Sensory Modulation Disorders: General

DESCRIPTION

"Modulation" is a term used to describe the central nervous system's ability to regulate its own activity. In relation to the sensory systems, modulation "refers to the tendency to generate responses that are appropriately graded in relation to incoming sensory stimuli rather than underreacting or overreacting to them" (Parham and Mailloux 1996, 324). Sensory modulation problems are believed to form a continuum from hyperresponsivity at one end to hyporesponsivity at the other.

Hyperresponsivity occurs in sensory defensiveness, which is observed when a child is overwhelmed by ordinary sensory input and thus reacts defensively to it. The defensive behavior may take the form of fight or flight behavior and/or the exhibition of negative emotions. Although technically any sensory system or combination of systems may be involved in sensory modulation problems, the most is known about tactile defensiveness and gravitational insecurity. The person is overwhelmed by ordinary sensory input and reacts defensively to it. The sympathetic nervous system may activate the fight or flight response, and there may be a display of strong negative emotions. The term "sensory defensiveness" was first used by Knickerbocker in 1980 and later by Wilbarger and Wilbarger in 1991.

At the hyporesponsive end are sensory registration problems, which include failure to attend to stimuli, poor focus of attention, or overfocused attention on irrelevant stimuli. Both under- and overattention can result in sensory dormancy or poor registration.

CAUSE

The mechanism of sensory modulation is not fully understood, but there is an assumption that the limbic system is involved in mediating sensory stimuli. Whether a dysfunctional limbic system is the only cause of sensory modulation problems or whether other central nervous system structures are also dysfunctional has not been resolved. The cause is assumed to be a failure of the central nervous system to modulate the incoming stimuli to a level acceptable to the person.

ASSESSMENT

Areas

- tactile
- auditory
- vestibular/gravity
- movement level
- oral arousal
- olfactory arousal
- visual arousal
- attention level
- postrotary nystagmus
- sensitivity to movement
- proprioceptive sensitivity
- emotional level

Instruments

The diagnosis of sensory defensiveness is made primarily from the report of caregivers and by using a checklist of behaviors associated with sensory defensiveness.

Instruments Developed by Occupational Therapy Personnel

- *DeGangi-Berk Test of Sensory Integration* (DBTSI) by G.A. DeGangi and R.A. Berk, Los Angeles: Western Psychological Services, 1983.
- *FirstSTEp Screening Test for Evaluating Preschoolers* by L.J. Miller, San Antonio, TX: The Psychological Corporation, 1993.
- *Leiter International Performance Scale—Revised* by G.H. Roid and L.J. Miller, Wood Dale, IL: Stoelting Co., 1997.
- *Miller Assessment for Preschoolers* (MAP) by L.J. Miller, San Antonio, TX: The Psychological Corporation, 1988.
- Sensory Integration and Praxis Tests by A.J. Ayres, Los Angeles: Western Psychological Services, 1989.
- *Sensory Profile* by W. Dunn, San Antonio, TX: Therapy Skill Builders, 1999.
- *The Sensory Rating Scale for Infants and Young Children* by B. Provost and P. Oetter, in The Sensory Rating Scale for Infants and Young Children: Development and reliability, *Physical and Occupational Therapy in Pediatrics* 13, no. 4 (1993): 15–37.

* *Test of Sensory Functions in Infants* (TSFI) by G.A. DeGangi and S.I Greenspan, Los Angeles: Western Psychological Services, 1989.
* *Toddler and Infant Motor Evaluation* (TIME) by L.J. Miller and G.H. Roid, San Antonio, TX: Therapy Skill Builders, 1994.

Instruments Developed by Other Professionals and Used by Occupational Therapy Personnel

* *Bayley Scales of Infant Development-II* (BSID-II) by N. Bayley, San Antonio, TX: The Psychological Corporation, 1993.
* *The Beery-Buktenica Developmental Test of Visual-Motor Integration* (VMI-4), 4th ed. by K.E. Beery and N.A. Buktenica, Parsippany, NJ: Modern Curriculum Press, 1997.
* *Bruininks-Oseretsky Test of Motor Proficiency* (BOTMP) by R. Bruininks, Circle Pines, MN: American Guidance Services, 1978.
* *Peabody Developmental Motor Scales* by M.R. Folio and R.R. Fewell, Austin, TX: Pro-ed, 1983.

PROBLEMS

Self-Care
* The person may not tolerate clothing and food with certain textures.
* The person may object to having his or her hair brushed or cut.
* The person avoids or is very slow going up and down stairs.

Productivity and Leisure
* The person has delays in reading, writing, and speech.
* The person has poor play skills.

Sensorimotor
Sensory Defensiveness
* tactile
  1. The person has an adverse reaction to diaper or clothing changes (whimpers, tries to push item off, pushes caregiver's hand away, tries to move away).
  2. The person has an adverse reaction to bathing and towel drying.
  3. The person has an adverse reaction to hair washing, hair combing, or hair cutting.
  4. The person dislikes changes in texture of foods and changes in nipples or spoons.
  5. The person dislikes having fingernails or toenails cut.
  6. The person dislikes being touched by another person.
  7. The person reacts negatively to light touch.
  8. The person perceives light touch as painful or irritating.
  9. The person may not tolerate touch from certain types of clothing, objects, animals, or people.
* gravitational
  1. The person dislikes or avoids being moved through the air by caregivers.

2. The person dislikes riding in cars and sitting in swings and rockers.
3. The person dislikes hanging upside down or being placed in an inverted position.
4. The person may show real fear, anxiety, or intense emotional reaction in response to movement situations that should require only alerting or changes in body or head position.

- auditory
  1. The person may startle upon hearing intrusive noises such as the telephone, doorbell, vacuum cleaner, or whistle.
  2. The person does not habituate to familiar sounds.
  3. The person may be overly distracted by noises.
  4. The person may become upset at or appear annoyed by sounds at normal levels.
- movement level
  1. The person appears to be moving constantly as though unable to stand still.
- movement sensitivity
  1. The person tolerates very little rotary or angular acceleration without having autonomic nervous system responses such as nausea or "feeling funny" in the abdomen.
- oral arousal
  1. The person may be overly sensitive to the texture of items placed in the mouth.
  2. The person may refuse to eat many foods because of texture, not taste.
  3. The person may dislike having objects in his or her mouth such as a toothbrush, dentist's fingers, or drill.
  4. The person may use heavy chewing to calm him- or herself.
  5. The person may chew on inappropriate things such as blankets, hands, and clothes.
- olfactory arousal
  1. The person may become upset or nauseous at the smell of certain odors.
  2. The person may have "flashbacks" upon smelling certain odors.
- visual
  1. The person looks away from or avoids gazing at complex visual stimuli such as a face or pattern such as a checkerboard.
  2. The person avoids bright lights that others enjoy.
  3. The person fails to visually explore surroundings.
  4. The person has difficulty habituating to visual stimuli.
  5. The person orients persistently to objects that are common in the visual field.
- attention
  1. The person appears to be reacting constantly to stimuli.
- postrotary nystagmus
  1. The person becomes overly dizzy after rotary movement called prolonged postrotary nystagmus.
- proprioceptive sensitivity
  1. The person may be overly sensitive to joint and muscle movement provided externally.
  2. The person may be very aware of movements of arms or legs.
- emotional arousal
  1. The person becomes upset by situations that might be considered trivial by others.

Sensory Dormancy
- somatosensory dormancy (tactile, mechanoreceptors)

1. The person continues to mouth most objects after nine months of age.
2. The person tends to use excessive force with tools, pencils, or crayons.
3. The person lacks normal responses to light touch or pain. He or she often appears not to feel pain and is oblivious to bumps, bruises, or other small injuries.
4. The person may bang the head or self-mutilate (in severe cases).
5. The person does seem to differentiate among different types of touch (e.g., light, firm).
- vestibular response dormancy (gravitational)
   1. The person has absent or delayed postural and balance reactions such as righting, protective, and equilibrium (without diagnosed neuromotor deficits such as cerebral palsy).
   2. The person seeks excessive and exaggerated amounts of vestibular input, such as long periods of jumping, spinning, or rocking.
   3. The person demonstrates a hyporesponsive elicited nystagmus during or after rotary activity.
   4. The person is not afraid of heights, falling, or moving fast.
- auditory response dormancy
   1. The person does not have or has delayed orienting responses to sudden or loud noises.
   2. The person does not startle to loud noises.
   3. The person has delayed responses to verbal requests due to slow auditory processing.
- movement level
   1. The person moves more slowly than others of the same age.
   2. The person appears to be conserving energy.
- oral arousal
   1. The person will put anything into the mouth.
   2. The person seems unaware that mouthing food or objects is socially inappropriate after a certain age.
- olfactory arousal
   1. The person does not seem to notice odors.
   2. The person does not identify odors.
- visual system
   1. The person does not respond to changes in the visual field, even though visual acuity is normal.
   2. The person does not appear to notice when objects enter the visual field.
   3. The person does not seem to notice changes in movement or color.
- attention level
   1. The person appears to pay little or no attention to environmental changes that require an active intervention or response.
- postrotary nystagmus
   1. The person does not show dizziness or shows decreased dizziness after rotary movement (called depressed postrotary nystagmus).
- sensitivity to movement
   1. The person tolerates excessive amounts of rotary or angular acceleration without an autonomic nervous system response.
- proprioceptive sensitivity
   1. The person does not appear to "feel" or have an internal awareness of some limb and muscle positions or movement.

- emotional arousal
  1. The person shows a decreased level of emotional response.

Psychosocial
Sensory Defensiveness
- The person may have an aversion to being held.
- The person may have an aversion to being handled.

Sensory Dormancy
- The person may cling to the caregiver.

TREATMENT/INTERVENTION

Sensorimotor
General
- Increase ability to calm self and cope with external stimuli.
- Decrease the general arousal level in the autonomic nervous system.
- Provide specific, controlled sensory input in one sensory channel known to inhibit (compete with) afferent flow in another.

Sensory Defensiveness
   The goal of therapy for sensory defensiveness is to inhibit or calm down response level.
- Vestibular: Speed should be slow; rhythms should be predictable; planes of movement should be horizontal or vertical, but not both in rapid succession; direction should be linear; range should be limited; frequency/amplitude should be high or low but not both in rapid succession; position should be upright, flexion, facing forward to movement. Examples: slow rocking, slow swinging, oscillating water bed, slow vertical oscillation.
- Proprioception: Pressure should be moderate to deep, location should be total body or proximal joints, duration should be over period of time of stimulus, position of the body should be flexed, amount of effort on joints should be heavy work. Examples include swaddling or "make a taco"; sustained joint compression ("make a pizza" or "make a hot dog"); pulling on Thera-Band; pushing or pulling play partner on equipment; lifting and carrying groceries, boxes, or furniture.
- Tactile: Speed should be slow; pressure should be moderate to deep skin depression; predictability should be high; location should be on the back, dorsolateral surfaces of extremities or face. Examples include slow massage with long, sustained stroke in one direction on the skin.
- Visual: Illumination should be low; colors should be pastels or deep tones; contrast should be low; space should be small, closed in, or with clear boundaries; environment should be simple and uncluttered. Examples include a small treatment room, tent, "hideout," "womb," or "mother" environment with bare walls.
- Auditory: Volume should be low; rhythm should be speed of heartbeat or slower; frequency should be low; types should be vibration, music, or rhyming speech. Examples include music with heartbeat rhythm, recited nursery rhymes, and soft, lyrical music.

- Gustatory and oral sensory-motor: Flavor should be sweet or mildly salty; viscosity should be moderate; temperature should be warm; texture should be smooth; and pattern should be suck, blow, bite, and crunch. Examples for sucking include a pacifier or hard candy; for blowing, a musical toy; for biting or crunching, carrots, celery, or potato chips.

Sensory Dormancy

- Vestibular: Speed should be moderate to fast; rhythmicity should be dysrhythmic and unpredictable; planes of movement may be horizontal, vertical, orbital, axial, or diagonal; position may be inverted or backward in space; range of activity may be wide; frequency/ amplitude should go from low to high. Examples including jumping on a trampoline; swinging in a helicopter swing, "whale" swing, or bolster swing; jumping through space; hanging on trapeze bar.
- Tactile: Speed should be rapid, pressure can be light touch, predictability should be random, locations should be ventromedial surfaces of extremities and periorbital area. Examples include playing in ball pit, light brushing to periorbital area, "swimming" through a fabric tunnel.
- Vision: Illumination should be moderate, colors should be bright, contrast should be high, space should be open with few boundaries, scene may be busy or cluttered. Working in a bright, sunny, large area such as a gym and having many pictures on a bulletin board or objects on walls would be helpful.
- Auditory: Volume should be moderate, rhythm depends on volume (hard rhythm and high volume tend to be arousing), frequency can be moderate to high, and type can be music with lyrics. Examples include listening to music with a loud, driving beat and reciting loud jump-rope rhymes or raps.
- Gustatory/oral sensory-motor: Flavor can be sour, spicy, bitter, or smoked; viscosity can be low; texture can be chewy, hard, or irregular; pattern should be chew, lick. Examples include drinking lemonade in sport bottle, licking popsicle or sucker, and chewing licorice rope.

PRECAUTIONS

- When assessing a child with a history of neglect or abuse, be aware that atypical responses to touch may occur.
- The ventral trunk area or any ticklish area should be avoided when using brushing or light touch stimuli.
- Avoid high-stimulus intensities that can lead to autonomic shutdown.
- Before using hard candies that may cause choking, be sure the person has enough oral motor skills to keep the candy away from the throat.

PROGNOSIS AND OUTCOME

- The person is able to tolerate sensory input with adjustments for sensitivities, if necessary.
- The person is able to perform daily living tasks independently according to developmental age.
- The person is able to participate in play or leisure tasks with peers.
- The person is able to attend school with peers without behavioral problems noted by teachers or staff.

• The person is able to use effective coping skills at home and school.

REFERENCES

Knickerbocker, B.M. 1980. *A Holistic Approach to the Treatment of Learning Disorders*. Thorofare, N.J: Charles B. Slack.

Parham, L.D., and Z. Mailloux. 1996. Sensory integration. In *Occupational therapy for children*, 3rd ed., eds. J. Case-Smith et al., 307–356. St. Louis, MO: Mosby.

Wilbarger, P., and J.L. Wilbarger. 1991. *Sensory Defensiveness in Children Aged 2–12: An Intervention Guide for Parents and Other Caretakers*. Denver, CO: Avanti Educational Programs.

BIBLIOGRAPHY

Dunn, W., and C. Brown. 1997. Factor analysis on the Sensory Profile from a national sample of children with disabilities. *American Journal of Occupational Therapy* 51, no. 7: 490–495.

Miller, L.J., and D.N. McIntosh. 1998. The diagnosis, treatment, and etiology of sensory modulation disorder. *Sensory Integration Special Interest Section Quarterly* 21, no. 1: 1–3.

Stallings-Sahler, S. 1998. Sensory modulation disorders. In *Pediatric occupational therapy and early intervention*, 2nd ed., ed. J. Case-Smith, 233–243. Boston: Butterworth-Heinemann.

Wilbarger, J., and T.M. Stackhouse. 1998. *Sensory modulation: A review of occupational therapy literature*. Littleton, CO: The KID Foundation.

Wilbarger, P. 1995. The sensory diet: Activity programs based on sensory processing theory. *Sensory Integration Special Interest Section Newsletter* 18, no. 2: 1–4.

Williams, M.S., and S. Shellenberger. 1994. The alert program for self-regulation. *Sensory Integration Special Interest Section Newsletter* 17, no. 3: 1–3.

Williams, M.S., and S. Shellenberger. 1996. *"How Does Your Engine Run?": A Leader's Guide to the Alert Program for Self-Regulation*. Albuquerque, NM: TherapyWorks, Inc.

Sensory Defensiveness

Baranek, G.T. et al. 1997. Sensory defensiveness in persons with developmental disabilities. *Occupational Therapy Journal of Research* 17, no. 3: 173–185.

Kinnealey, M. et al. 1995. A phenomenological study of sensory defensiveness. *American Journal of Occupational Therapy* 59, no. 5: 444–451.

Papadopoulos, R.J.B. 1997. Occupational therapy assessment of neurodevelopmentally disordered children and adolescents. *Occupational Therapy in Mental Health* 13, no. 1: 23–36.

Pertler, J.W., and J. Kundert. 1995. Overcoming sensory defensiveness. *Occupational Therapy Forum* 14, no. 8: 8–9.

Provost, B., and P. Oetter. 1993. The Sensory Rating Scale for Infants and Young Children: Development and Reliability. *Physical and Occupational Therapy in Pediatrics* 13, no. 4: 15–37.

Reisman, J.E., and A.Y. Gross. 1992. Psychophysiological measurement of treatment effects in an adult with sensory defensiveness. *Canadian Journal of Occupational Therapy* 59, no. 2: 248–257.

Sensory Dormancy

Parham, L.D., and Z. Mailloux. 1996. Sensory integration. In *Occupational therapy for children*, 3rd ed., eds. J. Case-Smith et al., 307–356. St. Louis, MO: Mosby.

Stallings-Sahler, S. 1998. Sensory dormancy and poor sensory registration. In *Pediatric occupational therapy and early intervention*, 2nd ed., ed. J. Case-Smith, 237–243. Boston: Butterworth-Heinemann.

Sensory Integrative Dysfunction— Sensory Modulation Disorders: Tactile Defensiveness

DESCRIPTION

Tactile defensiveness is an adverse reaction to touch, such as a feeling of discomfort and a desire to escape the situation when presented with certain types of tactile stimuli. Responses may be excessive emotional reactions, hyperactivity, or other behavior problems.

CAUSE

The cause is unknown but was assumed originally by Ayres (1972) to be a failure of the protective tactile system and the discriminative tactile system to attain a natural balance, leaving the protective system predominant. Current theory suggests a failure of the inhibitory or modulating system in the brain.

ASSESSMENT

Areas

- two-point discrimination
- locationalization of stimulus
- stereognosis
- graphesthesia
- social skills (especially those where physical contact may occur)
- dressing and undressing
- eating
- grooming
- play skills

Instruments

- *Sensory Integration and Praxis Tests* by A.J. Ayres, Los Angeles: Western Psychological Services, 1989. (Especially the subtests Graphesthesia [GRA] and Localization of Tactile Stimuli [LTS])
- *Tactile Sensitivity Behavioral Responses Checklist* by B.A. Bauer, *American Journal of Occupational Therapy* 31, no. 6 (1977): 357–361.
- *Touch Inventory for Preschoolers* (TIP) by C.B. Royeen, *Physical and Occupational Therapy in Pediatrics* 7, no. 1 (1987): 29–40.
- *Touch Inventory for Elementary-School-Aged* by C.B. Royeen, *American Journal of Occupational Therapy* 44, no. 2 (1990): 155–159.

PROBLEMS

Self-Care

- The person may react strongly to certain grooming activities, such as having the face washed, hair combed or cut, teeth brushed, or nails cut.
- The person may refuse to wear clothing made of certain fabrics.
- The person may have difficulty getting dressed because of a reaction to clothing against the skin.
- The person may push up pant legs or shirt (blouse) sleeves.
- The person may frequently adjust clothing as though the items do not fit properly, although the items are the correct size.
- The person may refuse to go barefoot or hate to wear shoes.
- The person may refuse to eat foods with certain textures.

Productivity

- The person may avoid certain play activities, such as playing in the sand.
- The person may become a behavioral problem in the classroom because of reactions to accidental or intentional physical contact with others.

Leisure

- The person may avoid certain leisure interests that require getting dirty or handling items with a variety of textures.

Sensorimotor

- The person may exhibit hyperactivity or an increase in skeletal movements.
- The person may strike out, hit, or fight anyone who accidentally brushes against him or her or whom the person accidentally brushes against.
- The person may run (take flight) from a situation in which light tactile stimuli occurred.
- The person may react by trying to rub or scratch out light tactile stimuli.
- The person may avoid being touched or having physical contact even with people that he or she likes.
- The person may avoid touching certain textures, such as sand, paste, or finger paints, and certain surfaces, such as blankets, carpets, or toys.
- The person may prefer to keep arms and legs covered with clothing even when warm.
- The person tends to react strongly to stimuli to the face, hands, and feet.

Cognitive

- The person may have a short attention span and become easily distracted.

Psychosocial

- The person may be accused of lacking self-control because of strange behavior when touching some objects or being touched.
- The person may act fearful, angry, or uncomfortable when approached or touched.
- The person may verbally express feelings of discomfort or a desire to escape.

- The person may be accused of exhibiting antisocial behavior because he or she withdraws or hits people who accidentally touch him or her or even stand too close.

TREATMENT/INTERVENTION

Treatment is based on the model of sensory integration. (See section on sensory motor activities in resources for additional activities.)

Self-Care
- Encourage the person to perform self-care activities independently, such as washing face and hands and brushing hair and teeth.

Productivity
- Alert parents or supervisor to the defensive/hypersensitive behavior and encourage creative solutions. The person can be assigned other chores or use gloves.

Leisure
- The person will select leisure activities that are acceptable to him or her. Parents, caregivers, or friends should not push or encourage the person to perform a leisure activity that produces discomfort or other defensive/hypersensitive behavior.

Sensorimotor
- Have the person crawl on all fours or belly crawl on various textured surfaces or through an obstacle course.
- Have the person play animal (assume position of the animal) games, such as snake, duck, crab, or dog while traversing various terrains (various textures of carpets, blankets, or mats).
- Apply firm pressure using cloth materials of various textures ranging from soft, such as fake fur, to rough, such as corduroy. Play hot dog. The person is the hot dog. Add ketchup (put a blanket, large towel, or fake fur over the person and press firmly to body). Add mustard (add another layer and press). Add pickles (add another layer and press). Add relish (add another layer and press). Place in a bun (roll up edges of the mat and press). Variations of the game include ham sandwich or deli sandwich.
- Use pairs of texture boards or cards covered with various materials, such as cotton, fur, corduroy, terry cloth, wool, or sandpaper. The person matches like pairs. Start with only two or three pairs of textures that are easy to discriminate. Add pairs as defensiveness decreases and matching skill improves.
- Use a large plastic tub or washbasin filled with Cheerios, uncooked rice, small beans, small pasta, small plastic beads, uncooked Cream of Wheat, or sand. Have the person search for objects, toys, or shapes hidden in the Cheerios (or other substance).
- Use a small cloth bag or box. Place an object, toy, or shape in the "feely bag" or "feely box." The person reaches in the bag or box, feels the item, and tries to guess what it is or match the item with an item in a group of objects on the table.
- Make craft projects from materials that have various textures or shapes, such as a collage or mosaic of cloth, felt, yarn, string, macaroni, beans, or papier-mâché.

- Use books with tactile or "touch me" panels that the person is encouraged to touch and feel.
- Have the person rub his or her body parts with various cloth textures, lotion, or powder. Start with the hands (usually the least defensive), then the arms and legs. The face, neck, anterior trunk, and soles of feet are usually the most sensitive. Play the swimming pool game. A mat is the swimming pool. The person "dives" into the pool (onto mat), swims (belly crawls), gets out, and dries off with a towel.
- Finger painting with sand or uncooked Cream of Wheat added for texture provides longer contact as the person becomes less defensive.
- Trace letters, shapes, roadways, or figures marked on sandpaper, felt board, corrugated cardboard, or other textured surface.

Cognitive
- Teach parents or caregivers to use firm pressure when dressing, washing, or assisting the person with an activity or task.

Psychosocial
- Provide instruction in relaxation techniques, such as slow rocking, rolling in a blanket, taking a lukewarm bath, or deep breathing.
- Alert teachers or group leaders to the defensive/hypersensitive behavior. The person may need to be first or last in line. The person may need a specific seating assignment.

PRECAUTIONS
- Usually treatment should begin on areas of the skin that are least defensive, such as the arms or backs of the hands.
- Avoid brushing against the direction of hair growth.
- Avoid crossing the midline of the body during early phases of treatment.

PROGNOSIS AND OUTCOME
- The person responds less defensively to touching or being touched.
- The person has an improved attention span.
- The person is able to participate in group activities without withdrawing or striking out.
- The person is able to perform self-care activities without discomfort.

REFERENCE
Ayres, A.J. 1972. Tactile defensiveness and related behavioral responses. In *Sensory integration and learning disorders*, 207-20. Los Angeles: Western Psychological Services.

BIBLIOGRAPHY
Baranek, G.T. et al. 1997. Tactile defensiveness and stereotyped behaviors. *American Journal of Occupational Therapy* 51, no. 2: 91–95.
Baranek, G.T., and G. Berkson. 1994. Tactile defensiveness in children with developmental disabilities: Responsiveness and habituation. *Journal of Autism and Developmental Disorders* 24, no. 4: 457–471.

Bennett, J.W., and C.Q. Peterson. 1996. The Touch Inventory for Elementary-School-Aged Children: Test-retest reliability and mother-child correlations. *American Journal of Occupational Therapy* 49, no. 8: 795–801.

Case-Smith, J. 1995. The relationship among sensorimotor components, fine motor skill, and functional performance in preschool children. *American Journal of Occupational Therapy* 49, no. 7: 645–652.

Murphy, J. 1995. Out of touch: Treating people with tactile hypersensitivity. *Advance for Occupational Therapists* 11, no. 23: 20, 46.

Parush, S. et al. 1996. A comparison of self-report and informant report of tactile defensiveness amongst children in Israel. *Occupational Therapy International* 3, no. 4: 274–283.

Sears, C.J. 1994. Recognizing and coping with tactile defensiveness in young children. *Infants and Young Children* 6, no. 4: 46–53.

Tupper, L.C., and K.E. Klostermann-Miesler. 1995. Sensory systems. In *School hardening: Sensory integration strategies for class and home*, eds. L.C. Tupper and K.E. Klostermann-Miesler, 9–16. Tucson, AZ: Therapy Skill Builders.

Sensory Integrative Dysfunction— Sensory Modulation Disorders: Gravitational Insecurity

DESCRIPTION

Gravitational insecurity is characterized by an abnormal anxiety or distress that arises when the gravity receptors of the vestibular system are stimulated by head position or movement, especially when the person's feet are not on the ground (Ayres 1979). The person fears a sudden change of head position or of the body's center of gravity, changes in head and body alignment, or the feet suddenly leaving the ground. The fear is especially evident whenever there is movement backward or upward through space. A person with gravitational insecurity often is also hypersensitive to movement and becomes dizzy or nauseated quickly.

CAUSE

The cause is unknown. The brain is unable to inhibit or modulate vestibular impulses by the macular receptors within the otoliths of the inner ear, which respond to linear acceleration.

ASSESSMENT

Areas

- response to movement in space initiated by others or the action of objects
- emotional reactions
- posture in relation to gravity
- balance and equilibrium

- muscle tone

Instruments
- *Sensory Integration and Praxis Tests* by A.J. Ayres, Los Angeles: Western Psychological Services, 1989.

PROBLEMS

Self-Care
- The person may have difficulty performing activities that require antigravity movements, such as standing on a stool to reach a water faucet, climbing the stairs to get ready for bed, sitting in a chair in which the feet do not reach the floor, or leaning the head back to get soap rinsed out of hair.

Productivity
- The person's play skills in cooperative play may be delayed because of fears related to climbing, sudden movements, spinning, or rapid changes of balance.
- The person may refuse to participate in certain play activities such as bicycle riding, ice skating, in-line skating, skateboarding, skiing, or hiking.

Leisure
- The person may prefer solitary activities in which he or she remains in control of head and body positions.
- The person will not participate in games that require climbing, sudden movements, spinning, or rapid changes of balance.

Sensorimotor
- The person is usually hypersensitive to movement such as spinning, frequent changes in direction and speed, or unusual body positions.
- The person becomes dizzy or nauseated quickly during any type of vestibular stimulation.
- The person tends to avoid having the head upside down (e.g., in somersaults, when hanging from a bar, when tumbling).
- The person tends to avoid situations requiring jumping through space (e.g., jumping from a higher surface to a lower surface, jumping from one platform to another).
- The person is slow at performing unusual movements, such as climbing from the front seat to the back, walking up and down an unfamiliar hill, or walking on uneven ground.
- The person tends to avoid walking on a raised surface (e.g., a balance beam, a railroad track, a curb) even if the surface is only a few inches off the ground.
- The person does not like to be pushed backward or raised upward.
- The person has difficulty moving his or her body in antigravity positions.
- The person prefers the upright position to reduce the impact of gravitational forces on the body.
- The person prefers sitting close to the ground in stable positions such as W sitting.
- The person tends to avoid sliding down a playground slide and insists on holding on to the sides of the slide.

- The person tends to avoid climbing or riding equipment or toys that require the feet to leave the ground, such as a jungle gym or merry-go-round.
- The person's muscle tone may increase rapidly in response to a perceived threat of falling, regardless of the actual risk.
- The person tends to ride passively on moving toys or equipment, such as in a wagon or on a merry-go-round.
- The person does not enjoy rotary movements such as spinning or turning around repeatedly for fear of losing balance.
- The person tends to avoid rotational movements of the body, preferring instead to "fix" the body and move by turning the feet.
- The person may try to avoid climbing stairs or taking escalators or elevators.
- The person's postrotary nystagmus is hyperreactive.
- The person may have been slow to learn to walk up and down stairs and may use the banister.
- The person may have poor awareness of his or her body scheme.
- The person may show poor ability to plan body movements within space and thus bump into things, trip and fall over objects, or lose balance.
- The person may have poor proprioception and difficulty identifying positions of body parts in space without using his or her eyes.

Cognitive
- The person is usually cognitively unaware of the sources of the responses although the cognitive capacity is normal.

Psychosocial
- The person is extremely fearful about heights and anxious about falling.
- The person shows fear of any sudden change of position, such as when riding in a car that turns a corner rapidly.
- The person tends to avoid roughhousing with others.
- The person may grasp the therapist tightly or clutch the therapist in response to a perceived threat of falling, regardless of actual risk.
- The person may become rigid and refuse to move or start to cry in response to a perceived threat from movement in space.
- The person may try to control and manipulate a situation to avoid distressing sensations, which may make the person appear obstinate and uncooperative.
- The person may be very shy and withdrawn.
- The person may appear anxious and tense, with shoulders elevated and close to the head.

TREATMENT/INTERVENTION
Treatment is based on the model of sensory integration therapy.

Self-Care
- The therapist may suggest to parents alternate ways of performing self-care activities that do not elicit gravitational insecurity, such as permitting the person to wash hands in a bowl of water placed at the person's height, flexing the head over a sink while standing on the floor to have the hair rinsed, or putting a stool under the feet.

Productivity

- The therapist may suggest that the person be excused from play situations that require climbing, jumping, bouncing, or swinging until the gravitational insecurity is reduced.

Leisure

- No special suggestions are available. The person will not willingly pursue leisure activities that produce feelings of gravitational insecurity. Therefore, unless gravitational insecurity is reduced, activities that might elicit leisure skills are of little value.

Sensorimotor

- Treat people by using a slow, deliberate, and gradual approach to the introduction of movements.
- Provide vestibular stimulation beginning with activities that use linear movements (back and forward, side to side) that permit the person to keep his or her feet on the floor and head in the upright position, such as in a rocking chair. Other techniques include having the therapist hold the person during early activities and providing helmets, mats, and pillows to increase a sense of security. Gradually some of the supports can be withdrawn.
- Activities may include (1) bouncing, or jumping from a kneeling position or from standing on an inner tube, partially inflated large ball, trampoline, or spring or shock cord suspended from the ceiling; (2) obital swinging (face remains in one direction) on a glider or platform swing, hammock, T-swing, sit-'n-spin, bolster swing, or barrel swing.
- Use deep pressure activities to facilitate organization of movement through touch and slow movements.

Cognitive

- Help person anticipate movement before it occurs by explaining what is happening next and letting the person see a demonstration before trying it.

Psychosocial

- Reduce fear of movement by encouraging self-initiated linear vestibular stimulation.
- Use nonthreatening positions, beginning with feet on the floor and slow speeds, small amplitude, and short durations that are tolerable to the person and within the person's control.
- Reassure the person that he or she will not be asked or required to assume any position or engage in any movement that makes the person feel uncomfortable, initiates a fear response, or increases anxiety.

PRECAUTIONS

- Do not require or force the person to assume any position or engage in any movement that makes the person feel uncomfortable, initiates a fear response, or increases anxiety.
- If the person has cerebral palsy or other brain injury, therapists should follow the following guidelines:
  1. The person should avoid the supine position if it increases extensor spasticity.
  2. Jumping or bouncing on the balls of the feet should be avoided if the positive support reaction is elicited or there is an increase in extensor spasticity.

3. The person should avoid positions that increase internal rotation, adduction of the hips, and retraction of the shoulder.

• Never overarouse or overstimulate the person with vestibular stimulation. Stop immediately if the person asks to stop, becomes sick, feels dizzy, flushes, shows pallor, or begins sweating. In linear acceleration, overarousal or overstimulation is most likely to occur in response to rapid reversal of movement, inversion of the head, or rapid acceleration or deceleration.

• Stimulation should be stopped if the person becomes withdrawn, destructive, anxious, or resistant.

• The intensity should be reduced if the person experiences sleep disturbances, such as nightmares or sleeplessness.

• Equipment must be kept in good working order. Regular checks of suspension units should be made to be sure the devices can withstand the combined weight of the person and the force of the swinging motion.

PROGNOSIS AND OUTCOME

• The person is able to tolerate the inverted position.
• The person is able to tolerate sudden acceleration and deceleration.
• The person is able to tolerate rotational movement.
• The person is not afraid of falling in normal situations.
• The person is able to maintain balance while moving from one surface to another.
• The person is able to perform activities or tasks that require climbing or stepping off the ground or floor, such as climbing onto a stepstool or climbing a ladder.

REFERENCE

Ayres, A.J. 1979. *Sensory integration and the child*, 62, 182. Los Angeles: Western Psychological Services.

BIBLIOGRAPHY

DeGangi, G.A. et al. 1994. Treatment of vestibular deficits in children with developmental disorders. In *Vestibular rehabilitation*, ed. S.J. Herdman, 360–377. Philadelphia: F.A. Davis.
Parham, L.D., and A. Mailloux. 1996. Sensory integration. In *Occupational therapy for children*, eds. J. Case-Smith et al., 307–356. St. Louis, MO: Mosby.

Sensory Integrative Dysfunction— Adaptive Movement Response Disorders: Vestibular Processing Disorder

DESCRIPTION

Vestibular processing disorder, called also postural and bilateral integration disorder, vestibular-bilateral disorder, vestibular-postural deficits, or vestibular-proprioceptive-based postural dysfunction, is characterized by deficits in coordinating the two sides of the body, poor equilibrium reactions, low muscle tone, and difficulties in communication, organization of behavior, and modulation of arousal (Baloueff 1998, 548). Vestibular processing disorders have been observed among children with learning disorders, developmental coordination disorder, and autism.

CAUSE

This disorder is caused by underreactive vestibular responses and inadequate maturation of postural reactions mediated by the brainstem that interfere with interhemispheric integration and result in limited lateralization of function by the cerebral hemispheres. The disorder is often not apparent until school age.

ASSESSMENT

Areas
- reflexes and reactions: protective, righting, and equilibrium
- postural responses on the ground: shifting weight in preparation for kicking a ball, positioning upper body for catching a ball
- postural responses in the air: being picked up, held, and handled
- bilateral integration: crawling movements, arm thrust, creeping patterns, stair climbing, jumping, ability to use hands together at midline, catching a ball with two hands, hand-to-hand transfer
- laterality: asymmetrical movement, hopping on one foot, holding an object with one hand while manipulating with the other

Instruments
Instruments Developed by Occupational Therapy Personnel
- *DeGangi-Berk Test of Sensory Integration* (DBTSI) by G.A. DeGangi and R.A. Berk, Los Angeles: Western Psychological Services, 1983.
- *A Guide to Testing Clinical Observations in Kindergartners* by W. Dunn, Bethesda, MD: American Occupational Therapy Association, 1981. (Out of print)

Characteristics of Vestibular Disorders

Vestibular Hypersensitivity
- Tends to be overwhelmed by movement and gets motion sickness in a car, or an airplane, in an elevator, or on carnival rides.
- Is fearful of falling and of height.
- Does not enjoy most playground equipment.
- Avoids roughhousing.
- Is anxious when feet leave the ground, as in jumping, climbing, swinging, or doing somersaults.
- Dislikes hanging with head upside down from a bar or leaning over backwards to wash hair.
- Moves slowly when getting onto equipment or riding toys.
- Was slow to learn to walk up or down stairs.
- Relies on railing to climb stairs longer than other children of same chronologic age.
- Dislikes trying new movement activities and/or has difficulty learning them.
- Dislikes irregular or unexpected movement.
- Dislikes low-to-ground positions such as prone or supine and prefers upright postures.
- Shows real fear, anxiety, or intense emotional reaction in response to movement situations that should only require alerting or changes in body/head position.
- Tries to control and manipulate situations to avoid distressful sensation, which may make child appear to be obstinate and uncooperative.
- May cling to a parent or caregiver for support.

Vestibular Hyposensitivity
- Craves movement and does not feel dizziness when other children do.
- Likes to climb too high.
- Is in constant motion, rocking or running about.
- Likes to swing very high and/or for long periods of time.
- Enjoys being upside down.
- Has little or no respect for heights, falling, or moving fast or moving in ways that may be dangerous and unsafe, even if caution is warranted.
- Has little sense of limits or controls.

Source: Adapted with permission from G.A. DeGangi, M.M. Goodin, and S. Wietlishach, Treatment of Vestibular Deficits in Children with Developmental Disorders, in *Vestibular Rehabilitation*, S.J. Herdman, ed., p. 365, © 1994, F.A. Davis Company.

- *Miller Assessment for Preschoolers* (MAP) by L.J. Miller, San Antonio, TX: The Psychological Corporation, 1988.
- *Sensory Integration and Praxis Tests* by A.J. Ayres, Los Angeles: Western Psychological Services, 1989. (Low scores on standing balance with eyes open or closed and similar scores on motor accuracy, bilateral motor coordination, space visualization, contralateral use, and other tests of right vs. left indicate this disorder.)
- *Test of Sensory Functions in Infants* (TSFI) by G.A. DeGangi and S.I. Greenspan, Los Angeles: Western Psychological Services, 1989.
- *Toddler and Infant Motor Evaluation* (TIME) by L.J. Miller and G.H. Roid, San Antonio, TX: Therapy Skill Builders, 1994.

Instruments Developed by Other Professionals and Used by Occupational Therapy Personnel
- *Bayley Scales of Infant Development-II* (BSID-II) by N. Bayley, San Antonio, TX: The Psychological Corporation, 1993.
- *Chandler Movement Assessment of Infants* by L. Chandler, M. Swanson, and M. Andrews, Rolling Bay, WA: 1988.
- *The Infanib* by P.H. Elison, San Antonio, TX: The Psychological Corporation/Therapy Skill Builders, 1994.
- *Peabody Developmental Motor Scales* by M.R. Folio and R.R. Fewell, Austin, TX: Pro-ed, 1983.

PROBLEMS

Self-Care
- The person may have difficulty performing self-care activities that require laterality or directionality. Buttoning is often a problem.

Productivity
- Reading and mathematics skills are usually below grade level. The person may read words backward.
- The person may write letters backward or upside down.
- The person may have specific academic problems such as dysgraphia or dyslexia.

Leisure
- The person is not good at many games and sports and may avoid them.

Sensorimotor
- Regulatory problems: The person may have sleep difficulties, poor self-calming skills, and hypo- or hyperactivity.
- Neuromotor development: The person may be slow in attaining motor milestones and have delayed development of gross and fine motor skills.
- Postural and motor control: The person may have low muscle tone, especially in the extensor muscles; poor balance and equilibrium reactions; poor joint stability, especially in the proximal joints; and poor bilateral coordination of the two sides of body. Note: Low muscle

Clinical Assessment of Vestibular Processing Problems

Sensorimotor

Infant Problems

- The infant is unable to calm self.
- The infant makes arrhythmic movements, not in synchrony with speech or music.
- The infant has fear of new activities that involve leaving the ground, such as being held up in the air or playing on slides, swings, or merry-go-rounds.
- The infant has aversion to new textures on body or to new textures or tastes in mouth.

Toddler or Childhood Problems

- The child has poor posture: lordotic (swayed lower back) or kyphotic (rounded upper back).
- The child's posture may be stiff, with little or no truck rotation.
- The child walks with a board-based gait beyond normal limits.
- The child walks on his or her toes.
- The child lacks smooth transition or grading of movements. Movements may be jerky or exaggerated.
- The child may have an aversion or hypersensitivity to smells, with possible lack of differentiation among odors.
- The child is clumsy, with poor balance.
- The child has trouble with motor planning: has difficulty imitating others' movements, figuring out how to climb down, or maneuvering around objects.
- The child is able to do an activity one day but is unable to do it the next.

Cognitive

- The child hurries from one activity to another and seems unable to stay with one activity more than a few seconds.
- The child's speech is difficult to understand after age three.

Psychosocial

Infant Problems

- The infant has passive, nonexpressive facial features.
- The infant has difficulty with transitions, such as leaving caregiver or going from one activity to another.

Toddler or Childhood Problems

- The child may be overly aggressive or passive.
- The child has poor social interaction skills with peers.

Source: Reprinted with permission from G.A. DeGangi, M.M. Goodin, and S. Wietlishach, Treatment of Vestibular Deficits in Children with Developmental Disorders, in *Vestibular Rehabilitation*, S.J. Herdman, ed., p. 366, © 1994, F.A. Davis Company.

Guidelines for Vestibular Stimulation Activities

- The child should always be actively involved in the vestibular activity. Examples include pushing him- or herself on the equipment or telling the therapist when to stop or start the motion.
- Incorporate vestibular stimulation within the context of the child's movement problems such as postural control, bilateral integration, or attention and self-calming.
- Select activities that provide ocular input, because the vestibular system works optimally in conjunction with visual input. Example: dim the lights while the child navigates through a tunnel on a scooter board with a flashlight.
- Enhance proprioceptive input through the use of weighted objects, firm pressure to joints, movement against gravity, traction, or resistive activities.
- Promote adaptive movement by providing vestibular stimulation and movement in all planes and in all directions.
- Vestibular stimulation can also be varied in terms of speed, frequency, and timing.

Source: Adapted with permission from G.A. DeGangi, M.M. Goodin, and S. Wietlishach, Treatment of Vestibular Deficits in Children with Developmental Disorders, in *Vestibular Rehabilitation*, S.J. Herdman, ed., p. 366, © 1994, F.A. Davis Company.

tone may lead to poor endurance, a tendency toward slouching, or difficulty in keeping the head upright. Impaired balance and equilibrium reactions may affect riding a bicycle, rollerskating, skiing, playing hopscotch, and other functions due to a lack of centering of the trunk. If proximal musculature is not well developed, the person may be unable to maintain body postures. Poor bilateral integration may affect activities such as cutting with scissors, buttoning a shirt, or doing jumping jacks.

- Perceptual motor development: The person may have poor motor planning skills, poor lateralization, difficulty with left and right, difficulty with sequencing of motor actions.
- Observations (DeGangi et al. 1994, 370):
  1. Extraneous body movements may occur when the person attempts to hold a stable body posture due to weak muscle cocontraction.
  2. There may be fixations of the neck, trunk, and shoulders during skilled motor activities.
  3. There may be weakness of the trunk and neck when assuming antigravity posture such as prone extension and supine flexion.
  4. The person may have poor distal prehension with lack of fine fingertip prehension and controlled wrist rotation.
  5. There may be poor integration of primitive reflexes such as the asymmetrical tonic neck reflex.

Types of Equipment Useful in Providing Vestibular Input

Standing/Kneeling
- large inner tube lying flat on the floor not fully inflated
- trampoline (Note: Do not tighten fully, keep some slack.)
- glider swing
- platform swing

Sitting
- net hammock suspended from a single point (A variant is to place a ball inside the hammock. The child sits astride the ball.)
- inverted T-swing (Two bolsters placed perpendicular to each other in the shape of an upside down T-swing are suspended from the leg of the T.)
- bolster swing
- standard swing that may be adapted to provide back or side support
- glider and platform swings can be used in the sitting position also

Quadruped (All Fours)
- glider or platform swings

Prone or Supine (Lying on Stomach or Back)
- barrel suspended at both ends
- scooter board
- wheelchair or gurney
- glider
- platform swing
- net hammock
- bolster

Useful in Encouraging Equilibrium Reactions
- tilt board
- large therapy ball
- barrel lying on its side
- inflatables
- various sizes of bolsters
- ramp
- stairs
- balance board

6. The person may have ocular-motor problems including poor eye convergence and quick localization of the eyes.
7. The person may have shortened duration of postrotary nystagmus.
8. The person may have difficulty doing tasks requiring both sides of the body, lack hand dominance, not cross the midline, and confuse right and left.

Cognitive
- The person usually has difficulty with projected action sequences involving anticipation of how to move in relationship to changes in the environment, such as when moving to kick a ball or catch a ball.
- The person may have attention deficits or be easily distracted.
- The person may have difficulty following directions due to lack of laterality or poor sense of direction.
- The person may have language delays.

Psychosocial
- The person may have low stress tolerance.
- The person may have a poor self-image due to repeated failure in performing adaptive responses.
- Language and communication skills may be below age level.

TREATMENT/INTERVENTION
Treatment is based on the model of sensory integration. Vestibular stimulation is used to influence balance, muscle, oculomotor responses, movement against gravity, postural adjustments, and activity level. Linear movement such as walking and jumping are assessed to assist in determining the person's ability to acclimate to the environment by facilitating the development of an understanding of body position and movement in space. Rotary and irregular movement such as spinning, accelerating and decelerating, and playing in an unusual position are assumed to provide strong input to the system for arousal and alertness (DeGangi et al. 1994, 365).

Productivity and Leisure
- Encourage the person to try out different play activities and explore the play environment.

Sensorimotor
- Improve integration of vestibular-proprioceptive processing.
- Improve postural mechanisms.
  1. Facilitate postural tone (stability) around proximal joints and trunk flexor, oblique, and extensor groups. If the person has very low muscle tone, use compression over the shoulders while the person is placed in a prone extension posture. Use a variety of materials such as stretchy ropes, resistive therapy bands, or heavy, weighted toys.
  2. Facilitate mature righting and equilibrium reactions. Use a large ball or tilt board.
  3. Facilitate development of antigravity postural control. Use heavy work patterns involving the abdominal and neck flexors together with proximal limb muscles (e.g., climbing,

jumping, holding onto a suspended tire in a flexed position, pulling up on a chin-up bar, putting together pop beads, or using other resistive toys).

4. Facilitate use of muscle cocontraction. Use games requiring "freezing" (e.g., Simon says, make like a statue) or do activities requiring carrying weighted boxes or pushing heavy objects.

- Promote total body extension against gravity using pivot-prone and prone-extension patterns such as lying in a hammock or bolster swing or lying on a scooter board. Add acceleration in a linear direction by riding down a ramp.
- Improve weight shifting and trunk rotation with extension in response to postural challenges beginning with segmental rolling, resisted diagonal movements against gravity, rotating from prone to supine to sitting up, and resisted rolling up a ramp.
- Facilitate postural orientation and ocular convergence patterns toward midline of the body.
- Enhance midline functions of the upper extremity: increase frequency of hands coming together at midline of body to hold and explore objects using toys and activities that require power gripping (e.g., squeezing a toy) or having feet in a controlled midline position (e.g., walking in a straight line). Encourage concurrent stabilization and manipulation of toys with two hands (e.g., reaching up and across body for object held in space).
- Facilitate emergence of a preferred hand for manipulation and use of that hand to cross the midline into contralateral space.
- Promote coordination of the two sides of the body starting with activities requiring symmetric body movement (e.g., using a rolling pin, jumping on a trampoline, throwing a large ball, pushing oneself from a wall surface while swinging in a hammock).
- Move to contrast the two sides of the body in alternating movement or reciprocal patterns, such as drumming the hand in rhythms, riding a tricycle or bicycle, or walking on hands in a wheelbarrow walk.
- Move to differentiate the two body sides so that one side is used for skilled actions while the other side acts as a stabilizer using activities such as buttoning, scissor cutting, stringing beads, writing, or kicking a ball.

Cognitive

- Specific therapy is not directed at cognitive functions since the assumption of sensory integrative therapy is that improved cognitive skills will follow improved sensorimotor integration.

Psychosocial

- Permit the person to direct his or her own therapy. The therapist assists, clarifies, suggests, and provides instructions as needed but does not direct or control.

PRECAUTIONS

- Do not overstimulate the person. Avoid sensory overload.
- Keep all equipment in good working order. Make sure suspended items are well anchored in the ceiling and can take the force of the person's weight and the force of the swing motion combined.
- Keep mats or mattresses on the floor to cushion trips and falls.

- If the person has a seizure disorder, confer with a physician before using vestibular stimulation.
- To avoid injury, go slowly when challenging the equilibrium reactions.

PROGNOSIS AND OUTCOME

- The person demonstrates improved performance in daily living tasks.
- The person demonstrates improved academic performance.
- The person demonstrates an increased level of play skill.
- The person demonstrates improved motor planning skills when performing unlearned motor tasks.
- The person demonstrates improved sensory processing skills.
- The person demonstrates increased attention span and focus of attention.
- The person demonstrates improved self-control and an improved ability to organize his or her behavior to interact with people and the physical environment.

REFERENCES

Baloueff, O. 1998. Sensory integration. In *Willard and Spackman's occupational therapy*, 9th ed., eds. M.E. Neistadt and E.B. Crepeau, 546–550. Philadelphia: J.B. Lippincott. 1998.
DeGangi, G.A. et al. 1994. Treatment of vestibular deficits in children with developmental disorders. In *Vestibular rehabilitation,* ed. S.J. Herdman, 360–377. Philadelphia: F.A. Davis.

BIBLIOGRAPHY

Ellison, P.H., and J.L. Horn. 1985. Construction of an Infant Neurological International Battery (INFANIB) for the assessment of neurological integrity in infancy. *Physical Therapy* 65: 1326.
Haak, L. et al. 1993. Relationship of ocular motor skills to vestibular-related clinical observations. *Physical and Occupational Therapy in Pediatrics* 13, no. 4: 1–13.
Le Postollec, M. 1998. The sounds of healing: Therapists use the Tomatis method to stimulate the brain and improve function. *Advance for Occupational Therapy Practitioners* 14, no. 32: 34–35.
Parham, L.D., and Z. Mailloux. 1996. Sensory integration. In *Occupational therapy for children,* 3rd ed., eds. J. Case-Smith et al., 307–356. St. Louis, MO: Mosby.
Stallings-Sahler, S. 1998. Vestibular-proprioceptive-based postural dysfunction. In *Pediatric occupational therapy and early intervention*, 2nd ed., ed. J. Case-Smith, 243–246. Boston: Butterworth-Heinemann.

Sensory Integrative Dysfunction— Adaptive Movement Response Disorders: Dyspraxia

DESCRIPTION

Dyspraxia refers to a condition characterized by difficulty with praxis—the ability to conceptualize, plan, and execute a nonhabitual motor act—that cannot be explained by a medical diagnosis or developmental disability and that occurs despite ordinary environmental opportunities for motor exercises (Parham and Mailloux 1996, 329). Dyspraxia is a difficulty with the planning and execution of movement patterns of a skilled or nonhabitual nature, originating in childhood (Baloueff 1998, 548). Dyspraxia is also called developmental apraxia, developmental dyspraxia, or motor planning disorder.

Motor planning involves generating an idea for a nonhabitual task, sequencing the idea, and executing the sequence efficiently and smoothly without thinking or watching the movement. For example, a child sees a riding toy for the first time and thinks about how to interact with it. Next the person moves toward the toy, mounts it, and begins to move. Finally the person successfully carries out the idea of interacting with the toy (Arkwright 1998, 15).

CAUSE

The cause is unknown. The person's brain is dysfunctional so that it hinders the organization of tactile, vestibular, and proprioceptive sensation and interferes with the ability to plan motor activities. The problem begins early in life and may continue into adulthood.

ASSESSMENT

Areas
- reflex development and maturation
- constructional praxis (ability to put parts together to form a unified single object, often a three-dimensional model, also called visuomotor ability, perceptuomotor ability, or visuoconstructive ability)
- design copying praxis (ability to reproduce or copy a design; sometimes used as an alternate term for constructional praxis, but two-dimensional as opposed to three)
- postural praxis (ability to imitate positions)
- oral praxis (ability to imitate movements and positions of tongue, mouth, and cheek)
- manual expressions or symbolic praxis (ability to pretend to use objects while looking at pictures of the objects).
- sequencing praxis (ability to order a sequence of movements or make transitions from one position to another)
- verbal command praxis (ability to perform learned gestures purely on verbal command)
- vestibular processing (ability to use postural reflexes)
- tactile processing (ability to use stereognosis and finger or joint localization)
- proprioceptive processing (ability to use postural control)
- visual and auditory processing (ability to use figure-ground perception)
- daily living skills
- play skills

Instruments
Instruments Developed by Occupational Therapy Personnel
- *DeGangi-Berk Test of Sensory Integration* (DBTSI) by G.A. DeGangi and R.A. Berk, Los Angeles: Western Psychological Services, 1983.

- *FirstSTEp Screening Test for Evaluating Preschoolers* by L.J. Miller, San Antonio, TX: The Psychological Corporation, 1993.
- *Hawaii Early Learning Profile* (HELP), rev. ed. by S. Furuno et al., Palo Alto, CA: VORT Corporation, 1985.
- *In-Hand Manipulation Test* by C.E. Exner, in Content validity of the In-Hand Manipulation Test, *American Journal of Occupational Therapy* 47, no. 6 (1993): 505–513.
- *Miller Assessment for Preschoolers* (MAP) by L.J. Miller, San Antonio, TX: The Psychological Corporation, 1988.
- *Pediatric Evaluation of Disability Inventory* by S.M. Haley et al., Boston: New England Medical Center Hospital, 1992.
- *Sensory Integration and Praxis Tests* by A.J. Ayres, Los Angeles: Western Psychological Services, 1989. (Low scores on postural praxis, sequencing praxis, oral praxis, praxis on verbal command, finger identification [FI], graphesthesia, localization of tactile stimuli [LTS], and manual form perception [MFP] indicate dyspraxia. Crossing midline of body [CML] score is often better than the crossing midline of body with the hand score [CMLX].)
- *Test of Sensory Functions in Infants* (TSFI) by G.A. DeGangi and S.I. Greenspan, Los Angeles: Western Psychological Services, 1989.

Instruments Developed by Other Professionals and Used by Occupational Therapy Personnel

- *Bayley Scales of Infant Development-II* (BSID-II) by N. Bayley, San Antonio, TX: The Psychological Corporation, 1993.

PROBLEMS

Types

There are many different types of dyspraxia.

- somatodyspraxia: a sensory integrative deficit that involves poor praxis as well as impaired tactile and proprioceptive processing (Parham and Mailloux 1996, 329)
- postural dyspraxia: the inability to plan and imitate large body movements and meaningless postures
- sequencing dyspraxia: difficulty making transitions from one motor action to another and sequencing movements
- oral and verbal dyspraxia: inability to produce oral movements on verbal command or in imitation, a skill that affects speech articulation
- constructional dyspraxia: inability to create and assemble three-dimensional structures
- graphic dyspraxia: inability to plan and execute drawings (DeGangi et al. 1993, 373)

Self-Care

- The person may have difficulty performing some activities of daily living or be delayed in acquiring such skills as putting on and taking off clothes and using fasteners such as buttons and zippers.

Productivity and Leisure

- The person tends to have poor manipulatory play skills (often ends up breaking or damaging toys).

- The person may have difficulty organizing play activities when alone.
- The person cannot do activities or tasks in a group situation without help from adults.
- The person has trouble with toys that are designed to be assembled, such as construction toys.

Sensorimotor
- The person may have awkward body movements.
- The person may seem clumsy.
- The person cannot identify the exact place on the body where he or she has been touched when vision is occluded.
- The person has difficulty imitating body postures.
- The person may lack body awareness.
- The person may seem weak and have low endurance.
- The person has trouble sequencing movements, such as in jumping jacks.
- The person has difficulty planning and making drawings.

Cognitive
- The person may be easily distracted from a task or seem to have difficulty maintaining attention to and concentration on task.
- The person may have poor ideational or concept formation skills.
- The person may have poor skills in planning ahead, including sequencing and timing.
- The person may have difficulty following verbal instructions, especially when given a series of instructions or when a single instruction requires that a series of tasks be performed.
- The person may have difficulty with problem solving.
- The person may have difficulty learning motor games and sports.
- The person may have difficulty learning new tasks.
- The person may have messy handwriting.
- The person may have difficulty with reception and understanding of language.

Psychosocial
- The person tends to be accident prone.
- The person may be easily hurt emotionally.
- The person may not tolerate changes in plans and expectations.
- The person tends to be stubborn, inflexible, or uncooperative.
- The person may have poor coping skills.
- The person usually has a poor self-concept and lacks a sense of mastery.
- The person may be emotionally labile.
- The person may need more protection than others do.

Environment
- When placed in a new situation, the person may not show interest in exploring the surroundings.

TREATMENT/INTERVENTION
Therapy for this condition is based on the model of sensory integration. Techniques are aimed at improving ideation and planning. Improvements in execution are assumed to follow.

Self-Care
- Guide parents to expect performance within the person's ability level, starting with the simplest activities the person can perform and increasing the level of difficulty.
- Help parents learn to model or demonstrate.

Productivity
- Guide teachers to expect performance within the person's ability level.
- Play activities may need to be modified to include the person.

Leisure
- Leisure skills should improve as praxis skills improve.
- Assist the person in exploring leisure interests.

Sensorimotor
- Somatodyspraxia: Use novel activities such as jumping off a low stool into a big pillow.
- Postural dyspraxia: Use whole body motor patterns, such as total flexion, total extension, rotation, and gross diagonal rotary patterns. Activities include going through an obstacle course or tunnel on a scooter board and aiming an object to knock down a tower.
- Sequencing dyspraxia: Use motor activities with differing demands for timing and sequencing of movements and observe the person's transition from one position or aspect of a task to another.
- Dyspraxia on verbal command: Speak slowly, use simple phrases (key words), and ask the person to verbalize what is to be done in the activity and what was done after the activity.
- Oral dyspraxia: General sensory stimulation may be given with various textured objects placed against the skin, such as cloths and brushes. Vibrators, popsicles, and honey dippers may be used in the mouth. Licking stickers and blowing bubbles may be used for orofacial tasks.
- Constructional dyspraxia: Use activities for postural dyspraxia, resetting the obstacle course or rebuilding the tower, for instance.
- Design copying dyspraxia: Practice with tracing, going from dot to dot, outlining, or coloring hidden figures.
- Provide tactile, vestibular, and proprioceptive input selectively and in combination. For sensory dysfunctions such as gravitational insecurity, tactile defensiveness, and vestibular-bilateral disorder, see specific sections for treatment programs.
- Focus visual direction on the body part by pointing, tapping, or offering verbal reminders.

Cognitive
- Help the person develop the conceptual organization of the skill or task.
- Help the person select and plan activities by modeling or demonstrating, asking questions, offering solutions, or suggesting alternatives (i.e., work toward independent problem solving).
- Help the person execute the plan.

Psychosocial
- Provide tasks that are challenging but can be completed successfully (i.e., support the development of a positive self-image and a sense of mastery).

- Interact with the person as a helper or assistant, not as an authority figure.
- Interact with the person to observe whether the task is too easy or difficult.
- Reward success but do not punish failure. Examine failure to determine what modifications are needed to provide success.

PRECAUTIONS

- Always monitor during tactile and vestibular stimulation for signs of overload.
- Do not attempt to change hand dominance if the person shows a preference for one hand over the other.

PROGNOSIS AND OUTCOME

- The person is able to perform self-care activities independently.
- The person is able to organize a play situation or leisure activity without assistance.
- The person demonstrates improved praxis (motor planning) skills.
- The person demonstrates improved performance of gross motor skills, such as running, jumping, hopping, and skipping.
- The person demonstrates improved performance of fine motor skills, including manipulation and dexterity.
- The person has established a preference for use of one eye, hand, foot, or side of body and consistently uses that eye, hand, foot, or side of body in performing the same or similar tasks.
- The person's processing of sensory information is in the normal range.
- The person is able to follow a series of instructions.
- The person is able to tolerate changes in plans or expectations without becoming upset; coping skills are improved.
- The person is able to perform tasks in a group setting without supervision.

REFERENCES

Arkwright, N. 1998. *An Introduction to Sensory Integration.* San Antonio, TX: Therapy Skill Builders.
Baloueff, O. 1998. Sensory integration. In *Willard and Spackman's occupational therapy,* 9th ed., eds. M.E. Neistadt and E.B. Crepeau, 546–550. Philadelphia: J.B. Lippincott. 1998.
DeGangi, G.A. et al. 1993. A comparison of structured sensorimotor therapy and child-centered activity in the treatment of preschool children with sensorimotor problems. *American Journal of Occupational Therapy* 47, no. 9: 777–786.
Parham, L.D., and Z. Mailloux. 1996. Sensory integration. In *Occupational therapy for children,* 3rd ed., eds. J. Case-Smith et al., 307–356. St. Louis, MO: Mosby.

BIBLIOGRAPHY

Chia, S.H. 1997. The child, his family, and dyspraxia. *Professional Care of Mother and Child* 7, no. 4: 105–107.
Cool, S.J. 1994. Praxis, lapsis, and sensorimotor integration. *Sensory Integration Special Interest Section Newsletter* 17, no. 4: 3–4.
Coster, W. et al. 1995. Therapist-child interaction during sensory integration treatment: Development and testing of a research tool. *Occupational Therapy Journal of Research* 15, no. 1: 17–35.

Dewey, D. 1995. What is developmental dyspraxia? *Brain and Cognition* 29: 254–274. (Author is not an occupational therapist.)

Exner, C.E. 1993. Content validity of the In-Hand Manipulation Test. *American Journal of Occupational Therapy* 47, no. 6: 505–513.

Hawley, V. 1992. Sensory integrative therapy and the dyspraxic child: A single case study. *Sensory Integration Special Interest Section Newsletter* 15, no. 4: 7–8.

Jarus, T., and D. Gol. 1995. The effect of kinesthetic stimulation on the acquisition and retention of a gross motor skill by children with and without sensory integration disorders. *Physical and Occupational Therapy in Pediatrics* 14, no. 3/4: 59–73.

Lai, J. et al. 1996. Construct validity of the Sensory Integration and Praxis Tests. *Occupational Therapy Journal of Research* 16, no. 2: 75–97.

Missiuna, C., and H. Polatajko. 1995. Developmental dyspraxia by any other name: Are they all just clumsy children? *American Journal of Occupational Therapy* 49, no. 7: 619–627.

Poole, J.L. et al. 1997. The mechanisms for adult-onset apraxia and developmental dyspraxia. *American Journal of Occupational Therapy* 51, no. 5: 339–346.

Stahl, C. 1995. The ongoing debate over sensory integration. *Advance for Occupational Therapists* 11, no. 25: 11, 17.

Stallings-Sahler, S. 1998. Emergent developmental dyspraxia. In *Pediatric occupational therapy and early intervention*, 2nd ed., ed. J. Case-Smith, 246–248. Boston: Butterworth-Heinemann.

Sensory Integrative Dysfunction— Sensory Discrimination and Perceptual Disorders

DESCRIPTION

Sensory discrimination is the ability to distinguish between different sensory stimuli. The term usually refers to the ability to make fine distinctions between stimuli of one sensory modality, such as discriminating between two points of tactile contact or differentiating between similar sounds (Parham and Mailloux 1996, 353). Perception is described as the organization of sensory data into meaningful units of information (Parham and Mailloux 1996, 353). Examples include stereognosis, which is a type of tactile input that permits a person to recognize an object by touching or feeling the object, usually with the fingers or hand, although other parts of the body can be used.

Discrimination and perception allow for refinement of the organization and interpretation of sensory input. Problems in discrimination and perception lead to inefficient or inaccurate organization and/or interpretation of the sensory information. Although problems in discrimination and perception often coexist with problems in sensory modulation, the two sets of problems are not inherently tied together. A person may have problems in discrimination or perception without showing signs of sensory modulation disorders (Parham and Mailloux 1996, 327).

Often perception is related to motor activity since motor output may confirm the efficiency or accuracy of the perception. Therefore, other terms that cover similar problems presented in this section are perceptual-motor, perceptomotor, and visual-perceptual-motor.

Visual perception includes visual discrimination, visual memory, visual spatial relationships, form constancy, sequential memory, figure-ground, and closure (Erhardt and Duckman 1997, 138).

CAUSE

Disorders associated with discrimination and perceptual disorders in children are autism, cerebral palsy, learning disabilities, prematurity, psychiatric disorders, traumatic head injury, stroke, and tumor.

ASSESSMENT

Areas

- sensory awareness and responsiveness
- visual attention: alertness, selection attention, ambient/peripheral attention, vigilance, shared attention
- visual memory: short-term and long-term memory
- visual discrimination/pattern recognition
- visual recognition: matching, categorization
- visual form (object) perception: form constancy, visual closure, figure-ground
- visual imagery (visualization)
- spatial perception: position in space, depth perception, topographical orientation
- auditory discrimination and perception
- tactile discrimination and perception
- proprioceptive discrimination and perception
- vestibular discrimination and perception
- gustatory discrimination and perception
- olfactory discrimination and perception
- integration skills: visual motor integration (eye-hand coordination)

Instruments

There is no instrument for directly measuring proprioception. Problems in proprioception must be inferred from clinical observation. No specific tests for measuring auditory, tactile, proprioception, vestibular, gustatory discrimination, and perception were identified.

Instruments Developed by Occupational Therapy Personnel

- *Checklist of Observable Clues to Classroom Vision Problems* by C.M. Schneck, in Visual perception, *Occupational therapy for children,* 3rd ed., eds. J. Case-Smith, A.S. Allen, P.N. Pratt, 365, St. Louis, MO: Mosby, 1996.
- *Erhardt Developmental Vision Assessment,* rev. ed. by R.P. Erhardt, San Antonio, TX: Therapy Skill Builders, 1990.
- *Observational Checklist of Visual Symptoms Associated with Visual Problems* by M.J. Bouska, N.A. Kauffman, and S.E. Marcus, in Disorders of the visual perceptual system, *Neurological rehabilitation*, 2nd ed., ed. D.A. Umphred, 711, St. Louis, MO: Mosby, 1990.

- *Pediatric Clinical Vision Screening for Occupational Therapists* by M. Scheirman, Elkins Park, PA: Pennsylvania College of Optometry, 1997.
- *Sensorimotor Performance Analysis* by E. Richter and P. Montgomery, San Antonio, TX: Therapy Skill Builders, 1989.
- *Sensory Integration and Praxis Tests* by A.J. Ayres, Los Angeles: Western Psychological Services, 1989.

Instruments Developed by Other Professionals and Used by Occupational Therapy Personnel

- *The Beery-Buktenica Developmental Test of Visual-Motor Integration* (VMI-4), 4th ed. by K.E. Beery and N.A. Buktenica, Parsippany, NJ: Modern Curriculum Press, 1997.
- *Benton Visual Retention Test* by A.L. Benton, San Antonio, TX: The Psychological Corporation, 1974.
- *Crane-Wick Test* by A. Crane and B. Wick, Houston, TX: Rapid Research Corporation, 1987.
- *Developmental Test of Visual Perception-2* (DTVP-2) by D.D. Hammill, N.A. Pearson, and J.K. Voress, Austin, TX: Pro-ed, 1993.
- *Matching Familiar Figures Test* by E. Cairns and T. Cammock, *Developmental Psychology* 14 (1978): 555.
- *Memory for Designs Test—Revised* by F.K. Graham and B.S. Kendall, *Perceptual Motor Skills* (Monograph Supplement 2-VII) 11 (1960): 11–20.
- *Motor-Free Visual Perception Test–Revised* by R.P. Colarusso and D.D. Hamill, Novato, CA: Academic Therapy Publications, 1996.
- *Reversals Frequency Test* by R.A. Gardner, Cresskill, NJ: Creative Therapeutics, 1978.
- *Test of Pictures-Forms-Letters-Numbers-Spatial Orientation & Sequencing Skills* by M.F. Gardner, Hydesville, CA: Psychological and Educational Publications, 1992.
- *Test of Visual-Perceptual Skills—Revised* (TVPS-R) by M.F. Gardner, Hydesville, CA: Psychological and Educational Publications, 1996.
- *Visual Screening Based on Classroom Behaviors by Optometric Extension Program Foundation,* reproduced in C.M. Schneck, Intervention for visual perception problems, *Occupational therapy: Making a difference in school system practice,* ed. J. Case-Smith, lesson 5:16. Bethesda, MD: American Occupational Therapy Association, 1998.

PROBLEMS

Note: Although the problems are presented individually by sensory modality, they often appear together. Visual and tactile problems are a common combination.

Self-Care

- The person has difficulty performing self-care tasks. For example, the person may be unable to button a shirt or blouse without using vision to compensate for poor tactile discrimination.

Productivity and Leisure

- The person has difficulty with building things and doing puzzles.

Sensorimotor

- visual discrimination and perception
  1. The person may bump into things.
  2. The person may lack personal space boundaries.
  3. The person has a disorganized position in space (e.g., runs out of space on paper and has difficulty lining up numbers).
  4. The person may have difficulty maintaining eye contact.
  5. The person may have difficulty with depth perception.
  6. The person may have difficulty recognizing and drawing letters, numbers, and shapes.
  7. The person has difficulty moving around and between objects guided by vision.
  8. The person may have difficulty with eye-hand or eye-foot coordination when guided by vision.
  9. The person may have difficulty with reach, grasp, and release (prehension) skills when guided by vision.
- auditory discrimination and perception
  1. The person may be hyper- or hyposensitive to sounds.
  2. The person may not be able to focus on foreground sounds while blocking out extraneous background sounds.
  3. The person may have difficulty with temporal or spatial relations.
  4. The person may have poor ability to use auditory system for information gathering in spite of normal hearing.
- tactile or haptic discrimination and perception
  1. The person may have difficulty differentiating objects haptically or identifying objects accurately by touch.
  2. The person may have poor two-point discrimination.
  3. The person may have poor conscious proprioception (kinesthesia).
  4. The person may have poor differentiation of touch for information gathering.
- proprioception discrimination and perception
  1. The person does not receive reliable information about body position.
  2. The person may appear clumsy, distracted, or awkward.
  3. The person has difficulty judging or is unable to judge force, velocity, or direction of movements accurately.
  4. The person tends to misjudge personal space and bump into others.
- vestibular (gravity) discrimination and perception
  1. The person may have difficulty when changes are needed in head or body orientation.
  2. The person may have difficulty when changes are needed in equilibrium/balance responses.
- other problems
  1. The person may have a sensory modulation problem. In particular, sensory defensiveness may be present.
  2. The person may have perceptual problems in more than one sensory system. Visual and tactile perceptual problems, for instance, often coexist.
  3. The person's motor skills, especially fine motor skills, may be affected by the sensory discrimination and perceptual problems.

Cognitive
- The person has poor handwriting.
- The person may confuse the letters *b* and *d*, *b* and *p*, or *d* and *q* and words such as *was* and *saw*, *on* and *no*.
- The person may avoid reading, writing, or drawing.
- The person has difficulty pronouncing words.
- The person has difficulty using prepositions correctly in speech (words such as *in front, through, under, beside*).
- The person may have difficulty remembering and sequencing multi-step directions.
- The person may appear inattentive or confused.
- The person may have difficulty with sequencing of verbal direction.
- The person may confuse words that sound similar, such as *doll* and *tall*.

Psychosocial
- The person may have trouble hearing in a group situation because of difficulty with focusing auditory attention.

Environment
- The person may get lost easily.

TREATMENT/INTERVENTION

Models of treatment interventions include sensory integration, developmental approaches, perceptual-motor approaches, auditory integration training, motor control theory, neurodevelopmental treatment, and the model of human occupation. Teachers, optometrists, neurophysiologists, and psychologists have all developed models of intervention for discrimination and perceptual training.

Sensorimotor
- Facilitate development of visual perception by working on foundational skills.
  1. tactile perception and manipulation such as drawing in sand, feeling shapes, and identifying objects by looking at them
  2. vestibular input such as moving over, under, through, and around objects, stimulating gravity receptors
  3. proprioceptive input such as having the client lie prone on a scooter board going down a ramp
- Facilitate specific visual perceptual skills.
  1. organization of forms in space activities, including fitting small objects into containers of different sizes
  2. visual memory activities, including showing the person an object, shape, or symbol for five seconds, then covering it and asking the person to name the objects or identify a similar object from among several items
  3. visual sequencing activities, including stringing beads from a picture of a sequence of beads
  4. visual motor activities, including following a pattern to make a design

5. visual motor integration activities, including throwing at a target (balls, darts), kicking at a target, jumping and landing on a target (hopscotch or "parachute jump"), and playing parachute games (running into the open space)
6. figure-ground discrimination activities, including picking out all of one color or shape from a box of assorted pegs, beads, or shapes; arranging blocks of one color in a pattern surrounded by blocks of another color; putting together puzzles with backgrounds that compete with the foreground; or locating hidden figures in line drawings
7. form and shape constancy activities, including sorting buttons by shape, color, or size; stringing beads of one shape that vary in size or color; using form board puzzles that outline shapes or objects; and copying Peg-Board forms or dot-to-dot forms
8. position-in-space activities, including stringing beads in a specified sequence, copying a set of blocks (four, six, or nine) with colors in the correct position, doing puzzles that require rotation to get the pieces to fit in the space, copying Peg-Board designs that emphasize left versus right or top versus bottom, and playing games such as dominos or tanograms
9. spatial relations activities, including copying pattern cards showing different shapes and sizes, copying pattern cards showing three-dimensional block designs, putting together interlocking puzzles, and copying abstract designs
10. body schema activities, including using obstacle courses, playing Simon says, doing the hokeypokey, and passing a beanbag behind the back or under the knee

- Facilitate auditory skills.
  1. Simplify directions. Give one direction at a time. Use short, simple phrases when giving directions. Make physical and visual contact with the person, wait for a response, and then have the person repeat the directions that were given.
- Facilitate proprioception skills.
  1. Use a variety of postures, such as being prone, side lying, sitting, and standing.
- Facilitate vestibular skills.
  1. Facilitate vestibular system with activities such as swinging, bouncing, spinning, bending over to touch toes, and swaying side to side with arms overhead like tree limbs.
  2. Provide vestibular stimulation through activities such as rocking or jumping on inner tubes.

Cognitive

- Teach the person to be an active and effective problem solver by encouraging experimentation and analysis.
- Provide opportunities for information processing from all sensory channels.
- Emphasize beginnings (initiation) and endings (termination) of movements.
- Assist person in judging movement patterns based on discrimination and perception by using terms like "efficient" or "inefficient" rather than "right" or "wrong."
- Facilitate generalization of tasks through variations in speed, direction, weight, size, shape, texture, and context.

Psychosocial

- Increase person's sense of independence and self-control by gradually reducing verbal and manual assistance.

- Increase person's ability to self-evaluate performance by tapering off external feedback and reinforcement by others.
- Increase the person's sense of competence by requiring practice in a variety of environments.

PRECAUTIONS

- Watch for signs of overstimulation.
- Watch for signs of overstressed coping skills, such as frustration behavior.
- Perceptual problems in children are not consistent from day to day. Expect to see uneven performance—performance that is better one day and worse the next. Illness frequently increases, temporarily, the severity of the perceptual disorder.
- Perceptual disorders in vision may distort perception of height. Make the person aware of heights from which it is unsafe to jump.

PROGNOSIS AND OUTCOME

The degree of progress is variable because of the variety of possible problems.
- The person demonstrates improved ability to perform self-care tasks independently.
- The person demonstrates improvement in play skills such as increased variety of play activities.
- The person demonstrates improved performance in academic tasks.
- The person shows improved ability to discriminate in selected sensory systems.
- The person shows improved performance on tasks requiring perceptual skills.
- The person is able to use compensatory techniques as taught.

REFERENCES

Erhardt, R.P., and R.H. Duckman. 1997. Visual-perceptual-motor dysfunction. In *Functional visual behavior: A therapist's guide to evaluation and treatment options*, ed. M. Gentile, 133–195. Bethesda, MD: American Occupational Therapy Association.
Parham, L.D., and Z. Mailloux. 1996. Sensory integration. In *Occupational therapy for children,* 3rd ed., eds. J. Case-Smith et al., 307–356. St. Louis, MO: Mosby.

BIBLIOGRAPHY

Arkwright, N. 1998. *An Introduction to Sensory Integration*. San Antonio, TX: Therapy Skill Builders.
Burpee, J.D. 1997. Sensory integration and visual functions. In *Functional visual behavior: A therapist's guide to evaluation and treatment options*, ed. M. Gentile, 87–104. Bethesda, MD: American Occupational Therapy Association.
Efferson, L. 1995. Disorders of vision and visual perceptual dysfunction. In *Neurological rehabilitation*, 3rd ed., ed. D.A. Umphred, 769–801. St. Louis, MO: Mosby.
Frick, S.M., and N. Lawton-Shirley. 1994. Auditory integrative training from a sensory integrative perspective. *Sensory Integration Special Interest Section Newsletter* 17, no. 4: 1–3.
Kimbell, J.G. 1993. Sensory integrative frame of reference. In *Frames of reference for pediatric occupational therapy*, eds. P. Kramer and J. Hinjosa, 87–175. Baltimore: Williams & Wilkins.

Loikith, C.C. 1997. Visual perception: Development, assessment, and intervention. In *Functional visual behavior: A therapist's guide to evaluation and treatment options*, ed. M. Gentile, 197–247. Bethesda, MD: American Occupational Therapy Association.

Okoye, R. 1997. Neuromotor prerequisites of functional vision. In *Functional visual behavior: A therapist's guide to evaluation and treatment options*, ed. M. Gentile, 55–86. Bethesda, MD: American Occupational Therapy Association.

Penso, D. 1993. *Percepto-Motor Difficulties*. London: Chapman & Hall.

Schneck, C.M. 1996. Visual perception. In *Occupational therapy for children*, 3rd ed., eds. J. Case-Smith et al., 357–386. St. Louis, MO: Mosby.

Schneck, C.M. 1998. Intervention for visual perception problems. In *Occupational therapy: Making a difference in school system practice: A self-paced clinical course*, ed. J. Case-Smith, Lesson 5. Bethesda, MD: American Occupational Therapy Association.

Wallen, M., and R. Walker. 1995. Occupational therapy practice with children with perceptual motor dysfunction: Findings of a literature review and survey. *Australian Occupational Therapy Journal* 42, no. 1: 15–25.

Part II

Sensory Disorders

Back Pain

DESCRIPTION

The most common site of back pain is in the low lumbar, lumbosacral, or sacroiliac region. It is often accompanied by sciatica, pain radiating down one or both buttocks or legs in the distribution of the sciatic nerve. *Regional low back pain* generally refers to pain to the leg above the knee and includes diagnoses of lumbar, lumbosacral, or sacroiliac pain plus strain, sprain, myofascial syndrome, musculoligamentous injury, soft tissue injury, spondylosis, and other diagnoses for pain believed to originate in the discs, ligaments, muscles, or other soft tissues of the lumbar spine or sacroiliac joints. *Radicular pain, with or without regional low back pain, with static or no neurologic deficit* refers to pain in the leg below the knee believed to originate with irritation of a nerve root in the lumbar spine and includes the diagnoses of sciatica; lumbar or lumbosacral radiculopathy, radiculitis, or neuritis; displacement or herniation of intervertebral disc with myelopathy, radiculopathy, radiculitis, or neuritis; and spinal stenosis with myelopathy, radiculopathy, radiculitis, or neuritis. *Radicular pain, with or without regional low back pain, with progressive neurologic deficit* refers to low back pain when there is a history of progressive deterioration in the neurologic symptoms and physical findings that include worsening sensory loss, increasing muscle weakness, or progressive reflex changes. Cauda equina syndrome is characterized by lack of sensation in the buttocks, genitalia, or thigh and accompanied by dysfunction of the bowel and bladder (Larson 1996).

CAUSE

Many factors may produce low back pain. It may be caused by acute ligamentous (sprain) or muscular (strain) problems, which tend to be self-limited. More chronic conditions include fibromuscular, osteoarthritic, or ankylosing spondylitic processes of the lumbosacral area. Back pain can be influenced by chronic poor-quality or deficient sleep, fatigue, physical deconditioning, or psychosocial problems and conflicts that alter the person's perception, behavior, and reporting of pain as well as the resultant degree of dysfunction, disability, and response to therapy. The prevalence of low back pain tends to increase with age, reaching 50 percent in persons 60 years and older (Merck 1999, 475–476).

ASSESSMENT

Areas

- self-care skills
- work and productivity
- leisure skills and interests
- motor skills: range of motion, muscle strength, gross coordination and movement
- postural control: postural alignment
- physical endurance and tolerance to activity

- soft tissue integrity
- location of pain
- role performance
- interpersonal skills
- self-expression
- self-control
- coping skills
- time management skills
- physical and social environment

Instruments

Instruments Developed by Occupational Therapy Personnel

- *Oswestry Low Back Pain Disability Index* by J.C.T. Fairback et al., *Physiotherapy* 66 (1980): 271–273.

Instruments Developed by Other Professionals and Used by Occupational Therapy Personnel

- *Chronic Disability Index* by G. Waddell and C.J. Main, in Assessment of severity in low-back disorders, *Spine* 9 (1984): 204–208.
- *Coping Strategy Questionnaire* by A.K. Rosestiel and F.J. Keefe, in The use of coping strategies in chronic low back pain patients: Relationship to patient characteristics and current adjustment, *Pain* 17 (1983): 33–44.
- *Movement and Pain Perceptions Scale* by J.R. Council et al., in Expectations and functional impairment in chronic low back pain, *Pain* 33 (1988): 323–331.
- *Pain Disability Index* by R.C. Tait, J.T. Chinall, and S.J. Krause, in The pain disability index: Psychometric properties, *Pain* 40 (1990): 171–182.

PROBLEMS

Self-Care

- The person is unable to perform specific activities of daily living independently.
- The person's overall health status may be worse than before.

Productivity

- The person may be unable to serve as a provider, as a parent, as a homemaker, or in another role.
- The person is often unable to do the lifting required by his or her job.
- The person may be unable or barely able to perform job duties or participate in vocational activities.
- The person may be unable to seek a job.

Leisure

- The person cannot perform leisure activities that he or she used to enjoy regularly.

Sensorimotor

- The person may have loss of or decrease in motor skills, muscle strength, and range of motion.
- The person may have difficulty maintaining postural control and alignment.
- The person may have decreased physical endurance for handling materials.
- The person may experience loss of functional mobility.
- The person may use more force and exertion than is needed to perform tasks, which adds to fatigue, and fail to follow safe handling techniques.
- The person may experience poor proprioception.

Cognitive

- The person is usually aware of a change in status but may not have the flexible thinking strategies needed to resolve problems.

Psychosocial

- The person may experience low self-esteem as a result of loss of independence.
- The person may become depressed over loss of roles and income.
- The person may have reduced coping skills.
- The person may experience a loss of self-control.
- The person may experience conflicts with family and friends.

Environment

- The person may experience criticism from family members, friends, coworkers, or employers who do not understand the decreased physical abilities and ongoing pain.
- The person may experience difficulty with time management.

TREATMENT/INTERVENTION

Treatment of low back pain often involves an interdisciplinary team using a biomechanical, compensatory, or cognitive/behavioral approach. Specific treatment programs include work conditioning and work hardening. Work conditioning/tolerance uses physical conditioning and functional activities related to the person's job. Work hardening is designed to restore an individual's physical, behavioral, and vocational functions using an interdisciplinary model. Work hardening addresses issues such as productivity, safety, physical tolerance, and work behavior (Larson 1996).

Self-Care

- Teach the person to kneel or use a half-kneeling position when performing self-care activities that require static bending in the standing position, such as brushing teeth at the bathroom sink.
- Teach the person safe lifting techniques at home (e.g., how to safely lift grocery bags from the trunk of a car or back of a van).
  1. Visually assess the load before attempting to lift it to ensure the load is of a manageable size and weight.
  2. Stand close to the load, facing the direction to be traveled, with feet slightly apart (or one slightly ahead of the other) and toes angled outward.

3. Keep the head up and the back straight (no tail raising).
4. Bend at the hips and knees using the hip extensors.
5. Grasp the load firmly at the base and center it as close to the body as possible.
6. Test the weight by raising the load slightly before making the full lift. If it is too heavy, rearrange the load or get help.
7. Lift by straightening the knees.
8. Keep the back straight at all times, and do not twist when bending, lifting, or setting load down.
9. Carry load close to the body using the arms to hold the items at waist height. If two loads are carried, distribute weight evenly as close to the sides of the body as possible.

- Teach good lying-down postures and explore sleeping habits with the person to arrive at the best sleeping positions and right amount of sleep per night.
- Teach good sitting posture and explore if some self-care tasks could be done in sitting rather than standing position.
- Teach good sitting posture for driving a car and techniques for getting into and out of the car.
- Teach the person how to use assistive devices to increase independence in activities of daily living.

Productivity
- Assist the person in determining safe changes of position during meal preparation in the kitchen. Also consider helping the person select quick and easy-to-prepare meals that save energy and time but provide adequate nutrition. Meals can be prepared ahead for days when the person does not feel like fixing anything.
- Teach energy conservation, pacing skills, and work simplification techniques.
- Consider rearranging storage of home items to avoid bending, twisting, and lifting as much as possible.
- Teach the person how to be safe while performing job-related tasks.
- Encourage the person to review work patterns at the job or at home to reduce lifting and improve work efficiency. Consider if sitting, sliding, pushing, pulling, or using an external lifting device could safely replace manual lifting. Consider if repositioning the person or task could reduce the amount of reaching required. Consider if reordering the sequence of tasks or moving tasks to another location would reduce the energy requirement. Consider ways to counteract boredom and reduce loss of task focus by changing positions or alternating tasks more frequently.
- Explore with the person possible work modifications such as using a lighter mophead, an extended handle on a mop or broom, and a trashcan with wheels to eliminate lifting.
- Teach the person how to have effective, long stretching breaks and how frequently the breaks should occur.
- Encourage the person to take brief stretching breaks every 20 minutes when performing repetitive tasks such as vacuuming.
- Consider if ergonomic principles and ergonomically designed furniture and work areas would reduce low back pain.
- Use task simulation to teach the person how to minimize spinal stress and assess tolerance for work tasks.

Leisure
- Help the person return to previously enjoyed leisure activities or explore new ones that may reduce the possibility of reinjury or aggravation to the low back.
- Have the person report participation in one leisure activity each time the person is seen in the clinic.

Sensorimotor
- During acute phase of illness or after surgery, the person may need to learn how to maintain or to avoid certain postures and positions.
- Teach good body mechanics for tasks that require lifting and turning, such as getting a child out of a car seat. Show the difference between faulty body mechanics and poor postures, with specific tasks and practice to correct techniques.
- Teach good body mechanics or alternate strategies for tasks requiring bending and stooping.
- Encourage the person to use just the right amount of force and exertion to perform a given task.
- Increase muscle strength, range of motion, and endurance to improve performance through progressive repetitive tasks.
- Improve postural alignment and postural control to enhance performance.

Cognitive
- Help the person to apply safe work practices in other environments, such as the yard, garden, golf course, shopping center, or community center.
- Help the person focus less on pain and more on functional movement.

Psychosocial
- Help the person identify and reduce psychological and socioeconomic pressures that might interfere with recovery.
- Increase the person's confidence, self-esteem, and self-concept by showing the person that tasks can be performed with no or minimal pain and maximum safety.
- Help the person identify important roles and role performance criteria.
- Improve the person's coping skills and sense of self-control by teaching relaxation techniques.
- Encourage the person to interact with family by requiring the person to report at least one interaction each time the person is seen in the clinic.

Environment
- Encourage the person and his or her spouse to attend an educational session on sexuality and back pain.
- Teach work safety to all employees at the person's work site.
- Teach the person time management skills by helping him or her develop a daily and weekly calendar of tasks and check off when the tasks are completed.
- Help the person decide on the best times to do activities during the day (e.g., when energy is greatest and medication reduces pain the most).
- Help the person evaluate furniture and other devices to determine if another item would enable the person to have better posture, offer better support, or reduce fatigue and pain.

PRECAUTIONS
- Unresolved low back pain may lead to failure of the person to resume work activities and/ or a decrease in productivity. Addressing all aspects of the individual's life is important.
- Pain may have become the dominant factor in the person's life. Focusing on work and productivity takes the emphasis away from pain.
- Be aware that pain medications may make the person drowsy and decrease motivation to do anything, including eat. Medications may also be interfering with sleep cycles.

PROGNOSIS AND OUTCOME
- The person is able to perform self-care activities without pain or aggravation of existing condition.
- The person is able to work at least part-time or participate in a volunteer activity.
- The person reports that he or she has participated in leisure activities.
- The person demonstrates safe lifting techniques at work, at home, and in community settings.
- The person demonstrates good postural alignment and control in performance of daily tasks.
- The person demonstrates use of energy conservation, work modification, and work simplification techniques.
- The person performs expected roles to the satisfaction of the person and others.
- The person demonstrates effective coping and stress management skills.

REFERENCES
Beers, M.H., and R. Berkow, eds. 1999. *The Merck Manual of Diagnosis and Therapy*, 17th ed. Whitehouse Station, NJ: Merck Research Laboratories.
Larson, B.A. 1996. *Occupational Therapy Practice Guidelines for Adults with Low Back Pain*. Bethesda, MD: American Occupational Therapy Association.

BIBLIOGRAPHY
Callahan, D.K. 1993. Work hardening for a client with low back pain. *American Journal of Occupational Therapy* 47, no. 7: 645–649.
Cicinelli, L. 1996. Back pain. In *Occupational therapy and physical dysfunction: Principles, skills, and practice*, eds. A. Turner et al., 667–690. New York: Churchill Livingstone.
Gibson, L., and J. Strong. 1996. The reliability and validity of a measure of perceived capacity for work in chronic back pain. *Journal of Occupational Rehabilitation* 6: 159–175.
Gibson, L., and J. Strong. 1998. Assessment of psychosocial factors in functional capacity evaluation of clients with chronic back pain. *British Journal of Occupational Therapy* 61, no. 9: 399–404.
Klinger, J.L. 1997. The client with back pain or chronic pain. In *Meal preparation and training: The healthcare professional's guide*, 87–90. Thorofare, NJ: Slack.
Large, R., and J. Strong. 1997. The personal constructs of coping with chronic low back pain: Is coping a necessary evil? *Pain* 73, no. 2: 245–252.
Moran, M., and J. Strong. 1995. Outcomes of a rehabilitation programme for patients with chronic back pain. *British Journal of Occupational Therapy* 58, no. 10: 435–438.
Smithline, J. 1997. Low back pain. In *Occupational therapy: Practice skills for physical dysfunction*, 4th ed., ed. L. Pedretti, 715–734. St. Louis, MO: Mosby.

190   QUICK REFERENCE TO OCCUPATIONAL THERAPY

Strong, J. et al. 1994. An investigation of the dimension of chronic low back pain: The patients' perspective. *British Journal of Occupational Therapy* 57, no. 6: 204–208.
Strong, J. et al. 1994. Chronic low back pain: An integrated psychosocial assessment model. *Journal of Counseling and Clinical Psychology* 62: 1058–1063.
Strong, J. et al. 1994. Function and the patient with chronic low back pain. *Clinical Journal of Pain* 10: 191–196.
Strong, J. et al. 1995. International replication study of the integrated psychosocial assessment model for patients with chronic low back pain. *Clinical Journal of Pain* 11: 296–306.
Strong, J., and R.G. Large. 1995. Coping with chronic low back pain: An ideographic exploration through focus groups. *International Journal of Psychiatry in Medicine* 25: 361–377.
Wilson, D.J. et al. 1997. Lumbar spinal moments in chronic back pain patients during supported lifting: A dynamic analysis. *Archives of Physical Medicine and Rehabilitation* 78, no. 9: 967–972.

Body Scheme Disorders

DESCRIPTION

Body scheme is the awareness of body parts and the position of the body and its parts in relation to themselves and objects in the environment (Quintana 1995, 206). Body scheme develops through the integration of proprioceptive, tactile, and pressure input making up the neural postural model. This scheme is the neural foundation for perception of body position and the relationships of the body and its parts (Van Deusen 1993, 117). Dysfunction is the result of one or more neural lesions and related psychological or sociological problems (Van Deusen 1993, 118).

The concepts of body scheme and body image are frequently confused or interchanged. "Body scheme" refers to the neural processing of somatic sensory information, while "body image" refers to the subjective feelings an individual has about him- or herself and his or her body (Corbett and Shah 1996, 326). Body image is a dynamic synthesis of the sensory body scheme and those environmental inputs providing relevant emotional and conceptual components (Van Deusen 1993, 118). Body image disorder is the inability to perceive the appearance of one's own body (Grieve 1993, 108). Body image disorder refers to the disturbances in the synthesis of the neural body scheme and its psychological representation that relate to performance problems (Rubio and Van Deusen 1995, 552).

One hypothesis about body knowledge processing suggests that there are four kinds of representations necessary: (1) semantic and lexical information about body parts, including the names of body parts, the functional relations between body parts, and the functional purpose of body parts; (2) category-specific visuospatial representations of an individual's own body and of bodies in general, including a structural description of where body parts are located, the proximity relationships between body parts, and the boundaries that define each body part; (3) the emergent, dynamic body-reference system that gives information about the position and changes in position of body parts relative to each other and to external space; and (4) the motor representations that contribute to the construction of a spatial representation of the body (Zoltan 1996, 73).

CAUSE

Damage to the somesthetic affect system, the thalamus, and the posterior parietal or temporal lobes may produce body scheme disorders. Lesions in the left hemisphere may produce a bilateral body scheme disorder, which can be identified through a verbal examination. In contrast, a lesion in the right hemisphere may be manifested behaviorally as a unilateral body scheme disorder (Corbett and Shah 1996, 327).

Van Deusen covers stroke, anorexia nervosa, phantom limb pain, mastectomy, burns, spinal cord injury, and rheumatoid arthritis in her book. Many other disorders—such as tumors, lupus, scleroderma, neurofibromas, or any disorder that changes the neural sensory system—could also be included.

ASSESSMENT

Areas

- anosognosia: severe form of neglect in which the person fails to recognize or denies the presence or severity of paralysis; usually transient
- finger agnosia: confusion in naming the fingers on command or knowing which one was touched
- right-left discrimination: selective incapacity to apply the right-left distinction to symmetrical parts of the body
- somatognosia: the lack of awareness of body structure and the failure to recognize one's parts and their relationship to each other
  1. macrosomatognosia: seeing the whole body or part of it as abnormally or exceptionally large
  2. microsomatognosia: seeing the whole body or part of it as abnormally small
- unilateral body neglect: inability to integrate and use perceptions from one (usually left) side of the body (see section on unilateral neglect)

Instruments

There are several categories of assessments: self-report instruments, examiner-administered paper and pen tests, computer-assisted instruments, psychophysical methods, and functional tools.

General

- *Behavioural Inattention Test* (BIT) by B.A. Wilson, J. Cockburn, and P.W. Halligan, Bury St. Edmunds, Suffolk, England: Thames Valley Test Co., 1987. (Distributed in the United States by Northern Speech Services–National Rehabilitation Services, Gaylord, MI)
- *Chessington Occupational Therapy Neurological Assessment Battery* (COTNAB) by R. Tyerman et al., Nottingham, England: Nottingham Rehab., 1986.
- *Rivermead Perceptual Assessment Battery* (RPAB) by S. Whiting et al., Windsor, Berkshire, England: NFER-Nelson, 1985. (Distributed in the United States by Western Psychological Services, Los Angeles)

Anosognosia
  There is no formal test. Simply record spontaneous behavior.

Finger Agnosia
* finger locationization (Zoltan 1996, 85–86)
* finger identification (Zoltan 1996, 86)
* imitation (Zoltan 1996, 86)

Right-Left Discrimination
* Ayres' Right-Left Discrimination Test (Zoltan 1996, 83)
* point to body parts on command (Zoltan 1996, 83–84)
* Piaget Test of Left/Right Concepts (Scheiman 1997, 101)

Somatognosia
* body revisualization (Zoltan 1996, 76)
* body visualization and space concepts (Zoltan 1996, 75–76)
* draw-a-man (Zoltan 1996, 76–77)
* face puzzle (Zoltan 1996, 79)
* human figure puzzle (Zoltan 1996, 78)
* point to body parts—imitation (Zoltan 1996, 75)
* point to body parts on command (Zoltan 1996, 74–75)

PROBLEMS

Self-Care
* The person has difficulty performing self-care activities correctly, especially dressing, bathing, and other activities requiring functional mobility.

Productivity and Leisure
* The person may have difficulty with reading and writing.

Sensorimotor
* The person may have difficulty using both arms or both legs together in tandem or reciprocal actions.
* The person may assemble a puzzle composed of body parts in a random or nonsensical pattern.
* The person may draw a person whose body parts are not in the right places.
* The person may consistently confuse left and right directions. (Note: Normal people often confuse left and right directions when facing a person or if an unusual orientation is presented. Left-right confusion should be part of a group of problems, not the only problem.)
* The person may have poor balance and equilibrium reactions.
* The person may have inaccurate movements even though proprioception is normal.

Cognitive

- The person may report that an arm or a leg is very large or very small (macro- or microsomatognosia).
- The person may state that an arm or a leg belongs to someone else, such as the examiner.
- The person may give the arm or leg a different name.
- The person may deny the arm or leg exists.
- The person may appear to ignore a command to move the arm or leg.
- The person may have difficulty establishing a reference point to the outside world using him- or herself, another person, or an object.

Psychosocial

- The person may have difficulty differentiating between his or her own body parts and those of other people.

TREATMENT/INTERVENTION

Treatment may involve a sensory integration, neurodevelopmental therapy, transfer of training, or functional approach—or a combination of these. Sensory integration and neurodevelopmental approaches assume that the body scheme is formed through sensory experience and maturation of the central nervous system. According to these approaches, remediation can occur by reintroducing the sensory experiences and maturational activities. Transfer of training and functional approaches such as adaptation and compensation are based on the assumption that there is an innate neural representation of the body that is not dependent on sensory feedback. Thus, it may be helpful to use practice techniques that focus on teaching or relearning previously known information about the body scheme or the application of techniques designed to reduce the impact of body scheme disorder (adaptation and compensation).

Self-Care

Adaptive or Compensatory Approach

- Place food and utensils on the unaffected side.
- Give all instructions from the unaffected side.
- Repetitive practice and cuing may also be helpful (e.g., identifying the left by the presence of a ring or watch).

Productivity and Leisure

- Place work materials on the unaffected side.

Sensorimotor

Sensory Integrative or Remedial Approach

- Increase the person's awareness of the neglected side through tactile stimulation such as brushing, icing, or rubbing the arm or leg before dressing or grooming.
- Have the person wear a weight cuff on one side during treatment to provide increased proprioception input while calling attention to the side.
- Use of pressure and cutaneous stimulation may be helpful.

- Use activities that focus attention on the neglected side (e.g., placing work materials on the affected side and approaching the person from the affected side).
- Increase somatognosia or body scheme training to increase awareness of the relationship between body segments using games (Simon says) or obstacle courses.

Neurodevelopmental Approach
- Provide bilateral weight bearing with handling techniques.
- Begin with rolling over and progress to prone-on-elbows posture.

Cognitive
Transfer of Training
- Touch the person's body parts, then identify the part of the body that has been touched.
- Have the person practice assembling human figure puzzles.
- Quiz the person on body parts, asking questions such as "Where is your left knee?"

Psychosocial
- Family members and friends could be taught to use one or more of the approaches.

PRECAUTIONS
- Be alert to signs of spasticity if rubbing is used.
- Be alert to safety issues. The person may get lost easily, especially with left-right confusion. The person may be unaware of heat and get burned.
- Be aware that a person with dressing difficulties may put pants on one leg only, put a shirt on one arm only, or dress in other socially inappropriate ways.

PROGNOSIS AND OUTCOME
Prognosis and outcome depend on the problem's type, severity, and location. People with severe anosognosia and a lesion in the right hemisphere are likely to have a poor outcome even several months later. Those with mild finger agnosia and a lesion in the left hemisphere may recover within a few weeks.
- The person is able to perform self-care tasks correctly with prompting or use of adaptive strategies.
- The person is able to correctly identify body parts when asked to point to them on him- or herself and others.
- The person will be able to distinguish right from left using the left ring finger for cuing.
- The person is able to identify fingers correctly when touched with vision occluded.

REFERENCES

Corbett, A., and S. Shah. 1996. Body scheme disorders following stroke and assessment in occupational therapy. *British Journal of Occupational Therapy* 59, no. 7: 325–329.
Grieve, J.I. 1993. Spatial deficits—disorders of body image and body scheme. In *Neuropsychology for occupational therapists: Assessment of perception and cognition,* ed. J.I. Grieve, 108–109. Boston: Blackwell Scientific Publications.

Quintana, L.A. 1995. Evaluation of perception and cognition: Body scheme. In *Occupational therapy for physical dysfunction*, 4th ed., ed. C.A. Trombly, 206–207. Baltimore: Williams & Wilkins.
Rubio, K.B., and J. Van Deusen. 1995. Relation of perceptual and body image dysfunction to activities of daily living of persons after stroke (review). *American Journal of Occupational Therapy* 49, no. 6: 551–559.
Scheiman, M. 1997. *Understanding and Managing Vision Deficits: A Guide for Occupational Therapists.* Bethesda, MD: American Occupational Therapy Association.
Van Deusen, J. 1993. Introduction to body image dysfunction. In *Body image and perceptual dysfunction in adults,* ed. J. Van Deusen, 117–121. Philadelphia: W.B. Saunders.
Zoltan, B. 1996. Body scheme disorders. In *Vision, perception and cognition: A manual for the evaluation and treatment of the neurologically impaired adult,* ed. B. Zoltan, 73–90. Thorofare, NJ: Slack.

BIBLIOGRAPHY

Quintana, L.A. 1995. Remediating perceptual impairments: Body scheme. In *Occupational therapy for physical dysfunction*, 4th ed., ed. C.A. Trombly, 530–531. Baltimore: Williams & Wilkins.
Van Deusen, J. 1993. Conclusions: Adult body image, visual, and somesthetic dysfunction. In *Body image and perceptual dysfunction in adults,* ed. J. Van Deusen, 231–241. Philadelphia: W.B. Saunders.

Body Scheme Disorders— Unilateral Neglect

DESCRIPTION

Unilateral neglect is defined as the failure to report, respond to, or orient to stimuli in the space contralateral to the site of the brain lesion (Grieve 1993, 123). Although unilateral neglect can occur from lesions in either hemisphere, lesions in the right usually cause more severe problems than those on the left. Unilateral body neglect is a subcategory of unilateral neglect and refers to the inability to integrate and use perceptions from one side of the body (Zoltan 1996, 80). In other words, the person with unilateral body neglect ignores one-half (usually the left side) of the body. The deficit may occur independently of visual field deficits such as hemianopsia, or other sensory impairments, or be compounded by those deficits.

A person with unilateral neglect may show extinction to two touch stimuli applied simultaneously, one on either side of the body. For example, if both hands or both sides of the face are touched while the eyes are closed, the person will report the stimulus on only one side, such as the right. In auditory neglect, the person does not respond to sounds on the neglected side, even though the hearing is normal. In tactile neglect, the person does not explore one side of space.

Unilateral neglect may exist with or without hemianopsia since unilateral neglect involves hemispatial problems while hemianopsia is a hemiretinal disorder. Assessment for hemianopsia should be done separately from assessment for unilateral neglect because treatment approaches are different (Golisz 1998, 13). Also, a person with just hemianopsia is usually aware of the problem.

Unilateral neglect is also called hemi-inattention, unilateral inattention, hemispatial neglect, unilateral spatial agnosia, unilateral akinesia, or unilateral extinction. The terms "neglect" and "inattention" are actually misnomers. The neglect and inattention are not conscious acts to ignore or avoid. The person is often totally unaware of neglecting or failing to attend or becomes aware only after the situation has occurred. A major goal of treatment is to close the gap between awareness and action.

CAUSE

The cause is considered to be a lesion in the brain. Most commonly, lesions occur in the temporoparietal lobe, but lesions of the frontal lobe, inferior parietal lobe, cingulate gyrus, thalamus, and striatum may also result in unilateral neglect. Damage or lesions in the right hemisphere appear to cause more severe problems than lesions in the left hemisphere.

ASSESSMENT

Assessment may be static (quantitative), qualitative, or dynamic. Static assessments are most helpful in determining the presence and severity of neglect but may underestimate the severity of the symptoms because a single "snapshot" view may miss problems that evolve in an ongoing situation. Qualitative approaches such as interviews allow the examiner to predict similar task difficulties but provide little data for making a prediction about the potential for improvement through intervention. Dynamic assessment allows the examiner to determine the array of problems demonstrated within the neglect syndrome by combining exploration of a person's awareness of neglect, use of strategies to cope, and responsiveness to cues or task modification.

Areas
- self-care tasks, especially eating, dressing, and grooming
- productivity tasks, especially reading and writing
- sensory functions, especially visual, tactile, touch, and auditory
- perceptual functions, especially spatial relationships, including horizontal (left-right), radial distance (near-far), and vertical (up-down)
- cognitive functions, especially attention and alertness

Instruments
Instruments Developed by Occupational Therapy Personnel
- *Chessington Occupational Therapy Neurological Assessment Battery* (COTNAB) by R. Tyerman et al., Nottingham, England: Nottingham Rehab., 1986.
- *Rivermead Perceptual Assessment Battery* (RPAB) by S. Whiting et al., Windsor, Berkshire, England: NFER-Nelson. 1985. (Distributed in the United States by Western Psychological Services, Los Angeles)

Instruments Developed by Other Professionals and Used by Occupational Therapy Personnel

- *Behavioural Inattention Test* (BIT) by B.A. Wilson, J. Cockburn, and P.W. Halligan, Bury St. Edmunds, Suffolk, England: Thames Valley Test Co., 1987. (Distributed in the United States by Western Psychological Services, Los Angeles)
- *The Bells Test* by L. Gautheir, F. DeHaut, and Y. Joanette, in The Bells Test: A quantitative and qualitative test for visual neglect, *Journal of Clinical Neuropsychology* 11, no. 2 (1989): 49–54.
- *Benton Visual Retention Test* by A.B. Sivan, San Antonio, TX: The Psychological Corporation, 1992.
- *Boston Diagnostic Aphasia Examination* (Parietal Lobe Test) by H. Goodglass and E. Kaplan, in *Assessment of aphasia and related disorders*, Philadelphia: Lea & Febiger, 1972.
- *Indented Paragraph Test* by B. Caplan, in Assessment of unilateral neglect: A new reading test, *Journal of Clinical and Experimental Neuropsychology* 9 (1987): 359–364.
- *Line Bisection Test* by T. Schenkenberg, D.C. Bradford, and E.T. Ajaz, in Line bisection and unilateral visual neglect in patients with neurological impairment, *Neurology* 30 (1980): 509–517.
- *Rey-Osterrieth Complex Figure* by J. Meyer and K. Meyer, Odessa, FL: Psychological Assessment Resources, 1995.
- *Weintraub Mesulam Cancellation Tests,* in M.M. Mesulam, *Principles of Behavioral Neurology: Tests of Directed Attention and Memory*, Philadelphia: F.A. Davis, 1985.

PROBLEMS

Self-Care
- The person usually has difficulty performing self-care activities. For example, the person may shave only one side of the face, brush the hair on only one side, or apply makeup to only half the face.
- The person may eat only the food that appears to the right of midline.
- The person has difficulty locating items that appear in the left field of body orientation. If the field of vision is changed to allow the same items to appear in the right field of body orientation, the person may locate the items quickly and easily by tactile exploration or visual search.

Productivity
- The person may be unable to return to work because of safety factors or difficulty performing job duties where work functions involve simultaneous attention to both sides of the body or space (e.g., reading directions from left to right of midline).
- The person may have difficulty performing homemaking skills such as shopping because items to the left side of midline may not be seen and thus not be purchased.
- The person may write or draw on or read only one-half of a page.

Leisure
- The person may be unable to enjoy leisure activities that require simultaneous attention to both sides of the body or space (e.g., sports).

Sensorimotor
- The person may bump into things on the affected side because of visual inattention or extinction.
- In the acute phase, the person may have marked deviation of the head, eyes, and trunk away from midline and to the side away from the lesion as though pulled by a magnet.
- Even after the acute phase has ended, the person may drift to the right when walking along a straight path because of residual effects of neglect.
- The person may have single or multiple sensory modality extinction, motor extinction, and oculomotor impersistence.
- The person may bisect a line asymmetrically because of visual neglect of part or all of the left visual field.
- The person may frequently roll a wheelchair to the left and into the wall because the right arm is doing most or all of the work, even if the left arm is capable of pushing.

Cognitive
- The person may lack awareness that neglect behaviors are occurring.
- In severe cases, the person may fail to recognize that the contralateral extremity is part of his or her body.
- If asked to describe a picture, the person may report details only from the right side of the picture, largely ignoring the left side.

Psychosocial
- The person may fail to respond to or notice persons on the affected side.
- The person may experience emotional changes, such as flattened affect or heightened anxiety.

Environment
- The person may get lost easily because he or she does not turn to the neglected side.
- The person's performance may be affected by the stimulus or task characteristics, resulting in uneven performance.

TREATMENT/INTERVENTION

There are two major models for treatment of unilateral neglect (Golisz 1998, 12). The first assumes that unilateral (sensory) neglect is an attentional-arousal disorder in the orienting response usually mediated by the right hemisphere. In other words, the right hemisphere is underaroused and needs arousal techniques. The second model assumes that neglect is primarily a disorder of spatial exploration involving both tactile and visual search strategies. In other words, the problem is one of imagery skills (seeing or feeling in one's mind) being disrupted or perhaps damaged and in need of cuing, refocusing, or other compensatory techniques.

In occupational therapy, the models include the multicontext treatment approach, functional training, and lateralization tasks. The multicontext treatment approach is based on the dynamic interactional model of cognition, which views cognitive impairments as deficits in the application of underlying strategies that can affect task performance (Golisz 1998, 19). The functional approach emphasizes the performance of the task, not the underlying skills. Adaptation and compensatory techniques are used if the task can be performed normally. The lateralized task approach involves use of hemisphere-specific tasks to modify the interhemispheric imbalance using cognitive-perceptual remediation or retaining techniques.

Self-Care

- Have the person practice dressing, grooming, and eating tasks under supervision and provide immediate feedback about results.

Productivity

- Practice a variety of tasks that the person does regularly (e.g., working at a desk, vacuuming, or caring for a child).

Leisure

- Use tasks selected from the person's leisure interests.

Sensorimotor

- Grade the visuospatial tasks from simple to complex or from few distractors to many. Block design and cancellation tasks are often used.
- Use visuospatial tasks to activate the right hemisphere or verbal stimuli to activate the left hemisphere.
- A multisensory approach might include a stereognosis task with abstract shapes, a jigsaw puzzle, and classical or jazz music for the right hemisphere; and a stereognosis task with three-dimensional alphabet letters, a crossword puzzle, and reading aloud for the left hemisphere.
- Patch the right eye to force the left eye to explore more of the environment.

Cognitive

- Use dynamic cuing. In a cancellation exercise with numbers in random order, the cues might be the following:
  1. Check and verify an answer: "Are you sure you found all the number 5s?"
  2. Provide general feedback: "There are still some number 5s remaining. Can you find them?"
  3. Provide specific feedback: "There are still some number 5s remaining on the left side."
  4. Structure the task: "Try beginning on the left side. Go slowly and use your finger to point to each number."
  5. Modify the task: Reduce the number of items or establish a boundary line with red tape on the left side of the worksheet.
- Use other cuing techniques such as the following:
  1. Anchoring: Place a digit or sticker at the beginning of a line and draw the person's attention to the digit or sticker.

2. Tracing: Have the person trace a line of directions with a finger, for example, before reading the directions.
3. Anchoring and tracing combined: Place the anchor marker. Then have the person find the marker, trace the line of directions with a finger, and then read.
- Use cue cards with statements such as the following:
  1. Am I remembering to move my eyes all the way to the left?
  2. Am I searching for items in an organized manner (left to right, top to bottom)?
  3. Am I going too fast?
- Grade the task difficulty by changing task characteristics.
  1. *Surface characteristics* include stimulus type, type of task, presentation mode, environmental context, spatial arrangement, movement requirements, rules or directions, and variable stimulus attributes.
  2. *Conceptual characteristics* are the underlying skills and strategies required to perform the task (Golisz 1998, 20).
- Provide practice in transfer of training. Physically similar tasks are the easiest to transfer.
  1. near transfer: one or two surface changes in task characteristics
  2. intermediate transfer: three to six changes in surface characteristics
  3. far transfer: tasks that are conceptually the same but physically different
  4. very far transfer: tasks that require the strategy transfer to everyday functioning
- Incorporate metacognitive training that includes two interrelated aspects:
  1. knowledge concerning one's own cognitive processes and capacities
  2. ability to monitor one's own performance

The person must be able to move from a cued environment to an uncued condition, which requires internalized ability to estimate and self-monitor performance (Golisz 1998, 21).
- Have the person predict performance by self-questioning.
  1. How difficult is this task going to be?
  2. Should I use an anchor on the left side to help orient me?

Psychosocial

- Increase visual scanning techniques by encouraging the person to "look to the left."
- Use a videotaped performance of the person doing some tasks where neglect is evident, and use the tape as a basis for discussion.

PRECAUTION

- Be aware of safety issues involving the side of the body that is being neglected. The person may not attend to a real danger if the danger appears on the neglected side. The person could be burned with a heating pad or place his or her hand on a hot burner. The person could push the wheelchair down stairs. The person might not notice broken glass. The person might not notice that a hand rail is available on the left side.

PROGNOSIS AND OUTCOME

Prognosis and outcome are largely dependent on the severity of the symptoms. Mild symptoms usually disappear in a few weeks. More severe problems may continue for many months.

- The person is able to perform self-care tasks without supervision using cue cards or other reminders.
- The person is able to perform productivity activities without supervision.
- The person is able to engage in leisure activities.
- The person is able to use compensatory strategies successfully to cope with new tasks or situations.

REFERENCES

Golisz, K.M. 1998. Dynamic assessment multicontext treatment of unilateral neglect. *Topics in Stroke Rehabilitation* 5, no. 1: 11–28.

Grieve, J.I. 1993. Disorders of attention. In *Neuropsychology for occupational therapists: Assessment of perception and cognition*, ed. J.I. Grieve, 123–131. Boston: Blackwell Scientific Publications.

Zoltan, B. 1996. Body scheme disorders. In *Vision, perception and cognition: A manual for the evaluation and treatment of the neurologically impaired adult*, ed. B. Zoltan, 73–90. Thorofare, NJ: Slack.

BIBLIOGRAPHY

Cermak, S.A., and K. Lin. 1994. Assessment of unilateral neglect in individuals with right cerebral vascular accident. *Topics in Geriatric Rehabilitation* 10, no. 2: 42–55.

Golisz, K.M., and J.P. Toglia. 1998. Evaluation of perception and cognition—unilateral inattention. In *Williard and Spackman's occupational therapy*, 9th ed., eds. M.E. Neistadt and E.B. Crepeau, 270–272. Philadelphia: J.B. Lippincott.

Kagayama, S. et al. 1994. Neglect in three dimensions. *American Journal of Occupational Therapy* 48, no. 3: 206–210.

Lin, K-C. 1996. Right hemispheric activation approaches to neglect rehabilitation poststroke (review). *American Journal of Occupational Therapy* 50, no. 7: 504–515.

Lin, K-C et al. 1996. Effects of cuing on line bisection in post-stroke patients with unilateral neglect. *Journal of the International Neuropsychological Society* 2, no. 5: 404–411.

Quintana, L.A. 1995. Evaluation of perception and cognition: Unilateral neglect. In *Occupational therapy for physical dysfunction*, 4th ed., ed. C. Trombly, 207–210. Baltimore: Williams & Wilkins.

Quintana, L.A. 1995. Remediating perceptual impairments: Unilateral neglect. In *Occupational therapy for physical dysfunction*, 4th ed., ed. C. Trombly, 531–534. Baltimore: Williams & Wilkins.

Roden, W. 1997. Reducing neglect in adult hemiplegia: Recent findings and implications for treatment. *British Journal of Occupational Therapy* 60, no. 8: 347–351.

Tam K, and R. Tegner. 1997. Video feedback in the rehabilitation of patients with unilateral neglect. *Archives of Physical Medicine and Rehabilitation* 78, no. 4: 410–413.

Van Deusen, J. 1993. Unilateral neglect from brain lesion. In *Body image and perceptual dysfunction in adults*, ed. J. Van Deusen, 123–147. Philadelphia: W.B. Saunders.

Chronic Pain

DESCRIPTION

Chronic pain persists, constantly or intermittently, past the normal time of healing and serves no useful adaptive role or biological purpose. In other words, the pain persists beyond what is expected for a disease or injury or it recurs at various times for months or years. The International Association for the Study of Pain considers the demarcation point between acute and chronic pain to be three months. Pain-related disorders most often seen by occupational therapy personnel are headache, low back, arthritis, cancer, myofascial, and extremity pain.

Chronic pain can be classified based on the underlying pathophysiology.

- *Nociceptive pain* (tissue irritation) is due to activation of pain-sensitive nerve fibers, either somatic or visceral, and produces an aching or pressure sensation, as seen in arthritis and cancer.
- *Neuropathic pain* arises from injury to neural structures and includes deaffent pain, sympathetic response pain, and peripheral pain.
  1. *Deaffent pain* is due to injury in the central nervous system (e.g., brachial plexus avulation or lesion pain).
  2. *Sympathetic response pain* is due to activity in the sympathetic nervous system efferents (e.g., reflex sympathetic dystrophy).
  3. *Peripheral pain* is due to changes in the peripheral nerves (e.g., abnormal sprouting of injured nerves that causes a neuroma). The pain is often a burning or lancinating sensation.
- *Psychogenic or idiopathic pain* occurs in the absence of a known organic lesion but does include malingering or Munchausen's syndrome. The types of pain sensation are much more varied.

Chronic pain can also be classified based on temporal factors (Engel 1998, 454).

- *Chronic, periodic pain* is acute but intermittent (e.g., migraine headaches).
- *Chronic, intractable, nonmalignant pain* is present most of the time, with varying intensity (e.g., low back pain; see also section on back pain).
- *Chronic, progressive pain* is often associated with malignancies.

CAUSE

The cause of chronic pain is not completely understood. The oldest and primary theory is the gate control theory of pain, which assumes that within the dorsal horn of the spinal cord a gatelike mechanism exists. That mechanism can be opened or shut to peripheral nerve impulses going to the brain. Impulses allowed though the gate, assumed to be the substantia gelatinosa neurons within the dorsal horn cell, are relayed to the transmission cells for projection to the brain, which interprets the type and degree of pain. Inhibitory influences supposedly can occur from the brainstem and the periphery. Although research has shown the gate control theory has many flaws, no better theory has been proposed to date.

ASSESSMENT

Areas

- daily living skills and performance
- productivity (functional capacity evaluation, occupational history, work skills, interests, and values)
- leisure interests and skills
- roles and habits
- functional status: range of motion, muscle testing, endurance, and physical fitness
- pain (note description, individual's perception, responses, location, intensity, and motions or activities that cause it)
- personal attitudes and beliefs about health and illness
- self-perception and self-efficacy
- coping skills
- affective state
- support skills
- time management
- cultural views of pain and suffering

  Other types of assessment may be needed depending on the location and type of pain.

Instruments

Instruments Developed by Occupational Therapy Personnel

- *NPI Interest Checklist* by J. Matsutsuyu, in The interest checklist, *American Journal of Occupational Therapy* 23, no. 6 (1969): 368–373. Modified by J. Rogers, The NPI interest checklist, in *Mental health assessment in occupational therapy: An integrative approach to the evaluation process*, ed. B.J. Hemphill, Thorofare, NJ: Slack, 93–114.
- *Occupational History* by L. Moorhead, in The occupational history, *American Journal of Occupational Therapy* 23, no. 4 (1969): 329–338. Modified by G. Kielhofner et al., The reliability of a historical interview with physically disabled respondents, *American Journal of Occupational Therapy* 40, no. 8 (1986): 551–556.
- *Occupational Performance History Interview II* (OPHI-II) by G. Kielhofner et al., Chicago: University of Illinois at Chicago, 1999. (Available through the American Occupational Therapy Association, Bethesda, MD)
- *Role Checklist*, 2nd ed. by F. Oakley, Bethesda, MD: Occupational Therapy Service, National Institutes of Health, 1982.
- *Schultz Upper Extremity Pain Assessment* by K.S. Schultz, in The Schultz structured interview for assessing upper extremity pain, *Occupational Therapy in Health Care* 1, no. 3 (1994): 69–82.
- *Self-Efficacy Gauge* by M. Gage et al., in Measuring perceived self-efficacy in occupational therapy, *American Journal of Occupational Therapy* 48, no. 9 (1994): 783–790.
- *24-Hour Log* by G. Larrington, in An exploratory study of the temporal aspects of adaptive functioning, Unpublished master's thesis, University of Southern California, 1970.

Instruments Developed by Other Professionals and Used by Occupational Therapy Personnel

- *Activity Diary* by W.E. Fordyce et al., in Pain measurement and pain behaviour, *Pain* 18 (1984): 53–69.
- *Functional Assessment Screening Questionnaire* by R.W. Millard, in The functional assessment screening questionnaire: Application for evaluating pain-related disability, *Archives of Physical Medicine and Rehabilitation* 70 (1989): 303–307.
- *McGill Pain Questionnaire* by R. Melzak, in The McGill Pain Questionnaire: Major properties and scoring methods, *Pain* 3 (1975): 277–299.
- *Pain Beliefs and Perceptions Inventory* by D.A. Williams and B.E. Thorn, in An empirical assessment of pain beliefs, *Pain* 36 (1989): 351–358.
- *Pain Disability Index* by R.C. Tait, J.T. Chinall, and S.J. Krause, in The pain disability index: Psychometric properties, *Pain* 40 (1990): 171–182.
- *Sickness Impact Profile* by M. Bergner et al., in The sickness impact profile: Development and final revision of a health status measure, *Medical Care* 19 (1981): 787–805.
- *Survey of Pain Attitudes Revised* by M.P. Jensen, P. Karoly, and R. Huger, in The development and preliminary validation of an instrument to assess patients' attitudes toward pain, *Journal of Psychosomatic Research* 31 (1987): 393–400.

In addition to formal tests, three types of self-reporting forms are used: the Verbal Rating Scale, the Numerical Rating Scale, and the Visual Analog Scale.

PROBLEMS

Self-Care
- The person may avoid performing certain activities of daily living to avoid associated pain.
- The person may experience sleep disorders.
- The person may complain of having decreased appetite and complain about the loss of sense of taste for food.
- The person's eating habits may have changed so that the person eats more or less food than he or she did before the chronic pain.
- The person or his or her spouse may report diminished sexual activity.

Productivity
- The person may be unable to perform job tasks because pain interferes.
- The person may avoid performing some household tasks because of pain.
- The person may have difficulty with parenting because of pain.

Leisure
- The person may lack the energy to participate in leisure activities.
- The person may avoid leisure activities to avoid associated pain.

Sensorimotor
- The person may have an asymmetrical posture as a result of "favoring" the painful area.
- The person's spine may be misaligned, flattened, or generally asymmetrical.

- The person's gait may be abnormal, and his or her balance reactions may be reduced.
- The person may have disuse atrophy and general deconditioning.
- The person may protect joints to avoid pain that accompanies movement involving those joints.
- The person may lose passive or active range of motion, develop contractures or crepitus, and become uncoordinated due to failure to move or exercise joints.
- The person may experience motor loss such as suddenly dropping things or falling without warning.
- The person may have autonomic responses such as sweating, flushing, or tachycardia.
- The person may experience muscle spasms, tightness, hardness, ropelike muscles, or twitch responses.
- The person's reflexes may become exaggerated or diminished or be absent.
- The person's skin temperature may increase or decrease.
- The person's vascular system may have abnormal responses (e.g., discoloration, diminished or absent hair growth, ulcerations).
- The person may have lassitude and lack of energy and have decreased physical activity.
- The person may have pain that is described as aching, pressing, burning, lancinating, tingling, or otherwise painful.
- The person's pain may be poorly localized and projected.
- The person may have sensory impairment.
- The person's tolerance to pain often has decreased.

Cognitive
- The person may be unable to concentrate because pain interrupts.
- The person may be preoccupied with thoughts about pain.

Psychosocial
- The person usually has blunted affect.
- The person may experience loss of self-esteem as his or her performance decreases.
- The person may feel hopelessness or helplessness and a sense of futility.
- The person may report or demonstrate emotional distress such as anger, irritability, anxiety, emotional lability, or depression.
- The person may withdraw from social situations.
- The person may have loss of libido.
- The person may experience loss of normal roles and role performance but may acquire the role of a sick person.

Temporal
- The person spends much of the time dealing with pain.

TREATMENT/INTERVENTION
Treatment models for managing chronic pain often use a multidisciplinary team approach. Practice models used in occupational therapy include the biopsychosocial model, the occupational behavior model, the model of human occupation, the appraisal model of coping, behavior modification, and the attitudes-beliefs-intentions-behavior model (Strong 1996,

158–159). The biopsychosocial model addresses the biological, psychological, and social aspects of the person and his or her pain. The occupational behavior model focuses on the person's competence in performing self-care, work, rest, and play roles and attempts to maximize performance in spite of pain. The model of human occupation considers the person in relation to volitional, habituation, and performance systems and attempts to maximize the individual's occupational behavior in all systems. The appraisal model of coping focuses on the individual's self-efficacy beliefs and their relationship to coping with pain, illness, and disability. Behavior modification uses environmental reinforcers for developing and promoting well behaviors while minimizing behaviors that promote illness. The attitudes-beliefs-intentions-behavior model focuses on recognizing the role of attitudes and beliefs held by the individual with pain and organizing treatment around those attitudes and beliefs.

Self-Care
- Encourage the person to maintain or increase independence in performing activities of daily living.
- Assist the person to adjust to living with chronic pain.

Productivity
- Provide work hardening, if needed, to assist in return to work.
- Provide opportunities for the person to explore career options, if needed.
- Provide opportunities for the person to practice home management skills.

Leisure
- Explore with the person leisure activities, including old and new interests.

Sensorimotor
- To avoid or reduce immobilization, encourage the person to participate in a graded activity program, beginning with the level of activity the person can tolerate before pain becomes a factor.
- Focus away from sensory registration and processing of pain onto functional activities and a balanced lifestyle (distraction or diversion).
- Increase amount of physical activity as the primary means of increasing range of motion, muscle strength, and physical endurance.
- Cutaneous stimulation modalities such as transcutaneous electrical nerve stimulation, massage, thermotherapy (hydrocolator packs, paraffin therapy, ultrasound, diathermy, whirlpool, aquatic therapy), cryotherapy, and vibration may be useful. (Note: Most occupational therapy personnel will need postgraduate education, continuing education courses, or inservice training to use physical modalities safely and effectively in pain management.)

Cognitive
- Help the person learn to manage or organize time rather than pain. Take rest breaks, not pain breaks. Rest before pain becomes a factor. Make rest, not pain, the reward.
- Educate the person about the relationships among pain, stress, tension, and thought processes. Help the person replace negative thoughts about events with more positive thoughts.

Psychosocial
- To counteract depression, increase the person's level of activity.
- Encourage participation in activity task groups to help the person reestablish a sense of self.
- Use individual activities in creative crafts or competitive games to help the person reestablish a sense of mastery.
- Have the person identify enjoyable rewards that can be used when personal goals are obtained. Charting activity is one measure the person can use to see progress by engaging in activity rather than responding to pain.
- If pain is related to stressors in the person's life, provide training in relaxation techniques or biofeedback to help the person relax the major skeletal muscle groups. Repeating phrases about the ideal state (autogenic training) or focusing on images to achieve a desired goal (guided imagery) may also be done.
- Encourage the person to resume roles and role functions within the family and society.
- Participation in group discussion can assist in identifying stressors that lead to pain and provide the opportunity to learn how others deal with chronic pain.
- Help the person's family stop responding to pain behavior. Encourage other kinds of interaction such as engaging in purposeful and enjoyable activities.

PRECAUTION
- Be aware of changing theories of pain causation and corresponding changes in treatment techniques. Pain causation is still poorly understood.

PROGNOSIS AND OUTCOME
- The person is able to perform self-care and daily living activities independently using self-help devices if needed.
- The person demonstrates performance of productive activities.
- The person demonstrates performance of leisure activities.
- The person is able to manage and control pain.
- The person demonstrates ability to solve problems and make decisions.
- The person demonstrates ability to follow a time management plan.
- The person demonstrates a positive self-image.
- The person demonstrates internal locus of control.
- The person has a dependable social support system.

REFERENCES

Engel, J.M. 1998. Treatment for psychosocial components: pain management. In *Willard and Spackman's occupational therapy*, eds. M.E. Neistadt and E.B. Crepeau, 454–458. Philadelphia: Lippincott-Raven.
Strong, J. 1996. *Chronic Pain: The Occupational Therapist's Perspective*. New York: Churchill Livingstone.

BIBLIOGRAPHY

Berg, J. 1997. The touch that heals. *OT Week* 11, no. 44: 18–19.

Borg, B., and M.A. Bruce. 1997. Quality of life. In *Occupational therapy stories in practice*, eds. B. Borg and M.A. Bruce, 63–76. Thorofare, NJ: Slack.

Carruthers, C. 1997. Developing a pain management programme. *British Journal of Occupational Therapy* 60, no. 5: 221–222.

Edwards, H. 1993. Chronic pain. In *Conditions in occupational therapy: Effect on occupational performance,* eds. R.A. Hansen and B. Atchison, 173–203. Baltimore: Williams & Wilkins.

Engel, J.M. 1993. Children's compliance with progressive relaxation procedures for improving headache control. *Occupational Therapy Journal of Research* 13, no. 4: 219–230.

Engel, J.M. 1996. Pediatric pain management. *Rehab Management* 9, no. 1: 43–46.

Engel, J.M. et al. 1994. The durability of relaxation training in pediatric headache management. *Occupational Therapy Journal of Research* 14, no. 3: 183–190.

Gilmore, R., and J. Strong. 1998. Pain and multiple sclerosis. *British Journal of Occupational Therapy* 61, no. 4: 169–172.

Haglund, L., and C. Henriksson. 1994. Testing a Swedish version of OCAIRS on two different patient groups. *Scandinavian Journal of Caring Science* 8, no. 4: 223–230.

Henahan, K., and L.D. Baruch. 1994. Physical and occupational therapy in the prevention and management of pain in the intensive care unit. In *Handbook of critical care pain management,* eds. R.J. Hamill and J.C. Rowlingson, 251–268. New York: McGraw-Hill.

Herbert, P., and R.L. Rochman. 1998. Dealing with pain: Treating the physical, psychological, and emotional aspects of patients with chronic pain. *TeamRehab Report* 11, no. 5: 56, 58–59, 96.

Hettinger, J. 1995. Pain: The silent epidemic grows. *OT Week* 9, no. 33: 20–22.

Kerr, T. 1995. CARF standards update: New pain programs for 1995. *Advance for Occupational Therapists* 11, no. 33: 15.

Low, J.F. 1997. Religious orientation and pain management. *American Journal of Occupational Therapy* 51, no. 3: 215–219.

Marmer, L. 1996. Researching the effect of occupation on pain level. *Advance for Occupational Therapists* 12, no. 40: 18, 50.

McCormack, G.L. 1993. *Pain Management: Mind-Body Techniques for Treating Chronic Pain Syndromes.* Tucson, AZ: Therapy Skill Builders.

Ross, R.G., and P.C. LaStayo. 1997. Clinical assessment and pain in occupational therapy and physical therapy. In *Assessment in occupational therapy and physical therapy,* eds. J. Van Deusen and D. Brunt, 123–133. Philadelphia: W.B. Saunders.

Solet, J.M. 1995. Transcending pain. *OT Week* 9, no. 33: 22–23.

Strong, J. et al. 1992. The measurement of attitudes towards and beliefs about pain. *Pain* 48: 227–236.

Thiers, N. 1994. When the pain won't stop. *OT Week* 8, no. 34: 22–24.

Trumble, E.A., and M.P. Krengel. 1996. Functional evaluation. In *Pain medicine: A comprehensive review*, ed. P.P. Raj, 106–113. St. Louis, MO: Mosby.

Unruh, A.M. 1996. Gender variations in clinical pain experience. *Pain* 65: 123–167.

Wincent, M.M., and J.M. Engel. 1994. Vestibular-proprioceptive abilities in children experiencing recurrent headaches. *Physical and Occupational Therapy in Pediatrics* 14, no. 2: 63–65.

Hearing Loss—Child

DESCRIPTION

Hearing loss means difficulty in hearing normal speech or common sounds in the environment. Normal hearing requires the ability to perceive sounds in the speech range of 500 to 2000 hertz (the frequency or number of sound vibrations per minute) or sound waves measured at approximately 0 decibels to 25 decibels (the distance a sound moves an air particle). Hearing loss occurs when a person loses 15 decibels or more within the range of most speech sounds. A person is described as *prelingually deaf* if he or she did not have or lost the ability to hear prior to the development of speech and *prevocationally deaf* if he or she lost the ability to hear before reaching age 19. Adult deafness refers to hearing loss occurring after age 19.

A hearing test called an audiogram is used to evaluate hearing status. Hearing impairment includes mild loss (25 decibels to 40 decibels), moderate loss (40 decibels to 55 decibels), moderate to severe loss (55 decibels to 70 decibels), severe loss (70 decibels to 90 decibels), and profound loss (90 decibels or more). A high tone loss means the person can hear lower tone sounds, including vowel sounds, but may miss some consonants, which have higher tone sounds. A low tone loss means the person hears the consonants but misses the vowels. A flat tone loss means all frequencies are equally affected.

CAUSE

Two major causes are (1) a lesion in the external auditory canal or the middle ear (conductive hearing loss) or (2) a lesion in the inner ear or the eighth cranial nerve (sensorineural hearing loss). Hearing loss may occur as a result of structural problems, genetic conditions, ototoxic drugs, infections, and disease syndromes. The major disorder resulting in conductive hearing loss in children is otitis media and its sequelae. Onset may occur at any age. The major disorders resulting in exogenous congenital sensorineural hearing loss are anoxia during birth, congenital rubella, congenital cytomegalic inclusion disease, congenital toxoplasmosis, congenital syphilis, neonatal herpes simplex infection, Rh incompatibility, or ototoxic drugs given to the mother. However, in many cases the exact disorder that caused the hearing loss is unknown.

ASSESSMENT

Because the ability to hear, listen, and understand instructions is often a prerequisite to many standardized tests, assessment using such tests may be difficult and unproductive with children or adolescents with moderate, profound, or severe hearing loss. Observations, interviews, and actual task performance may provide more useful information in such cases.

Areas

- daily living skills, especially functional communication
- play skills

Risk Indicators of Hearing Loss

- The newborn has no startle (Moro) reflex.
- At 3 months, the infant does not alert and orient to the sound of human voices or sound-producing toys.
- At 6 months, the infant stops cooing.
- Between 8 months and 12 months, the child does not turn when someone whispers.
- At 1 year, the child does not say any words such as "mama", "bye-bye," and "doggie."
- At 2 years, the child is not using words to communicate basic needs or during interactions.
- At 2 years, the child does not respond to verbal requests such as "Show me the keys."
- At 3 years, the child's speech is mostly unintelligible and consists primarily of vowel sounds.
- At 3 years, the child does not use two- and three-word sentences.
- The child also seems to frequently have a cold or the sniffles.

Source: Adapted with permission from E. Snow, Services for Children with Visual or Auditory Impairments, in *Occupational Therapy for Children*, 3rd ed., J. Case-Smith, A.S. Allen, and P.N. Pratt, eds., pp. 717–742, © 1996, Mosby-Year Book, Inc.

- leisure skills and interests
- motor skills: gross motor and bilateral integration skills
- fine motor coordination, manipulation, dexterity (especially finger dexterity if manual communication methods are being used)
- balance and postural control, muscle tone
- sensory awareness and discrimination in visual, tactile, proprioceptive, kinesthetic, and vestibular systems
- praxis and motor planning
- attention span and concentration
- sequential learning
- self-perception
- coping skills
- social skills
- language development

Instruments
- *Battelle Developmental Inventory* by J. Newborg et al., Itasca, IL: Riverside Publishing, 1984.
- *Bayley Scales of Infant Development-II* (BSID-II) by N. Bayley, San Antonio, TX: The Psychological Corporation, 1993.
- *Bruininks-Oseretsky Test of Motor Proficiency* (BOTMP) by R. Bruininks, Circle Pines, MN: American Guidance Services, 1978.

- *The Beery-Buktenica Developmental Test of Visual-Motor Integration* (VMI-4), 4th ed. by K.E. Beery and N.A. Buktenica, Parsippany, NJ: Modern Curriculum Press, 1997.
- *Hiskey Nebraska Test of Learning Aptitude Forms* by M.S. Hiskey, Austin, TX: Pro-ed, 1986.
- *Leiter International Performance Scale—Revised* by G.H. Roid and L.J. Miller, Wood Dale, IL: Stoelting Co., 1997.
- *Test of Visual-Perceptual Skills—Revised* (TVPS-R) by M.F. Gardner, Hydesville, CA: Psychological and Educational Publications, 1996.

PROBLEMS

Self-Care
- The person may be delayed in developing daily living skills.
- The person's functional communication skills may be delayed.

Productivity
- The person may have poorly developed play skills, especially in peer or interaction play.
- The person usually lags behind peers in developing reading and writing skills due to language deficits. Handwriting may be difficult to read.
- The person may experience job discrimination and other work-related difficulties as a young adult.
- The person may lack skills in homemaking and home management if he or she has lived in an institution.

Leisure
- The person may have only a few leisure interests, and they are likely to be underdeveloped.

Sensorimotor
- The person may be clumsy and uncoordinated, especially in bilateral coordination.
- The person may have poor or inadequate muscle tone and cocontraction.
- The person may have difficulty with fine motor skills, which would limit his or her ability to perform the rhythmic sequencing of fingers and hands necessary for signing.
- The person may have difficulty with praxis (motor planning).
- The person may have inadequate postural reflex integration (equilibrium reactions) or antigravity postural control.
- The person may have poor bilateral integration.
- The person may be hyperactive.
- The person may have poor oral motor functions—including controlling saliva, sucking, chewing, swallowing, and using tongue for sound production—and absent or hyperactive gag reflex.
- The person may have problems with eye motility, such as fixation, scanning, or tracking.
- The person may have visual-perceptual problems related to visual spatial perception, form constancy, and visual-sequential memory. These problems could interfere with learning letters, copying letters correctly in sequence, and spelling.

- The person may have prolonged or depressed postrotary nystagmus. (Note: A child with hearing impairment may have superior visual concentration and refocusing ability because of dependence on visual input. Vestibular testing should include balance tests as well to determine whether there is vestibular dysfunction.)
- The person may be tactilely defensive, which interferes with wearing a hearing aid.
- The person may have difficulty organizing multisensory input.

Cognitive

- The person may have poor attending behavior due to visual and/or auditory distractibility.
- The person may have difficulty planning ahead.
- The person may have difficulty with problem solving and decision making.
- The person may have delays in developing conceptualization and categorization skills.

Psychosocial

- The person may have poor self-perception and sense of mastery.
- The person may have low self-identity and self-esteem.
- The person may feel isolated and rejected.
- The person may have low motivation due to overprotection at home.
- The person may lack self-control and be impulsive.
- The person may have behavior problems such as temper tantrums, stubbornness, or inflexibility.
- The person may fail to develop or have delayed development of interpersonal language skills, including talking with parents and caregivers.
- The person usually is delayed in development of social skills such as taking turns and interacting with peers.
- The person may be overdependent on others.
- The person often experiences stereotyping and prejudice in the community.

Environment

- The family usually experiences grief or mourning after the initial diagnosis.
- The family may respond to the guilt by overprotecting the person.
- Family relations may be strained.

TREATMENT/INTERVENTION

Models of treatment are based primarily on sensory integration and secondarily on neurodevelopmental therapy and behavior modification. Occupational therapy personnel should also be aware that the teachers of the deaf are divided as to whether children who are deaf should be taught only through oral or auditory language (in which case manual sign language is prohibited), manual sign language only, or a mix of oral and manual sign language called total communication. If both language systems are encouraged, occupational therapy personnel will need to learn sign language to work effectively with this population.

Self-Care

- Help the person to develop age-appropriate daily living skills.

Productivity
- Provide handwriting practice or consider using the computer keyboard for written class assignments.
- Provide work-related experiences to teach good work habits, cooperating with peers, following directions, and applying for a job, including filling out an application and interviewing.
- Provide opportunities for practicing skills in homemaking, home management, and independent living through simulated or actual experiences, such as shopping for groceries.

Leisure
- Provide opportunities to explore leisure interests and develop skills.

Sensorimotor
- Promote attainment of development motor milestones, if needed.
- Improve balance of muscle tone between flexion and extension.
- Develop fine motor and hand coordination skills. Activities might include use of finger puppets, rubber band exercises, computer touchscreen activities, or games using clothespins, binder clips, or electrical clips.
- Enhance sensory processing of kinesthetic, proprioceptive, tactile, and visual systems through activities that stimulate each sensory modality.
- Improve bilateral integration, if needed. (See section on vestibular disorders.)
- Increase postural security and balance, especially in antigravity positions, if needed.
- Improve motor planning skills, if needed. (See section on dyspraxia.)
- Improve eye motility skills, if needed.
- Improve visual-perceptual skills, especially form constancy and spatial relationships, if needed.
- Decrease tactile defensiveness, if present. (See section on tactile defensiveness.)
- Moderate vestibular response if hyper- or hyporesponsiveness is present. (See section on gravitational insecurity.)

Cognitive
- Increase attending behavior and attention span, if needed.
- Improve problem-solving and decision-making skills by permitting choice.
- Improve sequential relationship skills through the use of activities and games that have steps or a series of tasks to complete.
- Increase time management skills by planning and following a schedule of activities.

Psychosocial
- Improve self-perception through creative activities such as arts, crafts, music, drama, and dance.
- Increase coping skills through a stress management program.
- Assist in developing the person's language skills. (Note: The most common communication technique is American sign language, or ASL, in conjunction with finger spelling and speech reading. This technique is called total communication.)
- Improve group interaction skills through use of group tasks or activities.

- Use role playing to develop social skills and check for generalization to community activities.

Environment
- Consider use of assistive technology to facilitate communication.
- Provide family with community resources designed for the person with hearing impairments.

PRECAUTIONS
- Vestibular dysfunction may be difficult to identify without the assistance of an audiologist or neurologist because of compensatory behavior through the visual system.
- Communication must be established prior to testing or treatment. The therapist may need to learn signing or use alternate communication symbol systems, such as Bliss symbols, in order to communicate with the child or adolescent.
- Some deaf children are extremely sensitive to rotation. Watch carefully for signs.
- Generally, shouting, talking loudly, or exaggerating mouth movements are not helpful in improving communication. Use other communication techniques.

PROGNOSIS AND OUTCOME
- The person is able to coordinate the use of two hands to sign.
- The person is able to perform gross motor skills, including jumping, hopping, and skipping.
- The person is able to maintain balance and postural control in static (standing balance) and dynamic situations.
- The person is able to perform motor planning tasks when presented with activities that are unfamiliar.
- The person's response to visual, tactile, proprioceptive, and vestibular stimuli is within normal range.
- The person's attention span is within normal range.
- The person demonstrates the ability to plan and complete a task that requires organizing a sequence of steps or tasks.
- The person is able to plan and follow a daily activity schedule.
- The person demonstrates improved self-perception.
- The person demonstrates knowledge of stress management techniques.
- The person has functional communication skills using oral and/or signing techniques.
- The person is able to interact in group situations within his or her age range.
- The person is able to perform activities of daily living independently within his or her age range.
- The person is able to perform productive activities within his or her age range.
- The person is able to perform leisure activities within his or her age range.

BIBLIOGRAPHY

Bilger, C.R. 1997. Small miracles. *OT Week* 11, no. 24: 14–15. (Dual diagnosis)

Orr, C. 1998. Improving oral imitation in preschool children with and without hearing impairment. *Physical and Occupational Therapy in Pediatrics* 18, no. 3/4: 97–107.

Porr, S.M. 1998. The visual and auditory systems: Hearing impairments. In *Pediatric therapy: A systems approach*, eds. S.M. Porr and E.B. Rainville, 254–266. Philadelphia: F.A. Davis.

Sikora, D.M., and D.S. Plapinger. 1994. Using standardized psychometric tests to identify learning disabilities in students with sensorineural hearing impairments. *Journal of Learning Disabilities* 27, no. 6: 352–359.

Snow, E. 1996. Services for children with visual or auditory impairments. In *Occupational therapy for children,* 3rd ed., eds. J. Case-Smith et al., 717–742. St. Louis, MO: Mosby.

Stahl, C. 1997. Developing the skills for refined sign-language expression. *Advance for Occupational Therapists* 13, no. 20: 14–15.

Low Vision—Adult

DESCRIPTION

Low vision is defined as bilateral subnormal visual acuity or abnormal visual field resulting from a disorder in the visual system that results in decreased visual performance. Low vision means there is a visual impairment severe enough to interfere with successful performance of activities of daily living but allowing some usable vision. The range of low vision is from 20/80 to 20/1000. Vision at the 20/80 range provides nearly normal performance with magnification or other aids to enlarge or provide better lighting. Vision at the 20/1000 range creates problems in orientation and mobility and limits reading unless aids are used. Low vision is the third most common disability in the United States after arthritis and cardiac disease. Approximately one in six adults who are 45 years to 74 years of age and older report moderate or severe visual impairment. After 75 years of age, the number is one in four. Usually the person also has at least one other chronic condition (Warren 1998, 3).

CAUSE

There are multiple causes, including reduced light transmission through the cornea, loss of retinal receptors, and changes in the eye membrane. Diseases associated with low vision include macular degeneration, glaucoma, diabetic retinopathy, optic atrophy, degenerative myopia, vitreal hemorrhage, retinal detachment, and retinitis pigmentosa. Other conditions causing low vision include stroke, head trauma, Parkinson's disease, multiple sclerosis, myasthenia gravis, and Alzheimer's disease. Cataracts is no longer included as a cause of low vision because successful surgery can correct the problem.

The person with low vision experiences difficulty using vision due to one or more of the following four deficits: inability to focus the visual image on the retina, inability of the retina to accurately encode or record the visual image, inability of the optic nerve or pathways to transmit the visual image with the central nervous system, or inability of the central nervous system to analyze the visual information and integrate it with other sensory input to form perceptions and make decisions (Warren 1998, 9). Specific problems may include macular scotoma, ocular pain, blurred vision, diplopia or double vision, distortion of vision, photophobia, flashing lights, halos around lights, abnormal color vision, visual hallucination, night blindness, and inability to see details.

ASSESSMENT

Areas

- self-care: applying makeup, applying toothpaste, eating neatly (including seasoning foods and applying toppings), managing medication, mending clothes, caring for nails, selecting clothes, using the telephone
- meal preparation: cooking, cutting, pouring liquids, measuring ingredients, reading recipes and instructions, setting appliance dials, setting timers, slicing
- home management: cleaning, ironing, maintaining car, maintaining yard, performing minor household repairs such as changing lightbulbs
- shopping: accessing transportation, locating correct aisle or item, making shopping list, paying for items and checking change received, reading prices
- money management: addressing envelopes, maintaining checkbook or ledger, reading bills or financial statements, writing checks or money orders
- community activities: accessing transportation, avoiding collisions, eating out in restaurants, locating public restrooms, negotiating curbs and steps, orienting to unfamiliar places
- productivity history, skills, interests, and values
- leisure activities and skills
- visual system: near and far acuity, contrast sensitivity function, color perception, visual field, oculomotor and pupillary function, and visual processing, including visual attention and memory
- functional mobility
- sensory acuity, registration, and modulation
- sensory processing and perceptual skills
- problem-solving and coping skills
- self-perception and self-concept
- environment: amount of illumination, glare, pattern, and contrast within the visual environment

Instruments

Instruments Developed by Occupational Therapy Personnel

- *Checklist of Pertinent Clinical Observation* by T.A. Williams, in *Adults with developmental disabilities: Current approaches in occupational therapy,* eds. M. Ross and S. Bachner, 158–162, Bethesda, MD: American Occupational Therapy Association.

Instruments Developed by Other Professionals and Used by Occupational Therapy Personnel

- *Minnesota Low Vision Reading Test* by G.E. Legge, J. Ross, and A. Luebker, *Optometry and Vision Science* 66 (1989): 843–853.

Pepper Visual Skills for Reading Test, 2nd ed. by G.R. Watson, S. Whittaker, and M. Steciw, Lilburn, GA: Bear Consultants, Inc., 1995.

PROBLEMS

Self-Care
- The person may experience a decrease in his or her ability to perform activities of daily living (e.g., eating, dressing, grooming, toileting, bathing) independently.
- The person may experience difficulty with mobility and increased loss of balance or falls inside or outside the home.
- The person may be unable to read the letters and numbers on the telephone or in the telephone book.

Productivity
- The person may experience difficulties in performing home management activities such as cooking, doing the laundry, or doing light housecleaning.
- The person may retire from work or quit volunteering because of changes in visual acuity or field of vision.

Leisure
- The person may discontinue some leisure activities or interests because of loss of visual acuity or changes in field of vision.

Sensorimotor
- The person has decreased ease of mobility.
- The person has increased incidence of fractures, burns, or other injuries.
- The person frequently has loss of visual discrimination (contrast perception) of detail versus background.
- The person may lose macular vision, which reduces the ability to focus directly on an object or person.
- The person may lose peripheral vision, which reduces the ability to scan the visual field.
- The person may have night blindness, the inability to see in dim or faint light.
- The person may have color vision defects, reduced ability to see the saturation of light necessary to accurately identify colors.
- The person may lose depth perception, the ability to orient oneself and objects in space and judge the distance between oneself and objects.
- The person may have increased sensitivity to glare and be unable to see in certain lighting conditions.

Cognitive
- Cognitive abilities are not directly affected by the disorder.
- Some indirect consequences may be the loss of opportunities to learn or relearn information because visual conditions were not suited to the person's special needs.

Psychosocial
- The person usually loses self-esteem and self-confidence.
- The person may feel hopeless and helpless.
- The person may feel anxious and demonstrate increased stress reactions.
- The person may become depressed or angry.
- The person may lack motivation and be apathetic.
- The person may become dependent on others.
- The person may experience a sense of loss and may mourn the loss of good sight.
- The person may reduce social interactions because of difficulty participating with others who have better vision.
- The person may relinquish roles or experience a change of roles in the family.

TREATMENT/INTERVENTION

The primary treatment model is to teach compensatory strategies, environmental adaptation, and use of assistive technology. The person must decide which compensatory strategies to use. One person may wish to let someone else such as the spouse do certain tasks while the individual does other, more enjoyable tasks. Another person will want to complete the task without assistance no matter how long it takes or how many assistive devices may be needed. Allowing personal choice is important to successful management of low vision.

Self-Care
- Explore with the person activities of daily living that have become more difficult to perform and suggest approaches that might improve performance, overcome fear of performing, or make the task easier to do.
- Determine if self-help devices and optical or nonoptical aids may be useful to the person and suggest that the person try using the devices to read medication and food labels and to dial the telephone.
- Work with orientation and mobility specialists regarding the need for a cane or electronic travel aids.

Productivity
- Explore with the person any home management activities that may have become more difficult to perform and suggest approaches, including the use of optical or nonoptical aids, that might improve performance or make the task easier to do.
- Help the person practice writing legibly with the aid of lined paper or stencils.
- Encourage the person to engage in other productive activities, such as volunteering.
- Assist in assessment of the person's ability to drive. Generally, the person should have best corrected visual acuities between 20/40 and 20/200 or a visual field of less than 140 degrees in the horizontal plane, or needs to be evaluated by a qualified driving evaluator.

Leisure
- Encourage the person to explore old interests that could be renewed and to develop new interests.

Examples of Optical and Nonoptical Aids

- magnifiers
- telescopes
- gooseneck lamps that adjust to a variety of positions to increase illumination
- large print clocks and watches
- checks with bold lines
- acetate filters to increase contrast between background and foreground
- large-print books
- large-print playing cards
- color-coded marks on stoves or ranges to indicate temperature

---

- Suggest modifications, such as the use of optical or nonoptical aids, that might make the activities more fun.

Sensorimotor
- Help the person identify situations in mobility that are difficult to negotiate safely and suggest solutions, such as small risers on outside stairs that might be difficult to see on a bright sunny day. A cane can be used to determine the depth and the slope of a railing.
- Provide the person with opportunities to practice using new visual equipment or optical aids that may be prescribed.
- Provide practice in using other senses to substitute or compensate for low vision, especially tactile and hearing senses.

Cognitive
- Instruct the person in the possibility of using other senses to substitute or compensate for low vision.
- Dispel stereotypical fears of blindness. Few people are completely blind, and few are completely helpless; a decrease in visual acuity is not a death sentence.
- Encourage the person to use creative problem-solving and coping skills for his or her life situation that are satisfactory to him or her and family members.

Psychosocial
- Provide opportunities for the person to improve self-perception through the use of creative activities, such as art, crafts, drama, music, and dance.
- Encourage the person to express feelings about decreasing vision and talk about what situations or tasks are most difficult to perform.
- Encourage the person to participate in group situations with other people who have low vision or are blind to learn how others cope and to trade hints for solving problems.

- Help the family sort out roles in the family unit and encourage the person with low vision to adopt an active role.
- Encourage the person and family to seek out resources in the community and use the resources as needed.

Environment

- Instruct the person and family on how to make the living environment safer by improving or increasing contrast, illumination, and pattern. The following steps will help:
  1. increasing lighting but avoiding glare (Halogen, full spectrum, and fluorescent lighting are usually better choices than incandescent lighting.)
  2. providing better contrasts between light and dark surfaces
  3. removing items that might trip the person, such as throw rugs, power cords, or small footstools
  4. avoiding extreme light to dark changes
  5. choosing colors carefully for maximum contrast of hue
  6. using solid colors rather than patterns to improve contrast
  7. reducing clutter in the room
- Assist the person and family in identifying local and national resources that can provide information, services, and devices to persons with low vision (e.g., talking books from the library).

PRECAUTIONS

- Always be alert to safety hazards.
- Always be alert for possible changes in or loss of tactile sensitivity.

PROGNOSIS AND OUTCOME

- The person is able to perform self-care tasks independently, including eating, dressing, toileting, and bathing.
- The person is able to manage medication independently, including reading and checking labels for instructions.
- The person is able to manage homemaking tasks independently, including meal preparation, doing laundry, and regulating the temperature of the living quarters.
- The person is able to go shopping at a store independently.
- The person is able to manage finances accurately, including writing checks for the correct amount, reading price tags, and identifying bills and coins correctly.
- The person is able to use optical devices successfully to compensate for loss of vision.
- The person can perform productive activities using assistive technology.
- The person engages in a variety of leisure activities.
- The person is knowledgeable about community and equipment resources available to people with low vision.
- The person is knowledgeable about ways to alter or adapt the environment to increase visibility and safety.

REFERENCE

Warren, M. 1998. *Occupational Therapy Practice Guidelines for Adults with Low Vision.* Bethesda, MD: American Occupational Therapy Association.

BIBLIOGRAPHY

Bachelder, J.M., and D. Harkins Jr. 1995. Do occupational therapists have a primary role in low vision rehabilitation? *American Journal of Occupational Therapy* 49, no. 9: 927–930.

Beaver, K.A., and W.C. Mann. 1995. Overview of technology for low vision. *American Journal of Occupational Therapy* 49, no. 9: 913–921.

Broadway, K. 1997. Using clinical reasoning in vision treatment. *Advance for Occupational Therapists* 13, no. 45: 15, 46.

Christenson, M.A. 1996. Adaptations for vision changes in older persons. *OT Practice* 1, no. 1: 30–33.

Colenbrander, A., and D.C. Fletcher. 1995. Basis concepts and terms for low vision rehabilitation. *American Journal of Occupational Therapy* 49, no. 9: 865–869.

Cooper, B.A. et al. 1993. Exploring the use of color cuing on an assistive device in the home: Six case studies. *Physical and Occupational Therapy in Geriatrics* 11, no. 4: 47–59.

Dugan, M.C., and P. McGrann. 1993. Testing vision rehab services in a long-term care setting. *OT Week* 7, no. 22: 14–15.

Hettinger, J. 1995. A focus on vision. *OT Week* 9, no. 32: 20–21.

Horowitz, B.P. 1997. Gerontic occupational therapy practice. In *Functional visual behavior: A therapist's guide to evaluation and treatment options*, ed. M. Gentile, 461–491. Bethesda, MD: American Occupational Therapy Association.

Kern, T., and N.W. Miller. 1997. Occupational therapy and collaborative intervention for adults with low vision. In *Functional visual behavior: A therapist's guide to evaluation and treatment options*, ed. M. Gentile, 493–536. Bethesda, MD: American Occupational Therapy Association.

Kerr, T. 1996. Treating the psychosocial effects of vision loss. *Advance for Occupational Therapists* 12, no. 1: 18.

Lampert, J., and D.J. Lapolice. 1995. Functional considerations in evaluation and treatment of the client with low vision. *American Journal of Occupational Therapy* 49, no. 9: 885–890.

Lange, M.L. 1995. Aiming high. *TeamRehab Report* 6, no. 9: 26–30.

Lange, M.L. 1995. High-tech solutions for low vision. *OT Week* 9, no. 46: 14–15.

Powell-Schrepfer, J. 1993. Co-treatment lessens the impact of low vision. *OT Week* 7, no. 21: 18–19.

Rosenthal, S.B. 1995. Living with low vision: A personal and professional perspective. *American Journal of Occupational Therapy* 49, no. 9: 861–864. (Case report)

Schuchard, R.A. 1995. Adaptation to macular scotomas in persons with low vision. *American Journal of Occupational Therapy* 49, no. 9: 870–876.

Stahl, C. 1997. Occupational therapy for macular deficits: Handling vision loss. *Advance for Occupational Therapists* 13, no. 45: 14.

Warren, M. 1995. Nationally speaking: Including occupational therapy in low vision rehabilitation. *American Journal of Occupational Therapy* 49, no. 9: 857–860.

Warren, M. 1995. Providing low vision rehabilitation services with occupational therapy and ophthalmology: A program description. *American Journal of Occupational Therapy* 49, no. 9: 877–883.

Warren, M. 1999. Treating low vision. *Advance for Occupational Therapy Practitioners* 15, no. 13: 7, 25.

Warren, M., and J. Lampert. 1994. Considerations in addressing the daily living needs in older persons with low vision. In *Low Vision and Vision Rehabilitation*, eds. A. Colenbrander and D.C. Fletcher, 187–195. *Ophthalmology Clinics of North America* 7.

Williams, T.A. 1995. Low vision rehabilitation for a patient with a traumatic brain injury. *American Journal of Occupational Therapy* 49, no. 9: 923–926. (Case report)

Vestibular Diseases

DESCRIPTION

The vestibular system provides the brain with information that controls balance through postural reflexes, stabilizes eye gaze through the vestibulo-ocular reflexes so the person sees clearly, codes spatial coordinates for object orientation and navigation, and contributes to autonomic responses, which prepare the person for "fight or flight."

Symptoms of vestibular diseases and disorders may include dizziness or vertigo, disequilibrium or apraxia, unsteady gait, blurred vision, nystagmus, hearing loss in one or both ears, tinnitus, nausea, and vomiting. The disorders can be divided into three groups: peripheral, central, and systemic. Note that several have multiple names. *Peripheral disorders* include benign paroxysmal positional vertigo/positional vertigo/postural vertigo/canalithiasis/ cupulolithiasis, acute labyrinthitis/vestibular neuronitis, purulent labyrinthitis/chronic vestibulopathies, Ménière's disease/endolymphatic hydrops, Lermoyez' variant of Ménière's disease, and bilateral vestibulopathies. *Central disorders* include vestibular schwannoma/ acoustic neuroma/acoustic neurinoma/eighth nerve tumor, Wallenberg's syndrome/lateral medullary syndrome, migraine headache, multiple sclerosis, head injury, cerebellopontine angle tumor, cerebellopontine angle infarct/brainstem infarct or hemorrhage, and disequilibrium of aging. Systemic disorders include diabetes and connective tissue disorders.

Benign paroxysmal positional vertigo, called also positional vertigo, postural vertigo, canalithiasis, or cupulolithiasis, is a violent vertigo lasting more than 30 seconds and is induced by certain head positions such as tilting the head backward to look up or lying on one ear or the other.

Acute labyrinthitis, called also vestibular neuronitis, is a disorder characterized by sudden onset of severe vertigo that is persistent at first, then paroxysmal. The disease is considered to be a neuronitis involving the vestibular division of the eighth cranial nerve.

Purulent labyrinthitis, also called chronic vestibulopathies, is characterized by severe vertigo and nystagmus that invariably results in complete hearing loss and is often followed by facial paralysis.

Ménière's disease is associated with generalized dilation of the membranous labyrinth (endolymphatic hydrops) and is characterized by recurrent prostrating vertigo, sensory hearing loss, and tinnitus. In *Lermoyez' variant* of Ménière's disease, hearing loss and tinnitus precede the first attack of vertigo by months or years.

Vestibular schwannoma, called also acoustic neuroma, acoustic neurinoma, or eighth nerve tumor, is a benign tumor that develops from the Schwann cells forming the sheaths of the vestibular nerves. The tumor usually arises in or immediately medial to the internal auditory canal and as it grows, presents as a cerebellopontine angle mass. As it grows into the cerebellopontine space, it begins to compress the cerebellum and brainstem. The fifth and later the seventh cranial nerves may become involved. In young children and adults, the tumor is usually surgically removed, but in older adults, radiation may be used.

Wallenberg's syndrome, also known as lateral medullary syndrome, is due to the occlusion of the posterior interior cerebellar artery and is marked by ipsilateral loss of temperature and pain sensations of the face and contralateral loss of these sensations in the extremities and trunk, ipsilateral ataxia, dysphagia, dysarthria, and nystagmus.

CAUSE

The cause of most vestibular disorders is unknown. Viruses and viral infections are thought to be involved. In benign paroxysmal positional vertigo, some possible etiologic facts appear to be spontaneous degeneration of the utricular otolithic membranes, labyrinthine concussion, otitis media, ear surgery, and occlusion of the anterior vestibular artery. Acute neuronitis is thought to be viral in origin because of its frequent epidemic occurrence, particularly among adolescents and young adults. Purulent labyrinthitis is caused by the invasion of bacteria into the inner ear. The cause of Ménière's disease is unknown, but it may result from overproduction or decreased absorption of endolymph, which causes endolymphatic hydrops or endolymphatic hypertension, with consequent degeneration of the vestibular and cochlear hair cells. Ménière's disease may also stem from autonomic nervous system dysfunction that produces a temporary constriction of blood vessels supplying the inner ear. Vestibular schwannomas are derived from Schwann cells.

ASSESSMENT

Areas

Screening

- dizziness
  1. Vertigo is an abnormal sensation of rotary movement associated with difficulty with balance, gait, and navigation in the environment.
  2. Oscillopsia, or oscillating vision, is a condition in which objects seem to move back and forth, to jerk, or to wiggle. It occurs in multiple sclerosis.
  3. Lightheadedness must be considered to rule out vestibular disorders. Lightheadedness usually indicates a stress disorder, anxiety, or a reaction to a medication.
- balance
  1. equilibrium during standing or movement
  2. spatial orientation during movement
  3. vision during movement

Comprehensive

- self-care tasks: observation of performance and client/family/caregiver report
- productivity: observation of performance and client/family/caregiver report
- leisure: observation of performance and client/family/caregiver report
- sensorimotor
  1. active and passive range of motion of the neck, limbs, and trunk
  2. muscle tone
  3. muscle strength
  4. postural control in static and dynamic positions (sitting, standing, transfers, and transitions)

5. postural alignment
6. gross coordination of the body in movement tasks
7. gait abnormalities such as wide-based gait, instability or sway in lateral or anteroposterior directions, uneven cadence, and "high guard" of the hands and upper extremities
8. oculomotor responses including the vestibulo-ocular reflex, optokinetic responses, smooth pursuit, saccades, gaze holding, and convergence/divergence
9. spatial orientation, including upright orientation, perception of vertical orientation to gravity, spatial localization such as accurate pointing, and spatial navigation such as walking a straight line
10. self-motion perceptual awareness such as dizziness, vertigo, or lightheadedness
11. perceptual illusions such as oscillopsia or optokinetic-induced illusions
12. vestibular function, including balance tests and canal function tests
13. dynamic visual acuity
14. tactile sensation
15. proprioception

Instruments

Instruments Developed by Other Professionals and Used by Occupational Therapy Personnel

- *Berg Balance Scale* (BBS) by K.O. Berg et al., in Measuring balance in the elderly: Preliminary development of an instrument, *Physiotherapy Canada* 41 (1989): 304–310.
- *Dynamic Visual Acuity While Walking* by E.J. Hillman et al., in Dynamic visual acuity while walking in normals and labyrinthine-deficient patients, *Journal of Vestibular Research* 9 (1999): 49–57.
- *Falls Efficacy Scale* (FES) by M.E. Tinetti, D. Richman, and L. Powell, in Falls efficacy as a measure of fear of falling, *Journal of Gerontology: Psychological Science* 45 (1990): P239–P243.
- *Falls Reach* (FR) by P.W. Duncan et al., in Functional reach: A new clinical measure of balance, *Journal of Gerontology: Medical Sciences* 45 (1990): M192–M197.
- *Get Up and Go* (GUGT) by S. Mathias, U.S.L. Nayak, and B. Isaacs, in Balance in elderly patients: The "Get up and Go" test, *Archives of Physical Medicine and Rehabilitation* 67 (1986): 387–389.
- *Tinetti Performance-Oriented Assessment of Mobility* (POAM) and subscale *Performance-Oriented Assessment of Balance* (POAB) by M.E. Tinetti, in Performance-Oriented Assessment of Mobility problems in elderly patients, *Journal of the American Geriatric Society* 34 (1986): 119–126.

PROBLEMS

Self-Care

- The person experiences falls or disequilibrium during performance of self-care tasks such as transfers from sitting to standing or getting in and out of the bathtub or shower.
- The person has difficulty sleeping.

Productivity
- The person has difficulty driving.
- The person exhibits impaired performance in occupational roles.

Leisure
- The person has reduced his or her participation in community or social activities.

Sensorimotor
- The person has difficulty performing tasks requiring good visual acuity, such as reading or working at a computer.
- The person complains of stomach awareness or nausea.
- The person may be deconditioned and have low endurance.
- The person may appear unsteady while sitting, standing, walking, or climbing stairs.

Cognitive
- The person may state that he or she is unable or unwilling to do certain tasks, perform certain routine activities, or go certain places because of dizziness or balance problems.
- The person may express concern about or fear of falling.
- The person may express concern or embarrassment about falling in public places.
- The person may express concern that others perceive him or her as drunk because of "unsteady" or "stumbling" gait.

Psychosocial
- The person may have agoraphobia.
- The person may show signs of depression.
- The person may show signs of anxiety.
- The person may be socially withdrawn.
- The person may be unable to fulfill occupational roles to his or her satisfaction.
- Others view the person as having difficulty meeting performance demands or expectations for social activities at home, at work, or in the community.
- Others view the person as disabled.
- Others view the person as not meeting or fulfilling role expectations.

Environment

Information about the person's environment may be reported by the person or by others.

Physical
- The person may have difficulty walking on sloping or uneven walkways and sidewalks.
- The person may have difficulty adjusting vision to reduced or changing illumination, such as moving from shade to sunlight, or glare.
- The person may have difficulty negotiating steps with or without handrails.
- The person may have difficulty with visual distractors such as dotted or patterned floor coverings, movement of other people in the environment, open spaces with nothing to touch or "hang on to," and glassed-in walkways or walls.

- The person may have difficulty negotiating some supported surfaces such as shag or pile carpeting, foam or rubbery surfaces, slippery surfaces, or rough terrain.

Temporal

The person may have difficulty crossing the street in the allotted walk time.

TREATMENT/INTERVENTION

Treatment/intervention involves two major perspectives. One deals with safety issues and compensatory strategies. The other deals with protocols for direct intervention with specific types of vestibular disorders. Education and training in safety issues and compensatory strategies are learned as part of the standard educational program in occupational therapy. Use of direct intervention protocols requires specific training in the remediation of vestibular disorders, which would usually be acquired through continuing education or through specialized field work in a clinical setting that serves persons with vestibular disorders.

Self-Care

- Recommend appropriate safety equipment for the home such as bathroom grab bars, tub seats, and safety mats; flooring materials that provide a flat surface with an even pattern that does not reflect glare; and lighting that provides an even distribution pattern while avoiding dark and light spots in traffic areas.
- Adapt self-care skills to reduce potential for falls (e.g., wearing flat shoes with nonskid soles, dressing in a sitting position).

Productivity

- Adapt meal preparation by using carts to carry dishes and heavy pans in the kitchen.
- Incorporate work simplification techniques to counteract deconditioning.

Sensorimotor

- Select and administer exercises recommended for specific vestibular disorders. For benign paroxysmal positional vertigo, techniques include the Epley maneuver for canalithiasis and the Semont maneuver for cupulolithiasis and various adaptations of the basic maneuvers called modified Epley maneuver, modified Epley maneuver with augmented head rotations, and modified Semont maneuver. The Epley maneuver begins with the Dix-Hallpike maneuver, then the head is turned to the opposite side before sitting up, with 6- to 13-second intervals between position changes. The Semont maneuver begins by facing the head opposite from the involved side. Then the head is tilted backward with the face up and toward the involved side while still facing away from the involved side and then the patient sits up, with two to three minutes between position changes.
- Use purposeful activities incorporating head movement.
- Practice transfer training for transitions from sit to stand, stand to sit, and floor to stand (to get up safely from a fall).
- Provide opportunities for balance retraining, including weight shifting, moving and negotiating in space, and carrying and manipulating objects while moving.
- Practice balance retraining exercises in different physical environments with different lighting conditions, different support surfaces, and different visual cues.

- Use activities and exercises graded to increase muscle strength, especially in the neck, trunk, legs, and feet.
- Use activities and exercises graded to increase flexibility in joint mobility, especially in the neck, trunk, legs, and feet.
- Use activities and exercises graded to increase physical endurance.

Cognitive

- Explain vestibular anatomy and function.
- Relate the person's symptoms to functional deficits based on scientific knowledge.
- Explain the rationale for treatment based on scientific knowledge.
- Provide information about other resources such as patient advocacy groups, community resources, publications, and Internet resources.

Psychosocial

- Encourage participation in social activities.

PRECAUTION

- Use short treatment sessions for exercises and active participation tasks.

PROGNOSIS AND OUTCOME

Prognosis and outcome depend on the type of vestibular disorder.

- The person is able to perform daily activities independently without assistance.
- The person is able to engage in a productive occupation, whether paid or unpaid.
- The person is able to engage in specific leisure occupations within limits of the disorder.
- The person demonstrates knowledge of the disorder and methods to control or eliminate the major symptoms.
- The person demonstrates coping skills.

BIBLIOGRAPHY

Cohen, H. 1993. Occupational therapy in vestibular rehabilitation. In *Dizziness and balance disorders: An interdisciplinary approach to diagnosis, treatment, and rehabilitation,* ed. I.K. Arenburg, 751–757. New York: Kugler.

Cohen, H. 1994. Vestibular rehabilitation: How neuroscience relates to occupational therapy. *Israel Journal of Occupational Therapy* 3, no. 4: E97–E112.

Cohen, H. 1994. Vestibular rehabilitation improves daily life function. *American Journal of Occupational Therapy* 48, no. 10: 919–925.

Cohen, H. 1999. Special senses 2: The vestibular system. In *Neuroscience for rehabilitation,* 2nd ed., ed. H. Cohen, 149–167. Philadelphia: Lippincott Williams & Wilkins.

Cohen, H. et al. 1993. Research report: A study of the Clinical Test of Sensory Interaction and Balance. *Physical Therapy* 73, no. 6: 346–351.

Cohen, H. et al. 1995. Disability in Meniere's disease. *Archives of Otolaryngology—Head and Neck Surgery* 121, no. 1: 29–33.

Cohen, H. et al. 1995. Occupation and visual/vestibular interaction in vestibular rehabilitation. *Otolaryngology—Head and Neck Surgery* 112, no. 4: 526–532.

Cohen, H. et al. 1995. Oscillopsia and vertical eye movements in Tullio's phenomenon. *Archives of Otolaryngology—Head and Neck Surgery* 121, no. 4: 459–462.

Cohen, H. et al. 1995. Vestibular rehabilitation with graded occupations. *American Journal of Occupational Therapy* 49, no. 4: 362–367.

Cohen, H. et al. 1996. Changes in sensory organization test scores with age. *Age and Ageing* 25, no. 1: 39–44.

Cohen, H.S., and J.A. Gavia. 1998. A task of assessing vertigo elicited by repetitive head movement. *American Journal of Occupational Therapy* 52, no. 8: 644–649.

Cohen, H.S., and J. Jerabek. 1999. Efficacy of treatment for posterior canal benign paroxysmal positional vertigo. *Laryngoscope* 109: 584–590.

Donato, S.M., and K.H. Pulaski. 1998. Overview of balance impairments: Functional implications. In *Stroke rehabilitation: A function-based approach,* eds. G. Gillen and A. Burhardt, 90–108. St. Louis, MO: CV Mosby.

Hillman, E.J. et al. 1999. Dynamic visual acuity while walking in normals and labyrinthine-deficient patients. *Journal of Vestibular Research* 9: 49–57.

Nakamura, D.M. et al. 1998. Measures of balance and fear of falling in the elderly: A review. *Physical and Occupational Therapy in Geriatrics* 15, no. 4: 17–32.

Sherlock, J. 1996. Getting into balance. *Rehab Management* 9, no. 1: 33, 35–36, 38.

Stahl, C. 1995. OT takes leading role in vestibular treatment. *Advance for Occupational Therapists* 11, no. 10: 13, 54.

Vision Disorders—Adult

DESCRIPTION

Vision disorders or visual impairment may occur in visual acuity, visual fields, extraocular eye movements such as diplopia (double vision) and nystagmus (involuntary rapid oscillation of the eyeballs), ptosis (drooping eyelid), exophthalmos (blinking), and oculovestibular reflexes. The retina and macula may be affected by changes within the brain such as papilledema, optic atrophy, vascular disease, retinitis, or other disorders.

Disorders of vision can occur through two modes: focal control or attentive vision; and ambient, peripheral, or preattentive vision. Focal vision provides attention to important features of an object that is being perceived and distinguished. Ambient vision works with the other sensory systems to organize and stabilize the visual field, to detect events in the environment, to determine the location in space and distance from the individual, to monitor verticality of objects, and to align the body with those objects. Finally, ambient vision is the mode of vision used in functional mobility.

Disorders of vision are not limited to the visual system itself and thus may reflect problems in other parts of the nervous system as well. Disease in the brainstem, cranial nerves, or cerebellum may lead to specific disturbances in ocular motility (eye movements) and pupillary reactivity to changes in light conditions. Disorders in the autonomic system may be indicated by ptosis and loss of pupillary dilation.

Vision disorders involve reception components including visual acuity; ocular alignment; oculomotor control, including visual fixation, pursuit eye movements or tracking, and

saccadic eye movements; visual scanning; visual convergence/divergence; visual fields; and visual skills, including visual accommodation, binocular vision, and stereopsis vision.
- visual acuity: the capacity to pick out fine details of objects in the visual field both near (reading a book) and far (reading a street sign)
- ocular alignment or phoria: even horizontal and vertical alignment of eyes
- oculomotor control: responsible for the reception of visual stimuli
  1. visual fixation: ability to focus gaze on a specific stationary object or target
  2. pursuit eye movements or tracking: used to focus continuously on a moving object so the image is maintained continuously on the fovea. Tracking may occur with eyes and head together or with eyes moving independently of the head.
  3. saccadic eye movements: rapid change of fixation from one point in the visual field to another
- visual scanning: awareness of the visual field and any new or novel stimulus that appears in the field
- visual vergence (convergence/divergence): the ability to move the eyes inward toward the nose or outward toward the temporal aspect of the face
- visual fields: the amount of visual space (measured in degrees) that one or both eyes can see while fixating on a point so as not to move the eyes; includes peripheral and focal vision. The visual field includes approximately 65 degrees upward, 75 degrees downward, 60 degrees inward, and 95 degrees outward when the eye is looking straight forward.
- visual skills
  1. visual accommodation: the process of obtaining clear vision that allows the person to focus on objects at varying distances
  2. binocular vision: the ability to mentally combine the images from the two eyes into a single perception
  3. stereopsis or depth perception: binocular depth perception or three-dimensional vision (covered under visual perception)

For the purpose of this handbook, visual impairments are related primarily to changes in the anatomy (structure) and physiology (functions or abilities) of the eye (visual) system and/or the brain's loss of ability to control various functions of the eye system. Visual perceptual disorders, discussed separately, relate to the brain's difficulty in organizing the input from the eye system so the information can be processed and codified. Some authors do not make a distinction between the eye system as a discrete unit of the brain and use of the input from the eye system that is accessed, processed, and evaluated by many areas of the brain at both the subconscious and conscious (cognitive) levels.

CAUSE

The causes of visual disorders can be direct, such as injury to the eye, or indirect, due to conditions within the body such as diabetes, which may lead to diabetic retinopathy. Some visual disorders are congenital, and others are acquired through mechanical changes such as fractures to the face or tumor growth against the optic nerve, pressure changes produced by increased spinal fluid or edema, vascular insufficiency, lesions in the visual structures, and disturbances in the autonomic system.
- refractive error:
  1. Myopia: The eye is too long, so the focused image falls in front of the retina.

2. Hyperopia: The eye is too short, so the focused image falls behind the retina.
3. Astigmatism: The eye is not perfectly spherical, causing the image to be distorted.
4. Insufficiency of accommodation: There is a reduced ability to focus on objects at normal distances. The objects or the head must be farther away or closer.
5. Fusion: Fusion is the ability of the eyes to focus on the same target at the same time.
6. Stereognosis or depth perception: These are the ability of the eyes to focus on the same target at the same time.

- ocular alignment or phoria: the natural positioning of the eyes
  1. Esophoria: The eyes are postured in front of the point of focus.
  2. Exophoria: The eyes are postured in back of the point of focus.
  3. Hyperoria: The eyes are postured above the point of focus.
  4. Hypo-oria: The eyes are postured below the point of focus.
- strabismus: the visible turning of one eye, which affects fusion and depth perception
  1. Esotropia strabismus: One eye turns in.
  2. Exotropia strabismus: One eye turns out.
  3. Hypertropia strabismus: One eye turns up relative to the other (more normally positioned) eye.
  4. Hypotropia strabismus: One eye turns down relative to the other (more normally positioned) eye.
  5. Intermittent strabismus: The person is sometimes strabismic and sometimes phoric (fusing).
  6. Alternating strabismus: The person switches from using one eye to using the other.
  7. Constant strabismus: One eye (always the same one) always turns in or out.
  8. Concomitant strabismus: The amount of eye turn is the same regardless of whether the person is looking up, down, right, left, or straight ahead.
  9. Nonconcomitant strabismus: The amount of eye turn changes depending on which direction the eyes are looking.
- oculomotor dysfunction: difficulty with activities that require smooth pursuits, tracking, and convergence and divergence. For example, during reading tasks the person may lose his or her place, skip lines, or reread lines. Other problems might be poor ball-handling skills, poor eye-hand coordination, decreased balance, and clumsiness.
- cortical blindness: a marked decrease in visual acuity causing severe blurring that is uncorrectable with lenses because destruction of the visual cortex (area 17) has occurred
- age-related changes
  1. cataracts: loss of clarity of vision due to loss of transparency of the crystalline lens of the eye
  2. age-related macular degeneration: loss of central vision due to fluid leaking from the deeper layers of the retina, pushing the retina up and detaching it from the nourishing layer
  3. arteriosclerosis: hardening of the retinal arteries leading to ischemia and retinal death due to lack of oxygen
  4. diabetic retinopathy: collection of sorbitol within the lens, which causes an osmotic gradient of fluid into the lens and leads to disruption of the lens matrix and loss of transparency

---

Screening Questions for Visual Impairment

- Have you noticed any difference in your vision?
- Do you see double?
- Did your prescription (for visual correction) change?
- Do you experience headaches?
- Have you noticed any differences in your ability to read?
- Have you noticed any differences in your ability to drive?

---

5. glaucoma: increased intraocular pressure, which interferes with blood flow and nutrients to the optic disc

ASSESSMENT

Areas
- self-care skills and performance
- productivity skills and performance
- leisure skills and performance
- visual processing skills: visual acuity, ocular alignment, visual fixation, visual fields, oculomotor control, saccadic eye movement, ocular or visual pursuit, ocular or visual scanning, convergence, phoria, strabismus, cortical blindness, age-related changes
- cognitive skills: alertness, attending behavior, attention span
- psychosocial skills: coping skills, problem-solving skills

Instruments
There are multiple terms for many visual functions. A single accepted classification system was not identified. Where possible, synonyms and related terms are noted.
- visual acuity (Aloisio 1998, 277; Zoltan 1996, 29–31)
  1. Far: Use eye charts such as the Snellen, "tumbling" E, Landot C, or Lighthouse Picture symbols set at a distance of 20 feet and an occluder or eye patch.
  2. Near: *Pepper Visual Skills for Reading Test*, 2nd ed. by G.R. Watson, S. Whittaker, and M. Steciw, Lilburn, GA: Bear Consultants, Inc., 1995. Near distance can be up to 16 inches.
- ocular alignment (teaming, binocularity) and mobility (movement): Hirschberg or penlight technique (Aloisio 1998, 277; Zoltan 1996, 32)
- visual fixation: Warren Test of Visual Fixation (Zoltan 1996, 33)
- visual fields: confrontation testing with eye patch (Aloisio 1998, 278–279; Zoltan 1996, 35–36)
- oculomotor control (ocular range of motion) and saccadic eye movement (Aloisio 1998, 278; Zoltan 1996, 37–39)
  1. King-Devick Tests
  2. Warren Test of Saccadic Eye Movements

3. *Bouska Test of Saccadic Eye Movement* by M.J. Bouska, N.A. Kauffman, and S.E. Marcus, in Disorders of the visual perceptual system, *Neurological rehabilitation,* 2nd ed., ed. D.A. Umphred, St. Louis, MO: CV Mosby, 1990, 722.
4. Pepper Visual Skills for Reading Test (see reference under "visual acuity" above)
- ocular pursuit (Zoltan 1996, 41)
  1. direction of gaze
  2. ocular pursuit test
- ocular scanning (Zoltan 1996, 41–42)
  1. *Scanboard Test* by M.L. Warren, in Identification of visual scanning defects in adults after cerebrovascular accident, *American Journal of Occupational Therapy* 44 (1990): 391–399.
- convergence and divergence (Aloisio 1998, 277; Zoltan 1996, 43–44)
  1. Warren Test of Convergence
  2. *Visual Evoked Potentials* by W.V. Padula, S. Argyris, and J. Ray, in Visual evoked potential: Evaluating treatment for post-trauma vision syndrome in patients with traumatic brain injuries, *Brain Injury* 8, no. 2 (1994): 125–133.
- visual spatial attention (see Zoltan 1996, 45–48)
  1. *Behavioural Inattention Test* (BIT) by B.A. Wilson, J. Cockburn, and P.W. Halligan, Bury St. Edmunds, Suffolk, England: Thames Valley Test Co., 1987. (Distributed in the United States by Northern Speech Services–National Rehabilitation Services, Gaylord, MI)
  2. line crossing
  3. star cancellation
  4. article reading
  5. coin sorting
  6. line bisection test
- stereopsis (Aloisio 1998, 278)
  1. viewer-free random dot test
- accommodation (Aloisio 1998, 278)
  1. isolated letters and occluder or eye patch

PROBLEMS

Self-Care
- The person may have difficulty in performing self-care skills, blurred vision, loss of visual focus and concentration, visual field loss, or confusion.
- The person may have difficulty reading text or numbers (e.g., telephone numbers or newspaper articles) close up.
- The person's ability to maneuver safely in the environment may be impaired due to problems with visual awareness, loss of depth perception, and visual scanning of the visual field.

Productivity
- The person may find it difficult to drive safely because of blurred vision, diplopia, loss of depth perception, or difficulty focusing attention and maintaining concentration.

- The person may have difficulty performing certain work tasks because of blurred vision, visual fatigue, or difficulty focusing attention and maintaining concentration.

Leisure
- The person may abandon leisure activities because of blurred vision, visual fatigue, or difficulty focusing attention and maintaining concentration.
- The person may have difficulty enjoying new leisure activities due to difficulty with visual acuity, visual attention and concentration, or diplopia.

Sensorimotor
- The person with *exophoria, exotropia, hyperopia,* or *hypo-opia* may experience the following: eyes drift apart, eyes constantly struggle to achieve alignment, binocularity is impaired, depth perception is impaired, ability to achieve and maintain convergence is impaired, a problem occurs in the mismatch between the way the individual sees the world and the way the world is, diplopia (double vision) can occur constantly or intermittently, and fusion is a struggle, resulting in mental and visual confusion (Arnsten 1994, 4).
- The person with a problem with *eye teaming (binocularity)* has an inability to focus both eyes, via the eye muscles, on the same spot at the same time because of muscle tone imbalance, which results in failure of the eye muscles to pull (contract) at the same degree of strength in the vertical or horizontal plane. These are vision disorders.
    1. The person may misalign numbers or words in columns due to difficulty in maintaining vertical or horizontal visual alignment.
    2. The person may have double vision or diplopia due to decreased range of motion of one eye.
    3. The person may lack depth or distance perception due to lack of focus of one eye.
    4. The person may squint (partially close) one eye or cover the eye altogether.
- The person with *convergence insufficiency* may experience the following: difficulty focusing; decreased depth perception; difficulty and confusion in interpreting space; decreased eye-hand coordination in self-care and hygiene; difficulty in driving, sports, and ambulation because the eyes do not help the brain stay focused; and slow speed of convergence (Aloisio 1998, 274; Arnsten 1994, 4).
- The person with *accommodation insufficiency* may have blurred vision, inattention, poor concentration, eye strain, and visual fatigue. The person's ability to shift from far to near may be impaired, and the person may demonstrate slow or absent pupillary responses (Aloisio 1998, 274; Arnsten 1994, 4).
- The person with *impaired oculomotor motility (ocular motility, ocular control,* or *eye movement control)* may have excessive head movement and reduced saccades; poor attention span; and difficulty reading (frequently losing his or her place and skipping lines of text), writing (slow copying speed), driving, tracking or visually pursuing objects in the environment, and focusing on details (Aloisio 1998, 274; Arnsten 1994, 4).
- The person who has a problem with eye movements (ocular motility) has an inability to move the eyes, via the eye muscles, in a smooth, coordinated manner that permits tracking (following a specific target) and scanning (looking, observing the visual scene to determine if the object is present). These are vision disorders.
    1. The person may neglect, be unaware of, or ignore objects in his or her left field of vision (visual field neglect, unilateral field neglect).

2. The person may be unable to locate (see, identify) objects in half of the visual field (hemianopia, visual extinction).
3. The person may have difficulty maintaining his or her place while reading, writing, or copying (tracking).
4. The person may skip lines or repeat lines while reading, writing, or copying (tracking).
5. One or both eyes may "jump" when crossing the midline or center of the visual field while moving horizontally or vertically (tracking).
6. The person may be unable to move one or both eyes across or up and down the visual field without moving the head (paralysis of gaze).
7. The person may be unable to locate objects visually in space, especially when the body is moving (scanning and fixation).
8. The person may be unaware of objects moving into the field of vision from the periphery due to difficulty in scanning.

- The person with *visual field loss* (visual field cut) may start reading in the middle of the page, ignore food on one half of the plate, have difficulty maneuvering in the environment, and have loss of awareness of peripheral visual fields (Aloisio 1998, 274; Arnsten 1994, 4).
- A person may experience *decreased blink rate* as a result of an imbalance of the autonomic system leading to dry eyes, an impaired ability to focus, and staring into space (Arnsten 1994, 4).
- The person with *decreased visual acuity* may experience blurred vision in one or both eyes consistently or inconsistently with visual fatigue and task incompletion for near or distant tasks (Aloisio 1998, 274).
- The person with *decreased functional scanning* may omit letters, words, or numbers; lose his or her place when returning to the next line of text; have exaggerated head movements; and hold work very close to his or her eyes (Aloisio 1998, 274).
- The person with *loss of color perception* may report that colors are muddy or impure; that color fades out; and that it is difficult finding items by color (Aloisio 1998, 274).
- The person with *loss of stereopsis* usually will have deficits in three-dimensional perception and decreased spatial judgment, especially in fine motor tasks (Aloisio 1998, 274).
- The person with *loss of eye movement* (paralysis) may be unable to move eyes to the right or left and up or down or have difficulty moving eyes from a fixed gaze position.
- The person with *age-related macular degeneration* will experience difficulty with all near-point activities of daily living (e.g., reading, sewing, cooking), compromise safety, and decrease mobility in the environment.

Cognitive

- The person may have a decrease in alertness, a shortened attention span, and a decreased ability to focus attention on specific tasks.
- The person may have signs of confusion and disorientation because the eyes are not providing accurate and complete information to the brain.

Psychosocial

- The person may not notice a friend or relative if that individual approaches or stands in the area of visual field loss.
- The person may exhibit signs of frustration at not being able to perform tasks.

Environment
- The person may experience difficulty with mobility and work activities in environments with poor contrast, glare, and poor illumination.

TREATMENT/INTERVENTION

Treatment and intervention include both bottom-up and top-down approaches. The bottom-up approaches are remedial or restorative, sensory integration, neurodevelopmental, and Affolter. The top-down approaches are adaptive, occupational performance, functional, and dynamic interactional approach. The remedial approach focuses on promoting new neural connections and recovering function using repeated drills and exercises. Sensory integration (SI) focuses on the organization of sensation for use in meaningful perception during the execution of an adaptive response. Neurodevelopmental therapy (NDT) focuses on stimulation of sensory systems through handling, development of normal postural movement and body scheme, "forced use" techniques to change functional capacity, and functional activities to promote movement organization, interaction with the environment, and cognitive processing. Affolter focuses on the sensory systems as the key to problem solving that leads to learning and independence through experiential learning situations and interaction with the environment. SI, NDT, and Affolter all start with tactile and kinesthetic input as a means of building a base of information for vision and visual input. The adaptive approach promotes adjustment to the environment by maximizing the person's skills in compensation techniques to perform occupational behaviors. Occupational performance focuses on the development of a person's sense of competency, mastery, and self-esteem through the performance of activities, tasks, and roles in self-care, play, leisure, and work. The functional approach uses adaptation and compensation techniques directly focused on the occupational tasks the person needs to perform by either changing the person to better perform the occupation or changing the environment to better suit the person's performance. In the dynamic interactional approach (DIA), the person practices performance in a variety of situations or contexts that is designed to promote generalization and use of information and strategies across a variety of tasks and occupations.

Occupational therapy personnel frequently work with optometrists or functional optometrists in the treatment of visual impairments. Other professionals may include a neurologist, psychologist, neuropsychologist, ophthalmologist, and neuro-ophthalmologist.

Self-Care
- Use self-care objects and activities in visual training exercises whenever possible.
- Suggest using available services for some tasks such as going to the beauty parlor for hair washing and setting or going to a podiatrist for toenail cutting if the task is too difficult.

Productivity
- Household, work, and leisure objects and activities can be integrated into visual training activities.
- If possible, practice visual training activities in the home or work setting.

Leisure
- If possible, practice visual training exercises using favorite leisure tasks and activities.
- Show the person that leisure interests can be maintained or altered.

Sensorimotor

See Zoltan (1996) for additional treatment ideas.

General
- Support use of glasses or prisms, if they are prescribed, by insisting that they be worn during treatment sessions.
- Educate the person and family as to how visual impairments interfere with daily functioning.
- Include movement in visual training exercises to integrate vision and motor actions.
- Include the person's cognitive thinking strategies in planning visual activities.

Visual Acuity
- If correction with optical lenses is insufficient, help the person learn techniques for enlarging print, reduce the density or "clutter" of the stimulus situation or task, increase the contrast between stimulus figure and ground, and improve the lighting conditions and reduce glare.
- For continuing problems of low contrast or illumination, the following environmental adaptations may be helpful:
  1. Increase contrast by using brightly or boldly colored tape on the edge of stair surfaces, paint doors bright colors, put bright labels on prescriptions, and label canned goods with different colors for different types of foods. Paint walls a light color and use dark furniture, light switches, plugs, and electrical outlets. Vertical blinds and shades can be used to control the amount of light in the room.
  2. Increase light using halogen or fluorescent lights. Make sure lighting is even; avoid shadows as much as possible. Recommend use of nonglare paper. Visors and side shields may also be helpful. Encourage the person to place the light source on the side of the best eye when doing close work.
  3. Encourage the person to use solid colors for bedspreads, countertops, dishes, rugs, tablecloths, and towels. Avoid patterns, which can blend into the background, making identification more difficult.
  4. Encourage the person to reduce clutter in cabinets and closets and on countertops and tables. Recommend ways to organize household items for easier identification and location.
- An occupational performance frame of reference can be used by focusing on
  1. performing self-care and homemaking activities independently, using efficiency, safety, and assistive devices as needed
  2. performing writing and communication tasks legibly, using lined paper and brightly colored pens as needed
  3. performing financial management and transactions independently with aids as needed
  4. performing leisure and community activities with assistive devices as needed

Ocular Alignment (Remedial Approach)
- Eye range of motion exercises that have been ordered should be done in the direction of the paresis.
- Double vision may be controlled by using a patch to occlude one eye or by encouraging fusion by starting at the most distant point where the person can maintain fusion and slowly moving the target further away until fusion is maintained at all distances.
- Ask the person to follow (track) a brightly colored object while it is moved horizontally, vertically, and diagonally.

Visual Field Deficits
- remedial approach
  1. Begin by placing self-care items and food and performing leisure activities on the side with the visual field deficit and with "forced use" make the person look to that side. Then progressively move the items toward and across the midline.
  2. The person should be taught to be aware of the deficit through the use of visual scanning. Teach the person to look to the left to check for objects in the left field, such as food on the left side of the plate or differences between the two sides, as would occur if only the right side of the face is shaved.
  3. Use verbal cues such as "Look over here" or "Look to the left," other auditory cues such as a bell or snapping fingers, or tactile cues such as rubbing to encourage the person to look toward the affected side.
  4. Use worksheets that require the person to cross the midline to complete the activity.
  5. Use a computer program designed to remediate visual field deficits.
- adaptive approach
  1. Place self-care items and food and perform leisure activities within the person's good field of vision (usually the right side).
  2. Educate the person and family about how visual field loss affects performance and how to minimize its impact on daily activities. Also stress the importance of safety.
  3. Assist the person in the development of compensatory strategies if he or she is aware of the deficit. Help the person practice these compensatory strategies in a variety of settings.

Oculomotor Deficits—Saccadic Eye Movements
- remedial approach
  1. Have the person call out or point to letters alternating between two columns on opposite sides of a page or chalkboard or printed on two sticks held several inches apart at reading distance. Vary the distance laterally and away from the eyes as the person improves. Vary the task with numbers, short two- to four-letter words, or line drawings.
  2. Add vestibular movement by having the person sit on a ball and read the letters by making a quarter-turn, then a half-turn, and then a three-quarter turn.
  3. Use a computer retraining program designed for remediation of oculomotor deficits.
- adaptive approach
  1. Use an anchor marker such as a red strip down the left margin for reading materials.
  2. Reduce the density of (or number of words on) the page during reading activities.

Visual Fixation and Scanning

- remedial approach
  1. Encourage the person to perform activities that require scanning, but do not concentrate on the scanning itself. Instead focus on the activity. Looking at a row of family photographs or sports trading cards requires scanning. Have the person find and identify certain photographs or cards. For variety, change to larger photographs or cards. Use retraining principles such as anchoring with a bright strip, slowing or speeding up the rate of scanning, reducing or increasing the density of items on the page, and providing positive feedback.
  2. Have the person cross out or cancel certain letters (e.g., all the *h*s) from a paragraph or page of a magazine or newspaper article.
  3. Use mazes, puzzles, or games that require scanning (e.g., 20 Questions).
  4. Gather a number of objects that the person uses every day (e.g., fork, toothbrush, keys, coins, pens) and have the person look for a specific item. Go to the grocery store, hardware store, or sports store and look for specific items. Scan the telephone book for a specific person or type of item. Scan the classified ads in the newspaper for specific items.
- adaptive approach
  1. Provide anchoring or cuing before beginning visual scanning or search activity.
  2. Remind the person about pacing the speed of visual scanning (e.g., "Go slowly and follow each line").
  3. Use audiotapes or posted lists to provide instructions for locating items of clothing or fixing a simple meal.
  4. Provide the family with information about scanning difficulties and their impact on daily living.

Convergence

- Remedial approach: Practice fusion exercises by beginning with the point where the person can hold fusion and gradually increasing the distance.
- Adaptation approach: Teach the person to use his or her best eye for focal vision for near vision tasks.

Visual Spatial Inattention

- remedial approach
  1. Patch the better eye to force the person to use the inattentive eye. Patching can be done alone or in combination with anchoring.
  2. Use dynamic stimuli such as flashing lights rather than static stimuli to increase alerting and attention responses.
  3. Increase orientation skills by asking the person to identify the beginning point of the task or some middle point.
  4. Use sensory cuing with verbal, auditory, and tactile activities.
  5. Use a computer program designed to remediate visual spatial inattention.
- adaptive approach
  1. Help the person learn to use head turning to compensate by leading the eyes from attended to unattended space.

2. As improvement occurs, change from head movements to eye movements and finally to scanning.
3. Begin with simple, familiar objects to locate in unattended space and gradually increase the number of items.
4. For daily activities, initially place all items within the person's good field of vision. Encourage the person to help identify compensatory strategies to increase functional independence.

Cognitive
- Ask the person to help plan visual activities.
- Ask the person to contribute ideas about what might be his or her best compensation strategies.

Psychosocial
- Help the person practice focusing or fixating vision on another person's face when that person is talking.
- Help the person practice turning toward the sound of a human voice, especially if the voice comes from the side of the visual field loss.

Environment
- Encourage family members to participate in treatment and learn what the person can do so independence can be maintained.
- Encourage family members to consider changes that will increase safety, mobility, and independence in the home.
- Encourage the person who insists on driving to limit driving to familiar areas, to avoid freeways, and to drive only during the day.
- Provide information and practice with public transportation or using delivery services if the person cannot drive.

PRECAUTIONS
- Be aware that visual impairments increase the likelihood of the person falling, whether or not there are obstacles. Hip fractures are a common result. Persons with vision worse than 20/100 are at greatest risk (Parthasarathy 1995, 14).
- Always consider how visual impairments affect the person's safety, especially when driving. Refer for driving evaluation if such equipment is not available.

PROGNOSIS AND OUTCOME
- The person is able to perform self-care and daily living tasks independently using aids (e.g., eyeglasses, prisms) as prescribed and compensatory techniques as needed.
- The person is able to perform home management or work-related tasks using aids as prescribed and compensatory techniques as needed.
- The person is able to perform and enjoy leisure pursuits using aids as prescribed and compensatory techniques as needed.

- The person is able to use his or her remaining visual processing skills effectively in the environment to accomplish occupational tasks.
- The person is able to use cognitive knowledge about visual impairments to figure out ways to compensate for the loss of vision.
- The person continues to interact with others and enjoy family and group activities.

REFERENCES

Aloisio, L. 1998. Visual dysfunction. In *Stroke rehabilitation: A function-based approach,* eds. G. Gillen and A. Burhardt, 267–284. St. Louis, MO: Mosby.

Arnsten, S.M. 1994. Vision therapy within occupational therapy. *Occupational Therapy Forum* 9, no. 24: 4–5, 10–11. (Case reports)

Parthasarathy, S.R. 1995. Rehab with a vision. *Advance for Occupational Therapists* 11, no. 45: 14–15.

Zoltan, B. 1996. Visual processing skills. In *Vision, perception, and cognition: A manual for the evaluation and treatment of the neurologically impaired adult,* 3rd ed., ed. B. Zoltan, 27–51. Thorofare, NJ: Slack.

BIBLIOGRAPHY

Beis, J-M et al. 1994. Detection of visual field deficits and visual neglect with computerized light-emitting diodes. *Archives of Physical Medicine and Rehabilitation* 75, no. 6: 711–714.

Breske, S. 1995. Opening eyes to vision deficits in rehab. *Advance for Occupational Therapists* 11, no. 25: 15, 54.

Buning, M.E., and J.R. Hanzlik. 1993. Adaptive computer use for a person with visual impairment. *American Journal of Occupational Therapy* 47, no. 11: 998–1008.

Cate, Y. et al. 1995. Occupational therapy and the person with diabetes and vision impairment. *American Journal of Occupational Therapy* 49, no. 9: 905–911.

Chaikin, L.E., and S. Downing-Baum. 1997. Functional visual skills. In *Functional visual behavior: A therapist's guide to evaluation and treatment options,* ed. M. Gentile, 105–131. Bethesda, MD: American Occupational Therapy Association.

Collins, L.F. 1996. Understanding visual impairments. *OT Practice* 1, no. 1: 27–29.

Connor, M., and W. Padula. 1997. Visual rehabilitation of the neurologically involved person. In *Functional visual behavior: A therapist's guide to evaluation and treatment options,* ed. M. Gentile, 295–319. Bethesda, MD: American Occupational Therapy Association.

Efferson, L. 1995. Disorders of vision and visual perceptual dysfunction. In *Neurological rehabilitation,* 3rd ed., ed. D.A. Umphred, 769–801. St. Louis, MO: Mosby.

Frymann, V.M. 1997. Evaluation and treatment of visual dysfunction. In *Functional visual behavior: A therapist's guide to evaluation and treatment options,* ed. M. Gentile, 251–266. Bethesda, MD: American Occupational Therapy Association.

Gianutsos, G. 1997. Vision rehabilitation following acquired brain injury. In *Functional visual behavior: A therapist's guide to evaluation and treatment options,* ed. M. Gentile, 267–294. Bethesda, MD: American Occupational Therapy Association.

Gianutsos, G., and I.B. Suchoff. 1997. Visual fields after brain injury: Management issues for the occupational therapist. In *Understanding and managing vision deficits: A guide for occupational therapists,* ed. M. Scheiman, 333–358. Bethesda, MD: American Occupational Therapy Association.

Hellerstein, L.F. 1997. Visual problems associated with brain injury. In *Understanding and managing vision deficits: A guide for occupational therapists,* ed. M. Scheiman, 233–248. Bethesda, MD: American Occupational Therapy Association.

Hellerstein, L.F., and B.I. Fishman. 1997. Visual rehabilitation for patients with brain injury. In *Understanding and managing vision deficits: A guide for occupational therapists,* ed. M. Scheiman, 249–282. Bethesda, MD: American Occupational Therapy Association.

Kerr, T. 1995. OTs teach "eccentric viewing" to clients with macular disorders. *Advance for Occupational Therapists* 11, no. 34: 14, 22.

Klinger, J.L. 1997. The client who has complete or partial loss of vision. In *Preparation and training: The healthcare professional's guide*, ed. J.L. Klinger, 105–112. Thorofare, NJ: Slack.

Peralta, C. 1999. A team approach to vision rehabilitation. *OT Practice* 4, no. 3: 46–48.

Scheiman, M. 1997. Management of refractive, visual efficiency, and visual information processing disorders. In *Understanding and managing vision deficits: A guide for occupational therapists*, ed. M. Scheiman, 153–216. Bethesda, MD: American Occupational Therapy Association.

Stahl, C. 1995. What you know about vision is important. *Advance for Occupational Therapists* 11, no. 47: 11.

Stancliff, B.L. 1996. Roundtable: Occupational therapy's role in vision impairment. *OT Practice* 1, no. 1: 18–19.

Titcomb, R.E. et al. 1997. Introduction to the dynamic process of vision. In *Functional visual behavior: A therapist's guide to evaluation and treatment options*, ed. M. Gentile, 3–39. Bethesda, MD: American Occupational Therapy Association.

Todd, V.R. 1993. Visual perceptual frame of reference: An information processing approach. In *Frames of reference for pediatric occupational therapy,* eds. P. Kramer and J. Hinjosa, 177–232. Baltimore: Williams & Wilkins.

Vicci Jr, V.R. 1995. Vision and rehab: Do you see what I see? *Advance for Occupational Therapists* 11, no. 45: 14, 46.

Warren, M. 1994. Visuospatial skills: Assessment and intervention strategies. In *AOTA self-study series: Cognitive rehabilitation*, ed. C.B. Royeen, Lesson 7. Bethesda, MD: American Occupational Therapy Association.

Warren, M., and S. Powell. 1998. Treatment of visual deficits. In *Physical dysfunction: Practice skills for the occupational therapy assistant*, ed. M.B. Early, 397–409. St. Louis, MO: Mosby.

Yuen, H.K. 1993. Improved productivity through purposeful use of additional template for a woman with cortical blindness. *American Journal of Occupational Therapy* 47, no. 2: 105–110.

Vision Disorders—Infant or Child

DESCRIPTION

An infant or child who loses vision early in life before most major stages of development have occurred is either blind or visually impaired. Blindness as a legal term means that corrected vision in the better eye is less than 20/200 (6/60 meters) or the visual field has a visual angle of 20 degrees or less (tunnel vision). An infant blind at birth is referred to as congenitally blind, but if the blindness occurs after birth, the person is referred to as adventitiously blind.

Components of Visual Reception

- *Visual reflexes* include the pupillary response, which decreases or increases depending on the amount of light available, and the blink reflex, which protects the eye by closing the eyelid.

- *Visual acuity* is the ability to resolve the fine details of objects in the visual field. This ability is measured in feet from the object, comparing the person to an average person (Schneck 1998, 6).
- *Accommodation* is the ability to change the focus of the eye so objects at different distances can be seen clearly (Schneck 1998, 6).
- *Oculomotor control and alignment* involve coordinated (control) actions in the same plane (alignment) of the extraocular muscles, innervated by the third, fourth, and sixth cranial nerves, which are responsible for automatic conjugate eye movements: lateral, vertical, and convergence (Schneck 1998, 3–4).
- *Convergence/divergence* is the ability of both eyes to turn toward and away from the medial plane (Schneck 1998, 6).
- *Visual fields* are the extent of physical space visible to an eye in a given position: the average is approximately 65 degrees upward, 75 downward, 60 inward, and 95 outward (Scheiman 1997, 401).
- *Visual skills* include binocular fusion and stereopsis. Binocular fusion is the ability to mentally combine the images from the two eyes into a single perception, whereas stereopsis is the ability of the binocular vision to determine depth perception or three-dimensional vision (Schneck 1998, 6).
- *Scanning* is the exploration of space by eye movement (Grieve 1993, 158).

Categories of Visual Impairment in Infants and Children

- *Ocular visual impairment* refers to conditions of the eyeball or to lesions of the anterior visual pathway, which runs from the retina to the lateral geniculate nucleus. Visual disorders include congenital cataracts, optic nerve atrophy or hypoplasia, retrolental fibroplasia, and retinopathy of prematurity.
- *Prenatal ocular conditions* involve congenital anomalies and the absence of part or all of the eye structure. These conditions include colobomas of the iris, congenital cataracts, congenital glaucoma, retinitis pigmentosa, and ocular albinism (Baker-Nobles 1997, 376).
- *Cortical visual impairment* (cortical blindness) is a bilateral loss of vision with normal pupillary response and no other abnormalities.
- *Eye muscle imbalance* is damage to one or more of the optic nerves or cranial nerves III, IV, or VI, or dysfunction of the association areas of the brain, especially the optic lobe. Strabismus is an example of muscle imbalance of the extraocular muscles resulting in deviation of one eye from parallelism with the other. The result is failure of one eye to converge properly on an image. Two major causes are (1) a specific oculomotor nerve lesion that results in paralysis of one or more ocular muscles (paralytic or nonconcomitant strabismus) or (2) a supranuclear defect within the central nervous system that results in unequal ocular muscle tone (nonparalytic or concomitant strabismus). Concomitant strabismus may be further divided into convergent (esotropia), divergent (exotropia), or vertical (hypertropia or hypotropia).

CAUSE

The most common cause of seeing disorders is prematurity that requires that oxygen be used for life support. About one-third of these infants will suffer retinopathy, especially retrolental fibroplasia. Other causes include congenital cataracts, optic atrophy, cortical blindness, Leber's congenital amaurosis syndrome, severe infectious diseases, and injuries. Examples of disorders with visual impairments are Apert syndrome, cerebral dysgenesis, cerebral palsy, CHARGE syndrome, cytomegalovirus (CMV), diabetes mellitus, Down's syndrome, head injuries, hemorrhage, herpes simplex virus, hydrocephalus, juvenile rheumatoid arthritis, microphthalmia, nystagmus, perinatal hypoxia-ischemia, prematurity, rubella measles, strabismus, syphilis, TORCH syndrome, toxoplasmosis, and trauma to the eye.

ASSESSMENT

Areas
- activities of daily living
- functional skills in play and self-care
- play skills development
- academic skills and achievement
- leisure skills and interests
- postural control: muscle tone and strength, reflex development and maturation, balance, stability, postural security, and endurance
- motor skills: gross motor development, skills, hand grasp functions, bilateral integration and coordination, controlled and isolated movement
- fine motor skills: development, dexterity, manipulation, and bilateral hand coordination
- motor planning or praxis skills
- sensory sensitivity, awareness, and orientation
- sensory processing and modulation: tactile, vestibular, proprioception (body schema and directionality, position in space), and auditory
- sensory discrimination and perceptual skills: tactile and auditory discrimination, identification of body parts and planes, spatial orientation
- visual reflexes: pupillary response, blink reflex
- visual acuity and accommodation
- oculomotor control (eye motility): alignment, fixation, ocular saccadics, and visual tracking (pursuit)
- visual motor skills
- visual fields
- visual skills: accommodation (eye focusing), binocularity (fusion), or monocularity (no fusion)
- convergence/divergence
- scanning
- problem-solving skills
- imitation and learning skills
- self-concept
- interpersonal relations, especially bonding to parents or caregiver
- social skills with peers, teachers, and other adults

Instruments
Instruments Developed by Occupational Therapy Personnel
- *Clinical Observation of Neuromuscular Development* by A.J. Ayres (adapted by M.P. Gilbert), *Sensory Integration Special Interest Section Newsletter* 5, no. 3 (1982): 4.

- *Erhardt Developmental Vision Assessment-Revised* (EDVA-R) by R.P. Erhardt, San Antonio, TX: Therapy Skill Builders, 1994.
- *Play History* by N. Takata, in *Play as exploratory learning: Studies in curiosity behavior*, ed. M. Reilly, Beverly Hills, CA: Sage, 1974.
- *Sensory History* by A.J. Ayres, Torrance, CA: Ayres Clinic, 1977.

Instruments Developed by Other Professionals and Used by Occupational Therapy Personnel

- *Denver Developmental Screening Test II* by W. Frankenburg, J. Dodds, and A. Fandal, Denver, CO: Denver Developmental Materials, 1990.
- *Developmental Programming for Infants and Young Children* by S.I. Rogers and D.B. D'Eugenio, Ann Arbor, MI: University of Michigan Press, 1977.
- *Family Needs Survey* by D. Baily and R. Simeonsson, Chapel Hill, NC: Frank Porter Graham Child Development Center, 1985.
- *Family Support Scale, Enabling and Empowering Families: Principles and Guidelines for Practice* by A. Dunston, M. Trivette, and S. Deal, Cambridge, MA: Brookline Books, 1988.
- *Functional Vision Inventory for the Multiply and Severely Handicapped* by B.M. Langley, Chicago: Stoelting Co., 1980.
- *Milani-Comparetti Motor Development Screening Test*, 3rd ed. rev. by W. Stuberg, Omaha, NE: Meyer Rehabilitation Institute, 1993.
- *Minnesota Rate of Manipulation Test* (MRMT), Circle Pines, MN: American Guidance Services, 1969.
- *Oregon Project Developmental Checklist* by D. Brown, V. Simmons, and J. Mathwin, Medford, OR: Jackson Education Service District, 1984.
- *Reynell-Zinkin Development Scales for Young Visually Handicapped Children* by J. Reynell and P. Zinkin, Wood Dale, IL: Stoelting Company, 1979.
- *Social Maturity Scale for Blind Preschool Children* by K.E. Maxfield and S. Bucholz, New York: American Foundation for the Blind, 1957.
- functional vision testing
- reflexes
  1. Pupillary responses to the presence of light should be quick and occur in both eyes at the same time to the same degree or size.
  2. Defensive blinking should occur when an object such as a finger is moved quickly toward the eyes.
- acuity and accommodation
  1. Snellen chart (optotype [letters or symbols] testing): The person reads the letters on the chart. The letters get progressively smaller on each line. The person is supposed to stand or sit 20 feet from the chart, which is the basis for the notation of 20/x, that is, a person standing 20 feet away can see what a person with normal vision can see at X distance.
  2. Contrast sensitivity testing: The person tries to detect differences in brightness levels between adjacent surfaces. Two types of tests exist. Sine wave grating tests use a series of pattern samples at varying spatial frequencies and contrast levels that the individual is required to detect by indicating the orientation of lines. Optotype tests assess peak contrast sensitivity rather than spatial frequencies.
- ocular control and alignment

1. Cover test: Have the person fix on a pencil or flashlight held in front of him or her. Alternately cover and uncover an eye. Watch for a shift in the eye that is being uncovered as that eye picks up fixation on the object. In esotropia, the eye that was covered will turn in to achieve fixation, while in exotropia the eye will rotate out to fixate.
   2. Tracking (ocular pursuit) test: Have the person watch the tip of a pencil or finger puppet held about 12 inches to 14 inches from the face. Move the pencil to the right and left, up and down, and diagonally. Note which eye is focusing and when the focus changes, if ever. Usually the change of focus occurs at the midline.
- visual-motor skills
   1. Observe a young child's eye-hand skills as he or she reaches for food or utensils, builds a block tower, or uses a crayon. Eye-foot skills can be observed as the person steps up or down small dropoffs or curbs.
   2. Indications of a problem include under- and overreaching, collisions with targets, missing targets, or over- and understepping (Lampert 1998, 18).
- visual field
   1. observation of eye position, head position, tone, and posture when objects are placed on a table
   2. observation of any lack of responses when targets are present in various areas and planes
- scanning
   1. For a younger child, present an array of toys and ask the child to locate a specific one. Difficulty can be graded by the number of items presented.
   2. For a younger child, present pictures or photographs and ask the child to point to specific items. Note the number of missed items.
   3. An older child may be presented with a letter or symbol cancellation test.
- interview of parents

PROBLEMS

Self-Care
- Self-feeding and -drinking are delayed because of a lack of hand-to-mouth skills.
- The person may avoid certain foods because of an odor or taste and become a picky or poor eater.
- Self-dressing skills are delayed due to lack of hand skills or to tactile defensiveness.

Productivity
- The person may have underdeveloped play skills, especially a lack of exploratory and creative play.

Leisure
- The person may have little, if any, interest in toys, games, or group activities.
- The person does not occupy him- or herself with play or vocalization.

Sensorimotor
- The person usually does not use his or her hands for exploring the environment and does not bring his or her hands to the mouth or together at midline. Rather, this person will tend to

**Comparison of Developmental Norms of Sighted
and Blind Children (mean ages)**

Behavior	Sighted (in Months)	Blind (in Months)
Makes midline reach in response to sound only	4 to 5	8.00
Elevates self by arms to prone on elbows position	2.1	8.75
Rolls from back to stomach	6.4	7.25
Crawls on all fours	7.1	13.25
Raises self to sitting position	8.3	11.00
Pulls up to stand	8.6	13.00
Walks with hands held	8.8	10.75
Walks alone across room	12.1	19.25

Source: Data from E. Adelson and S. Fraiberg, 1975, Gross Motor Development in Infants Blind From Birth, in *Annual Progress in Child Psychiatry and Child Development*, S. Chess and A. Thomas, eds., pp. 130–149, Brunner/Mazel Publishers and S. Fraiberg, *Insights from the Blind: Comparative Studies of Blind and Sighted Infants*, 1997, Basic Books, Inc.

hold the hands slightly fisted at shoulder height (high guard).
- The person usually does not like the prone position since vision does not motivate him or her to raise the head. The prone position also impedes breathing and freedom of motion.
- The person may have delays in elevating to prone, creeping, crawling, rising to sitting, pulling to standing, and walking (mobility skills) that are assumed to be related to lack of visual stimulation, which in turn delays the development of spatial and temporal relationships.
- Fine motor skills requiring manipulation and dexterity may be delayed because of lack of hand use. The use of Braille slows down learning.
- The person may avoid gross motor activities because of fear of movement. Thus, coordination and bilateral integration are poor and the person is earthbound, unable to jump, hop, or stand on one foot.
- Muscle tone may be poor (hypotonia), especially in prone extension and full flexion, but may be present throughout the body.
- Development of righting and equilibrium reactions may be delayed. Posture and balance may be poor.
- Other sensory systems may not be spontaneously explored as a means of learning about the environment. Intentional reaching may be delayed.
- The person may be tactilely defensive when picked up, during baths, or during diaper changes.
- The person may develop blindisms (self-stimulating mannerisms), such as head rolling; eye rubbing, pressing, or poking; hand fingering or rubbing; rocking or swaying the body; flicking or waving the hands in front of the eyes; and dropping the chin to the chest.
- The person may have difficulty with spatial or temporal tasks and become easily lost.
- The person may have poor body awareness, lateralization, and directionality.
- The person may be hyper- or hyporesponsive to vestibular stimulation.

- The person may be unable to replace a limb if it is passively moved to another position because proprioception is inadequate.
- The person may have a strong reaction to certain odors or smells.
- The person may be clumsy or have motor incoordination when visual perception is required.
- The person may have a history of delayed developmental milestones.
- The person may have visual perception dysfunctions (see section on visual perception).
- The person may have amblyopia (loss of visual acuity due to lack of proper stimulation).
- The person may have anisometropia (significant difference in magnitude of the refractive error between the two eyes).
- The person may have an astigmatism (blurred and distorted vision both near and far due to oval-shaped rather than spherical eye).
- The person may have strabismus (malalignment of the eyes all or part of the time).
- The person may have difficulty with oculomotor control.
- The person may have difficulty with fixation of gaze.
- The person may have difficulty tracking or pursuing an object from side to side or up and down, especially as the object crosses the midline.
- The person may lack saccadic eye movement, which will interfere with development of scanning skills.
- The person may have visual field loss.
- The person may have poor visual acuity.
- The person may have difficulty with visual skills.
- The person may have difficulty with accommodation.
- The person may have limited or no binocular vision.
- The person may have difficulty with convergence/divergence.
- The person may have difficulty with visual scanning.
- The person may have eye-hand incoordination or eye-foot incoordination.
- The person may have prolonged postrotary nystagmus.

Cognitive

- The person may have poor attending behavior and awareness of the environment.
- The person may have a tendency to use haptic memory rather than spatial or auditory memory. He or she has no concept of object permanence.

Psychosocial

- The person may have a tendency to be passive rather than active in his or her environment.
- The person may seem to withdraw from his or her environment.
- Bonding between the parent and the child may be delayed because the child does not take the initiative.
- Early nonverbal language, such as facial expressions and smiling, is delayed.
- The person may be fearful of unfamiliar voices or noises because visual identification is not available.
- Separation anxiety may be more severe and last longer than in other children.
- The person lacks visual feedback about socially approved behavior and nonverbal communication.
- The person may have loss of self-confidence and self-esteem because of repeated failure.
- The person may have feelings of being a failure, not being able to keep up with peers.

- The person may have feelings of being different, not like other kids.
- The person may experience rejection by peers, such as being told he or she is dumb, retarded, or klutzy, or become the class clown and take advantage of being different.
- Social interaction skills may be delayed.

TREATMENT/INTERVENTION

Models of treatment are based on sensory integration, stages of normal growth and development, and neurodevelopmental therapy.

Self-Care
- Promote learning and performance of daily living activities.
- Encourage hand-to-mouth skills by permitting the person to finger feed and be messy.

Productivity
- Promote development of play skills.
- Assist the person with school performance tasks.

Leisure
- Help the person explore and develop interests to build leisure skills.

Sensorimotor
- Encourage physical movement in space, such as rolling, amphibian crawling, creeping, and walking, using auditory sounds. (Note: Research suggests that mobility in the blind person is dependent on an ability to localize sound.)
- Promote reflex maturation through modulation of sensory sensitivities and the opportunity to experience various positions.
- Encourage use of hands to reach, explore, and manipulate the environment. Explore faces, foods, clothing, and common objects in the environment.
- Promote development of fine motor skills, beginning with self-feeding and holding a vibrator.
- Decrease fear of movement through a gradual introduction to vestibular and proprioceptive stimuli. (See sections on sensory integration disorders.)
- Encourage acceptance of the prone position by gradually introducing the position and using it with rocking or swinging in the parents' arms or on a bolster. Use a flashlight or other colored lights to attract any remaining vision. Slowly increase the length of time the person is in the prone position to facilitate development of extensor tone.
- Encourage sensory registration or awareness, starting with rocking and gently bouncing the child, massaging the child, singing to the child, or putting bells on the child's booties.
- Promote tactile sensory sensitivity and discrimination through the use of various textures or a feely bag, or by having the person locate objects hidden in sand.
- Decrease tactile defensiveness, if present, through the use of pressure, such as rolling in a blanket or being sandwiched between two mats.
- Promote vestibular sensitivity and discrimination through linear acceleration and deceleration on a bolster swing, platform swing, hammock swing, or net swing or by jumping, hopping, or bouncing on an inner tube or net swing that is hung from a large spring.

- Promote spatial and auditory relationships by having the person explore a room while creeping or walking. Use obstacle courses or mazes to refine his or her skills; these skills are necessary for the person to be able to use a cane.
- Maximize the use of residual vision through exploration of colored light sources from a flashlight, colored panels, or a string of Christmas tree lights. Add a bell to a penlight to encourage auditory and visual localization.
- Promote the person's response to sound and encourage localization of sounds through the use of bells on wrists or feet; crib toys that make a sound if rocked, pressed, or shaken in the hand; and music from a radio, cassette tape player, or toys with music disks. Increase the distance of sounds when the person is able to locate (turn to, touch, or grasp) sounds within arm's length.
- Maximize use of tactile perceptual, auditory perceptual, visual perceptual, and kinesthetic senses.
- Discourage blindisms by changing the person's behavior to some purposeful movement or activity, especially those related to vestibular or proprioceptive stimuli.
- Discourage eye pressing and poking, if present. Watch for infants sleeping with knuckles in the eye sockets. Encourage the person to keep fingers out of the eyes. Using arm splints to limit elbow flexion may be necessary to decrease this behavior.
- Encourage and provide opportunities for reach, manipulation of objects, movement, and exploration of the environment.
- Minimize tactile defensiveness, if present, and develop tactile perception.
- Provide vestibular and proprioceptive activities to promote body awareness in space and decrease self-stimulatory behaviors, if present.
- Develop the person's use of his or her remaining functional vision during movement and play.
- Improve the person's motor planning skills. Activities include throwing a ball or beanbag at a target at various distances, performing animal walks (frog, duck, inchworm, crab), or climbing a jungle gym.
- Improve balance and postural control. Activities include balancing on a t-stool while throwing a beanbag or kicking a ball, walking on stepping stones (carpet or colored squares placed at irregular intervals on the floor), or playing hopscotch.
- Activities for eye-hand coordination include hitting a target (start with large target and decrease size), stringing beads (start with large holes), and placing pegs (start with large pegs).

Cognitive

- Encourage concept development, including the concepts of object permanence, object recognition, sameness and difference, cause and effect, and conservation of mass.
- Show the person how to imitate to promote early learning.
- Improve spatial and auditory memory through repetitive practice and games.

Psychosocial

- Encourage the development of a sense of self.
- Promote exploration of and a sense of control (mastery) over the environment by providing toys that can be acted upon by holding, shaking, stacking, taking apart, nesting, pounding, or climbing into or upon.

- Assist parents in promoting bonding with the person by having parents place the person's hands on the parents' faces and encouraging the person to explore the parents' faces.
- Assist parents in learning to play with the person.
- Encourage language development by talking to the person about what is happening in the environment and what he or she is doing. Encourage parents to describe activities at home when the person is involved or present.

NOTES

- Adjusting the lighting in the room may enhance the person's visual performance. Lights, especially fluorescent lights, may need to be dimmed and windows shaded to reduce glare.
- Noise may also need to be controlled so the person can concentrate on the desired tasks without interference from other noises in the environment.
- Always talk to the person and explain activities at the person's level of understanding. Use normal vocabulary, including the words "look" and "see."
- Use materials with a strong contrast between foreground and background, such as black and white.

PRECAUTION

- The person should have a safe place in which to play that is free of physical hazards. Hang electrical cords and eye-catching objects that might be dangerous, such as Christmas lights, out of range of the person's hands.

PROGNOSIS AND OUTCOME

Surgical correction, optometric therapy, and the use of prisms and glasses may reduce the problems and severity of strabismus.
- The person is able to judge whether an activity can be performed safely to avoid injury.
- The person is able to perform self-care activities independently.
- The person is able to perform educational activities at the grade level expected for his or her chronological age.
- The person is able to participate in leisure activities.
- The person is able to feed himself or herself at least some foods.
- The person is able to participate in dressing or has gained some independent skills.
- The person has improved play skills.
- The person demonstrates use of his or her hands to explore the environment.
- The person demonstrates improvement in mobility skills and an increased level of development.
- The person demonstrates improvement in fine motor skills and an increased level of development.
- The person demonstrates increased muscle tone in prone extension.
- The person demonstrates improved righting and equilibrium reactions that lead to improved balance and posture.
- The person is able to localize sounds.
- The person spends less time using blindisms.

- The person tolerates vestibular stimuli and is less fearful of movement.
- The person has bonded to parents or caregivers.

REFERENCES

Baker-Nobles, L. 1997. Pediatric low vision: Ocular pathology and cortical visual impairment. In *Functional visual behavior: A therapist's guide to evaluation and treatment options,* ed. M. Gentile, 375–401. Bethesda, MD: American Occupational Therapy Association. (Case report)

Grieve, J.I. 1993. *Neuropsychology for occupational therapists: Assessment of perception and cognition.* Boston: Blackwell Scientific Publications.

Lampert, J. 1998. Working with students with visual impairment. In *Occupational therapy: Making a difference in school system practice: A self-paced clinical course,* ed. J. Case-Smith, 1–40. Bethesda, MD: American Occupational Therapy Association.

Scheiman, M. 1997. *Understanding and Managing Vision Deficits: A Guide for Occupational Therapists.* Bethesda, MD: American Occupational Therapy Association.

Schneck, C.M. 1998. Intervention for visual perception problems. In *Occupational therapy: Making a difference in school system practice,* ed. J. Case-Smith. Bethesda, MD: American Occupational Therapy Association.

BIBLIOGRAPHY

Baker-Nobles, L., and A. Rutherford. 1995. Understanding cortical vision impairment in children (review). *American Journal of Occupational Therapy* 49, no. 9: 899–903.

Benham, P. 1993. The child with visual deficits. In *Practice issues in occupational therapy: Intraprofessional team Building,* ed. S. Ryan, 27–34. Thorofare, NJ: Slack.

Downing-Baum, S. 1995. Exercises in pediatric vision therapy. *OT Week* 9, no. 24: 20–22.

Downing-Baum, S. 1995. OT and vision therapy in pediatrics: Finding pathways. *Occupational Therapy Forum* 10, no. 17: 14–17.

Downing-Baum, S., and D. Maino. 1996. Case studies show success in OT-OD treatment plans. *Advance for Occupational Therapists* 12, no. 44: 18, 46. (Case reports)

Dunlea, A. 1996. An opportunity for co-adaptation: The experience of mothers and their infants who are blind. In *Occupational science,* eds. R. Zemke and F. Clark, 229–241. Philadelphia: F.A. Davis.

Geniale, T. 1997. The treatment of the child with cerebral palsy and low vision. In *Functional visual behavior: A therapist's guide to evaluation and treatment options,* ed. M. Gentile, 403–440. Bethesda, MD: American Occupational Therapy Association.

Hyvarinen, L. 1995. Considerations in evaluation and treatment of the child with low vision. *American Journal of Occupational Therapy* 49, no. 9: 891–897.

Porr, S.M. 1999. The visual and auditory systems. In *Pediatric therapy: A systems approach,* eds. S.M. Porr and E.B. Rainville, 241–254. Philadelphia: F.A. Davis.

Roley, S.S. 1995. Visual impairments: Issues reflected through four children and their families, Part I. *Sensory Integration Special Interest Section Newsletter* 18, no. 3: 2–4.

Roley, S.S. 1995. Visual impairments: Issues reflected through four children and their families, Part II. *Sensory Integration Special Interest Section Newsletter* 18, no. 4: 1–4, 7.

Snow, E. 1996. Services for children with visual or auditory impairments. In *Occupational therapy for children,* 3rd ed., eds. J. Case-Smith et al., 717–742. St. Louis, MO: Mosby.

Todd, V.P. 1999. Visual information analysis: Frame of reference for visual perception. In *Frames of reference for pediatric occupational therapy,* 2nd ed., eds. P. Kramer and J. Hinojosa, 205–255. Philadelphia: Lippincott Williams & Wilkins.

Visual Perception Disorders—Adult

DESCRIPTION

Visual perception disorders involve difficulty perceiving and understanding information from the visual system because of dysfunction in the cortex. The visual perception components include visual attention, visual memory, visual discrimination, visual recognition, visual form perception, visual spatial perception, visual imagery, and integration of the visual stimulus with other sense modalities (Schneck 1998).

CAUSE

The usual cause of visual perception disorders in adults is injury or damage to the association areas of the brain or the nerve tracts leading to the association areas, especially the optic lobe. Injury or damage to the right hemisphere is thought to produce greater problems in visual perception than similar injury or damage to the left hemisphere. However, visual perception disorders can occur in both the left and right hemiplegia. Causes in adults are related to brain lesions that result from a cerebrovascular accident, a traumatic head injury, a tumor, viral encephalitis, multiple sclerosis, Parkinson's, Korsakoff's amnesia, dementia, or other causes.

ASSESSMENT

Areas

- visual attention (attending to a visual stimulus on verbal command)
    1. visual alertness (prepares the person to mobilize visual attention systems)
    2. visual focused attention (ability to respond to different kinds of visual stimulation, which requires skills in direction and orientation; Zoltan 1996, 125)
    3. selective visual attention (involves discrimination of stimulus information and differentiating responses, which allows activation and inhibition of responses selectively; Zoltan 1996, 125)
    4. ambient/peripheral attention (ability to look at visual field in general without focusing on any specific object)
    5. vigilance or sustained visual attention (ability to maintain attention for a long period of time, Zoltan 1996, 125)
    6. alternating or flexible attention (alternating back and forth between mental tasks while using vision to check on something else; Zoltan 1996, 125)
    7. shared or divided attention (ability to look at several things at once; Zoltan 1996, 125)
- visual memory
    1. long-term visual memory
    2. short-term visual memory
- visual form discrimination (ability to detect and differentiate between features such as color, texture, shape, and size of the stimuli)

1. abstract visual form discrimination (ability to identify or distinguish between different types of forms based on general criteria such as writing devices [e.g., pens, pencils, markers])
2. specific visual form discrimination (ability to identify specific criteria characteristic of one specific item from among others that may be similar, such as a favorite pen)

*   visual recognition or visual gnosia (ability to perceive, determine, or know what an object is or who a person is based on visual cues only)
    1. matching same and different objects or colors (ability to determine that two or more objects or colors are the same or different based on their physical properties)
    2. categorization (ability to recognize or discriminate between objects based on size, color, or shape)
*   visual form perception
    1. form constancy (recognition of objects based on their visual form or shape)
    2. visual-closure or part/whole discrimination (ability to perceive and determine that certain parts make up a whole or that a whole may be composed of identifiable parts)
    3. figure-ground discrimination (ability to distinguish the important object or detail from the background or unimportant details)
*   visual spatial perception or visual spatial relations (ability to perceive and deal with the relation of objects to each other or an object to the self or body using vision)
    1. position in space (ability to perceive, interpret, and act on concepts that deal with the position of objects in space, such as up, down, under, over, in, out, behind, in front of, or beside)
    2. depth, distance perception, or stereopsis (ability to interpret information from the environment that gives cues as to how deep, how low, how high, or how far away an object is in the environment)
    3. topographical orientation (understanding or remembering the relations of places to one another, which permits a person to negotiate space without becoming lost)
*   visual imagery or visualization (ability to see in one's mind an object or situation without the benefit of immediate visual input)
*   visual motor skills (visual motor integration, eye-hand coordination; related to the person's ability to integrate visual information processing skills with fine motor movement)

Instruments

Instruments Developed by Occupational Therapy Personnel

*   *Arnadottir Occupational Therapy Neurobehavioral Evaluation* (A-One) by G. Arnadottir, in *The brain and behavior: Assessing cortical dysfunction through activities of daily living,* St. Louis, MO: Mosby, 1990.
*   *Loewenstein Occupational Therapy Cognitive Assessment* by M. Itzkovich, B. Elezar, and S. Averbuch, Pequanock, NJ: Maddack, 1990.
*   *Motor-Free Visual Perception Test—Vertical Format* (MVPT-V) by L. Mercier et al., Novato, CA: Academic Therapy Publications, 1997.
*   *Ontario Society of Occupational Therapists Perceptual Evaluation* (OSOT), Toronto, Canada: Study Group on the Brain-Damaged Adult, 1977.

- *Rivermead Perceptual Assessment Battery* (RPAB) by S. Whiting et al., Windsor, Berkshire, England: NFER-Nelson, 1985. (Distributed in the United States by Western Psychological Services, Los Angeles)
- *Sensorimotor Integration Test for Evaluation of CVA* by J.E. Jongbloed, J.B. Collis, and W. Jones, in A sensorimotor integration test battery for CVA clients: Preliminary evidence of reliability and validity, *Occupational Therapy Journal of Research* 6, no. 3 (1986): 157–170.
- *St. Mary's CVA Evaluation* by D. Harlowe and J. Van Deusen, in Construct validation of the St. Mary's CVA Evaluation: Perceptual measures, *American Journal of Occupational Therapy* 38, no. 3 (1984): 184–186.
- *Structured Observational Test of Function* by A. Laver, Windsor, Berkshire, England: NFER-Nelson, 1995.

Instruments Developed by Other Professionals and Used by Occupational Therapy Personnel

- *Albert Test* by M.L. Albert, in A simple test of visual neglect, *Neurology* 23 (1973): 658–664.
- *Behavioural Inattention Test* (BIT) by B.A. Wilson, J. Cockburn, and P.W. Halligan, Bury St. Edmunds, Suffolk England: Thames Valley Test Co., 1987. (Distributed in the United States by Northern Speech Services-National Rehabilitation Services, Gaylord, MI)
- *Chessington Occupational Therapy Neurological Assessment Battery* (COTNAB) by R. Tyerman et al., Nottingham, England: Nottingham Rehab., 1986.
- *Color Perception Battery* by E. DeRenzi and H. Spinnier, in Impaired performance on color tasks in patients with hemispheric damage, *Cortex* 3 (1967): 194–216.
- *Dvorine Pseudo-Isochromatic (Color) Plates,* 2nd ed. by I. Dvorine, Baltimore: Waverly Press, 1953.
- *Embedded Figure Test* by O. Spreen and A.L. Benton, in *A compendium of neuropsychological tests*, eds. O. Spreen and E. Strauss, 291–296, New York: Oxford University Press, 1969, reprinted 1991. (Also available from Neuropsychological Laboratory, University of Victoria, Victoria, British Columbia, VSW 3P5)
- *Embedded Figures Test* by H.A. Witkin et al., Palo Alto, CA: Consulting Psychologists Press, 1971.
- *Facial Recognition* by A.L. Benton and M.W. Van Allen, Los Angeles: Western Psychological Services, 1968.
- *Hooper Visual Organization Test* by H.E. Hooper, Los Angeles: Western Psychological Services, 1958, revised 1983.
- *Ishibara Color Plates* by Kanehara & Company, Tokyo: 1977.
- *Judgment of Line Orientation* by A. Benton, Odessa, FL: Psychological Assessment Resources, 1973. (Also available from Western Psychological Services, Los Angeles)
- *Kohs Block Test* by S.C. Kohs, in Intelligence measurement. A psychological and statistical study based on the block design test, New York: McMillan, 1923.
- *Minnesota Paper Form Board—Revised* by R. Likert and W.H. Quasha, San Antonio, TX: The Psychological Corporation, 1970.
- *Mooney's Closure Faces Test* by C.M. Mooney, in Closure as affected by configural clarity and contextual consistency, *Canadian Journal of Psychology* 11 (1957): 1–11.

- *Raven's Progressive Matrices* by J.C. Raven, Los Angeles: Western Psychological Services, 1991.
- *Test of Everyday Attention* (TEA) by I.H. Robertson et al., Bury St. Edmunds, Suffolk, England: Thames Valley Test Co., 1994. (Available from Northern Speech Services-Northern Rehabilitation Services, Gaylord, MI)
- *Test of Facial Recognition* by A.L. Benton et al., Odessa, FL: Psychological Assessment Resources, 1973, reprinted 1994. (Also available from Western Psychological Services, Los Angeles)
- *Test of Three-Dimension Constructional Praxis* by A.L. Benton and M.L. Fogel, *Archives of Neurology* 7 (1962): 347–354.
- *Test of Visual-Perceptual Skills (Non-motor) Upper Level—Revised* by M. Gardner, Hydesville, CA: Psychological and Educational Publications, 1995.
- *Visual Form Discrimination* by A.L. Benton, Odessa, FL: Psychological Assessment Resources, 1973. (Also available from Western Psychological Services, Los Angeles)
- *Visual Object and Space Perception* (VOSP) by E. Warrington and M. James, Bury St. Edmunds, Suffolk, England: Thames Valley Test Co., 1991. (Available from Northern Speech Services-Northern Rehabilitation Services, Gaylord, MI)

PROBLEMS

Self-Care
- The person may fail to complete some tasks, such as eating food on only the left side of the plate or shaving only the left side of the face, due to a lack of awareness of items in the left field of vision.

Productivity
- The person may be unable to perform some job tasks, such as those of a visual inspector, because of perceptual disorders.
- The person may have trouble performing some home management activities (e.g., dusting) because of poor eye-hand coordination (breaking objects) or poor visual scanning to determine that dust has been removed.

Leisure
- The person usually avoids participation in leisure activities that require good performance of perceptual tasks that the person performs poorly.

Sensorimotor
- Visual attention: The person may have difficulty orienting him- or herself to receive incoming visual information.
- Visual memory: The person may have difficulty understanding and remembering the relationship of one place to another.
- Visual discrimination: The person may have difficulty finding, focusing on, and identifying an object (foreground) from the environment (background) in order to act on the object only.
- Visual recognition or visual agnosia: The person may have *visual agnosia,* the inability to recognize familiar and unfamiliar objects by sight even though the same objects may be

correctly identified by touch.
- Visual form perception: The person may be unable to identify part of an object and its relation to the whole (object) or place in the whole. Conversely, the person may be unable to perceive that a whole (object) is composed of parts.
- Visual spatial perception
  1. The person may have difficulty negotiating the environment due to problems with spatial relationships, which reduces the ability to perceive the environment (relation of objects to the self or body) and respond accordingly.
  2. The person may have difficulty judging the depth or height of a vertical surface or horizontal distance between the self and an object or between two objects.
  3. The person may have difficulty perceiving and interpreting spatial concepts, such as up, down, under, over, in, out, right, or left.
- Visual imagery or visualization: The person may be unable to see in the mind's eye, thus limiting imagery. Body image is an example. The person has difficulty *visualizing* an accurate image of the body.
- Integration of the visual stimulus with other sense modalities: The person has an inability to "steer" the body part in response to visual input. Problems may occur in the visual motor system or the extremity neuromuscular system or both.

Cognitive

- The person may have difficulty following (getting meaning from) written instructions because of the visual perceptual disorder.
- The person may have a short attention span because he or she is bothered by the eyes.
- The person may have difficulty with topographical orientation (locating the top left of a page to begin reading, writing, or copying; or becoming lost in space because of difficulty using environmental cues to orient him- or herself).
- The person may repeat the same error over and over again and not learn or have difficulty learning from the experience.
- The person may take an inordinately long time to complete a task or may quickly complete it without checking for accuracy.
- The person may exhibit poor organizational skills because he or she is unable to determine or remember what the pieces or parts of an object do and how they fit together.

Psychosocial

- The person may fear failure or ridicule.
- The person may have poor self-concept or low self-esteem.
- The person may have difficulty initiating or completing a task.
- The person may become easily frustrated and refuse to continue working on a task.
- The person may deny that anything is wrong with his or her functional skills or behavior or that any disability exists.
- The person may avoid social situations to avoid embarrassment because of clumsy behavior.

TREATMENT/INTERVENTION

Two types of treatment/intervention exist: adaptive and remedial. Adaptive techniques or methods teach coping skills to aid adjustment to the environment using the person's strengths or assets to "cover" or "work around" the problem areas. Remedial techniques or methods attempt to improve or increase the person's ability to function by retraining or reteaching previously known perceptual skills based on the assumption that the central nervous system is plastic and can reestablish connecting links that have been damaged or establish collateral or alternate links to bypass or substitute for damaged areas of the brain. Models of treatment include sensory integration or sensorimotor, neurodevelopmental therapy, transfer of training (learning theory), and functional training (compensation).

Self-Care
- Training in block design may help with organization of eating behavior.

Productivity
- Objects with which the person is familiar from home or work should be used in treatment sessions when possible.

Leisure
- Objects that the person is familiar with from leisure activities may be useful in treatment sessions.

Sensorimotor
Visual Attention
- remedial
  1. Provide cues to help the person access and use previous knowledge to organize new information.
  2. Use reward or token system to maintain attention for a predetermined length of time. The person should determine the reward.
  3. Identify which types of tasks and environments are most motivating to the person and use those tasks and situations to increase visual attention.
  4. Use computer programs designed to increase attending behavior.
- adaptive
  1. Encourage the person to use verbal mediation to compensate for attention deficit (e.g., "Look at Joe's face and focus attention on his eyes while he is speaking to me") or say steps of process aloud as the step is performed (e.g., "Put on your left sock").
  2. When instructions are given, ask the person to repeat information just provided.
  3. Reduce distractions. Remove clutter and reduce noise level in external environment and use of visual imagery to focus mental attention on the task.
  4. Emphasize important aspects of task by underlining, using a highlighter, printing in a different color, or enlarging the font.

Visual Memory
- remedial
  1. Help the person relearn rehearsal skills by asking the person to repeat information learned earlier (e.g., just a few minutes ago, an hour ago, several hours ago, yesterday).
  2. Help the person identify categories or events than can be used to encode or "file" information.

3. Vanishing cues or fade-out techniques can help the person remember in small increments.
*   adaptive
    1. Encourage the use of lists, schedules, and step-by-step instructions.
    2. Audiotapes can be used for persons with severe visual impairment.
    3. Have the person rehearse.
    4. Use association strategies where new information is associated with old information.
    5. Use pegging or mnemonic techniques where the letters of a word or phrase are used to organize a sequence.

Visual Discrimination

*   Remedial: Embedded figures may be useful in reestablishing foreground-background ability.
*   Compensation: Instruct the person to use other senses, such as touch, to examine objects rather than relying on vision.
*   Adaptation: Reduce the number of objects in the environment. Add color strips to objects to assist in identifying and locating them.

Visual Recognition—Remedial

*   Practicing with tasks involving block design, visual scanning, and visual cancellation (crossing out a particular letter every time it appears in a random list of letters) may assist with reading and writing.
*   Assemble a number of objects that are similar in shape or size or color and ask the person to identify each object.

Visual Form Perception—Remedial

*   Start with simple puzzles with few pieces and gradually increase the complexity of the puzzles.
*   Use objects with few pieces, such as a canister and lid. Have the person put the lid on the canister. Gradually increase the number of pieces until the person can reassemble a coffee pot or similar item with five to seven pieces.

Visual Spatial Perception—Remedial

*   Provide opportunities to reproduce designs to reestablish part-whole perception and position in space. Parquetry blocks, puzzles, and pegboards are useful.
*   For position in space, place three or four identical objects in the same orientation and one in a different orientation and ask the person to identify the one that is in a different orientation. The orientation may be up, down, right, or left. To confirm the selection, ask the person to place an object in the same orientation as the others.
*   For topographical disorientation, start with simple directions, asking the person to go from one place to another in a room, to another room, or outside. Gradually increase the complexity of the directions. Using familiar or expected patterns may support learning and remembering.
*   Frequently used routes may be marked with colored dots or other symbols to assist the person in locating a particular place. The symbols should be placed close together (inches apart) initially and then farther apart (feet apart, yards apart) as the learning occurs.

Visual Imagery—Remedial
- Start by having the person look at pictures of people and identify whether the people are fat, thin, or average.
- Have the person look at him- or herself and others in the mirror and indicate whether the people are fat, thin, or average.

Integration of the Visual Stimulus with Other Sense Modalities
- Games requiring gross motor actions with a ball and target may be useful to reestablish basic eye-hand or eye-foot coordination.

Cognitive
- Teach compensatory techniques to change how the person behaves: (1) Explain a problem and use simple directions to correct the problem, (2) establish and carry out a routine, (3) do each activity in a consistent manner, and (4) employ repetition as needed.
- Teach adaptation (alter the environment): Use color, such as colored ribbons, or sound, such as bells, to alert or increase attention to the involved side of the body or neglected visual field.
- Teach organization and sequence: Puzzles that illustrate the steps in a task may be used to facilitate relearning the organization and sequence of an activity.

Psychosocial
- No specific techniques were mentioned in the literature. Use of compensatory and adaptational techniques should reduce fear, frustration, and anxiety.
- Communication may be enhanced through the use of visual cues or demonstration.

PRECAUTIONS
- Persons with perceptual disorders should be watched carefully to avoid injury. The person may be unable to determine the height of a stair riser or small curb. The person with field neglect may not see a danger that is close.
- Perceptual disorders are not always readily apparent to family members, friends, supervisors, or coworkers. Small changes in the environment, such as decreases in lighting, may increase significantly the degree of dysfunction. People who live, work, and play with the person should be informed about the dysfunction to increase safety and reduce the likelihood that the affected person will get embarrassed.

PROGNOSIS AND OUTCOME
- The person is able to perform self-care and daily living activities independently.
- The person is able to perform productive activities to the level of satisfaction stated by the individual and family.
- The person is able to participate in leisure activities that are enjoyable to the individual.
- The person shows improvement in his or her scores on perceptual functions originally assessed as deficient.

REFERENCES

Schneck, C.M. 1998. Intervention for visual perception problems. In *Occupational therapy: Making a difference in school system practice*, ed. J. Case-Smith, lesson 5:3. Bethesda, MD: American Occupational Therapy Association.

Zoltan, B. 1996. Visual discrimination skills. In *Vision, perception, and cognition: A manual for the evaluation and treatment of the neurologically impaired adult*, 3rd ed., ed. B. Zoltan, 91–106. Thorofare, NJ: Slack.

BIBLIOGRAPHY

Arnadottir, G. 1999. Evaluation and intervention with complex perceptual impairment. In *Cognitive and perceptual dysfunction: A clinical reasoning approach to evaluation and intervention*, ed. C. Unsworth, 393–454. Philadelphia: F.A. Davis.

Borst, M.J., and C.Q. Peterson. 1993. Overcoming topographical orientation deficits in an elderly woman with a right cerebrovascular accident. *American Journal of Occupational Therapy* 7, no. 6: 551–554.

Cermak, S.A., and K-C Lin. 1997. Assessment of perceptual dysfunction in the adult. In *Assessment in occupational therapy and physical therapy*, eds. J. Van Deusen and D. Brunt, 302–333. Philadelphia: W.B. Saunders.

Chen Sea, M.J. et al. 1993. Patterns of visual spatial inattention and their functional significance in stroke patients. *Archives of Physical Medicine and Rehabilitation* 74, no. 4: 355–360.

Chen Sea, M.J. et al. 1993. Performance of normal Chinese adults and right CVA patients on the Random Chinese Word Cancellation Test. *Clinical Neuropsychologist* 7: 237–247.

Chen Sea, M.J., and A. Henderson. 1994. The reliability and validity of visuospatial inattention tests with stroke patients. *Occupational Therapy International* 1, no. 1: 36–48.

Fanthome, Y. et al. 1995. The treatment of visual neglect using the transfer of training approach. *British Journal of Occupational Therapy* 58, no. 1: 14–16.

Foss, J.J. 1993. Cerebral vascular accident: Visual perceptual dysfunction. In *Body image and perceptual dysfunction in adults*, ed. J. Van Deusen, 11–38. Philadelphia: W.B. Saunders.

Grieve, J.I. 1993. Introduction to assessment. In *Neuropsychology for occupational therapists: Assessment of perception and cognition*, ed. J.I. Grieve, 85–95. Boston: Blackwell Scientific Publications.

Grieve, J.I. 1993. Spatial deficits. In *Neuropsychology for occupational therapists: Assessment of perception and cognition*, ed. J.I. Grieve, 105–113. Boston: Blackwell Scientific Publications.

Grieve, J.I. 1993. Visual perceptual deficits and agnosia. In *Neuropsychology for occupational therapists: Assessment of perception and cognition*, ed. J.I. Grieve, 96–104. Boston: Blackwell Scientific Publications.

Hunt, L.A. et al. 1995. Review of the visual system in Parkinson's disease. *Optometry and Vision Science* 72, no. 2: 92–98.

Laver, A., and C. Unsworth. 1999. Evaluation and intervention with simple perceptual impairment (agnosias). In *Cognitive and perceptual dysfunction: A clinical reasoning approach to evaluation and intervention*, ed. C. Unsworth, 299–356. Philadelphia: F.A. Davis.

Lincohn, N.B. et al. 1997. Perceptual impairment and its impact on rehabilitation outcome. *Disability and Rehabilitation* 19, no. 6: 231–234.

Marshall, S.C. et al. 1997. Attentional deficits in stroke patients: A visual dual task experiment. *Archives of Physical Medicine and Rehabilitation* 78, no. 1: 7–12.

Matthey, S. et al. 1993. The clinical usefulness of the Rivermead Perceptual Assessment Battery: Statistical considerations. *British Journal of Occupational Therapy* 56, no. 10: 365–370.

Mercier, L. et al. 1995. Motor free visual perceptual test: Impact of vertical answer cards position on performance of adults with hemispatial visual neglect. *Occupational Therapy Journal of Research* 15, no. 4: 223–236.

Neistadt, M.E. 1994. Perceptual retraining for adults with diffuse brain injury (review). *American Journal of Occupational Therapy* 48, no. 3: 225–233.

Niestadt, M.E. 1994. Using research literature to develop a perceptual retraining treatment protocol. *American Journal of Occupational Therapy* 48, no. 1: 62–72.

Paul, S. 1996. Effects of computer assisted visual scanning training in the treatment of visual neglect: Three case studies. *Physical and Occupational Therapy in Geriatrics* 14, no. 2: 33–44.

Paul, S. 1997. The effects of video assisted feedback on a scanning kitchen task in individuals with left visual neglect. *Canadian Journal of Occupational Therapy* 64, no. 2: 63–69.

Quintana, L.A. 1995. Remediating perceptual impairments. In *Occupational therapy for physical dysfunction*, 4th ed., ed. C.A. Trombly, 529–538. Baltimore: Williams & Wilkins.

Su, C.Y. et al. 1995. Performance of older adults with and without cerebrovascular accident on the test of visual-perceptual skills. *American Journal of Occupational Therapy* 49, no. 6: 491–499.

Van Deusen, J. 1993. Alcohol abuse. In *Body image and perceptual dysfunction in adults*, ed. J. Van Deusen, 65–81. Philadelphia: W.B. Saunders.

Van Deusen, J. 1993. Introduction to perceptual dysfunction. In *Body image and perceptual dysfunction in adults*, ed. J. Van Deusen, 1–9. Philadelphia: W.B. Saunders.

Warren, M. 1993. A hierarchical model for evaluation and treatment of visual perceptual dysfunction in adult acquired brain injury (review). *American Journal of Occupational Therapy*, Parts 1 and 2, 47, no. 1: 42–66.

Warren, M. 1996. Evaluation and treatment of visual deficits. In *Occupational therapy: Practice skills for physical dysfunction*, 4th ed., ed. L.W. Pedretti, 193–212. St. Louis, MO: CV Mosby.

York, C.D., and S.A. Cermak. 1995. Visual perception and praxis in adults after stroke. *American Journal of Occupational Therapy* 49, no. 6: 543–550.

Part III

Nervous System Disorders

Amyotrophic Lateral Sclerosis

DESCRIPTION

Amyotrophic lateral sclerosis (ALS) is a motor neuron disease characterized by progressive degeneration of corticospinal tracts, anterior horn cells, and/or bulbar (brainstem) motor nuclei. Muscular weakness, atrophy, and signs of anterior horn cell dysfunction are usually first noticed in the hands while a person is performing fine motor tasks such as keyboarding or handling money, but sometimes they are first noticed in the feet during walking. The site of onset is random, and progression is usually symmetrical. Problems may be caused by either upper or lower motor neurons. Other signs and symptoms are cramps, fasciculations, spasticity, hyperactive deep tendon reflexes, extensor plantar reflexes, dysarthria, hoarseness, and dysphagia. Sensory systems, cognitive functions, and urinary sphincters are usually spared. There are two major subtypes of ALS: spinal (progressive) muscular atrophy and progressive bulbar palsy. Spinal muscular atrophy is characterized by lower motor neuron involvement such as weakness, atrophy, loss of reflexes, and fasciculation. Progressive bulbar palsy is characterized by upper motor neuron involvement and loss of muscles innervated by the cranial nerves. Most persons with ALS (50 percent) die within 3 years of onset, 20 percent live 5 years, 10 percent live 10 years, and some live up to 30 years (Merck 1999, 1486). The disease was first documented in 1868 by French neurologist Jean-Martin Charcot. Because the famous baseball player Lou Gehrig died of ALS in 1941, ALS is also known as Lou Gehrig's disease.

CAUSE

Although the cause is unknown, theories about the etiology of ALS include a slow-acting virus, a toxic reaction to the build up of glutamate in nerve cell synapses, an autoimmune disorder, a hormone abnormality, and an enzyme deficiency. About 10 percent have an inherited form that is transmitted on a dominant gene. People aged 40 to 70 are affected most frequently. Men are affected two to three times more frequently than women.

ASSESSMENT

Areas

- daily living, especially dysphasia, constipation, and insomnia
- productivity history, skills, interests, and values
- leisure skills and interests
- functional muscle strength and tone testing by groups of muscles
- active and passive range-of-motion testing
- gross and fine motor coordination
- signs of atrophy of hand muscles: thenar and hypothenar eminences
- muscle tone
- postural control and balance

Clinical Stages of ALS

- Stage 1: The person is able to perform normal activities of daily living. Minor limitations and some pain may be present. Endurance is less. Use of work simplification and energy conservation techniques can increase activity level.
- Stage 2: The person demonstrates muscle imbalance, decreased mobility and function, and increased muscle fatigue due to using more energy to perform activities of daily living. Self-help aids may be useful to reduce the energy expended.
- Stage 3: The person demonstrates progressive weakness of axial (trunk) muscles and greater loss of mobility and endurance. A wheelchair is essential to travel any distance. Assistance is needed to perform many activities of daily living.
- Stage 4: The person is totally dependent in activities of daily living, a respirator may be needed, and swallowing is difficult or impossible.

Source: Reprinted with permission from D.W. Janiszewski, J.T. Caroscio, and L.H. Wisham, Amyotrophic Lateral Sclerosis: A Comprehensive Rehabilitation Approach, *Archives of Physical Medicine and Rehabilitation*, Vol. 64, No. 7, pp. 304–307, © 1983.

- physical endurance
- skin integrity
- pain
- sensory registration and processing
- problem-solving and decision-making skills
- memory skills
- judgment of safety
- self-perception
- mood or affect: uncontrolled emotional outbursts, lability
- depression
- social skills
- roles and role performance
- architectural and environmental barriers

Instruments

No specific instruments were mentioned. Assessments that evaluate the following may be useful:
- activities of daily living, especially chewing and swallowing
- occupational history
- leisure activities
- muscle strength
- range of motion
- posture and balance

- hand functions
- roles and role performance

PROBLEMS

Self-Care
- The person may have difficulty with or be unable to perform activities that require fine motor skills, such as buttoning, zipping, and typing.
- The person may have difficulty with chewing and swallowing.

Productivity
- The person may be unable to continue working because of physical limitations.

Leisure
- The person may be unable to continue playing sports, playing an instrument, or enjoying other leisure activities that require muscle strength or fine motor skills.
- The person may not enjoy eating out because of chewing and swallowing problems.

Sensorimotor
- The person may have muscle weakness and atrophy (progressive muscular atrophy).
  1. intrinsic muscles of the hand
  2. upper arm and shoulder muscles
  3. lower limbs (usually in later stages), limiting mobility
- The person may have muscle spasticity and hyperreflexia (progressive muscular atrophy).
- The person may have muscle cramps in thigh muscles, which may result in falling.
- The person may have muscle fasciculations.
- The person may have brainstem signs (progressive bulbar palsy).
  1. dysarthria (difficulty articulating words when speaking due to tongue atrophy)
  2. dysphagia (difficulty with chewing and swallowing)
  3. dyspnea (difficulty in breathing due to respiratory muscle weakness)
- The person may have fatigue, with muscles that feel tired and heavy.
- The person may have reduced range of motion.
- Generally, sensation is spared except in some hereditary cases.

Cognitive
- Generally, cognition is intact, unless an Alzheimer-type dementia is also present.

Psychosocial
- The person may become depressed.
- The person may express feelings of hopelessness and despair.
- The person may feel helpless.
- The person may express suicidal thoughts.
- The person may lose his or her self-image because of altered body image.
- The person may become socially withdrawn.

TREATMENT/INTERVENTION

Treatment is based on symptoms and is aimed at maintaining an optimal level of function given the progressive, degenerative nature of the disease. Usually a multidisciplinary team is involved in the care and treatment of persons with ALS. Environmental adaptation and compensatory strategies are important models.

Self-Care

- Consider eating aids, grooming aids, and other devices that will increase the person's level of independence. Automated self-feeders should also be considered.
- Consider recommending changes in food consistencies (e.g., chopped and pureed foods) to facilitate swallowing.
- Facilitating swallowing techniques may be used before meals to aid swallowing effectiveness.
- Determine ability to operate environment-adapted aids that permit remote operation of lights, television, radio, and speakers. These aids may be useful as the disease progresses.
- Work with a speech pathologist to find the best alternative communication system as the disease progresses.
- Help the person select and learn how to use communication aids, including different types of telephones, eye-gaze charts, electronic scanners, and computer add-on boards.

Productivity

- Consider possible modifications of the work and home environments that might permit the person to continue working outside or inside the home.
- Consider possible alternative jobs or volunteer situations.
- In the early stages of the disease, energy conservation and work simplification techniques may help the person continue to be productive.
- Alternative keyboards or input devices (e.g., single switch control, head or mouth sticks, or eye gaze control) may be needed for the computer.

Leisure

- Consider possible modifications of leisure activities, such as assistive equipment or changes in rules, that might permit the person to continue to participate in some activities.
- Explore with the person new interests that would be within his or her physical capacity.

Sensorimotor

- If the person has muscle weakness, the following steps should be taken:
  1. Consider hand splints, neck supports, overhead slings, or mobile arm supports to maintain functional hand position, provide stabilization, and support weakened muscles. Splints might include a wrist cock-up, short opponens, soft cervical collar, or ankle-foot orthosis. Note: If item will be used only a short time, it may not be worth the money or time it would take to train the person to use it.
  2. To maintain functional performance, consider the use of self-help devices such as elongated handles, built-up handles, zipper pulls, button hooks, universal cuffs, Velcro closure cups with two handles, or plate guards.

3. If mild exercises are recommended, practice times should be short and the exercises should be done over several days to avoid fatigue. Strengthening should be done through functional activities such as the performance of self-care needs.
- If the person has muscle spasticity and muscle cramps, the following steps should be taken:
  1. Teach the person positions that reduce spasticity.
  2. Teach the person to change positions frequently.
  3. Teach the person to avoid situations that tend to increase spasticity, such as being in cold areas.
- If the person has brainstem symptoms, the following steps should be taken:
  1. If dysarthria becomes severe, consider alternate communication such as language boards with words, pictures, or letters.
  2. Consider recommending soft foods that require less chewing and/or moist foods to ease swallowing, eating slowly, and eating smaller bites. Increasing the number of meals and decreasing the size of the meals may also be useful.
  3. Encourage good posture when resting or sleeping.
- Maintain the person's physical endurance during the early stages through sports such as swimming or bicycling.
- Help the person select a wheelchair. Generally, the chair will need a reclining back, a headrest, an elevating padded leg rest, a padded armrest, and a safety belt. A lap tray and mobile arm supports may also be useful.
- An aquatics program may help the person maintain range of motion to prevent contractures, maintain endurance, and practice balance activities.
- As the disease progresses, passive stretching and range of motion exercises may be needed to prevent contractures.
- Assist the person in pain management (see section on chronic pain).

Cognitive
- Teach the person work simplification and energy conservation techniques.
- Teach the person safety considerations and tools for overcoming architectural barriers, such as grab bars, reachers, and shower chairs.

Psychosocial
- Provide opportunities for the person to maintain a positive self-concept through playing computer games, doing crafts, playing music, dancing, or doing other activities.
- Teach relaxation and deep breathing exercises to help deal with stress and maintain respiratory functioning.
- Discuss with the person's family how roles and responsibilities may change, and help the family adapt as the disease progresses.
- Encourage the person to maintain social interaction with relatives and friends.

Environment
- Encourage the family to participate in a self-help or support group if one is available.

- Teach the person and family about ALS and techniques for managing the progression of the disease. Discuss the person's and family's preferences regarding mechanical ventilation and tube feeding while the person is still functioning fairly well.
- Teach the family members or caregivers how to maintain good posture in bed, when sitting, and when reclining as the disease progresses.
- Teach the family members or caregivers how to use and maintain all assistive technology
- Work with the family to determine which home modifications may be needed to permit the person to stay at home as long as possible.

PRECAUTIONS

- Muscle strengthening through progressive-resistive exercises is usually not part of the treatment program since strengthening will not alter the course of the disease and may cause cramping and fatigue.
- The person should not engage in activities that can cause an overuse syndrome, which may result in loss of muscle strength.
- Watch for signs of reactive depression.
- Watch for signs of decreased respiratory function. Suctioning may be needed.
- The person should be protected from respiratory infections as much as possible.
- Watch for signs of swallowing difficulties and choking.
- Avoid fatigue.
- As the disease progresses and the person is less able to move, watch for signs of pressure sores.
- Consider the cost and appearance of any assistive device as well as how the family and person with ALS will accept it. The person's "gadget tolerance" should be determined to avoid overwhelming the person with equipment and devices.

PROGNOSIS AND OUTCOME

- The person demonstrates performance of self-care activities within the level of disease and dysfunction using assistive devices and technology as needed.
- The person performs productive activities using assistive devices and technology as needed.
- The person participates in leisure activities.
- The person is maintaining muscle strength within the level of disease.
- The person or the family members perform daily range-of-motion exercises.
- The person is maintaining physical endurance within the level of disease.
- The person is using proper positioning techniques to prevent deformity and contractures.
- The person is using adapted equipment, including splints or wheelchairs for positioning and self-help devices for self-care, productivity, or leisure, as needed.
- The person demonstrates knowledge of work simplification and energy conservation techniques.
- The person and family demonstrate knowledge of safety precautions and techniques to overcome architectural barriers.
- The person is able to perform activities and roles that provide self-satisfaction.
- The person and family are knowledgeable about community resources.

REFERENCE

Beers, M.H., and R. Berkow, eds. 1999. *The Merck Manual of Diagnosis and Therapy*, 17th ed. Whitehouse Station, NJ: Merck Research Laboratories.

BIBLIOGRAPHY

Appel, V., and M. Trail. 1997. Learning to live with ALS: Occupational therapy plays a major role. *Advance for Occupational Therapists* 13, no. 7: 17.

Appel, V., and M. Trail. 1997. When the diagnosis is ALS. *Advance for Occupational Therapists* 13, no. 5: 21.

Ber, P. 1998. Degenerative diseases of the central nervous system: Amyotrophic lateral sclerosis. In *Physical dysfunction: Practice skills for the occupational therapy assistant*, ed. M.B. Early, 484–486. St. Louis, MO: Mosby.

Beresford, S., and G. Hill. 1996. Motor neuron disease. In *Occupational therapy and physical dysfunction: Principles, skills, and practice*, eds. A. Turner et al., 481–496. New York: Churchill Livingstone.

Corr, B. et al. 1998. Service provision for patients with ALS/MND: A cost-effective multidisciplinary approach. *Journal of the Neurological Sciences* 160 (suppl. 1): S141–S145.

Murphy, N.M., and B. Thompson. 1994. Hospice: A family approach to amyotrophic lateral sclerosis. In *Amyotrophic lateral sclerosis: A comprehensive guide to management*, eds. H. Mitsumoto and F.H. Norris, 267–282. New York: Demos.

Newman, E.M. et al. 1995. Amyotrophic lateral sclerosis. In *Occupational therapy for physical dysfunction*, 4th ed., ed. C.A. Trombly, 741–742. Baltimore: Williams & Wilkins.

Pedretti, L.W., and G.L. McCormak. 1996. Amyotrophic lateral sclerosis. In *Occupational therapy: Practice skills for physical dysfunction*, 4th ed., ed. L.W. Pedretti, 842–844. St. Louis, MO: CV Mosby.

Pulaski, K.H. 1998. Adult neurological dysfunction: Amyotrophic lateral sclerosis (ALS). In *Willard and Spackman's occupational therapy*, 9th ed., eds. M.E. Neistadt and E.B. Crepeau, 672–673. Philadelphia: J.B. Lippincott.

Richer, C.B., and C.A. Bhasin. 1999. *Occupational Therapy Practice Guidelines for Adults with Neurodegenerative Diseases*. Bethesda, MD: American Occupational Therapy Association.

Trail, M. 1995. An activist follows his vision. *OT Week* 9, no. 6: 18–19. (Case report)

Trail, M. et al. 1993. ALS: Studying the fatigue factor. *OT Week* 7, no. 50: 20.

Zarrella, S. 1995. EEG-based brain-computer interface may enable communication in ALS and stroke. *Advance for Occupational Therapists* 11, no. 17: 14.

Cerebrovascular Disorder—Stroke

DESCRIPTION

A stroke is characterized by the sudden or gradual onset of neurologic symptoms caused by a diminished supply of blood to the brain. The range of disease is from little strokes, called transient ischemic attacks, in which the symptoms are reversible, to a complete stroke in which the symptoms may never completely go away. Brain infarctions or ischemic strokes account for about 75 percent of strokes, and intracerebral or subarachnoid hemorrhages for about 15 percent; the remainder are of other or unknown causes. Strokes can occur at any age, but the incidence increases with age and doubles with every decade after age 55 (Agency for Health Care Policy and Research Post-Stroke Rehabilitation, 1995, 23). The most common site of a stroke is the middle cerebral artery. Other sites are the internal carotid artery, anterior cerebral artery, posterior cerebral artery, cerebellar artery, or vertebrobasilar arteries. Stroke may also be called cerebrovascular accident (CVA) or apoplexy (an old term).

CAUSE

Ischemic strokes are typically caused by arteriosclerotic or hypertensive stenosis, thrombosis, or embolism (Merck 1999, 1471). Intracerebral hemorrhage usually results from rupture of an arteriosclerotic vessel that has been long exposed to arterial hypertension or made ischemic by local thrombosis but may be caused by a congenital aneurysm or vascular malformation. Subarachnoid hemorrhage usually occurs as a result of head trauma, aneurysm, arteriovenous malformation, or hemorrhagic disease (Merck 1999, 1424–1425). Contributing factors include arteritis; atherosclerosis; cigarette smoking; diabetes mellitus; elevated levels of cholesterol, lipoprotein, or triglyceride in the blood; a family history of stroke; heart disease; high-estrogen oral contraceptives in women; hypertension; polychythemia vera; and a sedentary lifestyle.

ASSESSMENT

Areas
- daily living skills
- functional capacities
- productivity history, skills, interests, and values
- leisure history, skills, and interests
- motor skills: muscle strength and tone, range of motion, gross motor coordination
- fine motor coordination, manipulation, and dexterity
- hand functions: grasp, hold, and release
- balance and postural control
- praxis and motor planning
- bilateral integration
- sensory registration
- sensory processing
- perceptual skills
- pain
- cognitive functions: level of awareness, concentration, orientation, memory, problem solving, learning skills, judgment of safety
- mood and affect
- self-perception
- language and communication
- roles and role functions
- social and family support

Instruments

Instruments Developed by Occupational Therapy Personnel

- *Arnadottir Occupational Therapy Neurobehavioral Evaluation* (A-One) by G. Arnadottir, in *The Brain and Behavior: Assessing Cortical Dysfunction through Activities of Daily Living,* St. Louis, MO: Mosby, 1990.
- *Assessment of Motor and Process Skills,* 2nd ed. by A.G. Fisher, Fort Collins, CO: Three Star Press, 1997.
- *Canadian Occupational Performance Measure,* 2nd ed. by M. Law et al., Ottawa, Canada: Canadian Association of Occupational Therapists, 1994.
- *Functional Test for the Hemiplegic/Paretic Upper Extremity* by D.J. Wilson, L.L. Baker, and J.A. Craddock, in *American Journal of Occupational Therapy* 38, no. 3 (1984): 159–164; or D.J. Wilson, Assessment of the hemiparetic upper extremity: A functional test, *Occupational Therapy in Health Care* 1, no. 2 (1984): 63–69.
- *Interest Checklist* by J. Matsasuya, in *American Journal of Occupational Therapy* 23, no. 4 (1969): 323–328.
- *Kohlman Evaluation of Living Skills,* 3rd ed. by L.K. Thomson, Bethesda, MD: American Occupational Therapy Association, 1992.
- *Loewenstein Occupational Therapy Cognitive Assessment* (LOTCA) by M. Itzkovich et al., Los Angeles: Western Psychological Services or Pequannock, NJ: Maddock, Inc., 1988.
- *Modified Interest Checklist* by J. Rogers, J. Weinstein, and J. Firone, in *American Journal of Occupational Therapy* 32, no. 10 (1978): 628–630.
- *Northwick Park ADL Index* by J. Benjamin, in *British Journal of Occupational Therapy* 39, no. 12 (1976): 301–306.
- *Nottingham Leisure Scale* by A.E.R. Drummond and M.F. Walker, in The Nottingham Leisure Questionnaire, *British Journal of Occupational Therapy* 7, no. 11 (1994): 414–418.
- *Nottingham 10-point ADL Scale* by D. Ebrahim, F.M. Nouri, and D. Barer, in Measuring disability after a stroke, *Journal of Epidemiology and Community Health* 39 (1985): 86–89.
- *Occupational Therapy Functional Assessment Compilation Tool* (OT FACT) by R.O. Smith, Bethesda, MD: American Occupational Therapy Association, 1990.

Instruments Developed by Other Professionals and Used by Occupational Therapy Personnel

- *Action Research Armtest* by R.C. Lyle, in A performance test for assessment of upper limb function in physical rehabilitation treatment and research, *International Journal of Rehabilitation Research* 4 (1981): 483–492.
- *Activities Index* by M. Holbrook and C.E. Skilbeck, in *Age and Ageing* 12 (1983): 170.
- *Barthel Index* by F.I. Mahoney and D.W. Barthel, in *Maryland State Medical Journal* 14 (1965): 61–65.
- *Behavioural Inattention Test* (BIT) by B.A. Wilson, J. Cockburn, and P.W. Halligan, Bury St. Edmunds, Suffolk, England: Thames Valley Test Co., 1987. (Distributed in the United States by Western Psychological Services, Los Angeles)
- *Brunnstrom Recovery Stages* by S. Brunnstrom, in *Movement Therapy in Hemiplegia,* New York: Harper & Row, 1970. (See also S.K. Shah, Reliability of the original Brunnstrom

recovery scale following hemiplegia, *Australian Occupational Therapy Journal* 31, no. 4 (1984): 144–151)

- *Child-Care Testing in Functional Training* by E. Cicenia, G. Stephenson, and C. Springer, in *Archives of Physical Medicine and Rehabilitation* 38 (1957): 651–655.
- *Frenchay Activities Index* by M. Holbrook and C.E. Skilbeck, in An activities index for use with stroke patients, *Age and Ageing* 12 (1983): 166–170.
- *Frenchay Arm Test* by L.H. DeSouza, R.L. Langton Hewer, and S. Miller, in Assessment of recovery of arm control in hemiplegic stroke patients I: Arm function tests, *International Rehabilitation Medicine* 2 (1985): 3–9.
- *Fugl-Meyer Assessment* (Brunnstrom-Fugl-Meyer Test) by A.R. Fugl-Meyer et al., in The post-stroke hemiplegic patient: A method of evaluation, *Scandinavian Journal of Rehabilitative Medicine* 7 (1975): 13–31.
- *Functional Independence Measure*, 4th ed. by Uniform Data System for Medical Rehabilitation, Buffalo, NY: Research Foundation, State University of New York at Buffalo, 1993.
- *Instrumental Activities of Daily Living Scale* by M.P. Lawton and E.M. Brody, in *Gerontologist* 9 (1969): 181.
- *Leisure Activities Blank* by G.E. McKechnie, Palo Alto, CA: Consulting Psychologists Press, 1975.
- *Mini Mental State Examination* by M.F. Folstein, S.E. Folstein, and P.R. McHugh, in Mini-mental state: A practical method for grading the cognitive state of patients for the clinician, *Journal of Psychiatric Research* 12 (1975): 189–198.
- *Modified Motor Capacity Assessment* by B. Lindmar and E. Hamrin, in Evaluation of functional capacity after stroke as a basis for active intervention, *Scandinavian Journal of Rehabilitation Medicine* 20 (1988): 103–109.
- *Motor Assessment Scale* by J.H. Carr et al., in Investigation of a new motor assessment scale for stroke patients, *Physical Therapy* 65 (1985): 175–180.
- *Ritchie Articular Index* by R.W. Bohannon and A. LeFort, in Hemiplegic shoulder pain measured with the Ritchie Articular Index, *International Journal of Rehabilitation Research* 9 (1986): 379–381.
- *Self-Assessment to Determine Child Care* by H. Anderson, in *The Disabled Homemaker*, Springfield, IL: Charles C Thomas, 1981.
- *Sodring Motor Evaluation of Stroke* (SMES) by T.B. Wyller et al., in Predictive validity of the Sodring Motor Evaluation of Stroke patients (SMES), *Scandinavian Journal of Rehabilitation Medicine* 28 (1996): 211–216.

PROBLEMS

Self-Care

- The person usually experiences some difficulty in performing daily living skills, especially eating, dressing, grooming, and toileting.
- The person may be incontinent.
- The person may have dysphagia or difficulty with swallowing.
- The person may have dysarthria or difficulty with pronunciation of words.

Productivity
- Many problems depend on whether the left or right side is involved.
- The person may be unable to use the involved hand.

Leisure
- The person may be unable to engage in leisure activities due to motor or sensory problems.
- The person may lack interest in leisure activities due to cognitive problems.

Sensorimotor
- The symptoms from a CVA vary in type and intensity depending on the type of stroke and the amount of tissue damage incurred.
- The person usually has hemiplegia and/or hemiparesis.
- The person may have low (hypotonicity), high (hypertonicity), or fluctuating muscle tone on the involved side.
- The person may have clonus.
- The person may have spasticity.
- The person may have flaccidity.
- The person may have ataxia.
- The person usually has motor skill deficits.
- The person may have motor perseveration or impersistence.
- The person may develop contractures.
- The person may have tendinitis.
- The person may have an impaired sense of balance and equilibrium.
- The person may have hyporesponsiveness (diminished or absent response to sensory input). (Note: Auditory sense is not usually affected by the stroke itself, but hearing may be decreased by the normal aging process, especially in men.)
- The person may have visual deficits, including loss of visual acuity, diplopia (double vision), and visual field deficits such as homonymous hemianopsis (visual spatial neglect). (Note: Color discrimination is usually not changed by the stroke itself but may be less acute due to changes occurring in the normal aging process.)
- The person may have visual perceptual problems, such as difficulty with figure-ground or depth perception and spatial relations.
- The person may have perceptual motor impairments, such as unilateral neglect, apraxia or dyspraxis, body awareness deficits, and agnosia. These topics are discussed in separate sections.
- The person may have disturbance of body image or prosopagnosia (difficulty in recognizing familiar faces).
- The person may have astereognosis (tactile amnesia).
- The person may experience numbness or decreased tactile sensation.
- The person may experience loss of proprioception (position sense).
- The person may experience loss of mechanoreception (deep pressure and vibration).
- The person may lose the ability to notice when the temperature changes.
- The person's sense of taste and smell may be dulled.
- The person may develop pressure sores.

- The person may develop pain (causalgia), especially in the shoulder.
- The person may develop shoulder-hand syndrome (see section on reflex sympathetic dystrophy syndrome).

Cognitive

- The person may have difficulty with starting and finishing tasks due to lack of motivation or drive.
- The person may have a decreased level of consciousness.
- The person may have decreased attending behavior and ability to concentrate.
- The person may be disoriented and confused.
- The person may have memory loss.
- The person may have difficulty with sequencing and organization of tasks. Categorization may also be affected.
- The person may have difficulty with abstract reasoning and problem solving.
- The person may have difficulty thinking in a flow of ideas that provides flexibility to find alternatives.
- The person may lack insight into deficits or dysfunctions that have occurred as a result of the stroke.
- The person may lack judgment or the ability to understand the consequences of actions, including the safety of him- or herself and others.
- The person may have difficulty generalizing learning from one situation to another.
- The person may have difficulty learning new information.
- The person may have difficulty monitoring performance for quality control. The same errors or omissions occur repeatedly.
- The person may experience cognitive fatigue, which may be manifested as increasing difficulty with attention and concentration, lethargy, distractibility, performance errors and decreased quality control, performance speed, and frustration tolerance.

Psychosocial

- The person may be impulsive.
- The person may perseverate or repeat meaningless actions many times until someone intervenes.
- The person may become depressed or express feelings of despair and hopelessness.
- The person may be labile, showing emotional instability or mood impairment.
- The person may be anxious or fearful about his or her health.
- The person may become hostile or angry.
- The person may have low frustration tolerance.
- The person may be easily irritated.
- The person may be apathetic or show a flat affect.
- The person may have poor self-concept and loss of self-esteem.
- The person may have communication problems (expressive or receptive aphasia).
- The person may experience changes in social role.
- The person may experience sexual dysfunction.
- The person may have difficulty with social activities.

TREATMENT/INTERVENTION

The treatment models include remedial, compensatory, functional, environmental adaptation, and prevention. Specific models of treatment include biomechanical, neurodevelopment therapy, stages of recovery, and motor relearning program.

Self-Care

- If the dominant side is the affected or involved side, teach compensatory techniques for self-care and activities of daily living. If return of function occurs, the person can decide whether compensatory techniques are still needed.
- Encourage functional mobility during self-care and activities of daily living with adaptive techniques.
- If the person has dysphagia (see also section on dyphagia), take the following steps:
  1. Assess palatal and pharyngeal reflexes.
  2. Elevate the person's head and turn it toward the unaffected side when feeding.
  3. Place food on the unaffected side of the mouth if the person is able to manage oral intake.
- If the person has trouble dressing, teach the person to put the garment on the affected side first, then the unaffected side.
- If the person has trouble transferring, take the following steps:
  1. Teach the person to put the unaffected leg under the affected leg and lift it to move the lower part of body or position the affected leg.
  2. Teach the person to use his or her unaffected arm to lift and position the affected arm.
- A variety of self-help devices may be useful, including button hooks, utensils, reachers, Velcro fasteners, extended handles, and enlarged handles for eating, writing, and grooming.

Productivity

- Evaluate the person's job requirements and determine the person's level of function.
- Look for possible environmental adaptations or modifications of job tasks that might enable the person to function satisfactorily in the job situation.
- Suggest possible alternative job situations if the person is unable to function satisfactorily in his or her current job.

Leisure

- Determine what leisure activities the person enjoyed before the CVA and whether the person will be able to continue those activities, with or without modification of the tasks or environmental adaptations.

Sensorimotor

- If the person has hemiplegia or hemiparesis (see also the section on hemiplegia), take the following steps:
  1. Provide range-of-motion exercises using facilitation techniques.
  2. Promote proper positioning and body alignment.
  3. Consider providing a splint to keep the person's wrist and hand in a neutral or slightly extended position to avoid wrist drop.
- If the person needs motor retraining, use sensorimotor or functionally based approaches that accomplish the following:

1. Encourage normal postural mechanisms.
2. Encourage normal movement patterns.
3. Use the affected side in functional activities as much as possible.
- If the person has clonus, placing pressure on the heel or standing with the heel down will stop the clonus.
- If the person has spasticity or high muscle tone, use facilitation techniques designed to decrease (inhibit or reduce) the tone in the flexor muscles of the upper extremity and the extensor muscles in the lower extremity.
- If the person needs bilateral integration, take the following steps:
  1. Increase tactile and visual input to encourage development of movement sense.
  2. Keep the involved extremity in the visual field and properly positioned.
  3. Use upper extremity activities with hands clasped, such as pushing a bag or sack across a table.
  4. Place the involved arm on a hemiskate. With the active hand, move the hemiskate in a figure eight pattern on a table.
  5. As improvement occurs, use the involved hand as a stabilizer and then as the initiator of tasks.
- If the person needs to increase strength and endurance, take the following steps:
  1. Note: Reduce spasticity first. Strengthen through resistive tasks only to point of spasticity.
  2. Grade endurance tasks and times, using those activities that are meaningful to the person (e.g., self-care, productivity, or leisure activities).
- If the person has flaccidity or low muscle tone, use facilitation techniques designed to increase muscle tone, such as tactile and proprioceptive input.
- If the person has ataxia, avoid letting him or her walk unassisted on rough or uneven surfaces without supervision, but work toward improving balance reactions.
- If edema occurs, use elevation and retrograde massage.
- If the person has motor perseveration, divert or refocus the individual's attention.
- If the person has shoulder-hand syndrome, provide massage, compression, elevation, proper positioning, and vigorous exercise (see section on complex regional pain syndrome).
- If the person has contractures, apply pressure in the direction opposite to the contracture, especially if the contractures resulted from an activity that required repetitive motions.
- If the person has subluxation, apply compression to the joint capsule and provide full support using pillows in bed and a lapboard or arm trough while sitting. Use of arm slings is controversial because the sling tends to increase the flexion, adduction posture while reducing sensory feedback but not reducing the subluxation. A sling may be needed temporarily for severe edema.
- If the person has tendinitis, see section on complex regional pain syndrome.
- If the person has visual deficits (see also section on visual perception disorders), such as
  1. hemianopsia, approach the person from the unaffected side, address him or her by name, and teach the person to move his or her head to compensate for the lack of visual field
  2. double vision (diplopia), patch one eye or cover one lens of his or her eyeglasses
  3. diminished visual acuity, encourage the person to wear eyeglasses if they were worn before the stroke, and provide good lighting.

- If the person has sensory input (touch, pressure, pain, temperature, proprioception) deficits, take the following steps:
  1. Touch the person firmly with your whole hand instead of a finger.
  2. Teach the person to protect the involved side from mechanical and thermal injuries.
  3. Teach the person to inspect skin for signs of injury or irritation.
  4. Provide opportunities for the person to handle objects of different weights, textures, and sizes. Stress recognition of differences.
  5. Teach the person to check body position visually to compensate for decreased position sense.
  6. Instruct the person about changes in taste and smell that could contribute to poor appetite, complaints about food having no flavor, failure to enjoy smelling fresh flowers, or concerns that the person would not notice if food has "gone bad."
  7. Instruct the person that reduced sensory awareness increases the potential for injury.
- If the person has the following perceptual deficits, take the steps listed below:
  1. body scheme disturbance (amnesia or denial of paralyzed extremities)
     - Direct the person's attention to the involved side and provide sensory input.
     - Teach the person to maintain hygiene for the involved side.
  2. disorientation to time, place, or other people
     - Provide a calendar, a clock, and pictures of family members to reinforce orientation.
     - Correct any of the person's misinformation.
     - Reorient the person as necessary.
     - Talk to the person about the environment.
     - Attempt to limit the amount of changes in the person's schedule.
  3. apraxia (loss of ability to perform purposeful actions)
     - Correct misuse of objects and demonstrate proper use.
     - Note incorrect sequence of actions or steps while the person is performing a task, and demonstrate the proper sequence.
  4. spatial orientation (deficits in locating objects in space, estimating size, or judging distance)
     - Reduce or remove stimuli that distract the person.
     - Have the person relearn skills by repeated practice.
     - Place necessary items such as tools and equipment where the person will see them.
     - Remind the person where these items are kept when not in use.
  5. right-left disorientation
     - As words or directions are spoken, point to the side of body that should be used.
     - As words or directions are spoken, point to the direction in space.
- If the person has pressure sores or decubitus ulcers, take the following steps:
  1. Prevention should be based on having the person avoid spending long periods in one position. Frequent turning or release of pressure every two hours is recommended.
  2. Skin surfaces over bony prominences should be inspected frequently.
- If the person has shoulder pain, take the following steps:
  1. Prevention should be based on having the person avoid uncontrolled abduction of the shoulder during exercises. Avoid using overhead slings or pulley exercises.
  2. Support the person's arm during range-of-motion exercises or skateboard exercises.

Cognitive

- If the person has loss of memory, take the following steps:
  1. Correct facts or information that are misremembered.
  2. Provide facts or information that cannot be remembered.
- If the person has a short attention span and is easily distracted, take the following steps:
  1. Remove or eliminate from the environment stimuli that tend to be distracting.
  2. Divide activities into simple, short steps.
  3. Work on new tasks when the person is rested.
  4. Provide motivation and praise the person for accomplishing or finishing a task.
- If the person has poor judgment or reasoning skills, take the following steps:
  1. Protect the person from injury (physical and psychological).
  2. Set realistic goals for the person to achieve.
  3. Give simple explanations or rationales for doing something in a particular way.
- If the person exhibits poor transfer of learning from one situation to another, take the following steps:
  1. Repeat instructions. Do not expect the person to remember.
  2. Explain similarities in situations simply and briefly.
- If the person has an inability to calculate, take the following steps:
  1. Review basic math skills.
  2. Suggest that the person use a small calculator.

Psychosocial

- If the person has lability, take the following steps:
  1. Disregard bursts of emotion.
  2. Explain to the person that emotional lability is part of the illness and that the condition will improve with time.
- If the person shows hopelessness and despair, take the following steps:
  1. Provide opportunities for success.
  2. Provide feedback on improvement by comparing the person's previous and current levels of performance when the level has improved.
- If the person shows reduced tolerance to stress, take the following steps:
  1. Control the amount of stress experienced by the person.
  2. Keep practice sessions short.
- If the person shows fear, hostility, frustration, and anger, take the following steps:
  1. Accept the person's behavior.
  2. Be supportive; allow the person to verbalize feelings.
- If the person shows confusion, take the following steps:
  1. Clarify misconceptions.
  2. Verify time, date, and place.
- If the person exhibits withdrawal and isolation, take the following steps:
  1. Provide stimulation and a safe, comfortable environment.
  2. Encourage contact with other people, especially family and friends.
- If the person shows depression, take the following steps:
  1. Try to involve the person in activities that he or she enjoys.
  2. Observe the person carefully for suicidal tendencies.

- If the person has the following communication problems, work with a speech pathologist, if available:
  1. expressive aphasia (anomia)
     - Provide alternate methods of communication, such as the alphabet or symbol boards.
     - Have the person repeat individual sounds of the alphabet.
     - Have the person identify common objects in the environment.
     - Be patient as the person tries to speak or gesture.
  2. receptive aphasia
     - Speak clearly and in simple terms, using gestures as needed.
     - Provide for alternate methods of communication.
  3. global aphasia
     - Determine what skills are intact.
     - Speak in very simple sentences.
     - Practice individual sounds of the alphabet.
     - Point to common objects, give them a name, and ask the person to repeat the name.
     - Have the person write simple words and simple sentences.
  4. dysarthria
     - Provide alternative forms of communication, such as the alphabet or picture boards.

Environment
- Educate the person and his or her caregiver about problems associated with stroke and recovery from stroke.

PRECAUTIONS
- Loss of sensation increases risk of injury. Monitor the person's safety.
- Watch for signs of reflex sympathetic dystrophy and treat immediately.
- Watch for signs of reactive or secondary depression.
- Watch for signs of contractures.
- Watch for signs of skin breakdown or pressure sores and treat immediately.
- Avoid abnormal postures and movements.

PROGNOSIS AND OUTCOME
   Major recovery of functional abilities occurs within the first six months after the stroke, but some recovery continues from six months to two years afterward. Of primary importance is the person's ability to learn because rehabilitation is a learning process. Also important are the multiple factors involved, including physical, psychological, and social functions that are intertwined and interrelated. The most frequent measure of recovery is the degree of independence the person has achieved in activities of daily living.
- The person has the functional skills needed to survive within his or her living situation.
- The person is able to participate in productive activities.
- The person is able to participate in leisure activities that provide satisfaction and enjoyment.
- Muscle strength in the upper extremities has improved in all muscle groups.
- Range of motion has improved in all joints of the upper extremity.

- Edema has decreased.
- The person demonstrates skill in performing self-ranging exercises to maintain the involved upper extremity.
- Sensation in the upper extremity has improved so that burns or injuries can be avoided.
- The person is able to compensate for lack of visual field, if needed.
- The person has improved balance and equilibrium reflexes and reactions.
- The person demonstrates knowledge of safety factors and judgment in selection of activities, tasks, or methods to avoid injury to him- or herself or others.
- The person has increased physical endurance and fitness.
- The person demonstrates coping skills needed to live with chronic disability.
- The person and his or her family or support group demonstrate an understanding of chronic disability and knowledge of resources needed to reduce the degree of handicap.
- The person is able to perform activities of daily living within limitations of residual disability.
- The person is able to use adapted equipment, if needed.

REFERENCES

Beers, M.H., and R. Berkow, eds. 1999. *The Merck Manual of Diagnosis and Therapy*, 17th ed. Whitehouse Station, NJ: Merck Research Laboratories.

Agency for Health Care Policy and Research Post-Stroke Rehabilitation. 1995. Post-stroke rehabilitation: assessment, referral, and patient management. Clinical practice guideline. *Quick Reference Guide for Clinicians* 16: 23.

BIBLIOGRAPHY

Acquaviva, J. 1996. *Occupational therapy practice guidelines for adults with stroke*. Bethesda, MD: American Occupational Therapy Association.

Alon, G. et al. 1998. Efficacy of a hybrid upper limb neuromuscular electrical stimulation system in lessening selected impairments and dysfunctions consequent to cerebral damage. *Journal of Neurologic Rehabilitation* 12: 73–80.

Bernspaing, B., and A.G. Fisher. 1995. Differences between persons with right or left cerebral vascular accident on the Assessment of Motor and Process Skills. *Archives of Physical Medicine and Rehabilitation* 76, no. 12: 1144–1151.

Bird, C., and R.C. Mahoney. 1994. Training in activities of daily living. In *Management of persons with stroke*, eds. M.N. Ozer et al., 346–367. St. Louis, MO: Mosby.

Brodie, J. et al. 1994. Cerebrovascular accident: Relationship of demographic, diagnostic, and occupational therapy antecedents to rehabilitation outcomes. *American Journal of Occupational Therapy* 48, no. 10: 906–913.

Brouwer, B.J., and P. Ambury. 1994. Upper extremity weight-bearing effect on corticospinal excitability following stroke. *Archives of Physical Medicine and Rehabilitation* 75, no. 8: 861–866.

Carey, L.M. et al. 1993. Sensory loss in stroke patients: Effective training of tactile and proprioceptive discrimination. *Archives of Physical Medicine and Rehabilitation* 74, no. 6: 602–611.

Cermak, C.A. et al. 1995. Performance of Americans and Israelis with cerebrovascular accident on the Loewenstein Occupational Therapy Cognitive Assessment (LOTCA). *American Journal of Occupational Therapy* 49, no. 6: 500–506.

Clarke, P.A. 1995. Occupational therapy for stroke patients at home. *Clinical Rehabilitation* 9: 91–96.

Clemson, L. et al. 1999. Family perspectives following stroke: The unheard stories. *Topics in Stroke Rehabilitation* 6, no. 1: 6077.

Colan, B.J. 1995. Post-stroke guidelines standardize care. *Advance for Occupational Therapists* 11, no. 39: 14.

Colan, B.J. 1995. Treatment protocols for stroke standardizing. *Advance for Occupational Therapists* 11, no. 40: 19.

Culler, K.H. et al. 1994. Child care and parenting issues for the young stroke survivor. *Topics in Stroke Rehabilitation* 1, no. 1: 48–64.

Dorfman, H., and C. Siebert. 1994. Occupational therapy: Making stroke patients feel at home. *Caring Magazine* 13, no. 2: 36–40.

Dove, C.A. et al. 1994. Metoprolol for action tremor following intracerebral hemorrhage. *Archives of Physical Medicine and Rehabiltation* 75, no. 9: 1011–1014.

Driessen M.J. et al. 1997. Occupational therapy for patients with chronic diseases: CVA, rheumatoid arthritis, and progressive diseases of the central nervous system. *Disability and Rehabilitation* 19, no. 5: 198–204.

Drummond, A.E.R., and M.F. Walker. 1994. The Nottingham Leisure Questionnaire. *British Journal of Occupational Therapy* 7, no. 11: 414–418.

Drummond, A.E.R., and M.F. Walker. 1996. Generalization of the effects of leisure rehabilitation for stroke patients. *British Journal of Occupational Therapy* 59, no. 7: 330–334.

Falconer, J.A. et al. 1994. Predicting stroke inpatient rehabilitation outcome using a classification tree approach. *Archives of Physical Medicine and Rehabilitation* 75, no. 6: 619–625.

Fransisco, G. et al. 1998. Electromyogram-triggered neuromuscular stimulation for improving the arm function of acute stroke survivors: A randomized pilot study. *Archives of Physical Medicine and Rehabilitation* 79, no. 5: 570–575.

Gainer, F.E. 1996. Developing a clinical pathway for stroke. *OT Practice* 1, no. 6: 30–33.

Galski, T. et al. 1993. Prediction of behind-the-wheel driving performance in patients with cerebral brain damage: A discriminant function analysis. *American Journal of Occupational Therapy* 47, no. 5: 391–396.

Gibson, J.W., and J.K. Schkade. 1997. Occupational adaptation intervention with patients with cerebrovascular accident: A clinical study. *American Journal of Occupational Therapy* 51, no. 7: 523–529.

Gillen, G., and A. Burkhardt. 1998. *Stroke Rehabilitation: A Function-Based Approach.* St. Louis, MO: Mosby.

Gitlin, L.N., and D. Burgh. 1995. Issuing assistive devices to older patients in rehabilitation: An exploratory study. *American Journal of Occupational Therapy* 49, no. 10: 994–1000.

Hachisuka, K. et al. 1997. Test-retest and inter-method reliability of the self-rating Barthel Index. *Clinical Rehabilitation* 11: 28–35.

Hartman-Maeir, A., and N. Katz. 1995. Validity of the Behavioral Inattention Test (BIT): Relationships with functional task. *American Journal of Occupational Therapy* 49, no. 6: 507–516.

Horner, R.D. et al. 1997. Racial differences in the utilization of inpatient rehabilitation services among elderly stroke patients. *Stroke* 289, no. 1: 19–25.

Jackson, S. 1996. Cerebrovascular accident. In *Occupational therapy and physical dysfunction: Principles, skills, and practice*, 4th ed., eds. A. Turner et al., 433–462. New York: Churchill Livingstone.

Joiner, C., and M. Hansel. 1996. Empowering the geriatric client. *OT Practice* 1, no. 2: 34–35, 37–39.

Jongbloed, L. 1994. Adaptation to a stroke: The experience of one couple. *American Journal of Occupational Therapy* 48, no. 11: 1006–1013.

Jongbloed, L. et al. 1993. Family adaptation to altered roles following a stroke. *Canadian Journal of Occupational Therapy* 60, no. 2: 70–77.

Karplus, D.L. 1994. Psychosocial impact of stroke on the family. *Occupational Therapy Forum* 9, no. 14: 4, 8–10.

Katz, N. et al. 1995. Construct validity of a geriatric version of the Loewenstein Occupational Therapy Cognitive Assessment (LOTCA). *Physical and Occupational Therapy in Geriatrics* 13, no. 3: 31–46.

Kempers, K. 1994. Preparing the young stroke survivor for return to work. *Topics in Stroke Rehabilitation* 1, no. 1: 65–73.

Kerr, T. 1996. Recovering from stroke together. *Advance for Occupational Therapists* 12, no. 39: 17.

Khader, M.S., and G.S. Tomlin. 1994. Change in wheelchair transfer performance during rehabilitation of men with cerebrovascular accident. *American Journal of Occupational Therapy* 48, no. 10: 899–905.

Klein, B.S. 1995. Reflections on . . . An ally as a partner in practice. *Canadian Journal of Occupational Therapy* 62, no. 5: 283–285.

Klein, B.S. 1996. Healing as a creative process: Rehabilitation from a client's perspective. *OT Practice* 1, no. 12: 32–35.

Kong, T.K. et al. 1995. Development of a hierarchical activities of daily living scale for Chinese stroke patients in geriatric day hospitals. *Aging in Clinical Experimental Research* 7, no. 3: 173–178.

Korner-Bitensky, N. et al. 1998. The impact of interventions with families poststroke: A review. *Topics in Stroke Rehabilitation* 5, no. 3: 69–85.

Larson, B.A., and P.M. Watson. 1993. The adult with a cerebral vascular accident. In *Practice issues in occupational therapy: Intraprofessional team building*, ed. S.E. Ryan, 137–144. Thorofare, NJ: Slack.

Lewinter, M., and S. Mikkelsen. 1995. Therapists and the rehabilitation process after stroke. *Disability and Rehabilitation* 17, no. 5: 211–216.

Lofgren, B.L. et al. 1997. In-patient rehabilitation after stroke: Outcomes and factors associated with improvement. *Disability and Rehabilitation* 20, no. 2: 55–61.

Logan, P.A. et al. 1997. A randomized controlled trial of enhanced social service occupational therapy for stroke patients. *Clinical Rehabiltation* 11: 107–113.

Mann, W.C. et al. 1995. A follow-up study of older stroke survivors living at home. *Topics in Geriatric Rehabilitation* 11, no. 1: 52–66.

Marmer, L. 1995. Group treatment works well in stroke recovery. *Advance for Occupational Therapists* 11, no. 39: 13.

Matyas, T.A., and K.J. Ottenbacher. 1993. Confounds of insensitivity and blind luck: Statistical conclusion validity in stroke rehabilitation clinical trials. *Archives of Physical Medicine and Rehabilitation* 74, no. 6: 559–565.

McLaughlin, C. 1995. Spreading the word about stroke care. *Advance for Occupational Therapists* 11, no. 42: 4.

Mew, M.M., and E. Fossey. 1996. Client-centered aspects of clinical reasoning during an initial assessment using the Canadian Occupational Performance Measure. *Australian Occupational Therapy Journal* 43, no. 3/4: 155–166.

Moseley, C.B. 1995. Rehabilitation potential among nursing home stroke patients. *Physical and Occupational Therapy in Geriatrics* 13, no. 4: 11–25.

Moseley, C.B. 1996. Rehabilitation effectiveness among long-term nursing home stroke residents. *Physical and Occupational Therapy in Geriatrics* 14, no. 4: 27–41.

Mukand, J. et al. 1998. Streamlining stroke care. *Advance for Occupational Therapists* 14, no. 15: 18–19.

Okkema, K. 1993. *Cognitive and perceptual treatment techniques in the stroke patient: A guide to functional outcomes in occupational therapy*. Gaithersburg, MD: Aspen Publishers.

Okkema, K. 1994. Self-care strategies following stroke. In *Ways of living: Self-care strategies for special needs*, ed. C. Christiansen, 227–234. Rockville, MD: American Occupational Therapy Association.

Ottenbacher, K.J., and S. Jannel. 1993. The results of clinical trials in stroke rehabilitation research. *Archives of Neurology* 50, no. 1: 37–44.

Parker, C.J. et al. 1997. The role of leisure in stroke rehabilitation. *Disability and Rehabilitation* 19, no. 1: 1–5.

Pedretti, L.W. et al. 1996. Cerebral vascular accident. In *Occupational therapy for physical dysfunction*, 4th ed., ed. L.W. Pedretti, 785–806. St. Louis, MO: CV Mosby.

Preston, L.A. 1998. Nerve blocks: OT's role in enhancing nerve blocks for spasticity. *OT Practice* 3, no. 10: 28–35.

Pulaski, K.H. 1998. Cerebrovascular accident. In *Willard and Spackman's occupational therapy*, 9th ed., eds. M.E. Neistadt and E.B. Crepeau, 668–670. Philadelphia: J.B. Lippincott.

Radomski, M.V. 1995. There is more to life than putting on your pants. *American Journal of Occupational Therapy* 49, no. 6: 487–490.

Royeen, C.B., ed. 1996. *Stroke: Strategies, treatment, rehabilitation, outcomes, knowledge, and evaluation* (Self-study course). Bethesda, MD: American Occupational Therapy Association.

Sabari, J.S. 1997. Motor recovery after stroke. In *Assessments in occupational therapy and physical therapy*, eds. J. Van Deusen and D. Brunt, 249–270. Philadelphia: W.B. Saunders.

Sabari, J.S. 1995. Carr and Shepherd's motor relearning programme for individuals with stroke. In *Occupational therapy for physical dysfunction*, 4th ed., ed. C.A. Trombly, 501–509. Baltimore: Williams & Wilkins.

Sachs, D. et al. 1995. A survey of treatment settings: Methods and modalities in occupational therapy treatment and evaluation of stroke patients. *Israel Journal of Occupational Therapy* 4, no. 4: E114.

Segal, M.E., and M. Gillard. 1997. Longitudinal assessment of stroke survivors' handicap. *Topics in Stroke Rehabilitation* 4, no. 1: 41–52.

Segal, M.E., and R.R. Schall. 1995. Assessing handicap of stroke survivors: A validation study of the Craig Handicap Assessment and Reporting Technique. *American Journal of Physical Medicine and Rehabilitation* 74, no. 4: 276–286.

Shiffman, L.M. 1998. Cerebrovascular accident. In *Physical dysfunction practice skills for the occupational therapy assistant*, ed. M.B. Early, 411–432. St. Louis, MO: Mosby.

Sim, T.C. et al. 1997. Outcome after stroke rehabilitation in Hong Kong. *Clinical Rehabilitation* 11: 236–242.

Smith, P.M. et al. 1996. Intermodal agreement of follow-up telephone functional assessment using the Functional Independence Measure in patients with stroke. *Archives of Physical Medicine and Rehabilitation* 77, no. 5: 431–435.

Stewart, M.J. et al. 1998. Peer visitor support for family caregivers of seniors with stroke. *Canadian Journal of Nursing Research* 30, no. 2: 87–117.

Strasser, D.C. 1997. Linking treatment to outcomes through teams: Building a conceptual model of rehabilitation effectiveness. *Topics in Stroke Rehabilitation* 4, no. 1: 15–27.

Thomas, K.S. et al. 1994. A pilot project for cognitive retraining with elderly stroke patients' learning of new motor skill patterns used in upper extremity dressing. *Physical and Occupational Therapy in Geriatrics* 12, no. 4: 51–66.

Trombly, C. 1995. Clinical practice guidelines for post-stroke rehabilitation and occupational therapy practice. *American Journal of Occupational Therapy* 49, no. 7: 711–714.

Unsworth, C. 1994. Discharge accommodation recommendations for stroke patients following rehabilitation: A study of clinician and team decisions. *Australian Occupational Therapy Journal* 41, no. 3: 143–144.

Unsworth, C. 1996. Clients' perspectives on discharge housing decisions after stroke rehabilitation. *American Journal of Occupational Therapy* 50, no. 3: 207–216.

Unsworth, C. 1997. Decision polarization among rehabilitation team recommendations concerning discharge housing for stroke patients. *International Journal of Rehabilitation Research* 20, no. 1: 51–69.

Wolfe, C.D.A. et al. 1997. The uptake and costs of guidelines for stroke in a district of southern England. *Journal of Epidemiology and Community Health* 51: 520–525.

Woodsen, A.A. 1995. Stroke. In *Occupational therapy in physical dysfunction*, 4th ed., ed. C.A. Trombly, 677–704. Baltimore: Williams & Wilkins.

Wyller, T.B. et al. 1995. The Barthel ADL Index one year after stroke: Comparison between relatives' and occupational therapist's scores. *Age and Ageing* 24: 398–401.

Wyller, T.B. et al. 1996. Predictive validity of the Sodring Motor Evaluation of Stroke patients (SMES). *Scandinavian Journal of Rehabilitation Medicine* 28: 211–216.

Yuen, H.K. 1996. Management of avoidance behaviors using direct and indirect psychological methods. *American Journal of Occupational Therapy* 50, no. 7: 478–482.

Coma

DESCRIPTION

Coma is a state in which a person is unarousable and any response to repeated stimuli is only a primitive avoidance reflex. In profound coma, all brainstem and myotatic reflexes may be absent. Stupor is unresponsiveness from which the person can be aroused only briefly by vigorous, repeated stimulation (Merck 1999, 1385).

CAUSE

Impaired consciousness can be caused by any of the following: (1) supratentorial mass lesions, (2) subtentorial lesions, (3) diffuse and metabolic cerebral disorders, or (4) psychiatric disorders.

ASSESSMENT

Areas

- reflexes
- muscle tone, especially spasticity
- range of motion
- balance and postural control
- praxis
- sensory registration
- sensory processing
- perceptual skills
- attending behavior
- attention span, concentration
- orientation
- ability to follow direction
- judgment of safety
- problem-solving skills
- daily living skills

Instruments

No specific instruments developed by occupational therapists were identified in the literature. The scales below are used frequently as reference points for persons recovering from comatose states.
• *Glasgow Coma Scale* (GCS) by G. Teasdale and B. Jennett, in Assessment of coma and impaired consciousness: A practical scale, *Lancet* 2 (1974): 81–83. See also B. Jennett and G. Teasdale, *Management of Head Injuries*, Philadelphia: F.A. Davis, 1981.
• *Innsbruck Coma Scale* (ICS) by A. Benzer, G. Mittschiffthaler, M. Marosi et al. Prediction of non-survival after trauma: Innsbrock coma scale, *Lancet* 338 (1991): 977–978.
• *Rancho Los Amigos Cognitive Functioning Scale* by C. Hagen, in Language disorders in head trauma, *Language disorders in adults: Recent advances*, ed. A.L. Holland, 257–258, San Diego, CA: College-Hill Press, 1984. See also D. Malkmus, B.J. Booth, and C. Kodimer, *Rehabilitation of the Head-Injured Adult: Comprehensive Cognitive Management*, Downey, CA: Professional Staff Association of Rancho Los Amigos Hospital, 1980.
• *Unified Stroke Scale* by J.M. Orgogozo, K. Asplundh, G. Boysen. A unified form for neurological scoring of hemispheric stroke with motor impairment, *Stroke* 23 (1992): 1678–1679.

PROBLEMS

Sensorimotor

Motor Responses

The following list of motor responses is based on the Glasgow Coma Scale:
• Level I (no response). No change to stimuli occurs, no movement occurs, no change in muscle tone occurs, the eyes do not open, and the face does not twitch.
• Level II (extensor response). The person responds with generalized movement patterns known as decerebrate rigidity or extensor posturing. The head retracts; the trunk extends; the shoulders and hips extend, adduct, and rotate internally; the elbows and knees extend; the forearm pronates; the wrist and fingers flex; and the feet plantar flex and invert. Spinal reflexes and lower brainstem reflexes may be present, such as the tonic labyrinthine reflex and asymmetrical tonic neck reflex.
• Level III (abnormal flexion). The person responds with generalized movement patterns known as decorticate rigidity or flexor posturing. The shoulders are slightly flexed, adducted, and internally rotated; the forearm is pronated; and the wrist and fingers are flexed. No change occurs in the lower extremities. Midbrain reactions, such as neck and body righting reactions, may be elicited.
• Level IV (withdraws). The person's response to stimulation is withdrawal of the entire limb even though only the hand or foot is touched. Spontaneous, nonpurposeful movements may occur without any apparent external stimulation.
• Level V (localizes). The person may brush away painful stimuli, move only the part of the body being stimulated, blink at a light shown in the eyes, turn away from strong light or sound, or follow a beam of light with the head. Cortical equilibrium reactions (protective extension) can be elicited.

- Level VI (obeys). The person is able to respond appropriately to stimuli and withdraws only from noxious or irritating stimuli. The person responds to simple requests and can initiate purposeful activity. Movements include limb abduction and movement away from the midline of the body.

Sensory Responses

The following list of sensory responses is based on the Rancho Los Amigos Cognitive Functioning Scale:
- Level I (no response). The person is unresponsive to any stimuli.
- Level II (generalized response). The person reacts inconsistently and nonpurposefully to stimuli in a nonspecific manner. The earliest response may be to deep pain.
- Level III (localized response). The person reacts specifically, but inconsistently, to stimuli. Responses are related directly to the type of stimulus presented. The person may turn his or her head toward a sound or focus on an object. The person may withdraw an extremity when presented with a painful stimulus.
- Level IV (confused/agitated). The person responds to discomfort by trying to remove restraints or the nasogastric tube. The person may respond out of proportion to the stimuli given, even after the stimuli are removed. The person does not discriminate among persons or objects.
- Level V (confused/inappropriate). The person continues to respond out of proportion to the stimuli presented.
- Level VI (confused/appropriate). The response to stimuli is appropriate. The person is able to tolerate unpleasant stimuli, such as the nasogastric tube, when the need for the stimuli is explained.

Cognitive

The following list is based on the Rancho Los Amigos Cognitive Functioning Scale:
- Level I (no response). The person shows no evidence of cognitive response.
- Level II (generalized response). Responses are nonspecific and may include physiologic changes, gross body movements, or vocalizations.
- Level III (localized response). The person may follow simple commands, such as "Close your eyes" or "Squeeze my hand." The person may respond inconsistently, in a delayed manner, and to some people but not to others.
- Level IV (confused/agitated). The person responds primarily to the internal rather than the external environment. Gross attention is very brief, and selective attention is usually nonexistent. The person is unaware of present events, lacks short-term recall, and may be reacting to past events.
- Level V (confused/inappropriate/nonagitated). The person appears alert and is able to respond to simple commands fairly consistently, but responses to complex commands may be nonpurposeful, random, or fragmented. He or she has gross attention to the environment but is highly distractible and lacks the ability to focus attention. Memory is severely impaired. He or she may perform previously learned tasks with structure but is unable to learn new information. Maximum supervision is required to ensure safety.
- Level VI (confused/appropriate). The person follows directions consistently and can perform familiar activities, especially those learned and practiced for many years. New learning is difficult and is not remembered. Attention to tasks is improved for structured

tasks but not for unstructured tasks. Past memory is better than recent memory. The person shows goal-directed behavior but is dependent on the external environment for direction. Moderate supervision is required. The person has vague recognition of some staff members.

- Level VII (automatic/appropriate). The person is oriented and able to function in a structured environment with a dependable routine. Learning new tasks is possible, but carryover is poor. Judgment of safety, insight into his or her condition, problem solving, and planning skills are still poor. Minimal supervision is still needed for safety reasons.
- Level VIII (purposeful/appropriate). The person is alert and oriented, can plan ahead, remembers the past, learns new tasks, and functions in an unstructured setting. Return to the community is possible, including working. However, some decrease in quality and rate of processing information may be evident, and the ability to reason abstractly may be decreased.

Psychosocial

Intrapersonal

- Level III (localized response). The person may have a vague awareness of him- or herself and his or her body, such as responding to discomfort by pulling at the nasogastric tube, catheter, or restraints.
- Level IV (confused/agitated). The person is detached from the present and responds primarily to internal agitation, confusion, and a heightened state of activity. Behavior may be bizarre and nonpurposeful to the immediate environment. The person may be euphoric or hostile.
- Level V (confused/inappropriate). The person may become agitated as a result of external stimuli. The person is unable to initiate tasks and may use objects inappropriately. The person responds best to family members.
- Level VI (confused/appropriate). The person is able to be responsible for his or her behavior. He or she has some self-awareness and awareness of basic needs.
- Level VII (automatic/appropriate). The person generally is aware of him- or herself, his or her body, family members, food, people, and interaction in the environment, but reality testing and reaction to stress are still poor.
- Level VIII (purposeful/appropriate). The person is functional in society but may still show decreased tolerance to stress.

Interpersonal

- Level IV (confused/agitated). Verbalization is frequently incoherent or inappropriate to the environment. Confabulation may be present.
- Level V (confused/inappropriate). With structure, the person may be able to converse on a social, automatic level for short periods of time. Verbalization may continue to be inappropriate at times, with confabulation. The person may be able to interact with family members.
- Level VI (confused/appropriate). The person can respond to familiar social situations.
- Level VII (automatic/appropriate). The person can initiate social responses and activities in which he or she has an interest.
- Level VIII (purposeful/appropriate). The person may continue to have difficulty interacting in some social situations.

Self-Care

- Levels I, II, and III. The person needs maximum assistance to perform self-care activities.
- Level IV (confused/agitated). The person is able to perform some self-care activities with direct assistance.
- Level V (confused/inappropriate). The person is able to perform self-care activities with assistance and may accomplish feeding with supervision.
- Level VI (confused/appropriate). The person can perform self-care activities with supervision.
- Level VII (automatic/appropriate). The person can perform self-care activities independently, but judgment remains impaired.
- Level VIII (purposeful/appropriate). The person is independent in performing all self-care activities.

Productivity

- Level VI (confused/appropriate). The person can perform repetitive work tasks in a structured setting.
- Level VII (automatic/appropriate). The person can participate in work evaluation and explore alternative careers if needed.
- Level VIII (purposeful/appropriate). The person can participate fully in work evaluation and determine a productive role for him- or herself.

Leisure

- Level VI (confused/appropriate). The person is able to participate in structured leisure activities.
- Level VII (automatic/appropriate). The person is able to initiate leisure activities in which the person has an interest.
- Level VIII (purposeful/appropriate). The person is able to develop new leisure interests.

TREATMENT/INTERVENTION

Only levels I through III of the cognitive levels are addressed here. For higher levels, see the section on head injuries. Models of treatment include neurodevelopmental treatment, movement therapy, proprioceptive neuromuscular facilitation, and sensory integration.

Sensorimotor

Motor

- Level I. Attempt to evoke voluntary motor responses to sensory stimulation. Techniques such as quick stretching, tapping over the muscle belly, approximating joints, and quick icing may be applied.
- Level II. Increase the variety of voluntary motor responses to sensory stimulation. The person's responses might include turning toward a noise, changing the facial expression in response to a particular smell, pushing an obnoxious stimuli away, or changing muscle tone.
- Level III. Increase the use of gross motor function and muscle tone through movement patterns and activities. Encourage the person to respond by verbally requesting the movement with a short command ("Look up," "Reach") and then helping the person to perform

the movement, if needed. Begin with head, neck, and trunk movement and progress from proximal to distal following normal development.

Sensory

The following steps apply to levels I, II, and III:
- Apply pressure on the fingernail bed or sternum.
- Use auditory stimulation, such as the actual or recorded voices of family members, familiar musical tapes, or loud noises (clap, ring bells, call the person's name, etc.). (Note: If a startle reflex occurs, stop this approach.)
- Use tactile stimulation, such as rubbing the person's face and body with various textures.
- Use temperature changes, such as wiping the skin with warm or cold towels.
- Use vibration with vibrators of various speeds.
- Use vestibular stimulation by changing the person's body position from supine to sitting, rolling, tilting, slow spinning or rocking, and inverting his or her head on a large therapy ball. (Note: This is contraindicated if person has a tracheotomy, increased cranial pressure, or seizures.)
- Use olfactory stimulation by placing noxious or pleasant smells under the person's nose.
- Use proprioceptive stimulation by moving the person's arms, legs, and body.
- Use visual stimulation by providing brightly colored objects, mobiles over the bed, mirrors, flashlights, photographs, and pictures.

Cognitive

- Level I. Attempt to promote awareness through use of various stimuli. Reduce extraneous background, visual, and auditory input as much as possible.
- Level II. Increase awareness of environment and promote attending behavior.
- Level III. Increase attention span and orientation and promote following directions.

Psychosocial

See head injury section.

Self-Care

- Levels II and III. The person needs maximum assistance to perform self-care activities, but encourage the person to assist by providing visual and verbal cues. Facilitate normal oral motor movements. Reduce hypersensitivity and abnormal tone.
- Level IV. Help the person perform self-care activities by providing verbal directions.

Productivity

See head injury section.

Leisure

See head injury section.

PRECAUTIONS

- Generally, sessions should be kept short, about 15 to 30 minutes. Note increases in posturing or fluctuations in status.

- Remember that responses may be delayed. Wait for a response and repeat the same stimulus before giving a new one.
- Use only one or two different types of stimuli per session to reduce confusion.
- Avoid posturing, such as arching of back and other extensor patterns. Rotate the person's shoulders opposite the hips, flex hips and knees, generally avoid the supine position, and exert pressure to the back of the head.
- If overstimulation occurs, use pressure to the abdomen, neutral warmth, or reflex inhibiting patterns.

PROGNOSIS AND OUTCOME

The length of coma is indicative of outcome. Comas of more than a few months do not lead to a positive prognosis. Few people recover fully.
- The person is able to control voluntary movements.
- The person is able to respond correctly to sensory stimuli in all senses.
- The person is able to respond correctly to verbal commands and follow simple directions.
- The person is oriented to person, place, and time.
- The person is able to perform basic self-care skills with assistance.

REFERENCE

Beers, M.H., and R. Berkow, eds. 1999. *The Merck Manual of Diagnosis and Therapy*, 17th ed. Whitehouse Station, NJ: Merck Research Laboratories.

BIBLIOGRAPHY

Kerr, T. 1995. Behind the veil of coma. *Advance for Occupational Therapists* 11, no. 29: 12–13. (Case report)
Kerr, T. 1995. Students compare coma scales to predict outcomes. *Advance for Occupational Therapists* 11, no. 29: 13, 46.
Sakzewski, L., and J. Ziviani. 1996. Factors affecting length of stay for children with acquired brain injuries: A review of the literature. *Australian Occupational Therapy Journal* 43, no. 3/4: 113–124.
Scott, A.D., and P.W. Dow. 1995. Traumatic brain injury. In *Occupational therapy for physical dysfunction*, 4th ed., ed. C.A. Trombly, 705–733. Baltimore: Williams & Wilkins.

Complex Regional Pain Syndrome

DESCRIPTION

Complex regional pain syndrome is a chronic pain state induced by soft tissue or bone injury (complex regional pain syndrome [CRPS] type I, or reflex sympathetic dystrophy [RSDS]), or by nerve injury (CRPS type II, or causalgia) in which pain is associated with autonomic changes such as sweating or vasomotor abnormalities and/or trophic changes such as skin and bone atrophy, hair loss, and joint contractures (Merck 1999, 1372). CRPS is more likely to involve sympathetically maintained pain than other types of chronic pain. Treatment may include a nerve block. RSDS was documented during the Civil War by Silas Weir Mitchell, a neurologist. Other names include minor or major traumatic dystrophy or shoulder-hand syndrome.

CAUSE

The precise cause is unknown, although several theories exist. The syndrome usually occurs secondary to a preexisting condition, such as stroke, traumatic injury to the head or spinal cord, major surgery, infection, fracture, pulmonary disease, myocardial infarction or other heart disease, repetitive motion disorder, or cervical disk degeneration. Onset usually is identified when the pain, edema, and trophic changes can no longer be attributed to the original cause. Both sexes and all age groups are affected, but the incidence is higher in women, and the most common age range is 45 to 65.

ASSESSMENT

Areas
- daily living activities
- productivity history, skills, interests, and values
- leisure skills and interests
- muscle strength, hand and grip strength
- range of motion
- hand functions
- functional capacities evaluation
- edema and swelling
- pain intensity
- sensory registration
- sensory processing

Instruments
- Circumferential measurement: The circumference of the widest point of swelling is measured in inches or centimeters.
- *Comprehensive Pain Evaluation Questionnaire* by R.N. Jaminson et al., in Cognitive-behavioral classification of chronic pain: Replication and extension of empirically derived patient profiles, *Pain* 57 (1994): 277–292. (Also printed in R. Williams, *RSD: Reflex Sympathetic Dystrophy,* Bethesda, MD: American Occupational Therapy Association, 1995.)
- *Symptom Checklist,* in R. Williams, *RSD: Reflex Sympathetic Dystrophy,* Bethesda, MD: American Occupational Therapy Association, 1995.
- Volar plate test: The test for joint tenderness is positive if there is increased pain with passive flexion of the joint, especially the proximal interphalangeal joints of the hand.
- Volumetry by K. Schultz-Johnson, in *Volumetrics: A Literature Review*, Santa Monica, CA: Upperextremity Technology. Also in G. Davidoff et al., Pain measurement in RSD, *Pain* 32 (1988): 27–34.

Stages of CRPS Type I (RSDS)

Stage 1
- duration: one to three months
- severe, burning pain in localized region
- localized edema—pitting and nonpitting
- hyperesthesia
- increased or decreased hair and nail growth
- stiffness
- muscle spasm
- loss of joint mobility
- vasospasm affecting color and temperature of skin
- skin changes—atrophy, dryness, scaling and shiny appearance
- possible pale, cyanotic, or red extremities
- possible hyperhydrosis, causing sweat to drip from the hands
- possible osteoporosis

Stage 2
- duration: three to six months
- more severe, diffuse pain
- edema: persistant and spreading beyond the initial site but not responding to traditional reduction techniques
- less hair growth and cracked, brittle, and grooved nails
- deossification apparent on X-ray
- joint thickened and stiff
- diminished muscle tone and strength
- muscle atrophy
- blue extremities
- pronounced sensitivity to touch
- advancing, diffuse osteoporosis

Stage 3
- duration: more than six months, possibly permanent
- irreversible trophic changes
- intractable pain, possibly spreading to include entire limb
- marked muscle atrophy
- severely limited mobility of affected area (joint ankylosing) and pericapsular fibrosis
- flexor tendon contractions and possible subluxations
- marked bone deossification that is more diffuse
- drawn, pale, dry, and shiny skin
- profound, diffuse osteoporosis

continues

continued

- decreased blood flow
- decreased skin temperature
- increased or decreased sweating
- loss of connective tissue
- possible constructures
- possible ankylasing of interphalangeal joints of the hand or foot as stiffness increases

PROBLEMS

Self-Care
- The person may avoid performing some daily living tasks to avoid aggravating pain response.

Productivity
- The person may avoid performing productive activities to avoid aggravating pain.

Leisure
- The person may stop performing some leisure activities to avoid aggravating pain.

Sensorimotor
- The person may have reduced range of motion.
- The person may have swelling.
- The person may have muscle atrophy.
- The person may have muscle cramping and spasms.
- The person may lose bone density (osteoporosis).
- The person may experience trophic changes, such as increased nail curvature, flattening of the cuticle base (rugae pattern), loss of pulp bulk, skin and hair changes, and tissue atrophy.
- The person may report that pain is severe, constant, and burning.
- The person may have muscle tenderness.
- The person may have skin and vasomotor changes, including rubor, pallor, and atrophy.
- The person may experience hyperesthesia.
- The person may have alternating vasodilation and vasoconstriction, resulting in alternating sensations of hot and cold.

Cognitive
- The person may have difficulty with problem-solving tasks because of preoccupation with pain or avoidance of pain.

Psychosocial
- The person may be emotionally labile.

- The person may be anxious, worried, or apprehensive about the condition.
- The person may exhibit signs of hysteria.
- The person may be defensive or hostile.
- The person may be dependent on others.
- Conversation tends to be dominated by the subject of pain or disability.

TREATMENT/INTERVENTION

Treatment often includes nerve blocks such as stellate ganglion blocks, sympathectomy, dorsal rhizotomy, and surgically implanted morphine pumps. Models of treatment are remedial in early stages but change to compensatory in later stages. Consensus on best treatment approaches is lacking, as the survey by Headley (1996, 12) demonstrates. Stress or tissue loading (Carlson 1996, 1), sensory integration/desensitization, physical agent modalities, functional restoration, and neuromuscular reeducation are frequently used approaches.

Self-Care

- Encourage performance of activities of daily living. Functional activities are a central part of any treatment program for CRPS or RSDS. Activities should be of sufficient intensity, duration, and frequency to create a change in the sympathetic reflex arc. A home exercise program is important.

Productivity

- Encourage the person to engage in work or homemaking activities.
- Work-related interventions such as ergonomic evaluation, work hardening, functional restoration and retraining, or employment preparation may be used.

Leisure

- Help the person to participate in some leisure activity, whether an old favorite or a new venture.

Sensorimotor

- A stress loading program may be useful in changing the sympathetic nervous system's effects, including contracture and fibrosis. Stress loading is defined as active sustained exercise requiring forceful use of the entire extremity, with minimal motion of painful joints (Carlson 1996, 1). Scrubbing and carrying are two examples of functional stress loading that should be done in a slow, rhythmic pattern. (Caution: Carlson states that stress loading should be used initially as the only technique to treat pain [Carlson 1996, 1]. Fibrosis may be treated after pain is decreased.)
- Compression and traction may be used alternately (stress loading). The person scrubs a plywood board while positioned on the floor on all fours. The person is told to scrub by applying as much pressure (compression) as possible using a back and forth motion while leaning on the affected arm. Sessions are three minutes long, three times per day. The person is also told to carry a weighted briefcase or purse in the affected hand (traction), with the arm

extended throughout the day. The weight is from 1 to 5 pounds and is determined in the initial visit.
- The Jobst intermittent compression unit is useful in reducing "pitting" edema in the early stage.
- Encourage active range of motion for the person's shoulder and elbow through the use of a skateboard or reciprocal pulley. A dowel or wand can also provide range-of-motion exercise for the forearm. Once shoulder movement is 90 degrees, place the hand flat on a wall and push against the wall for half a minute 10 to 15 times a day (Hareau 1996, 369).
- Increase muscle strength by adding weights to the skateboard, pulleys, dowels, or weight wells for progressive resistance exercises for the shoulder, elbow, forearm, wrist, and fingers.
- Splints may be used for positioning. Be alert to swelling. Make the splints adjustable.
- The use of warm, moist heat is helpful in reducing pain and hypersensitivity.
- Electrical stimulation such as a dorsal column stimulator may be useful. Work with physical therapists or physician regarding use of electrical stimulation unless fully trained in use of electrical modalities.
- Thermal modalities, including superficial heat and cold, may be helpful to counteract vasoconstriction or vasodilation. Coordinate use of thermal modalities with physical therapists or physician unless trained in use of thermal agents.
- Serial casting may be used to stress load but must be closely monitored so as to avoid a recurrence of RSDS.

Cognitive
- Explain the purpose of treatment and the treatment program in easy to understand language, and state what is expected of the person.
- Instruct the person on a home exercise program, providing a specific number of repetitions and the amount of resistance to be used.

Psychosocial
- Use highly structured, purposeful activities, such as making link belts, potholders, or latch rugs, that are highly repetitive and require few problem-solving skills but encourage the use of both hands.

PRECAUTIONS
- This syndrome can become a permanently disabling condition if early diagnosis and treatment are not provided. Therapists should be alert to early signs of the syndrome, such as constant complaints about pain, anxious behavior, or complaints about sweating or temperature changes in an extremity, especially the hands or feet.
- Be aware of side effects of medications, including local or systemic corticosteroids, muscle relaxers, alpha and beta blockers, analgesics, anti-inflammatories, tricyclics, and tranquilizers.
- Avoid eliciting pain during treatment. Use slow, gentle movements and start with movements that are less likely to be painful. For example, do not start with shoulder internal and external rotations.

PROGNOSIS AND OUTCOME

Early therapy is important, although not a guarantee of success. Remission and exacerbation may occur; however, less than 5 percent of cases recover spontaneously. Transcutaneous electrical nerve stimulation, nerve blocks, and sympathectomies plus therapy seem to offer the best treatment.

- The person is able to perform daily living skills independently.
- The person demonstrates performance of productive activities.
- The person is able to perform leisure activities.
- The person does not complain of pain.
- The person is able to move the affected part normally.
- The person is able to use the affected part to perform daily activities.
- The person does not complain or show continued evidence of temperature changes in the affected part.

REFERENCES

Beers, M.H., and R. Berkow, eds. 1999. *The Merck Manual of Diagnosis and Therapy*, 17th ed. Whitehouse Station, NJ: Merck Research Laboratories.
Carlson, L. 1996. The treatment of reflex sympathetic dystrophy through stress loading. *Physical Disabilities Special Interest Section Newsletter* 19, no. 2: 1–3.
Hareau, J. 1996. What makes treatment for reflex sympathetic dystrophy successful? *Journal of Hand Therapy* 9, no. 4: 367–370.
Headley, B. 1996. Consensus needed for RSD intervention. *Advance for Occupational Therapists* 12, no. 16: 12, 50.

BIBLIOGRAPHY

Baxter, T. 1996. Upper limb injuries—reflex sympathetic dystrophy. In *Occupational therapy and physical dysfunction: Principles, skills, and practice*, 4th ed., eds. A. Turner et al., 727–728. New York: Churchill Livingstone.
Burkhardt, A. 1998. Edema control. In *Stroke rehabilitation: A function-based approach*, eds. G. Gillen and A. Burkhardt, 153–154. St. Louis, MO: Mosby.
Kasch, M. 1996. Reflex sympathetic dystrophy. In *Occupational therapy: Practice skills for physical dysfunction*, 4th ed., ed. L.W. Pedretti, 680. St. Louis, MO: CV Mosby.
Kasch, M. et al. 1998. Acute hand injuries—reflex sympathetic dystrophy. In *Physical dysfunction practice skills for the occupational therapy assistant*, ed. M.B. Early, 585–586. St. Louis, MO: Mosby.
Leilich, S. 1995. Managing reflex sympathetic dystrophy. *Advance for Occupational Therapy* 11, no. 22: 13.
Letcavage, N. 1999. Feeling the burn. *Advance for Directors in Rehabilitation* 8, no. 4: 29–30, 48.
Phillips, C.A. 1995. Impairments of hand function. In *Occupational therapy for physical dysfunction*, 4th ed., ed. C.A. Trombly, 789–790. Baltimore: Williams & Wilkins.
Williams, R. 1995. *RSD: Reflex Sympathetic Dystrophy*. Bethesda, MD: American Occupational Therapy Association.

Guillain-Barré Syndrome

DESCRIPTION

Guillain-Barré syndrome is an acute, rapidly progressive form of inflammatory polyneuropathy characterized by muscular weakness and mild distal sensory loss that in about two-thirds of cases begins five days to three weeks after a banal infectious disorder, surgery, or immunization. In most cases, demyelination occurs along the peripheral nerves, spinal nerve roots, and selected cranial nerves. However, in severe cases, axonal degeneration occurs rather than demyelination. The typical pattern of symptoms begins with paresthesias, usually in the legs and progressing toward the arms. Muscle weakness is always more prominent than sensory abnormalities and may be most prominent in the proximal areas. Weakness of facial and oropharyngeal muscles occurs in 50 percent of cases. In 10 percent of cases, respiratory failure also occurs and can be life threatening when the medulla becomes involved. About 5 percent die. About 10 percent develop chronic relapsing polyneuropathy (Merck 1999, 1494). The disorder is also called infectious polyneuritis, infectious neuronitis, polyradiculoneuritis, postinfectious polyneuritis, acute inflammatory demyelinating polyradiculoneuropathy, Landry's syndrome, Landry's ascending paralysis, Landry-Guillain-Barré syndrome, or Landry-Guillain-Barré-Strohl syndrome. The disorder was first described in 1859 by Landry.

CAUSE

While the exact cause is unknown, the disorder may be a response to a virus in which the immune system attacks the peripheral nerves, causing inflammation and degenerative changes in both posterior (sensory) and anterior (motor) nerve roots. Wallerian degeneration occurs in the axon, resulting in a slow recovery period. Onset occurs most commonly between the ages of 30 and 50. The disorder has three stages: (1) acute onset, which begins when the first symptoms appear and ends when no further symptoms are noted (usually one to three weeks), (2) a plateau period, when no significant change occurs, which lasts from several days to two weeks, and (3) a recovery phase, when remyelination and axonal regeneration occur, which may take up to two years.

ASSESSMENT

Areas

- muscle strength (Note: Testing is tiring and thus may have to be done over more than one session.)
- range of motion
- physical endurance
- gross motor control
- fine motor coordination, manipulation, and dexterity
- sensory registration or awareness

- sensory processing: discrimination of light touch, stereognosis, pain and temperature, proprioception, and two-point discrimination
- pain
- self-concept
- daily living skills
- productivity history, skills, interests, and values
- leisure interests and skills

Instruments

No comprehensive or specific test for assessing Guillain-Barré syndrome is mentioned in the occupational therapy literature. Testing may take several days because of low endurance and fatigue. The following may be useful:
- daily living assessment
- occupational history
- interest checklist
- manual and functional muscle tests (do not do both in same session)
- gross motor coordination as strength returns
- hand function test
- range of motion test
- sensory registration test: light touch, pressure, two-point discrimination, pain and temperature, proprioception, and stereognosis
- sensory sensitivity
- dysphagia test if swallowing and speech problems exist
- skin integrity

PROBLEMS

Self-Care

- The person in the acute stage will be unable to perform self-care activities. Thereafter, the person may experience difficulty in performing self-care tasks, depending on the progression of the disorder.
- In severe cases, the person may experience difficulty in speaking and eating due to deviation or paralysis of the tongue, which is controlled by the hypoglossal cranial nerves (XII).
- In severe cases, the person may experience difficulty swallowing, coughing, and gagging due to involvement of the glossopharyngeal (IX) and vagus cranial nerves (X).

Productivity

- The person is usually unable to work or manage a household until the disease has run its course.
- In severe cases, the person may have to reduce work or occupation and/or reduce performance of household tasks.

Leisure

- The person probably will not be able to engage in preferred leisure activities during acute stages.

- The person may not regain enough function to engage in preferred leisure sports and may need to consider other leisure pursuits.

Sensorimotor
- The person usually experiences muscle weakness (flaccid type) that generally begins in the lower extremities and proceeds up the body to the trunk and cranial nerves (VII, IX, X, XI, XII).
- The person usually has substantial loss of range of motion.
- The person may have loss of respiratory control and decreased respiratory volume.
- The person may lose the ability to smile, frown, whistle, or drink with a straw due to involvement of the facial cranial nerves (VII).
- The person will have hypotonia in involved areas of the body.
- The person may be uncoordinated because strength may return unevenly at first.
- The person may lose superficial and deep reflexes, such as stretch reflexes, abdominal reflexes, and plantar reflexes.
- The person usually fatigues easily until respiratory sufficiency is fully restored.
- The person may develop contractures from lack of active movement.
- The person usually has temporary loss of sensation of touch below the point of the body affected by the disorder. Loss of tactile sensation may include facial muscles if the whole body is involved.
- The person may have loss of sensation of proprioception.
- The person may experience increased pain in proximal muscle groups in the thighs, shoulders, and trunk.
- The person may experience pain on passive range of movement.
- The person may experience tenderness when muscles are palpated.

Cognitive
- Cognitive faculties are not affected directly by the disorder.

Psychosocial
- The person may fear becoming dependent.
- The person may express anxiety about the degree of recovery.
- The person may express feelings of frustration at being helpless.
- The person usually has limited tolerance for social interaction during early recovery.

TREATMENT/INTERVENTION
Treatment is usually done by a comprehensive rehabilitation team. The model of treatment is primarily remedial, although compensatory techniques may be used to permit earlier performance of some activities. Careful grading of activities in terms of strength and endurance factors is important. Assistive technology should be used sparingly and only on a temporary basis for most clients.

Self-Care
- Help the person relearn activities of daily living and regain independence as soon as strength permits. Begin with sedentary activities such as grooming and move to dressing and bathing as strength and endurance increase.

- Assistive devices, such as arm supports or slings, may be useful for short periods of time to permit earlier function.
- Protective splints may be needed for short periods of time.

Productivity

- Temporary modification of the work environment and simplification of some work tasks may permit the person to return to work earlier.
- Temporary modification of the home environment or simplification of homemaking tasks may permit the person to function at home earlier. Activities can included preparing meals, doing laundry, and doing light housekeeping.

Leisure

- Consider which of the person's existing interests can be incorporated into a total management program. Begin with passive interests.
- Explore new interests that can be developed within the total management program.
- Sedentary and nonresistive leisure interests can be used as treatment when the person has enough strength and endurance to sit for short intervals.
- The person will not be able to participate in strenuous leisure activities until full recovery occurs.

Sensorimotor

- Maintain the person's passive range of motion and encourage active range of motion as motor control returns in descending pattern. Stay within pain tolerance.
- Maintain good positioning while lying in bed and sitting up.
- Increase muscle strength and endurance through gentle, nonresistive activities and games until muscle innervation is normal. Continuous passive motion may be useful when active motion is limited by muscles graded at or below fair. Muscles should be graded fair-plus or better before resistive activities are used. Begin with passive motion in proximal joints. As tolerance level increases, active range of motion and light exercises may be started. Note any muscle imbalance.
- Stress joint protection while working with the person and to all staff.
- Decrease joint stiffness and prevent muscle atrophy or contractures through gentle, nonresistive activities and games.
- Consider splinting to prevent deformity and contractures from atrophy and disuse during the acute stage and to maintain functional position during the early recovery period.
- Increase coordination and integration of the two sides of the body.
- Increase hand manipulation and dexterity through the use of crafts or games that require frequent grasp and release.
- Increase physical tolerance by slowly increasing therapy or work time.
- Provide opportunities for sensory stimulation as the person's sensory system function returns.
- Tactile, proprioceptive, and vestibular stimulation can be used as the person regains function.

Cognitive

- Assist in instruction about the course of the disease to decrease the person's anxiety and fear.
- Instruct the person in energy conservation and work simplification.
- Instruct the person in joint protection.
- Instruct the person in stress management.
- Discuss with the person the need to avoid overexertion, which may result in a setback.

Psychosocial

- Provide positive encouragement, reassurance, and assistance to decrease the person's fear, anxiety, and feelings of frustration and helplessness.
- Provide training in relaxation techniques to reduce fear and anxiety.
- Provide opportunities for socialization. Talking to the person about his or her interests can be done during passive range-of-motion exercises. As strength returns, the interests can be incorporated into the treatment program.

PRECAUTIONS

- Watch for redness over bony areas of the body and change the person's position every two hours.
- Watch the person for signs of fatigue. Do not continue activity if signs of fatigue are present. Also, watch for signs of substitution. Use of suspension slings or mobile arm supports may permit hand activities to continue without fatigue to shoulder and upper arms. Alternate resistive and nonresistive activities.
- Have the person maintain good posture and positioning at all times to protect joints while muscles are weak.
- Never range muscles past the point of pain.
- Avoid irritation of inflamed nerves. Go slowly on exercise program.
- Do not recommend that the person purchase expensive self-care or mobility aids unless the physician has determined that full or substantial recovery will not occur. Rental or loan of equipment may be justified if equipment will assist the person to regain functional performance earlier.

PROGNOSIS AND OUTCOME

Most people recover in a few weeks to a few months. About 95 percent recover completely within six months to two years.

- The person is able to perform daily living activities independently.
- The person is able to perform productive activities.
- The person is able to perform leisure activities.
- The person is able to walk independently.
- The person has regained muscle strength within good to normal range.
- The person has full or nearly full range of motion in all joints.
- The person is able to perform all basic hand functions.
- The person has normal or near normal sensation in tactile, vestibular, and proprioceptive senses.

• The person has resumed social contacts and community activities.

REFERENCE

Beers, M.H., and R. Berkow, eds. 1999. *The Merck Manual of Diagnosis and Therapy*, 17th ed. Whitehouse Station, NJ: Merck Research Laboratories.

BIBLIOGRAPHY

Drastal, S., and C. Nead. 1997. Norman's conquest: An ECU opens up the possibilities. *TeamRehab Report* 8, no. 4: 15–16. (Case report)

Kerr, T. 1996. Treating the complexities of Guillan-Barré syndrome. *Advance for Occupational Therapists* 12, no. 27: 13, 46. (Case report)

McCormack, G.L., and L.W. Pedretti. 1996. Guillain-Barré. In *Occupational therapy: Practice skills for physical dysfunction*, 4th ed., ed. L.W. Pedretti, 750–751. St. Louis, MO: CV Mosby.

McCormack, G.L. et al. 1998. Motor unit dysfunction—Guillain-Barré. In *Physical dysfunction: Practice skills for the occupational therapy assistant*, ed. M.B. Early, 558–559. St. Louis, MO: Mosby.

Pulaski, K.H. 1998. Guillain-Barré syndrome. In *Willard and Spackman's occupational therapy*, 9th ed., eds. M.E. Neistadt and E.B. Crepeau, 677–678. Philadelphia: Lippincott-Raven Publishers.

Hemiplegia

DESCRIPTION

Hemiplegia is defined as loss of sensorimotor function of both limbs on one side of the body. The arm is usually affected more severely than the leg.

CAUSE

The cause of this disorder is brain injury involving the sensorimotor pathways. The injury may occur before birth, as in cerebral palsy, or after birth, as in cerebrovascular disorders or blunt trauma.

ASSESSMENT

Note: The ability to respond to communication varies among persons with hemiplegia. Determine whether the person responds best through words, pantomime, or written instructions.

Areas

• daily living skills
• productivity history, skills, interests, and values
• leisure skills and interests

- range of motion
- muscle strength
- muscle tone
- fine motor coordination (note speed and precision), manipulation, dexterity
- hand functions
- balance and postural tone
- bilateral integration
- praxis, motor planning
- sensory registration
- sensory processing: shape, texture, point localization and discrimination, proprioception
- perceptual skills
- ability to follow simple verbal or pantomimed instruction
- memory (ability to remember what is said and taught)
- problem-solving ability
- attention span
- organized and sequenced tasks or steps in a task
- ability to learn new skills
- judgment (relating to safety) in home management skills
- language and communication skills

Instruments

Instruments Developed by Occupational Therapy Personnel

- *Functional Test for the Hemiplegic/Paretic Upper Extremity* by D.J. Wilson, L.L. Baker, and J.A. Craddock, in *American Journal of Occupational Therapy* 38 (1984): 159–164; or D.J. Wilson, Assessment of the hemiparetic upper extremity: A functional test, *Occupational Therapy in Health Care* 1, no. 2 (1984): 63–69.
- *Hemiplegia Evaluation* by B. Baum et al., Occupational Therapy Department, Massachusetts Rehabilitation Hospital, Boston, 1979.

Instruments Developed by Other Professionals and Used by Occupational Therapy Personnel

- *Action Research Armtest* by R.C. Lyle, in A performance test for assessment of upper limb function in physical rehabilitation treatment and research, *International Journal of Rehabilitation Research* 4 (1981): 483–492.
- *Brunnstrom Fugl-Meyer Test* by A.R. Fugl-Meyer, L. Jaasko, and I. Leyman, in The post-stroke hemiplegic patient, *Scandinavian Journal of Rehabilitation Medicine* 7 (1975): 13–31.
- *Brunnstrom Recovery Stages* by S. Brunnstrom, in *Movement Therapy in Hemiplegia*, New York: Harper & Row, 1970. (See also S.K. Shah, Reliability of the original Brunnstrom recovery scale following hemiplegia, *Australian Occupational Therapy Journal* 31, no. 4 (1984): 144–151)
- *Evaluation of the Hemiplegic Subject* by F. Guarna et al., in *Scandinavian Journal of Rehabilitation Medicine* 20 (1988): 116.
- muscle tone tests—elbow and shoulder (see Worley 1993, 1996)
- dynamometer and pinch meter

Comparison of Left and Right Hemiplegia

Left Hemisphere	*Right Hemisphere*
Normal	
Dominant for language	Dominant for visuospatial tasks
Analyzes details	Synthesizes wholes
Organizes data in conceptual similarities	Organizes data in structural similarities
Uses reason and attention to detail	Uses intuition and imagination
Good at verbal memory	Good at figural memory
Following damage	
Aphasia common (lack of expressive or receptive speech)	Aprosodia common (lack of variation in pitch and rhythm of speech)
Reaction is catastrophic	Reaction is indifference
Difficulty processing information in auditory modality	Difficulty processing information in visual modality
Profits more from nonlanguage cues such as pantomine, gestures, and visual images	Profits more from language cues such as verbal elaboration

Source: Adapted with permission from L.A. Quintana, Evaluation of Perception and Cognition, in *Occupational Therapy for Physical Dysfunction*, 4th ed., C.A. Trombly, ed., p. 204, © 1995, Williams & Wilkins.

- goniometer
- aesthesiometer (tests two- or three-point discrimination)

PROBLEMS

Self-Care

- The person may have difficulty with hand-to-mouth activity.
- The person may have difficulty in dressing, grooming, and toileting.

Productivity

- The person may be unable to perform tasks due to problems produced by hemiplegia.
- Other aspects of productivity are discussed in the section on cerebrovascular disorders.

Leisure

- The person may be unable to perform some favorite leisure activities due to problems produced by hemiplegia.
- Other aspects of leisure activities are discussed in the section on cerebrovascular disorders.

Sensorimotor

- loss of body symmetry and trunk stability
  1. Body posture and position usually become asymmetrical due to lack or decrease of sensory motor feedback on the involved or affected side.
  2. Trunk instability usually occurs during the flaccid stage because the trunk weight is shifted to the affected side. The spastic phase of recovery usually includes trunk instability due to shifting of weight to the unaffected side to avoid falling.
  3. The head is usually flexed toward the affected side but rotated away from it.
  4. The affected arm is usually held close to the body with the scapula retracted, shoulder adducted, and the elbow, wrist, and fingers flexed.
  5. The pelvis is usually retracted and elevated; the hip is internally rotated, adducted, and extended; the knee is extended; the ankle is plantar flexed and supinated; and the toes are flexed.
  6. The shoulder and pelvis usually approach each other due to flexor spasticity.
  7. In standing and walking, the person usually leads with the unaffected side and drags the affected side toward the unaffected. The effect is that the person moves in a diagonal pattern rather than a vertical (straight forward) pattern.
- loss of range of motion (Waters et al. 1995, 1405)
  1. A functional shoulder range less than 100 degrees of flexion, 90 degrees of abduction, 30 degrees of external rotation, and 70 degrees of internal rotation will reduce ability to perform daily living tasks.
  2. Functional elbow range is 120 degrees of flexion and 30 degrees of extension.
  3. Functional forearm range is full pronation and 60 degrees of supination.
  4. Functional wrist range is –30 degrees of extension.
  5. Functional finger range is –30 degrees of flexion at the metacarpophalangeal and promotion interphalangeal flexion.
  6. A functional thumb should abduct to 30 degrees and have full extension in the interphalangeal joint.
- changes in muscle tone on affected side
  1. Muscle tone usually shows flaccidity in early recovery followed by spasticity.
  2. Muscle tone may change depending on body position.
  3. Typical hypertonus or spasticity in the upper extremity results in retraction and depression in the shoulder girdle, internal rotation and adduction of the shoulder, elbow flexion, forearm pronation, wrist and finger flexion, and thumb adduction.
- loss of skilled voluntary movement patterns on affected side
  1. The person usually has loss of gross motor skills in the shoulder and elbow.
  2. The person usually has loss of fine motor manipulation and dexterity if any spasticity is present.
  3. The person usually has loss of hand functions, such as grasp and pinch, if moderate or severe spasticity is present.
- increase in mass movement patterns on affected side
  1. The person may have flexion synergy (scapular retraction and/or elevation, shoulder abduction, and external rotation; elbow flexion; forearm supination; and wrist and finger flexion), especially during sitting or standing, due to lack of normal reciprocal inhibition, which relaxes the flexors during extension.

2. The person may have extension synergy (scapular protraction, shoulder adduction, and internal rotation; elbow extension; forearm pronation; and finger and thumb extension).
3. The person may have stereotypical movements.

- loss of automatic reflexes or reactions
  1. The person may have persistent primitive reflexes.
  2. The person may have loss of righting and equilibrium reflexes or reactions that impair a sense of balance.
- loss of bilateral integration of the two sides of the body
  1. The person usually has loss of gross motor coordination, such as bilateral skills and reciprocal skills.
  2. The person usually has loss of fine motor coordination of the hands and fingers to perform activities, such as typing with both hands or playing the piano.
- loss of motor planning skills
  1. The person may have difficulty executing a motor act and appear clumsy.
  2. The person may have difficulty with sequential movements.
- edema (dependent) and swelling due to vasomotor changes
- lost or reduced sensation on the involved side
  1. The person may have loss of two-point discrimination in the fingertips and palms.
  2. The person may have loss of proprioception (position sense).
  3. The person may have loss of stereognosis.
  4. The person may have loss of light touch and deep pressure.
  5. The person may have loss of temperature sense.
  6. The person may have loss of sense of position in space.
  7. The person may have visual neglect problems, including homonymous hemianopsia of half of the visual field.
  8. The person may have visual distortion of verticality.
  9. The person may have homonymous hemianopsia.
  10. The person may have unilateral neglect of one side of the body, especially of the upper extremity, which may be ignored.
  11. The person may lack proprioceptive or kinesthetic awareness of the relationship of body parts to one another.
  12. The person may lack the ability to interpret the relation of body parts in space.*
- increased pain
  1. The person may have pain in the back and neck related to postural strain.
  2. The person may have pain in the upper extremity such as glenohumeral subluxation, shoulder-hand syndrome, spasticity, central pain, degenerative changes about the shoulder, and referred pain resulting from cervical spondylosis.

Cognitive
- Cognitive disabilities are discussed in the section on cerebrovascular disorders.

Psychosocial
- The person may deny that the involved side of the body exists (unilateral neglect).

Note: According to Waters et al. 1995, the person will not use the affected hand unless proprioception is intact and discrimination between two points is less than 1 cm apart.

Order of Return of Voluntary Movement in the Upper Extremity

- flexion of the shoulder (initially results in flexion of the elbow, wrist, and fingers)
- flexion of the elbow (initially may result in flexion of the shoulder, wrist, and fingers)
- flexion of the wrist
- flexion of the fingers
- supination of the forearm
- extension of the shoulder
- extension of the elbow
- flexion of the shoulder independent of the elbow, wrist, and fingers
- flexion of the elbow independent of the shoulder, wrist, and fingers
- alternate flexion and extension of all fingers together
- selective flexion and extension of the index finger, then the middle
- thumb opposition to lateral side of the index finger (key pinch)
- thumb opposition to the fingertips

Source: Reprinted with permission from R.L. Waters, P.J. Wilson, and C. Gowland, Rehabilitation of the Upper Extremity after Stroke, in *Rehabilitation of the Hand: Surgery and Therapy*, 4th ed., J.M. Hunter, E.J. Mackin, and A.D. Callahan, eds., pp. 1404–1405, Copyright © 1995, W.B. Saunders Company.

- The person may have loss of receptive or expressive language that interferes with communication.
- Other intrapersonal and psychological problems are discussed in the section on cerebrovascular disorders.

TREATMENT/INTERVENTION

Traditionally models of treatment were based on compensatory or substitutive techniques (using one hand, changing dominance) and biomechanical/orthopaedic techniques (muscle strengthening, increasing endurance and range of motion). Popular models include the sensorimotor approach, neurodevelopmental treatment, movement therapy, and proprioceptive neuromuscular facilitation. Contemporary models include motor relearning, the contemporary task-oriented approach, and assistive technology. The ideas presented below are general. See Trombly (1995, 433–527) for an overview of specific models.

Self-Care

- Self-care activities can be integrated into a motor and sensory retraining program as described above. Dressing, bathing, grooming, and feeding all provide motor and sensory tasks.
- To facilitate function, use self-help devices such as universal cuffs to hold spoons and other objects while grasp is poor, enlarged handles to promote grasp, and bilateral handles on cups or glasses to encourage use of both hands.

Productivity

- Specific homemaking tasks can be used in the therapy program, such as washing dishes (use nonbreakable ones), putting groceries away, folding laundry, dusting and polishing, setting or clearing the table, and ironing.
- Work tasks that are useful in therapy include sorting and counting, stocking shelves, folding letters and putting them in envelopes, wrapping packages, and pushing a cart.

Leisure

- Many crafts can be adapted to facilitate the therapy program, such as holding paintbrushes with both hands, putting handles on block prints, or turning a table loom around to use gross movement to beat the weft.
- Games can be adapted by enlarging the size of the pieces of a puzzle, using large diameter dowels as pegs, or using door handles to enlarge the grasp surface. Tick-tack-toe and checkers can be easily adapted.

Sensorimotor

- Improve, maintain, and restore body symmetry, positioning, and trunk stability.
  1. In bed, the person's head should be on a pillow to prevent lateral flexion. In a side-lying position on the affected side, the person's shoulder should be brought forward, the arm extended to a right angle with the body or on a diagonal, the affected hip extended, and the knee flexed. The person may perform simple craft activities or play simple games.
  2. If the person is sitting, use the back and seat of the chair to form a right (90-degree) angle. The person should be positioned at a right angle with both hips flexed and feet flat on the floor or footboard. If the chair is too deep, place a firm cushion behind the back. Weight should be evenly divided over the hips. Both arms should be kept on the table surface, and both hands should be within the visual field.
  3. To ensure trunk stability, have the person
     - Practice leaning forward with hands clasped and arms extended
     - Practice shifting weight from one hip to the other (shifting from the affected side back to the unaffected is harder) with hands clasped and extended
     - Practice diagonal weight shift using forward right, back left movement and then forward left, back right, with hands clasped and extended
     - Practice rotating from left to right, right to left, with hands clasped and extended
       Craft and game activities should be incorporated into movement patterns, such as block printing (hands clasp a dowel attached to the block print). Use equipment such as a half-lapboard or arm trough to maintain trunk alignment.
  4. To prevent contractures in the shoulder, elbow, and wrist, use proper positioning, range-of-motion exercises (done slowly), and electrical stimulation to the extensor muscles. (Note: Avoid pain because it increases spasticity.) If contractures have already occurred, serial casting may be used and should be changed once a week.
- Normalize muscle tone on the affected side.
  1. To inhibit the position for spasticity of the upper extremity, bring the scapula forward and upward by holding the person's upper arm in the axilla and rotate inward and upward on the medial border of the scapula. The shoulder is externally rotated, the elbow is extended, the forearm is supinated, the wrist is dorsiflexed, the fingers are

extended and abducted, and the thumb is abducted. Always feel for tone changes but do not force (stretch) spastic muscle. Tapping the muscle belly of a hypotonus (low-tone) muscle, placing weight on the palm of the hand (or heel of the foot), and gently but firmly pushing the distal end of a joint toward the proximal end are useful techniques for reducing the effect of hypertonus.

2. To promote the inhibiting position, use crafts or games that require gross motor functions. While spasticity is present, fine motor activities generally should be avoided, especially those that require that the activity be performed close to the body.

- Decrease mass movement (synergies or stereotypical) patterns while improving skilled movements.

1. Position the person in a correct posture and the upper extremity in an inhibiting pattern.
2. Use gross motor patterns combined with fine motor movements, such as using large pieces for prehension in selected crafts or games. Grade requirements for prehension as mass movement patterns become less dominant.
3. Have the person place the ulnar border of the hemiplegic hand and wrist in the palm of the uninvolved hand with the thumb in the palmar arch and the fingers clasping the dorsum of the hand, wrist, and ulnar side of the forearm. Straighten elbows and bring arms forward. The person can use this arm position for self-ranging activities in supine and sitting positions and for gross motor activities of rolling and transfers.
4. Begin treatment with scapula mobilization. With the person in the supine position, the person's arm should go between the therapist's body and arm. Using both hands, move the scapula up and down in elevation and depression and forward and back in abduction and adduction. If no resistance (spasticity) is felt, then movements into flexion and external rotation can be started, beginning with 30 degrees to 60 degrees of motion and gradually increasing movement if no resistance is present. Next, overhead movements can be started if no pain is reported. Stop if resistance or pain are reported and begin again.
5. Place and hold activities can begin if no spasticity is present. Move the person's arm, with the person's assistance, to a position and then ask the person to hold the position as the amount of holding assistance is gradually reduced.

- Improve the person's postural control, equilibrium, and balance.

1. In a sitting position on a bench, the person reaches over his or her head, to the front, to the left, and to the right for objects; then he or she reaches to the floor for objects in front, to the left, and to the right. The bench may be lowered at the beginning of the activity to facilitate reaching.
2. In a standing position, the person performs the same activities and self-care activities, such as dressing and homemaking, that require items to be put on a high or low shelf and then removed. For the low shelf, vary the position from bending over to stooping.

- Increase bilateral integration of the two sides of the body.

1. Activities begin with bilateral movement of both arms and hands doing the same activity. The affected arm or hand may be held by the unaffected hand or tied to a handle or dowel.
2. The next activities are performed unilaterally with the affected arm or hand. Unilateral activities may begin with holding objects while bearing weight on the palm that the unaffected hand can manipulate; then have the person hold objects using the grasp of the

affected hand that the unaffected hand can manipulate; and finally have the person manipulate (reach, grasp, and release) objects with the affected hand (with no assistance from the unaffected hand).

3. The next activities are performed with both hands in parallel (both hands reach, grasp, and release) or in alternating (right-left, right-left) patterns.

- Improve praxis and motor planning.
  1. Familiar objects that can be taken apart and put back together provide excellent practice for motor planning. Examples include a coffeepot, meat grinder, or vegetable chopper.
  2. Preparing and serving a meal provides a variety of motor planning opportunities.
- Decrease edema and swelling.
  1. Place the person's arm in an elevated position.
  2. Consider using continuous passive motion.
  3. Use resting or positioning splints, if needed.
- Increase tactile awareness, discrimination, and stereognosis.
  1. Select a variety of tactile sensations, such as hard, soft, wet, dry, smooth, and rough.
  2. Tactile retraining is best combined with motor activities, especially bilateral integration and self-care activities, such as washing and drying the affected side, but games of Feely Bag or "What's in the box?" may be added.
- Increase proprioceptive and kinesthetic awareness of position of body parts in relation to each other.
  1. Usually, no special activities are needed since proprioception and kinesthesia are inherent in most motor activities.
  2. Use hand games, such as "How far is this?"
- Improve eye motility and visual perceptual skills.
  1. Orient the person toward the affected side. Approach the person from the affected side.
  2. Position the person's hand on the affected side within the visual field. The person should position the affected arm or hand while in a sitting position. Do not perform this task for the person.
  3. Activities should be performed bilaterally, and the person should focus vision on the hands and the task. Remind the person to watch or pay attention if necessary.
- Improve body schema and awareness of the body in space.
  1. Encourage the person to initiate movement with both sides of the body, such as rolling, coming to a sitting position, and walking.
  2. The person should be encouraged to dress the affected side independently.
- Decrease shoulder pain and subluxation.
  1. Positioning is important. Use of a sling may be helpful but should be carefully considered. Note that research suggests that pain is not related to subluxation or to flaccidity but to uncontrolled abduction.
  2. Avoid using overhead sling or pulley exercises that permit uncontrolled abduction. Shoulder pain may be related to problems in muscle tone of the rotators and soft tissue damage, which are aggravated during abduction activity without support to the shoulder.

Cognitive

See section on cerebral palsy or cerebrovascular disorders.

Psychosocial

See section on cerebral palsy or cerebrovascular disorders.

PRECAUTIONS

- Contractures may occur if the flexion synergy pattern persists.
- Avoid abnormal movements. Reposition the person to inhibit or reduce engaging the abnormal movement patterns.
- Spasticity increases the possibility of contractures occurring.

PROGNOSIS AND OUTCOME

- The person demonstrates symmetrical posture in static positions.
- The person's muscle tone has normalized (spasticity has decreased).
- The person is able to perform gross motor movements with the affected side without effects of mass synergies. For example, the person is able to selectively extend the fingers and thumb without simultaneously extending the elbow or engaging mass extensory synergy.
- The person is able to perform hand skills (grasp and prehension) with the affected hand.
- The person is able to maintain static and dynamic balance.
- The person is able to perform bilateral and reciprocal movements using both sides of the body.
- The person is able to plan and execute motor activities that are unfamiliar.
- Edema and swelling are controlled.
- The person is able to use the visual system for fixation, gaze, scanning, and tracking throughout the visual field.
- The person is able to perform tasks requiring visual perception.
- The person is able to respond to, discriminate among, and identify tactile input.
- The person is able to accurately respond to changes in the position of body parts.
- The person is able to move his or her body through space without bumping into walls or falling over objects.

REFERENCE

Trombly, C.A. 1995. Remediating motor behavior through contemporary approaches. In *Occupational therapy for physical dysfunction*, 4th ed., ed. C.A. Trombly, 433–527. Baltimore: Williams & Wilkins. (Reviews Bass-Haugen and Mathiowetz, Bobath, Brunnstrom, Knott and Voss, Rood, and Shepard and Carr)
Waters, R.L. et al. 1995. Rehabilitation of the upper extremity after stroke. In *Rehabilitation of the hand: Surgery and therapy,* 4th ed., eds. J.M. Hunter et al., 1401–1412. St. Louis, MO: Mosby.

BIBLIOGRAPHY

Abreu, B.C. 1995. The effect of environmental regulations on postural control after stroke. *American Journal of Occupational Therapy* 49, no. 6: 517–525.
Boissy, P. et al. 1997. Characterization of global synkineses during hand grip in hemiparetic patients. *Archives of Physical Medicine and Rehabilitation* 78, no. 10: 1117–1124.

Boyd, E.A. et al. 1993. A radiological measure of shoulder subluxation in hemiplegia: Its reliability and validity. *Archives of Physical Medicine and Rehabilitation* 74, no. 2: 188–193.
Byrne, D.P., and E. Ridgway. 1998. Considering the whole body in treatment of the hemiplegic upper extremity. *Topics in Stroke Rehabilitation* 4, no. 4: 14–34.
Davis, J.Z. 1996. Neurodevelopmental treatment of adult hemiplegia: The Bobath approach. In *Occupational therapy: practice skills for physical dysfunction*, 4th ed., ed. L.W. Pedretti, 435–450. St. Louis, MO: CV Mosby.
Dirette, D., and J. Hinojosa. 1994. Effects of continuous passive motion on the edematous hands of two persons with flaccid hemiplegia. *American Journal of Occupational Therapy* 48, no. 5: 403–409.
Flinn, N. 1995. A task-oriented approach to the treatment of a client with hemiplegia. *American Journal of Occupational Therapy* 49, no. 6: 560–569.
Gillen, G., and A. Burkhardt. 1998. *Stroke rehabilitation: A function-based approach.* St. Louis, MO: Mosby.
Hall, J. et al. 1995. Validity of clinical measures of shoulder subluxation in adults with poststroke hemiplegia. *American Journal of Occupational Therapy* 49, no. 6: 526–533.
Hseih, C.L. et al. 1996. A comparison of performance in added-purpose occupations and rote exercise for dynamic standing balance in persons with hemiplegia. *American Journal of Occupational Therapy* 50, no. 1: 10–16.
Kennelty, S. 1997. Techniques for controlling upper extremity edema. *OT Practice* 2, no. 2: 24–26.
Koltin, S.E., and H.S. Rosen. 1996. Hemiplegia and feeding: An occupational therapy approach to upper extremity management. *Topics in Stroke Rehabilitation* 3, no. 3: 69–86.
Nelson, D.L. et al. 1996. The effects of an occupationally embedded exercise on bilaterally assisted supination in persons with hemiplegia. *American Journal of Occupational Therapy* 50, no. 8: 639–646.
Padilla, R.L. 1998. Working with elders who have had cerebrovascular accidents. In *Occupational therapy with elders: strategies for the COTA*, eds. H. Lohman et al., 213–223. St. Louis, MO: Mosby.
Pedretti, L.W. 1996. Movement therapy: The Brunnstrom approach to treatment of hemiplegia. In *Occupational therapy: Practice skills for physical dysfunction*, 4th ed., ed. L.W. Pedretti, 401–416. St. Louis, MO: CV Mosby.
Roden, P.W. 1997. Reducing neglect in adult hemiplegia: Recent findings and implications for treatment. *British Journal of Occupational Therapy* 60, no. 8: 347–351.
Rodriguez, A.A. et al. 1996. Gait training efficacy using a home-based practice model in chronic hemiplegia. *Archives of Physical Medicine and Rehabilitation* 77, no. 8: 801–805.
Runyan, C. 1995. Using neurodevelopmental treatment principles to prevent shoulder pain in adult hemiplegia. *Gerontology Special Interest Section Newsletter* 18, no. 1: 3–4.
Stern, H.I. 1994. A preliminary study using a daily living task to assess upper limb function: A single case study of upper limb hemiparesis. *British Journal of Occupational Therapy* 57, no. 8: 294–296.
Turton, A. et al. 1996. Contralateral and ipsilateral EMG responses to transcranial magnetic stimulation during recovery of arm and hand function after stroke. *Electroencephalography and Clinical Neurophysiology* 101: 316–338.
Van Dyck, W.R. 1999. Integrating treatment of the hemiplegic shoulder with self-care. *OT Practice* 4, no. 1: 32–37.
Worley, J.S. 1993. Relationships among three clinical measures of muscle tone in shoulders and wrists of patients with poststroke conditions. *Canadian Journal of Occupational Therapy* 60, no. 5: 253–261.
Worley, J.S. et al. 1996. Reliability of potential clinical measures of muscle tone in the elbows of patients after stroke. *American Journal of Occupational Therapy* 50, no. 7: 554–560.
Wu, S.H. et al. 1996. Effects of a program on symmetrical posture in patients with hemiplegia: A single-subject design. *American Journal of Occupational Therapy* 50, no. 1: 17–23.
Zorowitz, R. et al. 1996. Shoulder pain and subluxation after stroke: Correlation or coincidence? *American Journal of Occupational Therapy* 50: 194–200.

Multiple Sclerosis

DESCRIPTION

Multiple sclerosis (MS) is a slowly progressive disease of the central nervous system characterized by disseminated (scattered) patches of demyelination of nerves in scattered areas of the spinal cord and brain that result in multiple and various neurologic signs and symptoms that in most, but not all, cases appear and disappear (exacerbation and remission) (Merck 1999, 1474). Myelin is a fatty protein tissue that surrounds nerves and aids in transmission of nerve impulses to and from the brain. When the myelin is destroyed, the repair tissue (glial cells) forms fibrous gliosis (scarring), the sclerotic lesions or plaques that impede the transmission of nerve impulses.

The Multiple Sclerosis Society recognizes four types or patterns of progression and prognosis: (1) relapsing-remitting, (2) primary-progressive, (3) secondary-progressive, and (4) progressive-relapsing. In the relapsing-remitting type, which affects about 70 percent of persons with MS, there are clearly defined relapses, either with full recovery or with partial recovery and residual deficits but no disease progression between relapses. In the primary-progressive type, which affects about 15 percent of persons with MS, there is progressive disease from the onset, with no distinct relapses, although there may be occasional plateaus or temporary minor improvements. The secondary-progressive type of MS begins with a pattern of clear relapses and recovery but then progresses steadily over time, with continued worsening between occasional acute attacks. In the progressive-relapsing type, there is a steady progression from the onset, but with clearly defined relapses within the context of continued progression. Except for the progressive patterns or severe disability from disuse, the overall life expectancy is changed very little.

MS has been described by individuals throughout recorded history but was not formally identified and described until 1868, when Jean-Martin Charcot wrote about it.

CAUSE

The specific cause is unknown. Theories of etiology include allergies, decreased blood flow, vitamin deficiency, autoimmune reaction, a slow-acting virus, genetic susceptibility, and trauma. Environmental factors such as geomagnetic latitudes, climate, and dietary patterns are significant up to age 15. Thereafter, environmental factors appear to have no effect. The disease occurs most commonly in people between the ages of 15 and 50. More women than men are affected. Caucasians of European ancestry are affected more than people of any other race.

The type, intensity, and effect of specific symptoms depend on which part of the nervous system is involved. Basal ganglia or cerebellum involvement would cause intention tremors and ataxia. Corticospinal tract involvement would result in weakness and/or spasticity.

ASSESSMENT

It is important to note that no two cases of MS are the same. Therefore, the problems listed below are those found in groups of persons. Any given person may experience many or few of the identified problems. Also, in some patterns of MS, symptoms come (exacerbations) and

---

**Signs and Symptoms of Multiple Sclerosis,
by Role in the Disease Progress**

- primary (directly related to the demyelination): transient fatigue, double vision, optic neuritis, paresthesia, motor weakness, ataxia, unsteady gait, bowel and bladder dysfunction, pain, decreased cognition, spasticity, neuralgia, dysarthria, dysphagia
- secondary (complications of the primary symptoms): contractures, urinary tract infection, decubitus ulcers, pain, and cognitive impairments
- tertiary (result from reactions to the primary and secondary symptoms): emotional, social, and vocational impact of the disease on the person, family, and community

Source: Adapted with permission from P. Ber, Degenerative Diseases of the Central Nervous System—Multiple Sclerosis, in *Physical Dysfunction: Practice Skills for the Occupational Therapy Assistant,* M.B. Early, ed., pp. 478–481, © 1998, Mosby-Year Book, Inc.

---

go (remissions). Thus, some persons experience the same problems repeatedly while others experience a given problem only once or twice.

Areas
- daily living skills: feeding, dressing, bathing, grooming, and toileting
- productivity history, interests, values, and skills
- leisure interests and skills
- muscle strength
- physical endurance and fatigue
- muscle tone
- fine motor coordination, manipulation, and dexterity
- hand functions, grip strength, and dominance
- static and dynamic balance and postural control
- active, passive, and functional range of motion
- mobility and ambulation, with and without aids or assistive devices
- sensory registration, acuity, and awareness
- sensory processing, especially of the upper extremity sensibility: stereognosis, two-point discrimination, and proprioception
- perceptual skills, especially of the visual system
- cognitive skills: attending behavior, concentration, memory and retention of previous learning, ability to follow instructions
- problem-solving and decision-making skills
- self-concept
- coping skills
- language and communication skills
- architectural and environmental barriers
- home or work modification

Instruments

During initial evaluation, be aware that the person's performance may be negatively affected by anxiety and stress from the evaluation process itself. Carefully explain the reason for each assessment and provide rest times.

* functional range of motion

Instruments Developed by Occupational Therapy Personnel

* *Assessment of Motor and Process Skills*, 2nd ed. by A.G. Fisher, Fort Collins, CO: Three Star Press, 1997.
* *Box and Block Test* by P. Holser and E. Fuchs, Bolingbrook, IL: Sammons Preston, 1957.
* *Box and Block Test* by V. Mathiowetz et al., in Adult norms for the Box and Block Test of manual dexterity, *American Journal of Occupational Therapy* 39, no. 6 (1985): 386–391.
* *Canadian Occupational Performance Measure*, 2nd ed. by M. Law et al., Ottawa: Canadian Association of Occupational Therapists Publications, 1994.
* *Hand Grip Strength* by M. Kellor, J. Frost, and N. Silbert, in Hand strength and dexterity, *American Journal of Occupational Therapy* 22 (1971): 77–83.
* *Nine Hole Peg Test* by M. Kellor et al., Bolingbrook, IL: Sammons Preston, 1971.
* *Occupational Therapy Evaluation* by B. Wolf, in *Multiple sclerosis, Interdisciplinary rehabilitation of multiple sclerosis and neuromuscular disorders*, eds. F.P. Maloney, J.S. Burks, and S.P. Ringel, 106–109, Philadelphia: J.B. Lippincott, 1981.
* *Qual-OT* by R.H. Robnett and J.A. Gliner, in Qual-OT: A quality of life assessment tool, *Occupational Therapy Journal of Research* 15, no. 3 (1995): 198–214.

Instruments Developed by Other Professionals and Used by Occupational Therapy Personnel

* *Boston Naming Test* by E.F. Kaplan et al., San Antonio, TX: The Psychological Corporation, 1983.
* *Fatigue Impact Scale* (FIS) by J.D. Fisk et al., in Measuring the functional impact of fatigue, *Clinical Infectious Diseases* 18 (1994): 79–83.
* *Fatigue Severity Scale* by L.B. Krupp et al., in The Fatigue Severity Scale: Applications to patients with multiple sclerosis and systemic lupus erythematosus, *Archives of Neurology* 46 (1989): 1121–1123.
* *Functional Independence Measure* by Uniform Data Systems for Medical Rehabilitation, Buffalo, NY: State University of New York at Buffalo, 1993.
* *Incapacity Status Scale* (subsection of the MRD) by J. Mertin, L. Jones, and R. Trevan, in Critical evaluation of the Incapacity Status Scale, *Acta Neurologica Scandinavica Supplement* 70, no. 101 (1984): 68–71.
* *Kurtzke Disability Scale* (subsection of the MRD) by J.F. Kurtzke, in On the evaluation of disability in multiple sclerosis, *Neurology* 11, no. 8 (1961): 686–695.
* *Minimal Record of Disability* (MRD). This scale has been established as the worldwide standard measurement of multiple sclerosis. Therapists should be familiar with the instrument whether or not it is always used. It contains five parts: demographic information, neurologic functional systems of Kurtzke, disability status scale of Kurtzke, an incapacity status scale, and an environmental scale (obtainable from the National Multiple Sclerosis Society, 205 East 42nd Street, New York, NY 10017).

- *Mini Mental State Examination* by M.F. Folstein, S.E. Folstein, and P.R. McHugh, in Mini-mental state: A practical method for grading the cognitive state of patients for the clinician, *Journal of Psychiatric Research* 12 (1975): 189–198.
- *Modified Ashworth Scale* by R.W. Bohannon and M.B. Smith, in Interrater reliability of a modified Ashworth scale of muscle spasticity, *Physical Therapy* 67, no. 2 (1987): 206–207 (for muscle tone).
- *Muscle Testing*, 6th ed. by H.J. Hislop, Philadelphia: W.B. Saunders, 1995.
- *Symbol Digit Modalities Test* by A. Smith, Los Angeles: Western Psychological Services, 1982.

PROBLEMS

Self-Care
- During exacerbations of muscle weakness, the person may be unable to perform a variety of self-care tasks.
- Because the person fatigues easily, even self-care tasks may use up available energy.
- Visual disturbances may create problems in performing self-care tasks.
- Loss of touch, pain, or temperature sensation may cause safety concerns in avoiding injury or burns.
- Loss of position sense may lead to falls.
- The person may experience urinary frequency, urgency, hesitancy, nocturia, retention, or incontinence.
- The person may experience difficulty swallowing food (dysphagia).

Productivity
- The person may be forced to give up a job because of inconsistent performance or an inability to perform due to the exacerbations.
- If there is a loss of visual acuity or diplopia, the person may experience difficulty reading directions or instructions or seeing the computer screen.
- Because of fatigue, the person may have difficulty doing even light housekeeping tasks.

Leisure
- The person may be unable to participate safely in favorite leisure occupations because of periodic motor or sensory dysfunction.
- Because of fatigue, the person may not enjoy leisure activities.

Sensorimotor
- The person usually experiences motor problems such as intermittent muscle weakness, intermittent paralysis, spasticity and/or flaccidity, gross and fine motor incoordination, or clumsiness.
- The person usually has low endurance and fatigues easily.
- The person may have problems in joint mobility such as loss of range of motion, stiffness, and contractures.

- The person may experience symptoms of cerebellar ataxia such as intermittent ataxia and gait disturbances (tripping or stumbling) or ataxic symptoms such as intention tremor.
- The person may experience paresthesia or dyesthesia.
- The person may have partial or total loss of vibratory sense, temperature sensation, pain sensation, sense of touch, position sense (proprioception), or joint sensibility (kinesthesia).
- The person may experience changes in tactile awareness such as numbness, disturbances in pain sensation, or hypersensitivity.
- The person may experience vertigo.
- The person may experience problems of ocular motility such as nystagmus (rapid alternating movements of the eyes) or disconjugate gaze.
- The person may experience episodes of diplopia (double vision), blurred or dimmed vision, partial blindness (scotoma) or total loss of visual acuity, or partial or total loss of color vision for various amounts of time.
- The person may experience episodes of acute pain.
- The person may experience Lhermitte's sign (shocks that feel electric spreading down the body when the head is flexed forward).

Cognitive
- The person may be inattentive and distractible at times, have a short attention span, or have difficulty with concentration.
- The person may show signs of short-term memory loss or disturbance in recent memory.
- The person may experience difficulty learning and retrieving new information.
- The person may have difficulty learning or forming new concepts, especially those requiring abstract reasoning.
- The person may have a reduced capacity to solve problems or deal with complex ideas.
- The person may have difficulty with verbal fluency, especially in pronunciation, called dysarthria.

Psychosocial
- The person may appear apathetic or demonstrate apparent indifference (la belle indifference).
- The person may demonstrate episodes of poor judgment and impulsivity.
- The person may demonstrate emotional lability.
- At times, the person may experience dysarthria or slurred speech (difficulty pronouncing words correctly because of tongue weakness).
- At times, the person may demonstrate scanning speech (syllables are separated by pauses).
- The person may experience depression and loss of self-worth because he or she is unable to keep up work or homemaking roles.
- The person may quit going to social functions because of fear of embarrassing him- or herself or his or her family.

Environment
- Family and friends may have difficulty understanding why the person is able to do something one day and not the next. They may think the person is faking illness or disability.

TREATMENT/INTERVENTION

Models of treatment include remedial, compensatory, maintenance, prevention, and environmental adaptation. During mild symptoms of the disorder, remedial, maintenance, preventive, and simple environmental adaptations may be needed. During moderate symptoms, more environmental adaptations will be needed, along with compensatory techniques. During severe symptoms, environmental adaptations will be a primary model of treatment. If very severe symptoms are present, the person would require that a caregiver be present at least 12 hours a day.

Self-Care

- Teach energy conservation, pacing, work simplification, and good body mechanics for performing self-care tasks.
- Provide adaptive equipment for self-care tasks and instruction in use, as needed.
- Provide instruction in safe transfers, especially from bed to (wheel)chair, and in and out of the tub or shower.
- Instruct the person in the safe use of a wheelchair, if needed.
- Make recommendations to increase safety, such as using grab bars and nonskid tape in the bath or shower, eliminating throw rugs, and using a railing or banister on stairs.

Productivity

- Make recommendations for modifications of the home or living environment that will facilitate performance of basic homemaking tasks.
- Recommend modification of work environment or task performance if the person is able to continue employment. An example might be communicating by using a computer rather than writing by hand.
- If the person can no longer work at a job, encourage him or her to volunteer, take classes, or help with homemaking tasks to continue feeling productive.
- Teach the person work simplification, pacing, and energy conservation techniques for work and home tasks.

Leisure

- Recommend leisure activities based on individual preferences and abilities.
- Explore the person's interests to determine what leisure activities might replace those that cannot be continued because of disability.

Sensorimotor

- Maintain or increase the person's upper extremity strength through progressive resistance exercises within the person's limits of fatigue.
- Maintain or improve coordination and reduce tremor through such techniques as cooling the extensor surface of the upper extremity muscles, rest-and-exercise programs, adding weight to the affected limb, and learning or relearning movement strategies.
- Maintain or increase endurance through a rest-and-exercise program that alternates cycles of rest with cycles of exercise.
- Prevent contractures through range-of-motion exercises and gentle stretching of tight muscles by using manual methods and mechanical methods (splints).

- Increase the skill of tactile senses to substitute for loss of sight, if needed.
- Teach use of sight inspection to substitute for loss of touch, pain, or position sense in order to reduce the risk of injury to skin or joints, if needed. Note: If vision is unreliable, modification of the person's environment may be necessary.

Cognitive

- Improve cognitive strategies for coping with the disease, such as planning activities in advance, providing for rest cycles, and seeking assistance from others instead of doing it all.
- Encourage the person to keep a personal calendar to assist in memory tasks and cognitive changes. A family calendar may be helpful.
- Increase knowledge of safety to avoid injury.
- Provide repeated opportunities to practice new learning to compensate for possible memory and learning deficits.
- Instruct the person in time management, which focuses on energy conservation, pacing, and work simplification while performing self-care, productivity, and leisure activities.

Psychosocial

- Provide stress management training to improve emotional control and coping behavior.
- Facilitate emotional adjustment to the disability by helping the person establish realistic life goals and take control of a personal rehabilitation program.
- Suggest participation in group self-help programs to provide the opportunity to share problems and solutions with others.
- Encourage the person to involve family members in the rehabilitation and management program in order to encourage family cooperation and support.
- Discuss with the person and family changes in role performance that may be required or that may conserve energy for other occupations that the family values. For example, the children or spouse could bring in the groceries and help put them away. As a result, the person has energy for leisure activities with the children or spouse.

Environment

- Teach the person and family about the disorder and how it affects performance. Clarify misconceptions the individual and family may have. Discuss how physicians may have labeled the person in the past (e.g., the person has a "psychological problem" or is "hysterical").
- Discuss with the person and family how assistive devices function and how to maintain them.
- Work with the person, family, and architect on home modifications that increase safety and simplify self-care and homemaking tasks.
- Explore how using public transportation (instead of driving) might help the person conserve energy and avoid safety problems related to vision.
- An educational program focused on fatigue management may be useful (Bowcher and May 1998 and Welham 1995).

PRECAUTIONS

- There are no known techniques proven to be effective in improving motor control or coordination in persons with cerebellar dysfunction and accompanied spinal motor tract involvement. Each person must be studied to determine which, if any, technique seems to provide some relief from tremor and overall improvement of function.
- Remissions do not mean that the function will suddenly and completely return. The person and therapist should understand that some decrement in function can be expected after each exacerbation.
- Inactivity probably causes more severe disability than the disorder itself (except in the progressive type). The person needs to keep active.
- Stress, heat, pain, fatigue, and exacerbations are all known to change the functional status of the person with MS from day to day. These factors must each be considered when assessing the functional status of the individual on any given day. The treatment program for a particular day may need to be modified as a result.
- Monitor use of progressive resistive exercise carefully to avoid fatigue, increased weakness, and potential injury—all of which may defeat the purpose of using the technique in the first place.
- Use of vision to compensate for loss of tactile, pressure, and temperature sensation may be unsuccessful with MS because vision is also affected. Environmental changes may be necessary to reduce or eliminate such risks. For example, do not use thermal-type physical agents, especially those using heat.
- Persons with coordination, balance, and gait problems must be monitored closely during transfers because of increased risk of falling.

PROGNOSIS AND OUTCOME

- The person maintains maximum muscle strength within the progressive stage of the disease.
- The person demonstrates use of compensatory techniques for loss of sensory functions (visual and tactile).
- The person demonstrates knowledge and performance of safety factors needed to avoid injuries due to decreased visual and tactile acuity and discrimination.
- The person demonstrates knowledge of good body mechanics and positioning.
- The person demonstrates ability to use adaptive equipment correctly.
- If a wheelchair is used, the person demonstrates mobility techniques and knowledge of routine maintenance of the chair and its parts.
- The person demonstrates knowledge of energy conservation and work simplification techniques.
- The person has organized a daily schedule that provides a balance of self-care, productivity, and leisure activities appropriate for the person's level of energy.
- The person has identifiable roles within the family or living unit that are satisfying to the individual.
- The person participates in social situations and activities.
- The person independently performs self-care activities, using adaptive devices if necessary.

- The person demonstrates the ability to seek assistance when needed and can instruct others regarding the type of care needed.
- The person demonstrates productive work and leisure skills.

REFERENCES

Beers, M.H., and R. Berkow, eds. 1999. *The Merck Manual of Diagnosis and Therapy*, 17th ed. Whitehouse Station, NJ: Merck Research Laboratories.

Bowcher, H., and M. May. 1998. Occupational therapy for the management of fatigue in multiple sclerosis. *British Journal of Occupational Therapy* 61, no. 11: 488–492.

Welham, L. 1995. Occupational therapy for fatigue in patients with multiple sclerosis. *British Journal of Occupational Therapy* 58, no. 12: 507–509.

BIBLIOGRAPHY

Ber, P. 1998. Degenerative diseases of the central nervous system—multiple sclerosis. In *Physical dysfunction: Practice skills for the occupational therapy assistant*, ed. M.B. Early, 478–481. St. Louis, MO: Mosby.

Bhasin, CA. Understanding MS. *TeamRehab Report* 6, no. 8 (1995): 20–23.

Chiara, T., et al. 1998. Cold effect on oxygen uptake, received exertion, and spasticity in patients with multiple sclerosis. *Archives of Physical Medicine and Rehabilitation* 79, no. 5: 523–528.

Crist, P. 1993. Contingent interaction during work and play tasks for mothers with multiple sclerosis and their daughters. *American Journal of Occupational Therapy* 47, no. 2: 121–131.

Doble, S.E., et al. 1994. Functional competence of community-dwelling persons with multiple sclerosis using the Assessment of Motor and Process Skills. *Archives of Physical Medicine and Rehabilitation* 75, no. 8: 843–851.

Fernie, G.R., et al. 1994. Increasing the accessibility of a conventional cooking range for wheelchair users. *American Journal of Occupational Therapy* 48, no. 5: 463–466.

Frankel, D. 1995. Multiple sclerosis. In *Neurological rehabilitation*, ed. D.A. Umphred, 588–605. St. Louis, MO: Mosby.

Hietpas, J., et al. 1996. Multiple sclerosis. In *Occupational therapy: Practice skills for physical dysfunction*, 4th ed., 837–841. St. Louis, MO: CV Mosby.

Jensen, D., and R. Linroth. 1993. The adult with multiple sclerosis. In *Practice issues in occupational therapy: Intraprofessional team building*, ed. S.E. Ryan, 121–128. Thorofare, NJ: Slack.

Kerr, T. 1995. How hi tech simplifies life for people with MS. *Advance for Occupational Therapists* 11, no. 49: 14.

Kerr, T. 1997. Living with MS: Occupational therapy for people with multiple sclerosis. *Advance for Occupational Therapists* 13, no. 46: 20–22, 24.

LaBan, M.M., et al. 1998. Physical and occupational therapy in the treatment of patients with multiple sclerosis. *Physical Medicine and Rehabilitation Clinics of North America* 9, no. 2: 603–614.

Lundmark, P., and I.B. Branholm. 1996. Relationship between occupation and life satisfaction in people with multiple sclerosis. *Disability and Rehabilitation* 18, no. 9: 449–453.

Mozdzierz, T. 1993. Multiple sclerosis. In *Conditions in occupational therapy: Effect on occupational performance*, eds. R.A. Hansen and B. Atchinson, 347–364. Baltimore: Williams & Wilkins.

Newman, E.M., et al. 1995. Degenerative diseases—multiple sclerosis. In *Occupational therapy for physical dysfunction*, 4th ed., ed. C.A. Trombly, 743–745. Baltimore: Williams & Wilkins.

Richer, C.B., and C.A. Bhasin. 1999. *Occupational therapy practice guidelines for adults with neurodegenerative diseases*. Bethesda, MD: American Occupational Therapy Association.

Robnett, R.H., and J.A. Gliner. 1995. Qual-OT: A quality of life assessment tool. *Occupational Therapy Journal of Research* 15, no. 3: 198–214.

Roush, S.E. 1995. The satisfaction of patients with multiple sclerosis regarding services received from physical and occupational therapists. *International Journal of Rehabilitation and Health* 1, no. 3: 155–166.

Roush, S.E. 1996. Examining the relationship between physical and occupational therapists and their patients with multiple sclerosis. *International Journal of Rehabilitation and Health* 2, no. 3: 125–137.

Sephton, S. 1998. Living with MS: New treatment and current research promise improved function. *Advance for Occupational Therapy Practitioners* 14, no. 40: 36–37.

Stahl, C. 1995. Biofeedback teaches MS patients bodily awareness. *Advance for Occupational Therapists* 11, no. 5: 19, 54.

Stahl, C. 1995. MS foundation chronicling reported effects of alternative therapies. *Advance for Occupational Therapists* 11, no. 5: 19.

Teague, S.J. 1995. An analysis of multiple sclerosis: The potential of desferoxamine mesylate. *Journal of Occupational Therapy Students* 9, no. 1: 19–25.

Thiers, N. 1993. Computer camp exposes people with MS to technology. *OT Week* 7, no. 25: 20–21.

Tipping, L. 1996. Multiple sclerosis. In *Occupational therapy and physical dysfunction: Principles, skills, and practice*, eds. A. Turner et al., 497–513. New York: Churchill Livingstone.

Zarella, S. 1995. Outpatient program optimizes care for MS patients. *Advance for Occupational Therapists* 11, no. 30: 22.

Parkinson's Disease

DESCRIPTION

Parkinson's disease is an idiopathic, slowly progressive, degenerative disorder of the basal ganglia in the central nervous system. The disease is characterized by slow and decreased movement, muscular rigidity, resting tremor, and postural instability (Merck 1999, 1466). It affects about 1 percent of those 65 years and older and 0.4 percent of those over 40 years of age. It may begin in childhood or adolescence (juvenile parkinsonism).

Parkinson's disease affects all races and people in all geographic regions of the world but is more common in men than in women. Also called shaking palsy, Parkinson's disease is named for James Parkinson, a British physician who first wrote about the disorder in 1817.

CAUSE

The cause of primary Parkinson's is not known. In primary Parkinson's, the pigmented neurons of the substantia nigra, locus coeruleus, and other brainstem dopaminergic cell groups are lost, which results in depletion of the neurotransmitter dopamine.

Secondary parkinsonism, the term given to related disorders, results from a loss of or interference with the action of dopamine due to degenerative disease, drugs, or toxins. The most common cause is ingestion of antipsychotic drugs or reserpine, which produces parkinsonism by blocking dopamine receptors. Administration of an anticholinergic drug can reduce the symptoms (Merck 1999, 1466–1467).

Stages of Parkinson's Disease

- Stage 1: There is unilateral involvement only with no or minimal functional impairment; the major symptom usually is resting tremor.
- Stage 2: There is midline or bilateral involvement without impairment of balance, and mild functional impairment related to trunk mobility and postural reflexes, such as difficulty turning in bed and getting in and out of the car.
- Stage 3: There is impairment of balance (postural instability) and mild to moderate functional impairment.
- Stage 4: There is increased impairment of balance, but the person is still able to walk; functional impairment increases, especially difficulties with manipulation and dexterity, which interferes with eating, dressing, and washing.
- Stage 5: The person is confined to a wheelchair or bed.

Source: Adapted with permission from M.M. Hoehn and M.D. Yahr, Parkinsonism: Onset, Progression and Mortality, *Neurology*, Vol. 17, No. 5, pp. 427–442, © 1967, Lippincott-Raven.

ASSESSMENT

Areas
- daily living skills
- productivity history, skills, interests, and values
- leisure interests and skills
- muscle strength, including grip and pinch strength
- range of motion, active and passive
- muscle tone, especially degree of rigidity
- fine motor control, including eye-hand coordination, manipulation, and dexterity
- gross motor control, including rolling, turning, walking, climbing, coming to a sitting or standing position, and making transfers
- physical tolerance and endurance
- movement speed (slow or normal)
- posture and postural control, especially flexion posture
- balance, equilibrium, and protective reactions
- mobility (ease of movement) of the body and face
- ambulation, including gait pattern and speed, especially festinating gait and propulsion
- praxis and motor planning skills
- sensory registration and processing, especially vision
- cognitive skills, especially memory and problem solving
- self-concept
- affect or mood (especially note signs of depression)
- coping skills
- social and family support

- role performance
- architectural and environmental barriers

Instruments

The literature mentions only one specific instrument for the evaluation of Parkinson's disease. Some mention general areas such as activities of daily living, upper and lower extremity status, cognitive skills, and sensory perceptual skills.

- *Assessment of Motor and Process Skills* (AMPS), 2nd ed. by A.G. Fisher, Fort Collins, CO: Three Star Press, 1997.
- daily living skills
- occupational history
- leisure interest checklist
- manual muscle testing, dynamometer, pinch meter
- goniometry
- handwriting samples
- timed movements with a stopwatch, such as sitting and standing tolerance and standing balance with eyes open and eyes closed
- observing ability to walk forward and backward and cross one leg over in front of the other (braiding)
- oral-motor skills
- ocularmotor control skills and saccades (Note: This area is controversial; see Lazaruk 1994.)
- proprioception

PROBLEMS

Self-Care

- The person may have increasing difficulty with activities of daily living due to the progression of the disease, especially increasing postural instability and slowed movements.
- Cutting food and chewing may be very slow due to akinesia or bradykinesia and loss of proprioceptive information.
- The person may experience difficulty in swallowing (dysphagia), with episodes of choking and drooling.
- The person usually experiences increasing loss of independence related to problems of postural instability.
- The person may be unable to write legibly. Often, handwriting becomes very small (micrographic).
- The person may have difficulty reading because the eyes do not move together.
- The person complains of fatigue and develops a sedentary lifestyle.

Productivity

- The person usually has increasing difficulty performing work tasks in the home and on the job due to postural instability and slowed movement.

- The person may have to retire early from work and avoid volunteer positions due to concern about postural stability and difficulty with movement.

Leisure
- The person may have restricted or curtailed favorite leisure activities due to problems in gross and fine movements and postural control, or concern about appearance, such as drooling in public.

Sensorimotor
- The person usually has bradykinesia (slow movements).
- The person usually has akinesia and hypokinesis (difficulty and slowness in initiating movement).
- The person usually has a resting tremor in the forearm and elbow, with pill-rolling movements between the fingers and thumb. Later, tremors may appear in the legs, trunk, face, lips, tongue, and neck.
- The person usually has rigidity (increased muscle tone) in the muscles of the neck, trunk, and forearm, which may respond to passive stretching with a series of jerky (cogwheel), giving movements or lead pipe movements in which there is slow, smooth resistance.
- The person usually has a characteristic posture, especially when walking, in which the neck, thoracic spine, hips, and knees are flexed. There is also a loss of the natural arm swing.
- The person usually has a masklike face (fixed expression) that does not accurately reflect the person's actual emotions.
- The person's speech may be slow, of diminished volume, and without inflection.
- The person may have a shuffling or short step gait, with acceleration as walking continues forward (festination) and in a reverse direction (retropulsion).
- The person may have a reduction of motor activity level due to movement difficulties, with a corresponding decrease in endurance, physical fitness, and muscle strength from disuse. Respiratory function is also compromised.
- The person may have loss of coordination, manipulation, and dexterity (fine motor coordination). The grasp, lift, and release sequence may become ineffective and slow.
- The person may lose gross motor skills related to trunk muscles, especially rotation and segmental rolling (difficulty rotating or turning the body, such as rolling over in bed or turning the upper torso while standing).
- The person may have difficulty initiating movements (motor planning).
- The person may have difficulty executing movements with any speed.
- The person may have difficulty with sequential movement and rhythmic flow of movement due to loss of automatic movement sequences.
- The person may have motor restlessness (akathisia) or an inability to lie or sit quietly.
- The person usually has postural instability due to loss of righting reactions, including tilt, or protective and equilibrium reactions.
- The person may have abnormal posture; the neck, if flexed forward of the spine, is fixed, and arm swing is lost during walking.
- The person may experience fluctuations in the severity of symptoms over a 24-hour period, especially before and after taking medication.
- The person may have decreased saccades in visual tasks and diminished oculomotor control.

Cognitive

- The person may have dementia and memory loss. (Note: The literature is mixed as to whether the dementia is directly related to Parkinson's disease or a coexisting disorder.)
- The person may lose spatial orientation.

Psychosocial

- The person may have loss of self-esteem.
- The person may express feelings of uselessness and hopelessness.
- The person may become depressed because of increasing disability.
- The person may express suicidal thoughts.
- The person may have monotone speech.
- The person may have decreased interest in social activities.

TREATMENT/INTERVENTION

Treatment is based on accommodative, remedial, compensatory, preventive, and environmental adaptation models. Accommodative techniques involve learning to identify the fluctuations in the symptoms and adjusting or grading the activities accordingly.

Self-Care

- Assist the person in developing a routine for performing self-care activities within the limitations of functional mobility.
- Teach adaptive techniques to reduce the effects of tremor, such as using both hands with arms close to the body to lift a glass or cup or using the elbow as a pivot to raise a fork from a plate to the mouth.
- Encourage the person to maintain maximum functional level in all activities of daily living as long as possible. Discourage caregivers from assisting too much.
- Discuss with the caregivers how to balance the need for the person to handle self-care independently with the need for the person to have energy remaining for productive and leisure activities.
- Provide practice in writing to increase the size and legibility of handwriting or have the person use a computer.

Productivity

- Encourage the person to continue productive activities as long as possible.
- Explore alternative productive activities if previous ones cannot be continued. Consider volunteer, student (there are classes for older citizens), and homemaking activities.

Leisure

- Encourage the person to maintain and pursue leisure interests that are within his or her physical capacity.
- Encourage the person to develop new interests that can substitute or replace interests that cannot be continued safely.

Sensorimotor

- Maintain or increase the person's active and passive range of motion, especially extension.
- Prevent contractures by stretching tight muscles.
- Improve speed and flexibility using sports and games.
- Maintain or improve dexterity and coordination through repetitive motions, such as sorting tasks.
- Improve gait, with emphasis on increasing step length, widening the base of support, increasing the range of hip flexion, enhancing reciprocal arm movements, and improving stops, starts, and turns.
- Maintain mobility through the use of rhythm, music, singing, and dancing to initiate movement.
- Improve motor planning and increase speed by adding visual cues, such as looking at others or in a mirror, and adding auditory cues, such as music with a pronounced rhythm, a metronome, verbal suggestions, and reinforcement from the therapist.
- Increase manipulation and dexterity (as measured by speed and accuracy) through the use of games, puzzles, writing exercises, and hand crafts, such as mosaics, link belts, felt craft, and origami.
- Improve movement patterns through proprioceptive neuromuscular facilitation patterns, especially for trunk rotation.
- Enhance awareness of problems in posture and balance and suggest methods to prevent falls, such as removing throw rugs, using banisters or hand rails when climbing stairs, and wearing flat shoes.
- Provide an opportunity for safe practice of static and dynamic balance activities in a group exercise class. Clients can hold hands to increase stability while standing on one leg, rocking back and forth on heels and then toes, or doing the grapevine step (alternating placing leg in front and then in back while moving to the right or left).
- Consider the use of music or a metronome to provide a beat or rhythm for practicing posture and balance activities.
- Assist the person in establishing a repertoire of adaptive and compensatory techniques to reduce the impact of immobility and maximize sensory stimulation.
- Teach the person relaxation and stretching exercises.

Cognitive

- Teach concepts of energy conservation and work simplification.
- Teach concepts of home safety, especially those safety considerations that may reduce the possibility of falling, such as nonskid mats, grab bars in the bathroom, and strong railings or banisters.
- Assist in teaching the person and family about Parkinson's disease and about useful treatments.
- Teach the person techniques for visual tracking, such as focusing on the left side or using an anchor or start point.

Psychosocial

- Promote relaxation by teaching deep breathing and imagery. Include slow rocking, inverted position, and other inhibitory techniques to decrease tone.

- Maintain or increase self-esteem by recognizing special skills or talents and rewarding good effort.
- Encourage vocalization to increase voice volume through speaking and singing activities.
- Provide support to the family as needed, including instruction for better treatment management.
- Use a group approach to achieve therapy objectives, especially exercise and teaching groups to improve mood (decrease depression) and increase socialization.
- Encourage the person to discuss roles within the family and living unit. Change only those roles that the person cannot safely do, but maintain as many roles as possible.
- Encourage the family to participate in the treatment program.

Environment
- With the person and family, determine what in the home or work environment could be changed to reduce the impact of immobility and reduced postural security while maximizing sensory stimulation. For example, using a bar stool for sitting can be helpful.
- Encourage the person and family to participate in a self-help or support group.
- Help the person and family to explore the community for resources.

PRECAUTIONS

- The person is prone to loss of balance and may fall on objects. Maintain safety procedures at all times.
- Observe the person for signs of side effects from medication, such as dystonic movements, orthostatic hypotension, mental disturbances, cardiac arrhythmias, or gastrointestinal disturbances.
- Observe the person for signs of severe depression.

PROGNOSIS AND OUTCOME

Parkinson's disease is a progressive, degenerative disorder. Treatment can slow the degree of disability but not the course of the disease.
- The person is able to perform activities of daily living at the maximum level of independence possible given the current stage of the disease.
- The person demonstrates improvement in ease of movement in trunk muscles.
- The person demonstrates improvement in postural control and balance.
- The person demonstrates improvement in motor planning abilities.
- The person demonstrates improvement in manipulation and dexterity (fine motor coordination).
- The person demonstrates improvement in gross motor coordination.
- The person has the level of endurance needed to perform functional activities.
- The person has increased range of motion to permit performance of functional activities or has learned to use adapted equipment.
- The person demonstrates knowledge of safety considerations.

- The person demonstrates knowledge of energy conservation and work simplification techniques.
- The person and family demonstrate knowledge of support services available in the community.

REFERENCES

Beers, M.H., and R. Berkow, eds., 1999. *The Merck Manual of Diagnosis and Therapy*, 17th ed. Whitehouse Station, NJ: Merck Research Laboratories.

Lazaruk, L. 1994. Visuospatial impairment in persons with ideopathic Parkinson's disease: A literature review. *Physical and Occupational Therapy in Geriatrics* 12, no. 2: 37–48.

BIBLIOGRAPHY

Beattie, A. 1996. Parkinson's disease. In *Occupational therapy and physical dysfunction: Principles, skills, and practice*, eds. A. Turner et al., 535–570. New York: Churchill Livingstone.

Ber, P. 1998. Degenerative diseases of the central nervous system—Parkinson's disease. In *Physical dysfunction: Practice skills for the occupational therapy assistant*, ed. M.B. Early, 481–484. St. Louis, MO: Mosby.

Fox, C.M., and R.N. Alder. 1999. Neural mechanisms of aging. In *Neuroscience for rehabilitation*, 2nd ed., ed. H. Cohen, 401–418. Philadelphia: Lippincott Williams & Wilkins.

Grogan, G. 1994. The personal computer: A treatment tool for increasing sense of competence. *Occupational Therapy in Mental Health* 12, no. 4: 47–70.

Hariz, G.M. et al. 1998. Assessment of ability/disability in patients treated with chronic thalamic stimulation for tremor. *Movement Disorders: Official Journal of the Muscular Dystrophy Society* 13, no. 1: 78–83.

Hooks, M.L. 1996. Parkinson's disease. In *Occupational therapy: Practice skills for physical dysfunction*, 4th ed., ed. L.W. Pedretti, 845–851. St. Louis, MO: Mosby.

Hunt, L.A. et al. 1995. Review of the visual system in Parkinson's disease. *Optometry and Vision Science* 72, no. 2: 92–98.

Jain, S.S., and G.E. Francisco. 1993. Parkinson's disease and other movement disorders. In *Rehabilitation medicine: Principles and practice*, 3rd ed., ed. J.A. DeLisa, 1035–1056. Philadelphia: J.B. Lippincott.

Kerr, T. 1995. Getting the right connection. *Advance for Occupational Therapists* 11, no. 41: 15.

Kerr, T. 1995. Pallidotomy: Making a comeback as Parkinson treatment. *Advance for Occupational Therapists* 11, no. 38: 17.

Marmer, L. 1995. Relaxation improved function in Parkinson patients. *Advance for Occupational Therapists* 11, no. 32: 16.

Melin-Eberhardt, K., and J.E. Walker, Jr. 1993. The elderly with Parkinson's disease. In *Practice issues in occupational therapy: Intraprofessional team building*, ed. S.E. Ryan, 147–152. Thorofare, NJ: Slack.

Newman, E.M. et al. 1995. Parkinson's disease. In *Occupational therapy for physical dysfunction*, 4th ed., ed. C.A. Trombly, 745–747. Baltimore: Williams & Wilkins.

Pulaski, K.H. 1998. Parkinson's disease. In *Willard and Spackman's occupational therapy*, 9th ed., eds. M.E. Neistadt and E.B. Crepeau, 671. Philadelphia: J.B. Lippincott.

Schwartz, A.W. 1994. Activities of daily living. In *The comprehensive management of Parkinson's disease*, eds. A.M. Cohen and W.J. Weiner, 63–73. New York: Demos.

Thibeault, R. 1997. A funeral for my father's mind: A therapist's attempt at grieving. *Canadian Journal of Occupational Therapy* 64, no. 3: 107–114.

Postpolio Syndrome

DESCRIPTION

Postpolio syndrome (or postpoliomyelitis syndrome) is characterized by muscle fatigue, pain, and decreased endurance, often accompanied by weakness, fasciculations, and atrophy in selected muscles, which may occur many years after paralytic poliomyelitis, particularly in older persons and in those who were more severely affected initially (Merck 1999, 2342). The condition was first described in 1979 in the *Rehabilitation Gazette*.

CAUSE

Persons must have a past history of poliomyelitis. The exact cause of current symptoms is unclear, and many explanations have been proposed. The symptoms may be related to further loss of anterior horn cells due to aging in a population of neurons already depleted by earlier poliovirus infections (Merck 1999, 2342). Another explanation is that the symptoms are due to a superimposed second condition, such as diabetes mellitus, disk herniation, or degenerative joint disease (Merck 1999, 1486). The latter cause may be related to chronic mechanical strain of weakened musculature and ligaments and loss (degenerative joint disease or arthralgia) or dropout or dysfunction of axon terminals of reinnervated motor units (muscle overuse, myofascial pain, or compressive neuropathy).

ASSESSMENT

Areas
- daily living activities
- productivity history, skills, interests, and values
- leisure skills and interests
- muscle strength (Note: Muscles may not be as efficient as their strength suggests and may vary greatly in strength throughout the range of motion.)
- range of motion (functional)
- muscle tone (Note tightness in muscle groups.)
- pain in muscles or joints
- myoclonus
- physical tolerance and endurance
- sense of self-concept and self-worth
- coping and stress management skills
- role performance: family, social, work, and so on
- types of self-help devices being used
- architectural and environmental barriers

Instruments

No specific tests developed by occupational therapists were identified for this disorder. The following types of tests should be useful:
- activities of daily living scale
- occupational history
- leisure checklist
- manual muscle test
- goniometry
- physical capacities
- coping skills
- time management

PROBLEMS

Self-Care
- The person may have increased difficulty performing activities of daily living, especially bathing, grooming, dressing, swallowing, and controlling bladder and bowels.
- The person may have increasing difficulty with ambulation, transfers, and driving.

Productivity
- The person may experience increased difficulty performing job tasks, such as those requiring walking distances within a building or between buildings.
- The person may experience difficulty performing homemaking tasks.

Leisure
- The person may be unable to continue some leisure activities because of decreased muscle strength and increased pain.

Sensorimotor
- The person usually has decreased physical tolerance and endurance.
- The person usually has progressive muscle weakness and atrophy in muscles affected and unaffected by polio, called progressive postpolio muscular atrophy.
- The person may have fasciculations and myoclonus.
- The person may have respiratory insufficiency.
- The person may have increasing loss of ambulation skills, especially stair climbing.
- The person may awaken with headaches.
- The person may have difficulty swallowing and may choke.
- The person may have transient fatigue, muscle weakness, or pain after exercise, which are early signs of the postpolio syndrome.
- The person may have signs of nerve entrapment syndromes.
- The person may have degenerative arthritis as a coexisting condition.
- The person may have loss of temperature control in the affected limb(s).
- The person may experience pain in the muscles, joints, or back.
- The person may experience increased sensitivity and intolerance to cold.

- The person may have loss of sensation.

Cognitive
- The person may experience difficulty in concentration.

Psychosocial
- The person is likely to deny there is any major problem or concern.
- The person usually has increased feelings of helplessness.
- The person may become depressed.
- The person may have feelings of anxiety and fear about becoming increasingly disabled.
- The person may express feelings of anger at being unable to perform certain activities.
- The person may refuse to believe that changes in lifestyle may be necessary.
- The person may have decreased participation in social activities due to decreased endurance.

TREATMENT/INTERVENTION
Models of treatment are not well established since this aspect of polio has been documented fairly recently. There are models in remedial (limited), compensatory, preventive, and environmental adaptation. Consultation, supportive education, and collaborative problem solving are important in helping the person examine his or her life situation realistically, determine values and priorities, and make lifestyle modifications that permit maximum function consistent with his or her current health status. A team approach is often used.

Self-Care
- Introduce the person to the self-help devices that were not available when the person received rehabilitation. Work collaboratively with the person to determine which devices might be helpful and save energy for other important activities. Be sure to provide proper training in use.
- Devices that may have been used for many years should be checked to determine if they still function, fit properly, are needed to do a task, and are the best solution for the task.
- Help the person determine the best balance of work, play, relaxation, and rest. Teaching the person about the metabolic costs of various tasks may be useful in developing a priority list of what is most important and what can be let go.

Productivity
- Discuss and make recommendations for possible changes and adaptations in job tasks or the physical work environment.
- Discuss and make recommendations for possible changes and adaptations in the living environment to increase safety and accommodate reduced endurance.
- Teach the person energy conservation, pacing, and work simplification techniques.
- The person may need adaptations to make driving a car easier or may need to change to a van that will easily accommodate a wheelchair.

Leisure
- Explore existing leisure activities for possible adaptations that might permit continued participation, such as adapted bowling or using a cart for golf.

- Explore interests to determine possible new leisure activities that are within the person's physical limitations.

Sensorimotor
- Encourage the person to try aerobic exercises to strengthen weakened muscles and maintain cardiovascular fitness. Swimming or doing exercises with a group sitting in chairs would be good examples. Avoid fatigue and pain. The key is to use a mild exercise program in which resistance can be applied gradually with adequate rest time between exercises.
- Provide training in the use of a wheelchair or motorized scooter, if indicated, especially in relation to the job and home.
- Assist in training the person to adjust to a new orthosis (a leg brace, for example) if indicated.
- Provide padded gloves or elbow pads to the person with compression injuries resulting from the use of a cane, crutch, or wheelchair.
- Teach principles of joint and muscle protection, especially where muscle imbalances are present. Splinting may be useful to protect joints, keep them in proper alignment, prevent muscle stretch, and improve mechanical advantage of weak muscles.
- Biofeedback may be helpful in increasing temperature control and pain management.
- If the person is overweight, work with a dietician to develop a sound weight reduction program.

Cognitive
- Teach energy conservation, pacing, and work simplification techniques.
- The person may need to learn new eating habits to lose weight and increase his or her energy level.
- Provide the person with an opportunity to solve problem situations that are of greatest concern to the person.
- Teach time management skills to permit cycles of rest and activity.

Psychosocial
- Encourage the person to speak about his or her feelings. A self-help support group may be useful to encourage the sharing of feelings.
- Teach stress management techniques, including relaxation training.
- Encourage the person to continue social activities but suggest possible modifications, such as shorter outings.

Environment
- Discuss with the person and family if modifications to the home would be helpful.
- Help the person and family learn about the condition and what to expect in relation to function and performance.
- Encourage the person and family to participate in support groups and network among persons with postpolio, such as through the International Polio Network in St. Louis, Missouri, the newsletter *Polio Network News,* or an Internet group.
- Help the person and family maintain a regular routine that stresses comfort and safety.

PRECAUTIONS

- Most polio survivors have become overachievers, as if compensating for the polio. Helping an individual to learn that it is all right to slow down may be the most important step toward helping that person accept the new limitations imposed by his or her body. Such a person does not want to be considered disabled and has prided him- or herself on being able to pass as completely able-bodied or has minimized the disability by using adaptive equipment or compensatory strategies. Introduce small changes slowly so the person can adjust a little at a time.
- Make sure the person avoids the overuse weakness that occurs following strenuous exercise or activities and results in a loss of maximum muscle strength lasting for days or weeks.
- Do not use a vigorous strengthening exercise program and warn the person of the danger of damaging weak muscles and joints if such a program is undertaken at a local gym.

PROGNOSIS AND OUTCOME

Prognosis and outcome depend on the degree to which the individual is able to change his or her lifestyle to function within physical limitations instead of overextending the limits. Functional independence using adaptive devices as needed is also a key factor, along with successful management of psychological stress.

- The person is able to perform self-care activities independently using self-help devices, if needed.
- The person is able to perform productive activities with job modifications, if needed.
- The person is able to perform leisure activities with adaptations, if needed.
- The person has maintained or increased muscle strength.
- The person has maintained or increased range of motion.
- The person has maintained or increased physical tolerance and endurance.
- The person has maintained or increased functional mobility by modification of crutches or use of a wheelchair.
- The person demonstrates knowledge of stress management techniques.
- The person demonstrates knowledge of energy conservation, pacing, and work simplification techniques.
- The person demonstrates knowledge of time management techniques to balance self-care, productivity, leisure, and rest.

REFERENCE

Beers, M.H., and R. Berkow, eds. 1999. *The Merck Manual of Diagnosis and Therapy*, 17th ed. Whitehouse Station, NJ: Merck Research Laboratories.

BIBLIOGRAPHY

Agree, J.C. et al. 1996. Low-intensity alternate-day exercise improves muscle performance without apparent adverse effect in postpolio patients. *American Journal of Physical Medicine and Rehabilitation* 75, no. 1: 50–58.

Marmer, L. 1996. Post-polio syndrome: Getting the word out. *Advance for Occupational Therapists* 12, no. 20: 13, 46.

McCormack, G.L., et al. 1998. Motor unit dysfunction—poliomyelitis and post-polio. In *Physical dysfunction: Practice skills for the occupational therapy assistant*, ed. M.B. Early, 556–558. St. Louis, MO: Mosby.

McCormak, G.L., and L.W. Pedretti. 1996. Postpolio syndrome. In *Occupational therapy: Practice skills for physical dysfunction*, 4th ed., 749–750. St. Louis, MO: CV Mosby.

Newman, E.M. et al. 1995. Postpolio syndrome. In *Occupational therapy for physical dysfunction*, 4th ed., ed. C.A. Trombly, 747–749. Baltimore: Williams & Wilkins.

Rodriguez, A.A. et al. 1995. Electromyographic and neuromuscular variables in post-polio subjects. *Archives of Physical Medicine and Rehabilitation* 76, no. 11: 989–993.

Westbrook, M., and D. McIlwain. 1996. Living with the late effects of disability: A five-year follow-up survey of coping among post-polio survivors. *Australian Occupational Therapy Journal* 43, no. 2: 60–71.

Part IV

Cardiopulmonary Disorders

Cardiovascular Disease—Adult

DESCRIPTION

Cardiovascular disease affects the blood supply, tissues, and muscles in and around the heart and the vascular system of the body. Diseases include arterial hypertension, orthostatic hypotension, syncope, arteriosclerosis, coronary artery disease, heart failure, shock, arrhythmias, cardiac arrest, valvular heart disease, endocarditis, pericardial disease, diseases of the aorta and its branches, and peripheral vascular disorders. Corrective surgery includes percutaneous transluminal coronary angioplasty for angina, coronary artery bypass grafting for blocked arteries, intraaortic balloon pump to increase cardiac output, and valve replacement for valvular heart disease. Complications following surgery may be a myocardial infarction or stroke. Descriptions below are from Merck 1999, 1629–1784.

Hypertension is elevated systolic blood pressure at or above 140 mm of mercury and/or diastolic blood pressure at or above 90 mm of mercury. Hypertension is usually treated with drugs known to lower blood pressure.

Orthostatic hypotension is an excessive fall of blood pressure typically greater than 20 mm systolic or 10 mm diastolic of mercury on assuming the upright posture and thus is not an actual disease but a manifestation of abnormal regulation.

Syncope is a sudden, brief loss of consciousness, with loss of postural tone (fainting).

Arteriosclerosis is a generic term for several diseases in which the arterial wall becomes thickened and loses elasticity. Atherosclerosis is the most common type of arteriosclerosis and is characterized by patchy subintimal thickening (atheromas or plaques) of medium and large arteries, which can reduce or obstruct blood flow.

Coronary artery disease includes angina pectoris and myocardial infarction. *Angina pectoris* is a clinical syndrome due to myocardial ischemia typically precipitated by exertion and relieved by rest or nitroglycerin. *Myocardial infarction* or ischemic myocardial necrosis usually results from abrupt reduction in coronary blood flow to a segment of myocardium or heart muscle.

Heart failure or congestive heart failure is symptomatic myocardial dysfunction resulting from a pattern of hemodynamic, renal, and neurohormonal responses in which the plasma volume increases and liquid accumulates in the lungs, abdominal organs such as the liver, and peripheral tissues.

Shock is a state in which blood flow to and perfusion of peripheral tissues are inadequate to sustain life because of insufficient cardiac output or maldistribution of peripheral blood flow.

Arrhythmias include bradyarrhythmias, or slow arrhythmias, and tachyarrhythmias, or fast arrhythmias. Most arrhythmias are not clinically significant unless they are sustained enough to cause symptoms such as dizziness or syncope.

Cardiac arrest is the absent or inadequate ventricular contraction that immediately results in systemic circulatory failure. It is a medical emergency.

Valvular heart disease occurs when the mitral, tricuspid, and aortic heart valves fail to function properly.

Endocarditis is an inflammation of the endocardium of the heart.

Classes of Cardiac Disease

- Class I: These patients have cardiac disease but not the resulting limitations of physical activity. Ordinary physical activity does not cause undue fatigue, palpitation, dyspnea, or anginal pain.
- Class II: These patients have cardiac disease resulting in slight limitation of physical activity. They are comfortable at rest. Ordinary physical activity results in fatigue, palpitation, dyspnea, or anginal pain.
- Class III: These patients have cardiac disease resulting in marked limitation of physical activity. They are comfortable at rest. Less than ordinary physical activity causes fatigue, palpitation, dyspnea, or anginal pain.
- Class IV: These patients have cardiac disease resulting in an inability to carry on any physical activity without discomfort. Symptoms of cardiac insufficiency or of the anginal syndrome may be present even at rest. If any physical activity is undertaken, discomfort is increased.

Source: Reproduced with permission, *Nomenclature and Criteria for Diagnosis of Disease of the Heart and Great Vessels, 8th ed.*, 1979. Copyright American Heart Association.

Pericardial disease includes congenital anomalies and acquired disorders.
Diseases of the aorta include aneurysms, aortic dissection, inflammation, and occlusion.
Peripheral vascular disorders affect the arteries, veins, and lymphatics of the extremities.

CAUSE

The causes of cardiovascular disease include blood clots (thrombus or embolus), thickening of the artery walls (arteriosclerosis), bacterial infections (bacterial endocarditis) that result in damage to the valves, high blood pressure, arrhythmias, and other contributing or lifestyle factors, such as diet and nutrition, lack of exercise, high-stress jobs, and poor health habits. The cause of primary or essential hypertension is unknown, although many theories exist. Secondary hypertension is caused primarily by renal disorders and/or certain drugs. Orthostatic hypotension is caused by gravitational stress, which in turn is due to impaired autonomic reflex mechanisms as a result of certain neurologic disorders and drugs. Atherosclerotic plaque consists of accumulated intracellular and extracellular lipids, smooth muscle cells, connective tissue, and glycosaminoglycans that occur in conjunction with several risk factors, including age, male sex, family history, abnormal serum lipid levels, hypertension, smoking, obesity, physical inactivity, certain metabolic diseases such as diabetes mellitus, and chlamydia pneumoniae infection. Coronary artery disease is most often due to atheromas, coronary spasm, or an embolus in a coronary artery. The most common cause of myocardial infarction is an acute thrombus that occludes an artery previously partially obstructed by an atherosclerotic plaque. Heart failure usually starts with left ventricular failure due to coronary artery disease, hypertension, or congenital defects of the heart. Shock is associated with hypertension and oliguria. Cardiac arrest results from electrical dysfunction or mechanical failure of the cardiac system. Valvular heart disease is due to incompetency, insufficiency, or obstruction of one or more heart valves. Endocarditis is caused by microbial infections or trauma to the endocardium. Pericardial disease may be caused by congenital conditions such as pericardial cysts or absence of the parietal pericardium or acquired conditions caused by infection, inflammation, trauma, or neoplasms. Diseases of the aorta may be due to congenital disorder, degenerative changes, infections, or blockages of the aorta or its branches. Peripheral vascular disorders may be caused by occlusion, inflammation, arteriole spasm or vasospasm, dilation, and unknown causes.

ASSESSMENT

Areas

- daily living activities
- productivity history, interests, skills, and values
- job analysis, including the amount of dynamic and static work done, energy requirements in terms of metabolic costs, temperature stress, and psychological stress
- leisure interests and skills
- blood pressure (At-rest blood pressure should be less than 140/90 to be considered normal. Blood pressure readings greater than 140/90 indicate hypertension. If the systolic pressure is less than 90, the person is considered hypotensive.)
- heart rate (The pulse should be between 60 and 100 beats per minute.)
- rate pressure product (double product): Heart rate (HR) times systolic blood pressure (SBP) yields rate pressure product (RPP) with last two numbers dropped. Example: HR (90) × SBP (135) = 12,150 minus last two numbers = RPP (122).
- muscle strength
- range of motion
- gross and fine motor coordination
- sensation
- physical endurance
- work tolerance
- graded exercise testing, dynamic and static
- time management
- mood or affect
- self-concept
- self-control
- coping skills

Instruments

- *Rate of Perceived Exertion Scale* by G. Borg, in Perceived exertion as an indicator of somatic stress, *Scandinavian Journal of Rehabilitation Medicine* 2, no. 3 (1970): 92–98; or G. Borg, Psycho-physical bases of perceived exertion, *Medicine and Science in Sports and Exercise* 14 (1982): 377–381.
- count of pulse
- sphygmomanometer (to measure blood pressure)
- goniometer (to measure joint range of motion)
- dynamometer (to measure muscle strength)
- coping skills

- electrocardiogram (to observe heart function)
- electrocardiogram unit with oscilloscope (to monitor heart's electrical activity)
- oximeter (to measure percentage of hemoglobin saturated with oxygen)
- stethoscope
- arterial pressure line (to monitor blood pressure and gas)
- Holter monitor (a recording device that stores electrocardiogram tracings for a period of time)

PROBLEMS

Self-Care

- The person may be unable to perform some activities of daily living, especially those that require reaching overhead with upper extremities because of dyspnea (shortness of breath), chest pain, cyanosis, fatigue, dizziness, weakness, or lack of endurance.
- The person may deliberately stop performing daily living activities to avoid symptoms such as shortness of breath, chest pain, or fatigue.
- The person may be overweight, eat a poorly balanced diet, smoke, or engage in other risk factors that increase the risk of cardiovascular disease and symptoms.
- The person may become inactive in the mistaken belief that overactivity caused the attack.

Productivity

- The person may be unable to continue in his or her present occupation because of dyspnea, chest pain, cyanosis, fatigue, dizziness, weakness, lack of endurance, or job activities that require exertion beyond safe limits.
- The person may be unable to return to some jobs because of regulations that prevent a person who has ischemic cardiac disease from returning to such employment.

Leisure

- The person may be unable to continue some leisure activities because of chest pain, dyspnea, cyanosis, fatigue, dizziness, weakness, lack of endurance, or activities that require exertion beyond safe limits.

Sensorimotor

- The person may have poor physical tolerance and endurance—deconditioning.
- The person may have muscle weakness.
- The person may fatigue quickly.
- The person may have disuse atrophy.
- The person may have decreased speed and accuracy in fine motor manipulation and dexterity.
- The person may have pain in the chest or arm upon exertion.
- The person may have dyspnea or difficulty breathing and shortness of breath.
- The person may have palpitations.
- The person may experience a sense of lightheadedness and syncope.
- The person will be more tired from doing upper extremity activities than from doing lower extremity activities.

- The person may develop orthostatic hypotension.
- Pain associated with myocardial infarction in men is initially substernal, visceral pain described as an ache or pressure and may radiate to the back, jaw, or left arm.

Cognition

- Cognitive faculties are usually not affected, but decreased blood supply to the brain may result in ineffective use of cognitive skills.

Psychosocial

- The person may experience anxiety and fear about becoming an invalid or dying.
- The person may become agitated.
- The person may be depressed.
- The person may experience loss of self-confidence.
- The person may have feelings of hopelessness and helplessness.
- The person may deny there are any problems.
- The person may withdraw from family and friends.
- The person may become demanding.
- The person may become dependent.
- The person may lack a social support system.
- The person is usually apprehensive and anxious.
- The person may feel distressed and fearful.
- The person may feel a loss of self-esteem.
- The person may be passively dependent and want to be treated rather than participate in the treatment process.
- The person may be obsessive-compulsive and tend to overdo treatment recommendations.
- The person may be irritable when his or her health and career become the focus of concern.
- The person may have a history of stressor factors, such as excessive work and responsibilities, job dissatisfaction, family problems, and life dissatisfaction.
- The person may have poor coping skills and/or a Type A personality that results in a chronic stress response.
- Family roles may change.
- Family members may become overprotective.

TREATMENT/INTERVENTION

The primary medical treatment model in cardiac rehabilitation programs is usually a multidisciplinary team approach based on the biomedical model, which focuses on physical reconditioning. Occupational therapy practitioners focus on models that consider the milieu and environment. Treatment models include the occupational behavior model of work, play, and rest, and SABRES, which is a British occupational therapy program that focuses on psychological factors. The acronym stands for sleep, arousal, breathing, rest and effort, and self-esteem.

Four Phases of Cardiac Rehabilitation Programs

- Phase I is the inpatient stage. Goals include early mobilization, psychological support, and some eduction to prepare and condition the person for the physical and psychosocial demands required for adjustment to the roles after discharge. Methods include range-of-motion exercises, sitting, standing, and walking; resumption of usual personal care activities; and basic education about how the disease process affects physical and functional status as well as immediate issues regarding recovery. Occupational therapy can be focused on self-care and graded activity as well as teaching principles of energy conservation, pacing, and work simplification.
- Phase II is the early postdischarge stage. Goals include optimizing physical conditioning, assessing risk factors, doing continuing education and counseling, and facilitating return to work and leisure tasks. Methods include initiation of a supervised exercise program based on exercise test results, risk factors, and medical history; provision of ongoing education and counseling to address disease process; risk factor modification; discussion of psychological reactions; and resumption of functional and vocational tasks and life roles. Occupational therapy can be focused on increasing independence in self-care and work roles.
- Phase III is outpatient management. Goals include stabilizing physical conditioning of cardiovascular system and physiological responses to exercise and reinforcing risk factor modification. Methods include continuation of supervised exercise or initiation of unsupervised exercise and continuation of comprehensive education focusing on maintenance of risk factor modification and return to productive occupations. Occupational therapy can be focused on encouraging progression toward higher energy levels for return to work and leisure pursuits or, in the case of persons with severe cardiac disease, adaptation of tasks or physical surroundings may be necessary to enable the achievement of maximal levels of function.
- Phase IV is long-term management. Goals include long-term maintenance of physical conditioning and psychosocial support system and of secondary prevention, especially lifestyle changes. Methods include encouraging participation in cardiac support groups, educational workshops, or social outings. Occupational therapy can be focused on continuing to teach and encourage change in personal behaviors and reinforce risk factor modification principles in all life roles.

Source: Adapted with permission from L. Tooth and K. McKenna, Contemporary Issues in Caridac Rehabilitation: Implications for Therapists, *British Journal of Occupational Theapy*, Vol. 59, No. 3., pp. 133–140, © 1996, College of Occupational Therapists Ltd.

SABRES Program

- Person should
  1. Be honest about functional capabilities
  2. Have a healthy respect for fatigue
  3. Know when to go forward, change course, and back off
  4. Keep a reserve of energy on hand for contingencies and emergencies
- Person should
  1. Examine exhausting and time-wasting habits
  2. Learn to conserve energy
  3. Pace and space daily activities to avoid time pressure
  4. Stop trying to do several things at once
- Person should
  1. Avoid angina
  2. Become familiar with effects on self of different levels of varieties of exercise
  3. Self-check effects of emotional tension and effort
  4. Learn to use a sphygmomanometer
  5. Learn to count heart rate
- Person should
  1. Increase general mobility and body awareness through graded walking program
  2. Focus on stamina rather than speed
  3. Not exercise after a large meal
- Person should
  1. Do fitness training if it is pleasurable
  2. Warm up before exercising
  3. Learn to stay at 60 percent to 70 percent of maximum heart rate
  4. Avoid sports that put sudden, severe demands on the left ventricle upon isometric effort or sports that involve exposure to cold
  5. Learn and follow the phrase "Train, don't strain"

Source: Adapted with permission from J.C. King and P.G. Nixon, A System of Cardiac Rehabilitation: Psychophysiological Basis and Practice, *British Journal of Occupational Therapy*, Vol. 51, No. 11., pp. 378–384, © 1988, College of Occupational Therapists Ltd.

Self-Care

- Instruct the person in work simplification, pacing, and energy conservation techniques. For example, the person can sit while grooming him- or herself instead of standing.
- Provide adapted equipment, such as elongated handles, to reduce the need for raising the arm above the shoulder and to assist in the performance of activities of daily living, if needed.
- Instruct the person to monitor performance of self-care daily living tasks for signs of cardiac stress. Tasks that have previously caused the person pain or discomfort should be monitored.
- Provide opportunities to practice selecting foods and planning and preparing meals that follow the recommended diet.

Productivity
- Explore work interests if the person is unable to continue in his or her present paid employment.
- Help the person maintain or increase home management activities.
- Provide a work tolerance or work hardening program to increase work tolerance or the length of time the person can function in a job situation.
- Provide work simulation environment to assist in determining whether the person can return to the same job situation and work setting.
- If the person must change jobs, help him or her explore career interests and options in cooperation with vocational rehabilitation, if it is available.

Leisure
- Help the person modify existing leisure activities to fit within permitted energy expenditure levels.
- Encourage the person to explore and develop old or new interests that are within the safe limits of his or her cardiac capacity.
- Encourage the selection of leisure activities that involve physical and social participation and a balance of leisure activities.

Sensorimotor
- Increase the person's physical and work tolerance within safe limits (such as diastolic blood pressure under 120 mm) through graded activity, such as games and exercises performed individually or in groups. Grading is done according to the amount of time, frequency of performance, degree of resistance (weight), or position of the task. Grading may also be accomplished by combinations of static and dynamic activities, such as carrying (holding) a given weight load while walking.
- Help the person avoid loss of muscle strength through participation in graded resistive activity within safe limits.
- Analyze activity or task performance to reduce or avoid situations that result in pain and encourage work simplification, energy conservation, or time management.
- Help the person learn to function within the limits of his or her pain and monitor heart rate and blood pressure.

Cognition
- Teach the person to analyze tasks in relation to the concepts of energy conservation, pacing, and work simplification such as setting priorities, combining tasks, eliminating nonessentials tasks, and following work–rest cycles.
- Reinforce concepts of good nutrition through discussion of and practice in the preparation of foods with less salt and saturated fats but more fiber.
- Teach the concept of energy levels required or demanded to perform various tasks using the metabolic equivalent table (MET) system. One MET is the energy consumed at rest, approximately equivalent to 3.5 milliliters of oxygen per kilogram of body weight per minute (i.e., the basal metabolic rate).
- Teach the person to develop a time management schedule that organizes cycles of rest and activity and a more balanced lifestyle of self-care, productivity, and leisure.

- Assist in teaching the person about lifestyle modification, including avoiding or reducing risk factors associated with diet, smoking, and physical activity.
- Instruct the person in the use of good body mechanics, such as proper lifting techniques.

Psychosocial

- Provide instruction and training in stress management, including relaxation techniques.
- Improve self-concept and self-esteem through the use of creative activities, such as art, crafts, drama, music, and games.
- Increase the person's sense of self-control and decrease anxiety and depression through information aimed at increased understanding of the condition, especially the monitoring of activity levels.
- Encourage the person to express feelings, thoughts, and needs through group discussion sessions.
- Permit the family and the person to discuss their roles and who will assume various roles during the recovery phase.

Environment

- Encourage the person to change his or her lifestyle using the substitution approach (e.g., remove three "bad" foods and include three "good" foods). Make lifestyle less sedentary by increasing the number of leisure interests and the time spent pursuing such interests.
- Suggest possible modifications, based on ergonomics, in the home or work environment that might reduce the cardiac stress.

PRECAUTIONS

- Watch for the Valsalva maneuver: the person holds his or her breath while performing a task such as shaving or lifting a heavy object. The Valsalva maneuver increases intrathoracic pressure, which decreases venous return, slows the heart rate, and increases blood pressure. The person should be taught to avoid using the Valsalva maneuver.
- Symptoms to be avoided are angina pain or chest discomfort, dizziness or faintness, dyspnea or difficulty breathing, fatigue, claudication pain in the legs, and palpitations. The person should stop activities if symptoms appear and report symptoms to the physician.
- Signs to be avoided are arrhythmias, ataxic gait, cold sweat, glassy stare, high systolic or diastolic blood pressure, irregular pulse, low blood pressure during exercise, and pallor.
- Stop activities if any of the following signs appear: pallor, excessive sweating, ataxic gait, glassy stare, irregular pulse, pulse above 120 beats per minute, extreme elevation of systolic or diastolic blood pressure, low blood pressure, or electrocardiogram changes, such as arrhythmias, ischemia, or heart blocks. Report signs to the physician.
- Symptoms of ischemia or decreased blood flow to the brain include ataxic gait, dizziness, faintness, and glassy stare.
- Signs of pump failure include pallor and lowered blood pressure on exercise.
- Signs of sternal instability after surgery are a feeling of shifting or snapping of the sternum. Arm motions that cause clicking, such as shoulder abduction, should be avoided.
- One-sided pulling or pushing actions with the arms, such as getting out of bed or up from a chair, should be avoided for six weeks to eight weeks after a sternotomy (cutting the sternum to get access to the heart).

METs and Activities

METs	Activities

METs   *Activities*

1–2 METs
4–7 ml O_2/min/kg

Doing sedentary leisure tasks with arms supported (reading, writing, playing cards, sewing, knitting, doing needlework, embroidering, painting, watching television, listening to a radio or CD player, doing puzzles, doing mind teasers).

At 1.5 METs, leather lacing, making a kink belt, turkish knotting, doing basketry or macrame, weaving, copper tooling, clay building, light wood sanding.

Standing for up to 5 minutes or walking at a rate of 1 mile (1.6 kilometers) per hour

Eating a meal

Transferring from bed to chair

Taking care of personal hygiene while sitting: shaving, brushing teeth, combing hair

Toileting using urinal, bedpan, or bedside commode

Doing homemaking tasks such as washing dishes or ironing

Automobile driving, flying, and riding a motorcycle

Keyboarding on a computer

2–3 METs
7–11 ml O_2/min/kg

Standing for 5 minutes to 30 minutes with intermittent upper extremity tasks

Performing sustained upper extremity activity (2 minutes to 30 minutes)

Taking care of personal hygiene while standing: shaving, brushing teeth, combing hair

Total body bathing at sink (sponge bath)

Dressing and undressing

Total body mobility: bending for small objects, reaching for objects, walking at a rate of 2 miles (3.25 kilometers) per hour

Doing homemaking tasks such as scrubbing pans, unpacking groceries, vacuuming, sweeping, and mopping

Doing jobs such as repairing automobiles, radios, or televisions; doing janitorial work; and bartending

Participating in moderate leisure activities such as woodworking; making ceramics; metal hammering; floor loom weaving; playing checkers; leather tooling; using small power tools; bicycling on level ground; playing billiards, skeet, or shuffleboard; playing golf using a power car; horseback riding while horse walks;

continues

continued

	playing the piano or most other musical instruments; light woodworking
3–4 METs 11–14 ml O$_2$/min/kg	Walking 3 miles (5 kilometers) per hour Doing total showering tasks (hair and total body washing, drying, and dressing) Doing homemaking tasks, including preparing meals, doing hand laundry, changing bed linens, and washing the floor on hands and knees Climbing stairs at a rate of 24 feet per minute Using energy conservation techniques with activities such as bricklaying, plastering, using a wheelbarrow, doing machine assembly, driving a truck in traffic, doing basic welding, cleaning windows, doing light janitorial work, bartending, and pressing Doing leisure activities such as cycling, horseshoe pitching, volleyball, pulling a golf cart, doing archery, sailing, fly fishing, trotting on horseback, playing badminton doubles, and playing a musical instrument Playing with children
4–5 METs 14–18 ml O$_2$/min/kg	Walking 3.5 miles (5.5 kilometers) per hour Doing jobs such as painting masonry, hanging wallpaper, doing light carpentry, and pushing a light power mower Having a bowel movement Doing leisure activities such as playing table tennis, carrying golf clubs, dancing a foxtrot, playing badminton singles, playing tennis doubles, raking leaves, hoeing, and doing most calisthenics
5–6 METs 18–21 ml O$_2$/min/kg	Walking 4 miles (6.5 kilometers) per hour Doing jobs such as digging in a garden, shoveling light dirt/soil Having sexual intercourse Walking up stairs (30 feet per minute) Doing leisure activities such as cycling 10 miles (16 kilometers) per hour, canoeing 4 miles (6.5 kilometers) per hour, horseback riding (posting to trot), stream fishing, ice or in-line skating
6–7 METs 21–25 ml O$_2$/min/kg	Walking 5 miles (8 kilometers) per hour Shoveling for 10 minutes with loads of 22 pounds (10 kilograms) Doing jobs such as splitting wood and lawn mowing Doing leisure activities such as cycling at 11 miles (17.5 kilometers) per hour, playing singles tennis,

continues

continued

	folk (square) dancing, light downhill skiing, ski touring, waterskiing
7–8 METs 25–28 ml O_2/min/kg	Jogging 5 miles (8 kilometers) per hour Cycling 12 miles (19 kilometers) per hour Doing jobs such as digging ditches, carrying 175 pounds (80 kilograms), hand sawing hardwood Doing leisure activities such as galloping a horse, downhill skiing, playing basketball, mountain climbing, playing ice hockey, playing touch football, playing paddleball, and canoeing 5 miles (8 kilometers) per hour
8–9 METs 28–32 ml O_2/min/kg	Shoveling for 10 minutes with loads of 31 pounds (14 kilograms) Running 5.5 miles (9 kilometers) per hour, cycling 13 miles (21 kilometers) per hour, ski touring in loose snow, playing social games of squash or handball, fencing, playing vigorous basketball
10+ METs 32+ ml O_2/min/kg	Shoveling for 10 minutes with loads of 35 pounds (16 kilograms) Running at a rate of 6 miles (10 kilometers) per hour or faster Ski touring at greater than 5 miles (8 kilometers) per hour in loose snow Playing competitive handball or squash

Source: Data from Atchison, 1995, Cragg et al, 1998, Matthews et al, 1996, Wilde et al, 1995, and Wilke et al, 1995.

- A heart rate that is greater than 125 beats per minute when only minimal effort is being exerted should be reported to the physician.
- If a shunt is present for renal dialysis, blood pressure readings should be done on the side opposite the shunt.
- Equipment must be moved carefully. Know the techniques for dealing with arterial pressure lines, oximeters, and monitors.
- The person should never exceed a maximum heart rate that is roughly computed by subtracting the person's age in years from 220. True maximum heart rate can be determined by a symptom-limited graded exercise test. Usually, a percentage such as 75 percent of the computed value is stated as the maximum heart rate allowed.

PROGNOSIS AND OUTCOME

- The person demonstrates knowledge of a safe level of upper extremity activity as monitored by heart rate, blood pressure, rate pressure product, time, or other measurement.

- The person demonstrates knowledge and use of energy conservation, pacing, and work simplification techniques in performing his or her daily routine.
- The person demonstrates knowledge of time management and can plan a schedule of activities that conforms with his or her known safe level of activity as monitored by heart rate, blood pressure, rate pressure product, or other measurement.
- The person is able to perform activities of daily living within his or her maximum level of independence within safe limits of his or her cardiac status.
- The person demonstrates the physical fitness, endurance, tolerance, and psychosocial skills needed to maintain the highest level of functional activities within safe limits of his or her cardiac status.
- The person demonstrates strength, endurance, and tolerance to perform productive activities.
- The person is able to select and perform leisure activities within a safe level of activity.
- The person engages in a balance of activities within the daily schedule and routine.
- The person demonstrates the ability to monitor all tasks and routines to stay within safe limits of his or her cardiac status.
- The person demonstrates role performance that is satisfactory to him- or herself and his or her family.

REFERENCE

Beers, M.H., and R. Berkow, eds. 1999. *The Merck Manual of Diagnosis and Therapy*, 17th ed. Whitehouse Station, NJ: Merck Research Laboratories.

BIBLIOGRAPHY

American College of Sports Medicine. 1986. *Guidelines for graded exercise testing and prescription*, 3rd ed. Philadelphia: Lea & Febiger.

American Heart Association. 1979. *The exercise standards books*. Dallas, TX.

Atchison, B. 1996. Cardiopulmonary diseases. In *Occupational therapy for physical dysfunction*, 4th ed., ed. C.A. Trombly, 875–886. Baltimore: Williams & Wilkins. (Case reports)

Cook, M. 1996. Chronic cardiac failure. In *Occupational therapy and rehabilitation: Principles, skills, and practice*, eds. A. Turner et al., 797–815. New York: Churchill Livingstone. (Case report)

Cragg, J.K. et al. 1998. Working with elders who have cardiovascular conditions. In *Occupational therapy with elders: Strategies for the COTA*, eds. H. Lohman et al., 257–265. St. Louis, MO: Mosby.

Dougherty, S.M. et al. 1993. Physiologic responses to snow shoveling and thermal stress in men with cardiac disease. *Medicine and Science in Sports and Exercise* 25, no. 7: 780–795. (Erratum appears in *Medicine and Science in Sports and Exercise* 25, no. 9 [1993]: 1088.)

Ferraro, R. 1998. Cardiopulmonary dysfunction in adults. In *Willard and Spackman's occupational therapy*, 9th ed., eds. M.E. Neistadt and E.B. Crepeau, 693–701. Philadelphia: Lippincott-Raven.

Huntley, N. 1998. Reading the signs of heart disease. *OT Practice* 3, no. 6: 38–41. (Case reports)

King, J.C. 1996. Acute cardiovascular disorder and disease. In *Occupational therapy and rehabilitation: Principles, skills, and practice*, eds. A. Turner et al., 779–796. New York: Churchill Livingstone. (Case reports)

King, J.C. 1996. Introduction to cardiac rehabilitation. In *Occupational therapy and rehabilitation: Principles, skills, and practice*, eds. A. Turner et al., 769–777. New York: Churchill Livingstone.

Matthews, M.M. 1998. Cardiac dysfunction and chronic obstructive pulmonary disease. In *Physical dysfunction: Practice skills for the occupational therapy assistant*, ed. M.B. Early, 505–518. St. Louis, MO: Mosby. (Case reports)

Matthews, M.M. et al. 1996. Cardiac dysfunction. In *Occupational therapy: Practice skills for physical dysfunction*, 4th ed., ed. L.W. Pedretti, 693–709. St. Louis, MO: Mosby. (Case reports)

New York Heart Association. 1979. *Nomenclature and Criteria for Diagnosis of Diseases of the Heart and Great Vessels*, 8th ed. Boston: Little, Brown & Co.

Parmely, W.W. 1986. Position report on cardiac rehabilitation: Recommendations of the American College of Cardiology. *Journal of the American College of Cardiology* 7: 451–453.

Sheldahl, L.M. et al. 1994. Snow blowing and shoveling in normal and asymptomatic coronary artery diseased men. *International Journal of Cardiology* 43, no. 3: 233–238.

Sheldahl, L.M. et al. 1996. Responses of people with coronary artery disease to common lawn-care tasks. *European Journal of Applied Physiology* 72, no. 4: 357–364.

Thomas, J.J. 1996. Comparison of patient education methods: Effects of knowledge of cardiac rehabilitation principles. *Occupational Therapy Journal of Research* 16, no. 3: 166–178.

Tooth, L., and K. McKenna. 1996. Contemporary issues in cardiac rehabilitation: Implications for therapists. *British Journal of Occupational Therapy* 59, no. 3: 133–140.

Tooth, L. et al. 1993. Prediction of compliance with a post-myocardial infarction home-based walking programme. *Australian Occupational Therapy Journal* 40, no. 1: 17–22.

Whyte, N. 1997. T'ai Chi for clients in cardiac rehabilitation. *OT Practice* 2, no. 10: 38–41.

Wilde, C.K., and J.A. Hall. 1995. Occupational therapy in cardiac rehabilitation. *Physical Medicine and Rehabilitation Clinics of North America* 6, no. 2: 349–372.

Wilke, N.A. et al. 1993. Baltimore Therapeutic Equipment work simulator: Energy expenditure of work activities in cardiac patients. *Archives of Physical Medicine and Rehabilitation* 74, no. 4: 419–424.

Wilke, N.A. et al. 1995. Energy expenditure during household tasks in women with coronary artery disease. *American Journal of Cardiology* 75, no. 10: 670–674.

Chronic Obstructive Pulmonary Disease

DESCRIPTION

Chronic obstructive pulmonary disease (COPD) is a disease characterized by chronic bronchitis or emphysema and airflow obstruction that is generally progressive, may be accompanied by airway hyperreactivity, and may be partially reversible (Merck 1999, 568). Included in COPD are chronic bronchitis, emphysema, and asthma. Chronic bronchitis is characterized by chronic productive cough for at least three months in each of two successive years for which other causes (such as infection, cancer, and chronic heart failure) have been excluded. Emphysema is characterized by abnormal permanent enlargement of the airspaces distal to the terminal bronchioles with destruction of their walls and without obvious fibrosis. Asthma is characterized by airway inflammation that is manifested by airway hyperresponsiveness to a variety of stimuli and by airway obstruction that is reversible spontaneously or in response to treatment but may not be completely reversible in some patients (Merck 1999, 568).

CAUSE

The causes include infections, allergens, skeletal problems such as scoliosis, obesity, or nervous system diseases that affect the muscles that assist breathing. Any factor that leads to chronic alveolar inflammation, such as smoking, may lead to COPD. Diagnosis is usually made in midlife, but symptoms may have developed much earlier.

ASSESSMENT

Areas

- daily living activities and skills
- productivity history, skills, interests, and values
- home and community skills
- leisure activities
- vital capacity (may include information from pulmonary function tests, auscultation, and blood gas studies)
- range of motion
- muscle strength, especially in the hands and upper extremities
- physical fitness, endurance, and activity tolerance, especially of the upper extremities
- postural control and balance
- mobility
- perceptual skills (space, form, depth, praxis, figure-ground, body scheme, part-whole integration)
- cognitive skills (orientation, memory, abstract reasoning, judgment and problem solving, attention span, comprehension, intelligence)
- affect or mood (anxiety, depression, denial, passivity)
- coping skills
- social support
- architectural and physical barriers
- environmental safety and adaptability

Instruments

No named assessment instruments were identified. The following items may be helpful:
- activities of daily living scale
- occupational history
- leisure checklist
- goniometer
- dynamometer
- manual muscle test
- perceived exertion test
- heart rate
- respiration rate
- medical chart

PROBLEMS

Self-Care

- The person may be unable to perform some activities of daily living because of decreased endurance and physical tolerance due to decreased lung function, abnormal atrial blood gases, and decreased oxygen.
- The person may be unable to perform some self-care activities because of architectural or physical barriers, such as inaccessible doorways or shelves that are too high.
- The person may have difficulty taking medications from inhalers or nebulizers due to limited shoulder motion or weak thumb.

Productivity

- The person may be unable to continue occupations that expose the person to fumes, gases, or air particles, such as dust or pollen.
- The person may be unable to continue productive occupations because of shortness of breath and fatigue.

Leisure

- The person may be unable to continue leisure activities that require great physical exertion.
- The person may be unable to enjoy outside activities during certain times of year because of particles in the air.

Sensorimotor

- The person usually has decreased physical tolerance and endurance.
- The person usually has shortness of breath upon exertion.
- The person may have decreased range of motion.
- The person may have decreased muscle strength.
- The person may have poor posture.
- The person may have a nonproductive cough and complain of extreme fatigue.
- The person may have cyanosis or a blue tinge to the skin, especially around the mouth.
- The senses are not directly affected.

Cognition

- The person may experience confusion and impaired judgment due to lack of oxygen.
- The person may complain of difficulty concentrating.
- The person may have limited knowledge of the disease and its problems.
- The person may have limited knowledge of or judgment about safety hazards in the home.

Psychosocial

- The person may have feelings of hopelessness and helplessness.
- The person may become depressed or anxious.
- The person may withdraw from social activities.
- The person may become dependent on his or her spouse or other caregiver.
- The person may lack a social support system.

TREATMENT/INTERVENTION

Usually a team approach is used. Treatment models include the occupational behavior model of work, play, and rest.

Self-Care

- Encourage the person to use energy conservation, pacing, and work simplification techniques. Encourage maintenance of activities of daily living through use of task analysis to conserve energy, including prioritizing tasks, pacing activities, and economizing motion. For example, using a kitchen cart can reduce fatigue and strain caused by carrying objects.
- Provide adaptive equipment and training to assist the person in the performance of activities of daily living, if needed. Examples might include a long-handled reacher, a long-handled shoe horn, a sock aid, elastic shoelaces, a long-handled bath sponge, or a bath mitt.
- Make modifications so the person can more easily use dispensers for medications such as inhalers and nebulizers (Copley-Nigro 1995).
- Reduce the number of possible irritants in self-care products. Example: Recommend that the person use pump-style or roll-on hygiene or grooming products instead of sprays.
- Recommend that the person wear warm, lightweight coats (with goose down filler) in cold weather instead of heavy ones made of wool and wear a scarf or face mask to cover the face.

Productivity

- Suggest modifications in the work setting, if needed.
- Help the person to explore work interests if previous work activities cannot be continued because of health limitations.
- The person may want to wear a face mask or a dampened cloth when doing homemaking tasks that stir up dust such as sweeping, dusting, or vacuuming.
- Using an electric stove may be helpful. Nitrogen dioxide from gas burners can aggravate breathing problems.
- Recommend good ventilation in the work and home environments. The addition of ceiling fans or personal fans may be helpful. Also consider adequacy of ventilation while commuting or running errands in the car. A battery-operated fan can be useful in a car.

Leisure

- Help the person select leisure activities that are within his or her physical capacities.
- Explore interests to develop new activities if previous leisure activities must be abandoned.

Sensorimotor

- Increase the person's strength and endurance by using gravity-resistive exercises, especially for the upper extremities. Do not use weight training.
- Increase or maintain range of motion through performance of normal activities whenever possible.
- Provide the person with opportunities to practice breathing exercises while performing other activities.
- Encourage the person to maintain correct posture to maximize breathing. In the sitting position, the person should bend forward slightly at the waist while supporting the upper

body by leaning the forearms on a table. When standing, the person should lean forward and prop the body on a counter or shopping cart.

- Encourage the person to use the pursed lip breathing technique if shortness of breath occurs. The person should inhale deeply through the nose, purse the lips as though whistling, and slowly exhale through the pursed lips. Some resistance should be felt. Exhaling should take twice as long as inhaling.
- Diaphragmatic breathing uses an increase in the excursion of the diaphragm to improve chest volume. When a small object such as a paperback book is placed on the abdomen, the action of the diaphragm can be observed. As the person inhales, the object should rise, and as the person exhales, the object should fall.

Cognition

- Teach the person energy conservation, prioritizing, pacing, and work simplification. Help the person learn problem-solving techniques, using the least energy to perform everyday activities, such as sitting instead of standing. Decide what is most important to do and what can wait or be done by others. Decide when to rest or take a break within and between tasks. Decide which are the critical steps or tasks in a routine and which can be eliminated or combined.
- Teach good posture and proper body mechanics in lifting, carrying, reaching, pushing and pulling, brushing hair, shampooing, and showering.
- Teach recognition of possible hazardous materials that might cause additional breathing problems, such as dust, pollens, sprays, cleansers, or polishes, and suggest possible alternatives such as roll-ons or pumps instead of sprays. Changing air filters frequently and keeping air conditioning in good working order may be useful. Use of a mask while vacuuming may be helpful.
- Assist in teaching the person about medications, including their effects, side effects, dosages, schedules, and time intervals, so the person can self-medicate.
- Assist in teaching and managing techniques the person may need to facilitate breathing, such as postural drainage. For example, when and how should time for postural drainage be worked into the daily schedule?
- Assist in teaching the person about the safe use and care of various equipment for facilitating breathing. Consider whether an oximeter should be left with the person. Constant checking may increase anxiety and stress.
- Teach the person time management and activity scheduling to balance and pace self-care, productivity, and leisure. Peak performance is usually after a breathing treatment or medication absorption. Priority tasks should be scheduled for peak performance periods.
- Teach the person about safety and fall prevention in the home and community.
- Teach the person how to manage anxiety and panic attacks.
- Assist in teaching the person about good nutrition.

Psychosocial

- Provide training in stress management, including relaxation exercises using visual imagery to control anxiety and panic attacks.
- Encourage a sense of independence and autonomy within the limitations of the disease.
- Encourage socialization through group activities, such as a self-help group.

- Encourage the person to maintain a role as a responsible, active, and functioning member of the family and household.
- Communicate with the family members to inform them of the person's limitations, but emphasize the person's abilities and assets within the limitations of a chronic disability.
- Communication with some family members should include a discussion of sexual functioning and a recommendation to have a physician evaluate the individual (e.g., for erectile dysfunction and concerns about shortness of breath).

Environment
- Provide information on modifying the home to permit the person to contribute to home management.
- Recommend modifications of the home to increase safety, efficiency, and independence. The person may need to be relocated during home modification.
- Recommend modifications of work areas if the person is employed.

PRECAUTIONS
- The person should avoid irritants such as smoke, dust, and odors from solvents, powders, or spray aerosols such as cooking sprays, cleaners, and deodorants. If such items must be used or encountered, suggest that the person wear a face mask or use a dampened cloth over the nose and mouth.
- The person should wait at least one hour after eating before exerting him- or herself since digestion draws blood with oxygen away from muscles, including the diaphragm.
- Be sensitive to feelings of depression and isolation, especially if the person moved to another climate in hopes of gaining better health. The loss of social support may offset the gain in health.
- Intervention should be stopped if the person becomes nauseous, dizzy, or fatigued; has shortness of breath; or has chest pain.
- If oxygen equipment is necessary, the person should be informed and aware of safety issues related to this equipment.

PROGNOSIS AND OUTCOME
COPD is a chronic disorder that cannot be totally reversed or corrected. The objective is to continue to maximize function within the limitations of the disorder. Outcome depends on the present clinical status, recent functional history, and response to current activity.
- The person demonstrates physical endurance, muscle strength, and range of motion to perform functional activities.
- The person is able to perform activities of daily living to the maximum level of function consistent with the limitations of the disorder.
- The person demonstrates the ability to breathe properly during performance of activities.
- The person has been provided self-help devices and training in their use to assist in the independent performance of functional activities.
- The person demonstrates knowledge of energy conservation, pacing, and work simplification.

- The person demonstrates knowledge of precautions that avoid further compromising his or her breathing.
- The person is able to reduce reactions to stress through relaxation techniques.
- The person has been provided with information on modifying the home to increase the opportunity to perform self-care and home management.
- The person demonstrates knowledge of community resources.
- If a child, the person is able to perform developmental tasks at an age-appropriate level.

REFERENCES

Beers, M.H., and R. Berkow, eds. 1999. *The Merck Manual of Diagnosis and Therapy*, 17th ed. Whitehouse Station, NJ: Merck Research Laboratories.
Copley-Nigro, J. 1995. OT for individuals with COPD. *Advance for Occupational Therapists* 11, no. 26: 19.

BIBLIOGRAPHY

Ambrosino, N., and E. Clini. 1996. Evaluation in pulmonary rehabilitation. *Respiratory Medicine* 90, no. 7: 395–400.
Atchison, B. 1996. Cardiopulmonary diseases. In *Occupational therapy for physical dysfunction*, 4th ed., ed. C.A. Trombly, 886–892. Baltimore: Williams & Wilkins. (Case report)
Bach, J.R. 1998. Rehabilitation of the patient with respiratory dysfunction. In *Rehabilitation medicine: Principles and practice*, 3rd ed., ed. J.A. DeLisa, 1359–1383. Philadelphia: J.B. Lippincott.
Bendstrup, K.E. et al. 1997. Out-patient rehabilitation improves activities of daily living, quality of life, and exercise tolerance in chronic obstructive pulmonary disease. *European Respiratory Journal* 10, no. 12: 2801–2806.
Ferraro, R. 1998. Chronic obstructive pulmonary disease. In *Willard and Spackman's occupational therapy*, 9th ed., eds. M.E. Neistadt and E.B. Crepeau, 701–712. Philadelphia: Lippincott-Raven.
Gomes, E.G., and D. Thornhill. 1993. Home treatment of chronic obstructive pulmonary disease. *Gerontology Special Interest Section Newsletter* 16, no. 3: 3–4.
Hogan, B.M. 1995. Pulse oximetry for an adult with a pulmonary disorder. *American Journal of Occupational Therapy* 49, no. 10: 1062–1064.
Klinger, J.L. 1997. The client who has chronic obstructive pulmonary disease. In *Meal preparation and training: The healthcare professional's guide*, ed. J.L. Klinger, 103–104. Thorofare, NJ: Slack.
Klinger, J.L. 1997. If you have chronic obstructive pulmonary disease. In *Mealtime manual for people with disabilities and the aging*, ed. J.L. Klinger, 39–41. Thorofare, NJ: Slack.
Matthews, M.M. 1998. Cardiac dysfunction and chronic obstructive pulmonary disease. In *Physical dysfunction: Practice skills for the occupational therapy assistant*, ed. M.B. Early, 505–518. St. Louis, MO: Mosby.
Peralta, A.M., and S. Powell. 1998. Working with elders who have pulmonary conditions. In *Occupational therapy with elders: Strategies for the COTA*, eds. H. Lohman et al., 266–270. St. Louis: Mosby. (Case report)
Stahl, C. 1998. Teaching patients to reorganize their lives. *Advance for Occupational Therapists* 14, no. 5: 19.

Part V

Injuries

Amputation of a Lower Extremity—Adult

DESCRIPTION

Amputation in an adult results from the removal of a limb or other appendage or outgrowth of the body (Dorland's 1988, 66). There is no consistent list of terms used to describe the site of amputation. Each of the classification systems below has a slightly different organization and terminology. A major variation is whether the bone or joint is used as the reference point. Thus, transradial amputation (bone) is similar to below-elbow (joint) amputation. Several classification systems mix reference to a bone or joint.

Classification System by Level (Pasquenelli 1996, 601)
- complete phalange
- partial tarsal
- complete tarsal or Syme's amputation
- partial leg (upper 1/3, middle 1/3, lower 1/3)—below knee
- complete lower leg—knee disarticulation
- partial thigh (upper 1/3, middle 1/3, lower 1/3)—above knee
- complete thigh
- complete hip

Classification System by Level (Colburn and Ibbotson 1996, 644)
- partial foot (Chopart)
- Syme's
- standard below-knee
- short below-knee
- through-knee disarticulation
- standard above-knee level
- short above-knee
- through-hip disarticulation
- hindquarter or hemipelvectomy

CAUSE

Major causes of amputation of the lower extremities are peripheral vascular disease (PVD), especially diabetes; peripheral vasospastic diseases and chronic infections, such as gas gangrene and osteomyelitis; and malignant tumors. Other causes include trauma, such as motor vehicle accidents and chemical, thermal, or electrical injuries (Pasquenelli 1996, 599). Specific factors leading to amputation include duration of diabetes, history of leg or foot ulcers, hypertension, and smoking (Colburn and Ibbotson 1996, 647).

ASSESSMENT

Areas
- daily living skills, including activities of daily living (ADLs)and instrumental ADLs
- productivity history, interests, skills, and values

- leisure skills and interests
- mobility
- transfer techniques
- range of motion, active and passive
- muscle strength, upper and lower
- phantom limb sensation
- phantom limb pain
- visual acuity and perceptual skills
- hyperesthesia
- cognition, especially attention, concentration, memory, organization
- coping skills
- driving skills

Instruments

- *Activity Pattern Indicator* by Diller, L., W. Fordyce, D. Jacobs, and M. Brown. 1981. New York: Rehabilitation Indicators Project, New York Medical Center.
- *Dallas Pain Questionnaire* by Lawlis, G.F., R. Cuencas, D. Selby, and C.E. McCoy. 1989. The development of the Dallas Pain Questionnaire. *Spine* 14(5):511–516.
- *Pain Disability Index* by Pollard, C.A. 1984. Preliminary validity study of pain disability index. *Perceptual and Motor Skills* 59:974. (Scale reprinted in Van Deusen 1993, 182–183.)
- ADL assessment
- home and kitchen assessment
- work evaluation
- leisure checklist
- motor testing
- sensory testing
- neuromuscular testing
- cognitive testing
- psychosocial testing
- prosthetic checkout

PROBLEMS

Self-Care

- The person may have difficulty with dressing, transferring, and other ADLs that require balance or weight shift.
- The person will need to learn how to perform many self-care skills over again, especially for higher-level amputations, because the dynamics of the body have changed as a result of the amputation.

Productivity

- The person may have difficulty performing specific work tasks that require balance and mobility.
- The person may have difficulty performing specific homemaking tasks that require balance and mobility, such as meal preparation, house cleaning, and bed making.

Leisure

- The person may be unable to perform some leisure activities unless modifications are made.

- The person may be not be motivated to continue specific leisure activities.

Sensorimotor

- The person has loss of push-off force using the great toe, unless only toe digits 2–5 have been amputated.
- The person's center of gravity is changed in relation to loss of body mass, which affects balance and righting reactions.
- The person loses the automatic walking ability of the normal person, which means that walking will require more energy.
- The person may have difficulty with protective and equilibrium responses to maintain balance.
- The person may have difficulty with transfers.
- The person may have difficulty accommodating to uneven ground or surfaces, due to loss of inversion and eversion (accommodation).
- The person may have limited power and mechanical leverage of the leg if the amputation is a short above-knee type.
- The person may have loss of visual acuity and perception to retinopathy in diabetes.
- The person may lose position sense (kinesthesia and proprioception of the knee joint) if the amputation is above the knee.
- The person may develop hyperesthesia in the residual portion of the limb.
- The person loses body image in relation to the missing limb.
- The person may become deconditioned, due to bed rest.

Cognitive

- Cognition is not impacted directly by the amputation of one or both lower extremities but coexisting conditions, such as uncontrolled diabetes or head trauma from a motor vehicle accident, may cause cognitive dysfunction.

Psychosocial

- The person may have difficulty adjusting to the loss of limb, such as "why me?"
- The person may have hostile reactions that can be directed to the self or to the medical team.
- The person may be oversolicitous or friendly to mask hostility.
- The person usually mourns the loss of the limb and may become depressed over the loss.
- The person may express fears about returning to family, social, vocational, and sexual roles.

Environment

- The home may present architectural barriers.
- Safety considerations in the home may require assistive technology to be performed safely.
- The work environment may restrict the person's movement and safety.
- The person usually cannot drive a vehicle safely without equipment modification.

TREATMENT/INTERVENTION

Treatment is usually provided through a team approach including the physician, physical therapist, nurse, prosthetist, and occupational therapy personnel. Others may include a recreational therapist, psychologist, social worker, and vocational counselor. The primary frame of reference is biomechanical.

Self-Care

- Review performance of ADLs, such as bed mobility, dressing, bathing, grooming, transfer techniques. Instrumental ADLs should include meal preparation, purchasing food, cooking, serving, cleaning, doing laundry, stripping and making a bed, cleaning house, and working at various heights.

- Begin dressing lower extremity from a sitting position and grade difficulty to a standing position. Socks and shoes should be put on while sitting. A sock aid and elastic shoelaces may make the task easier. A footstool may be helpful.
- Wash the stump and residual limb daily, using a mild soap, and pat dry with a soft towel. Inspect the skin with a mirror for redness or cracks. Also check the unaffected foot for abrasions, cuts, or scratches. Clip toenails regularly.

Provide practice in transfers from bed, toilet, furniture, and vehicle, with and without the prosthesis. In bed, practice rolling from side to side and bridging activities, using knee and hip flexion and remaining foot to push body up from the bed to facilitate lower extremity dressing. Transfer training should include standing pivot transfer (90-degree pivot) toward the existing limb when possible and the 180-degree pivots toward the amputated side to increase independence in restrictive environments. Transfers using sliding boards may also be practiced, especially for bilateral amputees. If a wheelchair is used, it should have a zippered or removable back to allow for transfers by sliding backward to a surface and sliding forward to return to the wheelchair.

- Provide practice in putting on and taking off the prosthesis.
- Review dietary restriction, if necessary, such as for a person with diabetes.

Productivity

- If the person will be using a wheelchair, provide opportunity for negotiating a kitchen while preparing a meal.
- The person may need practice in negotiating work setting safely, whether using prosthesis or wheelchair.
- Work with the vocational evaluator or counselor if the person needs job retraining, including discussion and testing of interests and achievements, job analysis, job modifications, and follow-up.

Leisure

- Assist the person's ability to return to previous leisure interests and activities if possible.
- Assist the person to explore new interests to replace those no longer feasible or to add to existing interests and activities.
- Discuss modifications needed to participate in existing or new interests and activities.
- Provide resources and discuss with the person available prostheses for sports such as golf, swimming, or skiing.
- Specialized prostheses such as the energy-storing prosthetic foot (ESPF) may be used for sports requiring foot action, such as running or playing basketball.

Sensorimotor

Preprosthetic Training

- Promote skin healing and conditioning. The primary cause of delays in treatment are due to skin problems, including delayed healing, extensive skin grafting, skin breakdown, ulcers, neuromas, "corns," and infected sebaceous cysts. If an ulcer appears, it should be treated by rest, elevation, and hot compresses.
- Provide upper-extremity strengthening exercises.
- Prevent contractures, especially in the above-knee amputation (AKA), including flexion, external rotation, and abduction contracture of the affected hip. In below-knee amputation,

the most common contractures are external rotation deformity of the hip and flexion of the knee. Sleeping in the prone position can prevent hip flexion contractures.

- Prevent decubiti by teaching the person to inspect skin and change positions every two hours. If the person is using a wheelchair, techniques for weight shifting or wheelchair push-ups should be taught.
- Reduce dependent edema by proper positioning when person is in a wheelchair. Edema may also occur if the proximal end of the socket is too tight or due to an ill-fitting sock. Revision of the socket and a new or better fitting sock should reduce the edema. Ace-wrapping may also be used, which is done using diagonal bandaging beginning distally and the application of firm, even pressure distally, which decreases as the wrap is applied proximally. Some clinics prefer shrinker socks to Ace bandages. The sock is put on so that the bulky seam is on the outside; the top of the sock is folded back on itself about two-thirds of the way; the sock is stretched so that it fits smoothly on the end of the residual limb and pulled up over the limb (Pasquenelli 1996, 604).
- Provide endurance training and activity tolerance, especially if deconditioning has occurred.
- Desensitize the residual limb by tapping and gentle massage.
- Wearing a temporary or permanent prosthesis can reduce phantom sensation.

Postprosthetic Training
- Practice balance activities in sitting and standing positions.
- Use weight-bearing activities to avoid atrophy and increase weight transference and balance reactions. A temporary prosthesis may be used until the permanent one is available.
- Encourage the person to walk on uneven surfaces and up and down inclines or hills, to climb and descend from curbs, and to get into and out of elevators and onto and off escalators and through revolving doors.
- Increase the person's awareness and use of visual and remaining proprioceptive feedback to compensate for loss of tactile, kinesthetic, and proprioceptive feedback provided by the amputated limb.
- Assist the person to develop a new body image with prosthesis.

Cognitive
- Provide instruction in washing and caring for the stump.
- Provide instruction in the care and maintenance of the prosthesis.
- If a wheelchair is used, provide instruction in wheelchair propulsion and management. Instruction in care of other mobility aids, such as a walker, cane, or axillary crutches, should also be included if these devices are used by the person.
- Provide instruction in safety precautions, especially with bilateral lower-extremity amputees or use of a wheelchair.
- Instruct person in energy conversation, pacing, and work simplification techniques.
- Consider and discuss with the person his or her use of assistive devices, such as a cart, a high stool to sit on, or long handles to reach objects.
- Discuss prevention and health promotion routines for the unaffected leg, especially in cases of diabetes because the same factors that caused one leg to be amputated may be present for the other leg.
- Provide opportunity to practice problem solving, especially in the home and community.
- Assure the person that phantom sensation is common, especially in crush injuries.

Psychosocial
- Assist the person in adjustment to loss of limb through listening and discussion about the loss and the changes in roles that may or may not occur in relation to family, society, vocation, and sex.

- Counteract hostility and depression by focusing on rehabilitation process and return to former occupational roles.
- Encourage the person to consider attending a support group for amputees to learn how others manage and solve problems.
- Provide group activities so that the person can participate in social situations.

Environment
- If possible, a home visit, community visit, or visit to work place can assist in determining the needs of the person and can provide on-site instruction in managing issues or problems.
- Discussions with the person and his or her family about home modification may be needed to remove architectural barriers and improve safety, such as adding a ramp for a wheelchair or hand rails on both sides of stairs.
- Discussions with the person and his or her family about modifications to the kitchen may be necessary to facilitate access to cabinets.
- Discussions with the person and his or her employer about modifications to the work setting may be needed, such as eliminating steps to the entrance or rearranging the furniture or fixtures to create aisles that accommodate a wheelchair.
- The family or support system should be educated about transfer techniques and basics of managing the prosthesis.
- The vehicle driven by the person, if any, may need modifications, such as a left foot accelerator bar if the person has a right leg amputation or hand controls if both legs have been amputated.
- The person should be given instruction in the use of any assistive devices attached to the vehicle and checked out in driving safety.

PRECAUTIONS
- Do not place pillows beneath the knee in a below-knee amputation or under the stump in an AKA.
- The use of lotions or alcohol is not recommended in stump care.
- Do not wash the stump in the morning to avoid softening before prosthetic use. Stump hygiene should be performed in the evening.
- Avoid tight elastics and stretch socks, which might impair circulation.
- Avoid slip-on shoes or sandals, which might slip off the prosthesis.
- Always wear a sock and shoe on the unaffected limb to reduce swelling and edema.
- Always check the sock when putting it on for twists, wrinkles, or poor fit.
- Always check water temperature to avoid water that might scald or blister the skin.

PROGNOSIS AND OUTCOME
Good prognosis and outcome for use of the prosthesis requires cognitive skills, motivation, effective training, and proper maintenance. Good prognosis and outcome for the person depends on the cause and treatment of the original condition that resulted in the amputation. Diseases such as diabetes mellitus or cancer may shorten the person's life. Reckless driving or disrespect for safety rules at work could also cause additional injury or loss of life.

REFERENCES
Colburn, J. and V. Ibbotson. 1996. Amputation. In *Occupational Therapy and Physical Dysfunction: Principles, Skills, and Practice*, ed. A. Turner, M. Foster, and S.G. Johnson, 635–650. New York: Churchill Livingstone.
Dorland, W.A. 1988. *Dorland's Illustrated Medical Dictionary*, Philadelphia: W.B. Saunders Company.

Pasquenelli, S. 1996. Lower extremity amputations and prosthetics. In *Occupational Therapy: Practice Skills for Physical Dysfunction*, 4th ed., ed. L.W. Pedretti, 599–612. St. Louis: Mosby (Case reports).
Van Deusen, J. 1993. Phantom limb pain. In *Body Image and Perceptual Dysfunction in Adults*, ed. J. Van Deusen, 173–190. Philadelphia: WB Saunders.

BIBLIOGRAPHY

Celikyol, F. 1995. Amputation and prosthetics. In *Occupational Therapy for Physical Dysfunction*, 4th ed., ed. C.A. Trombly, 870–871. Baltimore: Williams & Wilkins.
Gillin, M. 1998. Above-elbow amputation: A case study in restoring function. *Journal of Hand Therapy* 11(4):278–283.
Morris, P.A. and L. Muhn. 1998. Amputation and prosthetics. In *Physical Dysfunction Practice Skills for the Occupational Therapy Assistant*, ed. M.B. Early, 468–476. St Louis: Mosby (Case report).

Amputation of an Upper Extremity—Adult

DESCRIPTION

Amputation in an adult results from the removal of all or part of an extremity, digit, organ, or projecting part of the body. There is no consistent list of terms used to describe the site of amputation. Each of the classification systems below has a slightly different organization and terminology. A major variation is whether the bone or joint is used as the reference point. Thus, transradial (bone) amputation is similar to below-elbow (joint) amputation. Several classification systems mix references to a bone or joint.

Classification by Level (Atkins 1994, 278)

- unilateral partial hand amputation—includes the loss of part or all of a single digit (finger or thumb) or any combination of digits, up to and including part of palm
- unilateral wrist disarticulation
- unilateral elbow amputation
- unilateral above-elbow amputation
- unilateral shoulder disarticulation amputation
- bilateral partial hand amputation
- bilateral wrist disarticulation
- bilateral below-elbow amputation
- bilateral above-elbow amputation
- bilateral shoulder disarticulation amputation

Classification by Level (Celikyol 1995, 850)

- transmetacarpal
- transcarpal
- transradial (includes wrist disarticulation, long below-elbow, short below-elbow, very short below-elbow)
- transhumeral (includes elbow disarticulation, standard above-elbow, short above-elbow, humeral neck above elbow)
- shoulder disarticulation
- intrascapulothoracic (forequarter)

**Component Parts for a Conventional Below-Elbow,
Body-Powered Prosthesis**

- Terminal device, such as a voluntary opening hook, which uses rubber bands for hook closing
- Wrist unit
- Housing base plate (distal)
- Forearm socket
- Flexible hinge
- Cable housing and cable
- Housing base plate or housing retainer (proximal)
- Triceps cuff
- Cable to control attachment strap
- Invented Y strap
- Control attachment strap
- Northwestern University (NU) ring or other standard ring
- Axilla loop
- Figure-of-eight harness

Source: Data from E.A. Spencer, Upper Extremity Amputation, in *Willard and Spackman's Occupational Therapy*, 9th ed., M.E. Neistadt, et al., eds. p. 688, © 1998, Lippincott-Raven; and F. Celikyol, Amputation and Prosthetics, in *Occupational Therapy for Physical Dysfunction*, 4th ed., C.A. Trombly, ed., p. 857, © 1995, Williams & Wilkins.

Classification by Level (Colburn and Ibbotson 1996, 651)
- partial hand
- through-wrist
- standard below-elbow
- short below-elbow
- elbow disarticulation
- above-elbow
- shoulder disarticulation
- forequarter

Classification by Level (Rock 1996, 569; Morris and Muhn 1998, 458)
- partial hand
- wrist disarticulation
- long below-elbow
- short below-elbow
- elbow disarticulation
- long above-elbow
- short above-elbow
- shoulder disarticulation
- forequarter
- bilateral amputation

Classification by Level (Spencer 1998, 686)
- transmetacarpal and partial hand

- wrist disarticulation
- long below-elbow
- short below-elbow
- very short below-elbow
- elbow disarticulation
- standard above-elbow
- short above-elbow
- shoulder disarticulation
- shoulder forequarter

Classification by Level (Theisen 1997, 254)

- wrist disarticulation
- long below-elbow
- short below-elbow
- very short below-elbow
- elbow disarticulation
- standard above-elbow
- short above-elbow
- humeral neck
- shoulder disarticulation

CAUSE

The two most common causes are trauma, such as from a cut, tear, burn, or freezing, and surgery performed to remove a diseased or useless part of the body. Common sources of trauma are motor vehicle and machinery accidents, gunshot wounds, and electrical burns. Common diseases that lead to amputation are peripheral vascular disease and diabetes mellitus.

ASSESSMENT

Evaluation must be considered in two parts. The first is centered on assessing the person's remaining functional abilities and level of function without the missing part. The second area of evaluation concerns the use of prosthetic devices to replace some of the lost functions.

Areas

- daily living skills
- productivity history, interests, skills, and values
- leisure skills and interests
- muscle strength in remaining body parts
- range of motion in joints proximal to amputation
- functional gross and fine motor skills available without prosthesis
- phantom limb sensation
- phantom limb pain
- hypersensitivity in stump
- body image and perception of self

- self-concept
- self-esteem
- attitude of acceptance
- coping skills
- driving skills

Instruments

Although the need for evaluation is discussed in several book chapters, only one protocol form was identified.

- self-care assessment
- manual muscle test
- goniometry
- sensory testing
- tape measure to record limb length and circumference
- driving evaluation
- *Prosthetic Evaluation* (Celikyol 1995, 862–863)

PROBLEMS

In general, the higher the level of amputation, the more problems occur in using a prosthesis because there are few joints to use as points of control.

Self-Care

- If the dominant hand is lost, tasks such as writing, handling money, and eating will be affected, as will two-handed tasks, such as dressing, grooming, and bathing.
- If the nondominant hand is lost, the primary problems involve two-handed activities in which the nondominant hand has been used in parallel (lifting, pushing, or pulling a heavy load or holding a large tool, such as a jackhammer) or to hold and manipulate objects, such as in holding a jar to unscrew the lid, opening an umbrella, or selecting correct change from a handful of coins.

Productivity

- Problems of productivity are related to the job tasks performed, but some common problems are loss of dominant hand skills and loss of two-handed activities that require coordination and dexterity. Assess what limitations and assets the individual may face in regaining productive skills.
- If job tasks involve highly skilled hand functions where speed and accuracy are key factors, such as in playing a violin or piano, painting, keyboarding, or electrical writing, the person may be unable to continue in his or her occupation.

Leisure

- The person may be unable to engage in some favorite leisure activities without modifications.
- The person may be unwilling to continue participation in some leisure activities because of appearance and changed body image.

**Typical Component Parts of Standard Above-Elbow,
Body-Powered Prosthesis**

- Terminal device (TD)—hook or hand, VO = voluntary opening, VC = voluntary closing
- Terminal device thumb
- Wrist unit—types include friction-held, locking, wrist flexion, and oval
- Terminal device housing and cable
- Forearm socket
- Lift loop
- Internal lock elbow unit
- Turntable
- Cable for locking elbow
- Socket
- Elastic anterior support strap
- Control attachment strap
- Lateral support strap
- NU ring
- Axilla loop

Source: Data from L.M. Rock, Upper Extremity Amputations and Prosthetics-Section 1: Amputations and Body Powered Prostheses, in *Occupational Therapy: Practice Skills for Physical Dysfunction*, 4th ed., L.W. Pedretti ed., pp. 567–585, (c) 1996, Mosby Year-Book Inc., P.A. Morris and L. Muhn, Amputation and Prosthetics, in *Physical Dysfunction Practice Skills for the Occupational Therapy Assistant*, M.B. Early ed., pp. 456–468, (c) 1998, Mosby Year-Book, Inc., and F. Celikyol, Amputation and Prosthetics, *Occupational Therapy for Physical Dysfunction*, 4th ed., C.A. Trombly, ed., pp. 849–874, (c) 1995, Williams & Wilkins.

Sensorimotor

- The person usually has loss of range of motion.
- The person may have loss of muscle strength.
- The person usually has loss of coordination, manipulation, and dexterity associated with the missing part.
- The person has loss of touch and tactile sensation provided by the missing part.
- The person has loss of proprioception and kinesthesia associated with the missing part.
- The person may experience phantom pain (pain from the missing part).
- The person's body scheme and self-image change.

Cognitive

- In cases where trauma is the cause, consideration should be given to checking to determine whether cognitive ability may also be involved.
- No changes in cognitive or cognitive-perceptual ability result directly from the amputation. However, any cognitive or cognitive-perceptual limitations present before the amputation may complicate the treatment program, such as difficulty in learning how to care properly for the stump or learning to use a prosthesis.

Psychosocial

- The person may express frustration at not being able to perform tasks as before.

- The person may suffer from loss of self-esteem, self-worth, and self-confidence ("I'm not the person I used to be").
- The complexity of hand functions used by the individual is often a factor.
- The person may express feelings of self-hatred and self-deprecation.
- The person may have a sense of mutilation, emasculation, or castration.
- The person may view the self as less attractive and less desirable as a mate.
- The person and family may view the amputation as a form of punishment or atonement for past sins or misdeeds.
- The person may express feelings of being viewed by others as a freak, a cripple, or a misfit.
- The person may feel anger ("Why me?") or guilt ("If only I had. . .") regarding the amputation.
- The person may be fearful of the future, expressing anxiety or panic as to what (bad thing) will happen next.
- The person may express feelings of grief, self-pity, despair, or suicidal impulses.
- The person may experience periods of depression, accompanied by feelings of helplessness and hopelessness.
- The person may avoid social situations in fear of rejection, being stared at, or being seen as different.
- The person may feel awkward (loss of self-confidence) in public situations, especially when tasks demand performance of skills lost because of the amputation, such as writing, handling change, or eating with utensils.

TREATMENT/INTERVENTION

Treatment and management of amputation requires a team approach. The primary team members are the physician, nurse, prosthetist, physical therapist, and occupational therapy personnel. Others may include the psychologist, social worker, and vocational counselor.

There are two phases of treatment: preprosthetic therapy and postprosthetic therapy. In the former, the person is learning to manage the stump and regain lost strength and endurance. In the latter, the person is learning to function with one or more prostheses. An early-fit prosthesis (before the final prosthesis is available) can be made if occupational therapy personnel have the equipment and time (see Maiorano and Byron 1995, 1211–1221 for instructions).

Models of treatment are based on the biomechanical (Trombly) and orthopedic models.

Self-Care
Preprosthetic Training
- If dominant hand has been amputated, consider change of dominance activities, such as writing.
- If only one upper extremity is amputated, have the person practice one-handed techniques so that some performance is possible without a prosthesis.
- If both extremities have been amputated, assist the person to learn to perform as much as possible without prostheses to encourage self-sufficiency. For example, a cuff with a pocket can be made that is put on with the stumps. Using the teeth, a spoon or toothbrush can be inserted into the pocket.

Considerations in Selecting a Prosthesis

- The person's preference for function versus comesis (see box on Hook vs. Myoelectric)
- The person's choice of control mechanisms: body-powered using cables, externally powered with either myoelectric or microswitch, passive with no active motion, or hybrid with a combination of body and electric power
- The person's life tasks and occupations at home, work, school, and community, including leisure interests
- The physical characteristics of the residual limb and stump, including the length of the limb, mobility, strength, and skin integrity
- The financial coverage for the prosthesis, such as workers' compensation or other third-party payment, or private payment
- The person's motivation, attitude, and coping skills
- The person's cognitive abilities to learn and grasp concepts of the prosthesis and its component controls

Source: Data from F. Celikyol, Amputation and Prosthetics, in *Occupational Therapy for Physical Dysfunction*, 4th ed., C.A. Trombly, ed., p. 854, © 1995, Williams & Wilkins.

- Maximize the person's ability to be independent in self-care activities.
- Explore use of assistive devices to facilitate self-care.

Postprosthetic Training
- Provide the person with opportunities to practice ADLs, including cutting food, eating, dressing, using scissors, opening jars and bottles, washing dishes, making change, signing one's name, using household tools (such as a hammer), and driving.
- Have the person practice in social situations, not just in a clinic, room, or home.
- Consider which assistive devices may promote or improve performance.

Productivity
Preprosthetic Therapy
- Review with person what job skills are needed.

Postprosthetic Therapy
- Encourage the person to practice skills necessary for the individual to be a productive person, such as driving with hand controls, learning to operate equipment with a prosthesis, and taking lecture notes or recording a lecture.
- Help the person to explore possible productive activities.
- Explore use of assistive technology, home modifications, and ergonomics to facilitate productivity.

Leisure

Preprosthetic Therapy

• Explore the person's interests and aptitudes for possible leisure pursuits.

Postprosthetic Therapy

• Provide opportunities for the person to practice various possible choices.
• Provide information on resources available for participation in sports and recreation for persons with amputations, such as golf, skiing, boating, fishing, bowling, etc.
• Consider adaptations of equipment that might facilitate performance of various leisure activities.

Sensorimotor

Preprosthetic Therapy

• Maintain or increase joint mobility through daily range of motion therapy to prevent contractures and prepare movements needed to use the prosthesis. Especially important are scapular abduction, humeral flexion, elbow flexion and extension, and forearm pronation and supination.
• Assist in reduction of edema through stump wrapping.
• Maintain skin integrity and facilitate wound healing through daily cleaning.
• Prevent or reduce scarring through application of creams to suture sites and massage.
• Assist in pain control (at site of incision and phantom pain) through desensitization techniques such as massage, percussion or tapping, vibration, wrapping, or weight bearing (constant pressure) on the distal end of amputated limb into various surfaces (clay, cotton, felt, rice, or terrycloth).
• Increase muscle strength, especially if deconditioning has occurred.
• If a myoelectric prosthesis will be used, assist in testing and selecting the muscle(s) to be used for controlling the prosthesis.

Postprosthetic Therapy

• Do a prosthetic checkout with the person, including: checking prosthesis against the prescription, checking comfort and fit of the prosthesis, checking operation of the components, and checking appearance of the prosthesis on the person.
• Practice grasp and release activities. A form board with objects of various shapes, sizes, and densities may be used.
• Teach the person to preposition prosthesis as needed to approach an object correctly in a manner that is as normal to the observer as possible.
• Help the person learn to use vision to gauge the strength needed to pick up an object. For example, a Styrofoam cup requires much less grip strength to pick up than does a ceramic cup.
• Teach the person to use the prosthesis to perform one-handed activities, such as picking up, placing, and releasing objects of various sizes, shapes, textures, and composition.
• Teach the person to use the prosthesis to assist the other hand (or prosthesis, if he or she is a bilateral amputee) in activities that require two hands, such as lifting large objects.

Considerations in Selecting a Hook vs. a Myoelectric Hand

Hook	*Myoelectric*
Better function	Better cosmetic appearance
Lighter weight	Less harnessing
Ease of seeing object being manipulated	Improved ability to work overhead
Less expense	Better grip strength
Greater durability/reliability	Ability to grasp large objects
Better sensory feedback	Stronger prehension force
Better precision	Minimal body movement and
Fits into small spaces	effort needed for control

Source: Data from D.J. Atkins, Managing Self-Care in Adults with Upper Extremity Amputations, in *Ways of Living: Self-Care Strategies for Special Needs*, p. 280, © 1994, American Occupational Therapy Association.

- Teach the person limitations of the prosthesis as a sensory-gathering tool.
- Teach the person to substitute the other hand, arm, or other parts of the body to gather such information.

Cognitive

Preprosthetic Therapy

- Instruct the person in limb hygiene and care: Limb should be washed daily with mild soap and dried thoroughly. Creams may be used to massage the suture lines to reduce scarring.
- Instruct the person in wrapping the limb to facilitate limb shrinkage unless cognitive or perceptual disability is severe. An Ace bandage, tubular bandage, or shrinker sock may be used. (See Rock 1996, 575 for illustration of wrapping technique.)
- Inform the person and his or her family about prostheses in general: Be realistic about what they can and cannot do.
- Discuss with the person and his or her family the types of prostheses available, demonstrate use if possible, provide information on the pros and cons of the various types, and permit the person to participate in the decision making about which type to select. (See box on differences between hook and myoelectric types.)

Postprosthetic Therapy

- Teach the person the names of the parts of the prosthesis and what each part does. Five components are common to all body-powered prostheses: socket, harness, cable, terminal device, and wrist unit, so they form a basic unit of training.
- Teach the person how to put on and take off the prosthesis. There are two methods, called the *coat* and *sweater* methods because the actions resemble putting on a coat or sweater. The coat method has two variations. Rock (1996, 580–581) discusses each method and provides illustrations.
- Discuss with the person a schedule for wearing the prosthesis, beginning with 15- to 30-minute intervals. If no skin problems exist, the wearing time can be increased.

> **Prosthetic Appliance Developers and Manufacturers**
>
> - Alternative Prosthetic Services, Brooklyn, NY
> - Army Prosthetics Research Laboratory (APRL), no longer operating
> - Child Amputee Prosthetic Project (CAPP), University of California at Los Angeles (UCLA)
> - Hosmer-Dorrance (HD), Campbell, CA
> - Liberty Mutual Research Center ("Boston elbow"), Hopkinton, MA
> - Motion Control ("Utah elbow"), Salt Lake City, UT
> - Otto-Bock Orthopedic Industry, Minneapolis, MN
> - Ross Prosthetics, White Plains, NY
> - Therapeutic Recreation Systems (TRS), Boulder, CO
>
> *Source:* Data from F. Celikyol, Amputation and Prosthetics, in *Occupational Therapy for Physical Dysfunction*, 4th ed., C.A. Trombly, ed., p. 873, © 1995, Williams & Wilkins.

- If the prosthesis is myoelectric, the battery pack should also be discussed regarding length of life and recharging, if necessary. When the prosthesis is stored, the battery should be in the off position. Also, the hand should be fully open to keep the web space stretched.
- Teach proper care and maintenance of the prosthesis, including the glove, if used.
- Teach the person concepts of work simplification, pacing, and energy conservation.
- Encourage the person to learn new ways to accomplishing tasks that were lost, including the use of a prosthesis.

Psychosocial
- Provide emotional support by exploring the feelings of the person and his or her family. The person and his or her family must learn to adjust to disability by talking about feelings.
- Assist the person in revising self-image and accepting that image with the prosthesis by helping the person to view the prosthesis as a means of meeting personal needs and goals.
- Explore with the person and his or her family what role changes may occur and how the person and family will cope with those changes.
- Encourage the person to participate in social activities.
- Provide resource information about and encourage the person to participate in a support group for amputees.

Environment
- Explore with the person and his or her family options for financing prosthesis and training. Social workers, if available, may also assist.

PRECAUTIONS
- The person should always check the stump for signs of skin breakdown and report any problems to the physician immediately.
- The person should always check the prosthesis to be sure it is in good working order.

- Make sure that the person knows how to contact the prosthetist for repair and maintenance.
- Do not wring out wrapping materials; this shortens the life of the elastic property.
- Watch for compensatory movements of the body, which should be accommodated for by repositioning the prosthesis, not the body. The person should maintain an upright posture and not engage in awkward or unusual movements.

PROGNOSIS AND OUTCOME

- The person has regained normal muscle strength in the remaining muscle groups.
- The person demonstrates proficiency in stump care and can perform stump care independently.
- The person demonstrates knowledge of the parts of the prosthesis and the function of each part.
- The person is able to put on and take off the prosthesis independently.
- The person is able to operate the prosthesis to perform a variety of tasks.
- The person demonstrates knowledge and performance of the safe use of the prosthesis to avoid damage to the prosthesis and injury to him- or herself or to others.
- The person can perform ADLs independently, using the prosthesis.
- The person can perform productive activities, using the prosthesis.
- The person can perform leisure activities, using the prosthesis.

REFERENCES

Atkins, D.J. 1994. Managing self-care in adults with upper extremity amputations. In *Ways of Living: Self-Care Strategies for Special Needs,* ed. C.H. Christiansen, 277–304. Rockville, MD: American Occupational Therapy Association.

Celikyol, F. 1995. Amputation and prosthetics. In *Occupational Therapy for Physical Dysfunction*, 4th ed., ed. C.A. Trombly, 849–874. Baltimore: Williams & Wilkins.

Colburn, J. and V. Ibbotson. 1996. Amputation. In *Occupational Therapy and Physical Dysfunction: Principles, Skills, and Practice,* ed. A. Turner, M. Foster, and S.G. Johnson, 635–644, 650–665. New York: Churchill Livingstone.

Maiorano, L.M. and P.M. Byron. 1995. Fabrication of an early-fit prosthesis. In *Rehabilitation of the Hand*, 4th ed., ed. J.M. Hunter, E.J. Mackin, and A.D. Callahan, 1211–1221. St. Louis: Mosby.

Morris, P.A. and L. Muhn. 1998. Amputation and prosthetics. In *Physical Dysfunction Practice Skills for the Occupational Therapy Assistant,* ed. M.B. Early, 456–468. St Louis: Mosby.

Rock, L.M. 1996. Upper extremity amputations and prosthetics, Section 1: Amputations and body powered prostheses. In *Occupational Therapy: Practice Skills for Physical Dysfunction*, 4th ed., ed. L.W. Pedretti, 567–585. St. Louis: CV Mosby.

Spencer, E.A. 1998. Upper extremity amputation. In *Willard and Spackman's Occupational Therapy*, 9th ed., ed. M.E. Neistadt and E.B. Crepeau, 685–689. Philadelphia: Lippincott-Raven.

Theisen, L. 1997. Preprosthetic management of upper extremity amputation. In *Hand Rehabilitation: A Practical Guide.* 2nd ed., ed. G.L. Clark, E.F.S. Wilgis, B. Aiello, D. Eckhaus, and L.V. Eddington, 253–255. New York: Churchill Livingstone.

BIBLIOGRAPHY

Atkins, D.J. 1993. TIRR myoelectric prosthesis project enters second year. *OT Week* 7(31):8. (See Atkins, Heard and Donovan for survey results.)

Atkins, D.J. 1996. Upper extremity amputations and prosthetics, Section 2: Electric-powered prostheses. In *Occupational Therapy: Practice Skills for Physical Dysfunction*, 4th ed., ed. L.W. Pedretti, 685–694. St. Louis: CV Mosby.

Atkins, D.J., D.C.Y. Heard, and W.H. Donovan. 1996. Epidemiological overview of individuals with upper-limb loss and their reported research priorities. *Journal of Prosthetics and Orthotics* 8(1):2–11.

Belkin, J. and P.M. Byron. 1997. Upper extremity orthotics and prosthetics. In *Assessment in Occupational Therapy and Physical Therapy,* ed. J. Van Deusen, D Brunt, 216–246. Philadelphia: WB Saunders.

Canelon, M.F. 1993. Training for a patient with shoulder disarticulation. *American Journal of Occupational Therapy* 47(2):174–178 (Case report).

Fraser, C. 1993. A survey of users of upper limb prostheses. *British Journal of Occupational Therapy* 56(5):166–8.

Klein, D. and A. Campbell. 1995. The CQI pathway. *Rehab Management.* 8(4):89–95.

Meredith, J.M. 1994. Comparison of three myoelectrically controlled prehensors and the voluntary-opening split hook. *American Journal of Occupational Therapy* 48(10):932–937.

Myers, J.B. 1994. Psychological adjustment after amputation. *Journal of Occupational Therapy Students* 8(1):48–53.

Olivett, B.L. 1995. Conventional fitting of the adult amputee. In *Rehabilitation of the Hand,* 4th ed., ed. J.M. Hunter, E.J. Mackin, and A.D. Callahan, 1223–1240. St. Louis: Mosby.

Rock, L.M. 1995. Adult upper extremity prosthetic rehabilitation. *Physical Disabilities Special Interest Section Newsletter* 18(1):1–2.

Stahl, C. 1998. Renee Katz remembers. *Advance for Occupational Therapy Practitioners* 14(37):32 (Case report).

Stahl, C. 1997. Occupational therapy improves use of UE prostheses. *Advance for Occupational Therapists* 13(37):15,50.

Thiers, N. 1994. Institute explores progress in artificial arm technology. *OT Week* 8(5):22–23.

Van Deusen, J. 1993. Phantom limb pain. In *Body Image and Perceptual Dysfunction in Adults,* ed. J. Van Duesen, 173–190. Philadelphia: WB Saunders.

Ware, L.C. 1997. Digital amputation and ray resection. In *Hand Rehabilitation: A Practical Guide.* 2nd ed., ed. G.L. Clark, E.F.S. Wilgis, B. Aiello, D. Eckhaus, and L.V. Eddington, 245–251. New York: Churchill Livingstone.

Yuen, H.K, D.L. Nelson, C.Q. Peterson, and A. Dickinson. 1994. Prosthesis training as a context for studying occupational forms and motoric adaptation. *American Journal of Occupational Therapy* 48(1):55–61.

Amputation of an Upper Extremity—Child

DESCRIPTION

Amputation in a child is defined as loss of part or all of one or both arms, through either errors of fetal development or surgical removal of the extremity after birth in children ages 0–12. In transverse deficiencies, all elements distal to a certain level are absent, and the limb resembles an amputation stump. In longitudinal deficiencies, specific maldevelopments occur, such as complete or partial absence of the radius, fibula, or tibia. Other coexisting conditions may include hypoplastic or bifid bones, synostoses, duplications, dislocation, or other bony defects (*Merck Manual* 1999, 2221). In the United States, boys are more often affected than are girls for both congenital and noncongenital or acquired amputations.

CAUSE

The causes of congenital amputations or limb deficiencies are due to primary intrauterine growth inhibition or secondary intrauterine destruction of normal embryonic tissues (*Merck Manual* 1999, 2221). Two known causes are teratogenic agents (such as thalidomide) and amniotic bands. Specific diseases or disorders include influenza, measles, or rubella; immune reactions, such as releasing hormone (Rh) incompatibility; endocrine diseases, such as diabetes; intrauteral factors, such as an obstructed or twisted umbilical cord or the position of the fetus; toxins; radiation; or nutritional excesses or deficiencies. The causes of noncongenital or acquired amputations in young children include traumatic injury, thermal injury, electrical injury, and tumors. Examples of traumatic injuries include accidents involving lawn movers; farm equipment; automatic meat grinders; and train, boat, and automobile accidents (Joe 1994, 16).

ASSESSMENT

Areas
- muscle strength
- gross motor development and skills
- fine motor skills, dexterity, and coordination
- sensory registration
- learning skills
- coping skills
- daily living skills
- play skills
- prosthetic checkout

Instruments
- Interview questions in Hubbard, S. 1995. Myoprosthetic management of the upper-limb amputee. In *Rehabilitation of the Hand*, 4th ed., ed. J.M. Hunter, E.J. Mackin, and A.D. Callahan, 1247. St. Louis: Mosby.
- ADL scale
- play history assessment
- prosthetic checkout form
- assistive technology needs assessment

PROBLEMS

Sensorimotor
- Child may lack range of motion.
- Child may have decreased muscle strength.
- Child may lack hand skills.
- Child may have developmental delay in gross motor skills.
- Child lacks tactile sensation from the missing part.

Cognitive
- Generally, amputees do not differ in levels of intelligence from nonhandicapped children.
- In some cases, the child may have mental retardation or learning and perceptual disorders, depending on the cause of the amputation. An example would be a traumatic automobile accident in which brain injury also occurred.

Psychosocial
- Child's parents may react to congenital deficiencies with feelings of guilt, anger, fear, repulsion, shock, or shame.
- Child's parents may react by abandoning the child, isolating him or her, or rejecting the child.
- Child's parents may express the wish that the child would die.
- Child will become aware of being different.
- Child may experience rejection from peers.
- Child may avoid certain activities or situations to escape possible rejection or ridicule.
- Child may become dependent on others to perform certain activities and not attempt to perform the activities for him- or herself.

Self-Care
- Child may have difficulty performing some self-care activities, especially if one or both hands are missing or malformed.

Productivity
- Child may experience difficulty manipulating and exploring objects in the play environment if one or both hands are missing or malformed.

Leisure
- Child may have limitations in the types of leisure interests to pursue if one or both hands are missing or malformed.

TREATMENT/INTERVENTION
Generally, a team approach is used. Team members might include the parents, physician, nurse, prosthetist, and occupational therapy personnel. Other members may include a physical therapist, social worker, and psychologist. Occupational therapy treatment approaches are biomechanical and developmental models.

Note 1: If the amputation is unilateral, the partial limb and prosthesis will always be primarily the assisting or holding limb. If the amputation is bilateral, the therapist can assist in determining which limb and prosthesis will be used as the dominant side.

Note 2: A prosthetic unit should always be checked regularly to determine that it is fitted properly, is the correct size, is comfortable, permits performance of the desired actions, is in good mechanical or electrical order, and operates as quietly as possible. Initially, the prosthetic checkout will be the therapist's or prosthetist's responsibility. The child can be taught to assist in the checkout and to become responsible for continuing checks of the same prosthesis. A new prosthesis should always be checked out first by the therapist or prosthetist.

Note 3: The trend is toward earlier fitting of the first prosthesis in congenital amputees. In general, sitting balance (in the first six or seven months of the child's life) is considered a prerequisite, but earlier fittings have been reported. Usually, the first prosthesis is passive. It can be used to grasp an object by placing the object in the jaw but cannot be opened with shoulder movements because no control line is attached.

Note 4: Occupational therapy personnel can assist in determining the best prosthesis for the child, using an expert system computer program (Stelzer and Creighton 1997, 70–73).

Self-Care

- Provide instruction, if needed, on how to perform self-care activities with or without the prosthesis. Generally, it is useful to know how to perform basic self-care activities without the prosthesis, in case the prosthesis is malfunctioning or being repaired. Self-care tasks may include drinking from a cup, eating from a plate, dressing, combing the hair, using the telephone, operating a light or appliance switch, writing, and keyboarding.
- Instruct child in basic mobility without prosthesis, such as getting in and out of bed.

Productivity

- Work with teachers to integrate the child into the classroom. It may be necessary to visit the school to see first-hand the situation in the classroom to make effective recommendations for the child to function in the school situation.
- An older child could be introduced to basic office skills, automobile repair, and household activities, such as food preparation, cleaning, vacuuming, making beds, and general maintenance.

Leisure

- Encourage the development of leisure interests within the limitations, if any, of the child's skill level. Examples include gardening, craft work, and woodworking.
- The child may be eligible to attend a myocamp (Stahl 1998 20–22, 40).

Sensorimotor

- If the child is a below-elbow amputee:
  1. Promote normal growth and development. The child is a person first and an amputee second. Periodic measurement of overall growth and development is important to determine the child's level of performance.
  2. Help the child to use compensatory skills to perform tasks or activities for which limb or hand function is not available, such as using the chin and shoulder to hold an object, placing the object between the knees, or pressing the object against the body.
  3. If a body-operated prosthesis is worn, the child needs to learn to operate the terminal device when a control line is added to the child's prosthesis to open, grasp, close, and release. If a myoelectric hand (Cookie Crusher prehensor) is used, the same actions should be mastered. The normal age for acquiring these skills is about 15 months for release function but 24–30 months for grasp at midline.
  4. Help the child to use the prosthesis to perform motor tasks, including picking up, holding, and manipulating objects of varying size, shape, texture, and density, as well as bilateral activities. Wrapping the terminal device or myoelectric prehensor with Coban may provide better grip or the child may use gloves with friction grids on the pads of the

fingers. Examples of large-sized objects include picking up towels, large square blocks, large dowels, sponges, and beanbags. Smooth-textured surfaces could include pens, pencils, or plastic utensils and toys. Bilateral activities might include holding a bag and getting a cookie out of it, holding a small cup and filling it with water, and catching and throwing a ball. General activities might include simple crafts; coloring, cutting, and pasting; placing cards, making jewelry; and playground activities.

- If the child is a shoulder-level amputee:
  1. Promote growth and development. Be aware that developmental patterns will be different from those of children with upper extremities intact. Delays in sitting and walking are common as a result of mechanical differences, due to lack of arms to use as props and balancing aids and hands to grasp furniture in pulling to a standing position. The child will scoot on his or her bottom rather than creep. The child will use his or her feet to develop fine motor skills.
  2. No age criteria are suggested for starting the use of a passive prosthesis. Factors to consider include the child's need to use his or her upper extremities, the parents' and child's acceptance, and the child's development level.
  3. Help the child to use a passive prosthesis by placing objects in the terminal device. For feeding, a swivel spoon is useful as a substitute for wrist and forearm movements. The elbow unit is unlocked, and the child can be taught to use body movements to scoop food onto the spoon. Then the child leans the forearm against the table, forcing the elbow to flex and bringing the terminal device and spoon to the mouth.
  4. Help the child to use a control cable. Generally, a thigh strap is used because the child can obtain full opening by flexing his or her trunk to open the terminal device and standing upright to close it. As the child gains skill, shoulder elevation motion can be substituted, then a motor unit, if desired. A hook is preferred because of greater visibility.
- Provide activities to toughen the skin and reduce pain sensation.
- Assess the prosthesis and stump sock for signs of skin irritation and discomfort due to poor fit, heat, or perspiration.

Cognitive

- Instruct the parents and child on the care and maintenance of the prosthesis.
- Instruct the parents and child on stump hygiene.
- Instruct the parents and child on the steps for putting on and removing the prosthesis.
- Instruct the parents and child on the functional operation of the prosthesis.
- Instruct the child in problem solving techniques and provide opportunity to practice so that novel situations not covered in the training sessions can be dealt with effectively.
- Teach the parents and child the basic concepts of energy conservation and work simplification to account for the increased energy used to operate a prosthesis.

Psychosocial

- Encourage an older child to discuss his or her anxiety about failure of the appliance to perform or the child's own failure to control the appliance, which may lead to an embarrassing situation, such as dropping a glass.
- Provide information to team members to design or modify the prosthesis so that it performs as well as possible to meet the needs of the child.

- Develop a home program for the parents and child to carry out between visits.

Environment
- Provide emotional support to parents.
- Instruct parents about prosthetic devices and what the devices can and cannot do. Video tapes may be useful.
- Instruct parents in normal growth and development and how the amputation may affect the child's growth and development. Video tapes are helpful.

Terminology in the Frantz-O'Rahilly Classification System

Major divisions
- Terminal anomaly—the distal portion of the limb is missing. The end of the portion that is present may be deformed.
- Intercalary defect—the middle portion of the limb is deficient, but the proximal and distal portions are present.
- Transverse limb deficiency—the defect extends across the entire width of the limb.
- Longitudinal limb deficiency—only the preaxial or postaxial portion is absent.

Subdivisions
- Terminal transverse limb deficiencies:
  1. amelia—absence of a limb
  2. hemimelia—absence of the forearm and hand or the leg and foot
  3. partial hemimelia—part of the forearm or lower limb is present
  4. acheiria or apodia—absence of the hand or foot
  5. complete adactylia—absence of all fingers, and thumb or toes, including the metacarpals or metatarsals
  6. complete aphalangia—absence of one or more phalanges from the fingers, thumb, or toes
- Terminal longitudinal limb deficiencies:
  1. complete paraxial hemimelia—complete absence of one of the bones in the forearm (radius or ulna) or leg (fibula or tibia) and corresponding portion of the hand or foot
  2. incomplete paraxial hemimelia—partial absence of one of the bones in the forearm or leg
  3. partial adactylia—absence of one to four fingers or toes, including their metacarpals or metatarsals
  4. partial aphalangia—absence of one to four phalanges in the fingers or toes
- Intercalary transverse limb deficiencies:
  1. complete phocomelia—hand or foot attached directly to the trunk

---

continues

continued

2. proximal phocomelia—hand and forearm or foot and leg attached directly to the trunk
3. distal phocomelia—hand or foot attached directly to the arm or thigh
- Intercalary longitudinal limb deficiencies:
  1. complete paraxial hemimelia—complete absence of one of the bones in the forearm or leg, but the hand or foot is more or less complete
  2. incomplete paraxial hemimelia—partial absence of one of the bones in the forearm or leg, but the hand or foot is more or less complete
  3. partial adactylia—absence of all or part of a metacarpal or metatarsal from one or more fingers or toes
  4. partial aphalangia—absence of the proximal or middle phalanx or both from one or more fingers or toes

Source: Data from C.H. Frantz and R. O'Rahilly, Congenital Skeletal Limb Deficiencies, *Journal of Bone and Joint Surgery,* © 1961, Vol. 43A, pp. 1202–1224.

PRECAUTIONS

- A prosthesis is not the solution for every child amputee. The therapist should understand and support a family's decision not to opt for a prosthesis or to discontinue the use of a prosthesis.
- A myoelectric prosthesis should not be worn in water, sand, or dirt. The child should also avoid using it in situations involving heavy lifting or excessive vibration.
- A cosmetic glove is vulnerable to rough or sharp objects and stains easily when exposed to materials such as clothing dyes, newsprint, grease, paint, and ink.

PROGNOSIS AND OUTCOME

Most children with congenital amputations lead normal lives. Children with amputations due to disease or trauma will have various prognoses, depending on their situation.

- The child is able to operate the prosthesis to perform motions of opening, grasping, holding, and releasing, if he or she chooses to use a prosthesis.
- The child and family demonstrate knowledge of how the prosthesis works and how to care for it.
- The child can perform self-care activities with or without the prosthesis at an age-appropriate level.
- The child can perform play and school activities at an age-appropriate level.
- The child can demonstrate leisure activities appropriate to his or her age level.

REFERENCES

Beers, M.H., and R. Berkow, eds. 1999. *The Merck Manual of Diagnosis and Therapy,* 17th ed. Whitehouse Station, NJ: Merck Research Laboratories.

Hubbard, S. 1995. Myoprosthetic management of the upper-limb amputee. In *Rehabilitation of the Hand*, 4th ed., ed. J.M. Hunter, E.J. Mackin, and A.D. Callahan, 1241–1252. St. Louis: Mosby.

Joe, B.E. 1994. RIC's amputee program: A family affair: A family affair. *OT Week* 8(4):16–17.

Stahl, C. 1998. My, my, what goes on at myocamp! Shriners' popular outdoor adventure is occupation at its best. *Advance for Occupational Therapy Practitioners* 14(48)20–22, 42.

Stelzer, L.M. and C, Creighton. 1997. Developing a computer based expert system for pediatric prosthetic training: A pilot study. *American Journal of Occupational Therapy* 51(1):70–73.

BIBLIOGRAPHY

Meredith, J.M., J.E. Uellandal, and R.D. Keagy. 1993. Successful voluntary grasp and release using the cookie crusher myoelectric hand in 2-year-olds. *American Journal of Occupational Therapy* 47(9):825–829.

Stahl, C. 1997. Occupational therapy improves use of UE prostheses. *Advance for Occupational Therapists* 13(37):15,50.

Tapper, B. 1994. Putting cosmetic prostheses to work. *OT Week* 8(4):14–15.

Athletic Injuries to the Upper Extremity

DESCRIPTION

Athletic injuries may be defined as injuries to the upper extremity as a result of participation in sports activities, including training and playing in games. Sports may include badminton, baseball, canoeing, cycling, football, golf, gymnastics, hockey, javelin throwing, kayaking, mountain biking, rock climbing, roller hockey, rowing, skiing, softball, squash, tennis, volleyball, weight lifting, and others.

The challenge of rehabilitating the athlete with upper extremity injury is to devise a mutually agreeable plan of treatment that is safe, effective, and accepted by the sport authorities. Any protective device must not compromise the healing of the injury, put the player at risk of reinjury before healing is complete, or increase the likelihood of injury to other players during practice time or competition.

CAUSE

Injuries occur as a result of high-speed objects or external forces that impact the upper extremity and produce contusions or shearing and repetitive stress.

ASSESSMENT

Areas

- daily living skills, including ADLs and instrumental ADLs
- productivity skills and values

Materials Used in Making Splints for Athletic Injuries

- Thermoplastics
- Plaster
- Fiberglass
- GE RTV-11 Silicone Cast
- Temper Stick Foam (Kees Goebel Medical Supply, Hamilton, OH)

Source: Data from S. Sailor and S.B. Lewis, Rehabilitation and Splinting of Common Upper Extremity Injuries in Athletes, *Clinics in Sports Medicine,* © 1995, Vol. 14, No. 2, pp. 412–413.

- leisure interests and skills
- range of motion, passive and active
- muscle strength and power
- endurance
- flexibility and tissue mobility
- general physical conditioning
- edema
- grip and hand strength
- hand function (precision grasp and pinch)
- light touch and pinprick
- two-point discrimination

Instruments
- goniometry
- volumetry
- manual muscle testing
- dynamometer and pinch meter
- Finkelstein's test—passively abduct and flex the first metacarpal and flex the metacarpophalangeal (MCP) joint of the thumb to reproduce the pain
- Tinel's sign
- Froment's sign
- Weber two-point discrimination
- Dellon moving two-point discrimination

PROBLEMS

Leisure
- The person may be unable to participate in the sport until his or her injury heals.
- The person may be unable to continue participating in the sport because of the severity of the injury.

Sensorimotor

General Problems

- The person may experience lack of range of motion.
- The person may lose muscle strength.
- The person may have skin tightness.
- The person may have stiffness and lack of joint flexibility and mobility.
- The person may lack endurance.
- The person may be generally deconditioned.
- The person may have edema, with or without inflammation.
- The person may have pain.
- The person may experience temporary or permanent sensory loss of tactile, proprioceptive, or kinesthetic sensation.
- The person may experience hyperesthesia or hypersensitivity at or around the site of injury.

Elbow

- The person may have *lateral epicondylitis* or "tennis elbow," which involves the origin of the extensor carpi radialis brevis (ECRB), occasionally the anterior edges of the extensor communis, the underside of the extensor carpi radialis longus, and, rarely, the origin of the extensor carpi ulnaris (Sailor and Lewis 1995, 435).
- The person may have *medial epicondylitis* or "golfer's elbow," which usually involves the origin of the flexor carpi radialis (FCR) and the pronator teres at the medial epicondyle but may involve the entire flexor origin (Sailor and Lewis 1995, 436).
- The person may have *triceps tendinitis* or "posterior tennis elbow," which is tendinitis of the triceps at its attachment to the olecranon. This type of tendinitis is uncommon (Sailor and Lewis 1995, 436).
- The person may have *cubital tunnel syndrome,* which is caused by a combination of direct trauma, as well as stretching of the nerve through repetitive elbow flexion and prolonged elbow flexion posturing, such as with pitching or weight lifting (Sailor and Lewis 1995, 436)
- The person may have a *medial collateral ligament injury* of the elbow, which results from chronic overload or in conjunction with damage to other elbow structures by traumatic injury (Sailor and Lewis 1995, 438).
- The person may have an *elbow dislocation,* which usually occurs when there is rupture of the medial collateral ligament (Sailor and Lewis 1995, 439).
- The person may have a *fracture to the head of radius* (Sailor and Lewis 1995, 441).
- The person may have distal humerus articular lesions, also known as *osteochondritis dissecans of capitellum of humerus* (Wright and Rettig 1995, 1827).

Forearm

- The person may have *radial tunnel syndrome,* which is a compression of the radial nerve in the forearm sometimes associated with weight lifting (Sailor and Lewis 1995, 431).
- The person may have *intersection syndrome,* which is characterized by pain and swelling at the point where the second dorsal compartment tendons are crossed by those of the first dorsal compartment (Sailor and Lewis 1995, 432).

- The person may have *pronator syndrome,* which is a compression of the median nerve in the forearm caused by forceful, repetitive pronation, combined with tight gripping in sports, such as baseball, racquetball, and tennis (Sailor and Lewis 1995, 433).

Wrist

- The person may have *tendinitis* in the wrist—especially from playing golf—due to the repetitive motions of palmar flexion and dorsiflexion of the right wrist, and the combination of radial deviation and ulnar deviation with extreme range of supination and pronation of the right forearm, but the musculotendinous units tend to "overload" (Wright and Rettig 1995, 1811).
- The person may have a wrist sprain caused by falls or twisting injuries (Sailor and Lewis 1995, 430).
- The person may incur *a wrist fracture of the radius* caused by a high-energy fall on the outstretched hand (Sailor and Lewis 1995, 429).
- The person may have *fractures of scaphoid carpal bone* (Sailor and Lewis 1995, 426).
- The person may have *stenosing tenosynovitis* (de Quervain's disease) of the first dorsal compartment of the wrist, which involves the abductor pollicis longus and the extensor pollicis brevis sheaths at the radial styloid process as they pass through the first dorsal compartment. Injury is common in racquet sports, such as squash and badminton, fly fishing, and mogul skiing because of the repetitive ulnar deviation required (Sailor and Lewis 1995, 422).
- The person may have *triangular fibrocartilage complex* (TFCC) *tear* injury. The most common type of tear is detachment of the triangular fibrocartilage near the attachment to the sigmoid notch of the radius (Wright and Rettig 1995, 1828).
- The person may have *flexor carpi ulnaris* (FCU) *tendinitis,* which produces pain and tenderness in the region of the pisiform or over the FCU tendon just proximal to the pisiform (Sailor and Lewis 1995, 425).
- The person may have *flexor carpi radialis* (FCR) *tendinitis,* which presents as pain over the FCR tendon, just proximal to the wrist flexor creases on the volar radial wrist (Sailor and Lewis 1995, 425).
- The person may have *Guyon's canal syndrome* or "handlebar palsy" as a result of repetitive impact of the volar ulnar aspect of the wrist against the handlebar and lack of protective covering of the palmar fascia (Wright and Rettig 1995, 1825).
- The person may have an *occult dorsal carpal ganglion* (Sailor and Lewis 1995, 421).

Thumb

- The person may have *Bennett's fracture* of the thumb in which the abductor pollicis longus muscle pulls the metacarpal proximal while a small bony fragment remains attached to the medial aspect of the volar ligament; or Rolando's fracture, which involves a large dorsal fragment in addition to the fragment on the volar ligament. The fracture is at the base of the first metacarpal and is actually a fracture with subluxation of the first metacarpal trapezial joint (Wright and Rettig 1995, 1823).
- The person may have an *ulnar collateral ligament injury* (*skier's thumb or gamekeeper's thumb),* which is complete or partial rupture of the ulnar collateral ligament (UCL) at the

MCP joint of the thumb, due to forceful abduction, torsion in combination with abduction and hyperextension, or a combination of stressed abduction and flexion, often resulting from falling on an outstretched hand. Causes include ski poles, lacrosse sticks, or hockey sticks (Sailor and Lewis 1995, 420).

Fingers

- The person may have *fractures* of the MCPs or phalanges. One common fracture in football is a unicondylar fracture in which one condyle is displaced (Wright and Rettig 1995, 1824).
- The person may have a *jersey finger* injury, an avulsion of the flexor digitorum profundus (FDP), which occurs when an athlete grabs an opponent's jersey and forcibly extends the distal phalanx, usually the ring finger (Wright and Rettig 1995, 1824). There are three types: (1) retraction of the ruptured tendon to the area of the proximal interphalangeal (PIP) joint, (2) retraction of the avulsed tendon into the palm, and (3) rupture of the tendon with an attached fragment of bone. Type II is most common and serious.
- The person may have *boutonnière deformity*, which is a slit in the dorsal covering of the PIP joint that occurs where the central slip of the extensor mechanism is avulsed or ruptured from its insertion on the dorsal base of the middle phalanx, which results in loss of PIP flexion (Wright and Rettig 1995, 1825).
- The person may have *pseudo boutonnière deformity*, which is damage to the proximal membranous portion of the volar plate, usually created by a hyperextension force or twisting injury to the PIP joint (Wright and Rettig 1995, 1825).
- The person may have *dorsal dislocation* (displacement) of the PIP joint, usually due to hyperextension stress and longitudinal compression. The volar plate is frequently disrupted at its distal membranous portion. Common injury in football (Wright and Rettig 1995, 1823).
- The person may have *volar dislocation* (displacement) of the PIP joint in which the extensor mechanism may be partially disrupted and, frequently, the head of the phalanx button-holes through the extensor mechanism between the central slip and the lateral bands (Wright and Rettig 1995, 1824).
- The person may have an unstable dorsal PIP dislocation with fracture (Wright and Rettig 1995, 1824).
- The person may have *mallet finger* injury, which occurs when a ball, helmet, or other equipment strikes or is stricken by an extended fingertip, forcing the distal interphalangeal (DIP) into flexion while the extensor mechanism is actively extended. The injury involves the rupture of the extensor mechanism of the proximal phalanx or fracture of the dorsal base of the distal phalanx with attached extension mechanism (Wright and Rettig 1995, 1824). There are five types of mallet finger injuries: (1) fibers of the extensor mechanism may be stretched but without complete division, (2) the extensor tendon may rupture or avulse from the dorsal base without bony involvement, (3) the tendon avulsion may include a small bony attachment, (4) a true fracture with significant involvement of the articular portion of the collateral ligament of the distal joint, and (5) a fracture dislocation of the epiphyseal plate, seen only in children.
- The person may have *tendinitis* from chronic overstretching or initiation of unaccustomed motion or activity.
- The person may have pain in the wrist, hand, or specific digits.

- The person may have numbness or loss of feeling in the wrist, hand, or specific digits.
- The person may have decreased or lost tactile sense, kinesthesis, or proprioception.

Cognitive
Athletic injuries do not directly affect cognitive functioning.

Psychosocial
- The person may express fear of repeated injuries, disability, or pain.
- The person may express concern for "letting the team down" during the time that the person is unable to participate, due to injury and rehabilitation.
- The person may experience tension and stress in relation to the injury and rehabilitation process.
- The person may express anger at being injured.
- The person may become depressed due to the injury itself, if severe, and due to length of the rehabilitation process.
- The person may go through a grief process if injury is severe or threatens to end a sports career, including disbelief, denial, and isolation; anger; bargaining; depression; and, finally, acceptance (Skerker and Schulz 1995, 25).

TREATMENT/INTERVENTION
Treatment is based primarily on the biomechanical model. The primary goals are to decrease pain and inflammatory response; reduce edema; maximize range of motion; improve muscle control and coordination; and increase strength, endurance, and proprioceptive awareness (Skerker and Schulz 1995, 23–24). The primary purpose of splints or casts in athletes is "to immobilize only the joints directly involved in quieting the inflamed tissue, thereby preventing weakness and stiffness of nearby joints, yet allowing the greatest function" (Sailor and Lewis 1995, 413, 416). Skerker and Schulz (1995, 30–33) outline a five-phase program for sports rehabilitation, including the acute injury phase, initial rehabilitation phase, progressive rehabilitation phase, integrated functions phase, and return to sport phase.

Self-Care
- Self-care activities can be used as gentle range of motion exercises following immobilization.
- Self-help or assistive devices may be useful during early rehabilitation.

Leisure
- Activities based on movements used in the sport may be adapted or used normally when resistive or unrestricted movements are permitted.
- Training schedule may be modified, such as by more frequent breaks or rest periods, by permitting only specific activities or exercises or having them done only with a splint or cast, restricting one or more joint actions.

Sensorimotor
General Considerations
- Modalities, such as icing, ice massage, pneumatic compression, paraffin wax, electrical stimulation, low-output laser, ultrasound, iontophoresis, phonophoresis, and heat have been

used in treating athletic injuries. Occupational therapy personnel need to be knowledgeable about licensure laws or regulations regarding use of physical agent modalities in occupational therapy. Some restrictions or additional training may be required.
- If splints are used, two may be necessary: one highly protective with padding for practice and competition, and one less restrictive for the rest of the time (Sailor and Lewis 1995, 412).

General Program for Fractures and Ligamentous Injuries
- If there is inflammation, gentle range of motion exercises may be performed twice daily to prevent stiffness and loss of range of motion. Such exercises are most comfortably done after bathing, when tissue temperature is elevated. Removable splints make exercising easier. Consider replacing the rigid, nonremovable immobilization devices with removable splints, once early healing has occurred. For stiff joints, joint mobilization techniques include traction and volar/dorsal glides may be used before range of motion exercises are begun. Static progressive splinting can be used to increase joint range of motion if other joint mobilization techniques are insufficient. Turnbuckles, hinges with adjustable stops, and Velcro tabs are means of applying static progressive tension, as opposed to dynamic tension applied by rubber bands and springs (Sailor and Lewis 1995, 419).

General Program for Overuse Syndromes and Tendinitis
- The hierarchy for exercise regimens is usually active range of motion (AROM) only (the person performs the joint movement without outside assistance), then isometric exercise (muscle contraction that does not produce joint motion), followed by isotonic exercises (muscle contraction that produces joint motion) and, finally, isokinetic exercises, which are characterized by flexed speed and accommodative resistance. After 30 nonrestrictive repetitions of a previously painful motion, the person can progress to isometric exercises. When isometric exercises can be performed without pain or inflammation, the person can progress to isokinetic exercises. Isotonic exercise can be either concentric (a shortening contraction) or eccentric (a lengthening contraction), depending on desired result. Isotonic exercises may include the use of free weights or resistive devices, such as Thera-Band or Thera-Tube (Smith and Nephew Rolyan, Inc.). Isokinetic exercises may include equipment such as the Cybex, Lido (Loredan) or Orthotron machines. Slowing training speeds focuses on strength, whereas high training speed enhances power and endurance. Proprioceptive neuromuscular facilitation (PNF) may be used as a strengthening program. The rotational and diagonal patterns are similar to many motions in sports activities, and the training focuses on groups of muscles, rather than individual ones. If tissue is tight, flexibility and mobilization of tissues is maintained and improved by gentle stretching exercises. Usually, a heat modality is used first to enhance connective tissue extensibility and increase vascularization to the area. Stretching exercises are usually done three times a day (Sailor and Lewis 1995, 417–418; see also Wright and Rettig 1995, 1834–1836).

Elbow
- *Lateral epicondylitis.* Treatment during the acute inflammatory stage may include a wrist immobilization splint in 30–45 degrees of wrist extension, which relieves tension on the extensor carpi radialis brevis muscle and other wrist extensors. After the acute inflammation has subsided, a counterforce brace can be worn in place of the wrist splint, provided that there is no nerve involvement around the elbow. The counterforce brace compresses the

involved muscle, which decreases the muscle's ability to expand normally, thereby decreasing the muscle force produced and elbow angular acceleration. It is worn just distal to the lateral epicondyle over the common extensor mass. Several commercial versions of counterforce braces are available. Consumer education is also advisable regarding the size of the racket handle, composition of the racquet, string tension, modification of the tennis stroke, and use of new balls to reduce the possibility of future injury. Full recovery may take 8–12 months, and small setbacks may occur (Sailor and Lewis 1995, 433–435; see also Wright and Rettig 1995, 1816–1819).

- *Medial epicondylitis.* Treatment may include a wrist immobilization splint in 10 degrees of palmar flexion to relieve tension in the flexor mass. If the flexor carpi radialis muscle is involved, the splint should include 10 degrees of radial deviation, as well as 10 degrees of palmar flexion. In severe cases, a Muenster-type splint may be used, which includes the elbow joint in the splint to decrease use of the pronator teres muscle. Once the acute inflammation has subsided, gentle flexibility activities may be started, followed by a carefully monitored progressive exercise program. Full recovery may take 8–12 months, and small setbacks may occur (Sailor and Lewis 1995, 436).
- *Triceps tendinitis.* Treatment may include an elbow splint positioned in 45 degrees of flexion to assist in resolving the inflammation. Rest and elimination of activities that aggravate the condition are recommended. Amount of time needed for rest before returning to sports activity is not given (Sailor and Lewis 1995, 436).
- *Cubital tunnel syndrome.* Treatment for mild symptoms includes fitting the person with an elbow pad to be worn over the posterior medial aspect of the elbow to protect the ulnar nerve from direct pressure or trauma. The pad may also be worn at night but with it turned so that the bulk of the pad is on the anterior aspect of elbow, thus limiting elbow flexion. In severe cases, a rigid thermoplastic splint may be fabricated to position the elbow at less that 45 degrees of flexion. Initially, the splint is worn at all times but as symptoms subside, the splint may be worn only at night. In construction, the volar approach is easier to fabricate but an elbow pad over the posterior medial elbow should be included, rather than splinting over the cubital tunnel. If the posterior approach is used, the splint should be constructed to avoid direct pressure on the ulnar nerve by using the technique of "bubbling out" the area over the nerve. Strengthening exercises using isometric or isotonic actions should be limited to 0–45 degrees of elbow flexion. Consumer education should stress learning to avoid exercises and activities in which the elbow is resting on the surface. Full recovery may take 3–6 months (Sailor and Lewis 1995, 437).
- *Medical collateral ligament injury.* Treatment for mild cases involves wearing a sling to rest the elbow. After the inflammation subsides, stretching and strengthening is initiated for all muscles around the elbow. In more severe cases requiring surgery, the person is splinted for 10 days in a position of 90 degrees of elbow flexion and neutral rotation. Mild gripping exercises may be initiated as soon as the pain subsides. Shoulder range of motion exercises continue throughout the rehabilitation period to maintain flexibility. Active range of motion for the wrist and forearm can begin at 10 days and strengthening at 4–6 weeks. At 6 weeks, elbow strengthening can begin. Thereafter, rehabilitation depends on the sport in which the person participates. Pitchers report that full recovery takes 18–24 months (Sailor and Lewis 1995, 438–439).
- *Elbow dislocation.* Treatment may include a posterior splint of thermoplastic or plaster to protect the elbow. The recommendation regarding the angle of splint is controversial. Some

therapists recommend almost full extension; others recommend 90 degrees of flexion for the first week. The more extended position is supposed to minimize the possibility of flexion contractures of the elbow. For more unstable elbows, a hinged elbow brace with an extension stop may be a better choice if varus and valgus control is required to maintain the reduction. Range of motion exercises for the shoulder, wrist, and hand should begin as soon as possible. As the pain and swelling decrease, gentle active elbow flexion can be started within the splint. To reduce edema, an elastic sleeve may be used. The splint can be removed at about 3 weeks to permit passive range of motion (PROM), except for situations where reinjury might recur. Instead, a neoprene sleeve can be used for light support around the elbow. After 4 weeks, progressive strengthening exercises can be initiated unless a fracture is also involved. A static-progressive or dynamic extension splint may be required to obtain full extension because extension is often difficult to obtain. A hinged elbow splint with an adjustable tension device can be used or a splint made from thermoplastic can be used and reheated according to a schedule to progressively extend the elbow (Sailor and Lewis 1995, 439–440).

- *Fracture of the head of the radius.* Fractures that are classified as simple, nondisplaced, or minimally displaced do not usually require therapy intervention. If surgery is required, therapy is indicated. Especially important is early motion, which requires collaboration between the surgeon and therapist and motivation of the person. Obstacles to early motion are instability and pain. A hinged elbow brace with stops positioned to limit flexion and extension may be used. The brace should also provide control for forearm rotation position and provide varus and valgus stability. The splint may be prefabricated or specially made to fit the special needs of the person. Transcutaneous electrical nerve stimulation (TENS) and icing may be used to alleviated pain. Heat and gentle stretch can increase comfort and achieve greater range of motion, once edema subsides. Soft tissue mobilization and scar massage can facilitate soft tissue extensibility, which will improve range of motion. A forearm rotation splint may also be needed to increase supination and sometimes pronation, because the radial head is a key component of forearm rotation. Exercises to strengthen supination and pronation may also be needed. The sequence of therapy requires an individualized protocol based on the fracture stability, surgical procedures used, amount of pain, motivation level, and clinical judgment (Sailor and Lewis 1995, 441–442).

- *Osteochondritis dissecans.* Treatment involves rest, icing, and biceps strengthening to control elbow hyperextension. Surgery may be required when loose bodies (chondral fragments) cause "locking" of the joint (Wright and Rettig 1995, 1828).

Forearm

- *Radial tunnel syndrome.* Lateral epicondylitis should be ruled out first. Conservative treatment includes a volar wrist immobilization splint in 30–45 degrees of extension for 3–6 weeks. The proximal strap should be slightly distal to the site of the radial nerve compression to avoid additional compression. A Muenster-type splint that comes over the elbow is used in severe cases. After inflammation has resolved, a program to improve range of motion and strengthening is begun. Resolutions may require several months. Consumer education to prevent a repeat of the injury should be stressed (Sailor and Lewis 1995, 431–432).

- *Intersection syndrome.* Conservation treatment is a splint that immobilizes the tendons of the first and second dorsal compartments. Thus, immobilization should include a forearm-based thumb spica splint with the wrist in slight extension, the thumb in palmar abduction, and the interphalangeal (IP) joint free. Wearing time is typically 3–6 weeks until the inflammation is resolved. After immobilization, range of motion and strengthening is initiated, as well as education to prevent reinjury (Sailor and Lewis 1995, 432–433).

* *Pronator syndrome.* Carpal tunnel syndrome (CTS) must be ruled out first. Treatment includes rest and avoidance of aggravating activity until symptoms resolve. Then a stretching and strengthening program for the elbow and forearm musculature can be started. Careful attention should be paid to the flexor pronator group. A Muenster-type splint may be worn for severe injury. Paresthesia and sensory changes may occur along the medial nerve distribution in severe cases (Sailor and Lewis 1995, 433).

Wrist

* *Wrist tendonitis.* A volar wrist splint with wrist in neutral position is worn continuously for 10–14 days, except for intermittent passive stretching. Pain is monitored closely. Cryotherapy, transverse and muscle massage, and stretching are the primary treatment components. When pain subsides, an eccentric strengthening program is started to facilitate muscle lengthening. Consumer education should stress proper warmup, flexibility exercises, and weight-training activities to avoid or reduce repeated episodes of tendonitis. In addition, a wrist brace may be recommended, such as the Nirschl R-U wrist brace and changing the grip of the golf club by using a curved grip club, such as the Bio-curve. The curved grip club is not accepted for tournament play by the United States Golf Association but may be used in practice (Wright and Rettig 1995, 1811–1813).
* *Wrist sprains* from falls or twisting injuries should be carefully evaluated to exclude carpal fractures, dorsal carpal impingement, occult dorsal carpal ganglions, or subtle scapholunate instability. Minor ligament injuries can heal with a wrist immobilization splint until pain and inflammation subside. Progressive range of motion and strengthening exercises can be used to regain full wrist function (Sailor and Lewis 1995, 430–431).
* *Wrist fracture of radius.* Usually, operative fixation or closed reduction is required before casting. When the fracture is stable, the person can be fitted with a volar wrist splint in a function wrist position. For return to play, a dorsal piece can be added for extra protection. When there is union of the fracture, light range of motion exercises can be started to reduce residual stiffness, followed by a strengthening program. A static-progressive dynamic wrist splint may be used to restore functional range of motion, if needed (Sailor and Lewis 1995, 429–430).
* *Scaphoid fracture.* Fracture is immobilized in a long- or short-arm thumb spica cast until healed. Time depends on the location of the fracture. When healing or fracture fixation has occurred, the person can be fitted with a forearm-based thumb spica splint with the wrist in neutral position. When sufficient healing has occurred, the splint can be removed for range of motion exercises to decrease stiffness. A playing cast may be used to allow return to play in some sports. After solid fracture healing has occurred, the person can progress to more range of motion and a strengthening program (Sailor and Lewis 1995, 426; see also Wright and Rettig 1995, 1819–1822, 1831–1833).
* *Stenosing tenosynovitis* (de Quervain's disease, de Quervain's tenosynovitis). The wrist should be immobilized in a splint that provides slight wrist extension, the thumb carpometacarpal joint in palmar abduction, and the metacarpophalangeal joint slightly flexed for 3–6 weeks. The IP joint of the thumb can be left free to permit light functional use of the

hand. The splint may be a total forearm-based thumb spica splint or radially based (only the radial side of the forearm) thumb spica splint. The radial side only splint has the advantage of leaving the ulnar border of the hand free to allow greater ease in writing and other light hand functions. The disadvantage is less rigidity, which is undesirable for a person who is very active (Sailor and Lewis 1995, 422–424).

- *Triangular fibrocartilage complex without dislocation or subluxation.* Conservative treatment is first attempted by immobilizing the forearm and wrist in long-arm cast or splint in neutral forearm rotation and wrist for 3–6 weeks. A Muenster-type splint can be used, in which the wrist and forearm are immobilized. The splint starts proximally over the epicondyles of the humerus and continues over the posterior elbow but allows elbow flexion and extension. A rigid thermoplastic material is used, and padding is placed inside the elbow area over the epicondyles to reduce friction. As healing occurs and pain lessens, the proximal portion of the splint can be trimmed to below the elbow, allowing forearm rotation but continuing wrist immobilization. After the area surrounding the injury is nontender during movement of the wrist and forearm, a program of progressive strengthening exercises is started for the forearm, wrist, and grip strength. If dislocation, subluxation, continued pain or failure to heal occurs, surgery may be required first. For additional information, see Sailor and Lewis 1995, 425; see also Wright and Rettig 1995, 1828–1830.
- *FCU tendinitis.* Splint the wrist in 10 degrees of palmar flexion and slight ulnar deviation to relieve tension on the FCU. After pain and inflammation have resolved, progressive range of motion and strengthening exercises can be initiated. Also provide, or refer to another professional to provide, consumer education regarding modification of technique in performing sport activities to avoid reinjury (Sailor and Lewis 1995, 425).
- *FCR tendinitis.* Splint the wrist in 10 degrees of palmar flexion and slight radial deviation to relieve tension on the FCR. After pain and inflammation have resolved, progressive range of motion and strengthening exercises can be initiated. Also provide, or refer to another professional to provide, consumer education regarding modification of technique in performing sport activities to avoid reinjury (Sailor and Lewis 1995, 425,426).
- *Guyon's canal syndrome.* Therapy includes a volar wrist splint to protect the inflamed structures and immobilize the wrist. If a specific type 1, 2, or 3 lesion can be determined, padding can be applied to the splint, proximal or distal to the area of nerve compression, to minimize direct pressure over the involved area. Joint mobilization techniques for the pisiform have been suggested, as have anterior and posterior glides to the individual carpals. Myofascial release may be used to decrease the tightness of the muscle and fascia; massage may be used to improve circulation and cryotherapy to decrease inflammation. Symptoms usually resolve in 2–4 weeks but may require more time to abate in chronic cases. The cyclist can achieve therapy by riding with "hands free." Next, the rider places hands on handlebars while wearing padded gloves for 10-, then 20-, then 30-minute intervals. At the same time, the rider can experiment with different hand positions. Weight training is encouraged to improve upper-body strength and hand strengthening, with emphasis on the intrinsic muscles (Wright and Rettig 1995, 1825–1827).
- *Occult dorsal carpal ganglion.* Usual treatment includes a steroid injection and a wrist immobilization splint in a position of comfort for the person. The splint is used until pain subsides, which may occur between 10 days and 3 weeks. A gradual program of mobilization and strengthening is then initiated. Surgical treatment may be required if there is frequent recurrence of symptoms that interfere with performance and function. Following

surgery, the wrist is immobilized for 1–2 weeks. Following immobilization, stretching and range of motion exercises are begun immediately and done frequently, such as every waking hour. Static-progressive or dynamic wrist splinting in flexion can be used if flexion is not restored with regular exercises programs. Use of scar mobilization techniques and scar pressure pads can be helpful to remodel the incisional scar and assist in regaining wrist flexion (Sailor and Lewis 1995, 431).

Thumb

- *Bennett's fracture.* Treatment includes closed reduction and percutaneous pin fixation or open reduction and internal fixation. A protective playing device (not specified in text) may permit return to play as early as 2–3 weeks if the participation does not involve throwing. For participants who throw, such as a quarterback, the return usually required is 6–8 weeks (Wright and Rettig 1995, 1823).
- *UCL injury, skier's thumb,* or *gamekeeper's thumb.* Grade I and II injuries (microscopic or incomplete ligament tears, nondisplaced bony avulsions, and no loss of ligament integrity) are immobilized in a hand-based (in the hand) fiberglass or plaster splint to reduce stress on the ligament at the MCP joint. Then a thermoplastic hand-based thumb spica splint is made using 1/16 inch thermoplastic material. The carpometacarpal joint (CMC) is splinted in palmar abduction, the MCP joint in slight flexion, and the IP joint is free. The splint should be worn at all times for 6 weeks, then part time for up to 2 or 3 months. Taping the UCL before athletic events provides light protection and may reduce reinjury. Grade III injuries (complete tears, displaced bony avulsions) need surgery first. A plaster-reinforced bulky dressing is used for a few days to allow swelling to decrease before fitting the thumb with a fiberglass hand-based thumb spica cast, which should be worn for 3–4 weeks. Then a thermoplastic hand splint can be made. For participation in aggressive sports, such as skiing or football, a removable extension on the thumb to cover the IP joint may be desirable. See Sailor and Lewis (1995, 420–422) and Wright and Rettig (1995, 1813–1815) for additional details.

Fingers

- *Finger fracture of the PIP joint.* Open reduction and internal fixation (ORIF) and occasional percutaneous pinning is usually required. No therapy is mentioned. The athlete can return to play within 1–2 weeks (Wright and Rettig 1995, 1824).
- *Jersey finger.* Type II injury, in which the avulsed tendon is retracted into the palm, must be repaired within 7–10 days because of the scarring that rapidly occurs. Types 1 and III, in which the tendon retracts close to the PIP joint, can wait to be repaired for up to 8 weeks, although earlier repair is recommended. Therapy depends on the athlete's age, level of play, and future plans. Failure to repair will cost the person about 15% of the digit's function. For young players, the repair should be made, but for older athletes, less aggressive therapy may be recommended. If the person has another career that involves fine motor skills, such as dentistry, music, or surgery, repair should be made, regardless of age. No specific therapy is discussed (Wright and Rettig 1995, 1824).
- *Boutonnière deformity.* Therapy involves splinting the PIP joint in extension. An exercise program should begin by holding the PIP extended and the DIP flexed to advance the lateral bands. Early mobilization of the extensor mechanism is encouraged. Splinting should continue for 6–8 weeks. Splinting the athlete for the remainder of the season is recommended during practice and play (Wright and Rettig 1995, 1825).

- *Pseudoboutonnière deformity.* Therapy involves splinting the finger in extension with a safety pin splint. A neoprene dynamic finger extension splint may also be used. The length of wearing time is not specified (Wright and Rettig 1995, 1825).
- *Dorsal dislocation of the PIP joint.* After the joint is reduced, it is usually stable. It should be splinted for 3–5 days, using an extension block splint, for example, followed by buddy taping. The person can return to playing (Wright and Rettig 1995, 1823).
- *Volar dislocation of the PIP joint.* Open reduction may be needed to reduce the dislocation. The extensor mechanism is usually repaired at the PIP, and that joint needs to be splinted in 0 degrees of extension for about 6 weeks. With the splint, the athlete may return to play as soon as symptoms permit or about 1–2 weeks (Wright and Rettig 1995, 1824).
- *Unstable dorsal PIP dislocation with fractures.* After closed or open reduction and pinning, an extension block splint is used. Early controlled mobilization is important to avoid loss of PIP joint flexion. Treatment usually requires 4–6 weeks unless the person can play with a boxing-glove type of playing cast on the hand, which effectively eliminates ball-handling activities (Wright and Rettig 1995, 1824).
- *Mallet finger.* The DIP joint should be splinted in extension using a Stack splint or dorsal or volar thermoplastic splint. Occasionally, open reduction is required. With the splint, the athlete may return to practice immediately (Wright and Rettig 1995, 1824–1825). For a unique splint that permits finger pad sensation to be used and permits hyperextension while the splint is on, see Johnson (1995, 18), as well as Paynter and Schindeler-Grasse 1993, 216).
- *Nerve compression injuries.* See the sections on carpal tunnel syndrome (CTS), median nerve injuries, ulnar nerve injuries, and radial nerve injuries.

Cognitive
- Instruct the person in preventive methods, such as the use of gloves, splints, padded handle bars, or other protective devices to prevent injury and reduce repetitive stress.
- Instruct the person in proper warmup, stretching, and cool-down after sports activity for the specific injury.
- Provide realistic information regarding the rehabilitation process.
- Inform the athlete of the severity of the injury and the expected length of time for recuperation.

Psychosocial
- Teach coping strategies as part of the rehabilitation program.
- Provide sense of control of the rehabilitation process by explaining the rationale for the rehabilitation approach and offering alternatives for implementing a specific program.

PRECAUTIONS
- Splints should be fabricated from material that protects the player but does not cause injury to opposing players. Generally, splints and casts constructed of thermoplastics, plaster, or fiberglass are not allowed in competitive sports. The GE RTV-11 playing cast is made primarily of silicone and is accepted by many, but not all, sports officials. For basic instructions on making a GE RTV-11 cast, see Sailor and Lewis (1995, 414–416).

- Watch for a skin rash under a splint, which may occur from exercise perspiration. A stockinet liner may be needed to absorb perspiration or holes may be made in the splint at random intervals. Be sure that the holes do not weaken the splint.
- A "playing cast" should be worn only during competition because there is no porosity to allow aeration of the skin and, over prolonged periods of time, the skin may develop maceration and dermatitis.
- Sports organization may require that, during the game, any hard casting material be covered with padding, such as a high-density, closed-cell polyurethane or similar material.
- Examine splints frequently for signs of structural fatigue (cracks or bending) and oxidation.
- Watch for edema or skin redness under and around the splint.
- Always have the person report any pain or numbness associated with the splint.
- Be aware of athletic rules regarding use of protective splints on the playing field. Rules differ for interscholastic, intercollegiate, and professional sports.

PROGNOSIS AND OUTCOME

- Person is free of pain and edema.
- Person has recovered full or nearly full range of motion.
- Person has recovered full muscle strength, including grip or hand strength.
- Person has recovered normal gross coordination of the body.
- Person has recovered normal bilateral coordination and dexterity of the hands.
- Person has recovered normal sequence of motions and timing.
- Person uses protective devices during athletic events, if recommended, to prevent additional or recurrent injury.

REFERENCES

Johnson, C.W. 1995. A new splint for mallet finger. *OT Week* 9(26):18–19.
Paynter, P. and P Schindeler-Grasse. 1993. Techniques for improving distal interphalangeal motion. *Journal of Hand Therapy* 6(3):216–217.
Sailor, S. and S.B. Lewis. 1995. Rehabilitation and splinting of common upper extremity injuries in athletes. *Clinics in Sports Medicine* 14(2):411–446.
Skerker, R.S. and L.A. Schulz. 1995. Principles of rehabilitation of injured athlete. In: *Upper Extremity Injuries in the Athlete,* 23–42. New York: Churchill Livingstone.
Wright, H.H. and A.C. Rettig. 1995. Management of common sports injuries. In *Rehabilitation of the Hand,* 4th ed., ed. J.M. Hunter, E.J. Mackin, and A.D. Callahan, 1809–1838. St. Louis: Mosby.

BIBLIOGRAPHY

Benaglia, P.G., F. Sartorio, and R. Ingenito. 1996. Evaluation of a thermoplastic splint to protect the proximal interphalangeal joints of volleyball players. *Journal of Hand Therapy* 9(1):52–56.
Canelón, M.F. and A.J. Karus. 1995. A room temperature vulcanizing silicone rubber sport splint. *American Journal of Occupational Therapy* 49(3):244–249.
Canelón, M.F. 1995. Silicone rubber splinting for athletic hand and wrist injuries. *Journal of Hand Therapy* 8(4):252–257.

Clements L.G. and S. Chow. 1993. Effectiveness of a custom-made below elbow lateral counterforce splint in the treatment of lateral epicondylitis (tennis elbow). *Canadian Journal of Occupational Therapy* 60(3):137–44.

Groth, G.N., D.M. Wilder, and V.L. Young. 1994. The impact of compliance on the rehabilitation of patients with mallet finger injuries. *Journal of Hand Therapy* 7(1):21–24.

Arthroplasty—Fingers

DESCRIPTION

Arthroplasty is a surgical procedure designed to reform a joint. Flexible implant prostheses made of silicone or silastic are used to replace the PIP, DIP, or MCP joints. Technically, the implants act as spacers or hinges, rather than as a joint, to maintain alignment during the process of encapsulation, whereby the body develops a fibrous joint capsule. Swanson et al. (1995, 1351), who developed the implant in the 1960s, describe the implant as a "flexible hinge implant [that] acts as a dynamic spacer to maintain internal alignment and spacing of the reconstructed joint and as an internal mold that supports the healing capsuloligamentous system around the implant while early motion is started."

Indications for arthroplasty in the fingers are chronic pain, stiffness, deformities, instability about a joint, or loss of cartilage (Theisen 1997b, 355). An example is the ulnar drift of the fingers and subluxation of the MCP joint seen in rheumatoid arthritis. Arthroplasty becomes the treatment of choice when more conservative measures fail, such as antiinflammatory medications, splinting, joint protection, ergonomic education and counseling, and steroid injection (Brown and Steen 1997, 62).

Arthrodesis is an alternative to arthroplasty. The advantage of arthroplasty is joint movement, especially in the PIP joints. Loss of movement in the DIP joints is less incapacitating.

CAUSE

Arthritic changes occurring in rheumatoid arthritis are the most common cause but osteoarthritis and trauma to the hand, such as a crushing injury, are also candidates for arthroplasty of the fingers.

ASSESSMENT

Areas

- range of motion, active and passive
- grip strength

Instruments

- goniometer
- modified blood pressure cuff or "bulb" type dynamometer

PROBLEMS

Sensorimotor

- The person may have joint instability.
- The person may have joint stiffness.
- The person may have loss of joint cartilage.
- The person may have edema.
- The person may have rotational deformities and nonalignment of the joints.
- The person may be slow to heal.
- The person usually has scarring.
- The person may experience skin tightness.
- The person may experience pain.

TREATMENT/INTERVENTION

For a detailed explanation of the surgery and development of the spacer, see Swanson et al. (1995, 1351). Primary treatment model is biomechanical.

Self-Care

- Self-care tasks can be used as general exercises.

Sensorimotor

- Monitor wound healing. Delay in wound healing may be due to medical conditions and nonsteroidal antiinflammatory drugs (NSAIDS) or steroids. Mobilization of tissue 3–4 weeks postoperatively assists in the development of greater tensile strength.
- Decrease and control edema using ice, compressive dressing, and elevation above the heart.
- Prevent scar adherence.
- Maintain rotational and angular stability and prevent rotational deformities and instability. If rotation of the MCP joint occurs, additional outriggers to provide counterforce may be needed. The action of the outrigger must be equal to the rotational force. Therefore, if the rotational deformity is medial or pronated, the opposite force must be lateral or supinated.
- Prevent contractures through early mobilization and gentle range of motion.
- Provide protective splinting during the postoperative period.
- Decrease joint stiffness and increase flexibility and AROM in flexion and extension or sagittal plane.
- Maintain capsular integrity in the ulnar and radial direction or frontal plane.
- Continuous passive movement may be used as an adjunct to treatment.
- Increase strength, especially grip strength.
- Monitor postoperative pain. Note: Greater than expected pain may be related to a flare-up in rheumatoid arthritis condition itself.

Specific Treatment for MCP Joint (Theisen 1997a, 349–354)

- Bulky dressing is removed 2–6 days postoperative and dynamic MCP extension splint applied. The finger slings should pull in approximately 15 degrees to the radial side to counteract ulnar pull. At the PIP interphalangeal extension, blocks or troughs are included

to prevent PIP flexion during active MCP flexion exercises. A static splint may be worn at night but the hand should be splinted continuously.
- Dynamic flexion splinting may be started for intermittent use at between the 2nd and 3rd week. The flexion splint should not pull the fingers in an ulnar direction.
- The schedule for wearing the dynamic MCP extension splint can be tapered off beginning 6 weeks postoperatively, unless there is MCP extension lag or flexion contracture.
- Mild isometric resistive exercises may be started at 8–10 weeks postoperatively. Continue to avoid ulnar forces.

Specific Treatment of the PIP joints (Theisen 1997b, 355–361; Brown and Steen 1997, 60, 62–65)
- A splinted compression dressing with plaster slab may be applied postoperatively. The bulky dressing may be removed the next day and a slight compressive dressing applied (Brown and Steen 1997, 62–63).
- A thermoplastic (1/16 or 1/8 inch) static extension splint should be applied and worn continuously, except during exercises, for up to 6 weeks. The PIP and DIP should be in full extension; the MCP may be flexed in natural hand position and no lateral force should be permitted. An alternative is a dynamic PIP extension splint with intermittent active flexion; however, as with the extension splint, no lateral force should be permitted (Theisen 1997b, 356–357). The splint may be applied on the volar or dorsal side. Theisen (357) shows a volar-based splint, Brown and Steen (1997, 63) mention a dorsal-based splint. Note: Brown and Steen (1997, 63) change to hook and loop buddy splint 4 days after surgery. A buddy splint is shown in Theisen (1997b, 359).
- After the 3rd postoperative week, a dynamic flexion splint may be worn to gain 70 degrees (Theisen 1997b, 357).
- Begin AROM of the PIP joint 3–5 days postoperatively but do not allow any lateral deviation (Theisen 1997b, 356). The AROM should emphasize blocked, isolated PIP joint flexion and assisted extension (Brown and Steen 1997, 63). Note: Brown and Steen (1997, 62) also stated that AROM may be initiated at 3–5 days if the central slip (terminal extensor tendon) was not detached. If the central slip was detached (cut), it needs to be protected and treated in a manner similar to a tendon repair.

Specific Treatment for DIP Joints (Theisen 1997b, 355–361)
- If the person has had Kirschner wire (K-wire) fixation, he or she should have 3–4 weeks of fixation, followed by another 4 weeks of DIP extension splinting. After fixation is removed, gradual AROM exercises should be started to 30 degrees of DIP flexion. An extension splint should be worn for 2 months after fixation is removed.
- If the person does not have K-wire fixation, both PIP and DIP joints are positioned in extension for 2 weeks. After 2 weeks, AROM is initiated with the PIP joint but the DIP joint continues in extension for an additional 2 weeks. Gentle flexion exercises should be performed gradually, progressing to 30 degrees of flexion. A night extension splint is worn for an additional 6 weeks.

Cognitive
- Involve the person in the treatment plan to encourage cooperation.
- Provide initial or continued consumer education program on joint protection.

PRECAUTIONS

- Be aware of any medications that may interfere with healing process, such as steroids; or those that predispose the person to additional problems, such as osteoporosis.
- Be aware that pain may not be related to the surgery or rehabilitation but to a flare-up of the underlying or pre-existing rheumatoid arthritis disease.
- Splints and exercises should avoid ulnar direction forces, so as to avoid reinforcing the ulnar drift.
- Watch for signs of medial rotation of the MCP joint (also called *pronation deformity*).
- Watch for extension contractures, especially in the fifth digit.
- Watch for signs of dislocation or fracture of the implant.
- Watch for signs of joint instability following surgery. Consult physician before beginning any therapy.
- Be aware of whether any additional surgery was done at the same time as the arthroplasty that might delay or interfere with therapy, such as ligament repair, tendon repositioning or reconstruction, tenolysis, or volar plate release.
- In the fingers, watch for signs of boutonniére or swan neck deformities.
- Specific precautions for PIP arthroplasty are flexor tendon adherence, malalignment, extension lag, fracture of the prosthesis, and synovitis.
- Stress loads must be kept minimal or moderate to avoid erosion of the silicone.
- Specific precautions for DIP arthroplasty are malalignment, mallet finger, fracture of the prosthesis, and synovitis.

PROGNOSIS/OUTCOMES

- The person will have active MCP and PIP flexion to 70 degrees.
- The person will have active MCP, PIP, and DIP extension to neutral.
- The person will have active flexion of the DIP to 30 degrees.
- The person will have neutral (normal) alignment of proximal phalangeals with corresponding metacarpal.

REFERENCES

Brown, L.G. and T.M. Steen. 1997. Rehabilitation following hand arthroplasty. *Rehab Management* 10(5):60, 62–5 (Case report).
Swanson, A.B., G.G. Swanson, and J.B. Leonard. 1995. Postoperative rehabilitation programs in flexible implant arthroplasty of the digits. In *Rehabilitation of the Hand*, 4th ed., ed. J.M. Hunter, E.J. Mackin, and A.D. Callahan, 1351–1375. St. Louis: Mosby.
Theisen, L. 1997a. Metacarpophalangeal joint arthroplasty. In *Hand Rehabilitation: A Practical Guide.* 2nd ed., ed. G.L. Clark, E.F.S. Wilgis, B. Aiello, D. Eckhaus, and L.V. Eddington, 349–354. New York: Churchill Livingstone.
Theisen, L. 1997b. Proximal interphalangeal and distal interphalangeal joint arthroplasty. In *Hand Rehabilitation: A Practical Guide.* 2nd ed., ed. G.L. Clark, E.F.S. Wilgis, B. Aiello, D. Eckhaus, L.V. Eddington, 355–362. New York: Churchill Livingstone.

BIBLIOGRAPHY

Schwartz, D.A. and C.A. Peimer. 1998. Distal interphalangeal joint arthroplasty in a musician. *Journal of Hand Therapy* 11(1):53–54.
van Veldhoven, G. 1995. The proximal interphalangeal joint swing traction splint. *Journal of Hand Therapy* 8(4):265–268.

Brachial Plexus Injuries and Disorders

DESCRIPTION

Brachial plexus injuries and disorders produce a mixed motor and sensory disorder in the corresponding limb. Injury or dysfunction in the brachial plexus does not fit the distribution of individual roots or nerves. Disorders of the rostral or upper brachial plexus (C5,6) produce disability about the shoulder and elbow, whereas those of the caudal or lower brachial plexus (C7,8; and T1) produce dysfunction in the forearm, wrist, and hand. In infants, injury to the rostral brachial plexus (C5,6) is called *Erb's palsy*, the most common type, whereas injury to the caudal portion (C8, T1) is called *Klumpke's palsy*. Involvement of spinal nerves C5 through TI is called *Erb-Duchenne-Klumpke palsy*. If only part of the brachial plexus is involved, sensory functions usually remain intact, but if the entire brachial plexus is involved, sensory loss often occurs (*Merck Manual* 1999, 2132–2132; Hogan 1995, 19). About 80% of Erb's palsy conditions resolve spontaneously in 12–18 months. Therapists see only the cases that do not resolve spontaneously.

In upper brachial plexus injury, the muscles affected are usually the deltoid, infraspinatus, teres minor, biceps, brachialis, brachioradialis, rhomboids, coracobrachialis, subscapularis, teres major, supraspinatus, and the supinator. Movements affected are shoulder adduction and internal rotation, elbow extension, forearm pronation, and wrist flexion. Lower brachial plexus injury involved the intrinsic muscles of the hand, the wrist flexors, and long flexors of the fingers. In addition, TI spinal nerve involvement may produce Horner's syndrome, which includes ptosis of the eyelid and contraction of the pupil on the affected or homolateral side. If the total arm is involved, there will be flaccidity of the entire arm with significant sensory loss (Hogan 1995, 19).

Hogan (1995, 19) illustrates four of brachial plexus lesions: praxis, neuroma, rupture, and avulsion. In praxis or neuropraxia, the nerve is damaged but not actually torn. In the neuroma form, scar tissue forms around a nerve. A rupture or neuromesis occurs when the nerve is torn but not at the location of the spine. An avulsion occurs when the nerve is actually torn away from the spine. Rupture or avulsion may require nerve grafts.

Brachial plexus injuries have been described for over 200 years by William Smellie but the ideas were refined by Guillaume Duchenne in 1872, Wilhelm H Erb in 1874, and A. Dejuerine Klumpke in 1885. Erb's palsy is also called *obstetrical palsy* or *Erb-Duchenne palsy*.

CAUSE

In infants, brachial plexus injuries may be caused by traction, friction, contusion, compression, or penetration in utero. The traction or stretching may occur in shoulder dystocia, breech extraction, or hyperabduction of the neck in cephalic presentation. Other causes include hemorrhage around a nerve, tearing of the nerve or root, avulsion of the roots with associated cervical cord injury, or radiation treatment for cancer, called *radiation-induced brachial plexopathy*, in which edema and fibrous tissue are thought to constrict the brachial plexus, resulting in loss of myelin. In adults, the most common causes are trauma resulting from fractures of the clavicle or humerus, subluxation of the shoulder or cervical spine, or invasion of metastatic cancer into the areas near the brachial plexus. The person may sustain concurrent vascular or skeletal injuries, which may delay treatment of the brachial plexus injury if the other injuries are life-threatening (Lowe and O'Toole 1995, 647).

ASSESSMENT
Areas
- daily living tasks
- productive skills, tasks, interests, values
- leisure
- edema
- motor control
- joint mobility
- extensor system function
- posture and positioning of the affected limb and body
- sensibility (sensory acuity and gnosia): light touch, proprioception, skin temperature
- soft tissue changes
- pain
- arm and hand functions
- roles and role performance

Instruments
Instruments Developed by Occupational Therapy Personnel
- developmental testing for children.
- *Sensorimotor Performance Analysis* by Richter, E. and P. Montgomery. 1989. Hugo, MN: PDP Products or San Antonio, TX: Therapy Skill Builders/The Psychological Corporation.

Instruments Developed by Other Professions and Used by Occupational Therapy Personnel
- goniometery; range of motion testing. Kendal, F.P. and E.K. McGreary. 1983. *Muscles: Testing and Function*, 3rd ed. Baltimore, MD: Williams & Wilkins. Note: In testing shoulder abduction, do not go beyond 90 degrees abduction; observe for subluxation during anterior and inferior movements and use care in moving limb in coronal abduction combined with lateral rotation.
- manual muscle testing. Kendal, F.P. and E.K. McGreary. 1983. *Muscles: Testing and Function*, 3rd ed. Baltimore, MD: Williams & Wilkins. Flow sheet for recording results appears in Lowe and O'Toole, 562–563.
- dynamometer and pinch meter
- volumetry to measure edema
- stereognosis. Gibson, J.J. 1962. Observation on active tough (Stereognozic test). *Physiology Review* 69:477–491.

- visual motor integration. Beery, K.E. and N.A. Buktenica. 1997. *The Beery-Buktenica Developmental Test of Visual-Motor Integration* (VMI-4), 4th ed. Parsippany, NJ: Modern Curriculum Press.
- hand sensitivity and function. Moberg, E. 1958. Objective methods for determining the functional value of sensibility in the hand (Moberg Pick-Up Test). *Journal of Bone and Joint Surgery* 40B:454–476. The Dellon modification is also widely used (Dellon 1981, 103–105). Note: The person with poor sensory return often does not incorporate the injured arm and hand spontaneously into routine tasks and skills, according to Lowe and O'Toole (1995, 648).
- sensory evaluation form for brachial plexus in Lowe and O'Toole, 1995, 549
- sensory evaluation for the hand in Lowe and O'Toole, 1995, 550
- asthesiometer (two-point)
- pain: visual analogue scale
- functional assessment form appears in Lowe and O'Toole, 1995, 656–657
- hand functions: Jebsen, R.H., N. Taylor, R.B. Trieschmann, M.J. Trotter, and L.A. Howard. 1969. An objective and standardized test of hand function. *Archives of Physical Medicine and Rehabilitation* 50(6):311–319.
- tone vibrator at 30 cycles per second (cps)

PROBLEMS

Self-Care

- The person may be unable to perform several or many self-help skills.

Productivity

- The person may miss several weeks of work.
- The person may be unable to return to previous job or modifications will be required.

Leisure

- The person may be unable to enjoy previous hobbies or avocational interests.

Sensorimotor

- The person usually has loss of functional skills due to edema, insensibility, muscle tightness, joint contractures, pain, and sometimes denial and inability to accept the injury (Lowe and O'Toole 1995, 663).
- The person usually has loss of motor control.
- The person usually has loss of normal joint mobility, especially the scapular and clavicular articulations of the glenohumeral joint (scapular and clavicular articulations), elbow joint, and joints of the forearm, wrist, and hand.
- The person usually has changes in the muscle extension system.
- The person usually has impaired hand and arm functions.
- The person may complain of fatigue due to heaviness of the affected extremity.
- The person may have decreased sensation.
- The person may have edema.
- The person may have decreased sensibility or sensation.

- The person may have pain due to deafferentation, to a tract force caused by the weight of the arm and/or subluxation. The pain may be described as burning, shooting, pins and needles, tingling, numbness, cramp, stiffness, frostbite, or tightness.

Cognitive
- Cognitive system is not directly involved.

Psychosocial
- The person may deny or refuse to accept the injury.
- The person may experience distress due to the injury.
- The person may become depressed.
- The person may experience difficulty in coping with the injury.

TREATMENT/INTERVENTION
Treatment usually requires a team approach. Team members may include physician(s), nurses, physical therapists, social workers, psychologists, the person's employer and family, in addition to occupational therapy personnel (Lowe and O'Toole 1995, 647). Models used in occupational therapy include biomechanical, neurodevelopmental therapy (called the *sensorimotor approach* in Shyur and Strutton 1993, 5), proprioceptive neuromuscular facilitation (PNF), and the Model of Human Occupation (MOHO). Other treatment approaches mentioned are manual therapy and craniosacral therapy, which would require additional training by most occupational therapy personnel (Hogan 1995, 20). Goals are to protect the limb from further harm, minimize edema, prevent contractures, and monitor and reintegrate sensorimotor recovery toward maximizing functional capability of the limb (Lowe and O'Toole 1995, 663).

Self-Care
- Selected ADLs that are meaningful and important to the person may be used in a home program.

Productivity
- Selected work or homemaking tasks that are meaningful and important to the person may be used in a home program.

Leisure
- Selected leisure or avocational interests that are meaningful and important to the person may be used in a home program.

Sensorimotor
- An integrated program that combines strength, endurance, and functional training using activities such as dancing or swimming provided to develop speed and coordination seems to provide the best program for facilitating motor control (Lowe and O'Toole 1995, 660).
- Minimize edema through use of massage, elevation, and pressure-gradient garments. Microelectrical neuromuscular stimulator (MENS), Coban wrap, Tubigrip sleeve, or a Jobst upper extremity pressure garment may be used. If edema is distal (from elbow down), a

Freedom GunSlinger splint can be used to reduce the dependency of the limb. If the entire limb is involved, an upper extremity abduction splint should be used to position the arm in forward flexion, abduction, and slight internal rotation. The splint is worn for 2 hours at a time (Lowe and O'Toole 1995, 655–656). Sadra (1995, 216–219) describes four different splints that have been used for brachial plexus injuries, including an elbow ratchet lock splint, a fail arm splint, a static elbow splint, and a universal arm splint. A universal sling may be helpful to reduce dependency of the limb, although use of slings is controversial. A sling was used by Bajuk, Jelnikar, and Ortar (1996, 400). Manual massage and mechanical lymph drainage may be used 30 minutes each during a day.

- Prevent myostatic contractures and muscle shortening through positioning, functional activities, and splints. In the hand, maintain first web space (between thumb and index finger), MCP and finger extension.
- Maximize functional motor ability using substitution and/or compensatory techniques.
- Encourage good posture, using a mirror to help the person see posture to compensate for poor proprioception.
- Posture is also important in maintaining muscular extensibility. Shortening of the upper trapezius can occur if the person is allowed to hold the limb in a poor posture or to use scapular substitution patterns. If the limb is expected to return to normal, the scapular musculature must be exercised. Contract-relax, hold-relax, or rhythmic stabilization performed at the scapular level can be useful (Lowe and O'Toole 1995, 661).
- Endurance training should precede strength training because endurance stimulates joints and muscle to adapt to new or unaccustomed activity (Lowe and O'Toole 1995, 659).
- Use functional patterns, including diagonal as well as the sagittal plane movements, rather than isokinetic exercises, to promote movement patterns (Lowe and O'Toole 1995, 659). A universal arm splint (Sadra 1995, 216–219) may be helpful in permitting use of residual movements to increase functional abilities.
- Use of Theraband to provide resistance to fair grade (3 out of 5) muscles is useful because resistance can be varied through the range. For muscles graded good or 4, weights can be incorporated to promote the eccentric contractions needed for limb control. Endurance training should be continued. Example: 10 repetitions with 2 lbs, 10 repetitions with 3 lbs, and 10 repetitions with 2 lbs.
- Weight bearing may be a useful exercise if there is adequate muscle support around the glenohumeral joint, especially in position of extension, which can stress the anterior capsule (Lowe and O'Toole 1995, 659).
- Use range of motion and joint mobilization techniques to counteract stiffness. Techniques should not use forceful motion. For supple joints, 10 minutes is enough, for stiff joints with loss of motor power, 15–20 minutes is needed. If pulleys are used, have the person supine so that weight of the body helps to stabilize the scapula. Joint gliding may be used at the MCP joints (Lowe and O'Toole 1995, 660).
- Avoid tightness, tendon shortening, and loss of muscular extensibility by using PNF techniques applied to the scapula. Techniques such as contract-relax, hold-relax, or rhythmic stabilization should be considered for the scapula. Watch for substitution patterns, such as use of scapula for weak glenohumeral musculature (Lowe and O'Toole 1995, 659).
- A ball bearing feeder orthosis or counter-balance sling may be used to promote proximal arm function. However, see precautions below.

- Biofeedback using audiovisual feedback may be used for reeducation and strengthening of muscles, including the biceps brachii and triceps brachii (Hogan 1995, 20).
- Functional splints may be used to facilitate lower arm function, such as a radial nerve splint to place wrist in neutral, thumb post splint to provide stable prehension surface, extension block splints to prevent hypertension and facilitate fingertip prehension, and tenodesis training splint if the person has good extensors to assist in prehension.
- Provide sensory reeducation based on Dellon's sequence of recovery of perception: pain and temperature, then touch, beginning first with 30-cps tuning fork, then moving-touch, constant touch, and 256-cps tuning fork (Dellon 1981, 117). Desensitization may be necessary before going to the early phase of sensory reeducation or concurrently with sensory reeducation. The early phase includes (1) reeducation of touch submodality-specific perceptions, such as 30-cps tuning fork, moving touch (also called *stroking*), constant touch, 256-cps tuning fork, and pressure, and (2) reeducation of any misdirected or incorrect localization of sensation. The protocol is that, first, the person directly observes the stimulus being applied, then the person shuts the eyes and concentrates on the stimulus as it is reapplied. The process is repeated several times, with the person concentrating attention and thought on the stimulus. The person should say to him- or herself, "I feel something moving on my index finger," "I feel constant touch on my middle finger," etc. The late phase of sensory reeducation begins when moving touch and constant touch can be perceived definitely and unambiguously at the fingertip with good location, which may take 6–8 months. The goal of the late-phase is recovery of tactile gnosis using object identification of familiar household objects of different shapes, size, and texture with eyes open, then shut while concentrating on the object (Dellon 1981, 213–221). A home program of sensory reeducation exercises is recommended four times daily for 15 minutes (Lowe and O'Toole 1995, 658).
- For a child, sensory stimulation is important. Placing a rattle in the involved hand can facilitate general awareness of the injured extremity. To increase proprioceptive input, place the child in the prone position. Maintain midline orientation and symmetry when positioning the child on the floor, in an infant carrier, or in the parent's arms. For other children, include bilateral upper-extremity play, moving from one position to another on the floor, upper-extremity placement, prehension and release, coordination, age-appropriate ADL activities, and strengthening (Hogan 1995, 20).
- If sensory recovery does not occur, compensatory techniques are taught, including good skin care, frequent skin inspection, avoidance of further injury or prolonged pressure to any one area of the skin, and increasing awareness of hot, cold, and sharp objects.
- Pain management is currently done with pharmacologic agents and surgery, if needed. The role of TENS is unclear for brachial plexus injury because of lack of controlled studies and the loss of or reduced sensibility. Bajuk, Jelnikar and Ortar (1996, 400) report that their patient did well. However, low-frequency pulsating magnetic field therapy was also used.

Cognitive

- Provide the person with information to allow the individual to make meaningful choices to achieve a better functional outcome.
- Provide instruction to the person about prevention of pressure sores, good skin care, frequent skin inspection, avoidance of further injury, and cognizance of hot, cold, and sharp objects. Such instruction is especially important if decreased sensibility is present.

- Instruct the person in adaptive techniques and assistive technology as needed.
- Parents should be instructed to approach the infant from the involved side to avoid unilateral neglect (Hogan 1995, 20).

Environment
- Provide the family with information about the disorder and choices to improve outcome.
- Encourage the person and family to participate in a self-help group.

PRECAUTIONS
- The person may have concurrent vascular and/or skeletal injuries that must be considered or addressed simultaneously.
- In children, PROM should not exceed 110 degrees of shoulder flexion or 90 degrees of shoulder abduction because the shoulder joint is still a fibrocartilaginous joint (Hogan 1995, 19).
- If pressure garments are worn, there should be visual inspection of the limb to note any possible constrictions at the axilla, elbow, wrist, or fingers caused by the edema or poor circulation. The person should be instructed to examine the color, capillary refill, and temperature of his or her figures, as well as checking radial pulse.
- If a splint is worn, the wearing time should be weighed against the deconditioning due to immobilization.
- Use of electrical stimulation is not recommended because of possible overuse syndrome, resulting in loss of muscle strength, amount of time required, and its cost (Lowe and O'Toole 1995, 659). The use with children is controversial (Hogan 1995, 20).
- Cost and difficulty of putting on orthotic devices should be weighed against possible benefits (Lowe and O'Toole 1995, 659).
- Weight-bearing training should be used only if there is adequate muscular support around the glenohumeral joint to avoid overstressing the anterior capsule (Lowe and O'Toole 1995, 659).
- Use of splint or sling to correct subluxation is not recommended (Lowe and O'Toole 1995, 660).
- Watch for muscular imbalances in the hand, such as first-web-space contracture, finger flexion contractures, and MCP hyperextension deformities (Lowe and O'Toole 1995, 662).

PROGNOSIS/OUTCOMES
- Recovery is variable but rarely is full recovery achieved.
- The person is able to perform self-care and ADLs independently using normal, adapted, or compensatory techniques or with assistive technology.
- The person is able to perform productive tasks with normal, adapted, or compensatory techniques or with environmental modifications.
- The person is able to perform leisure activities using normal, adapted, or compensatory techniques or with environmental modifications.
- Edema is minimized through the healing process or with massage, pressure garments, or other means.
- The person does not have contractures in soft tissue or joints.

- Pain management and control has been achieved.
- The person has normal sensibility or as much sensibility as can be expected, given the nature of the injury.
- The person has functional use of the extremity and hand to perform in an assistive or supportive role in task performance.
- The person is able to demonstrate use and maintenance of assistive technology, if provided.
- The person is able to explain and demonstrate continuing care of the extremity and precautions necessary to protect extremity from additional injury or dysfunction.

REFERENCES

Bajuk, S., T. Jelnikar, and M. Ortar. 1996. Rehabilitation of patient with brachial plexus lesion and break in axillary artery: Case study. *Journal of Hand Therapy* 9(4):399–403 (Case report).

Beers, M.H., and R. Berkow, eds. 1999. *The Merck Manual of Diagnosis and Therapy,* 17th ed. Whitehouse Station, NJ: Merck Research Laboratories.

Dellon, A.L. 1981. *Evaluation of Sensibility and Re-Education of Sensation in the Hand*, 117. Baltimore: Williams & Wilkins.

Hogan, L.J. 1995. OT with obstetric brachial plexus injuries. *Advance for Occupational Therapists* 11(35):19–20.

Lowe, C. and J. O'Toole. 1995. Therapist's management of brachial plexus injury. In *Rehabilitation of the Hand*, 4th ed., ed. J.M. Hunter, E.J. Mackin, and A.D. Callahan, 647–664. St. Louis: Mosby.

Sadra, H. 1995. Universal arm splint for brachial plexus injuries. *Canadian Journal of Occupational Therapy* 62(4):216–219.

Shyur, R.J. and R.J. Strutton. 1993. Erb-Duchenne-Klumpke palsy: A biomechanical and sensorimotor intervention comparison. *Physical Disabilities Special Interest Section Newsletter* 16(3)5–7 (Case report).

BIBLIOGRAPHY

Cooper, J. 1998. Occupational therapy intervention with radiation-induced brachial plexopathy. *European Journal of Cancer Care* 7(2), 88–92 (Case report).

Carpal Tunnel Syndrome

DESCRIPTION

Carpal tunnel syndrome is the name commonly given to compression neuropathies of the median nerve at the wrist. CTS comprises the largest percentage of the compression neuropathies and cumulative trauma disorders. The syndrome is usually the suspected diagnosis for any person who has hyperesthesia or paresthesia in the median nerve in the hand and/or in any person who has weakness or atrophy in the abductor pollicis brevis or opponens policis (Burke et al. 1994, 1241). CTS is not new: It was observed in 1717 by Ramazzini (Headley and Singer 1998, 21) and described by Sir James Paget in 1853 (Cicalis and Going 1995, 15).

Surgical management involves carpal tunnel release. Two techniques are common: open technique and endoscopic carpal tunnel release. The open technique is carried out using a curvilinear incision on the volar aspect of the wrist, which extends from the midpalm to about half an inch proximal to the wrist. Skin, subcutaneous tissue, palmar fascia, and the palmaris brevis have to be transected to reach the transverse carpal ligament. The endoscopic technique has two versions: the single-portal technique and the two-portal technique. Two versions of the two-portal technique are recognized: Chow technique and Resnick and Miller technique (Menon and Etter 1993, 139).

CAUSE

The cause of this syndrome is entrapment and compression of the median nerve in the volar aspect of the wrist between the longitudinal tendons of the forearm muscles that flex the hand and the transverse superficial carpal ligament. The floor of the carpal tunnel is formed by the carpal bones, and the roof is formed by the transverse carpal ligament. Eight flexor tendons for fingers and one flexor tendon for the thumb and median nerve all pass through the tunnel (Rice 1993, 38). The syndrome is more common in women and in workers with occupations that require repeated forceful wrist flexion. One or both wrists may be affected. Carpal tunnel syndrome can occur as a posttraumatic condition following a wrist or distal forearm fracture. Other causes include tumors or systemic disease. The age range of those affected is usually 40–60, but the syndrome can occur at any age.

ASSESSMENT

Areas
- daily living skills
- productivity history, skills, interests, and values
- leisure interests and skills
- range of motion
- grip and pinch tests
- muscle strength in the hand, wrist, and forearm
- hand functions
- fine motor coordination, manipulation, dexterity
- physical work tolerance, habits, patterns, and posture
- sensibility (acuity and gnosia)
- tactile sensation—light touch or pressure, two-point discrimination, stereognosis
- vibration
- temperature

Instruments
- Alderson-McGall Hand Function Questionnaire for patients with carpal tunnel syndrome: A pilot evaluation of a future outcome measure by Alderson and McGall (1999, 313–322).
- Automated Tactile Tester (ATT) by Horch, I., M. Hardy, S. Jimenez, and M. Jabaley. 1992. An Automated Tactile Tester for evaluation of cutaneous sensibility. *Journal of Hand Surgery* 17A:829–837. Tests touch-pressure, high-and low-frequency vibrations, warmth,

sharp-dull awareness, and two-point discrimination. Sensory abnormality in CTS is most easily detected by the low-frequency vibration and skin indentation tests (Jimenez et al. 1993, 128).
- Bio-Thesiometer—high-frequency vibration and temperature
- Disk-Criminator—static two-point discrimination
- dynamometer (Jamar) and pinch gauge
- Moberg Pick-Up Test by Moberg, E. 1958. Objective methods for determining the functional value of sensibility in the hand. *Journal of Bone and Joint Surgery* 40B:454–466. Modification by A.L. Dellon. 1981. Evaluation of sensibility and re-education of sensation in the hand,100–106. Baltimore, MD: Williams & Wilkins.
- Jebsen Hand Function Test. R.H. Jebsen, et al. 1969. An objective and standardized test of hand function. *Archives of Physical Medicine and Rehabilitation* 50:311–319.
- Nine-Hole Peg Test by V. Mathiowetz, K. Weber, N. Kashman, et al. 1985. Adult norms for the nine-hole peg test of finger dexterity. *Occupational Therapy Journal of Research* 5(1):24–38.
- Phalen's Sign in Phalen, G.S. 1996. The carpal tunnel syndrome: Seventeen years experience in diagnosis and treatment of 654 hands. *Journal of Bone and Joint Surgery* 48A:211–228.
- Purdue Pegboard Test by J. Tiffin. Lafayette, IN: Lafayette Instrument Co., 1948, revised 1960, 1999.
- Tinel's sign (see Percussion of the volar aspect of the wrist over the median nerve produces a tingling or prickling sensation. American Society for Surgery of the Hand. 1983. *The Hand: Examination and Diagnosis*, 2d ed., 81–83. Edinburgh, Scotland: Churchill Livingstone).
- Semmes-Weinstein Monofilaments (Bell, J.A. 1984. Light touch-deep pressure testing using Semmes-Weinstein monofilaments. In *Rehabilitation of the Hand*, 2d ed., ed. J.M. Hunter, et al., 399–406. St. Louis: C.V. Mosby).
- Southpaw Tactile Activity Kit by Southpaw Enterprises, Dayton, OH
- tuning forks, 30 cps and 256 cps
- Valpar Work Sample, Valpar Corporation, Tucson, AZ

PROBLEMS

Self-Care
- Activities requiring use of the wrist become more difficult to perform and more painful. Examples may include knitting, writing, driving, and telephoning (Vender et al. 1998, 84).

Productivity
- The person may be unable to continue his or her job if the tasks are causative factors in the disorder. Examples might include meat cutting, hammering, or using a screwdriver.

Leisure
- The person may be unable to continue leisure activities that aggravate the disorder. Examples might include digging in a garden; making punch, hooked, or latched rugs; and knitting or other needlework.

Sensorimotor

- The person may experience clumsiness and loss of fine motor control in the use of the affected hand, including dropping things, difficulty in holding small items, and difficulty in writing.
- The person may have edema of the fingers.
- The person may develop weakness or atrophy of the thenar muscles of the thumb.
- The person may experience decreased strength of palmar abduction of the thumb.
- The person may have decreased pinch and grip strength.
- The person may have decreased range motion.
- The person may have altered sensation, such as loss of feeling, tingling, numbness, and paresthesia in the palmar or radial aspect of the first three digits, wrist, or distal forearm along the distribution of the median nerve.
- The person may have pain upon flexion of the wrist, described as tingling or burning. The pain may disrupt sleep (nocturnal pain), which is one of the most significant symptoms of CTS.

Cognitive

Cognitive faculties are not directly affected by the injury.

Psychosocial

- The person may fear losing his or her job if unable to continue performing work tasks.
- The person may fear becoming permanently disabled.
- The person may refuse some social events because of the pain.

TREATMENT/INTERVENTION

Surgery, splinting, steroid injections, and activity modification have been more successful in modifying symptoms or correcting the disorder. Antiinflammatory medication does not appear to be of significant benefit in nerve disorders (Vender et al. 1998, 83). Models used in occupational therapy include the biomechanical model and ergonomics or human factors engineering.

Self-Care

- Encourage independence in performing ADLs.

Productivity

- Discuss with the person and his or her employer, if possible, job modifications that would reduce or eliminate postures that require frequent wrist flexion and activities that require repetitive wrist movements. Tool redesign may be helpful.
- A change of occupation may be useful or necessary to a job that does not require as much forceful use of the wrist or modification of existing job tasks.
- Provide work-tolerance or work-hardening training.
- Consider recommending that the person wear a splint when at work, if the person is returning to the same or a similar job situation.

Risk Factors and Non-Risk Factors for Carpal Tunnel Syndrome

- Acute trauma—Episodes of heavy lifting or pushing may contribute to the symptoms by causing soft tissue swelling or structural alteration, such as wrist fracture or ligament injury.
- Concept of use—Use of the hands per se is not a risk factor. Lack of use is more likely to be a problem, as is use of hands and upper extremities in a stressful, forceful, or awkward manner. Other risk factors may include vibration, pressure or compression of soft tissue, and wrist posture. The use is not related to employment versus unemployment, but to the manner of use.
- Deconditioning—Lack of fitness and general body conditioning seems to contribute to CTS.
- Deficit or lack of activity—Symptoms of CTS may appear initially but usually disappear when activity level increases.
- Developmental abnormalities—An unusually small cross-sectional area of the carpal tunnel may contribute to CTS. Abnormalities of tendons and muscle bellies may be related.
- Health habits—Obesity, alcoholism, and smoking seem to predispose a person to CTS.
- Preexisting disease—Diabetes, rheumatoid arthritis, and hypothyroidism may predispose a person to CTS. Gout, pseudogout, and tuberculosis can cause synovitis in the carpal tunnel.
- Repetitiveness—Repetition is not per se the problem because many methods of conditioning and maintenance of health activities require repetition, such as running, stair climbing, bicycling, or weight lifting. The pattern of use and medical conditions must be considered.
- Work setting— "if only work is considered, then only work will be found as the cause." Other factors should also be considered, such as lifestyle, habits of upper extremity use, and medical conditions.

Source: Data from M.I. Vender, et al., Upper Extremity Compressive Neuropathies, *Physical Medicine and Rehabilitation: State of the Art Reviews*, 1998, Vol. 12, No. 2, pp. 243–62; and V.J. Rice, Carpal Tunnel Syndrome: Can Prevention Be Brought? *Advance in Rehabilitation for Directors,* © 1993, Vol. 2, No. 6, p. 38.

Leisure
- Explore with the person whether some leisure interests may be contributing factors to CTS and need to be modified or discontinued.
- Encourage the person to explore and develop new interests.

Sensorimotor
- Increase the person's hand strength through the use of graded activities.
- Consider a static volar splint. Burke et al. (1994, 1241–1244) found that splinting in the neutral wrist position provided the most symptom relief, as opposed to splinting the wrist in

10–20 degrees of wrist extension (dorsal flexion) for 2 weeks. Note: The splint must be considered in relation to the person's hand use and symptoms. If the person will have to fight against the splint to perform a job, some other portion of the upper extremity will likely become involved. Likewise, if the person does not have night pain, a splint should not be worn at night (Vender 1998, 86). Despite the Burke finding, splinting in wrist extension is still illustrated and recommended by various authors (Margulies 1993, 17).

- Provide dexterity and coordination training.
- Maintain joint mobility through activities (crafts, games, cooking, etc.) that include flexion and extension of the wrist, circumduction of the wrist, opening and closing the hand, extending the thumb, and opposing the thumb and little finger.
- Use tendon-gliding exercises (Rozmaryn et al. 1998, 171–179 or Wehbe, 1987).
- Control edema after surgery using elevation and massage.
- Nerve gliding exercises may be needed after surgery.
- Use shoulder exercises to maintain range of motion. (Note: Persons with CTS may protect the wrist by not moving the arm, leaving the shoulder subject to inactivity.)
- Prevent adhesions after surgery.
- Provide sensory retraining, if necessary.

Cognitive
- Learn about the disorder and what activities aggravate the condition so that such activities can be avoided or reduced to a minimum, such as avoiding repetitive wrist flexion and extension motions, and pinching or gripping objects while the wrist is flexed.
- Learn joint protection concepts, such as lifting a box using the palms of the hands instead of the fingers.
- Instruct the person in activity modification to assist in symptom control, such as decreasing the amount of time spent in static holding positions, reducing extended reaching, and reducing ulnar deviation of the hand.

Psychosocial
- Encourage the person to express his or her feelings.
- Provide an opportunity for improving his or her self-image through creative activities, such as crafts, drama, and music.
- Encourage the person to participate in social activities.

Environment
- Split keyboards may be helpful for keyboard operators.
- Encourage the person to change positions frequently.
- Place frequently used tools within functional reach.
- Workstations should have adjustable features so that each can be adapted to the individual user, rather than the user being forced to adapt to the workstation.
- Arm rests may be useful to decrease the load on the neck and back musculature.
- Wrist supports may be helpful but the person should watch the amount of pressure applied to the wrist through the wrist support.

Treatment Schedule for Carpal Tunnel Repair

Week 0: Person is instructed in edema control by elevation of the hand above the heart, retrograde massage, and application of ice.

Weeks 1–3: Hand is immobilized in a volar splint for two weeks.

Week 2: Person is instructed in active range of motion exercises for entire upper extremity and three tendon glide exercises (the hook, the full fist, and the straight fist, followed by full finger extension). The goal is to perform the exercises 3 times per day, 10 repetitions each, but the number is increased slowly to avoid tenosynovitis. Complications such as reflex sympathetic dystrophy and infections are also explained.

Week 3: Variable, depending on person's recovery rate. Considerations include edema control, wound care, scar management, and need for nerve gliding exercises (3 times per day, 10 repetitions).

Source: Data from J. Menon and C. Etter, Endoscopic Carpal Tunnel Release-Current Status, *Journal of Hand Therapy*, 1993, Vol. 6, No. 2, p. 143.

PRECAUTIONS

- The symptoms leading to a diagnosis of CTS can be present in several other hand conditions. Careful diagnosis is important. The public is aware of CTS, and individuals may claim to have CTS when, in fact, another condition is present or coexists, such as cervical radiculopathy or de Quervain's tenosynovitis.
- Electrodiagnostic studies, such as electromyogram/nerve conduction studies (EMG/NCS), are the gold standard for verification of CTS. However, such studies are subject to many variables affecting reliability, including hand temperature, age, adherence to recognized standards, and the skill and experience of the examiner (Vender et al. 1998, 85). Occupational therapy personnel should be knowledgeable about the skills of the person doing the interpretation of the EMG/NCS and/or should seek expert medical opinion before assuming that the disorder is actual CTS.
- If a splint is applied, check to see that the splint maintains the normal hand arches and creases to permit fingers to bend but at the same time limits the thumb and wrist, and check for any redness or pressure sores at the wrist or thumb.
- Wrist supports should be worn only as part of a medically prescribed program.
- Warn the person that overuse may lead to tenosynovitis.
- Be aware of coexisting problems such as diabetes or low vision, which can require modifications to the treatment of CTS (Aquilante et al. 1996, 316–318).

PROGNOSIS AND OUTCOME

- Usually, the person is able to return to normal activities at about 3 weeks.
- The person is able to perform ADLs independently.

- The person is able to perform productive activities. Note: This outcome has many confounding variables, such as type of work, the motivation of the individual, chance of financial gain, availability of sick leave, and work location in the home (housework) or outside the home (Menon and Etter 1993, 143).
- The person is able to perform leisure activities.
- The person demonstrates normal hand strength, considering age, sex, and type of work.
- The person demonstrates improved hand grip, including pinch and grasp.
- The person demonstrates functional range of motion at the wrist and in fingers and thumb.
- The person demonstrates dexterity and coordination with the involved hand alone or bilaterally.
- The person has sensory awareness and discrimination in the hand.
- The person does not report postoperative pain or is pain free.

REFERENCES

Alderson, M. and D. McGall. 1999. The Alderson-McGall Hand Function Questionnaire for patients with carpal tunnel syndrome: A pilot evaluation of a future outcome measure. *Journal of Hand Therapy* 12(4):313–322.

Aquilante, K., T. Kern, and A. Coutney. 1996. Long-cane modification for carpal tunnel syndrome: A case report. *Journal of the American Optometry Association* 67(6):316–318.

Burke, D.T., M.M. Burke, G.W. Stewart, and A. Cambre. 1994. Splinting for carpal tunnel syndrome: In search of the optimal angle. *Archives of Physical Medicine and Rehabilitation* 75(11):1241–1244.

Cicalis, J. and T. Going. 1995. Carpal tunnel syndrome and return to work. *Occupational Therapy Forum* 10(5):14–17, 20–21.

Headley, B. and G. Singer. 1998. Carpal tunnel syndrome: Making the right diagnosis. *Advance for Occupational Practitioners* 4(14): 18, 21–22, 30.

Jimenez, S., M.A. Hardy, K. Horch, and M. Jabaley. 1993. A study of sensory recovery following carpal tunnel syndrome. *Journal of Hand Therapy* 6(2):124–129.

Margulies, J. 1993. Splinting for carpal tunnel syndrome. *Occupational Therapy Forum* 8(17):17.

Menon, J. and C. Etter. 1993. Endoscopic carpal tunnel release: Current status. *Journal of Hand Therapy* 6(2):139–144.

Rice, V.J. 1993. Carpal tunnel syndrome: Can prevention be brought? *Advance in Rehabilitation for Directors* 2(6);37–42.

Rozmaryn, L.M., S. Dovell, E.F. Rothman, K. Gorman, K.M. Olvey, and J.J. Bartko. 1998. Nerve and tendon gliding exercises and the conservative management of carpal tunnel syndrome. *Journal of Hand Therapy* 11(3):171–179.

Vender, M.I., K.L. Truppa, J.R. Ruder, and J. Pomerance. 1998. Upper extremity compressive neuropathies. *Physical Medicine and Rehabilitation: State of the Art Reviews* 12(2):243–262.

Wehbe, M.A. 1987. Tendon gliding exercises. *American Journal of Occupational Therapy* 41(3):164–167.

BIBLIOGRAPHY

Colan, B.J. 1996. Carpal tunnel syndrome: Ripping away the mask. *Advance for Occupational Therapists* 12(26):15–16.

Courts, R.B. 1995. Splinting for symptoms of carpal tunnel syndrome during pregnancy. *Journal of Hand Therapy* 8(1):31–34.

King, P.M. 1997. Sensory function assessment: A pilot comparison study of touch pressure threshold with texture and tactile discrimination. *Journal of Hand Therapy* 10(1):24–28.

Lalwani, P. 1996. Helping hands: Hand therapy for CTS. *Team Rehab Report* 7(4):40–43.

Ludlow, K.S., J,L. Merla, J.A. Cox, and L.N. Hurst. 1997. Pillar pain as a postoperative complication of carpal tunnel release: A review of the literature. *Journal of Hand Therapy* 10(4):277–282.

Marmer, L. 1996. The Washburn approach: An alternative to CT surgery. *Advance for Occupational Therapists* 12(3):12–13,50.

Peterson, M.L. 1997. Preventative education for the resources of carpal tunnel syndrome. *Journal of Occupational Therapy Students* 25–28.

Rosman, D.L. 1997. *Occupational Therapy Practice Guidelines for Adults with Carpal Tunnel Syndrome.* Bethesda, MD: American Occupational Therapy Association.

Skoff, H.D. and R. Sklar. 1994. Endoscopic median nerve decompression: Early experience. *Plastic and Reconstructive Surgery* 94:691–694.

Yoshida, T., H. Daikoku, H. Yamamoto, S. Saitoh, and H. Saitoh. 1993. A flexible dorsal wrist splint. *Journal of Hand Therapy* 6(4):323–325.

Cumulative Trauma Disorders

DESCRIPTION

Cumulative trauma disorder (CTD) is an umbrella term that describes a variety of diagnostic conditions involving soft-tissue structures, such as tendons, tendon sheaths, nerves, muscles and blood vessels. CTD can be characterized as (1) involving both mechanical and physiologic mechanisms, (2) affected by the intensity and duration of work, (3) related to a short, repetitive work cycle, to static work performed in an uncomfortable position or to a stressful work environment, (4) symptoms that tend to be poorly localized, nonspecific, and episodic, (5) insidious development that may occur after weeks, months, or years, and (6) slow recuperation that may require weeks, months, or years (Sanders 1997, 23–24). The soft-tissue injuries may be diagnosed as tendinitis, ganglionitis, bursitis, tenosynovitis, epicondylitis, peritendinitis, entrapment, compression, cervical syndromes, and myofascial pain. Others terms include *occupational cervicobrachial disorder* (OCD), *overuse syndrome, regional musculoskeletal disorder, repetitive strain injury* (RSI), *repetitive trauma disorders*, and *work-related disorders*. Sanders (1997, 25) and Fast (1995, 121) include the following conditions:

- Neck and shoulder problems
  1. Bicipital tendinitis
  2. Supraspinatus tendinitis
  3. Tension neck syndrome
  4. Thoracic outlet syndrome
- Elbow and forearm problems
  1. Cubital tunnel syndrome
  2. Lateral epicondylitis
  3. Medical epicondylitis
  4. Pronator teres syndrome

    5. Radial tunnel syndrome
    6. Tenosynovitis of the forearm muscles
- Wrist and hand problems
    1. Anterior interosseous syndrome
    2. Carpal tunnel syndrome—see earlier section
    3. de Quervain's syndrome
    4. Gamekeeper's thumb
    5. Ganglion cyst
    6. Guyon's tunnel syndrome
    7. Hand-arm vibration syndrome (Raynaud's syndrome or phenomenon, white finger)
    8. Hypothenar hammer syndrome
    9. Trigger digit

CAUSE

The exact cause or causes are unknown. Failure of cross-linkages within and between microfibrils in collagen molecules is considered a possible cause, as is excess loading of tendons (Lubaln et al. 1998, 466). The cause is likely to be multifactorial, involving personal, work-related and non–work-related factors. Fisher (1998, 297) and Kasch (1996, 681) list seven risk factors: high repetition, high force, awkward joint posture, direct pressure, vibration, prolonged static positioning, and insufficient rest. Occupation may be a causative factor. Performing artists such as musicians are an example (Dillinger [1997, 122] and Jacobs [1995, 121]). Other workers with high risk are waitresses; office workers; installers of overhead items, such as ceilings and light fixtures; fruit pickers; and some assembly jobs (Fisher 1998, 297). Factors cited by King (1995, 52), Howard and Derebery (1998, 98), Fast (1995, 121), and Melnik (1996, 149) include:
- Gender. Women are affected more often than men.
- Age. Body tissues may "wear out" and conduction through the median nerve may slow.
- Nutrition. Obesity is considered a risk factor for CTDs. Fluid retention from any systemic cause may increase symptoms.
- Strength. Greater upper body strength may protect some persons from CTDs.
- Medical history of trauma, previous injury, or reduced peripheral blood supply.
- Medical conditions, including diabetes, thyroid conditions, pregnancy, hormone therapy, and tumors.
- Environmental risks. Rapid work pace, leading to increased musculature tension in the hands and arms. Other work-related problems include extreme extension and flexion of the wrist, forceful pinching, gripping and manipulations greater than 2,000 times per hour, and use of vibratory hand tools.
- Sociologic and political risks. Labor and management relations, supervisor and supervisee relations, economic climate, the company's "bottom line."
- Physical stature. Small anatomical structures may predispose some people to injury.

ASSESSMENT
- Have the person list and describe his or her job tasks in detail. Having the person simulate specific job tasks may also be useful in clarifying problem areas.

Areas

- daily living skills
- productivity history, interests, values, and skills
- leisure interests, values, and skills
- functional range of motion of the upper extremities, active and passive
- functional muscle strength
- gross grasp and pinch strength
- edema
- fine motor coordination, manipulation, and dexterity
- work positions, posture, and movements
- sensibility, including tactile/touch and proprioception
- pain
- skin temperature
- sleep positions
- environments at home and work

Instruments

Instruments Developed by Occupational Therapy Personnel

- *Canadian Occupational Performance Measure*, 2nd ed., by Law, M. S. Baptiste, A. Carsell, M.A. McColl, H. Polatajko, and N. Pollock. 1994. Ottawa, Ontario, Canada: Canadian Association of Occupational Therapists.

Instruments Developed by Other Professionals and Used by Occupational Therapy Personnel

- *Crawford Small Parts Dexterity Test* by Crawford, J.E. and D.M. Crawford. 1956. San Antonio, TX: The Psychological Corporation, revised 1981.
- dynamometer and pinch meter—hand and pinch strength
- goniometry—joint motion and method of measuring and recording measurement by the American Academy of Orthopaedic Surgeons. Chicago, IL: The Academy, 1965.
- *LLUMC* (Loma Linda University Medical Center) *Activity Sort* by Work Evaluation Systems Technology. 1992. Long Beach, CA: WEST.
- manual muscle testing—muscle strength
- *Minnesota Manual Dexterity Test* by University of Minnesota Employment Stabilization Research Institute. 1969. Lafayette IN: Lafayette Instrument Company.
- *Minnesota Rate of Manipulation Test,* by University of Minnesota Employment Stabilization Research Institute. 1969. Circle Pines, MN: American Guidance Services.
- Moberg Pick-Up Test by Moberg, E. 1958. Objective methods for determining the functional value of sensibility in the hand. *Journal of Bone and Joint Surgery* 40B(3):454–476.
- Numerical Rating Scales by Jensen, L.B., L.A. Bradley, and S.J. Linton. 1989. Validation of an observation method of pain assessment in non-chronic back pain. *Pain* 29:267–274.
- Phalen's sign—wrist is held in maximum flexion for at least one minute (positive when pain or paresthesia is elicited).
- provocative testing, such as Tinel's sign—rules out compression syndromes
- Purdue Pegboard Test by J. Tiffin, Lafayette, IN: Lafayette Instruments, 1948, revised 1960, 1999.

- Semmes-Weinstein Calibrated Monofilaments. See Bell, J.A. 1987. The repeatability of testing with Semmes-Weinstein monofilaments. *Journal of Hand Surgery* [monograph] or Bell-Krotoski, J.A. 1990. Light touch-deep pressure-testing using Semmes-Weinstein monofilaments. *Rehabilitation of the Hand*, 3rd ed. ed. J.M. Hunter, et al., 585–593. St. Louis: C.V. Mosby).
- Sollerman Hand Function Test. By Sollerman, C. and A. Ejeskär. 1995. Sollerman hand function test: A standardized method and its use in tetraplegic patients. *Scandinavian Journal of Plastic Reconstructive Surgery and Hand Surgery* 29(2):167–176.
- Tinel's sign—percussion along the route of a nerve (positive when pain or hypersensitivity is elicited)
- tuning forks—30 and 256 Hz
- Visual Analogue Scale (VAS) by Huskinsson, E.C. 1974. Measurement of pain. *Lancet* 2(1):1127–1131.
- vibration—256-Hz tuning fork or vibrometer with a fixed frequency (120 Hz) and a variable amplitude, such as the Bio-Thesiometer by Bio-Medical Instrument Co., Newbury, OH.
- Von Frey monofilament testing
- volumetry—edema testing
- Two-point discrimination testing—Disk-Criminator or asthesiometer
- Weinstein Enhanced Sensory Test by Schulz, L.A. et al. 1998. Normal digit tip values for the Weinstein Enhanced Sensory Test (WEST). *Journal of Hand Therapy* 11(3):200–205.
- *West Tool Sort*, 3rd ed. by Work Evaluation Systems Technology. 1992. Long Beach, CA: WEST. Note: Dellon and Keller (1997, 493) discuss computerized testing for strength and sensory tests.

PROBLEMS

Self-Care
- The person may be unable to perform some ADLs because of pain, loss of hand function, or loss of sensation.

Productivity
- The person may have started a new job recently, been assigned additional work, or be working overtime, all of which may increase the workload and work time beyond the person's conditioning.
- The person may be unable to continue performing certain job tasks because of permanent disability.
- The person may be able to continue working only if performance requirements are changed or modifications in the work environment are made.
- The person may need vocational retraining to perform a different job.
- The person may suffer financial loss if not covered by workers' compensation or medical insurance, or if coverage is exhausted.

Leisure
- Participation in some sports or hobbies may contribute to or cause the CTD, especially if they require forceful or awkward movements or static postures and positions.

- The person may be unable to engage in leisure activities that require similar motions or body positions as those related to the cumulative trauma disorder.

Sensorimotor
- The person may have spasms, readiness swelling, or atrophy in the muscles.
- The person may have tenderness in the joints.
- The person may have changes in two-point discrimination, reflexes, and grip strength. Ability to alternate grip and release rapidly on the dynamometer suggests nonorganic cause of CTD.
- The person may have paresthesia or migratory pain that does not follow known anatomical distribution. CTD may be due to nonorganic cause.
- The person may have muscle fatigue that occurs more quickly with high force.
- The person may have inflammation of the tendon (tendinitis). (Tendon may become thickened, bumpy, or irregular. Some fibers may fray or tear apart.)
- The person may have excessive synovial fluid accumulation in the tendon sheath (tenosynovitis).
- The person may have constriction of the tendon sheath (de Quervain's disease).
- The person may have soreness or pain in the forearm or elbow (epicondylitis).
- The person may have burning or tingling pain in the shoulders (rotator cuff tendinitis).
- The person may have numbness, tingling, or "pins and needles" sensations in the hands or fingers that do not necessarily follow particular dermatomal or myotomal patterns (CTS or thoracic outlet syndrome).
- The person may have pale or ashen skin with intermittent numbness and tingling in the fingers (Raynaud's phenomenon).
- The person may have numbness or tingling in the elbow (ulnar neuritis).
- The person may have pain to extensor portion of the forearm or lateral epicondyle when resistance is applied to middle finger extension (radial tunnel syndrome).
- The person may have ulnar neuritis at the elbow (Howard and Derebery 1998, 99).

Cognition
- Cognitive faculties are not affected directly by CTD but cognitive concerns may contribute to CTD, especially when accompanied by psychological and emotional reactions.

Psychosocial
- The person may be dissatisfied with job, which can add to stress.
- The person may be concerned about job security, which may affect job performance.
- The person may have conflicts with the supervisor, which may add to stress.
- The person may fear being unable to work.
- The person may become angry or hostile about being unable to work.
- The person may become depressed after injury or depression may have contributed to the injury by decreasing person's attention and concentration.
- The person may be vindictive against employer for creating the situation in which the person was injured.
- The person may lose feeling of self-worth.
- The person may have poor coping skills to deal with injury.
- The pain may reduce effectiveness of judgment.

Considerations in the Physical Demands of a Job

- Lifting—weight to be lifted in pounds, size of the load in cubic inches, frequency of lifts per time unit, range through which objects are lifted in inches, use of two-hand (bilateral) lifts versus one-hand (unilateral)
- Carrying—weight to be carried in pounds, size of the load in cubic inches, frequency of carrying per time unit, distance through which objects are carried, two-handed versus one-handed carry, position of extremities in relation to the body, hand grasp pattern
- Reaching—range of reach in inches from the body horizontally, vertically, and diagonally, arc of reaching range in degrees, and frequency of reach per unit of time
- Pushing-pulling—position of body, frequency of push-pull per unit of time, two-handed versus one-handed
- Grasping—type of grasp required, repetitions of grasp per unit of time, position of hand in relation to wrist and arm

Source: Data from L.A. Bruening and D. Beaulieu, The Return to Work Phase for the Patient with Cumulative Trauma, in *Rehabilitation of the Hand*, 3rd ed., J.M. Hunter, E.J. Mackin, and A.D. Callahan, eds., p. 1194, © 1990, C.V. Mosby.

- The person may have a tendency to guard injured or painful body part.
- The person may make excuses for not participating in social activities because of pain or fatigue.

Environment
- Business may provide little protection for the worker and appear to be more interested in cost controls and profits.

TREATMENT/INTERVENTION
A multidisciplinary team is often used, which may include the physician, nurse, physical therapist, hand therapist (who may be an occupational therapist), employer, rehabilitation counselor, injured person, and occupational therapy personnel. In addition, treatment frequently is coordinated by workers' compensation or a private insurance company. Knowledge of workers' compensation regulations is important. Models of treatment in occupational therapy include the biomechanical model, behavior modification (operant conditioning), work stimulation testing and training, client-centered model, ergonomics or human factors engineering, and wellness education and chronic pain model.

Self-Care
- Gradually increase the person's performance of self-care and daily living activities.

Productivity
- Analyze the job duties and work site to make recommendations for job and tool modifications, if possible. An on-site job evaluation, videotaping, and photographs of the job as it is performed may be helpful.
- If the person's return to his or her present job is not possible, encourage management to provide alternate job placements and/or the person to explore other vocational interests.
- For mild CTD, the person can be treated on the job.
- If the person has already been off work, he or she may need or benefit from a work-hardening program before returning to the work setting.
- Any program or recommendations for a person at a work site need to be discussed with the employer to encourage the employer's support to assist the person with follow-through. The person is likely to get better results if the employer cooperates (Furth et al. 1994, 896–897).

Leisure
- The person may need to modify or, in rare instances, discontinue some leisure activities.
- Assist person in deciding how to manage or change performance of leisure interests. The same principles of pain control, ergonomics, and other models apply to leisure as they do for work.

Sensorimotor
- Reduce physiologic stresses due to positioning, force, intensity, repetition, etc. Biofeedback may be useful to help the person recognize tension and reduce the triggers.
- Improve posture in sitting and standing through use of videotaping, biofeedback, mirrors, and proprioceptive exercises.
- Encourage aerobic exercise and high-force, low-repetition activities, especially if the person has a high-repetition, low-force job, such as keyboarding (Derebery and Howard 1998, 219).
- Increase range of motion using stretching exercises for 1–2 minutes at a time to decrease tightness and discomfort (Derebery and Howard 1998, 220).
- During active use, limiting range of motion may be desirable, such as having person wear a tennis-elbow armband over the extensor muscle bellies to limit full excursion of the muscle (Kasch 1996, 681).
- Strengthening exercises should focus on the gross motor musculature using weight training 3 times a week for 10 minutes (Derebery and Howard 1998, 219–220).
- When using progressive resistive exercise, the resistance should be given at the end of the range (Kasch 1996, 681).
- Decrease edema and swelling.
- Reduce inflammation and pain by using icing, contrast baths, ultrasound phonophoresis, and interferential and high-voltage electrical stimulation (Kasch 1996, 681).
- Decrease muscle tightness in the hand using rubber or tennis ball exercises to squeeze and release. For fingers, rubber bands can be used.
- Improve posture and positioning using ergonomic principles to examine workstation and by recommending changes.
- Decrease the force while repetitions are maintained and provide adequate recovery time to reduce potential harm (Kasch 1996, 681)

- If a splint is used, the position should be neutral at the wrist. The splint should be removed three times a day for stretching the affected musculature to maintain or increase muscle length and avoid joint stiffness (Kasch 1996, 681).
- Increase endurance and work tolerance with aerobic conditioning, such as walking, running, biking, or using a ski machine 30 minutes at a time 3–5 days per week (Derebery and Howard 1998, 219).
- If person smokes, encourage person to stop.
- Desensitize hypersensitivity, if present.
- Reduce pain through use of paraffin bath, fluid therapy, whirlpool, heat packs, or other heat modality.
- Encourage activity that increases circulation to increase the pain threshold (Frost and Stricoff 1996, 1).
- If sleeping positions are contributing factors, work with person to change sleeping patterns.
- Stretch and strengthen the ulnar innervated muscles.
- Ulnar nerve glide exercise is done by positioning the shoulder in slight abduction, elbow in full flexion, and wrist in full extension.
- Padding at the elbow may be indicated to prevent direct pressure to the cubital tunnel.

Radial Tunnel Syndrome (Howard and Derebery 1998, 99, 100)
- Radial nerve guide exercise is done by positioning the shoulder in 80–90 degrees of abduction, fully extending the elbow, supinating the forearm, and radially deviating the wrist. The finger should curl naturally.

Thoracic Outlet Symptom/Syndrome (Howard and Derebery 1998, 99, 100)
- Deep tissue massage.
- Traction to release the compressed neurovascular bundle.
- Stretching exercises.
- A tennis ball may be used to perform acupressure for home relief.

Tendinitis (Howard and Derebery 1998, 99, 100)
- Decrease inflammation.
- Increase conditioning of the extremity.
- Reduce forearm or hand muscle spasm.
- Roll a tennis ball over the dorsal aspect of the forearm while extending and flexing the wrist to reduce the spasm.

Epicondylitis (Howard and Derebery 1998, 102)
- Regular exercise should include forearm and wrist stretching.
- Use of a tennis ball may be helpful in reducing muscle spasm.
- Icing affected muscles while on stretch helps to reduce spasms.

Vibration Syndrome (Howard and Derebery 1998, 102)
- Person should learn to avoid cold temperatures.
- If work involves prolonged and contracted muscle gripping, rest breaks, task rotation, and recognition of acceptable megahertz ranges, along with proper conditioning, can reduce symptoms.
- Person may also wear antivibratory gloves to reduce the impact.

Cognition

- Discuss all assessment findings with the person and assure the person that the condition can be corrected or alleviated and does not mean that the person will be permanently crippled (Howard and Derebery 1998, 219).
- Involve the person in the problem-solving process, such as taking note of activities at home and at work that seem to precipitate symptoms.
- Instruct the person about principles of good posture and body mechanics. Encourage muscle awareness.
- Instruct the person about energy conservation, pacing, and work-simplification concepts.
- Instruct the person in joint anatomy and joint protection principles.
- Instruct the person regarding concepts of good tool handling and machine operation.
- Instruct the person in use of stretching exercises to counteract static postures and positions, and short, tight muscles.
- A "tool box" may be used that includes a relaxation tape, written exercises, and educational literature (Frost and Stricoff 1996, 2).
- Instruct the person in a home exercise program.
- Instruct the person in the use of antivibration gloves, wrist supports, adapted work station or tools, and adapted computer keyboards, if these are prescribed or recommended.
- Instruct the person in new work habits, such as taking frequent rest breaks from repetitive tasks, exercising, and changing positions frequently. Support of the forearms and back when seated and support devices, such as forearm rests, lumbar supports, and foot rests, may also be recommended (Strause 1995, 2). Note: Strause discusses a number of different keyboards, including demiboards, which splint the keyboard into two halves, and chordal keyboards, in which a combination of seven keys is hit to form letters.
- Encourage the person to engage in aerobic exercises or activities.

Psychosocial

- Assist the person to reduce psychological stress by reducing tension through relaxation training.
- Assist the person to change negative emotions or reactions through discussion to clearly identify the problem, vent feelings, and examine possible solutions that the person might take to resolve the problem.

PRECAUTIONS

- Use of cold as a modality has produced mixed results and should be used with caution in dealing with pain. Some authors highly recommend ice, others highly recommend avoiding use of ice.
- Use of vibration is contraindicated because it may contribute to inflammatory problems (Kasch 1996, 681).
- Avoid giving the person a set number of repetitions to do. Help the person take responsibility for learning to listen and knowing his or her own body.
- Avoid forward head position, rounded shoulders with internal rotation, and wrist flexion.
- Avoid strengthening exercises that may add to fatigue and tension, especially in the distal extremity (Frost and Stricoff 1996, 2).

- Physical agent modalities, such as ultrasound, fluid therapy, and iontophoresis do not seem to be effective (Frost and Stricoff 1996, 2).
- Wearing a splint may lead to a false sense of security or the excessive force may be changed to another joint, which only adds to problems. A splint worn for a prolonged time period may contribute to atrophy, loss of mobility, and psychological dependence. Generally, wrist splints should be worn for no more than 1–2 weeks (Howard and Derebery 1998, 98).
- Be aware that CTD may be occurring because of psychological/emotional concerns of the workers and not to physical/physiologic problems. Try to locate the original source of the problem, which may not be directly observable (Howard and Derebery 1998, 98).
- Keep the number of treatment sessions to 2–6 to avoid the person becoming overly dependent on the occupational therapy services and personnel (Howard and Derebery 1998, 98).
- Avoid overreliance on modalities (Howard and Derebery 1998, 98).
- Observe signs of deconditioning or poor cardiovascular fitness. Exercise stimulates endorphin release, which increases feeling of well-being (Howard and Derebery 1998, 98).

PROGNOSIS AND OUTCOME
- The person is able to perform self-care and daily living activities independently with self-help devices, if needed.
- The person is able to perform productive activities, although a change of vocation may be necessary to avoid reinjury.
- The person is able to perform leisure activities.
- The person demonstrates normal muscle strength of the upper extremity for his or her sex, age, and occupation.
- The person demonstrates full range of motion of the upper extremity.
- The person demonstrates normal endurance.
- The person does not complain of pain in the upper extremity.
- The person demonstrates knowledge of good posture and body mechanics while performing activities.
- The person demonstrates knowledge of energy conservation and work-simplification techniques.
- Recommendations to the employer to modify the person's job or tools have been made.

REFERENCES

Dellon, A.L. and K.M. Keller. 1997. Computer-assisted quantitative sensorimotor testing in patients with carpal and cubital tunnel syndrome. *Annals of Plastic Surgery* 38(5):493–502.

Derebery, V.J. and L.L. Howard. 1998. Management of the painful arm: Cumulative trauma revised. *Physical Medicine and Rehabilitation: State of the Art Reviews* 12(2):215–224 (Case reports).

Dillinger, N.J. 1997. Experiences of professional orchestral musicians with chronic conditions. *Medical Problems of Performing Artists* 12:122–125.

Fast, C. 1995. Repetitive strain injury: An overview of the condition and its implications for occupational therapy practice. *Canadian Journal of Occupational Therapy* 62(3):119–126.

Fisher, T.F. 1998. Preventing upper extremity cumulative trauma disorders: An approach to employee wellness. *AAOHN Journal* 46(6):296–301.

Suggestions for Better Tool Design

- Bend the tool, not the wrist, to decrease the need for ulnar deviation.
- Keep the weight of the tool down when possible or provide a strap or harness to reduce the muscle strength needed to hold the tool.
- Keep the center of gravity of the tool aligned with the center of the hand grasp to reduce the unequal pull (contraction) of muscles.
- Adapt the tool to the task, rather than requiring the operator to use a general-purpose tool that does none of the tasks well.
- Design the tool for use by either hand to reduce the need for the left-handed person to adapt the body and hand to use a tool intended for right-handers.
- Handles should be designed for either power or precision grip. Power grip handles should permit the hand to wrap around the handle. Precision or pinch grip should permit the fingers to guide the action.
- Make the grip the proper size and shape. Size should be 1.25–1.75 inches and either cylindrical or oval. Flutes, ridges, or other texturing on the handle can improve torque. A T-shaped handle provides the best torque.
- Make the handle long enough—at least 4 inches—to permit the entire hand and all fingers to grip the handle. Short handles may be pressed into the palm to gain leverage and, thus, to press nerves and restrict circulation.
- Adjust the handle span for both men and women. Spans of 2.0–2.7 inches are good averages but some individuals may need larger or smaller spans to maintain maximum power.
- Form-fitted or finger-grooved handles should be examined carefully to determine whether the handles actually fit the person using the tool or fit only the tool's inventor.
- Spring-load pliers and scissors so that the tool opens automatically to reduce the pressure against the hand needed to open the tool manually.
- Make switches large enough to permit two or three fingers to start or stop the tool, thus reducing the pressure on any one finger.
- Handles should be nonporous, nonslip, and nonconductive.

Source: Data from V. Putz-Anderson, ed., *Cumulative Trauma Disorders: A Manual for Musculoskeletal Diseases of the Upper Limbs,* © 1988, Taylor & Francis.

Frost, L.D. and R. Stricoff. 1996. Respective strain injury: Is it its own diagnosis? *Physical Disabilities Special Interest Section Newsletter* 19(1):1–2.

Furth, H.J., M.B. Holm, and A. James. 1994. Reinjury prevention follow-through for clients with cumulative trauma disorders. *American Journal of Occupational Therapy* 48(10):890–898.

Howard, L.L. and V.J. Derebery. 1998. Occupational therapy and the management of cumulative trauma disorder. In *Occupational Hand and Upper Extremity Injuries and Diseases*, 2nd ed., ed. M.L. Kasdan, 97–101. Philadelphia: Hanley & Belfus (Case reports).

Jacobs, K. and K. Magglund. 1995. Musicians and overuse syndrome. *Rehab Management* 8(5):121–122.

Kasch, M.C. 1996. Cumulative trauma disorders. In *Occupational Therapy: Practice Skills for Physical Dysfunction*, 4th ed., ed. L.W. Pedretti, 681–682. St. Louis: C.V. Mosby.
King, J.W. 1995. Repetitive strain injuries. *Rehab Management* 8(2):51,52,56,58.
Lubaln, J.D., T.L. Wolfe, and M.S. DiPlacido. 1998. Team approach to rehabilitation in workers' compensation cases. In *Occupational Hand and Upper Extremity Injuries and Diseases*, 2nd ed., ed. M.L. Kasdan, 465–470. Philadelphia: Hanley & Belfus (Case reports).
Melnik, M.S. 1996. Upper extremity injury prevention. In *Industrial Therapy*, ed. G.L. Key, 148–180. St. Louis: Mosby.
Sanders, M.J. 1997. *Management of Cumulative Trauma Disorders*. Boston: Butterworth-Heinemann.
Strause, S. 1995. Cumulative trauma disorders in the workplace. *Work Programs Special Interest Section Newsletter* 9(2):1–4.

BIBLIOGRAPHY

Barthel, H.R., L.S. Miller, W.W. Deardorff, and R. Portenier. 1998. Presentation and response of patients with upper extremity repetitive use syndrome to a multidisciplinary rehabilitation program: A retrospective review of 24 cases. *Journal of Hand Therapy* 11(3)191–199 (Case reports).
Bear-Lehman, J. 1995. Upper extremity cumulative trauma disorders. In *Occupational Therapy for Physical Dysfunction*, 4th ed., ed. C.A. Trombly, 766–771. Baltimore: Williams & Wilkins.
Cederlund, R., A. Isacsson, and G. Lundbor. 1999. Hand function in workers with hand-arm vibration syndrome. *Journal of Hand Therapy* 12(1):16–24.
Kasch, M.C. 1995. Therapist's evaluation and treatment of upper extremity cumulative-trauma disorders. In *Rehabilitation of the Hand*, 4th ed., J.M. Hunter, E.J. Mackin, and A.D. Callahan, 1725–1737. St. Louis: Mosby.
Keller, K., J. Corbett, and D. Nichols. 1998. Repetitive strain injury in computer keyboard users: Pathomechanics and treatment principles in individual and group intervention. *Journal of Hand Therapy* 11(1):9–26.
Lawler, A.L., A.B. James, and G. Tomlin. 1997. Educational technique used in occupational therapy treatment of cumulative trauma disorders of the elbow, wrist, and hand. *American Journal of Occupational Therapy* 51(2):113–118.
Lindner-Tons, S. and K. Ingell. 1998. An alternative splint design for trigger finger. *Journal of Hand Therapy* 11(3):206–208.
Marks, P.H., J.J.P. Warner, and J.J. Irrgang. 1994. Rotator cuff disorders of the shoulder. *Journal of Hand Therapy* 7(2):90–98.
O'Connor, S.M. 1993. Hand therapy: Cumulative trauma disorders: Selling prevention. *OT Week* 7(31):16.
Ping, C.L.T.W., S.C.F. Keung, and P.L.W. Yee. 1996. Functional assessment of repetitive strain injuries: Two case studies. *Journal of Hand Therapy* 9(4):394–398.
Shackleton, T.L., K.L. Harburn, and S. Noh. 1997. Pilot study of upper-extremity work and power in chronic cumulative trauma disorders. *Occupational Therapy Journal of Research* 17(1):3–24.
Stahl, C. 1998. Hazardous harmony: Treatment and preventing UE injuries in musicians. *Advance for Occupational Therapists* 14(1):26, 29.
Talley, M. 1999. Vascular disorders of the hand: Therapist's commentary. *Journal of Hand Therapy* 12(2):160–163.
Walsh, M.T. 1994. Therapist management of thoracic outlet syndrome. *Journal of Hand Therapy* 7(2):131–44.
Williams, R. and M. Westmoreland. 1994. Occupational cumulative trauma disorders of the upper extremity (review). *American Journal of Occupational Therapy* 48(10):411–420.

Fractures of the Fingers

DESCRIPTION

Fractures can occur in the continuity of a bone, at the epiphyseal place, or in the cartilaginous joint surface. Fractures of the distal phalanx are the most frequent fracture (about 50%) and most often involve the thumb and middle finger. Middle phalanx fractures contribute about 10% of the total, and about 20% occur in the proximal phalanx. The remaining 20% occur in the metacarpals (Hritcko 1997, 319).

CAUSE

Common causes include industrial or work-related accidents, falls, and sports injuries.

ASSESSMENT

Areas

- daily living activities and tasks
- productivity history, skills, interests, and values
- leisure interests and skills
- occupation
- avocational interests
- hand dominance
- previous history of hand injury
- skin and nail integrity
- wound healing
- vascularity
- edema
- pain
- sensibility
- muscle strength
- range of motion
- tightness of the extrinsic and intrinsic muscles

Instruments

No specific assessment instruments were mentioned.

PROBLEMS

Sensorimotor

- Problems associated with treatment of finger fractures include scarring, decreased tendon gliding, PIP joint stiffness, and decreased range of motion at the MCP and DIP joints (Oxford 1996, 404).

TREATMENT/INTERVENTION

Treatment models in occupational therapy include the biomechanical model.

Self-Care

- Activities of daily living can provide purposeful activity to encourage gross grasp and fine motor prehension (Kearney and Brown 1994, 206).

Productivity

Work-hardening tasks can be implemented if the person is unable to meet the physical demands of his or her job (Kearney and Brown 1994, 206).

Sensorimotor

General Goals

- promote healing through maintaining/protecting reduction through immobilization splint
- maintain/increase ROM of noninvolved joints
- pain control
- edema control
- restore and maximize the functional return of the involved extremity and joint
- general complications include infection, delayed union, and malunion

Distal Phalanx—Tuft Fracture (Hritcko 1997, 321–322)

- A protective splint should be worn for 2–4 weeks until fracture site is nontender.
- Wound care depends on the injury mechanism.
- Active range of motion exercises can begin at 2–4 weeks in most cases. If the fracture is stable, exercises can begin during the first week.
- Passive range of motion (moving the finger through to the end of joint range) can begin at 5–6 weeks.
- Strength and endurance training can begin at 7–8 weeks.

Distal Phalanx—Shaft Fracture (Hritcko 1997, 322)

- A protective and immobilizing splint is worn for 3–4 weeks.
- Wound care as indicated.
- Active range of motion exercises can begin at 3–4 weeks.
- Passive range of motion can begin at 5–7 weeks.
- Strength and endurance training can begin at 8 weeks.
- Complications for distal phalanx fracture include infection, nailbed deformities, and hypersensitivity.

Middle Phalanx—Nondisplaced Fracture (Hritcko 1997, 322–323)

- Splint in "intrinsic plus" position. Immobilization should not exceed 3 weeks to avoid PIP stiffness. A buddy splint may be requested by some surgeons.
- Active range of motion exercise is initiated when pain and edema subside.
- For a stable fracture, AROM exercises can begin in 3–5 days.
- For an oblique or unstable fracture, exercises can begin at 3 weeks.
- Passive range of motion can begin at 4–6 weeks.

- Strength and endurance training can begin at 6–8 weeks.
- Complications to middle phalanx fractures include tendon adhesions and decreased excursion, and decreased joint mobility and stiffness.

Proximal Phalanx—Nondisplaced Extra-Articular Fracture (Hritcko 1997, 323)
- Splint with buddy tape.
- Begin AROM exercise immediately.
- Begin PROM at 5–7 weeks.
- Strength and endurance training can begin at 6–8 weeks.

Proximal Phalanx—Nondisplaced Intra-Articular Fracture (Hritcko 1997, 323)
- Splint in "intrinsic plus" position for 2–3 weeks.
- Active range of motion exercise can begin at 2–3 weeks.
- Passive range of motion exercise can begin at 4–8 weeks.
- Strength and endurance training can begin when clinical union is established, which usually occurs at 8–12 weeks.
- Complications for proximal phalanx fracture are stiffness and decreased joint mobility.

Distal Phalanx Fracture Postoperative Therapy (Hritcko 1997, 324)
- Shaft fractures are usually treated surgically with percutaneous K-wire for stabilization.
- Provide wound and pin care.
- Active range of motion for the PIP joint can begin in 3–5 days.
- Active range of motion for the DIP joint should begin when the K-wire is removed at 3–6 weeks.
- Protective extension splint should be worn from time of surgery to 2–6 weeks following removal of the K-wire.
- Strength and endurance training usually is initiated at 6–8 weeks.
- Complications include infection, nailbed deformities, and hypersensitivity.

Displaced Middle Phalanx Fracture (Hritcko 1997, 324)
- Surgeon may elect to stabilize the fracture site or rigidly fix the site, which will determine the type of therapy intervention.
- The hand should be splinted in the "intrinsic plus" position to support and protect the reduction site.
- Wound and pin care should be provided.
- Active range of motion should begin 5–15 days postoperatively, as specified by the surgeon, with gentle supported blocking exercise.
- Strength and endurance exercises should begin at 7–9 weeks.
- Complications include decreased tendon excursion and adhesions, stiffness, and decreased joint mobility.

Displaced Proximal Phalanx Fracture (Hritcko 1997, 324–325)
- Hand should be splinted in the "intrinsic plus" position to support and protect the reduction site.
- Wound and pin care should be provided.

- Active range of motion should be initiated at 5–15 days postoperatively, as determined by the surgeon and whether the site was rigidly fixed or stabilizing fixation was used.
- Passive range of motion can begin at 6–8 weeks.
- Strength and endurance exercises should begin at 8–10 weeks.
- Complications include associated soft tissue injuries, stiffness, and decreased joint mobility.

Intra-Articular Fractures (phalangeal fractures with articular surface involvement) (Kearney and Brown 1994, 199–209)

- Note any associated trauma present in the surrounding soft tissue or involved nerve, vascular supply, ligaments, flexor, and/or extensor tendons or the volar plate.
- Two splinting methods are commonly used. One is the *extension block splint,* which allows early active flexion of the PIP joint but prevents extension beyond a predetermined point because the joint may sublux or dislocate. Used most often for unstable volar fractures or fracture dislocations that involve 10–50% of the articular surface of the volar margin of the middle phalanx. Full extension of the PIP joint is blocked (stopped) at first, then progressively more extension is permitted as the weeks progress for 6–12 weeks of healing time. The second type of splint is a *dynamic traction splint,* using rubber band traction applied with the use of a transosseous K-wire placed transversely through the distal end of the bone immediately distal to the injured joint. In other words, if the PIP joint is injured, the wire is placed through the distal head of the middle phalanx. The traction force is called *ligamentotaxis,* which describes the traction forces exerted by the collateral ligaments and periarticular structure. The splint is composed of a splint base on the wrist and forearm, a 6-inch hoop attached to the base, which circumscribes the hand, size 19 rubber bands, transosseous wire through the digit for rubber band traction, and a moveable component with a tab on the hoop that can be changed to provide more extension or flexion as desired. The objective is to reduce the fracture fragments and maintain the reduction of any coexistent subluxation or dislocation. The fabrication of the dynamic traction splint is discussed and illustrated in the article. The splint is worn continuously for 6–8 weeks. The Chinchalker (1995a, 1995b) articles describe another splint developed for intra-articular fractures.
- After the splint is removed, range of motion and strength are increased.
- Serial casting may be used to obtain further range of motion for 2 weeks or longer. Casting is useful in reducing PIP and DIP soft-tissue contractures. A night case, such as the Dynamic Digit Extensor Tube (AliMed, Inc., Dedham, MA), may be used to maintain extension.
- Edema management should begin immediately with elevation. As healing permits, retrograde massage, wrapping with Coban (3M, St. Paul, MN) and elasticized finger sleeves, compression garments, such as the Jobst Cryotemp (Jobst Institute, Inc., Toledo, OH), which combines cold with intermittent pressure, or an inflatable air splint may be used.
- Scar management is influenced by movement, positioning, and pressure. An elastomer-type material, molded to the scar and changed as the scar changes, is useful. The material may be held in place with Coban to provide additional pressure. Active range of motion and mobilization of the scar and tissue assist in preventing adhesions and help to remodel scar tissue.
- Active range of motion exercises for all joints not limited by splinting or casting should begin immediately.
- Mobilization of joint just proximal and distal to the fracture site should begin when the fracture is stable. Continuous passive motion (CPM) is advocated by some surgeons and

therapists to reduce the detrimental effects of intra-articular adhesions and extra-articular contraction. Some persons find the "fixed" end range of motion and constant rate and force more reassuring than manual PROM (206). The CPM program is begun 3–4 times daily for 15–30 minutes, then increased in frequency and duration up to 8–24 hours daily from 1 to 3 weeks. See Kearney and Brown (1994, 207) for a chart of models of CPM units, their advantages, and their disadvantages.

- Active range of motion for the injured joint usually begins after 3 weeks of immobilization. The initial AROM exercises should be light, repetitive, and done frequently through the day. "Active range of motion and joint mobilization may be initiated earlier than end-range passive motion, because they are less stressful" (Kearney and Brown 1994, 206).
- Tendon guide exercises can be used to increase AROM, decrease edema, and decrease adhesions by providing maximum tendon excursion in relation to the bone. Both flexion and extension glide exercises should be used.
- Clinical activities or ADLs can be used to progress from gross grasp to fine motor prehension.
- Desensitization may be beneficial for DIP injuries. Lotion, graded materials and particle textures, and tapping or vibration may be used.
- Active motion tasks can be used to progress from light prehension to the addition of light resistance through the use of soft silicone putty, some settings of the BTE Work Simulation (Baltimore Therapeutic Equipment Co, Hanover, MD) or Lido Workset (Loredan Biomedical Inc, Davis, CA).
- Complications include limited passive and active joint mobility, adhesions, soft-tissue and joint contractures, instability, and persistent pain or edema.

Cognitive

- The person should be provided with specific written and verbal instruction regarding the splint, wearing time, changes in traction position for the dynamic splint, and proper care.
- The person should be given a written home exercise program.

Psychosocial

- Assist the person to have realistic expectations about the outcome of therapy based on the injury, surgery performed, if any, and therapy program (Russell 1999, 121).
- Allow the person to talk about concerns and prepare him or her for possible additional surgeries (Russell 1999, 121).

PRECAUTIONS

- Watch for associated concomitant soft tissue injury to the tendon or neurovascular structures.
- Watch for fracture stability that is influenced by the type of fracture, the rate of health, and the pain level.
- Watch for signs of nonunion or delayed union of fracture site.
- Intra-articular PIP joint fractures and metacarpal (MC) shaft fractures of the little finger are the most difficult currently to deal with effectively because of stiffness, continued pain, and cosmetic factors (Russell 1999, 122).

PROGNOSIS/OUTCOMES

- The person has a solid fracture union of finger bone.
- The person has healthy soft tissue.
- The person has full range of motion.
- The person has muscle strength sufficient to permit return to previous level of function.
- The person is pain free.

REFERENCES

Chinchalker, S.J., S.D. Patterson, D.C. Ross, and C.A. Weeks. 1995a. Results of dynamic traction and early mobilization of MCP and IP intra-articular fractures. *Journal of Hand Therapy* 8(1):50–1 (abstract).

Chinchalker, S.J., D. Ross, R.S. Richards, G.D. King, J.H. Roth, J. Laxamana, and M. LeBlanc. 1995b. Proceedings: The American Society of Hand Therapists: Management of MCP and IP joint peri- and intra-articular fractures using ORIF, dynamic traction, and early mobilization. *Journal of Hand Therapy* 8(1):49–50 (abstract).

Hritcko, G. 1997. Finger fracture rehabilitation. In *Hand Rehabilitation: A Practical Guide*. 2nd ed., ed. G.L. Clark, E.F.S. Wilgis, B. Aiello, D. Eckhaus, and L.V. Eddington, 319–328. New York: Churchill Livingstone.

Kearney, L.M. and K.K. Brown. 1994. The therapist's management of intra-articular fractures. *Hand Clinics* 10(2):199–209.

Oxford, K.L. 1996. Fracture bracing for proximal phalanx fractures. *Journal of Hand Therapy* 9(4):404–405.

Russell, C.R. 1999. Bone and joint injury in the hand: Therapist's commentary. *Journal of Hand Therapy* 12(2):121–122.

BIBLIOGRAPHY

Colditz, J.C. 1995. Functional fracture bracing. In *Rehabilitation of the Hand*, 4th ed., ed. J.M. Hunter, E.J. Mackin, and A.D. Callahan, 395–406. St. Louis: Mosby.

Fractures of the Wrist and Forearm

DESCRIPTION

The most common fracture of the forearm is to the distal end of the radius (Colles' fracture). A Colles' fracture occurs when the dorsal trabecular bone of the distal radius impacts into itself, resulting in angulation and shortening (Abrams et al. 1995, 89). The fracture is transverse and located about 1.5 inches from the radiocarpal joint (Barr 1994, 746). Presently, if the fracture site is extra-articular (not involving the articular portion of the bone), if the fragment is not comminuted, and if the fragment is pointing dorsally with the proximal portion of the fragment volar (apex of angulation is palmar), the fracture is called a *Colles' fracture*. If the displaced distal fragment points volar with the apex of angulation dorsal, the fracture is called a *Smith fracture* (Reiss 1995, 337). If either the dorsal or the volar articular margin of the radius is involved, the fracture is called a *Barton's fracture* (Reiss 1995, 337). Usually, the person presents with pain, tenderness, and swelling of the wrist. Colles' fracture was named for Abraham Colles, who first described the condition in 1814.

Other types of fractures to the wrist and forearm involve the ulna and carpal bones. Complex fractures involve the articular surfaces of the radius, ulna, and carpal bones.

Fractures of the distal radius can be divided into eight groups, using the Frykman classification system (Laseter and Carter 1996, 114; Reiss 1995, 338). Other classification systems are discussed and illustrated in Laseter and Carter (1996, 115–116).

I. Extra-articular (no involvement of the articular joint surface) distal radial fracture without distal ulnar styloid fracture

II. Extra-articular distal radial fracture with distal ulnar styloid fracture

III. Intra-articular distal radial fracture involving the radiocarpal joint without distal ulna fracture

IV. Intra-articular distal fracture involving the radiocarpal joint with distal ulna fracture

V. Intra-articular distal radial fracture involving the distal radioulnar joint without distal ulna fracture

VI. Intra-articular distal radial fracture involving the distal radioulnar joint with distal ulna fracture

VII. Intra-articular distal radial fracture involving both radiocarpal and distal radioulnar joint without distal ulnar fracture

VIII. Intra-articular distal radial fracture involving both radiocarpal and distal radioulnar joint with distal ulnar fracture

CAUSE

Typically, the cause of these fractures, especially a Colles' fracture, is falling on the extended or outstretched hand or a force of impact against the hand, as in an automobile accident. Usually, the person is an older female. Sports injuries, including crush injuries, are also possible causes.

ASSESSMENT

Assessment should concentrate on (1) determining the person's ability and skill in performing activities with the involved arm or exploring compensatory methods until function is restored and (2) preventing recurrent falls through analysis and correction of unsafe situations.

Areas

- daily living activities, including ADLs and instrumental ADLs
- range of motion, especially of the shoulder and digits
- hand functions—grasp, pinch, precision movement
- muscle strength
- edema
- structural alignment of bone and joint
- pain

- sensibility, functional
- skin sensitivity

Instruments

Note: Reiss (1995, 339) provides several interview questions and observations by the therapist for persons with Colles' fractures.
- Jebsen Hand Function Test by Jebsen, R.H., N. Taylor, R.B. Trieschmann, M.J. Trotter, and L.A. Howard. 1969. An objective and standardized test of hand function. *Archives of Physical Medicine and Rehabilitation* 50:311–319.
- Modified Clinical Scoring System (outcome for Colles' fracture) by Laseter and Carter (1996, 119).
- Point System to Evaluate End Results of Colles' Fracture (Reiss 1995, 339 and Laseter and Carter 1996, 118).
- Smith Hand Function Evaluation by Smith, H.B. 1975. Smith hand function evaluation. *American Journal of Occupational Therapy* 27:244–251.

PROBLEMS

Self-Care

- The person is unable to perform activities requiring hand grasp because of the cast initially, but also because of contractures or decreased wrist extension later on. Most problems occur when the dominant hand is involved.
- The person may have difficulty performing activities that require supination of the forearm because of the cast. Most problems occur in hand-to-face movements when the dominant hand is involved.
- The person may avoid performing some daily living activities, due to lack of knowledge about how to deal with the problem, such as not taking a shower because of lack of knowledge about how to keep the cast dry. (A plastic bag pulled over the cast and taped to the arm above the cast would keep it dry while showering.)

Productivity

- The person may have difficulty performing some job tasks that require hand grasp or supination of the forearm.
- The person may avoid doing some homemaking tasks for fear of further injuring the arm.

Sensorimotor

- The person may lose range of motion.
- The person may have tightness in wrist extension, which limits full range of motion in flexion.
- The person may have tightness in wrist flexion, which limits full extension.
- The person may have tightness in the interosseus membrane surrounding the radius and ulna, which limits supination and pronation.
- The person may have edema and swelling.
- The person may have finger and shoulder stiffness due to inabilities.
- The person may lose hand grasp functions.

- The person may lose forearm supination.
- The person may develop contractures.
- The person may have disuse atrophy.
- The person may have malunion.
- The person may experience pain with motion of the digits.

Cognitive

- Cognitive functions are usually not affected directly by the disorder, but cognitive disorders may be present due to other causes.

Psychosocial

- The person may fear loss of hand function.
- The person may fear loss of independence.
- The person may fear permanent disability.
- The person may be fearful of using the injured arm, due to lack of knowledge about safe and unsafe use during recovery.
- The person may withdraw from society to avoid explaining what happened.
- The person may become bossy and order others around.

TREATMENT/INTERVENTION

There are two major approaches to treatment of fractures. The first is *immobilization* of the joints above and below a fracture to stop all motion in those joints. The second is treatment using *functional bracing*, based on the idea that early motion facilitates bone healing (Colditz 1995, 395). Functional bracing reduces hospitalization and permits early return to function and employment. The principles of healing are based on primary and secondary healing. Primary healing occurs when fractures are rigidly immobilized. Secondary healing occurs when there is motion at the fracture site (Colditz 1995, 395–396). A functional fracture brace is created by applying a cylinder externally to the fracture site. The cylinder restrains soft tissue expansion, directing force equally in all directions internally during muscle contraction. As muscles contract within the space, their increased size is translated into compressive forces with the cylinder. This internal force mechanically stabilizes the fracture. Functional bracing works best in fracture sites where initial shortening is within acceptable limits because soft tissue is more effective in controlling angulation than rotation or length (Colditz 1995, 396).

There are two techniques for fixation: external and internal. In external fixation, the bone fragments are held together using transfixing metal pins through the fragments and a compression device is attached to the pins outside the skin. The pins and compression device are removed when the fracture site is healed. Internal fixation holds the fragments by use of smooth or threaded pins, K-wire, screws, plates attached by screws, or medullary nails that are applied directly to the bone after an incision is made through the skin and underlying tissue. The devices may be removed later or may remain in the body permanently (Ware 1997, 311–312).

The treatment model in occupational therapy is based on the biomechanical (Trombly) or orthopedic model.

**Techniques of Fracture Fixation for Wrist and
Distal Forearm Fractures**

- Percutaneous pin fixation
- Pins and plaster
- Closed reduction and external fixation (CREF)
- Open reduction and internal fixation (ORIF)
- Arthroscopic reduction and percutaneous external fixation

Source: Data from L.C. Ware, Internal/External Fixation of Wrist and Distal Forearm Fractures, in *Hand Rehabilitation: A Practical Guide*, 2ed ed., G.L. Clark, E.F.S. Wilgis, B. Aiello, D. Eckhaus, and L.V. Eddington, eds., p. 311, © 1997, Churchill Livingston.

Self-Care

- Recommend sleeping on the unaffected side with the affected arm placed on pillows or bolsters.
- Provide instruction in compensatory approaches, such as one-handed techniques when movement is required that the immobilized arm cannot perform, such as hand grasp or forearm supination.
- Encourage use of the immobilized arm for all activities in which active movement is possible and safe.
- Suggest adapted equipment that may be useful during immobilization and facilitate independence after recovery, such as elongated handles, elastic shoelaces, and nonskid materials.

Productivity

- A home program to encourage the person to use homemaking activities where possible can support therapy gains and facilitate the return to performing normal homemaking activities.
- A work-hardening program may be necessary to regain the movements and motions necessary to perform job tasks effectively and safely.

Leisure

- Leisure activities, such as crafts and games, may be useful in the therapy program to provide movements and motion patterns useful in regaining joint range, mobility, and strength.

Sensorimotor

- If internal fixation and dynamic external fixation are used to reduce and stabilize the fracture site, rehabilitation may begin during the first week (Ware 1997, 311).
- If static external fixation is used, rehabilitation does not begin until the sixth week at the earliest (Ware 1997, 311).
- Maintain full range of motion of all uninvolved joints (Ware 1997, 314).
- Prevent wound or pin tract infection (Ware 1997, 314).
- Provide mobilization or immobilization of fixated joint, depending on which type of fixation device was used (Ware 1997, 314).
- Prevent scar adhesions on extensor surface (Ware 1997, 314).

Isolated Ulna Fracture (distal one half)

- A functional brace composed of a cylinder of thin splinting material with overlapping edges is applied to the forearm while it is in the neutral position.
- Pressure is maintained on the interosseous membrane at both ends of the splint while the plastic material is hardening.
- Velcro straps are used so that the person may adjust the tightness of the cylinder (Colditz 1995, 400).

Double-Bone Forearm Fracture

- A functional brace can be applied after open reduction and plating to add strength.
- The brace is molded along the interosseous membrane to limit supination, pronation, and angular, torque forces (Colditz 1995, 400).

Colles' Fracture or Distal Radius Fracture

- Initial visit (Reiss 1995, 339–340)
  A. Review cast-wearing precautions.
  B. Check the immobilizing device for unnecessary restriction and tightness. The distal margin of the cast should not extend further than the distal palmar crease to avoid impeding range of motion of the MCP joints. Check that movement at the first carpometacarpal joint is possible so that web space can be maintained.
  C. Begin digital range of motion exercises.
  D. Begin shoulder range of motion exercises. Be aware that the cast may limit shoulder range and that full shoulder range will not be possible until the cast is cut down below the elbow.
  E. Offer assistive devices as necessary, depending on person's functional status.
  F. Provide specific instruction on care of the immobilizing device.
  G. Provide a home exercise program, including digital blocking exercises and tendon gliding exercises. Putty exercises and light gripping and pinching may be recommended. Exercises should be done both actively and passively on an hourly basis.
  H. Gentle ranging of the shoulder should be done initially by the therapist with emphasis on developing or maintaining normal scapulohumeral rhythm.
- Weeks 1–2
  A. Monitor for problems with the immobilizer and observe for any autonomic symptoms.
  B. Grade I and II distractions and posterior-anterior gliding exercises should be performed on all free joints.
  C. Include gentle MCP joint distractions, performed in conjunction with digital flexion exercises in the home program.
  D. Joint mobilization of the shoulder capsule may include anterior-posterior gliding, inferior gliding, and distraction of the humeral head, performed at the same time as physiologic moments.
- Weeks 3–4
  A. Usually, the cast is cut down at the elbow, which frees the joint so that elbow flexion and extension exercises can be started. Note: Resisted flexion is avoided to prevent the brachioradialis from pulling on the radial styloid.

    B. Gentle active exercises for pronation and supination are initiated. Note: Listen for clicks or pops at the radioulnar joint, indicating disruption of the joint.

    C. A sling is not recommended but may be used for geriatric persons. The result may be cervical and anterior chest tightness. Posture should be evaluated to determine whether the immobilizer is causing the arm to be carried at the side with the shoulder protracted and internally rotated while the trunk is leaning posterior or toward the opposite side.

    D. If postural deviations have occurred, they should be addressed. Neck retraction exercises and pectoral stretching for the anterior trunk can be performed.

    E. Loss of MCP flexion can be avoided by use of a padded MCP dorsal blocking splint extension, which is attached to the cast with Velcro.

    F. Reflex sympathetic dystrophy may be avoided by determining whether the vascular status is one of dilation or constriction. Use of modalities to counter the effect (constriction for dilation and dilation for constriction) to normalize the blood flow may be helpful.

- After immobilization is removed:

    A. Wrist range of motion is started.

    B. Before beginning passive stretching, determine with the physician the stability of the fracture site. In particular, do not begin passive wrist extension stretching, which might produce stress on the dorsal articular margin of the radius.

    C. Observe for deformities, especially loss of radial length. For distal radioulnar joint involvement, splint the forearm in neutral forearm pronation and supination but allow the wrist freedom to move. The splint is made of low-temperature plastic and begins on the volar aspect of the forearm just proximal to the wrist, loops around the elbow, which is in 90 degrees of flexion, to the posterior aspect of the forearm, then proximal to the radiocarpal joint.

    D. Compare wrist motion to noninvolved side. Check for hypermobility, clicking, or crepitus.

    E. Check for a volar intercalated segment instability (VISI) deformity, which occurs when there is disruption to the luno-triquetral ligament with the lunate maintaining a palmar flexed position. A distal intercalated segment instability (DISI) pattern occurs in the scapholunate ligament, which results in dorsiflexion of the lunate.

- Weeks 1–2 after immobilization:

    A. Focus is on reducing pain and restoring full motion and strength.

    B. A wrist control splint may be helpful to restore normal tenodesis and optimal length–tension relationships between the wrist extensors and digital flexors. The splint should be worn continually, except during exercise sessions and light ADLs for 2 weeks.

    C. Reduce stiffness. May begin by warming the joint and soft tissue, in fluid therapy or by light aerobic exercise, to improve elasticity, followed by joint mobilization techniques and low-load prolonged stretch.

    D. After the joint is warmed up, gentle stretching and joint mobilization techniques are used.

    E. The person can be instructed in self-PROM exercises to maintain gains made during therapy sessions. Putting the hands together as in prayer, called the *prayer stretch*, is an example.

- Weeks 3–4 after immobilization:

A. Focus on progressive strengthening of the wrist extensors after tenderness over fracture site has disappeared.
B. Resistance can be increased on the BTE (Baltimore Therapeutic Equipment).
C. PNF (proprioceptive neuromuscular facilitation) can be started to warm the entire extremity.
D. Active exercises can be started, such as wrist curls with free weights. Total upper extremity exercises against resistance should also be used.
E. Splinting may be needed to restore range of motion in wrist extension by using a dynamic wrist extension splint or static progressive splint.
F. For severe cases, CPM (continuous passive motion) may be necessary.
- Weeks 4–8 after immobilization:
  A. Work-hardening program may be started when pain-free range of motion is attained.
  B. Job tasks should be based on the person's job description.
  C. Pylometric exercises may be used to increase velocity of motion, such as twirling a baton or performing figure-eight turns via wrist motion by swinging a rope attached to a weighted ball.

Wrist and Forearm Postoperative Therapy—Internal Fixation (Ware 1997, 315)
- Week 1
  A. A thermoplastic splint or plaster cast is applied to immobilize the fixated fracture as per time period specified by the physician. Thermoplastic splints are easier to remove for bathing or dressing changes to associated soft tissue injury, if any. Be sure that the uninvolved joints are not restricted.
  B. Active range of motion should be started for all uninvolved joints. Note that uninvolved joint range of motion can be enhanced by good splinting.
  C. Edema control should be started.
- Week 2
  A. Gentle mobilization of the wrist can be started. Be sure that splint is worn when the person is not exercising.
  B. Scar control program should be started to prevent extensor adhesions.
- Weeks 6–12
  A. Splint may be discontinued when fracture site is healed and union is achieved.
  B. Joint mobilization and muscle strengthening activities are started.
- Post 6 months: Internal fixators may be removed or left in the body permanently.

Wrist and Forearm Postoperative Therapy—Static External Fixation (Ware 1997, 315–316)
- Week 1
  A. A thermoplastic splint is used to immobilize the fixated fracture for the time period directed by the physician.
  B. Active range of motion is begun for all uninvolved joints.
  C. Edema control program is started.
  D. The person is instructed on care of pin site.
- Weeks 6–12
  A. Physician removes the external fixator when fracture is healed.

    B. A protective wrist splint is applied.

    C. Scar control program is started.

    D. Mobilization and strengthening activities are started to regain full range of motion and muscle strength.

Wrist and Forearm Postoperative Therapy—Dynamic External Fixation (Ware 1997, 316)

- Week 1
  - A. Active and active assisted wrist flexion activities are started from the neutral position.
  - B. Scar control program is begun.
  - C. Active range of motion for uninvolved joints is started.
  - D. Edema control program should commence.
  - E. Person should be instructed on care of pin site.
- Week 4
  - A. Wrist and ulnar deviation activities are started.
- Weeks 8–10
  - A. Physician removes the external fixation device.
  - B. Scar control is started.
  - C. Mobilization and strengthening activities of the wrist are begun.
- Complications may include infection at the pin tract, fracture at the pin site, loosening of one or more pins, osteoarthritis, osteoporosis, reflex sympathetic dystrophy, adherence of tendons to the internal fixation device and scar, nerve compression, malunion and poor articular congruency, and refracture (Ware 1997, 312).

Ulnar Head Resection—Darrach Procedure, Bowers Hemisection-Interposition Technique, or Matched Ulnar Resection (DiGiovannantonio 1997, 300)

- The person is immobilized in a long arm cast in neutral forearm rotation for 7–10 days immediately after surgery.
- Cast is removed after 7–10 days and, if joint is stable, the person is placed in a short arm wrist splint with wrist at neutral to 30 degrees of extension.
  - A. At 2–4 weeks postoperatively, the person can begin moving safely within 45–60 degrees of wrist flexion and extension and forearm supination and pronation.
  - B. If person is pain free, wrist splint is discontinued during the 2- to 4-week period and the person may start normal range of motion activities and light ADLs, as tolerated.
  - C. Gradual muscle strengthening may be started for the hand, wrist, and forearm at 4–6 weeks, except for power grasp, which should be avoided until 8–12 weeks postoperatively.
  - D. At 6–10 weeks, more progressive strengthening and return to normal function may be initiated. Power grasp may be started at week 8 if the person is mostly pain free.
  - E. Active range of motion of all uninvolved joints should be started immediately.
- If cast is removed and joint is found to be unstable, the person is placed in a long arm splint in neutral forearm motion for about 4 weeks. This should be worn continuously.
  - A. At 7–10 days postoperatively, the person can begin AROM to within 45–60 degrees of wrist flexion and extension and do forearm supination and pronation. Note: Location of instability may limit type one or more motions.
  - B. Active range of motion should be limited to pain-free range of motion and performed only with occupational therapy personnel present.

C. The long arm splint may be discontinued after 4–6 weeks, and strengthening activities may be started, but avoid power grasp until 8–12 weeks postoperatively.
D. At 6–12 weeks, more progressive strengthening and return to normal function may be initiated. Power grasp may be started at week 8 if person is mostly pain free.
E. Active range of motion for all uninvolved joints should be started immediately.

Ulnar Head Resection—Sauve-Kapandji Procedure (DiGiovannantonio 1997, 300–301)

- Person is immobilized in a long arm cast for 7–10 days postoperatively.
- If K-wires were used to attain internal fixation, the person is placed in a long arm or Muenster-type splint over the elbow at neutral forearm rotation until 3–4 weeks postoperatively. The person may remove the splint to perform active supination and pronation exercises within 45–60 degrees. End of range activities must be avoided.
- If a screw was used to attain internal fixation, the person is placed in a wrist splint at 7–10 days postoperatively and active forearm supination and pronation within 45–60 degrees is started.
- For both types of fixation, range of motion at the wrist may be started 4 weeks postoperatively.
- The wrist splint should be worn between exercise periods for approximately 6 weeks postoperatively or until fusion between the radius and ulna is achieved, at which point, strengthening activities may be started. Avoid power grasp until week 8.
- At 8–12 weeks, progressive strengthening and return to normal function is initiated.
- Complications postoperatively include stylocarpal impingement, radioulnar impingement, regeneration of the distal ulna, radial deviation of the wrist, wrist instability, tendon rupture, nerve impairment, reflex sympathetic dystrophy, wrist synovitis, instability of the distal ulna, and inadequate bony resection.

Cognitive

- Teach the person the concept of one-handed techniques.
- Teach safety evaluation of the home and frequently traveled routes to reduce chances of another fall.

Psychosocial

- Encourage the person to verbalize concerns and provide realistic answers or solutions to allay the fears.
- Encourage the person to engage in social activities, such as group activities with persons who have upper extremity limitations.

PRECAUTIONS

- Watch for associated soft tissue loss.
- Watch for associated tendon injuries.
- Watch for associated nerve injuries.
- Watch for signs of peripheral nerve compression if the person's wrist is in flexion.
- Watch for signs of reflex sympathetic dystrophy or shoulder-hand syndrome.
- Listen for clicking or popping sounds in the wrist area during the early phases of range of motion activities. Alert the physician immediately and consider additional immobilization.

- Functional bracing cannot be used in the absence of bulky muscle tissues, where there is major soft-tissue injury or bone loss or where there is major displacement or angulation.
- A fracture that heals with poor articular congruency may lead to the development of traumatic arthritis (Reiss 1995, 337).
- Radial shortening (fracture heals without consideration for original length of the radius) can lead to ulnocarpal impingement, pain in the distal radioulnar joint, and decreased forearm rotation (Reiss 1995, 338).
- Changes in radial inclination of the articular surface alter grip strength (Reiss 1995, 338).

PROGNOSIS AND OUTCOME

Usually, the prognosis is good because the radius has a good blood supply and bone union can be expected. Disuse atrophy, bony malunion, peripheral nerve compression, reflex sympathetic dystrophy, and shoulder-hand syndrome are the major complications that may prolong the rehabilitation process and delay the return to functional activities and independent living.

- The person is able to perform daily living activities independently.
- The person is able to perform productive activities.
- The person is able to perform leisure activities.
- The person demonstrates functional range of motion in involved joints and full range of motion in uninvolved joints.
- The person demonstrates muscle strength necessary to perform daily activities.
- The person demonstrates basic hand functions.
- The person does not report chronic pain or swelling (edema) upon use of the arm or hand.
- The person demonstrates two-point discrimination and stereognosis.

REFERENCES

Abrams, W.B., M.H. Beers, and R. Berkow. 1995. *The Merck Manual of Geriatrics*, 2nd ed. Whitehouse Station, NJ: Merck & Co.

Barr, K. 1994. The use of air bag splints to increase supination and pronation in the arm. *American Journal of Occupational Therapy* 48(8):746–749.

Colditz, J.C. 1995. Functional fracture bracing. In *Rehabilitation of the Hand*, 4th ed., ed. J.M. Hunter, E.J. Mackin, and A.D. Callahan, 395–406. St. Louis: Mosby.

DiGiovannantonio, F. 1997. Ulnar head resection. In *Hand Rehabilitation: A Practical Guide,* 2nd ed., ed. G.L. Clark, E.F.S. Wilgis, B. Aiello, D. Eckhaus, and L.V. Eddington, 297–304. New York: Churchill Livingstone.

Laseter, G.F. and P.R. Carter. 1996. Management of distal radius fracture. *Journal of Hand Therapy* 9(2):114–128.

Reiss, B. 1995. Therapist's management of distal radial fractures. In *Rehabilitation of the Hand*, 4th ed., ed. J.M. Hunter, E.J. Mackin, and A.D. Callahan, 337–352. St. Louis: Mosby.

Ware, L.C. 1997. Internal/external fixation of wrist and distal forearm fractures. In *Hand Rehabilitation: A Practical Guide,* 2nd ed., ed. G.L. Clark, E.F.S. Wilgis, B. Aiello, D. Eckhaus, and L.V. Eddington, 311–318. New York: Churchill Livingstone.

BIBLIOGRAPHY

Jarus, T. and R. Poremba. 1993. Hand function evaluation: A factor analysis study. *American Journal of Occupational Therapy* 47(5):439–443.

Pesco, M.S. and P.C. Altner. 1993. Protective orthoplastic splint in the treatment of a patient with Colles' fracture by external fixation. *Journal of Hand Therapy* 6(1):39–41.

Thiers, N. 1993. Wrist research offers valuable clues for effective treatment. *OT Week* 7(31):14–15.

Weinstock, T.B. 1999. Management of fractures of the distal radius: Therapist's commentary. *Journal of Hand Therapy* 12(2):99–102.

Fractures of the Humerus

DESCRIPTION

The humerus may be fractured at the proximal end, in the middle portion, or at the distal end. Fractures of the proximal end are the most common (Murphy 1997, 259). The person with a proximal humeral fracture usually complains of shoulder pain and is unable to move the arm. On radiographic examination, the proximal humerus may show as many as four separate fragments: an articular fragment containing the humeral head, a greater tuberosity fragment, a lesser tuberosity fragment, and a distal fragment, including the humeral shaft. The fragments are prone to displacement because of muscle pull by the supraspinous, subscapularis, and pectoral muscles. Displaced fractures are classified according to the severity of the displacement into one of four patterns. About 80% of proximal humerus fractures are minimally displaced, with < 45 degree angulation and < 1 cm displacement of any fragment. Fractures in which a glenohumeral dislocation appears usually result from major trauma and constitute the most severe injuries (Abrams et al. 1995, 88).

Classification of Fractures (Neers, as cited in Murphy 1997, 260–261)

- One-part fracture—no segments are displaced more than 1 cm or angulation greater than 45 degrees.
- Two-part fracture—one segment is displaced in relationship to the other three.
- Three-part fracture—two segments are displaced in relationship to the other segments that are in opposition.
- Four-part fracture—all four segments are displaced.

Classification Based on Vascular Supply (American Orthopedic Association, as cited in Murphy 1997, 261)

- Type A fracture—the articular segment is not isolated from its vascular supply.
- Type B fracture—the fracture is partially isolated from its vascular supply.
- Type C fracture—the fracture is totally separated from its blood supply.

CAUSE

The most common cause of a proximal humeral fracture is a fall on an outstretched hand, but other types of trauma occur. The presence of osteoporosis and chronologic age past 40 are major contributing factors. The ratio of women to men is 2:1. In the younger population, proximal humeral fractures are often secondary to high-velocity injury and typically have greater displacement (Murphy 1997, 259).

ASSESSMENT

Areas
- daily living tasks
- activity of daily living assessment
- range of motion
- joint mobility
- edema
- sensory screening

Instruments
No specific instruments or tests were identified.

PROBLEMS

Sensorimotor
- The person may experience joint stiffness and loss of mobility.
- The person may have loss of range of motion.
- The person may have edema.

TREATMENT/INTERVENTION

Treatment depends on the number of fragments and extent of displacement. Once clinical unity has been obtained, rehabilitation can begin. Clinical unity is performed by the physician placing one hand on the humeral head and gently rotating the humerus in the other. When the fracture fragments move in unison, clinical unity has been attained. In nonoperative fractures, clinical unity occurs within 1–4 weeks in most cases. If internal fixation is used, clinical unity may occur immediately. Clinical union occurs when there is evidence of cancellous healing as seen on radiograph. Clinical union may occur at 6 weeks or shortly thereafter. The model used in occupational therapy is biomechanical.

Sensorimotor
- Stiffness should be treated with low-load prolonged stress (LLPS), using splints as opposed to high-load brief stress (LaStayo and Jaffe 1994, 122).

Proximal Humeral Fracture—Nonoperative (Murphy 1997, 259–164)
- Day 1
    A. A sling may be used to promote proximal stabilization.
    B. Use modalities such as heat to decrease shoulder pain.
    C. Maintain wrist and hand range of motion with exercise.
    D. Use techniques to reduce edema.

- Day 3–7
  - A. Decrease wearing time for sling. For example, when sitting, support the arm on a pillow on a supporting surface, such as an arm rest.
  - B. Initiate pendulum exercises: free swing of the shoulder while leaning forward from the waist.
  - C. Initiate range of motion for the elbow and forearm.
  - D. Continue edema control.
- Day 7 to 3 weeks:
  - A. In supine, gravity-eliminated position, begin PROM, active assistive range of motion (AAROM) of the shoulder with assisted elevation in the frontal plane, in the plane of the scapula, and external rotation.
  - B. A pulley system may be used for forward elevation.
  - C. Progress from gravity-eliminated position to PROM, AAROM while sitting with arm supported on a tabletop.
  - D. Splint should be discontinued.
- 3–4 weeks:
  - A. Begin PROM, AAROM in extension and internal rotation.
  - B. Begin isometric strengthening.
- 4–6 weeks:
  - A. Start place and hold AROM in supine position.
  - B. Start tabletop activities with the arm supported on a table while performing active reach activities, such as placing pegs in a pegboard, using a rolling pin, or dusting.
- 6–8 weeks:
  - A. Begin light function strengthening activities, such as copper tooling or sanding.
  - B. Continue with PROM, AAROM exercise to increase shoulder function and mobility.
  - C. Begin use of a work simulator and Theraband for progressive resistance.
- 8–12 weeks:
  - A. Continue stretching exercises to regain range of motion at end of the arc of motion at the shoulder.
  - B. Continue with progressive strengthening exercise and initiate the use of free weights starting with 1 lb and progressing to 5 lbs.
- Complications include a stiff and painful shoulder, distal edema and stiffness, delayed union, nonunion, degenerative arthritis, frozen shoulder, avascular necrosis, myositis ossificans, neurovascular injuries, and reflex sympathetic dystrophy.

Proximal Humeral Fracture—Postoperative (Murphy 1997, 264–265)

- A. The same treatment guidelines are used at a faster rate, once stabilization is achieved through surgery.
- B. Complications may include infection, hardware failure, failure to stabilize the fracture, soft tissue repairs, and other nonoperative complications.

Humeral Shaft Fracture (Colditz 1995, 397–399)

- A. A functional brace may be constructed from one piece of polyethylene applied circumferentially with Velcro closures and an overlapping long edge made of a 1/16-inch thick thermoplastic splinting material. The design must allow full shoulder and elbow range of motion and accommodated to the reduction of edema by allowing the fasteners to close tighter around the arm. Pressure must be maintained.

B. While applying the brace, ask the person to lean the trunk laterally toward the fracture site approximately 30 degrees from vertical, allowing the arm to hang vertically while providing room for the therapist to work between the arm and body. The person holds the hand in the lap with the noninvolved hand, allowing the elbow to assume a 90-degree angle.

C. The low-temperature thermoplastic materials can be molded directly to the person's arm, permitting good fit and correction of minor angulation.

D. Avoid positions that require external rotation of the distal fracture segment.

E. The brace must be removed daily for skin hygiene and application of a clean cotton stockinette liner. Corn starch may be applied to retard perspiration.

F. No specific rehabilitation program is provided.

Distal Humeral Fracture (Colditz 1995, 399)

A. Distal fractures usually require open reduction and internal fixation. A brace is used postoperatively for additional protection.

B. The humeral portion of the functional circumferential brace is made of one piece of polyethylene thin plastic, which is molded around the person's arm as far distally as possible without interfering with elbow range of motion.

C. The forearm portion of the circumferential brace is also made of one piece of plastic and applied with the forearm in neutral position.

D. A hinge is applied between the proximal and distal braces to hold them in place, which prevents varus, valgus, and translateral forces. Tape may be used to assist in determining the correct location of the hinge to permit elbow flexion and extension and correct naturally at the joint axis.

E. Closure should be on the anterior aspect of the arm and forearm to facilitate application and removal.

F. The hinge is applied on the posterior aspect.

G. A cotton stockinette sock is worn under the brace across the elbow joint.

H. No specific rehabilitation program is provided.

Cognitive

A. The person should be instructed in proper care of the brace or splint and in good skin care of the skin under the brace or splint. Failure to provide proper skin care can cause skin problems.

PRECAUTIONS

• Plastic materials such as those used in the brace cut off air circulation to the skin. The brace must be removed daily and the skin cleaned to avoid skin problems. Corn starch can reduce perspiration.

• Monitor edema closely. It should decrease as active motion returns. A Jobst pump or application of an elastic stockinette over the entire arm may be needed if the edema continues. Use of an elastic glove may be helpful if the edema is primarily in the hand.

PROGNOSIS/OUTCOMES

Prognosis depends on the number of fragments and the extent of displacement.
* The person will be able to perform daily living tasks.
* Joint alignment will be anatomically correct without the continuing need for external devices.
* The person will have full range of motion.
* The person's skin will be in good condition.

REFERENCES

Abrams, W.B., M.H. Beers, and R. Berkow. 1995. *The Merck Manual of Geriatrics*, 2nd ed., 88. Whitehouse Station, NJ: Merck & Co.

Colditz, J.C. 1995. Functional fracture bracing. In *Rehabilitation of the Hand*, 4th ed., ed. J.M. Hunter, E.J. Mackin, and A.D. Callahan, 395–406. St. Louis: Mosby.

LaStayo, P. and R. Jaffe. 1994. Assessment and management of shoulder stiffness: A biomechanical approach. *Journal of Hand Therapy* 7(2):122–130

Murphy, M.S. 1997. Proximal humeral fractures. In *Hand Rehabilitation: a Practical Guide,* 2nd ed., ed. G.L. Clark, E.F.S. Wilgis, B. Aiello, D. Eckhaus, and L.V. Eddington, 259–266. New York: Churchill Livingstone.

Fractures of the Hip and Hip Arthroplasty

DESCRIPTION

Fractures of the femoral neck are classified as occult, impact, displaced, or nondisplaced. The Garden classification describes the extent of impaction and dislocation, and the degree of disruption of the blood supply. Garden I is an impacted fracture showing the femoral head slightly tilted inward (valgus deformity) with an incomplete fracture line that leaves the medial cortex intact and, thus, is fairly stable. Garden II are nondisplaced fractures extending across both cortexes of the femoral neck and, thus, are more unstable. Garden III and IV show more displacement of the femoral neck. The person presents with groin pain and a shortened externally rotated leg that is too painful to move. Lack of blood supply can seriously impact healing, which may lead to osteonecrosis and nonunion (Abrams et al. 1995, 90–95).

Fractures of the intertrochanter are classified by the number of bony fragments and by the inherent stability. A two-part fracture typically shows a single break sloping obliquely between the greater and lesser trochanters . A three-part fracture also has a lesser trochanteric fragment, in addition to the oblique fracture, and is usually unstable. A four-part fracture has a greater and lesser trochanteric fragment, in addition to the oblique fracture, and is inherently unstable. Blood supply is usually maintained and, thus, osteonecrosis and nonunion are rarely problems (Abrams et al. 1995, 90–95).

There are five common sites of femoral fractures. Three occur at neck: subcapital, transcervical, and basilar. One occurs at the intertrochanter, called *intertrochanteric*. The fifth occurs in the shaft below the trochanters, called the *subtrochanteric* (Morawski et al. 1996, 737).

Hip arthroplasty is the surgical replacement, formation, or reformation of the hip joint. There are three types of surgical intervention: cup or modal arthroplasty, total hip arthroplasty (THA), and total hip surface replacement (Gower and Bowker 1993, 161). Of these most of the references deal with THA, which is also called total hip replacement (THR).

CAUSE

The most common cause of fractures is trauma caused by a fall, automobile accident, or a sudden rotational force. Factors contributing to falls are poor vision, orthostatic hypotension, poor balance, diminished mobility, side effects of medication, muscle weakness, neurologic diseases, reduced alertness, dementia, and environmental obstacles or hazards, such as poor lighting, throw rugs, or electrical cords (Coppard et al. 1998, 246, Clemson et al. 1996, 97). Degeneration of the head of the femur, such as necrosis or loss of bone strength as in osteoporosis, osteomalacia, osteoarthritis, or metastatic cancer contribute to the chance of a fracture. Fractures occur more frequently in men, due to occupational injuries during their 30s or 40s and in women past the age of 65. Femoral neck fractures occur more in older individuals. Hip fractures account for 90% of all fractures in persons over the age of 70 years (Coppard et al. 1998, 245). Subtrochanteric fractures occur in younger people.

Hip arthroplasty or replacement is considered when osteoarthritis, rheumatoid arthritis, ankylosing spondylitis, trauma, or other disease processes are involved.

ASSESSMENT

Areas

- daily living skills, including ADLs
- productivity history, skills, interests, and values
- leisure interests and skills
- muscle strength
- range of motion of the lower extremities
- physical endurance
- sensory registration and processing
- pain
- orientation (especially important in older persons)
- self-concept
- social support
- architectural and environmental barriers
- adaptive equipment and assistive devices (assistive technology)
- home safety
- knowledge of community resources.

Instruments
Instruments Developed by Occupational Therapy Personnel
- Home Activity Inventory by Gower, D. and M. Bowker. 1993. In *Practice Issues in Occupational Therapy: Intraprofessional Team Building*, ed. S.E. Ryan, 163. Thorofare, NJ: Slack.
- Klein-Bell ADL Scale by Klein, R. and B. Bell. 1982. *Archives of Physical Medicine and Rehabilitation* 63:335–338.
- Occupational Therapy Evaluation Form by Buddenberg, L.A. and J.K. Schkade. 1998. *Topics in Geriatric Rehabilitation* 13(4):52–68.
- Rehabilitation Services—Orthopedic-Occupational Therapy Initial Evaluation and Discharge Summary by DeKalb Medical Center. 1994. *American Journal of Occupational Therapy* 48(5):442–443.
- Westmead Home Safety Assessment by Clemson, L. Occupational Therapy Department, Westmead Hospital, Westmead, New South Wales 2145, Australia.

Instruments Developed by Other Professionals and Used by Occupational Therapy Personnel
- Functional Independence Measure, v. 4 by Uniform Data System for Medical Rehabilitation. 1990. Buffalo, NY: State University of New York at Buffalo.
- Orientation-Memory-Concentration Test by Katzman R., T. Brown, P. Fuld, A. Peck, R. Schechter, and H. Schimmel. 1983. Validation of a short orientation-memory-concentration test of cognitive impairment. *American Journal of Psychiatry* 140(6):734–739.
- Visual Analogue Scale by Huskinsson, E.C. 1994. Measurement of pain. *Lancet* 2:1127–1131.

PROBLEMS

Self-Care
- The person may have reduced his or her performance of ADLs to a minimum prior to surgery.
- The person may be using unsafe techniques for performing bathing and dressing activities.
- During recovery from hip fracture or arthroplasty, the person usually experiences difficulty to perform dressing, elimination, mobility, and hygiene, such as bathing or showering.

Productivity
- The person may have limited or stopped performing productive activities prior to surgery.
- The person may have numerous hazards in the home that may have contributed to the hip fracture.

Leisure
- The person may have given up many leisure activities prior to surgery.

Sensorimotor
- The person usually must limit hip flexion beyond 70–80 degrees for 6–8 weeks after surgery to permit soft tissue healing and avoid internal rotation or adduction of the hip. These precautions apply especially to hip replacement.

- The hip is frequently limited to 90 degrees of hip flexion in hip replacement.
- Out-of-bed activities usually can begin for fractures within 2–4 days after surgery.
- Crutches or a walker will be needed for 6–8 weeks and may be necessary for longer periods.
- Pain may continue to be present.
- Tactile sensation may be diminished.

Cognitive

- The person's thinking and problem-solving skills may be reduced, due to chronic pain.
- The person's cognitive skills may be decreased, and the decrease may be a contributing factor in the hip fracture.
- The person may have poor initiation of activity and diminished generalization of skills learned in rehabilitation (Buddenberg and Schkade 1998, 53).

Psychosocial

- The person may become depressed or anxious.
- The person may have lost self-esteem as an active, contributing member of society.
- The person may express feelings about being disabled and losing body image.
- The person many feel helpless and not in control of his or her own life and health status.
- The person may lose independence and autonomy, becoming dependent on others.
- The person may become a passive participant in the recovery process.
- The person may have stopped engaging in most social activities prior to surgery because of pain and limited mobility.

Environment

- Hospitalization may cause relocation trauma, presented as confusion, emotional lability, and disorientation.
- Encourage person to bring familiar objects from home and provide a calendar and current newspapers or magazines, which can be helpful in maintaining cognitive orientation.
- Hip fracture is a major cause of people being admitted to skilled nursing facilities (Buddenberg and Schkade 1998, 52).

TREATMENT/INTERVENTION

The goals of fracture treatment are to relieve pain, maintain good position of the fracture, allow for bony union for fracture healing, and restore optimal function to the person (Morawski et al. 1996, 736).

A team approach is often involved in caring for a person with hip fracture or hip replacement. Members may include an orthopedic physician, orthopedic nurse, physical therapist, nutritionist, pharmacist, social worker, and occupational therapy personnel.

The model of treatment is based on the rehabilitation or compensatory model, biomechanical model, and occupational adaptation.

Self-Care

- Provide self-help devices and opportunity to practice their use in activities that normally require hip flexion, such as putting on socks and shoes and picking up objects from the floor.

- Suggest that safety items, such as grab bars and nonskid tape, be installed in the bathroom to reduce the chance of falls.
- Recommend that dressing activities be done while sitting, when possible, to reduce problems of maintaining balance on one leg or with reduced vision as clothing is pulled over the head.
- Adapted equipment, such as a commode chair with armrests, a bench seat in the shower, and a bar stool for kitchen activities, may be recommended.

Total Hip Replacement—Posterolateral Approach (Morawski et al. 1996, 740–742)

- *Position* of hip stability is flexion, abduction and external rotation; position of hip instability is adduction, internal rotation, and flexion greater than 60 degrees.
- *Bed mobility*: Use a wedge or large pillow to support the operated leg and prevent internal rotation as the person sleeps on the nonoperated side. If possible, the person should sleep on the operated side.
- *Transfers*: Have person observe the proper technique before attempting it.
- *Chair*: The person should extend the operated leg and reach for the arm rests. Some weight should be born on the chair arms. The person then sits down slowly while maintaining some extension of the operated leg.
- *Commode chair*: An over-the-toilet chair with arm rests is recommended. The front legs should be one notch lower than the back legs.
- *Shower stall*: Nonskid strips or sticks should be placed on floor. When entering the shower, the walker or crutches and operated leg go in first, followed by the nonoperated leg. A shower chair may be recommended if balance is a problem. A soap-on-a-rope is useful to avoid the problem of dropping the soap.
- *Shower over tub*: The person stands parallel to tub facing fixtures. The knee is bent to clear the side of the tub, not the hip. If balance is a problem, a sponge bath at the sink may be the best solution.
- *Washing and drying lower extremities*: Use a long-handled bath sponge or back brush to reach the lower legs and feet. Wrap a towel around a reacher to dry the lower extremities.
- *Automobile or Truck*: The person should back up to the passenger seat, hold onto a stable part of the car, extend the operated leg, and slowly sit on the seat. Lean back, slide the buttocks toward the other side. The upper body and lower extremities should move as one unit as the person turns to face forward. Bench seats are recommended but not bucket seats in small cars. The seat should be positioned as far back as possible and the back of seat reclined. Pillows may be used to increase the height of the seat.
- *Dressing the lower body*: Assistive devices, such as a reacher or dressing stick, are helpful in putting on and taking off pants and shoes. Put pant leg on operated leg first, then on nonoperated leg.
- *Hair shampoo*: Stand or sit on a stool at the kitchen or bathroom sink to wash the hair until the person is able to use the shower. Always observe precautions for hip position.

Total Hip Replacement—Anterolateral Approach (Morawski et al. 1996, 742–743)

- *Position* of hip stability is flexion, abduction to neutral, and internal rotation; position of hip instability is adduction, external rotation, and hyperextension.
- *Bed mobility*: Recommended sleeping position is supine. Use a wedge or large pillow to support the operated leg and prevent internal rotation as the person sleeps on the nonoperated

side. In getting out of bed, the person should avoid adduction past midline and maintain extremity in internal rotation, initially moving toward the nonoperated extremity while getting out of bed.

- *Transfers*: Encourage the person to review the precautions before attempting the transfer itself.
- *Chair*: A chair with armrests is preferred that does not skid or slide as the person sits down or gets up. As the person is sitting down, the operated leg should be extended. The person puts part of the weight on the arm rests and sits down slowly. To stand up, the person first slides forward to the edge of the chair, then extends the operated leg and pushes off with the hands on the arm rests onto the nonoperated leg. Avoid low-seated chairs and soft or sling-seated chairs.
- *Toileting*: Usually, by the time of discharge, the person has enough hip mobility to use a standard toilet seat. Advise the person not to rotate the hip externally while wiping. The person should stand up and turn around to flush the toilet.
- *Shower stall*: Nonskid strips or stickers should be placed on the floor of stall and bottom of the tub. The person should place the walker or crutches in the stall first, then the operated leg, and finally the nonoperated leg.
- *Shower over tub*: Person should stand parallel to the tub and, using a walker or crutches, should transfer sideways by bending one knee at a time over the tub. If the person has poor balance, a sponge bath at the sink is recommended.
- *Washing and drying lower extremities*: Use a long-handled bath sponge or back brush to reach the lower legs and feet. Wrap a towel around a reacher to dry the lower extremities.
- *Automobile or Truck*: The bench seat is recommended, as opposed to bucket seats. The person should back up to the passenger seat, hold onto a stable part of the car, extend the operated leg, and slowly sit on the seat. The person should lean back, slide the buttocks toward the other side. The upper body and lower extremities should move as one unit as the person turns to face forward. Prolonged sitting in an automobile or truck is not recommended.
- *Lower body dressing*: Sitting in a chair or on the side of bed is recommended. The person should avoid full range of external rotation, such as crossing the legs to put on socks and shoes. Assistive devices, such as a reacher or dressing stick, are helpful in putting on and taking off pants and shoes. Put pant leg on operated leg first, then on nonoperated leg.
- *Hair shampoo*: Same as for posterolateral approach.

Productivity

- Assist the person to rearrange commonly used personal and homemaking items to decrease the need for bending, stooping, kneeling, or stretching overhead. For example, shoes can be put in hanging racks, and canned goods should be put within easy arm reach. Use work simplification techniques.
- The person should be cautioned against performing heavy housework, such as vacuuming, lifting more than 20 lbs, or making beds. Use energy conservation techniques.
- Remove clutter, cords, and scatter rugs to prevent tripping. Use home safety and precaution techniques.
- Organize activity schedule to provide periodic rest breaks. Use pacing technique.
- Sit in a firm, sturdy arm chair. Use good positioning and posture techniques.
- Use assistive technology where helpful.

Total Hip Replacement—Posterolateral or Anterolateral Approach (Morawski et al. 1996, 742)

- Heavy housework should be avoided.
- In the kitchen keep commonly used items at counter top level.
- An apron with large pockets can be used to help carry items.
- Slide, as opposed to lifting, objects across the counter when possible.
- A utility cart can be used on linoleum or wood floors to carry objects.
- A small basket or bag can be attached to a walker to help carry objects.
- The person can wear a fanny pack around the waist to carry objects.
- Reachers can be used to grasp items from low or high cupboards and to pick up items that fall on the floor.

Leisure

- Assist the person to define what leisure activities would be useful and which ones must be avoided. For example, short walks are good; outside gardening is bad. Substitute raising house plants.

Sensorimotor

- Strengthen the person's upper extremities for crutch walking and assisting in pushing up to rise from a chair or bed.
- Increase range of motion gradually through walking.
- Maintain or increase endurance and conditioning through physical activities.
- Help the person to monitor and control pain, if needed.

Cognitive

- Instruct the person how to avoid or correct architectural or environment barriers, such as low chairs, soft sofas, and throw rugs.
- The person should learn to avoid forcing hip flexion, as in reaching down to put on socks and shoes.
- The person should learn to avoid strenuous exercise.
- Assist the person to arrange a time schedule to permit activity and rest cycles.
- Instruct the person in concepts of energy conservation and work simplification.
- Discuss the need for evaluating his or her home or apartment for safety considerations; for example, mats or rugs should lie flat and not skid, railing and banisters should be sturdy and tightly in place.
- The effect of a rest or sleep period during the afternoon varies on persons' cognition. Most are drowsier after an afternoon nap period, but increased alertness is possible (Creighton 1995, 775).

Psychosocial

- Encourage the person to engage in activity that will maintain or increase self-esteem by assisting the individual to do familiar activities again, with modification if needed, and to learn new activities.
- Encourage the person to express feelings and discuss ways of coping with those feelings.
- The person should be encouraged to return slowly to social activities that are within safe limits.

- Encourage family members to participate in some treatment sessions to learn safe procedures and precautions.

Environment
- At least one family member or friend should learn the precautions to be observed, adapted techniques that can be employed, and assistive devices that are available when the person with a hip fracture or hip replacement is recovering.
- Instruction booklets are available on "life after a hip fracture or hip replacement" as reference materials for the person, family, and/or friends.
- Adapted equipment that is useful includes a Nelson bed, which can be tilted to 90 degrees to facilitate transfers, a reclining wheelchair with an adjustable back rest that can become a recliner, and a commode chair to facilitate safe transfers while maintaining precautions.
- Assistive devices that are useful include a large abduction wedge to be used to keep the lower extremities in the abducted position, dressing stick, reacher, long-handled sponge, long-handled shoe horn, elastic shoelaces, and sock aid.

PRECAUTIONS
- The person should be warned that infection in any part of the body should be treated promptly to decrease the chance of spreading to the hip joint.
- The person should be warned that strenuous activity, such as running, jumping, hopping, or lifting heavy objects, could result in reinjury of the hip.
- If the anterolateral approach is used in hip replacement, the person must be cautioned about external rotation, adduction, and extension for 6–12 weeks (Morawski 1996, 738).
- If the posterolateral approach is used, the person must be cautioned about flexion beyond 60–90 degrees, internal rotation, and adduction (Morawski 1996, 738).
- If bony ingrowth instead of cement is used to secure the prosthesis, weight bearing may be restricted for 6–8 weeks (Morawski 1996, 738).

PROGNOSIS AND OUTCOME
Recovery usually requires 2–3 months. A person who is independent before total hip surgery should be independent after surgery unless the individual prefers to have some assistance because independence is not a high priority (Gower and Bowker 1993, 161). However, Buddenberg and Schkade (1998, 52) state that most do not return to their previous level of functioning. Hoenig et al. (1997, 513) found that surgical repair with the first two days of hospitalization and more than five PT/OT sessions per week were associated with better health outcomes in a nationally representative sample of elderly persons with hip fracture.

During the recovery period, it is important that the person demonstrate knowledge and action relative to the specific hip movement precautions and bending restrictions applicable to the type of surgery performed.
- The person is able to perform ADLs independently.
- The person is able to perform productive activities, such as light housekeeping or volunteer work.

- The person is able to perform leisure activities of choice within restrictions imposed by the prosthesis. Generally, the prosthesis cannot withstand heavy-duty or prolonged static demands.
- The person demonstrates physical endurance to perform functional activities.
- The person demonstrates range of motion and muscle strength of hip necessary for walking, sitting, and climbing stairs.
- The person and his or her support group are aware of resources available, such as adapted equipment and assistive devices.
- The person demonstrates a knowledge of safety and an ability to minimize environmental barriers in the home, yard, and community.

REFERENCES

Abrams, W.B., M.H. Beers, and R. Berkow. 1995. *The Merck Manual of Geriatrics*, 2nd ed. Whitehouse Station, NJ: Merck & Co.

Buddenberg, L.A. and J.K. Schkade. 1998. A comparison of occupational therapy intervention approaches for older patients after hip fracture. *Topics in Geriatric Rehabilitation* 13(4)52–58.

Clemson, L., R.G. Cumming, and M. Roland. 1996. Case-control study of hazards in the home and risk of falls and hip fractures. *Age and Aging* 25:97–101.

Coppard, B.M., T. Higgins, and K.D. Harvey. 1998. Working with elders who have orthopedic conditions. In *Occupational Therapy with Elders: Strategies for the COTA*, ed. H. Lohman, R.L. Padilla, S. Byers-Connon, 245–256. St. Louis: Mosby.

Creighton, C. 1995. Effects of afternoon rest on the performance of geriatric patients in a rehabilitation hospital: A pilot study. *American Journal of Occupational Therapy* 49(8):775–779.

Gower, D. and M. Bowker. 1993. The elderly with a hip arthroplasty. In *Practice Issues in Occupational Therapy: Intraprofessional Team Building*, ed. S.E. Ryan, 161–168. Thorofare, NJ: Slack (Case report).

Hoenig, H., R. Sloane, R. Horner, L.V. Rubenstein, and K. Kahn. 1997. Hip fracture rehabilitation. *Archives of Internal Medicine* 158(1):100–101 Comments.

Morawski, D., K. Pitbladdo, E.M. Bianchi, S.L. Lieberman, J.P. Novic, and H. Bobrove. 1996. Hip fractures and total hip replacement. In *Occupational Therapy: Practice Skills for Physical Dysfunction*, 4th ed., ed. L.W. Pedretti, 735–746. St. Louis: CV Mosby (Case report).

BIBLIOGRAPHY

Bear-Lehman, J. 1996. Orthopaedic conditions—The hip. In *Occupational Therapy for Physical Dysfunction*, 4th ed., ed. C. Trombly, 761–764. Baltimore: Williams & Wilkins.

Butler, G.S., C.A. Hurley, K.L. Buchanan, and J. Smith-VanHorne. 1996. Prehospital education: Effectiveness with total hip replacement surgery patients. *Patient Education and Counseling* 29(2);189–197.

Coleman, S., D. Morawski, K. Pitbladdo, E.M. Bianchi, S.L. Lieberman, J.P. Novic, and H. Bobrove. 1998. Hip fractures and lower extremity joint replacement. In *Physical Dysfunction Practice Skills for the Occupational Therapy Assistant*, ed. M.B. Early, 491–504. St. Louis: Mosby (Case report).

Erickson, B. and M. Perkins. 1994. Interdisciplinary team approach in the rehabilitation of hip and knee arthroplasties. *American Journal of Occupational Therapy* 48(5):439–445.

Hagerty, J., J. Malka, P. Coll, and R. Lienby. 1993. Hip-replacement patients take path to rehab success. *OT Week* 7(5):14.

Hagsten, B.E. 1994. Occupational therapy after hip fracture: a pilot study of the clients, the care and the costs. *Clinical Rehabilitation* 8:142–148.

Hoenig, H., L.V. Robenstein, and K. Kahn. 1996. Rehabilitation after hip fracture - equal opportunity for all? *Archives of Physical Medicine and Rehabilitation* 77(1):58–63.

Hoenig, H., L.V. Rubenstein, R. Sloane, R. Horner, and K. Kahn. 1997. What is the role of timing in the surgical and rehabilitative care of community-dwelling older persons with acute hip fracture? *Archives of Internal Medicine* 157:513–530.

Kirkland, S. and T. Mitchell. 1995. Occupational therapy in an orthopaedic early discharge programme. *Australian Occupational Therapy Journal* 42(1):31–34.

Levi, S.J. 1997. Posthospital setting, resource utilization, and self-care outcome in older women with hip fracture. *Archives of Physical Medicine and Rehabilitation* 78(9):973–979.

Penrose, D. 1993. Total hip replacement and other hip surgeries. In *Occupational Therapy for Orthopedic Conditions*, ed. D. Penrose, 28–52. London: Chapman & Hall.

Platt, J.V. 1996. *Occupational Therapy Practice Guidelines for Adults with Hip Fracture/Replacement.* Bethesda, MD: American Occupational Therapy Association.

Spalding, N.J. 1995. A comparative study of the effectiveness of a preoperative education programme for total hip replacement patients. *British Journal of Occupational Therapy* 58(12):526–531.

Tinetti, M.E., D.I. Baker, M. Gottschalk, P. Garrett, S. McGeary, D. Pollack, and P. Charpentier. 1997. Systematic home-based physical and functional therapy for older persons after hip fracture. *Archives of Physical Medicine and Rehabilitation* 78(11):1237–1247.

Hand Injuries

DESCRIPTION

Hand injuries include the loss of functional abilities and sensation in the hand. The human hand is versatile and has multiple functions, such as fine prehensile action to powerful movement, a major organ of sensation, a means of tactile communication, use in nearly all ADLs, a means of self-protection, gesticulation during speech, a communication system with the deaf, and the "eye" of the visually handicapped (Penso 1993, 106) (see also sections on carpal tunnel syndrome, fractures, peripheral nerve injuries, finger injuries, tendon injuries, and tendon transfers).

CAUSE

The causes include amputation of any part of the hand, nerve injuries, joint deformities, joint dislocation, tendon injuries, contractures, cumulative trauma disorders, or fractures.

ASSESSMENT

Areas
- daily living skills
- productivity history, skills, interests, and values
- work capacity and tolerance

Types of Injuries to the Hand

- amputation (traumatic, congenital)
- bone fractures and dislocations
- joint injuries—puncture, infection, tearing of capsule
- joint dislocations
- joint deformities
- nerve compression
- nerve severance (partial or complete)
- muscle weakness
- muscle paralysis (temporary or permanent)
- skin and soft tissue injuries—puncture, infection, abrasions
- tendon injuries—rupture, tearing of sheath
- tendon dislocations
- thermal injuries to the skin and soft tissue (burns, freezing)
- transplantation or replantation

- leisure interests and skills
- range of motion, including active and passive, total activity movement (TAM) and total passive movement (TPM), and torque-angle
- joint play (accessory motions that are nonvoluntary, physiologic, and can be performed by someone else)
- extrinsic extensor or flexor tightness
- hand functions: dexterity, including gross and fine, manipulation
- grip/grasp and pinch strength
- muscle strength
- posture and attitude of wrist and hand, wrist slightly dorsiflexed, digits lie with increasing flexion toward the ulnar side of the hand
- physical capacity
- pain, including numbness and tingling
- sensitivity: response to light touch, two-point discrimination, pressure, point localization and proprioception, stereognosis, temperature, and vibration
- fine motor skills, manipulation, dexterity, and bilateral coordination
- skin color
- skin condition: note skin loss, previous injury resulting in scarring, thin or fragile skin
- edema: pitting edema (soft), brawny edema (hard)
- psychosocial reactions, such as fear and response to loss of control

Instruments
Categories of Tests (Kasch 1996, 664)
1. Modality tests for pain, heat, cold, vibration, and touch pressure.

Measuring Total Passive and Active Motion

Measuring total passive and total active motion is a method of recording joint range that is used to compare tendon excursion (active) and joint mobility (passive). Both are measurements of flexion minus extensor lag of the three joints in the fingers.

Total passive motion (TPM) is calculated by summing the angles formed by the MCP, PIP, and DIP joints in maximum passive flexion minus the sum of angles of deficit from complete extension at each of these three joints: (MCP + PIP + DIP flexion) – (MCP + PIP + DIP extension) = total flexion – total extensor lag TPM.

Total active motion (TAM) is calculated by summing the angles formed by MCP, PIP, and DIP joints in maximum active flexion, i.e., fist position, minus total extension deficit at the MCP, PIP, and DIP joints with active finger extension.

TPM and TAM are used to measure a single digit, to indicate the total motion of that digit in degrees, and to compare that information to subsequent measurements of the same digit or to the corresponding normal digit of the opposite hand in the same person to determine whether the person is gaining or losing motion.

Source: Data from M.C. Kasch, Hand Injuries, in *Occupational Therapy: Practice Skills for Physical Dysfunction*, 4th ed., L.W. Pedretti, ed., p. 677, © 1996, Mosby; and American Society for Surgery of the Hand, *The Hand: Examination and Diagnosis*, 3rd ed., pp. 122–123, © 1990, Churchill-Livingstone.

---

2. Functional tests to assess the quality of sensibility or tactile gnosis, such as two-point discrimination (static and moving) and the Moberg Pick-Up Test.
3. Objective tests that do not require active participation by the person, such as the wrinkle test, the Ninhydrin sweat test, and nerve conduction studies.

Signs (Kasch 1996, 664)

- sympathetic nervous system dysfunction signs: Skin does not wrinkle when held in water for 5 minutes; loss of ability to sweat; smooth, shiny skin; nail changes, "pencil-point" or tapering of the fingers.
- nerve compression and regeneration signs: provocative tests, such as Tinel's sign or Phalen's maneuver.

Types of Sensibility Tests (Kasch 1996, 665, 666)

- moving touch—measured by touch pressure
- discrimination—measured by static and dynamic (moving) two-point discrimination
- recognition or tactile gnosis—measures ability of the hand to perform complex functions by feel
- equipment used in assessment of the hand
- circumference tape (measure edema in the fingers)
- finger goniometer. See American Society for Surgery of the Hand. 1990. *The Hand: Examination and Diagnosis*, 3rd ed., 122–127. Edinburgh, Scotland: Churchill Livingstone.

- Disk-Criminator (static two-point discrimination). See Dellon, A.L., S.E. Mackinnon, and P.M. Crosby. 1987. Reliability of two-point discrimination measurements. *Journal of Hand Surgery* [AM] 12A:693–696.
- dynamometer. For positioning, see American Society for Surgery of the Hand. 1990. *The Hand: Examination and Diagnosis*, 3rd ed., 121–122. Edinburgh, Scotland: Churchill Livingstone. For values, see Stokes, H.M. 1981. The seriously injured hand: weakness of grip. *Journal of Occupational Medicine* 25:683–684.
- goniometer. Use the American Academy of Orthopaedic Surgeons values and the American Society for Surgery of the Hand reporting system.
- jeweler's rings (measure edema in the fingers)
- monofilaments. Semmes-Weinstein Calibrated Monofilaments (light touch-deep pressure). See Bell-Krotoski, J.A. 1995. Sensibility testing: Current concepts. In *Rehabilitation of the Hand,* 4th ed., ed. J.M. Hunter, 109–128. St. Louis: Mosby.
- pinch meter (finger strength). For norms, see Swanson, A.B., G. Swanson, and C. Goran-Hagert. 1990. Evaluation of impairment of hand function. In *Rehabilitation of the Hand*, 3rd ed., ed. J.M. Hunter. St Louis: Mosby-Year Book.
- ridge sensitometer. See Poppen, N.K., et al. 1979. Recovery of sensibility after suture of digital nerves. *Journal of Hand Surgery* 4:212–226.
- thermometer (measure skin temperature)
- tuning forks (measure vibration). Two forks are used. One vibrates at 30 cps or Hz (Hertz) and the other at 256 cps or Hz.
- vibrometer (measures vibration). Fixed frequency at 120 cps. Example is the Bio-Thesiometer.
- volumeter (measures edema). Instructions provided in Kasch (1996, 663).

Types of Tests

- Downey Hand Center Hand Sensitivity Test. See Yerxa, E.J., et al. 1983. Development of a hand sensitivity test for the hypersensitive hand. *American Journal of Occupational Therapy* 37(3):176–181 or Barber, L.M. 1990. Desensitization of the hand. In *Rehabilitation of the Hand*, 3rd ed., ed. J.M. Hunter et al., 1721–1729. St. Louis: CV Mosby. Also called the *Downey Community Hospital Hand Sensitivity Test.*
- finger and point identification (localization) or mapping. The finger is touched just enough to indent the skin with the point of a pencil. The person is asked to identify the finger that was touched and point to the finger where the pencil touched the skin (Malick 1996, 664).
- Jebsen Hand Function Test by Jebsen, R.H., et al. 1969. An objective and standardized test of hand function. *Archives of Physical Medicine and Rehabilitation* 50:311–319.
- manual muscle test by Lowett, R.W. and E.G. Martin. 1996. Certain aspects of infantile paralysis and a description of a method of muscle testing. *JAMA* 6:729–733. Current source of testing positions is Hislop, H.J. and J. Montgomery. 1995. *Daniels and Worthingham's Muscle Testing: Techniques of Manual Examination*, 6th ed. Philadelphia: WB Saunders or Kendall, F.P., E.K. McCreary, and P.G. Provance. 1993. *Muscle Testing and Function*, 4th ed. Baltimore, Williams & Wilkins. For comparison of muscle test grading systems, see Groth et al. (1998, 609–610).
- Moberg Pick-Up Test modified by A. Dellon (tactile gnosia, stereognosis). Dellon, A.L. 1981. *Evaluation of Sensibility and Re-Education of Sensation in the Hand*, 102–106. Baltimore, MD: Williams & Wilkins.

- Moving Two-Point Discrimination Test by Dellon, A. 1978. The moving two-point discrimination test: clinical evaluation of the quickly adapting fiber receptor system. *Journal of Hand Surgery* 3:474–481.
- McGill Pain Profile by Melzack, R. 1975. The McGill Pain Questionnaire: Major properties and scoring methods. *Pain* 1:277–299.
- ninhydrin sweat test (printing) test. See Groth et al. (1998, 616–617).
- O'Riain (also Orian) wrinkle test. See S. O'Riain. 1973. New and simple test of nerve function in the hand. *British Medical Journal* 3:615–616.
- palpation. Look for masses or nodules, changes in skin temperature, and texture of skin (i.e., dry, wet, soft, rough, or scarred)
- Quantitative Test of Upper Extremity Function by Carroll, D. 1965. A quantitative test of upper extremity function. *Journal of Chronic Diseases* 18:479-491.
- Sequential Occupational Dexterity Assessment (SODA) by Van Lankveld, W., P.V.P. Bosch, J. Bakker, S. Terwindt, M. Franssen, P. van Riel. 1996. Sequential occupational dexterity assessment (SODA): A new test to measure hand disability. *Journal of Hand Therapy* 9(1):27–32.
- Standardized sensory assessment for children of school-age by Cooper J., A. Majnemer, B. Rosenblatt, R. Birnbaum. 1993. A standardized sensory assessment for children of school-age. *Physical and Occupational Therapy in Pediatrics* 13(1):61–80.
- Smith Hand Function Evaluation by Smith, H.B. 1973. Smith hand function evaluation. *American Journal of Occupational Therapy* 25:77–83.
- Sollerman Test of Grip Function by Sollerman, C. 1984. *Assessment of Grip function: Evaluation of a New Test Method.* Sjobo, Sweden: Medical Innovation Technology (MITAB).
- tactile discrimination test. King, P.M. 1997. Sensory function assessment. *Journal of Hand Therapy* 10(1):24–28.
- tactile gnosia test. See the Moberg Pick-Up Test or King, P.M. 1997. Sensory Function Assessment. *Journal of Hand Therapy* 10(1):24–28.
- Tinel's sign. American Society for Surgery of the Hand, 1990. The hand: Examination and diagnosis, 3rd ed., 93–95. Edinburgh, Scotland: Churchill Livingstone.
- Three-Phase Hand Sensitivity Test. North Coast Medical, 1980. (Similar to the Downey Hand Center Sensitivity Test, listed above.)
- visual analogue test. Schultz, K.S. 1984. The Schultz structured interview for assessing upper extremity pain. *Occupational Therapy in Health Care* 1;1:69–82.
- commercial hand-finger coordination/dexterity tests:
  1. *Crawford Small Parts Dexterity Test*, revised, by Crawford, J.E. and D.M. Crawford. 1981. San Antonio, TX: The Psychological Corporation.
  2. *Hand-Tool Dexterity Test* by Bennett, G.K. 1965. Lafayette, IN: Lafayette Instrument.
  3. *O'Connor Finger or Tweezer Dexterity Tests* by O'Connor, J. 1926. Lafayette, IN: Lafayette Instrument.
  4. *Lafayette Grooved Pegboard.* 1977. Lafayette, IN: Lafayette Instrument.
  5. *Minnesota Manual Dexterity Test.* 1969. Lafayette, IN: Lafayette Instrument.
  6. *Minnesota Rate of Manipulation.* 1969. Circle Pines, MN: American Guidance Services.
  7. *Nine-Hole Peg Test.* 1971; 1985. Bolingbrook, IL: Sammons Preston.

8. *Pennsylvania Bi-Manual Work Sample* by Roberts, J. 1945. Circle Pines, MN: American Guidance Service.
9. *Purdue Pegboard Test* by Tippen, J. 1948, 1960, 1999. Lafayette, IN: Lafayette Instrument Company.
- *Valpar work sample series.* Tucson, AZ: Valpar Corporation.
  1. Valpar whole body range of motion work sample.
  2. Valpar upper extremity range of motion work sample.
  3. Valpar small tools (mechanical) work sample.
  4. Valpar eye-hand-foot coordination work sample.
  5. Valpar clerical comprehension work sample.

PROBLEMS

Self-Care
- The person usually is unable to perform some self-care and daily living tasks.

Productivity
- The person is usually unable to work during the acute phase of the disability.
- The person may be unable to continue employment in his or her current job.
- The person may be unable to perform some home-management tasks.

Leisure
- The person may be unable to engage in his or her favorite leisure activities.

Sensorimotor
- The person may have loss of range of motion.
- The person may have loss of joint mobility.
- The person may have loss of joint stability.
- The person may have loss of grip or pinch strength.
- The person may have loss of hand functions.
- The person may have loss of manipulation skills, dexterity, and bilateral coordination.
- The person may have vasomotor changes, such as changes in skin color and texture.
- The person may have edema and swelling.
- The person may have loss of sensory registration in tactile, proprioceptive, pressure, temperature, and vibrator senses.
- The person may have loss of sensory processing, including tactile discrimination and localization.
- The person may have loss of perceptual skills, such as stereognosis and graphesthesia.
- The person may have hypersensitivity, especially touch.

Cognitive
- Cognitive faculties are not usually affected directly by the hand disability, unless it is related to a closed or open head injury.

Psychosocial
- The person may fear disability or disfigurement.

- The person may be angry with his or her employer or him- or herself for causing the injury.
- The person may fear being unable to return to work.
- The person may experience loss of self-esteem.
- The person may grieve over loss of function.
- The person may become depressed.
- The person may fear changes in role identity.
- The person may withdraw from family or friends and social activities.
- The person may have changes in social roles.

TREATMENT/INTERVENTION

Models of treatment in occupational therapy are based on biomechanical and rehabilitative (compensatory) models.

Self-Care
- Encourage performance of self-care activities.
- Provide self-help devices and training, if needed.

Productivity
- Provide work tolerance or work-hardening programs, if needed.
- Provide opportunities to explore other vocational skills and interests if a return to the original job is impossible.
- Make recommendations to employers regarding job modifications that can reduce worker injury.
- Make recommendations for modification of homemaking activities to accommodate temporary or permanent disability.

Leisure
- Make recommendations for modifications of leisure activities for temporary or permanent disability.
- Assist the person to explore new or renew old interests to replace activities that cannot be continued, if necessary.

Sensorimotor
- Increase the person's range of motion through daily living activities, creative activities, or prescribed exercises.
- Improve joint mobility through joint mobilization techniques or daily living activities.
- Increase grip and pinch strength using exercises on the weighted dumbbells, Theraband, grippers, putty, spring-type clothes pins, or other household items and toys.
- Provide practice in the use of hand positions through activities or games that require various hand positions to perform a task.
- Increase coordination and dexterity through games or activities involving manipulation of small pieces or parts.
- Consider splinting to maintain the hand position, prevent deformity or contracture, or improve functional performance.

- Decrease edema through elevation, active and passive range of motion, retrograde massage, string wrapping, intermittent compression pump, air splints, heat and cold modalities, contrast bathers, high-voltage galvanic stimulation. Maintain reduction of edema through compression wrapping, pressure garments, and personal and caregiver education (Deshaies and Walsh 1997, 1-3).
- Provide pain management, if needed. (Doleys et al. 1997, 175–182).
- Provide sensory reeducation, if needed (Bentzel 1995, 424–427; Callahan 1995, 701–714).
  Description: A method that helps the person with a sensory impairment learn to reinterpret the altered profile of neural impulses reaching the conscious level.
  Application: Appropriate for persons with nerve injuries, replantations, toe-to-thumb transfers, skin grafts, and CVAs.
  Rationale: It is assumed that repeated stimuli are necessary to facilitate cortical reeducation to occur, which, in turn, results in improvement of sensation.
  Techniques:
  1. Treatment must include repeated sensory stimuli to those skin areas of sufficient intensity so that the person can feel the stimulus.
  2. Address in order tactile localization, two-point discrimination, and tactile gnosis.
  3. Graduation of sensory retraining activities is necessary, such as allowing compensation with vision at first but, as therapy progresses, the person must rely totally on tactile sensation. Initially, each task should be done with vision present and then with vision occluded.
  4. Sessions should be brief (10–15 minutes) because full concentration is needed. The environment should be free from distractions. Two to four session per day are recommended.
  5. Activities to increase tactile awareness: apply lotion, rub with a terrycloth towel, "draw" shapes on pile carpet, pick up objects with various textures with both hands and fingers interlaced, make a pattern with sand, knead dough, make objects from clay, stroke skin area with various textures, weave to macramé with sisal twine.
  6. When the person should be able to perceive moving touch and vibration at 30 Hz, the next goal is the differentiation of moving versus constant touch and to reeducate incorrect localization. To facilitate moving touch, the therapist can use the eraser end of a pencil to stroke up and down the area being reeducated while the person watches. The stroking is repeated with eyes closed while the person concentrates on feeling. The person can open the eyes again for reinforcement. For localization, stimulate one small area of skin at a time, using the eraser. As improvement occurs, use smaller stimuli, such as monofilaments.
  7. In tactile gnosis or discrimination, progress from gross to fine discrimination by asking for greater detail as the person shows progress. Objects may vary in size, shape, and texture, with finer discrimination required as improvement occurs. Levels of difficulty can be organized by starting with identification of same or different, asking the person to explain in what way the objects are the same or different and to identify the texture, object, or item. Examples include identifying geometric shapes made from Velcro strips mounted on cardboard; recognizing shapes and sizes of different wood blocks; recognizing different weights using sandbags and cotton bags; sorting a group of textures into rough and smooth or by

round versus square; counting the number of marbles in a box; increase the difficulty by adding other objects in with the marbles; identifying shapes cut out of cardboard; selecting a named object from a group of objects; determining which of two objects is heavier; locating objects hidden in a medium, such as sand, rice, unpopped popcorn, or Styrofoam particles; fit wood shapes into a puzzle; assemble wood letters into words or a message; identify whether two pieces of sandpaper or fabric are the same or different; identify number or geometric shapes traced on the person's skin; trace the path of a raised design maze formed with colored epoxy on cardboard; complete self-care and work tasks that require manipulation of objects without vision.

- Provide desensitization program, if needed (Bentzel 1995, 428–429; Waylett-Rendall 1995, 693–700).

  Description: Desensitization permits the person to learn to filter out unpleasant sensations (often interpreted as pain) and to respond with accurate perception to sensory input.

  Rationale: Desensitization is based on the belief that progressive stimulation will allow progressive tolerance to stimuli in situations where a person responds with hypersensitivity (pain response) to situations that would not normally cause pain.

  Application: Amputation stumps, neuromas, spinal cord injuries, brachial plexus injuries, nerve injuries, nerve compression, and soft tissue injuries.

  Techniques:
  1. Five-level program: Level 1 includes the use of vibration via a tuning fork, paraffin, and massage. Level 2 includes the use of vibration via a battery-operated massager, friction massage, and constant touch pressure. Level 3 includes the use of an electric vibrator and identification of textures. Level 4 includes the use of an electric vibrator and object identification. Level 5 includes the use of work and daily activities.
  2. Hierarchy of texture and vibration program: Each person arranges the 10 dowel textures, 10 immersion textures, and 9 vibration cycles in the order perceived as least to most irritating, which can be tolerated for 10 minutes, 3 or 4 times daily. The progress is recorded on the Downey Hand Center Hand Sensitivity Test form (see Instruments). The dowel textures are moleskin, felt, Quickstick (a splint padding material), velvet, semirough cloth, Velcro loop, Hard T-foam, burlap, rug back, and Velcro hook. The immersion textures are cotton, terrycloth pieces, dry rice, popcorn, pinto beans, macaroni, plastic wire insulation pieces, small BBs or buckshot, large BBs or buckshot, and plastic squares. The vibrations cycles are 83 cps near area; 83 cps near area, 23 cps near area; 83 cps near area, 23 cps intermittent contact; 83 cps intermittent contact, 23 cps intermittent contact; 83 cps intermittent contact, 23 cps continuous contact; 83 cps continuous contact, 53 cps intermittent contact; 100 cps intermittent contact, 53 cps intermittent contact; 100 cps intermittent contact, 53 cps continuous contact; and 100 cps continuous contact, 53 cps continuous contact.
  3. Other activities: continuous pressure using an Isotoner glove or weight-bearing pressure, massage, percussion, stroking, TENS, vibrometer, fluid therapy, acupuncture, compression distraction, ultrasound, graded textures, typing, washing hair, macramé, leather link belts, and a variety of work simulations.

- Provide compensatory education for the absence of protective sensation, if needed (Bentzel 1995, 429–430; Callahan 1995, 701–714).

Description: Treatment consists of education for the person and/or caregiver in precautions necessary to prevent injury.

Rationale: A person without protective sensory feedback in the fingers or hand has a high risk of burns, cuts, lacerations, and bruises. The mechanisms of damage include continuous, low pressure, which causes necrosis from lack of blood supply; high pressure, causing cutting or crushing by mechanical violence; excessive heat or cold, leading to burning or frostbite; repetitive mechanical stress of a moderate degree, causing inflammation and autolyis; and pressure on infected tissue that results in the spread of infection.

Application: For whatever reason, the person is unable to use or respond to protective sensory feedback from the fingers or hand.

Techniques:

1. Low pressure: need frequent position changes to avoid static pressure
2. High pressure: large handles on suitcases, drawers, and cupboards; large key holders
3. Heat: pot holders, utensils with wood or plastic handles, rather than metal
4. Cold: gloves or mittens
5. Repetitive pressure: lower the pressure or the number of repetitions, inspect the skin for signs of inflammation and give reddened skin areas total relief from pressure, wear soft shoe insoles, lose weight, wear gloves, use enlarged or padded handles on tools, walk shorter distances, use a variety of tools or alternate hands
6. Infection: rest infected body part completely; splint, bed rest, or other means of total immobilization may be necessary
7. Other techniques: substitute vision to prevent contact with sharp objects; use an insulated coffee cup; avoid exposure to extreme temperature; become aware of how much force is necessary in grasping objects; avoid small handles that concentrate forces on a small area of skin; apply lotion or oil daily; or apply a splint to active but insensate skin areas

Special Conditions:

- Camptodactyly—see Benson et al. (1994, 814–819). Splinting is effective with all three types of camptodactyly but is most successful with type 1 or congenital camptodactyly.
- Cancer, chemotherapy, and radiation—see Cook and Burkhardt (1994, 1141–1159).
- Capsulectomy—see Cannon (1995, 1173–1186).
- de Quervain's—see Canelón (1997, 144–153).
- Neuroma—see Spicher and Kohut (1996, 47–51).
- Replantation—see Buncke et al. (1995, 1075–1100). Includes protocols for digital, thumb, hand, and arm replantation on 1094–1095.
- Stiff hand—see Colditz (1995, 1141–1159).
- Swan neck deformity—see Eckhaus (1997, 151–156).
- Wrist arthrodesis—see Kozera (1997, 305–310).

Cognitive

- Provide instructions on a home program.
- Provide instruction in one-hand activities, if needed, during recovery period.
- Provide factual information on prognosis and outcome of specific injury or surgery.

Proposed Taxonomy of Hand Functions

Static hand tool functions
- **Grip or Grasp**: The hand holds an object by using large portions of the palmar surface of the fingers and/or thumb. Specific types include hook, cylindrical, palmar, or spherical grip or grasp.
- **Prehension**: The distal segments of one or more fingertip(s) and thumb tip hold small objects. Types include lateral (key), palmar, three-point (tripod, three-jaw chuck), and tip prehension.
- **Containment** (holding, storage): The hand holds more than one small-to-moderate sized object, such as peanuts, screws, coins, or nails, for later manipulation.
- **Stabilization**: A single object is held firmly or loosely in the hand, using one or a variety of grips or grasps, such as holding a hand pruner, a soldering iron, or an aspirin bottle.

Dynamic hand tool functions
- **Probe**: The fingertip(s), thumb tip or other portions of the fingers are used to push (using finger extension), pull (using finger flexion) or move laterally in order to move, support, or control an object or portion of an object, such as pushing a button through a button hole.
- **Translation**:
  1. Tip to palm: After grasping a small object with finger and thumb tips, the object may be slid or shifted from its initial position near the digit tips to the palm, such as picking up a coin and sliding it into the palm.
  2. Palm to tips: An object is moved from the palm to fingertips using probe or shift functions, such as picking a coin from several in the palm to put into a coin machine or eat peanuts from the hand.
  3. Across finger pads: Probe or shift functions are used to move the object across the palmar surface of the fingers in a radial ulnar direction from one finger to the next, such as dealing cards from a deck.
- **Rolling**: The thumb and finger(s) oppose each other to grasp an object with a tip or palmar prehension; they then move in a circular motion (thumb moving in a direction opposite to the fingers) while keeping contact with the object to form a ball or cylinder from a malleable object, such as clay, putty, or string.
- **Rotation**: The fingers are positioned so that their palmar surfaces may oppose one another and move in opposite directions to rotate an object. Rotation may occur on an axis that is parallel to metacarpals, parallel to palm and distal palmar crease, or perpendicular to palm. The action may move clockwise or counterclockwise as the object rotates, such as opening or closing a jar lid.
- **Shift**: The fingers, thumb, and palm, while maintaining contact with an object at several surfaces or points, alternately release, slide, or move, or

continues

continued

> otherwise change the surfaces of contact to allow the object to move in a more useful direction to accomplish a task, such as picking up a marking pen and shifting it into position to print or draw.
> • **Shift to Rotate**: The fingers, thumb, palm and remainder of the hand have several points or surfaces of contact with the object and move it generally 180 degrees, such as turning a pencil end for end to use the eraser.
>
> *Source:* Data from S. Worley, Evaluating and Training Adult Manipulative Hand Skills, *Physical Disabilities Special Interest Section Newsletter*, 1995, Vol. 18, No. 3, pp. 1–2; and C. Stahl, Taxonomy of Adult Hand Skills Aid Quality of Life, *Advances for Occupational Therapists,* © 1996, Vol. 12, No. 35, pp. 12–13.

Psychosocial

• Encourage the person to express feelings about the appearance of the hand and his or her fears for the future.
• Permit the person to express feelings of anger or guilt about the injury or the situation in which the injury occurred.
• Through scheduling or participation in a support group, encourage the person to share experiences with other clients who have had similar experiences.
• Encourage the person to continue participation in social activities. Provide ideas or techniques for adapting participation (in leisure activities, for example) if needed.

PRECAUTIONS

• Dynamometers must be recalibrated frequently to provide reliable data.
• When using a volumeter, the following decrease the accuracy of the reading: use of a faucet or hose that introduces air into the tank during filling, movement of the arm with the tank, inconsistent pressure on the stop rod, and use of the volumeter in various places (Kasch 1996, 663).
• A person without protective sensation (decreased proprioception and pressure feedback) tends to use too much force to perform simple activities, such as turning a key in a lock. The result is lacerations, abrasions, or other damage to soft tissue.
• A hand with decreased sensation may be used to grip or pinch objects repetitively beyond the point of tissue tolerance for which normal sensation would provide a warning (pain and redness). The result is blisters and bruises. Adapted grips are especially prone to cause such damage.
• Lack of sensation is usually accompanied by a lack of sweating. The result is dry, cracked skin, which is more likely to be damaged from daily use than skin that is soft and pliable.

PROGNOSIS AND OUTCOME

• The person demonstrates grip strength within normal range for his or her sex, age, and type of work. (Note: Right-hand-dominant people tend to have a 10% stronger grip in the right hand than the left, but left-hand-dominant people tend to have equal strength.)

- The person demonstrates functional range of motion in the fingers, thumb, wrist, and forearm.
- The person demonstrates functional hand positions, including pinch and grasp positions.
- The person demonstrates tactile awareness and discrimination.
- The person demonstrates dexterity and coordination using injured hand alone and bilaterally.
- The person is able to perform ADLs independently.
- The person is able to perform productive activities.
- The person is able to perform leisure activities.

REFERENCES

Benson, L.S., P.M. Waters, K.I. Kamil, S.P. Simmons, and J. Upton III. 1994. Camptodactyly: Classification and results of nonoperative treatment. *Journal of Pediatric Orthopaedics* 14:814–819.

Bentzel, K. 1995. Remediating sensory impairment. In *Occupational Therapy for Physical Dysfunction*, 4th ed., ed. C.A. Trombly, 423–432. Baltimore: Williams & Wilkins.

Buncke, H.J, R.L. Jackson, G.M. Buncke, and S.W. Chan. 1995. The surgical and rehabilitation aspects of replantation and revascularization of the hand. In *Rehabilitation of the Hand*, 4th ed., eds. J.M. Hunter, E.J. Mackin, and A.D. Callahan, 1075–1100. St. Louis: Mosby.

Callahan, A.D. 1995. Methods of compensation and reeducation for sensory dysfunction. In *Rehabilitation of the Hand*, 4th ed., eds. J.M. Hunter, E.J. Mackin, and A.D. Callahan, 701–714. St. Louis: Mosby.

Canelón, M.F. and E.M. Ervin. 1997. An on-site job evaluation performed via activity analysis. *American Journal of Occupational Therapy* 51(2):144–153.

Cannon, N.M. 1995. Postoperative management of metacarpophalangeal joint capsulectomies. In *Rehabilitation of the Hand: Surgery and Therapy*, 4th ed., eds. J.M. Hunter, E.J. Mackin, and A.D. Callahan, 1173–1186. St. Louis: Mosby.

Colditz, J.C. 1995. Therapist's management of the stiff hand. In *Rehabilitation of the Hand: Surgery and Therapy*, 4th ed., ed. J.M. Hunter, E.J. Mackin, and A.D. Callahan, 1141–1159. St. Louis: Mosby.

Cook, A. and A. Burkhardt. 1994. The effect of cancer diagnosis and treatment on hand function. *American Journal of Occupational Therapy* 48(9):836–839.

Deshaies, L.D. and M. Walsh. 1997. Comprehensive management of upper-extremity edema. *Physical Disabilities Special Interest Section Quarterly* 20(3):1–3.

Doleys, D.M., L. Marino, M. Howell, and B. Nicholson. 1997. Pain management program in hand therapy: A literature review and appraisal. *Journal of Hand Therapy* 10(2):175–182.

Eckhaus, D. 1997. Swan-neck deformity. In *Hand Rehabilitation: A Practical Guide*, 2nd ed., ed. G.L. Clark, E.F.S. Wilgis, B. Aiello, D. Eckhaus, and L.V. Eddington, 151–156. New York: Churchill Livingstone.

Groth, G.N., J. Guccione, P. Payner, E.C. Phillips, B. Sopp, M.B. Wulf, E.J. Walker, K.A. Mantz, and B.A. Kraemer. 1998. Therapy considerations following acute hand injuries. In *Manual of Acute Hand Injuries*, ed. Martin, D.S., E.D. Collins, 604–649. St. Louis: Mosby.

Kasch, M.C. 1996. Hand Injuries. In *Occupational Therapy: Practice Skills for Physical Dysfunction*, 4th ed., ed. L.W. Pedretti, 661–692. St. Louis: Mosby.

Kozera, B.F. 1997. Wrist arthrodesis. In *Hand Rehabilitation: A Practical Guide*, 2nd ed., ed. G.L. Clark, E.F.S. Wilgis, B. Aiello, D. Eckhaus, and L.V. Eddington, 305–310. New York: Churchill Livingstone.

Penso, D.E. 1993. *Perceptuo-motor Difficulties: Theory Strategies to Help Children, Adolescents and Adults.* London: Chapman & Hall.

Spicher, C. and G. Kohut. 1996. Rapid relief of a painful, long-standing posttraumatic digital neuroma treated by transcutaneous vibratory stimulation (TVS). *Journal of Hand Therapy* 9(1):47–51 (Case report).

Stahl, C. 1996. Taxonomy of adult hand skills aid quality of life. *Advance for Occupational Therapists* 12(35):12–13.

Waylett-Rendall, J. 1995. Desensitization of the traumatized hand. In *Rehabilitation of the Hand*, 4th ed., ed. J.M. Hunter, E.J. Mackin, A.D. Callahan. 693–700. St. Louis: Mosby.

Worley S. and G. Artis. 1995. Evaluating and training adult manipulative hand skills. *Physical Disabilities Special Interest Section Newsletter* 18(3):1–2.

BIBLIOGRAPHY

Artsberger, S.M. 1997. Edema control: New perspectives. *Physical Disabilities Special Interest Section Newsletter* 20(1):1–3.

Bear-Lehman, J. 1997. Functional evaluation of the wrist and hand. In *Musculoskeletal Disorders in the Workplace: Principles and Practice,* ed. M. Nordin, G.B.J. Andersoson, M.H. Pope, 450–457. St. Louis: Mosby.

Berman, K. and J.M. Failla. 1995. A method for converting a mallet finger splint into a Boutonnière splint. *Journal of Hand Therapy* 8(3):214.

Clark, G. 1993. An emotional journey. *TeamRehab Reports* 4(6):32–34.

Cooper, C. 1995. The geriatric hand patient: Special treatment considerations. In *Rehabilitation of the Hand*, 4th ed. ed. J.M. Hunter, E.J. Mackin, and A.D. Callahan, 1483–1491. St. Louis: Mosby.

Dannenbaum, R.M., L.A. Jones. 1993. The assessment and treatment of patients who have sensory loss following cortical lesions. *Journal of Hand Therapy* 6(2):130–138.

Daus, C. 1995. Traumatic hand injuries. *Rehab Management* 8(5):31–34.

Estes, J.P. 1993. Hand injuries. In *Conditions in Occupational Therapy: Effects on Occupational Performance*, ed. R.A. Hansen and B. Atchison, 81–97. Baltimore: Williams & Wilkins (Case reports).

Exner, C.E. 1995. Remediation of hand skill problems in children. In *Hand Function in the Child: Foundations for Remediation*, ed. A. Henderson, C. Pehoski, 197–222. St. Louis: Mosby.

Gilin, M. and B. Frown. 1995. The hands that keep the motor city rolling. *Advance for Directors in Rehabilitation* 4(7):55–56, 58.

Huebler, D. 1995. Outcomes in hand therapy. *Rehab Management* 8(3):109–111.

Jaffe, R., L.F. Chidgey, P.C. LaStayo. 1996. The distal radioulnar joint: Anatomy and management of disorders. *Journal of Hand Therapy* 9(2):129–138.

Johnson, S.L. 1993. Therapy of the occupationally injured hand and upper extremity. *Hand Clinics* 9:289–298.

Johnsone, B. and J. Duncan. 1998. Hand injuries in children. In *Atlas of Hand Surgery*, ed. W.B. Conolly, 135–146. New York: Churchill Livingstone.

Kasch, M.C., S.E. Poole, and M. Hiedl. 1998. Acute hand injuries. In *Physical Dysfunction: Practice Skills for the Occupational Therapy Assistant*, ed. M.B. Early, 566–588. St. Louis: Mosby.

Kenny, D. and E. Maday. 1994. Hand strengthening devices range from low-tech putty to computers. *Advance for Directors in Rehabilitation* 3(2):41–44.

Kenny, D. and E. Maday. 1994. Job simulation and hand rehabilitation. *Advance for Directors in Rehabilitation* 3(9):41–44.

King, P.M. 1997. Sensory function assessment: A pilot study of touch pressure threshold with texture and tactile discrimination. *Journal of Hand Therapy* 10(1):24–28.

Marmer, L. 1996. Making motionless hands move. *Advance for Occupational Therapists* 12(9):14–15,18.

O'Neill, G. 1995. The development of a standardized assessment of hand function. *British Journal of Occupational Therapy* 58(11):477–480.

Penrose, D. 1995. The hand. In *Occupational Therapy for Orthopedic Conditions*, ed. D. Penrose, 146–170. London: Chapman & Hall.

Philips, C.A. 1995. Impairments of hand function. In *Occupational Therapy for Physical Dysfunction*, 4th ed., ed. C.A. Trombly, 773–793. Baltimore: Williams & Wilkins.

Stewart, K.M. 1995. Therapist's management of the complex injury. In *Rehabilitation of the Hand*, 4th ed., ed. J.M. Hunter, E.J. Mackin, and A.D. Callahan, 1057–1074. St. Louis: Mosby.

Thompson, T. and P. Jolley. 1996. Wound care and management for a hand wound. *Physical Disabilities Special Interest Section Newsletter* 19(1):3–4.

Toth-Cohen, S., P.B. Petralia, and K.S. Miller. 1997. Therapists' experiences with computer-assisted instruction in hand therapy. *Journal of Hand Therapy* 10(1):41–45.

Walsh, W.W., N.N. Belding, E. Taylor, and J.A. Nunley. 1993. The effect of upper extremity trauma on handedness. *American Journal of Occupational Therapy* 47(9):787–795.

Hand Injuries—Tendon Injuries

DESCRIPTION

Tendon injuries are defined as lacerations, avulsion-type injuries, and crush injuries to the flexor or extensor tendons of the hand. The injury may occur primarily to the tendons, but more often it is accompanied by fractures, nerve injuries, and soft tissue damage. The type of injury often affects final outcome. Crushing or blunt injuries then lead to more scar formation. Laceration injuries often have a better prognosis (Stewart and van Strien 1995, 441).

Flexor tendon injuries usually occur between the distal palmar crease and the insertion of the flexor digitorum superficialis. The tendons lie in their sheaths beneath the fibrous pulley system, and any scarring causes adhesion.

Injuries to flexor tendons in Zone 1 can be functionally limiting because even a small amount of loss of excursion reduces the performance potential. The area designated Zone 2 used to be referred to as "no-man's land" because of the risk of permanent dysfunction in the hand after surgery, due to adhesions. However, current postsurgical management techniques have improved the outcome. Zone 3 lacerations are also susceptible to adhesion to adjacent tendons, lumbricals, and interossei, as well as overlying fascia and skin. Zone 4 injuries are at risk for adhesions to the synovial sheaths, to each other, and to the other structures lying within the carpal tunnel space. Zone 5 tendon injuries are prone to adhesions to the overlying skin and fascia (Stewart and van Strien 1995, 440–441).

Injury to extensor tendons may result in dorsal scar adherence during the healing process. If the dorsal extensor hood mechanism becomes adherent to the underlying structures, there will be limitations to normal excursion during flexion and extension. If zones V, VI, and VII (proximal to the MCP joints) become adherent, the result may be either incomplete extensions, also known as *extensor lag*, or incomplete flexion, which occurs from the loss of extensor tendon glide (Kasch 1996, 676).

If adhesions do not respond to conservative therapy, a surgical release technique called *tenolysis* can be used to salvage the tendon function (Schneider and Berger-Feldscher 1995, 463).

Factors Related to Skin Stress and Soft-Tissue Damage

Degree of stress (measured in degrees of force or pressure)
- low—most likely to be damaging if duration is continuous and ischemia results
- moderate—most likely to be damaging if repetitive
- high—usually damaging, but size is likely to be the critical factor

Duration of stress (measured in time units, such as seconds, minutes, hours, days)
- continuous short/long
- intermittent short/long

Repetition of stress (measured in number of repeated cycles)
- infrequent
- frequent
- constant

Direction of force of stress (measured in weight units, such as pounds, kilograms)
- direct (perpendicular to the surface)
- shear (lateral to the surface, may produce a tearing effect)

Size of stress (measured in surface units, such as inches, centimeters in diameter)
- localized
- large
- diffuse

Key locations of stress (described in relation to a body part)
- bony prominence in contact with a wrap, splint, or cast
- edges of a wrap, splint, or cast, including "windows" in casts

Source: Data from J.A. Bell-Krotoski, D.E. Breger, and R.B. Beach, Application of Biomechanics for Evaluation of the Hand, in *Rehabilitation of the Hand*, 3rd ed., J.M. Hunter, E.J. Mackin, and A.D. Callahan, eds., pp. 139–164 © 1990, Mosby.

CAUSE

The most frequent causes of these tendon injuries are work-related or sports activities; however, injuries resulting from knives, glass, or other sharp objects also occur. Injury may occur because the tendon is overstretched or ruptured; the tendon and part of its insertion onto the bone are avulsed or fractured; or the epiphysis is slipped from the bone shaft.

ASSESSMENT

Areas
- daily living tasks
- productivity history, skills, interests, and values
- leisure interests and skills

- range of motion (Measure AROM, PROM, total active motion for digits, and total passive motion for digits.)
- muscle testing
- grip and pinch strength
- wound care and management
- edema
- hand functions
- sensibility

Instruments
Equipment

- dynamometer (grip or grasp strength), see American Society for Surgery of the Hand, 1990. *The Hand: Examination and Diagnosis*, 3rd ed., 121–122. New York: Churchill Livingstone.
- goniometer (range of motion)
- pinch meter (finger strength)
- Semmes-Weinstein monofilaments (sensibility)
- volumeter (edema)
- tape measure or jewelry rings (edema)

Tests

- manual muscle test
- work assessment

PROBLEMS

Self-Care

- The person may be unable to perform some ADLs due to an inability to use the fingers in the normal or accustomed manner.

Productivity

- The person is usually unable to perform some productive activities due to an inability to use the injured fingers in the normal or accustomed manner.

Leisure

- The person may be unable to perform some favorite leisure activities due to an inability to use the injured fingers in the normal or accustomed manner.

Sensorimotor

Examples, not a comprehensive list:
- flexor tendon injuries of the hand
  1. Zone I (jersey finger)—lack of active flexion of the DIP joint, most commonly in the ring finger
  2. Zone II—lack of active flexion of the PIP joint
  3. Zones III, IV, and V—lack of active flexion of fingers at all joints

- extensor tendon injuries of the hand
  1. mallet finger
     a. inability to actively extend the DIP joint
     b. may have flexion deformity
  2. boutonnière deformity
     a. hyperextension of the MCP joint
     b. flexion of PIP joint
     c. hyperextension of the DIP joint
  3. dislocation of extensor digitorum communis hood
     a. incomplete active extension
- The person may have tenderness to touch.
- The person may experience pain with or without movement.

Cognitive
- There are no specific cognitive problems related directly to the tendon injury.

Psychosocial
- The person may express feelings of anger at his or her employer or at the situation that caused the accident.
- The person may feel guilty about causing an accident.
- The person may fear that his or her fingers will be unusable.
- The person may fear being unable to return to work.
- The person may fear that his or her hand and fingers will be disfigured.
- The person may have difficulty participating in some social activities during rehabilitation because of the injury or a requirement to wear a splint.
- The person may withdraw from social situations to avoid being seen with an injured hand or fingers in public.

TREATMENT/INTERVENTION
Models of treatment in occupational therapy are based on the biomechanical and rehabilitative (compensatory) models. The approaches to tendon management are most frequently called *immobilization, early passive mobilization,* and *early active mobilization.* There are many variations of the three approaches. Thus, the descriptions below should be considered representative but not comprehensive presentations of tendon management approaches.

Self-Care
- Consider providing self-help devices or adapted equipment for use until the hand or finger is healed.
- Consider instructing the person in the use of one-hand techniques to permit functional performance until the injured hand is healed or recovered from surgery.

Productivity
- Temporary job modification or reassignment may permit some persons to work during recovery.

- Provide simulated work and home-management activities to permit the person to try out the use of his or her hand or fingers in a controlled environment.
- Assist the person to explore alternative job or career choices if a return to his or her present job or vocation is not possible.

Leisure
- Suggest alternate techniques or equipment for performing leisure activities, if needed.
- Assist the person to explore new leisure interests if some favorite leisure activities cannot be continued, due to the nature of the injury.

Sensorimotor
- Prevent tendon rupture. Follow exercise precautions.
- Promote tendon healing through splinting.
- Encourage tendon excursion through use of tendon glide exercises.
- Prevent flexion contractures through selected exercises.
- Encourage tendon gliding while minimizing tendon gapping or extensor lag.
- Restore active and passive range of motion to involved digits; maintain full range of motion of all uninvolved joints of the affected extremity.
- Control edema: Elevate the hand above the level of the heart to minimize limb dependence. Cold packs may be applied 3–4 times per day, before exercise for 15–20 minutes. Coban may be applied without tension in a figure-of-eight distal to proximal digits with good vascularity. Isotoner gloves may be worn. Overhead (making a firm fist 10 times per hour) may be recommended if the hand can tolerate the active tendon excursion (Schneider and Berger-Feldscher 1995, 469).
- Increase grip and pinch strength through graded activities and progressive resistive exercises.
- The person may need a pain-management program. Transcutaneous electrical simulation or EMG biofeedback may be used.
- The person may need desensitization of the scar area.
- Splints used include:
  Blocking splint (Kasch 1996, 674)
  Dorsal forearm-based cynamic extension splint (Rivet 1997, 7)
  Dynamic outrigger splint (Kasch 1996, 675)
  Elastic traction splint to digital palmar crease (Steinberg 1997a, 110)
  Four finger method splint (Steinberg 1997a, 108)
  Kleinert splint (Rivet 1997, 7; Kasch 1996, 674, unlabeled)
  PIP/DIP flexion splint (Kasch 1996, 676)
  PIP extension splint made by LMB Hand Rehabilitation Products (Kasch 1996, 675)
  Plaster cylindrical splint for static PIP joint contracture (Kasch 1996, 675)
  Ring holding four rubber bands (Steinberg 1997a, 111)
  Splint with elastic traction (Rivet 1997, 7)
  Static dorsal DIP flexion splint (Rivet 1997, 7)
  Static postoperative protection splint (Rivet 1997, 7)
  Traction splint (Steinberg 1997a, 110)
  Volar splint (Steinberg 1997a, 109)
  Wristlet with rubber band traction (Steinberg 1997a, 112)

Flexor Tendon Repairs—Kleinert or Louisville Technique (and variations) for Controlled Mobilization of Acute Flexor Tendon Injuries

Called also *immobilization method* for Zones I through V of the hand (Kasch 1996, 675–676, Stewart and van Strien 1995, 446–454; Steinberg 1997, 105–107).

0–3 Weeks Postoperative

1. After surgery, rubber bands are attached to the nails with a hook held in place with cyanoacrylate glue or suture through the nail.
2. A dorsal blocking splint made from low-temperature thermoplastic splinting materials is applied to hold the wrist in 10–30 degrees flexion, the MCP joint in 40–60 degrees of flexion, and the IP joints are allowed to extend fully.
3. The rubber bands are placed over the hooks on the nails, held down with a safety pin in the palm (or wrist), and attached to another pin at the distal strap in the forearm. (Note: Some variations of the technique do not anchor in the palm or wrist.)
4. The rubber bands should provide enough tension to hold the PIP joints in 40–60 degrees of flexion without tension on the rubber bands themselves.
5. The IP joints must be able to extend fully with the splint to prevent joint contractures from occurring.
6. The splint is worn 24 hours a day for 3 weeks with instructions to the person to actively extend the fingers several times a day, which allows the rubber bands to pull the fingers into flexion. The finger extension exercise allows the tendon to glide through the tendon sheath and pulley system, which minimizes scar adhesion while enhancing nutrition and blood supply to the tendon.
7. The person is instructed to do range of motion on uninvolved joints and to keep the hand elevated.
8. The therapist provides protected PROM.
   a. Proximal interphalangeal motion: Passively flex and extend each PIP joint while passively moving the wrist, MCP, and flexing the DIP joint.
   b. DIP motion—passively flex and extend each DIP joint while passively moving the wrist, MCP, and flexing the PIP joint.
9. The therapist also provides wound care, edema control, and scar management.

3 Weeks Postoperative

1. The splint is changed to neutral wrist position 40–50 degrees of flexion and 0 degrees of IP flexion.
2. The splint is removed by the person hourly for exercise, using protected PROM with wrist at 10 degrees extension. Tendon gliding exercises include:
   a. Tenodesis: passively dropping the wrist into flexion with gravity assist.
   b. Hook fist with wrist in slight flexion.
   c. Flat fist with wrist in 10 degrees extension (DIPs are extended).
   d. Full fist with wrist in 10 degrees extension (DIPs are flexed).
   e. Place and hold (no resistance), position in tenodesis position.
   f. Place and hold (without resistance), grasp and release various sizes of dowels and cones.

3-1/2–6 Weeks Postoperative

1. The dorsal blocking splint is discontinued during the day but is worn at night and may be worn in crowded situations to avoid unexpected movements.

2. Decrease extrinsic flexor muscle tendon tightness by extending the wrist and fingers as much as possible. Serially adjust (one at a time) to accommodate increased extension position.
3. In therapy, continue protected PROM, tendon gliding, starting with passive, then place and hold exercises. Start gentle blocking (hold or restrict movement in all joints except the one being moved) for isolate flexor digitorum superficialis (FDS) and flexor digitorum profundus (FDP).

4-1/2–7 Weeks Postoperative

1. Evaluate tendon glide. If active flexion is improving, do NOT upgrade. If no improvement is noted, add towel walking finger exercise, light grasp and release, and gentle putty squeezing (not more than 10 repetitions of lightest grade putty).

5-1/2–8 Weeks Postoperative

1. Reevaluate tendon glide. If active flexion is improving, do NOT upgrade. If no improvement is noted, add sustained grip, such as light sanding with an adapted handle to maintain wrist and hand position, use Hand Helper exerciser with one rubber band, use heavier putty (grades light or medium), begin lifting with 1 lb and increase slowly to 10 lbs if the physician gives clearance.

10–12 Weeks Postoperative

1. Begin using heavy grade putty, lifting over 10 lbs, and job simulation of manual labor tasks.

Flexor Tendon Repairs—Duran and Houser Technique (and variations) of Controlled Passive Motion.

Called also *early passive motion methods* for Zones II to V of the hand (Kasch 1996, 674; Stewart and van Strien 1995, 446–454; Steinberg 1997, 107–111).

0 to 3–4 Weeks Postoperative

1. The wrist is positioned in 10 to 30 degrees of flexion and the MCP joints in 50 to 70 degrees of flexion in a dorsal blocking splint.
2. The IP joints may be:
   a. Strapped in extension in 0 degrees flexion with a Velcro (or similar) strap between exercise session and while sleeping. No rubber band or elastic traction is used.
   b. With rubber band or elastic traction.
      i. Four-finger method: A plaster cast or circumferential splint ending at PIP joint is applied, which allows full PIP and DIP extension. "Thick" rubber bands are allied to all four digits (regardless of number of fingers involved). A palmar pulley system is used, in which all four rubber bands are attached to a removable ring or anchor at the proximal end, volar surface of the forearm. A hand-based thermoplastic volar splint designed to maintain the IP joints in 0 degrees of flexion is added to the circumferential cast or splint while sleeping if no rubber band traction is used.
      ii. Modified Washington Method for involved digits only. A dorsal splint is applied to the end of the digits while allowing full PIP and DIP extension. Nylon fishing line is attached to two rubber bands through the palmar pulley. One rubber band is thick, and the other is cut in half to reduce resistance, or elastic thread may be used. Both rubber bands are attached to the proximal end of the volar forearm strap. During sleep, the rubber band traction may be loosen or removed.

3. Therapy is performed with 10–15 repetitions per hour.
   a. In the Modified Duran method (no rubber band traction), the person is instructed to do protected PIP and DIP PROM exercises (the joint not being exercised is held or blocked while the target joint is passively moved in flexion and extension). In addition, the person is instructed to do passive modified hook, flat and full fists, each alternating with active IP extension while passively blocking MCPs in flexion to maximize PIP and DIP extension.
   b. In the Modified Kleinhert (four-finger method or Washington regimen with rubber band or elastic traction) method, the person is instructed to flex all four IP digits passively by either removing the rubber bands from the proximal hook or removing the heavy rubber band while leaving the lighter rubber band or elastic thread in place.
   c. The therapist may, with splint removed, provide passive tenodesis, passive full fist with wrist at 10–30 degrees extension, alternating with passive wrist and MCP flexion and active IP extension. Passive flat fist with wrist in 10–30 degrees extension may be alternated with passive wrist and MCP flexion, along with active IP extension. Passive modified hook fist with wrist hyperflexed may be performed with MCPs at 0–20 degrees passive flexion and IP joints full passive flexion, alternating with passive wrist and MCP flexion, along with active IP extension.

3 Weeks Postoperative

1. The splint is changed to one with the wrist in neutral with or without rubber band or elastic traction.
2. The therapist evaluates tendon glide. If there is more than 50 degrees difference between full fist TAM (total active motion) and TPM (total passive motion), the program is upgraded by adding place and hold tenodesis to the home program, as well as nonresisted place and hold grasp and release. If there is less than 50 degrees of difference, the program is not upgraded. Place and hold tenodesis is done only in supervised therapy session.

4 Weeks Postoperative

1. The splint is worn only at night or in crowds, or a wrist band with elastic traction is used.
2. Exercises for extrinsic flexor muscle are started.
3. Therapy program is upgraded to guidelines under the immobilization method.

Flexor Tendon Repairs—Early Passive Mobilization in Zone 1 (Stewart and van Strien 1995, 454–455; Steinberg 1997, 111–113)

0–21 Days Postoperative

1. A dorsal static protective splint that extends to the fingertips is applied. The wrist is positioned in 30–40 degrees of flexion, the MCP joints are in 30 degrees of flexion, and PIP joints are fully extended. The affected DIP is placed in a static splint with 40–45 degrees of flexion. The splint will extend from the proximal motion of the middle phalanx to the tip of the finger but is taped only to the middle phalanx.
2. Therapy includes wound care, edema control, and scar management.
3. The person is responsible for 10–20 repetitions per waking hour with the splints on. The distal joint is passively flexed from 40 to 75 degrees (or full flexion). All fingers are passively placed in a full fist position and hook position. The MCP joints are passively hyperflexed by the uninvolved hand while the PIPs are actively extended to full extension.

The distal strap holds the unaffected fingers in extension while gentle place and hold active exercise for the superficialis muscle of the involved finger is done.

4. The therapist removes the dorsal protective splint while leaving on the dorsal digital splint. The fingers are passively flexed into the palm while the therapist extends the wrist to 10 degrees of extension. While the wrist is hyperflexed, the therapist places the fingers in a hook fist position with the MCP joint in full extension and the IP joints in full passive flexion.

3–4 Weeks Postoperative

1. The digital splint is discontinued while the dorsal protective splint continues to be worn.
2. In therapy, place and hold hook and full fist (within the splint) are added to the person's exercise program. Beginning with the fourth week, the person may remove the splint during exercise sessions to perform place and hold tenodesis, full fist, flat fist, and hook fist. Gentle blocked exercise for the profundus may be started.

4-1/2 Weeks Postoperative

1. A static digit extension splint may be worn.
2. In therapy, follow the guidelines for the immobilization method.
•   Early active motion (EAM) methods: Depend on the strength and quality of the repair procedures, time since the repair was done, ability and motivation of the person to cooperate with therapy, and the knowledge and skill of the therapist.

Indiana Method

1. Indications: The suture is four-strand Tajima with horizontal mattress repair (or equivalent four-strand repair procedure) with a running peripheral epitendinous suture. Therapy can begin within 48 hours of repair. The person has the ability and motivation to follow and perform the therapy program demonstrated by the therapist, and edema is minimal to moderate with no restrictions to passive flexion. There are minimal wound care complications, if any.
2. 24–48 hours postoperative:
    a. Splints: A typical dorsal blocking splint may be applied with the wrist in 20 degrees of flexion, the MCP joints in 50 degrees flexion, and the IP joints fully extended, OR a forearm-based tenodesis dorsal hinged splint is applied with the wrist hinge, allowing full wrist flexion and up to 30 degrees of extension. The MCP joints are in 60 degrees of flexion, and the IP joins are fully extended.
    b. Therapy. For the dorsal block splint, 15 repetitions per hour of individual passive flexion and extension to the PIP and DIP joints, followed by composite PIP/DIP PROM. For the hinged tenodesis splint, place and hold exercises are performed 25 times per hour while wearing the splint. The person passively flexes the fingers while simultaneously actively extending the wrist. This position is gently and actively held for 5 seconds. Afterward, the person relaxes and allows the wrist to drop into flexion, which allows the digits to straighten within the limits of the tenodesis splint.
3. 4 weeks postoperative:
    a. Splints: The hinged tenodesis splint is discontinued but the static dorsal block splint is worn all the time, except during exercise, until 6 weeks postoperative.

b. Therapy: With the dorsal block splint removed, the 25 repetitions every 2 hours of tenodesis place and hold exercises are performed plus active flexion and extension exercises of the digits and wrist with light muscle contraction. The person is instructed NOT to simultaneously extend the wrist and digits to avoid the potential of gapping or elongation of the sutures along the repair site.

4. 6 weeks postoperative:
   a. Splints: The dorsal block splint is discontinued.
   b. Therapy: Blocking exercises for index, middle, and ring fingers may be added if the digital active flexion is greater than 3 cm from the distal palmar crease. Note that no blocking is started for the little finger because the diameter and vascular supply to the profundus tendon are deficient, as compared with the other digits.

5. 7 weeks postoperative
   a. Passive extension exercises may be added to the therapy program.

6. 8 weeks postoperative
   a. Gentle strengthening exercises may be added to the therapy program.

7. 12–14 weeks postoperative
   a. The person may return to normal, unrestricted activity.

Minimum Active Muscle Tendon Tension (MAMTT) Method

1. Indications: Strength of suture, which must include epitendon running suture; the amount of edema; increase in flexion forces; time from surgical repair, which should be within 24–48 hours.

2. Guidelines:
   a. Splint: A removable dorsal block splint with or without elastic traction.
   b. Therapy: same as for early passive motion method, except:
      i. Person should perform place and hold exercise without therapist supervision.
      ii. The therapist should start working with the client 24–48 hours postsurgery, beginning with PROM. The splint is removed and the wrist is positioned in 20 degrees extension while passively flexing the MCP joint to 80 degrees, PIP joints to 75 degrees, and DIP joint to 40 degrees. The person holds this position, using no more than 20 grams of force. The person relaxes. The therapist then passively flexes the wrist and MCP joints while the person actively extends the IP joints.

Four-Finger Active Method

1. Indications: Suture with modified Kessler core suture and a new "cross-stitch" epitendon suture (or suture with similar strength), and therapy should begin within 48 hours of surgical repair.

2. 24–48 hours postoperative.
   a. Splint: A circumferential splint to cast should be applied with wrist in neutral and MCP joints and IP joints in rubber band traction with volar night splint.
   b. Therapy: Exercises are the same as for early passive motion four-finger method, except that the person actively holds full fist for 2–3 seconds after performing the passive full fist.

Extensor Tendon Repair for Zones V, VI, VII—Immobilization Method (Steinberg 1997, 93–102)

0–21 Days Postoperative

1. Splint: A volar splint is applied with wrist in 30–45 degrees extension, MCP joints and IP joints in 0 degrees extension. A removable volar component may be applied for sleeping and/or intermittently during the day to prevent PIP joint flexion contracture and/or extensor lag.
   a. Variation 1: If only the extensor indices proprius (EIP) or extensor digiti minimis (EDM) is involved, only the repaired tendon and digit need to be immobilized.
   b. Variation 2: If there is a simple injury to a single extensor digitorum communis (EDC), the repair site determines the type of splint. If the repair site is *proximal* to the interconnecting juncturae tendinum, all fingers are splinted in extension. If the repair site is *distal* to the interconnecting juncturae tendinum, only affected digit is splinted in full extension at the MCP and IP joints. The adjacent digits are splinted in 30 degrees of MCP flexion with IP joints free.
2. Therapy should include wound care, edema control, and range of motion.
   a. Metacarpophalangeal joint protective range of motion: The therapist supports the wrist and IP joints in full extension while gently moving the index and middle finger MCP joints from slight hyperextension to 30 degrees flexion, and the ring and small finger MCP joints from high hyperextension to 40 degrees flexion.
   b. Proximal interphalangeal and DIP joint protective range of motion: The therapist supports the wrist and MCP joints in full extension while passively moving each individual PIP and DIP joint through complete range of motion.

3 Weeks Postoperative

1. Splints: A volar splint is applied with the wrist in 20 degrees of extension, MCP at 0 degrees extension.
2. Therapy:
   a. Metacarpophalangeal AROM and AAROM with tenodesis: The MCP joints are extended with the wrist in neutral to slight flexion. The MCP joints are flexed (40–60 degrees with wrist in full extension).
   b. IP AROM and AAROM, PROM through complete range while wrist and MCP joints are supported in full extension.

4 Weeks Postoperative

1. Splints: Use a dynamic CP flexion splint as needed.
2. Therapy: Combine MCP/IP flexion with wrist extension, perform individual finger extension exercises, and isolate EDC extension exercise.

4-1/2–5 Weeks

1. Splints: Combination of MCP and IP traction may be initiated to decrease extrinsic extensor tightness.
2. Therapy: same as 3 and 4 weeks postoperative.

6–10 Weeks Postoperative

1. Composite finger and wrist flexion initiated when there is no extension lag present.

2. Add mild progressive strengthening, including wrist flexion and extension and forearm pronation and supination.

10–12 Weeks Postoperative

1. Add strong resistive exercise.

Early Passive Motion Method (Steinberg 1997, 93–102)

24 Hours to 3 Days Postoperative

1. Splint: Two-part dynamic splint with outrigger.
   a. Dorsal component: Wrist is held in 30–35 degrees static extension; MCP and IP joints in 0 degrees dynamic extension.
   b. Interlocking volar component: Wrist is the same as for dorsal component: MCP joints are permitted active flexion to 30 degrees for index and middle fingers and 40 degrees for ring and small fingers.
2. Therapy includes wound care, edema control, splint adjustments, and exercises.
   a. Controlled passive IP motion is the same as the first 3 weeks of the immobilization method for PIP and DIP joint protective range of motion.
   b. Person is responsible for exercising each hour. While maintaining IP joint extension, the person actively flexes digits at the MCP joints until fingers touch volar splint. Person releases digits, allowing extension loops to passively extend MCP joints to 0 degrees. For Zone VII injuries, while the loops support the other digits in extension, the person individually flexes the index finger MCP joint to the splint, small finger MCP to the splint, then the middle and ring fingers together to the splint. Person relaxes all digits to allow extension outrigger to passively extend MCP joints to 0 degrees.
   c. Wrist tenodesis:
      i. Zones V and VI: Simultaneous wrist extension with 30 degrees MCP flexion for the index and middle fingers and 40 degrees MCP flexion for the ring and little fingers, followed by simultaneous wrist flexion to 20 degrees with all digital joints held at 0 degrees.
      ii. Zone VII without wrist tendon involvement: Same as above except when digits are placed in 0 degrees, wrist is maintained in not less than 10 degrees of extension.
      iii. Zone VII with wrist tendon involvement: Same as above except when digits are placed in 0 degrees, the wrist is maintained in not less that 20 degrees extension.

3 Weeks Postoperative

1. Splints: Daytime: Volar block splint is removed but the dorsal dynamic splint is continued. Nighttime: Volar static splint is worn but adjusted to 30–45 degrees of wrist extension and 0 degrees of MCP and IP joint extension.
2. Therapy:
   a. Gradual active motion of MCP and IP joints is started with the dynamic extension splint.
   b. Modalities, dynamic splinting, and exercises are the same as management by immobilization from the 3-week period onward.

4–5 Weeks Postoperative

1. Splints: Continue to be worn.
2. Therapy: Therapist initiates composite finger flexion with wrist in extension.

6–23 Weeks Postoperative
1. Same as the immobilization method.

Wrist Extensors Without Finger Extensor Involvement (Zone VII) (Steinberg 1997, 93–102)
1. Splints: Wrist is splinted in 30–45 degrees extension with the MCP and IP joints free. Protective splinting is continued for up to 8 weeks.
2. Therapy:
   a. 3 weeks postoperative: Use gravity-eliminated active motion from 0 degrees to full wrist extension.
   b. 5–8 weeks postoperative: Slowly add increments of wrist flexion, plus radial and ulnar deviation.
   c. 8–12 weeks postoperative: Begin progressive strengthening exercises.

Thumb Extensors (Zones T-III, T-IV, T-V), Immobilization Method (Steinberg 1997, 93–102)

0–21 Days Postoperative
1. Splints: A volar protective splint is worn with wrist in 30 degrees extension; carpometacarpal (CMC) is in slight abduction; MCP and IP joints are in 0 degrees of extension.
2. Therapy includes wound care, edema control, and exercises.
   a. Metacarpophalangeal joint protective range of motion: The therapist supports the wrist and IP in full extension while gently moving the IP from full extension to 30 degrees flexion. Do not permit thumb to hyperextend at the MCP joint.
   b. IP joint protective range of motion: The therapist supports the wrist and MCP joint in full extension while gently moving thumb IP from full extension to 50 degrees flexion.

3–4 Weeks Postoperative
1. Splints: The splint is worn all the time except for exercise and showering. The splint may be shortened to allow for active flexion and extension of the IP joint:
   a. Variation 1: If there is IP joint extensor lag, add removable volar component.
   b. Variation 2: If there is an MCP extension contracture, intermittent gentle dynamic MCP flexion splinting may be used while supporting wrist and first metacarpal in extension.
2. Therapy:
   a. Begin supervised thumb abduction and MCP and IP joint flexion.
   b. Home program: For MCP mobility, support the wrist and IP in full extension and gently move the MCP joint from full extension to 30 degrees flexion. For IP mobility, support the wrist and MCP in full extension and gently move the thumb IP joint from full extension to 60 degrees flexion.

5 Weeks Postoperative
1. Splints: Combination of thumb abduction and MCP and IP flexion may be initiated.
2. Therapy: Add the combination of thumb abduction and MCP and IP flexion to the home program.

6–10 Weeks Postoperative
1. Splints: As needed.
2. Therapy: Begin composite of thumb and wrist flexion. Mild progressive strengthening may be started, including wrist flexion and extension and forearm supination and pronation.

10–12 Weeks Postoperative

1. Begin strong resistive exercise.

Thumb Extensors—Early Passive Motion Method (Steinberg 1997, 93–103)

0–21 Days Postoperative

1. Splints: A combined dorsal and volar splint.
   a. Dorsal splint: Wrist in 30 degrees of static extension and thumb MCP and IP joints in 0 degrees of dynamic extension.
   b. Volar splint: Static splint allowing 60 degrees of IP motion of the thumb.
2. Therapy:
   a. The person is responsible for active flexion to volar splint with passive extension via dynamic traction.
   b. The therapist performs maximal wrist extension with simultaneous MCP joint flexion to 30 degrees and wrist tenodesis with wrist in 0 degrees of extension and simultaneous thumb CMC, MCP, and IP extension alternating with full wrist extension and thumb CMC, MCP, and IP relaxed.

3–4 Weeks Postoperative

1. Splint: Continue to wear all the time except for exercise and showering.
2. Therapy: The therapist-led exercises of the first 3 weeks are added to the person's home program.

5–12 Weeks Postoperative

1. Splint and exercise program are the same as early immobilization method from 5 to 12 weeks.
- Flexor tenolysis surgery (removal of the peritendinous adhesions) (Schneider and Berger-Feldscher 1995, 463–475; Steinberg 1997, 119–126).
  1. Pulley reconstruction protection:
     a. Identify area(s) of pulley reconstruction
     b. Protect reconstruction area with a circumferential ring constructed from Velcro or a thermoplastic material until the edema is controlled, then continue use of thermoplastic ring.
     c. Ring should be worn for 6 months postoperatively.
  2. Tendon reconstruction program:
     a. 12–24 hours to 1 week postoperative (inflammation phase):
        i. Splint: A forearm-based progressive extension or static extension splint should be worn day and night for 2 weeks to prevent flexion contractures. The splint should be removed only for exercise and wound care.
        ii. Exercise: Active exercise should include 5–10 repetitions of each of the following exercises hourly each day: Place and hold, finger blocking, and finger extension. Passive exercise should include 5–10 repetitions 3 times per day, up to every hour if passive motion is limited. Perform gentle PROM to all joints (see box on page 488 for exercises).
        iii. Edema control: Technique not specified.
     b. 2–3 weeks postoperative (initiation of proliferation phase of wound healing):
        i. Splint: Wearing of static or progressive extension splint should be decreased during the day as AROM achieved intraoperatively by the surgeon is maintained

Types of Splints Illustrated in Chapters and Articles

- Bedford finger stall (Kasch in Pedretti 1996, 669)
- Blocking splint (Kasch in Pedretti 1996, 674)
- Buddy taping (Steinberg in Clark et al. 1997e, 136; Theisen in Clark et al. 1997, 359)
- Capener orthosis (Leveridge in Turner et al. 1996, 584, 586)
- Claw hand orthotic support (Leveridge in Turner et al. 1996, 587)
- DIP extension splint (Theisen in Clark et al. 1997, 360)
- Dorsal aluminum splint (Philips in Trombly 1995, 776)
- Dorsal blocking splint (Philips in Trombly 1995, 777)
- Dorsal protective splint (Steinberg in Clark et al. 1997c, 140)
- Dynamic extension for contracture splint (Steinberg in Clark et al. 1997c, 123)
- Dynamic extension splint for postoperative treatment (Theisen in Clark et al. 1997, 351)
- Dynamic finger extensor splint (Steinberg in Clark et al. 1997a, 97; Philips in Trombly 1995, 778)
- Dynamic flexion splint (Theisen in Clark et al. 1997, 358)
- Dynamic outrigger splint (Kasch in Pedretti 1996, 675)
- Dynamic PIP extension splint (Theisen in Clark et al. 1997, 357)
- Dynamic radial nerve orthosis (Leveridge in Turner et al. 1996, 585)
- Dynamic thumb extensor splint (Steinberg in Clark et al. 1997a, 101)
- Dynamic ulnar nerve splint (Kasch in Pedretti 1996, 672)
- Figure-of-eight splint (Steinberg in Clark et al. 1997e, 140); see also Tripoint splint
- Flail arm orthosis (Leveridge in Turner et al. 1996, 585)
- Flexion traction splint (Kasch in Pedretti 1996, 674)
- Forearm-based static extension splint (Steinberg in Clark et al. 1997e, 122)
- Four-finger method splint (Steinberg in Clark et al. 1997b, 108)
- Hand-wrist extension orthosis (Leveridge in Turner et al. 1996, 585)
- Immobilizing postoperative splint for fingers (Steinberg in Clark et al. 1997a, 96)
- Immobilizing postoperative splint for thumb (Steinberg in Clark et al. 1997a, 99)
- Intrinsic stretch splint (Steinberg in Clark et al. 1997e, 137)
- LMB Product—finger splint (Kasch in Pedretti 1996, 675)
- Low-profile radial nerve splint (Kasch in Pedretti 1996, 671)
- "Monkey palm" orthosis (Leveridge in Turner et al. 1996, 586)
- PIP/DIP flexion strap (Steinberg in Clark et al. 1997a, 137)
- PIP-DIP splint (Kasch in Pedretti 1996, 676)
- Plaster cylindrical splint (Kasch in Pedretti 1996, 675)

continues

continued

- Postoperative metacarpophalangeal joint arthroplasty splints (Philips in Trombly 1995, 780–781)
- Postoperative wrist arthroplasty splint (Philips in Trombly 1995, 782)
- Rolyan hand-based arthritis splint (Kurtz in Clark et al. 1997, 397)
- Semiflexible splint (Kasch in Pedretti 1996, 682)
- Serially applied thermoplastic splint (Steinberg in Clark et al. 1997e, 138)
- Static PIP extension splint (Theisen in Clark et al. 1997, 357)
- Static positioning splint (Theisen in Clark et al. 1997, 352)
- Tenodesis splints (Steinberg in Clark et al. 1997b, 114)
- Three-point extension splint (Steinberg in Clark et al. 1997e, 138)
- Thumb carpometacarpal (CMC) splint (Kurtz in Clark et al. 1997, 398)
- Thumb rotation strap (Leveridge in Turner et al. 1996, 586)
- Thumb stabilization splint (Kasch in Pedretti 1996, 671)
- Thumb web spacer (Leveridge in Turner et al. 1996, 583)
- Traction splints (Steinberg in Clark et al. 1997b, 110–112)
- Tripoint splint (Eckhaus in Clark et al. 1997, 154); see also Figure-of-eight splint
- Velcro "buddy" splint (Kasch in Pedretti 1996, 668); see also Buddy splint
- Volar splint (Steinberg in Clark et al. 1997b, 109)

        pain free. A dynamic extension splint to reduce flexion contractures may be worn for short periods during the day if the surgeon approves.

    ii. Exercise: Continue place and hold, finger blocking, and finger extension exercises. Add active tendon gliding exercises to be performed 3–10 times per hour. Have the person perform light ADLs that do not require resistive grasp and release.

  c. 4–6 weeks postoperative (proliferative phase ends as scar remodeling phase begins):

    i. Splint: Static or progressive extension splint should be worn in the daytime only, if needed, but continue night use for 6 months postoperatively. Wear dynamic extension splint as needed during the day. The person may exercise in flexion against resistance of splint.

    ii. Exercise: Continue exercises already outlined. Add graded isometric grip strengthening with physician approval but monitor closely. Continue ADLs but begin grading for difficulty.

  d. 8–12 weeks postoperative (scar remodeling continues):

    i. Gradually increase resistive exercises and activities so that there are no restrictions at 12 weeks.

Cognitive

- The person must be fully informed regarding the requirements of the program, the rationale for each exercise, the purpose of the splint, and the care and maintenance of the splint.

Exercises for Tendon Repair and Reconstruction

- Place and hold exercise
  1. With the uninvolved hand, passively manipulate the involved digit into the full flexion and actively maintain the digit in the position.
  2. Remove the uninvolved hand and hold the position in flexion without support, confirming active muscle contraction. Then actively extend all digits.
  3. For additional protection of the tendons, the wrist can be flexed to limit full excursion of the tendons.
  4. Comfort level determines the beginning number of repetitions that must be performed every waking hour. Repetitions should be increased until 10 can be performed each hour.
- Tendon gliding exercises (TGEs)
  1. Hook fist: The fingers should be in full extension in all joints. With the metacarpophalangeal (MCP) joints maintained in extension, actively flex the proximal interphalangeal (PIP) and distal interphalangeal (DIP) joints. The flexor digitorum superficialis (FDS) and flexor digitorum profundus (FDP) independently glide over each other most in this position.
  2. Straight fist: Begin by assuming the hook fist position, all fingers in full extension. Actively flex the MCP and PIP joints while maintaining the DIP joint in extension. (The FDS reaches its maximum excursion in this position.) End by fully extending the fingers.
  3. Full fist: Begin by assuming the hook fist position, then flex the MCP, PIP, and DIP joints fully, touching the distal palmar crease in the hand. (The FDP reaches its maximum excursion in this position.) End by fully extending the fingers.
  4. Wrist flexion with finger flexion
  5. Wrist extension with finger extension
- Protected passive range of motion (PROM) technique: Passively flex other digits and wrist while passively extending and flexing, in turn, the MCP, PIP, and DIP joints of all digits.
- Finger blocking exercise
  1. Block (hold) the MCP and PIP joints into extension, allowing isolated active DIP flexion.
  2. Block (hold) MCP into extension, allowing isolated PIP flexion.
- "Tabletop" position: The MCP joints are flexed at 90 degrees while the PIP and DIP joints are fully extended.
- Composite wrist and digit flexion: The wrist, MCP, PIP, and DIP joints are all flexed simultaneously.
- Composite wrist and digit extension: The wrist, MCP, PIP, and DIP joints are all extended simultaneously.

Source: Data from L.H. Schneider and B. Berger-Feldscher, Tenolysis: Dynamic Approach to Surgery and Therapy, in *Rehabilitation of the Hand*, 4th ed., J.M. Hunter, E.J. Mackin, and A.D. Callahan, eds., pp. 563–576, © 1995, Mosby; and B. Steinberg, Flexor Tenolysis, in *Hand Rehabilitation: A Practical Guide*, 2nd ed., G.L. Clark, et al., eds. pp. 119–126, © 1997, Churchill-Livingstone.

- The person must know the signs of problems in the healing process or skin damage caused by improper fit of the splint, and he or she must know how to report the problems promptly.

Psychosocial
- Permit the person to express feelings of anger or guilt about the injury or situation in which the injury occurred.
- Dispel fears of disfigurement, inability to use the hand, or inability to return to work by providing factual information on the prognosis and outcome of the specific injury or surgery.
- Encourage the person to continue participation in social activities. Provide ideas or techniques for adapting participation (in leisure activities, for example) if needed.

PRECAUTIONS

- In the Kleinert method, care must be taken to avoid contractures of the PIP joints due to too much tension on the rubber band(s) or incomplete IP extension available within the splint itself. If a flexion contracture occurs, a dynamic extension splint for the PIP joint should be applied during the week 5 or 6 postsurgery.
- Application of controlled stress to the healing tendon must be carefully evaluated, both in timing (number of days since surgery) and excursion of the tendon relative to the movement of the joint.
- Be aware that tendon repair does not occur in isolation. Always monitor soft-tissue healing and potential for bone and nerve involvement.
- Stress to the person the importance of following the exercise plan carefully to avoid active, heavy resistive movements until healing has occurred to reduce chances of tendon rupture.
- Complications of flexor tendon repair may include tendon rupture, minimal tendon gliding, flexion contractures, excessive scar formation, pain, severe edema, and infection.
- Complications of extensor tendon repair may include tendon rupture, excessive scar formation, active extensor tendon lag, and extrinsic extensor tendon tightness, limiting composite flexion.
- Complications for flexor tenolysis include pain, edema, bleeding, infection, excessive scar formation, auditory click or palpable crepitation, tendon rupture, flexion contractures, reconstructed pulley rupture, minimal gain or actual loss of motion, and person's inability to tolerate postoperative therapy.

PROGNOSIS AND OUTCOME

- The person is able to perform self-care skills independently.
- The person is able to perform productive activities.
- The person is able to perform leisure activities.
- The person has full range of motion in injured or surgically repaired tendons.
- The person has normal muscle strength in the affected muscles.
- The person has normal hand functions.
- The person has normal manipulation, dexterity, and bilateral coordination skills.
- The person does not report (or can manage) pain or hypersensitivity to touch.

Classification of Sensory Grade and Recovery of Sensibility

S0   Absence of sensation
S1   Recovery of deep pain sensibility
S1+   Recovery of superficial pain sensibility
S2   Recovery of pain and some touch sensibility
S2+   Recovery of pain and some touch sensibility but with overresponse
S3   Recovery of pain and touch sensibility with disappearance of overresponse; static two-point discrimination greater than 15 millimeters
S3+   Recovery of touch localization, static two-point discrimination 7–14 mm
S4   Complete recovery; static two-point discrimination 2–6 mm

Source: Data from K. Bentzel, Remediating Sensory Impairment, in *Occupational Therapy for Physical Dysfunction*, 4th ed., C.A. Trombly, ed., p. 427, © 1995, Williams & Wilkins.

REFERENCES

Kasch, M.C. 1996. Tendon injuries. In *Occupational Therapy: Practice Skills for Physical Dysfunction*, 4th ed., ed. L.W. Pedretti, 673–677. St. Louis: Mosby.

Rivet, L.B. 1997. *Occupational Therapy Practice Guidelines for Tendon Injuries.* Bethesda, MD: American Occupational Therapy Association.

Schneider, L.H. and B. Berger-Feldscher. 1995. Tenolysis: Dynamic approach to surgery and therapy. In *Rehabilitation of the Hand*, 4th ed., ed. J.M. Hunter, E.J. Mackin, and A.D. Callahan, 463–476. St. Louis: Mosby.

Steinberg, B. 1997a. Flexor tendon repair. In *Hand Rehabilitation: A Practical Guide.* 2nd ed., ed. G.L. Clark, E.F.S. Wilgis, B. Aiello, D. Eckhaus, and L.V. Eddington, 103–117. New York: Churchill Livingstone.

Stewart, K.M. and G. van Strien. 1995. Postoperative management of flexor tendon injuries. In *Rehabilitation of the Hand*, 4th ed., ed. J.M. Hunter, E.J. Mackin, A.D. Callahan, 433–462. St. Louis: Mosby.

BIBLIOGRAPHY

Byron, P. 1998. A multipurpose component. *Journal of Hand Therapy* 11(3):209–211.

Evans, R.B. 1995. An update on extensor tendon management. In *Rehabilitation of the Hand*, 4th ed., ed. J.M. Hunter, E.J. Mackin, and A.D. Callahan, 565–606. St. Louis: Mosby.

Evans, R.B. 1995. Immediate active short arc motion following extensor tendon repair. *Hand Clinics* 11(3):483–512.

Evans, R.B. and D.E. Thompson. 1993. The application of force to the healing tendon. *Journal of Hand Therapy* 6(4):266–284.

Maddy, L.S. and E.M. Meyerdierks. 1997. Dynamic extension assist splinting of acute central slip laceration. *Journal of Hand Therapy* 10(3):206–212.

May, E. 1994. Controlled mobilization after flexor tendon repair in the hand: Techniques, methods and results. *Australian Occupational Therapy Journal* 41(3):143 (Abstract).

Rose, H. 1996. MP/IP adjustable digit blocking splint. *Journal of Hand Surgery* 9(3):247–248.

Silfverskiold, K.L., E.J. May, and A. Oden. 1993. Factors affecting results after flexor tendon repair in zone II: A multivariate prospective analysis. *Journal of Hand Surgery*. 18A(4):654–662.

Silfverskiold, K.L., E.J. May, and A.H. Tornvall. 1993. Tendon excursions after flexor tendon repair in zone II: Results with a new controlled-motion program. *Journal of Hand Surgery*. 18A(3):403–410.

Skirven, T. and J. Trope. 1994. Complications of immobilization. *Hand Clinics* 10(1):53–61.

Steinberg, B. 1997b. Extensor tendon repair. In *Hand Rehabilitation: A Practical Guide*. 2nd ed., ed. G.L. Clark, E.F.S. Wilgis, B. Aiello, D. Eckhaus, and L.V. Eddington, 93–102. New York: Churchill Livingstone.

Steinberg, B. 1997c. Flexor tenolysis. In *Hand Rehabilitation: A Practical Guide,* 2nd ed., ed. G.L. Clark, E.F.S. Wilgis, B. Aiello, D. Eckhaus, and L.V. Eddington, 119–126. New York: Churchill Livingstone.

Steinberg, B. 1997d. Primary tendon grafts. In: *Hand Rehabilitation: A Practical Guide,* 2nd ed., ed. G.L. Clark, E.F.S. Wilgis, B. Aiello, D. Eckhaus, and L.V. Eddington, 127–132. New York: Churchill Livingstone.

Steinberg, B. 1997e. Staged tendon reconstruction. In *Hand Rehabilitation: A Practical Guide,* 2nd ed., ed. G.L. Clark, E.F.S. Wilgis, B. Aiello, D. Eckhaus, and L.V. Eddington, 133–142. New York: Churchill Livingstone.

Thomes, L.J. and B.J. Thomes. 1995. Early mobilization method for surgical repaired zone II extensor tendons. *Journal of Hand Therapy* 8(3):195–198.

Tottenham, V.M., K. Wilton-Bennett, and J. Jeffrey. 1995. Effects of delayed therapeutic intervention following zone II flexor tendon repair. *Journal of Hand Therapy* 8(1):27–31.

Wilson, G. 1995. Dynamic flexion splinting resolved scar adhesion after tendon repair. *Advance for Occupational Therapists* 11(22):19–20.

Hand Injuries—Tendon Transfers

DESCRIPTION

Tendons usually are transferred to improve the social, functional, and cosmetic needs of persons with upper extremity weakness due to injury or disorder (Mulcahey 1996, 419). Tendon transfer may interrupt a pattern of progressive deformity and dysfunction. The result tends to create a balance and stability of forces, such as between flexion and extension, more than strength in hand function (Hoard et al. 1995, 115, Eliasson 1998, 612). However, in the scapula and shoulder, proximal control and strength are two of the key elements of successful tendon transfers (Mulcahey 1996, 422). Generally, if two or more muscles perform the same movement, one of those muscles can be transferred to facilitate another movement without sacrificing the original movement (Mulcahey 1996, 419). An example is the transfer of the brachioradialis to the extensor carpi radialis brevis, which is performed to obtain or augment wrist extension strength and to provide useful tenodesis function of the hand.

In addition to the tendon transfers, augmentative procedures may be done to increase the effectiveness of the results, such as tendon and muscle lengthening, tendon or muscle releases, and tenodesis and arthrodesis procedures. Such combined procedures have been done on adults for many years but are now being done on children, as well (Mulcahey 1996, 607–637).

CAUSE

Common causes that lead to the tendon transfers are disorders such as peripheral nerve injury, spinal cord injury, and cerebral palsy. In the past, poliomyelitis was a common cause.

Special Precautions for Reduced Sensation in Hand

- Avoid heat, cold, and sharp objects; use gloves.
- Avoid applying more force than necessary to grip a tool or object; consciously monitor grip force.
- Avoid using small handles; build up the handles to increase distribution of pressure over grip surface.
- Avoid holding or using one tool for long periods of time; either change tools frequently or take rest breaks.
- Observe skin for signs of stress, such as redness, edema, or warmth. If blisters, lacerations, or other wounds occur, treat promptly.
- Follow skin care routine daily, using soaking and oil massage to keep moisture in skin.

Source: Data from A.D. Callahan, Methods of Compensation and Reeducation for Sensory Dysfunction, in *Rehabilitation of the Hand*, 3rd ed., J.M. Hunter, E.J. Mackin, and A.D. Callahan, eds., p. 614, © 1990, Mosby.

Specific movements requiring correction in spinal cord injury are MCP joint flexion, wrist extension and/or flexion, forearm pronation, and elbow extension (Mulcahey 1996, 420).

ASSESSMENT

Areas

- daily living skills
- productivity history, skills, interests, and values
- leisure interests and skills
- range of motion (Measure AROM, PROM, total active motion for digits, and total passive motion for digits.)
- muscle testing
- grip and pinch strength
- edema
- hand functions

Instruments

- Canadian Occupational Performance Measure (COPM), 2nd ed., by Law, M. et al. 1994. Ottawa, Ontario: Canadian Association of Occupational Thrapists.
- dynamometer and pinch meters (see American Society for Surgery of the Hand. 1990. *The Hand: Examination and Diagnosis*, 3rd ed., 121–122. Edinburgh, Scotland: Churchill Livingstone).
- goniometry by Norkin, C.C. and D.J. White. 1995. Measurement of joint motion: A guide to goniometry. Philadelphia: FA Davis.

- Froment's sign (forceful lateral pinch of the thumb against the lateral border of the index finger). American Society for Surgery of the Hand, 1983. *The Hand: Examination and Diagnosis*, 3rd ed., 29. Edinburgh, Scotland: Churchill Livingstone.
- *Functional Independence Measure*, v.4.0 by the Medical Research Foundation. 1994. Buffalo, NY: State University of New York at Buffalo.
- Grasp and Release Test by Stroh-Wuolle K.S., C.L. Van Doren, G.B. Thrope, M.W. Keith, and P.H. Peckham. 1994. Development of a quantitative hand grasp and release test for patients with tetraplegia using a hand neuroprosthesis. *Journal of Hand Surgery* 19A:209–218.
- Hand Function Assessment by Smith, B., M. Mulcahey, and R. Betz. 1996. Quantitative comparison of hand function with and without FES in adolescents with tetraplegia. *Paraplegia* 34:16–23.
- Hand Surgery Assessment—Preoperative. Bell-Krotoski, J.A. 1995. Preoperative and postoperative management of tendon transfers after ulnar nerve injury. In *Rehabilitation of the Hand*, 4th ed., ed. J.M. Hunter, E.J. Mackin, and A.D. Callahan, 738–739. St. Louis: Mosby.
- Hand-Tool Dexterity Test by Bennett, G. 1965. Lafayette, IN: Lafayette Instruments.
- Jebsen Hand Function Test by Jebsen, R.H., N. Taylor, R.B. Trieschmann, et al. 1969. An objective and standardized test of hand function. *Archives of Physical Medicine and Rehabilitation* 50:311–319. Childrens' version. Taylor, N., P.L. Sand, and R.H. Jebsen. 1973. Evaluation of hand function in children. *Archives of Physical Medicine and Rehabilitation* 54:129–135.
- manual muscle test. American Society for Surgery of the Hand. 1990. *The Hand: Examination and Diagnosis*, 3rd ed. Edinburgh, Scotland: Churchill Livingstone or Clarkson, H.M. 1999. *Musculoskeletal Assessment: Joint Range of Motion and Manual Muscle Strength*, 2nd ed. Baltimore: Lippincott, Williams & Wilkins.
- *Minnesota Rate of Manipulation Test*, Circle Pines MN: American Guidance Services, 1969.
- *Purdue Pegboard Test* by Tiffin, J. 1948, 1960, 1999. Lafayette, IN: Lafayette Instruments.
- volumeter.
- *WeeFIM*, v.4.0 by the Medical Research Foundation. 1993. Buffalo, NY: State University of New York at Buffalo.

PROBLEMS

Self-Care
- Problems in the performance of self-care activities are major factors in the decision to recommend a tendon transfer.

Productivity
- Problems in the performance of productive activities are major factors in the decision to recommend a tendon transfer.

Leisure
- Problems in the performance of leisure activities are considerations in the decision to recommend a tendon transfer.

Sensorimotor

- low median nerve palsy:
    1. paralysis of the thenar muscles (abductor pollicis brevis, opponens pollicis, flexor pollicis brevis, and lumbricals)
    2. inability of the thumb to abduct, pronate, flex, or oppose
    3. inability to use the thumb in opposition to grasp or release objects
- low ulnar nerve palsy:
    1. paralysis of the adductor pollicis (oblique and transverse fibers), deep head of the flexor pollicus brevis, lumbricals to the ring and small fingers, dorsal and volar interossei, and hypothenar muscles (adductor digiti quinti, flexor digiti quinti, and opponens digiti quinti)
    2. inability to pinch a piece of paper between the thumb and lateral border of the index finger (Froment's test)
    3. subluxation of the MCP joint and hyperflexion of the IP joint
- low median and ulnar nerve palsy:
    1. paralysis of all the lumbricals and dorsal and volar interossei muscles
    2. hand position is hyperextension of the metacarpal phalangeal joint and flexion of the IP joints
    3. when finger flexion is attempted, the IP joints must flex completely before the metacarpal phalangeal joints can be flexed
- high median and ulnar nerve palsy, such as C6–7 quadriplegia:
    1. paralysis of all the lumbricals and dorsal and volar interossei muscles
    2. loss of flexion of the IP joints of the thumb
    3. hand position is hyperextension of the metacarpal phalangeal joints and flexion of the IP joints
- dorsal tendon loss in the hand:
    1. paralysis of the extensors to the metacarpal phalangeal joints of the fingers and IP joints
    2. inability to actively extend the fingers
    3. inability to release objects by extending the fingers
- C5 quadriplegia—poor wrist extension:
    1. zero to fair strength in active wrist extensors
    2. fair-plus to normal deltoid and biceps strength
- C6 quadriplegia—poor elbow extension:
    1. lack of active elbow extension
    2. weak prehension strength
- Sensory registration of tactile two-point discrimination and moving touch, temperature, pressure, and proprioception may be decreased.

Cognitive

- Cognitive faculties are not specifically involved in the disorder, although overall intelligence is a consideration in the decision to transfer.

Psychosocial

- The person may be anxious about the surgery or outcome.
- The person may express fear of disfigurement.

TREATMENT/INTERVENTION

Self-Care
• Encourage the performance of self-care activities as healing permits.

Productivity
• Encourage the performance of productive activities as healing permits, including play, school, and work activities.

Leisure
• Encourage the performance of leisure activities as healing permits.

Sensorimotor
• Preoperative program:
  1. Maximize range of motion through exercises, mobilization, splinting, or serial casting.
  2. Implement a strengthening program.
  3. Instruct the person how to use the muscle in isolation, if possible.

Peripheral Nerve Injuries:
• Median nerve correction—surgical transfer of flexor digitorum sublimis tendon from the ring (fourth) finger around the flexor carpi ulnaris (which acts as a pulley) to the abductor pollicis brevis for insertion. (Note: Other transfers include use of the flexor digitorum sublimis to the base of the proximal phalanx, extensor indicus proprius to the proximal phalanx of the thumb, abductor digiti quinti to insertion on the abductor policis brevis, and palmaris longus to the radial side of the metacarpal joint.)
  1. No treatment for 3-1/2–4 weeks while hand remains in compressive dressing with the wrist in slight palmar flexion and the thumb in abduction.
  2. At 3-1/2–4 weeks, the person is fitted with a dorsal blocking splint with wrist in 30 degrees palmar flexion and thumb in 45 degrees of abduction, opposite to the index finger, and the person is encouraged to grasp light cylindrical objects (plastic cups or cones) and to perform isolated finger-to-thumb opposition exercises. Passive and active range of motion activities are to be performed every hour.
  3. At 6 weeks, the splint is removed and functional activities requiring grasp and release patterns are encouraged.
  4. At 8 weeks, functional hand use is encouraged through muscle strengthening and performance of hand activities related to the person's ADLs, work, and leisure.
• Ulnar nerve correction—surgical transfer of the extensor carpi radialis longus (ECRL) tendon routed through the third and fourth metacarpals and inserted into the adductor pollicis. (Note: Other transfers include transfer of the flexor digitorum sublimis to the base of the adductor pollicus and extensor pollicis longus, transfer of the extensor digiti quinti to the adductor pollicis and first dorsal interossei, and transfer of the extensor indicis proprius to the adductor pollicis.)
  1. No treatment for 4 weeks while the hand remains in compressive dressing with the wrist in slight dorsiflexion and the thumb in 30 degrees abduction.

2. At 4 weeks, a dorsal blocking splint is applied to hold the hand in the same position as the dressing (slight dorsiflexion of the wrist and 30 degrees abduction of the thumb). Passive and active range of motion activities are performed every hour, which require thumb adduction and lateral pinch to pick up and hold light objects.
3. At 6 weeks, the splint is removed and functional activities are graded to increase resistance to thumb adduction and lateral pinch.

- Low median and ulnar nerve correction—surgical transfer of the extensor carpi radialis longus elongated with a plantaris graft and split into four parts, which are slid through the carpal canal to the volar side of the hand, following the course of each lumbrical for insertion into the lateral bands of each digit except the index, which is inserted into the ulnar lateral band (Brand transfer). (Other transfers include the Stiles-Bunnell, Lasso procedure by Zancolli and Goldner.)
  1. No treatment for 4-1/2 weeks while the hand remains in compressive dressing with the wrist in 30–40 degrees flexion, the metacarpal phalangeal joints in full flexion, and the IP joints extended.
  2. At 4-1/2 weeks, a dorsal blocking splint is made to hold the wrist in 30 degrees flexion, the metacarpal phalangeal joints in 65–70 degrees of flexion, and the IP joints in extension. No passive flexion is permitted to avoid stretching the transfer insertion into the lateral band. Active range of motion is encouraged with the limits of the splint.
  3. At 6 weeks, the splint is reduced to a metacarpal phalangeal extension block and is worn between exercise periods and at night. Active and passive range of motion activities are performed with the wrist and fingers.
  4. At 8 weeks, the splint is discontinued. The person is encouraged to perform functional activities with the hand and to increase muscle strength.
- High median and ulnar nerve correction—surgical transfer of the extensor carpi radialis longus, which is brought radially around the forearm and inserted into the tendons of the flexor digitorum profundus, and surgical transfer of the brachioradialis into the flexor pollicis longus:
  1. No treatment for 3-1/2 weeks while the hand remains in postoperative dressing positioned in 30 degrees of wrist flexion, metacarpal phalangeal joints in 50 degrees flexion, and the IP joints in extension. The elbow should be in 90 degrees flexion.
  2. At 3-1/2 weeks, a dorsal blocking splint is made to hold the wrist flexed at 30 degrees, metacarpal phalangeal joints at 50 degrees, IP joints in extension, and the IP joints of the thumb in slight flexion. Active and passive range of motion activities are started.
  3. At 6 weeks, the splint is discontinued.
- Digital extension—surgical transfer of the flexor carpi ulnaris, which is brought around ulnarly and dorsally and inserted in the tendons of the extensor digitorum communis:
  1. No treatment for 4-1/2 weeks while the hand remains in postoperative dressing positioned in wrist and digit extension.
  2. At 4-1/2 weeks, an extension resting pan splint is made to position the wrist in 15 degrees of dorsiflexion, 10 degrees flexion at the metacarpal phalangeal joints, and extension of the IP joints.
  3. At 8 weeks, the splint is discontinued.

Spinal Cord Injuries

- General guidelines for combined transfer of the brachioradialis to the radial wrist extension and posterior deltoid-to-triceps transfer. Note: These two separate surgeries are often combined to save costs (Mulcahey 1996, 422).
  1. 1–4 weeks postoperative (immediate stage):
     a. After surgery, the upper extremity is immobilized in a bulky soft splint for 1–2 weeks. The extremity should be elevated to prevent edema.
     b. After the stitches are removed, a fiberglass or plaster cast is applied and immobilization continues.
     c. All joints not immobilized in the splint or cast should have range of motion exercises. The therapist should perform range of motion exercises on the shoulder while it is in the cast to prevent overuse and incorrect motions, and subsequent pain.
  2. 4–8 weeks postoperative:
     a. After the cast is removed, protective splinting, scar and retrograde massage, and active ROM (reeducation) activities are started.
     b. Splint should maintain the extremity in the postoperative position to protect the tendon transfers and prevent the recurrence of deformities. It should be lined with thin foam to protect insensate areas. With young children, buckles on the straps may be used instead of Velcro to make removal more difficult. For children, the splint should be removed only for therapy and bathing. For some adolescents and adults, daytime splinting may not be necessary. For some older individuals, the hand may be used for light ADLs and control of the powered wheelchair as soon as the person is able to begin.
     c. Retrograde massage should be started, which is performed distally to proximally.
     d. Scar massage is performed initially along the perimeter of the incision. After healing has occurred, scar massage should be performed over the surgical site. Firm pressure scar massage should be performed twice daily.
     e. Active range of motion and muscle reeducation are focused on teaching the person how to use the muscle in its new function. During the first 4 weeks after the cast is removed, AROM without resistance is performed. One useful activity for young children is placing the arm in water. Biofeedback or surface electrical stimulation to motor level threshold may be an effective adjunct to range of motion activities.
     f. If adhesions occur (see Precautions), scar massage, elastomer, ultrasound, and dynamic splinting can be used. If these fail, tendolysis may be performed (see chapter on tendon injuries).
  3. 9–11 weeks postoperative:
     a. Daytime splinting is usually discontinued at 9 weeks while nighttime splinting usually continues until the 12th week. However, when a deltoid-to-triceps transfer is performed, the splinting usually is maintained until the 11th week, and with arthrodesis procedures, the splinting may be continued until the 12th week.
     b. After daytime splinting is discontinued, the person is encouraged to use the tendon transfer through the day.

    c. The therapist should continue to evaluate functional performance and to modify treatment to avoid hand deformities or contractures. Should these occur, splinting should be immediately applied.

    d. At 9 weeks postoperatively, graded-resistive activities and ADL training should begin but passive stretching is avoided until 12 weeks postsurgery.

    e. Common goals for persons who have undergone tendon transfer for active grasp include writing, opening milk cartons, using scissors, using a pencil sharpener, self-catheterization, wheelchair mobility skills, and, for girls, applying makeup. For elbow extension transfers, the person should be able to extend the arms away from the face, reach surfaces above eye level, assist in transfers from chair to bed and back, improve wheelchair mobility skills, and be more effective in performing push-ups from the chair for pressure relief on the buttocks.

- Specific guidelines for deltoid to triceps transfer for elbow extension (Mulcahey 1996, 426–427)

    1. 0–4 weeks:

        a. The upper extremity is placed in a long-arm cast following surgery, with the elbow in no more than 20 degrees of flexion but the wrist and hand mobile.

        b. In bed, the arm should be elevated to reduce edema, and the shoulder should be abducted to 30 degrees.

        c. Passive range of motion of the hand is started the day after surgery and a wrist splint is made.

    2. 4–10 weeks:

        a. An elbow orthosis is used after the cast is removed to protect the transfer and prevent stretching or rupturing. The orthosis is locked in no more than 20 degrees of elbow flexion at the beginning and is increased 10 degrees each week. A hinged orthosis allows AROM with the brace itself.

        b. The orthosis is removed for twice-a-day therapy and skin checks. Therapy focuses on AROM of elbow extension with gravity eliminated. During AROM, the extremity should be supported and maintained, with the shoulder internally rotated to avoid compensatory patterns to occur. Active elbow flexion beyond the range of the orthosis is avoided.

        c. ADLs are integrated into the program.

        d. Scar reduction management and retrograde massage are begun.

    3. 10 weeks to 6 months:

        a. Progressive resistive exercises are started for elbow flexion.

        b. Wheelchair propulsion skills are integrated into the therapy program.

        c. A soft splint is worn at night to prevent elongation of the tendon for up to 6 months.

- Guidelines for flexor pollicis longus tenodesis (Moberg tenodesis) and transfer of the brachioradialis to wrist extensors for passive lateral pinch (Mulcahey 1996, 427–429)

    1. 0–4 weeks:

        a. Following surgery, the arm is immobilized for 4 weeks in 90 degrees of elbow flexion, 20 degrees of wrist extension, and flexion of the thumb and index MCP joints.

        b. While in bed, the person's arm is elevated to reduce edema.

    2. 4–8 weeks:

     a. A dorsal-based splint is made to position the wrist in 20 degrees of extension and the thumb and index MCP joints in flexion. The elbow is not incorporated into the splint but activities that require strenuous active elbow flexion, such as propelling a manual wheelchair and hooking the elbow over the back of the wheelchair, are not recommended.

     b. Scar reduction management and retrograde massage are begun.

     c. Active range of motion of wrist extension is begun but the thumb should be protected by positioning it between the index and middle fingers.

3. 8–16 weeks:

     a. Light ADLs are started at 8 weeks.

     b. Activities involving the thumb are begun between 8 and 10 weeks postsurgery.

     c. Daytime splinting is discontinued after the 11th week but nighttime splinting continues to 16 weeks.

     d. Wheelchair propulsion may be started at 12 weeks.

- Guidelines for rehabilitation of extensor carpi radialis longus to flexor digitorum profundus transfer for active finger flexion and brachialradialis to flexor pollicus longus transfer for active thumb flexion (Mulcahey 1996, 429–431)

1. 0–4 weeks:

     a. The arm is immobilized in a plaster cast for 4 weeks.

2. 4–8 weeks:

     a. A splint is worn during the day and night.

     b. After cast is removed, scar management and retrograde massage should be started.

     c. Active range of motion of wrist extension, finger flexion, and thumb flexion with the brachialradialis. During wrist extension, the thumb is positioned between the index and middle fingers to avoid resistance to the brachialradialis transfer. At the end of 6 weeks, wrist extension should approach presurgical range of motion

     d. At 6 weeks, reeducation of the ECRL for finger flexion and brachialradialis for thumb flexion should be emphasized. Resistance to finger and thumb flexion should be avoided until the end of the 10th week.

     e. At 7–8 weeks light grasp of objects and simple ADLs can be performed in therapy.

3. 8–11 weeks:

     a. Wheelchair propulsion with a splint can be started at about 10 weeks.

     b. Strengthening of pinch grasp also is started at about 10 weeks.

     c. Use of the hand to aid in transfers and mobility can be started at about 11 weeks.

- General guidelines for rehabilitation of tendon transfers for the two-stage approach for active grasp and release (Mulcahey 1996, 429–431)

1. Stage 1: Extensor stage.

     a. After 4 weeks, the cast is removed and AROM of the wrist flexors is started to activate passive tenodesis opening of the hand.

     b. Passive range of motion of the proximal and DIP joints is started.

     c. Scar management and retrograde massage is performed.

     d. At 6 weeks, muscle reeducation of the brachialradialis is started and AROM of the ECRL are initiated.

     e. At 8 weeks, strengthening activities are performed.

2. Stage II: Flexor stage.

Flexor Zones of the Hand

Zone I—includes the fingertips, DIP joint, and distal half between the DIP and PIP joints

Zone II—includes the proximal half between the DIP and PIP joints, the PIP joint, the MCP joint to the palmar crease

Zone III—includes the space between the palmar crease to a line drawn across the palm at the distal point where the thumb joins the hand

Zone IV—includes the space between the line drawn across the palm at the distal point where the thumb joins the hand to the crease at the wrist

Zone V—begins at the crease at the wrist up the forearm

Source: Data from B. Steinberg, Flexor Tendon Repair, in Hand Rehabilitation: A Practical Guide, 2nd ed., G.L. Clark, E.F.S. Wilgis, B. Aiello, D. Eckhaus, and L.V. Eddington, eds., p. 104, © 1997, Churchill Livingstone; and K.M. Steward and G. van Strien, Postoperative Management of Flexor Tendon Injuries, in Rehabilitation of the Hand, 4th ed., J.M. Hunter, E.J. Mackin, and A.D. Callahan, eds., p. 435, © 1995, Mosby.

---

a. At 7–10 weeks postoperatively, full wrist active and passive flexion is usually obtained. At this time, the ECRL is transferred to the flexor digitorum profundus (FDP) for active finger flexion and the pronator teres is transferred to the flexor pollicis longus (FPL) for active thumb flexion.

b. After 4 weeks in a cast, the cast is removed and therapy is started.
   i. Scar and retrograde massage is started.
   ii. Strengthening and AROM exercises are started.
   iii. Muscle reeducation is begun.

c. At 10 weeks, graded resistive activities are incorporated.

- With children, some modifications of the standard protocol may be needed, such as:
1. Prolonged protective splinting as a result of the child's difficulty in adhering to postoperative precautions
2. Use of biofeedback and other interactive activities to facilitate muscle reeducation because the child does not understand the reason for hand exercises

---

Extensor Zones of the Hand

Zone I—DIP joints of digits 2–5

Zone II—space between the DIP and PIP joints of digits 2–5

Zone III—PIP joints of digits 2–5

Zone IV—space between the PIP joints and the MCP joints of digits 2–5

Zone V—MCP joints

Zone VI—space between the MCP joints and the carpal bones of the wrist

Zone VII—carpal bones of the wrist

Source: Data from R.B. Evans, An Update on Extensor Tendon Management, in Rehabilitation of the Hand, 4th ed., J.M. Hunter, E.J. Mackin, and A.D. Callahan, eds., p. 566, © 1995, Mosby; and B. Steinberg, Extensor Tendon Repair, in Hand Rehabilitation: A Practical Guide, 2nd ed., G.L. Clark, E.F.S. Wilgis, B. Aiello, D. Eckhaus, and L.V. Eddington, eds., p. 94, © 1997, Churchill-Livingstone.

Extensor Zones of the Thumb

Zone T I—IP joint
Zone T II—space between the IP joint and the MCP joint
Zone T III—MCP joint
Zone T IV—space between the MCP joint and the carpal bones of the wrist
Zone T V—area of the carpal bones on the thumb side

Source: Data from R.B. Evans, An Update on Extensor Tendon Management, in Rehabilitation of the Hand, 4th ed., J.M. Hunter, E.J. Mackin, and A.D. Callahan, eds., p. 566, © 1995, Mosby; and B. Steinberg, Extensor Tendon Repair, in Hand Rehabilitation: A Practical Guide, 2nd ed., G.L. Clark, E.F.S. Wilgis, B. Aiello, D. Eckhaus, and L.V. Eddington, eds., p. 94, © 1997, Churchill-Livingstone.

---

3. Involvement of the parents in therapy to facilitate carryover of function at home and school (Mulcahey 1997, 50–51, Overview)
- Note: Functional electrical stimulation implants have been used to increase function (Davis et al. 1997, 307–312).

Cognitive
- Instruct the person in a home program.
- Provide instructions on one-handed activities, if needed, during recovery period.
- Assist the physician in providing factual information to the person about the recovery process of his or her particular tendon transfer procedure.

Psychosocial
- Permit the person to express concerns about how well the transfer will perform.

PRECAUTIONS
- Do not overstretch joints through PROM in early stages of postoperative recovery (about 3–6 weeks, depending on the type of transfer and rate of healing).
- Complications include adhesion, elongation, or detachment of the tendon.
- Adhesion may occur anywhere along the tendon transfer. Inspect the incision site for skin puckering and palpate the entire tendon to identify the presence of adhesions.
- In the hand, check joints for tendon gliding action, once extensor or dorsal blocking splints are removed. If gliding action is limited, consider initiating tendon gliding activities.

PROGNOSIS AND OUTCOME
- The person will have improved ability to perform self-care activities.
- The person will have improved ability to perform tasks in work settings.
- The person will have improved ability to perform functional tasks in leisure activities.
- The person will have functional range of motion for the movements expected as a result of the transplant.
- The person will have muscle strength within the range expected as a result of the transplant.
- The person will have joint stability expected as a result of the transplant.

Hand-Strengthening Equipment

Equipment	Measurable	Gradable
Spring-loaded clothespins with dowel rod stand	yes	4 grades
Hand exerciser with rubber bands	yes	color-coded rubber bands
Gross hand grippers	yes	yes
Digital Gross grasp hand exerciser	yes	yes
Hand and finger exercise system	yes	5 grades for gross grasp
Hand/wrist forearm table	yes	yes
Electric work simulator devices	yes	yes
Finger pulley exerciser	yes	graded finger weights
Thumb rubber bands and spring-resistant exerciser	limited	graded rubber bands and springs to 4 lbs
Elastic hand putty	no	yes, graded by color
Hand pump exercise	no	somewhat
Foam hand grippers	no	soft, medium, hard
Velcro board	no	somewhat, depending on size of roller
Rubber bands board	no	by using graded rubber bands
Elastic exercise tubing and strip	no	tubing—light to super heavy, strips—95–340 g
Velcro checkers	no	difficult

Source: Data from D. Kenny and E. Maday, Hand Strengthening Devices Range from Low-Tech Putty to Computers, *Advance for Directors in Rehabilitation*, © 1994, Vol. 3, No. 2, p. 42.

REFERENCES

Bell-Krotoski, J.A. 1995. Preoperative and postoperative management of tendon transfers after ulnar nerve injury. In *Rehabilitation of the Hand*, 4th ed., ed. J.M. Hunter, E.J. Mackin, and A.D. Callahan, 729–752. St. Louis: Mosby.

Davis, S.E., M.J. Mulcahey, R.R. Betz, and A.A. Weiss. 1997. Outcomes of upper-extremity tendon transfers and functional electrical stimulation in an adolescent with C-5 tetraplegia. *American Journal of Occupational Therapy* 51(4):307–312 (Case report).

Eliasson, A.C., C. Ekholm, and T. Carlstedt. 1998. Hand function in children with cerebral palsy after upper-limb tendon transfer and muscle release. *Developmental Medicine and Child Neurology* 40:612–621.

Hoard, A.S., J.A. Bell-Krotoski, and R. Mathews. 1995. Application of biomechanics to tendon transfer. *Journal of Hand Therapy* 8(2):115–123.

Mulcahey, M.J. 1996. Rehabilitation and outcomes of upper extremity tendon transfer surgery. In *The Child with a Spinal Cord Injury*, ed. R.R. Betz and M.J. Mulcahey, 419–448. Rosemont, IL: American Academy of Orthopedic Surgeons.

Mulcahey, M.J. 1997. An overview of the upper extremity in pediatric spinal cord injury. *Topics in Spinal Cord Injury Rehabilitation* 3(2):48–55.

BIBLIOGRAPHY

Mulcahey, M.J. 1997. Outcomes of upper-extremity tendon transfers and functional electrical stimulation in an adolescent with C-5 tetraplegia. *American Journal of Occupational Therapy* 51(4):307–312.

Mulcahey, M.J. et al. 1999. A prospective evaluation of upper extremity tendon transfers in children with cervical spinal injury. *Journal of Pediatric Orthopedics* 19(3):319–328.

Mulcahey, M.J., B.T. Smith, R.R. Betz, and A.A. Weiss. 1995. Outcomes of tendon transfer surgery and occupational therapy in a child with tetraplegia secondary to spinal cord injury (review). *American Journal of Occupational Therapy* 49(7):607–617.

Mulcahey, M.J., R.R. Betz, B.T. Smith, and A.A. Weiss. 1999. A prospective evaluation of upper extremity tendon transfers in children with cervical spinal cord injury. *Journal of Pediatric Orthopedics* 19(3):319–328.

Head and Brain Injuries—Adult

DESCRIPTION

Head injuries may result from penetration of the skull or from rapid acceleration or deceleration of the brain, which injures tissue at the point of impact, at the opposite pole (contrecoup), and along the frontal and temporal lobes. In addition, nerve tissue, blood vessels, and meninges may be torn or ruptured, resulting in disruption of neural transmission, intra- or extracerebral ischemia, hemorrhage, and cerebral edema (*Merck Manual* 1999, 1427).

Head injury causes more deaths and disability than any other neurologic condition before age 50 and occurs in > 70% of accidents, which are the leading cause of death in men and boys under 35 years of age. Mortality from severe injury approaches 50% (*Merck Manual* 1999, 1427).

A term closely associated with head injury is *traumatic brain injury,* which the National Head Injury Foundation defines as "an insult to the brain not of a degenerative or congenital nature but caused by an external physical force, that may produce a diminished or altered state of consciousness, which results in impairment of cognitive abilities or physical functioning. It can also result in the disturbance of behavioral or emotional function."

CAUSE

Automobile, motorcycle, or off-road vehicle accidents are the primary causes. Injuries are also possible from objects falling on the head or from a bullet entering the skull (*Merck*

The Thinking Corporation

- Administration (Frontal Lobe): decision making, fine motor control, goal setting, judgment, higher-level thinking, planning, problem solving.
- Purchasing and Inventory (Parietal Lobe): interprets form and space information; processes sensory information from senses, muscles, and joints; regulates input and information for organizing and processing.
- Communication (Temporal Lobe): auditory processing and expressive and receptive language; speech, some emotions, and dreams.
- Photography (Occipital Lobe): Processes visual information and integrates it with other centers.
- Personnel and Records (Limbic/Diencephalon): Regulation of emotions, alertness, and arousal; ability to organize and regulate information, memory, impulse control, appetite, sexual arousal, and body temperature. Assists in communication between departments.
- Transportation (Cerebellum): Responsible for large muscle control, posture, balance, equilibrium, and reflexes.
- Building and Maintenance (Brain Stem): Controls essential body functions, keeps basic operations going, regulates attention and incoming information.

Source: Data from T.A. Bell, Understanding Students with Traumatic Brain Injury: A Guide for Teachers and Therapists, *School System Special Interest Section Newsletter,* © 1994, Vol. 1, No. 20, p. 2.

Manual 1999, 1427). Traumatic brain injury can be caused by a penetrating injury through the skull (open) or a nonpenetrating injury in which no skull fracture is involved (closed). The damage to the brain is caused by localized contusions (focal damage) or diffuse axonal injury (diffuse damage). In addition to the primary damage, secondary damage may occur, including intracranial hematomas, cerebral edema, raised intracerebral pressure, hydrocephalus, intracranial infection, posttraumatic epilepsy, or ischemic (hypoxic) brain damage. Complications may include wound infection or osteomyelitis, pulmonary infection, hyperthermia, diabetes insipidus, inappropriate antidiuretic hormone secretion, heterotopic bone formation, and thrombophlebitis (Schlageter and Zoltan 1996, 808).

ASSESSMENT

Note: Head injuries rarely occur in isolation. Usually, there is trauma to other parts of the body, as well. Assessment may be complicated by the existence of additional injury sites.

Areas

- daily living skills
- productivity history, interests, values, and skills
- leisure interests and skills
- reflex/reaction integration
- postural control and balance

Women and Head Injury

- Behavioral Indicators

Women who have sustained a traumatic brain injury and report both alcohol and childhood sexual abuse histories are likely to:

Intrapersonal skills

1. Display behaviors indicative of decreased insight into personal feelings.
2. Display behaviors indicative of decreased insight into own needs.
3. Display behaviors indicative of decreased positive self-regard.
4. Display behaviors indicative of a decreased internal locus of control.

Interpersonal skills

1. Display poor social skills necessary to establish and maintain appropriate peer relationships.
2. Display difficulty recognizing unsafe situations and untrustworthy others.
3. Display seductive behaviors with clients, staff, and strangers.
4. Engage in unsafe sex practices.
5. Display a poor sense of interpersonal boundaries and limit setting.
6. Lack a supportive network of others who promote emotionally healthful behaviors.

- Directions for promoting positive change

Intrapersonal skills

1. Provide opportunities for women to identify and express their own emotions.
2. Provide opportunities for women to identify and learn to meet their own needs.
3. Provide opportunities for women to participate in activities that enhance self-respectful behaviors.
4. Provide opportunities for women to engage in activities that increase their internal locus of control.

Interpersonal skills

1. Provide opportunities for women to learn the social skills necessary to reduce anxiety in social situations without the use of alcohol.
2. Provide opportunities for women to learn the difference between using appropriate social behaviors and inappropriate seductive actions.
3. Provide opportunities for women to learn safe sex practices.
4. Provide opportunities for women to learn to recognize and respond to unsafe situations and untrustworthy others.
5. Provide opportunities for women to develop a sense of personal boundaries and engage in limit setting.
6. Provide opportunities for women to develop a supportive network of others who promote healthful behavior.

Source: Data from S.A. Gutman and P. Swarbrick, The Multiple Linkages between Childhood Sexual Abuse, Adult Alcoholism, and Traumatic Brain Injury in Women: A Set of Guidelines for Occupational Therapy Practice, *Occupational Therapy in Mental Health,* © 1998, Vol. 4, No. 3, pp. 33–65.

- range of motion and joint mobility
- muscle tone, abnormal tone
- gross motor skill coordination and mobility
- hand functions
- fine motor manipulation, dexterity, and bilateral coordination
- physical endurance
- sensory registration awareness and discrimination
- sensory processing
- perceptual skills, especially visual and auditory
- dysphagia
- arousal level and alertness
- attending behavior, attention span, and concentration
- orientation to time, person, place
- memory
- comprehension
- reasoning and problem-solving skills
- judgment of personal safety
- learning skills
- coping skills
- social interaction skills

Instruments

Instruments Developed by Occupational Therapy Personnel

- *Assessment of Motor and Process Skills* (AMPS), 2nd ed., by Fisher, A.G. 1997. Fort Collins, CO: Three Star Press.
- *Chessington Occupational Therapy Neurological Assessment Battery* (COTNAB) by Tyerman, R., A. Tyerman, P. Howard, C. Hayfield. 1986. Nottingham, England: Nottingham Rehab.
- *Loewenstein Occupational Therapy Perceptual Cognitive Assessment* by Najenson. T., L. Rahmani, B. Elazar, and S. Averbuch, 1983.
- *Motor-Free Visual Perception Test* (adult version) by Bouska, M.J. and E. Kwatny. 1983. *Manual for Application of the Motor-Free Visual Perception Test to the Adult Population*, 6th ed. Philadelphia: Author.
- *Motor-Free Visual Perception Test—Vertical Format (MVPT-V)* by Mercier, L., R. Hebert, R. Colarusso, and D. Hammill.1997. Novato, CA: Academic Therapy Publications.
- *Perceptual Evaluation Manual by the Study Group on the Brain-Damaged Adult.* 1977. Toronto, Canada: Ontario Society of Occupational Therapists.
- *Rabideau Kitchen Evaluation, Revised* by Neistadt, M. 1992. The Rabideau Kitchen Evaluation—Revised: An assessment of meal preparation skills. *Occupational Therapy Journal of Research* 12(4):242–255.
- *Rivermead Perceptual Assessment Battery* by Whiting, S. et al. 1985. Windsor, England: NFER-Nelson. In the United States, available from Western Psychological Services, Los Angeles, CA.
- *Role Checklist* by Oakley, F., G. Kielhofner, R. Barris, and R.K. Reichler. 1986. The role checklist: Development and empirical assessment of reliability. *Occupational Therapy Journal of Research* 6(3):157–170.

- *Routine Task Inventory* by Williams, L.R. and C.K. Allen. 1985. Research with a nondisabled population. In *Occupational Therapy for Psychiatric Diseases: Measurement and Management of Cognitive Disabilities*, ed. C.K. Allen, 315–338. Boston: Little, Brown & Co.

Instruments Developed by Other Professionals and Used by Occupational Therapy Personnel

- Barthel Index by Mahoney, F.I. and D.W. Barthel. 1965. Functional evaluation: The Barthel Index. *Maryland State Medical Journal* 14, 61–65.
- *Behavioural Inattention Test* by Wilson, B. and J. Cockburn. 1987. Gaylord, MI: Northern Rehabilitation Services.
- *Community Integration Questionnaire* by Willer, B. et al. 1993. Assessment of community integration following rehabilitation for traumatic brain injury. *Journal of Head Trauma Rehabilitation* 8(2):75–87.
- *Disability Rating Scale* by Rappaport, M., K.M. Hall, K. Hopkins, T. Belleze, and D.N. Cope. 1982. Disability rating scale for severe head trauma: Coma to community. *Archives of Physical Medicine and Rehabilitation* 63:118–123.
- *Functional Independence Measure* v. 4.0. Uniform Data System for Medical Rehabilitation. 1994. Buffalo NY: State University of New York at Buffalo.
- *Galveston Orientation and Amnesia Test* by Levin, et al. 1979. The Galveston Orientation and Amnesia Test. A practical scale to assess cognition after head injury. *Journal of Nervous and Mental Disease* 167:675–684.
- *Glasgow Coma Scale* by Teasdale, G. and B. Jennett. 1974. Assessment of coma and impaired consciousness: A practical scale. *Lancet* 2:81–83.
- *Glasgow Outcome Scale* by Jennett, B. and M. Bond. 1975. Assessment of outcome after severe brain damage. A practical scale. *Lancet* 1:480–484.
- *Luria-Nebraska Neuropsychological Battery* by Golden, C.J. 1980. Los Angeles: Western Psychological Service. Used mostly by neuropsychologists, but the results can be useful in occupational therapy program planning.
- *Mini Mental State* by Folstein, A.F., S.E. Folstein, and P.R. McHugh. 1975. Mini mental state: A practical method for grading the cognitive state of patients for the clinician. *Journal of Psychiatric Research* 12:189–198.
- *NYSOA King-Devick Test.* New York State Optometric Association. South Bend, IN: Bernell, n.d.
- *Rivermead Behavioural Memory Test* by Wilson, B., J. Cockburn, and A.D. Baddeley. 1985. Gaylord, MI: Northern Rehabilitation Services.
- Optic 2000 vision tester, industrial model. Stereo Optical Company. 1984. Chicago: Author.
- *Rey Complex Figure Test.* Visser, R. *Manual of the Complex Figure Test.* 1973. Amsterdam: Sweets and Seitlinger.
- dexterity, manipulation, and coordination tests:
  1. *Crawford Small Parts Dexterity Test*, revised by Crawford, J.E. and D.M. Crawford. 1981. San Antonio, TX: Psychological Corporation.
  2. *Jebsen Hand Function Test* by Jebsen, R.H. et al. 1969. *Archives of Physical Medicine and Rehabilitation* 50(6):311–319.

    3. *Minnesota Rate of Manipulation Test.* 1969. Circle Pines, MN: American Guidance
       Service (no specific author credited by publisher).
    4. *Purdue Pegboard Test,* Revised by Tiffin, J. 1948, 1960, 1999. Lafayette, IN: Lafayette
       Instrument Co.
- visual perception tests:
    1. *Motor-Free Visual Perception Test*, Revised by Colarusso, R.P. and D.D. Hamill. 1993.
       Novato, CA: Academic Therapy Publications.
    2. *Hooper Visual Organization Test*, 2nd ed., by Hooper, H.E. 1983. Los Angeles:
       Western Psychological Services.

PROBLEMS

Self-Care

- The person may be unable to perform certain ADLs because of spasticity, flaccidity, or limited range of motion. Spasticity may interfere with transfers, positioning in bed or in a wheelchair, and gait deviations that limit functional mobility.
- The person may have difficulty remembering how to do certain ADLs or other basic skills, such as simple math calculations.
- The person may start an activity and be unable to complete certain ADLs or be unable to start an activity but completes the activity with ease.
- The person may have difficulty with hygiene and grooming, kitchen skills, or reading or writing, due to visual or visual motor disturbances.
- The person may have difficulty with driving because of visual and motor disturbances.

Productivity

- Problems with decreased attention and concentration, memory, mental processing speed, interpersonal skills, awareness and judgment, emotion control, learning and cognitive flexibility, upper- and lower-extremity functioning speed and endurance may hinder a return to work (Skord and Ellexon 1996, 3).
- Personality changes may interfere with job performance.
- The person may have difficulty performing housekeeping and home management tasks.
- The person may be unable to perform child care tasks.

Leisure

- The person may be unable to continue previous leisure activities because of cognitive dysfunction.
- Interests may need to change because motor, perceptual, and cognitive skills are reduced as an outcome of the head injury.

Sensorimotor

- The person may have return of primitive reflexes, such as the tonic labyrinthine, asymmetrical tonic neck, symmetrical tonic neck, positive supporting, and grasp.
- The person may have impaired gross motor skills and coordination in rolling, sitting, or standing without support, rotating the trunk, and reciprocal movements of the arms and legs

---

Levels of Cognitive Functioning

- No response: unresponsive to any stimuli
- Generalized response: inconsistent and nonpurposeful response to a stimulus
- Localized response: specific but inconsistent response to a stimulus; may follow simple commands but performance is delayed
- Confused-agitated: incoherent verbalization, no independence in activities of daily living, becomes easily agitated, requires constant supervision for safety, short attention span, no short-term memory
- Confused-inappropriate: responds to simple commands, becomes agitated when presented with unfamiliar situations, performs activities of daily living with assistance, requires frequent supervision for safety, highly distractible, can converse at automatic level, memory is impaired, unable to learn new material
- Confused-appropriate: independent in performing activities of daily living but is dependent on external input for direction, follows simple directions, remote memory better than recent, requires minimal supervision for safety
- Automatic-appropriate: person appears appropriate and oriented within familiar environment, such as hospital or home, needs minimal supervision for learning and safety, can perform activities of daily living without prompting, judgment is impaired
- Purposeful-appropriate: person is alert and oriented, able to recall and integrate past and recent events, can function independently, needs no supervision, able to tolerate stress, uses judgment in unfamiliar situations

Source: Data from C. Hagen, Language-Cognitive Disorganization Following Closed Head Injury: A Conceptualization, in *Cognitive Rehabilitation: Conceptualization and Intervention*, L. Trexler, ed., pp. 138–139, © 1981, Plenum Press.

---

for walking. Functional skills, such as reaching, bending, and stooping, may also be affected.

- The person may have limitations in range of motion due to several factors, including increased muscle tone, myostatic contractures, heterotopic ossification, undetected fracture or dislocation, pain, or lack of cooperation from the person.
- The person may have muscle weakness in the extremities, due in part to decreased innervation and disuse atrophy.
- The person may have impaired hand functions and loss of fine motor manipulation, dexterity, and bilateral coordination skills, due to wrist tightness interfering with extension, hyperpronation of the forearm, and difficulty in releasing grasp.
- The person may have abnormal tone in trunk and extremities—hypertonicity (spasticity) or hypotonicity (flaccidity).
- The person may have impaired postural control and balance reactions. Posture in decerebrate rigidity is dorsiflexion of the neck, extension and internal rotation of the shoulders, and extension of the lower extremities. Posture in decorticate rigidity is flexion of the upper extremities and extension of the lower.

- The person may have impaired motor control due to the imbalance of muscle tone and muscle weakness. Often, one side of the body is more involved than the other.
- The person may have postural deficits, such as:
  1. Forward flexion or hyperextension of the head and neck. The head and neck may be flexed laterally to one side. Lateral flexion of trunk often accompanies lateral neck flexion.
  2. Scapula depression may be present with additional elements, such as protraction, retraction, and/or downward rotation. Some scapular muscles may be hypertonic, whereas others are hypotonic.
  3. Bilateral involvement of the upper extremities may occur with asymmetry between the two sides or involvement may occur only on one side.
  4. The trunk may be positioned in kyphosis or scoliosis with loss of lordosis, which are secondary conditions due to weak or spastic muscles, especially in the abdominals, spinals, and paraspinals.
  5. The pelvis has a posterior tilt, causing the person to sit on the sacrum, which facilitates the kyphosis position. Other problems in postural deviation include retraction of one side of the pelvis, which leads to the pelvis being oblique so that one side sits lower than the other.
  6. Extensor patterns are often seen in persons who are in a persistent vegetative state. Other postural problems in the lower extremities include hip adduction, knee flexion, plantar flexion, and inversion of the feet.
- The person may have decreased physical conditioning—tires easily, has low endurance and vital capacity.
- The person may have stiffness in joints—lack of flexibility, joint mobility, and range of motion.
- The person may show asymmetry of movement or abnormal movement patterns.
- The person may have ataxia, which involves abnormality of movement and disordered muscle tone. Ataxia in the trunk interferes with postural stability in sitting and standing.
- The person may have dysphagia (difficulty with swallowing) in any of the four states of swallowing: oral preparatory, oral, pharyngeal, and esophageal.
- The person may have constructional apraxia and other difficulties in motor planning and sequencing.
- The person may have decreased visual acuity.
- The person may have oculomotor disturbance involving visual tracking and scanning.
- The person may have difficulty with eye-hand coordination or eye-foot tasks, such as ambulation.
- The person may have visual neglect in field of vision.
- The person may have specific visual problems, including strabismus (eyes do not work together or team properly) with diplopia (double vision), insufficient convergence of the eyes for near tasks, accommodative dysfunction (causing blurred images), nystagmus, reduced blink rate, and lagophthalmos (incomplete lid closure).
- The person may have impaired hearing.
- The person may have impaired body awareness and body image.
- The person may have difficulty with discrimination tasks.
- The person may have loss of light touch and sharp/dull differentiation.

- The person may have impaired senses of taste and smell, due to involvement of cranial nerves.
- The person may have hypersensitivity to tactile, proprioceptive, vibratory, temperature, and vestibular stimuli.
- The person may have perceptual-motor problems, such as difficulty with figure-ground, position in space, size and/or shape discrimination, unilateral spatial inattention, part-whole integration, or visual organization.

Cognitive

- The person may be in a coma state. Levels of coma may include comatose, stupor, clouding, arousal to complete consciousness.
- The person may have reduced attention and concentration skills.
- The person may be easily distracted and unable to filter out distractions in the environment.
- The person may have lapses in immediate, short-term, and long-term memory.
- The person may have difficulty initiating a task but be able to complete task once it is started.
- The person may have decreased judgment regarding personal safety.
- The person may show delays in the processing of information. In assessing the person, it is important to differentiate between delayed processing and inability to perform.
- The person may have difficulty setting goals.
- The person may have decreased analytic skills, especially abstract skills. Information may be processed primarily in concrete terms.
- The person may have difficulty with sequencing tasks.
- The person may have difficulty organizing tasks.
- The person may have difficulty categorizing information.
- The person may have difficulty integrating information.
- The person may have difficulty learning or relearning skills.
- The person may demonstrate incomplete thought and action.
- The person may recognize that an error has occurred but be unable to take action that would correct the error.
- The person may have difficulty planning ahead in time.
- The person may have difficulty reasoning or thinking through the consequences of a particular action or set of actions.
- The person may have decreased judgment skills, including lack of personal safety.
- The person may have difficulty with problem solving and decision making.
- The person may show disorganization of verbal and nonverbal activity.
- The person may have slurred or dysarthric speech.
- The person may have impaired receptive language in reading comprehension, word recognition, or auditory comprehension (receptive aphasia).
- The person may have impaired expressive language in writing, word finding, fluency, or spelling (expressive aphasia).

Psychosocial

- The person may become agitated.
- The person may become combative, including kicking, biting, grabbing, or spitting.
- The person may become easily confused and disoriented.

Decision-Making Model in Treatment Planning for Head Injuries

- Are any of the person's basic cognitive abilities/skills impaired, such as attention, concentration, abstract thinking, information processing, problem solving, and memory?
- How are other related systems functioning, such as motor, visual, perceptual, sensory, or auditory?
- Does the person have the learning skills to be restimulated or retrained?
- Is a restimulation program enough to facilitate learning activities of daily living? If not, compensatory techniques should be used.
- Are there other conditions interfering with the cognitive retraining, such as emotional, behavior, or physical factors? If so, can the factors be reduced?
- Are other methods needed in addition to cognitive approaches?
- Can the person learn a compensatory strategy, such as use of a checklist?
- Should environmental restructuring be added to the treatment plan?
- Has the compensatory strategy been generalized from one daily living skill to another?
- Are the compensatory strategies effective and are the restimulation exercises beneficial? If so, continue; if not, change the program.

Source: Data from S.M. Schwartz, Adults with Traumatic Brain Injury: Three Case Studies of Cognitive Rehabilitation in the Home Setting, *American Journal of Occupational Therapy*, 1995, Vol. 49, No. 7, pp. 655–657.

- The person may have decreased inhibition (disinhibition) control. Behavior may include taking off clothes in public, shouting obscenities, or making unwelcome sexual advances.
- The person's personality may change from outgoing to introverted or vice versa.
- The person may change from totally independent to totally dependent, especially during early stages of recovery.
- The person may refuse to cooperate in treatment sessions. A differentiation between cognitive impairment and lack of interest in therapy should be determined.
- The person may be addicted to drugs or alcohol. A firm policy regarding substance abuse may be needed.
- The person may become depressed.
- The person may be anxious.
- The person may have low self-esteem or self-perception.
- The person may be nonassertive or demonstrate faulty assertion.
- The person may demonstrate aggressive behavior.
- The person may act inappropriately in social situations.
- The person may react differently to friends after the injury.
- The person may create family discord and disrupt family structure.
- The person may have sexual dysfunction.

Environment

- Roles within a family may be reversed and relationships changed.

- Modifications to the home may be necessary for the person to function, such as widening of a bathroom door to accommodate a wheelchair.

TREATMENT/INTERVENTION

Treatment and intervention are usually planned and implemented by a multidisciplinary team, including neuropsychology, physical therapy, speech language pathology, optometry, vocational counseling, recreational therapy, medicine, and counseling, as well as occupational therapy. Models of intervention include the cognitive behavioral model, cognitive organization, neurodevelopmental treatment, and Rancho Levels model. Models of practice in occupational therapy include the quadraphonic approach (Abreu 1998) cognitive rehabilitation model (Averbuch and Katz 1996, 99–124), neurofunctional approach (Giles 1996a, 135–147), dynamic interactional model (Toglia 1998, 5–50), Rancho Five Phase model (Tomas et al. 1993, 649–661), cognitive disabilities, model of human occupation and sensory integration.

Specific intervention goals should be encompassed with the general goals of providing a safe environment while minimizing the use of restrictive or restraint techniques and providing an environment that enables the person to participate in a comprehensive program that integrates caregivers into the process.

In addition to the head injury management program, other programs may be necessary, such as a drug and alcohol addiction program.

Self-Care

- Increase independent performance of self-care skills.
- Provide maximal assistance initially in the skills that are most deficient. Provide cues using sensory input through senses that are less involved.
- Provide moderate assistance using continuous verbal cueing and close supervision.
- Provide minimal assistance to ensure safety and provide intermittent cueing. The person should be able to perform at least half of the activity independently.
- Person performs self-care activities with setups (the objects needed are in sight and a list of steps may be visible). The therapist or family member checks to determine whether the activity was performed or assists if an unusual situation occurs.
- The person performs most self-care activities independently using self-help devices or adapted equipment if needed. No assistance is required except a final checkup.
- The person performs all self-care activities consistently without supervision or checkup by another person.

Productivity

- Improve the person's home-management skills. Grade activity based on amount of physical assistance needed, amount of on-site supervision needed, amount and type of cues needed, types of equipment used, the position in which the tasks are performed, and the amount of time needed to perform the tasks. The performance scale outlined in the self-care section above can be used to determine progression of the performance level.
- Improve work habits. Measure the person's ability to arrive on time, maintain attention and concentration, follow instructions, detect and correct errors, determine quality control, maintain a safe working environment, and work with others.

- Increase work tolerance. Determine the person's performance level in lifting, carrying, climbing, pushing, pulling, reaching, stooping, hand grasp and release, finger manipulation and dexterity, and bilateral hand and finger coordination.
- Consider industrial work settings as possible goals for employment because such settings are usually more routine, repetitive, and concrete with fewer tasks, fewer changes in work setting condition, and fewer demands for independent problem solving, cognitive flexibility, and good interpersonal skills (Skord and Ellexson 1996, 3).

Supported employment (place-train model) and work-hardening (physical conditioning model) programs may be useful

Leisure
- Reestablish old interests.
- Explore with the person new interests and provide opportunities for practice.

Sensorimotor
- Improve muscle tone for cocontraction, bilateral, reciprocal, and isolated movement.
  1. If low tone is a problem, use facilitating activities, such as irregular, rapid movements with sudden starts and stops, to increase tone.
  2. If high tone is a problem, use inhibitive or damping activities, such as rhythmic, slow, rocking movement, inverted position, weight bearing, neutral warmth, and rotation.
  3. Changing the position of the head (prone or supine) in relation to the body (extended, flexed, turned to right or left) may be used to change tone in bed and in sitting and standing positions.
- Increase gross motor skills and coordination.
  1. Use activities at the person's neuromuscular level of development.
  2. If rolling is a problem, use activities or games that emphasize rolling.
  3. If trunk rotation is a problem, use activities or games that emphasize rotating the trunk.
- Improve hand functions.
  1. Begin with activities requiring gross grasp and release (full hand) with forearm in middle position between supination and pronation.
  2. As extension of the wrist improves (release improves), decrease the size of objects so that radial fingers are used (three digits, then two digits).
- Increase fine motor manipulation, dexterity, and coordination.
  1. Use activities or games requiring one hand at a time.
  2. Move to activities or games in which the hands are used bilaterally.
  3. Then add activities or games that require reciprocal or alternating hand movements.
- Improve postural control and balance.
  1. Begin with head control in midline position using external support, inhibiting abnormal tone, facilitating righting reactions of head and neck, placing object of interest at eye level directly in front of person, or joint approximation applied through the head and neck.
  2. Facilitate postural alignment through adaptive postural reactions (rotation, weight shift, parachute or protective reactions, tilt or equilibrium reactions).
  3. Facilitate sensory integration of two sides of the body, crossing midline of body through the use of sensory integrative techniques (see section on adaptive response disorders).
- Increase the person's endurance.

1. Start with short, frequent sessions (15–20 minutes two or three times daily), then increase the length.
2. Provide a program to be carried out between occupational therapy sessions.
- Increase joint mobility and range of motion, especially in upper extremities.
  1. Use daily living activities, games, or dance that require use of range of motion, such as reaching high and low, throwing a ball, or placing objects left or right.
  2. Consider use of splints to maintain range of motion, such as a resting night splint, to avoid contractures.
  3. Consider use of casting to increase range of motion (Hill 1994, 219–224).
- Increase sensory registration, awareness, and arousal. Use the following modalities to provide sensory stimulation.
  1. touch (Rub skin with various textures.)
  2. tactile (Have the person explore or hunt for objects buried in sand, rice, or cereal.)
  3. vibration (Use a variety of vibrator heads and fast and slow vibration.)
  4. proprioception/kinesthesia (Have the person change positions from lying down to being on all fours, sitting, standing, walking, and maneuvering in an obstacle course.)
  5. equilibrium (Use tilt boards, balancing on inner tubes, and dance exercises.)
  6. sound (Listen to music with a variety of tempos or play rhythm instruments.)
  7. vision (Look at a family album or track moving objects or visual light, such as a flashlight.)
  8. smell—sweet (perfume, candy), acid (vinegar, lemon juice)
  9. taste—sugar, salt, spices, extracts.
- Improve sensory processing or sensibility.
  1. tactile (Provide experiences with objects of different textures [soft, hard, smooth, rough], size [large, small], shape [round, square], composition [cloth, metal], sharpness [sharp, dull].)
  2. temperature—hot, lukewarm, cold, frozen
  3. visual discrimination—shapes, sizes, colors, composition, or gestalt
  4. auditory (Distinguish among words, sounds, and noises.)
- Improve perceptual-motor performance.
  1. stereognosis (Use a "feely" bag with two or three common objects in it and gradually increase the number of objects or bury objects in rice, cream of wheat, or other small textured substances and have the person locate and identify objects.)
  2. body awareness or image
     a. Use movement in space and tactile stimulation to increase body awareness.
     b. Have the person name body parts in front of a mirror or name parts on another person or in a picture to increase body image.
  3. visual perception (see also section on visual perception disorders)
     a. Provide practice in visual fixation, tracking, and scanning.
     b. Provide practice in form constancy, figure-ground perception, visual memory, and visual integration with auditory and tactile (cross-modal transfer) perception.

Cognitive (see also chapter on cognitive dysfunction)
- arousal (Use modalities to provide sensory stimulation. See sensory registration above.)
- attention:
  1. Begin with simple tasks, such as copying simple designs with a pencil, pegs, or blocks.

2. Use simple crafts, such as link belts, pot holders, mosaic tile, embroidery, or leather lacing.
3. Use simple games or puzzles.
4. Slowly increase the complexity of the task, number of steps in the task, and the amount of time needed to complete the task.

- distractibility:
  1. Begin with a controlled environment (one on one in a small room with minimum visual, audio, or other distractions).
  2. Gradually increase the size of the room, the number of persons present, and the number of visual objects, sound levels, and smells.

- orientation:
  1. Begin with the person, place, and time.
  2. Gradually increase complexity of learning, such as increasing the size of the room, increasing the number of persons present, and increasing the number of visual objects, sound levels, and smells.
  3. Expand beyond the immediate environment to include all living quarters, the community, reading maps, and reading time schedules.

- memory and learning (see also section on memory disorders):
  1. Use consistent, concise instruction.
  2. Emphasize relevant information (use simple declarative sentences).
  3. Use compensatory techniques, such as memory books or notebooks, lists, diaries, planning or schedule books, and visual or tactile cues.
  4. Have the person repeat steps before performing the task, then perform the task, and repeat steps after performing the task.

- ability to follow commands or directions:
  1. Start with simple, single verbal commands, such as "pick up the spoon." Demonstrate as needed to provide multisensory input.
  2. Gradually increase the number of commands to be performed in a single location.
  3. Next, include commands to be performed in different locations around the room, in different rooms, or outside.
  4. Use cues or a demonstration at first, then fade out prompts.
  5. Use rehearsal (person repeats commands), performance (person performs commands), summary (person repeats actions performed), and comparison (person compares initial commands with those performed).

- executive functions—initiations of task
- executive functions—problem solving and decision making:
  1. Use real or simulated situations, such as the home, supermarkets, community recreational facilities, city streets.
  2. Use small group discussion.
  3. Use cues to structure the situation, such as pictures or writing each answer given on a large easel.
  4. Use a problem-solving outline (state the problem, list possible solutions, organize solutions into a hierarchy, select the best solution, implement the solution, evaluate the results, and try again).

- executive functions—sequencing of tasks and activities:

1. Grade the number of steps in the sequence, starting with three and increasing the number.
2. Repeat the same task or routine to increase mastery (practice).
3. Have the person outline the steps or sequence verbally or in writing.
4. Provide compensatory techniques, such as visual pictures or lists.

- executive functions—judgment of safety:
  1. Structure the environment at home or work to promote safety. This may require a visit to the living situation to determine potential safety hazards and recommend changes. Examples might include a cubicle bed, alarm system, walkie-talkie, helmet, and a safety checklist for the wheelchair.
  2. Use cues (visual, auditory, tactile) to alert the person to danger.
  3. Discuss possible consequences (ask "what if" questions) of an activity before starting that activity.
  4. Provide simulated dangerous situations and rehearse possible actions.
- executive functions—time management:
  1. The person follows a predetermined schedule.
  2. The person participates in developing a schedule.
  3. The person is responsible for developing a schedule and reporting how well he or she has been able to follow that schedule.
- energy conservation/work simplification (Instruct the person and family caregivers in concepts and techniques of energy conservation and work simplification.)

Psychosocial

- Increase the person's self-perception through creative activities, such as art, crafts, drama, music, or dance. Activities need to be simple and have cues and verbal support for people who function at a low cognitive level. Gradually increase the skill level required as the person's cognitive level improves.
- Improve coping skills and frustration tolerance through training in relaxation techniques and by talking about alternative strategies that are socially acceptable or through group discussions on handling frustration.
- Increase social interaction skills through participation in role playing or role simulation, small task groups, or large discussion groups. Encourage the family to take the person on short outings and to invite friends into the home first (familiar setting), then to accept invitations outside the home.
- Increase group participation skills through one-on-one sessions with the therapist, small groups (3–4 people in sessions), task groups (5–7 people), or large discussion groups (8–12 people). In Schulz (1994, 305–309), 11 factors emerged from group participation: socialization; finding out other people's perceptions and attitudes; expressing thoughts and feelings; receiving support; feeling something in common with other group members; gaining understanding, empathy, and acceptance through listening and sharing; getting perspective by learning about other people's limitations and strengths; helping others; getting help with problem solving; feeling hope; and learning information about head/brain injury. In Schwartberg (1994, 297–304), 10 factors emerged: telling others about one's own pain and suffering; actively listening to familiar pain and suffering in others; accepting that there is a problem with group recognition of the problem; grieving and laughing about daily

situations; perceiving validation from others' similar experiences; being accepted by others and having a respite from hiding one's disability; supporting the survivor's survival; giving and receiving practical suggestions; receiving and giving information from personal experiences; distinguishing between problems that result from the head injury and those that would exist without a head injury.
- Increase role performance.
  1. The person is able to identify various roles by observing a film videotape or by role playing.
  2. The person is able to participate in role performance with assistance, such as role-playing or working in a task group.
  3. The person is able to perform roles independently and critique his or her performance.
- Encourage the person and family to participate in a self-help group, if available.

PRECAUTIONS
- The person's response may vary from day to day. Recovery from head injury does not necessarily follow a smooth course. Expect some regression and plateaus in performance.
- Be aware of the drugs or medication that the person is taking and their possible side effects. Be especially aware of their possible influence on performance skills, balance, and thinking processes.
- If splints, orthotic devices, or casts are used, check the skin frequently for signs of pressure on pressure points, such as bony prominences.
- If the open head injury is greater than 5 centimeters square, the person should be wearing a helmet to prevent further injury to the brain (Schlageter and Zoltan 1996, 809).
- When a person is getting up for the first time, blood pressure, pulse rate, and oxygen saturation rate should be monitored closely and treatment stopped if the levels do not stay within parameters established by the physician (Schlageter and Zoltan 1996, 809).
- Watch for signs of changes in neurologic status, such as pupillary change, diaphoresis (excessive sweating), vomiting, behavioral changes, changes in postural reflexes, and changes in respiratory pattern or blood pressure and pulse (Schlageter and Zoltan 1996, 809, Scott and Dow 1995, 708).
- Vestibular stimulation is contraindicated for a person with a tracheostomy, elevated intracranial pressure, or seizures (Scott and Dow 1995, 715).

PROGNOSIS AND OUTCOME
   Common predictive measures include the score on the Glasgow Coma Scale (GCS), length of posttraumatic amnesia (PTA), and performance on the Glasgow Outcome Scale. Factors that best predict outcome for reintegration in the community are age, disability level, and cognition. Best predictors for return to work are length of PTA, cognition, disability levels, GCS, functional status, length of acute stay, and prior occupation (Fleming et al. 1999, 417). Recovery can continue for 6–12 months postinjury. For an example of a critical pathway approach, see Abreu et al. 1996, 420–421. An example of performance program profile is included in Liberto et al. 1993, 293–396.
- The person is able to perform ADLs independently.

- The person is able to perform productive activities at home, as a volunteer, or as a paid worker.
- The person is able to participate in leisure activities.
- The person is able to control muscle tone to permit movement throughout a range of motion with minimal or no spasticity.
- The person has functional range of motion in all joints.
- The person is able to perform gross motor skills, including rolling, trunk rotation, sitting, standing on one or two feet, walking, and climbing.
- The person is able to perform fine motor skills, including use of both hands in asymmetrical, bilateral, or symmetrical; and reciprocal or alternating movements.
- The person is able to adjust posture to maintain midline stability, head control, and balance in a variety of static and dynamic situations.
- The person is able to respond within normal range to all types of sensory input.
- The person is able to attend to tasks without becoming distracted.
- The person is oriented to time, place, and person.
- The person is able to take responsibility for personal safety.
- The person is able to learn and master new tasks.
- The person is able to initiate a task and monitor the task through to completion.
- The person is able to plan, organize, and complete tasks on a daily schedule.
- The person and family caregiver demonstrate knowledge of techniques of energy conservation, pacing, and work simplification.
- The person is able to participate in social activities, exhibiting socially acceptable behavior.
- The person is able to work cooperatively in a group situation.

REFERENCES

Abreu, B.C. 1998. The quadraphonic approach: Holistic rehabilitation for brain injury. In *Cognition and Occupation in Rehabilitation: Cognitive Models for Intervention in Occupational Therapy*, ed. N. Katz, 51–98. Bethesda, MD: American Occupational Therapy Association.

Abreu, B.C., G. Seale, J. Podlesak, and L. Hartley. 1996. Development of critical paths for post-acute brain injury rehabilitation: Lessons learned. *American Journal of Occupational Therapy* 50(6):417–427.

Averbuch, S. and N. Katz. 1996. Cognitive rehabilitation: a retraining model for clients following brain injuries. In *Cognition and Occupation in Rehabilitation: Cognitive Models for Intervention in Occupational Therapy*, ed. N. Katz, 99–124. Bethesda, MD: American Occupational Therapy Association.

Beers, M.H., and R. Berkow, eds. 1999. *The Merck Manual of Diagnosis and Therapy,* 17th ed. Whitehouse Station, NJ: Merck Research Laboratories.

Fleming, J., L. Tooth, M. Hassell, and W. Chan. 1999. Prediction of community integration and vocational outcome 2–5 years after traumatic brain injury rehabilitation in Australia. *Brain Injury* 13(6):417–431.

Giles, G.M. 1996a. A neurofunctional approach to rehabilitation following severe brain injury. In *Cognition and Occupation in Rehabilitation: Cognitive Models for Intervention in Occupational Therapy*, ed. N. Katz, 135–147. Bethesda, MD: American Occupational Therapy Association.

Gutman, S.A. and P. Swarbrick. 1998. The multiple linkages between childhood sexual abuse, adult alcoholism, and traumatic brain injury in women: A set of guidelines for occupational therapy practice. *Occupational Therapy in Mental Health* 14(3):33–65.

Hill, J. 1994. The effects of casting on upper extremity motor disorders after brain injury. *American Journal of Occupational Therapy* 48(3):219–224.

Liberto, L., K. Tomlin, K. Lutz, L. Nash, and S. Schapiro. 1993. Cognitive rehabilitation. In *Minor Head Trauma: Assessment, Management and Rehabilitation*, ed. S. Mandel, R.T. Staloff, and S.R. Schapiro, 290–305. New York: Springer-Verlag.

Schlageter, K. and B. Zoltan. 1996. Traumatic brain injury. In *Occupational Therapy: Practice Skills for Physical Dysfunction*, 4th ed., ed. L.W. Pedretti, 807–836. St. Louis: Mosby (Case report).

Schulz, C.H. 1994. Helping factors in a peer-developed support group for persons with head injury, part 2: Survivor interview perspective. *American Journal Of Occupational Therapy* 48(4):305–309.

Schwartzberg, S.L. 1994. Helping factors in a peer-developed support group for persons with head injury, part 1: Participant observer perspective. *American Journal of Occupational Therapy* 48(4):297–304.

Schwartz, S.M. 1995. Adults with traumatic brain injury: Three case studies of cognitive rehabilitation in the home setting. *American Journal of Occupational Therapy* 49(7):655–657 (Case reports).

Scott, D.A. and P.W. Dow. 1995. Traumatic brain injury. In *Occupational Therapy for Physical Dysfunction*, 4th ed., ed. C.A. Trombly, 705–734. Baltimore: Williams & Wilkins.

Skord, K. and M.T. Ellexson. 1996. Increasing industrial job placement among persons with severe traumatic brain injury. *Work Programs Special Interest Section Newsletter* 10(4):3–4 (Case report).

Toglia, J.P. 1998. A dynamic interactional model to cognitive rehabilitation. In *Cognition and Occupation in Rehabilitation: Cognitive Modes for Intervention in Occupational Therapy*, ed. N. Katz, 5–50. Bethesda, MD: American Occupational Therapy Association.

Tomas, E.S., M.F. Undzis, E.A. Shores, and M.R. Sidler. 1993. Nonsurgical management of upper extremity deformities after traumatic brain injury: The Rancho Los Amigos comprehensive treatment program. *Physical Medicine and Rehabilitation: State of the Art Reviews*. 7(3):649–661.

BIBLIOGRAPHY

Alon, G., D. Amit, D. Katz-Behiri, H. Weingarden, and R. Nathan. 1998. Efficacy of a hybrid upper limb neuromuscular electrical stimulation system in lessening selected impairments and dysfunctions consequent to cerebral damage. *Journal of Neurologic Rehabilitation* 12:73–80.

Annoni, J.M., D.G. Jenkins, and J. Williams. 1995. Four case reports illustrating the contribution of intensive cognitive rehabilitation in patients neuropsychologically handicapped as a result of brain damage. *Disability and Rehabilitation* 17(8):449–455 (Case reports).

Avery-Smith, W. and D.M. Dellaros. 1994. Approaches to treating dysphagia in patients with brain injury. *American Journal of Occupational Therapy* 48(3):235–246.

Banja, J.D. and L. Banes. 1993. Moral sensitivity, sodomy laws, and traumatic brain injury rehabilitation. *Journal of Head Trauma Rehabilitation*. 8(1):116–119.

Braverman, S., J. Spector, D.L. Warden, B.C. Wilson, T.E. Ellis, M.J. Bamdad, and A.M. Salazar. 1999. A multidisciplinary TBI inpatient rehabilitation programme for active duty service members as part of a randomized clinical trial. *Brain Injury* 13(6):405–415.

Bruno, J., G. Iles, and K. Yalamanchi. 1996. How shorter length of stays affect prescribed technology. *Advance for Occupational Therapists* 12(47):9.

Butrick-Wenger, D. 1998. Using SI techniques with adults with head injury. *OT Practice* 3(10):45–47 (Case report).

Chen, S.H., J.D. Thomas, R.L. Gleuckauf, and O.L. Bracy. 1997. The effectiveness of computer-assisted cognitive rehabilitation for persons with traumatic brain injury. *Brain Injury* 11(3):197–209.

Christiansen, C., B. Abreu, K. Ottenbacker, K. Huffman, B. Masel, and R. Culpepper. 1998. Task performance in virtual environments used for cognitive rehabilitation after traumatic brain injury. *Archives of Physical Medicine and Rehabilitation* 79(8):888–892.

Chin, M. 1996. Case report: Using MLD for shoulder problems. *Advance for Occupational Therapists* 12(37):14.

Colan, B.J. 1995. Interdisciplinary approach proves effective in treating incontinence in patients with TBI. *Advance for Occupational Therapists* 11(13):22–23.

Conti, G.E. 1993. Traumatic brain injury. In *Conditions in Occupational Therapy: Effects on Occupational Performance*, ed. R.A. Hansen and B. Atchison, 155–172. Baltimore: Williams & Wilkins.

Downing-Baum, S. and D. Maino. 1996. Case studies show success in OT-OD treatment plans. *Advance for Occupational Therapists* 12(44):18, 46.

Englander, J., S. Cleary, P. O'Hare, K.M. Hall, and L.D. Lehmkuhl. 1993. Implementing and evaluating injury prevention programs in the traumatic brain injury model systems of care. *Journal of Hand Trauma Rehabilitation* 8(2):101–113.

Fleming, J. and F. Mass. 1994. Prognosis of rehabilitation outcome in head injury using the Disability Rating Scale. *Archives of Physical Medicine and Rehabilitation* 75(2):156–163.

Fleming, J. and J. Strong. 1995. Self-awareness of deficits following acquired brain injury: considerations for rehabilitation. *British Journal of Occupational Therapy* 58(2):55–60.

Fleming, J.M., J. Strong, and R. Ashton. 1996. Self-awareness of deficits in adults with traumatic brain injury: How best to measure? *Brain Injury* 10(1):1–15.

Fleming, J.M., J. Strong, and R. Aston et al. 1997. A 1-year longitudinal study of severe traumatic brain injury in Australia using the Sickness Impact Profile. *Journal of Head Trauma Rehabilitation* 12:27–40.

Galski, T., H.T. Ehle, and J.B. Williams. 1997. Off-road driving evaluations for persons with cerebral injury: A factor analytic study of predriver and simulator testing. *American Journal of Occupational Therapy* 51(5):352–359.

Gilbert, C. and S. Giroux. 1993. Acute care rehabilitation of the traumatic brain injured. *Occupational Therapy Forum* 8(21):4–5.

Giles, G.M. 1994. Functional assessment and intervention. In *Brain Injury Rehabilitation: Clinical Consideration*, ed. M.A.J. Finlayson and S.H. Garner, 124–156. Baltimore, MD: Williams & Wilkins.

Giles, G.M. 1994. Illness behavior after severe brain injury: Two case reports. *American Journal of Occupational Therapy* 48(3):247–250 (Case reports).

Giles, G.M. 1994. The status of brain injury rehabilitation (review). *American Journal of Occupational Therapy* 48(3):199–205.

Giles, G.M. 1994. Why provide community support for persons with brain injury? (Editorial) (Review). *American Journal of Occupational Therapy* 48(4):295–296.

Giles, G.M. 1996b. *Coping with Brain Injury: A Guide for Family and Friends*. Bethesda, MD: American Occupational Therapy Association.

Giles, G.M. and J. Clark-Wilson. 1993. *Brain Injury Rehabilitation: A Neurofunctional Approach*. San Diego, CA: Singular Publishing Group.

Giles, G.M., J.E. Ridley, A. Dill, and S. Frye. 1997. A consecutive series of adults with brain injury treated with a washing and dressing retraining program. *American Journal of Occupational Therapy* 51(4):256–266.

Gutman, S.A. and D.L. Leger. 1997. Enhancement of one-to-one personal skills necessary to initiate and maintain intimate relationships: A frame of reference for adults having sustained traumatic brain injury. *Occupational Therapy in Mental Health* 13(2):51–67.

Gutman, S.A., and J. Napier-Klemie. 1996. The experience of head injury on the impairment of gender identity and gender role. *American Journal of Occupational Therapy* 50(7):535–544.

Haig, J. 1997. Assessment tools used by occupational therapists with head injured patients in a rehabilitation setting. *British Journal of Occupational Therapy* 60(12):541–545.

Hallet, J.D., N.D. Zasler, P. Maurer, and S. Cash. 1994. Role change after traumatic brain injury in adults. *American Journal of Occupational Therapy* 48(3):241–246.

Hanson, C.S. 1993. Traumatic brain injury. In *Body Image and Perceptual Dysfunction in Adults*, ed. J. Van Deusen, 39–63. Philadelphia: WB Saunders.

Hettinger, J. 1995. After a traumatic brain injury. *OT Week* 9(49):14–15.

Jackson, J.D. 1994. After rehabilitation: Meeting the long-term needs of persons with traumatic brain injury. *American Journal of Occupational Therapy* 48(3):251–255.

Jensen, R. and J. Tyler-Rice. 1997. Community re-entry vital after TBI. *Advance for Occupational Therapists* 13(30):5.

Katz, B. 1996. Service with a song. *Advance for Occupational Therapists* 12(32):15.

Kerr, T. 1996. Beating the odds: Educator fights way back to classroom after TBI. *Advance for Occupational Therapists* 12(18):15 (Case report).

Kerr, T. 1995. Exercise increases energy, confidence in TBI patients. *Advance for Occupational Therapists* 11(27):19.

Koba, M. and A. Brown. 1995. Addressing residual cognitive deficits in brain injury patients. *Advance for Occupational Therapists* 11(27):16–17.

Larsson, A., C. Nystrom, S. Vikstrom, T. Malfridsson, and I. Soderback. 1995. Computer-assistive cognitive rehabilitation for adults with traumatic brain damage: four case studies. *Occupational Therapy International* 2(3):166–189.

Leonard, J. 1996. The miracle in the kitchen. *Advance for Occupational Therapists* 12(18):14.

Lutz, K. and L. Nash. 1993. Community and vocational re-entry in minor head injury. In *Minor Head Trauma: Assessment, Management and Rehabilitation*, ed. S. Mandel, R.T. Staloff, and S.R. Schapiro, 306–317. New York: Springer-Verlag.

Mackay, L.E., P.E. Chapman, and A.S. Morgan. 1997. Occupational therapy for severe brain injury. In *Maximizing Brain Injury Recovery: Integrating Critical Care and Early Rehabilitation*, ed. L.E. Mackay, P.E. Chapman, A.S. Morgan, 304–330. Gaithersburg, MD: Aspen Publishers.

Mackay, S. and M. Wallen. 1996. Re-examining the effects of the soft splint on acute hypertonicity at the elbow. *Australian Occupational Therapy Journal* 43(2):51–59.

McWilliams, S. 1996. Head injury. In *Occupational Therapy and Physical Dysfunction: Principles, Skills, and Practice*, ed. A.M. Turner, M. Foster, and S.G. Johnson, 463–480. New York: Churchill Livingstone.

Meghji, C., E. Lonneberg, A.L. Bridgman, C. Malcolm, and B. Brown-Hall. 1995. Practice make perfect: An interdisciplinary community living skills group for person with brain injury. *Journal of Cognitive Rehabilitation* 13(6):4–7.

Neistadt, M.E: 1993. The relationship between constructional and meal preparation skills. *Archives of Physical Medicine and Rehabilitation* 74(2):144–148.

Neistadt, M.E. 1994. The effects of different treatment activities on functional fine motor coordination in adults with brain injury. *American Journal of Occupational Therapy* 48(10):877–882.

Neistadt, M.E. 1994. A meal preparation treatment protocol for adults with brain injury. *American Journal of Occupational Therapy* 48(5):431–438.

Neistadt, M.E. 1994. The neurobiology of learning: Implications for treatment of adults with brain injury (Review). *American Journal of Occupational Therapy* 48(5):421–430.

Neistadt, M.E. 1994. Perceptual retraining for adults with diffuse brain injury. *American Journal of Occupational Therapy* 48(3):225–234.

Nelson, D.L. and D.A. Lenhart. 1996. Resumption of outpatient occupational therapy for a woman five years after traumatic brain injury. *American Journal of Occupational Therapy* 50(3):223–228 (Case report).

Pulaski, K.H. and L. Emmett. 1994. The combined intervention of therapy and bromocriptine mesylate to improve functional performance after brain surgery. *American Journal of Occupational Therapy* 48(3):263–270 (Case report).

Radomski, M.V. 1996. *Occupational Therapy Practice Guidelines for Adults with Traumatic Brain Injury*. Bethesda, MD: American Occupational Therapy Association.

Schlageter, K., M.M. Matthews, and M. Tipton-Burton. 1998. Traumatic brain injuries. In *Physical Dysfunction: Practice Skills for the Occupational Therapy Assistant*, ed. M.B. Early, 608–621. St. Louis: Mosby.

Seale, G.S. and B.C. Abreu. 1999. Pathways to better care. *Rehab Management* 12(1):56–59.

Shamberg, S. and A. Shamberg. 1995. Reentry begins at home. *Rehab Management* 8(5):124–127.

Sietsema, J.M., D.L. Nelson, R.M. Mulder, D. Mervau-Scheidel, and B.E. White. 1993. The use of a game to promote arm reach in persons with traumatic brain injury. *American Journal of Occupational Therapy* 47(1):19–24.

Stahl, C. 1998. Metacognition and brain injury: When the person you see isn't you. *Advance for Occupational Therapists* 14(18):7–8.

Stahl, C. 1997. Job coaching should be viable option. *Advance for Occupational Therapists* 13(23):15.

Stahl, C. 1995. Undetected mild head injury can wreck lives. *Advance for Occupational Therapists* 11(8):13.

Thiers, N. 1993. When not-so-mild symptoms surface later. *OT Week* 7(19):14–16.

Wallen, M. and S. Mackay. 1995. An evaluation of the soft splint in the acute management of elbow hypertonicity. *Occupational Therapy Journal of Research* 15(1):3–16.

Yuen, H.K. 1993. Self-feeding system for an adult with head injury and severe ataxia. *American Journal of Occupational Therapy* 47(5):444–451 (Case report).

Yuen, H.K. 1994. Neurofunctional approach to improve self-care skills in adults with brain damage. *Occupational Therapy in Mental Health* 12(4):31–45 (Case report).

Zasler, N.D., K. Murphy, and A. Holiday. 1994. Neurorehabilitation following mild traumatic brain injury. *Rehab Management* 7(3):121–123 (Case report).

Head Injury—Child

DESCRIPTION

Head injury is the second most common form of trauma for which children are admitted to the hospital. The greatest incidence of head injuries occurs in children < 1 year and > 15 years of age. The number of head injuries in boys exceeds that of girls . Serious injury to the developing nervous system may result in residual impairment of physical, cognitive, and emotional functions for the rest of the person's life (*Merck Manual* 1999, 2265).

In 1990, the federal law, Individuals with Disabilities Education Act (IDEA) (Public Law 101-476) added traumatic brain injury to the list of disabilities that may qualify a student for special education. The Act specifically states that children with traumatic brain injury may not be classified as mentally retarded, emotionally disturbed, learning disabled, or any other inappropriate category (Bell 1994, 1).

CAUSE

The most common cause of head injury in children is a fall in or around the home. Other causes are bicycle accidents, especially when the child was not wearing a helmet, motor vehicle accidents, especially when the child was not in a car seat or wearing a safety belt, gun shots, forceful blows to the head, or banging against an object or wall (*Merck Manual*

1999, 2265). Additional causes noted in Sakzewski and Ziviani (1996a, 114) include abuse, assault, and pedestrian accident.

ASSESSMENT

Areas
- daily living skills
- developmental milestones
- gross motor skills
- fine motor dexterity, manipulation, and coordination
- attention and orientation
- memory
- social interaction

Instruments
- *Bruininks-Osertsky Test of Motor Proficiency* by Bruininks, R.H. 1978. Circle Pines, MN: American Guidance Services.
- *Child Behavior Checklist* by Achenbach, T.M. and C.S. Edelbrook. 1983. Burlington, VT: University of Vermont Department of Psychiatry.
- *Children's Orientation and Amnesia Test* (COAT) by Ewing-Cobbs, L., H.S. Lewin, J.M. Fletcher, M.E. Miner, and H.M. Eisenberg. 1990. The Children's Orientation and Amnesia Test: Relationship to severity of acute head injury and to recovery of memory. *Neurosurgery* 27:683–691.
- *Glascow Coma Scale* by Teasdale, G. and B. Jennett. 1994. Assessment of coma and impaired consciousness. *Lancet* 2:81–84.
- *Impact on Family Scale* by Stein, R.E.K. and C.K. Riessman. 1980. The development of an Impact-on-Family Scale: Preliminary findings. *Medical Care* 18:462–472.
- *Pediatric Evaluation of Disability Inventory* by Haley, S.M., W.J. Coster, L.H. Ludlow, J. Haltiwanger, and P. Andrellos. 1998. San Antonio, TX: Psychological Corporation/Therapy Skill Builders.
- *Slosson Intelligence Test and Oral Reading Test for Children and Adults* by Slosson, R.L. New York: Slosson Educational, 1985.

PROBLEMS

Self-Care
- The child may have poor hygiene habits.
- See adult section for additional items.

Sensorimotor
- The child may have partial paralysis.
- The child may have poor coordination.
- The child may lack body awareness.
- The child may have decreased endurance.

- The child may have decreased muscle strength.
- The child may have difficulty with gross motor tasks.
- The child may have difficulty with fine motor tasks, especially speed and dexterity.
- The child may have abnormal muscle tone.
- The child may have poor balance or equilibrium.
- The child may become easily fatigued.
- The child may have poor motor planning skills.
- The child may have visual field cuts (reduction of visual field).
- The child may have decreased ocular motor skills.
- The child may have difficulty with visual tracking.
- The child may have visual-perceptual deficits.
- The child may have loss of hearing.
- The child may have problems with tactile processing of information.
- The child may have poor oral motor skills.

Cognitive
- The child may have difficulty with memory.
- The child may have loss of attending behavior and concentration.
- The child may have poor judgment.
- The child may have difficulty with problem solving.
- The child may have difficulty with processing speed (usually, processing is slowed down).
- The child may be easily distracted.
- The child may have difficulty following directions.
- The child may have difficulty with tasks that require planning ahead.
- The child may have difficulty with tasks that require sequencing or are done in a specific order.
- The child may have difficulty with tasks that require reasoning.
- The child may have difficulty with situations that require flexibility (changing directions or plans because of changing circumstances).
- The child may have difficulty categorizing or grouping like objects or things together.
- The child may have difficulty generalizing information from one situation to another.
- The child may have poor goal-directed behaviors.
- The child may be unable to follow through with tasks.
- The child may have difficulty with communication and language, such as stuttering, perseverating, confabulation, tangentiality, aphasia, or dysarthria.

Psychosocial
- The child may become withdrawn or depressed.
- The child may have low frustration tolerance.
- The child may have poor motivation.
- The child may become irritable quickly.
- The child may be impulsive.
- The child may have acting out behaviors.
- The child may be disinhibited and display inappropriate behavior.
- The child may be aggressive.
- The child may perseverate.

- The child may act silly at inappropriate times.
- The child may deny that anything is wrong.

TREATMENT/INTERVENTION
- No specific models were identified.

Note that self-care, productivity, and leisure were not discussed. For general ideas, see section on head and brain injuries—adult.

Sensorimotor
- For motor issues, see section on head and brain injuries—adult.
- Adjust the work load to allow for rest periods—pacing.
- Limit the amount of visual stimulation on a page by covering parts of the page or using a cut-out window to single out the particular task.
- Teach the child to use a finger or guide to help with visual tracking.
- Allow extra time to examine visual input or repeat auditory instruction.
- Use symbols to mark margins, right/left and top/bottom.
- Slow down instruction and allow time when requesting a response.
- Color cue visual materials.

Cognitive
General
- Identify the use the child's best learning modality or modalities.
- Consider using one-on-one or small group instruction.
- Teach learning/study skills, such as highlighting, outlining, or paraphrasing.
- Be consistent in giving information and asking questions so that the child does not think a different subject is being addressed or a different response is required.

Attention/Concentration
- Keep instructions short and concise.
- Keep activities and materials relevant and stimulating.
- Keep the therapy or work area and environment organized and free of excessive distractions.
- Continually monitor and refocus as necessary.
- Use an external timer or alarm to structure "on-task" behavior.
- Place a symbol or picture card in view of the child as a reminder to stay on task.
- Use cue reminders of basic tasks, such as the alphabet, number line, steps to task completion.
- Regularly summarize information.

Orientation
- Have the child keep a log or journal of significant events.
- Use environmental cues or verbal cues to refocus the child.
- Use buddy system or peer helper.
- Teach problem-solving strategies that can be generalized to various situations.

Comprehension and Memory
- Use alerting signals before giving information; model, demonstrate, and use gestures in instruction.

- Simplify or rephrase explanations.
- Encourage the child to restate information in his or her own words.
- Teach the child to ask for clarification.
- Teach the child to identify key points, both before and after receiving information, such as use the "wh" questions (who, what, when, where, why) before doing a task.
- Use repetition and rehearsal.
- Use external aides, such as log books, checklists, tape recordings, journals.
- Use mnemonics, association, clustering.
- Use mental imaging.
- Go from general to specific, concrete to abstract, and nonverbal to verbal.

Executive Skills
- Provide organization techniques, including checklists, journals, schedules, assignment sheets, categorization and task analysis.
- Use diagrams or graphs to illustrate information.
- Project and describe situations in which target information will be needed or used.
- Assist in planning and sequencing events.
- Improve judgment through use of role playing, structured discussions, videotapes, questioning techniques.
- Teach and use problem-solving techniques.
- Provide ongoing feedback.
- Facilitate generalization by teaching the format or process, not just the task, and by using the format or process in a variety of tasks and situations.

Psychosocial
- Remember that denial, lack of motion, and apathy can be related to brain functioning rather than avoidance behavior.
- Help the child to understand the consequences of behavior, such as interrupting others.
- Use rewards for appropriate behavior.
- Teach social skills and reading social cues regularly.
- Use role playing to assist learning-appropriate responses to a given situation.
- Use a calm and friendly approach.
- Be sensitive to changes in the environment that may cause stress to the child.
- Prepare the child for changes and transitions.

Environment
- Refer to maps and landmarks for getting around the environment.
- Use calendars and timers for orientation of day and time, if needed.
- In the classroom, have the child sit up front.
- Prepare the child for tests and other situations in advance. Alternative testing situations may be necessary if timed tests are used routinely, such as using oral tests with short answers and multiple choices.
- Help peers to understand and accept neurologically based behaviors.

PRECAUTIONS
- See section on head and brain injuries—adult.

PROGNOSIS/OUTCOMES

If child was in a coma for longer than one month, the outcome tends to be poorer. Children under 7 years when injured have a worse social and school outcome than do older children. Damage to the brain may disrupt acquisition of skills, especially if the frontal lobe is damaged. Motor skills are recovered better than intellectual function (Parkin et al. 1996, 134). For specific outcomes, see section on head and brain injuries—adult.

REFERENCES

Beers, M.H., and R. Berkow, eds. 1999. *The Merck Manual of Diagnosis and Therapy,* 17th ed. Whitehouse Station, NJ: Merck Research Laboratories.

Bell, TA. 1994. Understanding students with traumatic brain injury: A guide for teachers and therapists. *School System Special Interest Section Newsletter* 1(2):1–4.

Parkin, A.E., F. Maas, and S. Rodger. 1996. Factors contributing to school for students with acquired brain injury: Parent perspectives. *Australian Occupational Therapy Journal* 43(3/4):133–141.

Sakzewski, J. and J. Ziviani. 1996a. Factors affecting length of hospital stay for children with acquired brain injuries: A review of the literature. *Australian Occupational Therapy Journal* 43(3/4):113–124.

BIBLIOGRAPHY

Chaplin, D., J. Deitz, and K.M. Jaffe. 1993. Motor performance in children after traumatic brain injury. *Archives of Physical Medicine and Rehabilitation* 74(2):161–164.

Coster, W.J., S. Haley, and M.J. Baryza. 1994. Functional performance of young children after brain injury: A 6-month follow-up study (review). *American Journal of Occupational Therapy* 48(3):211–218.

Sakzewski, J., J. Ziviani, and C. Swanson. 1996b. Impact of early discharge planning and case management on length of hospital stay for children with acquired brain injury. *Australian Occupational Therapy Journal* 43(3/4):105–112.

Peripheral Nerve Injuries— Upper Extremity

DESCRIPTION

Trauma to the peripheral nerves is categorized into three types. One is *neuropraxia,* which most often occurs as a result of blunt trauma or compression, causing a contusion of the nerve. Because the axons remain in continuity and, thus, there is no Wallerian degeneration, recovery usually occurs within a few days or weeks. The second type is *axonotmesis,* in which there is degeneration of the nerve fibers distal to the site of injury but the internal organization of the nerve remains intact. Recovery usually occurs within 6 months if the cell body remains alive and the fibers are able to grow down their original neurilemmal sheaths. The third type is *neurotmesis,* which occurs when the nerve is completely lacerated, divided, or irreparably damaged over a portion of its length. Because of the damage to the nerve, the reconnection of fibers and end-organs is less likely to be satisfactory (Leveridge 1996, 578; Kasch 1996, 669). Note: Compression-type injuries are discussed in the sections on carpal tunnel syndrome and repetitive strain injuries. Injuries to the brachial plexus are also discussed separately.

CAUSE

Causative factors include: (1) cervical cord and brachial plexus lesions, (2) complete or partial lacerations, fractures, and dislocations to the arm, forearm, wrist, or hand, (3) prolonged compressions, (4) callus formation around a fracture, or (5) mononeuritis.

ASSESSMENT

Areas

- daily living skills
- productivity history, skills, values, and interests
- leisure interests and skills
- range of motion, passive and active
- muscle strength, grip, and pinch strength
- hand functions and prehension skills
- fine motor coordination, manipulation, and dexterity
- sensibility, including tactile discrimination, stereognosis, proprioception, temperature, and vibration
- pain
- sympathetic functions: dryness, temperature, color, soft tissue atrophy, and nail changes

Instruments

Equipment

- goniometry
- manual muscle test
- Intrinsic-meter dynamometer. Mannerfelt, L. 1966. Studies on the hand in ulnar nerve paralysis. *Acta Orthopaedica Scandinavica* (Suppl 87):61–86.
- Jamar dynamometer. Mathiowetz, V., N. Kashman, G. Volland, K. Weber, M. Dowe, and S. Rogers. 1985. Grip and pinch strength; normative data for adults. *Archives of Physical Medicine and Rehabilitation* 66:69–74.
- Semmes-Weinstein Monofilaments (light touch-deep pressure). J.A. Bell-Krotoski. 1990. Light touch-deep pressure testing using Semmes-Weinstein monofilaments. In: *Rehabilitation of the Hand*, 3rd ed., ed. J.M. Hunter et al., 585–593. St. Louis: CV Mosby.
- tactilometry. Lundborg, G., A. Lie-Stenström, and C. Sollerman. 1986. Digital vibrogram: A new diagnostic tool for sensory testing in compression neuropathy. *Journal of Hand Surgery* 11A:693–699.
- tuning forks: 30 Hz and 256 Hz applied proximal to distal. Dellon, A.L. 1981. *Sensibility and Re-Education of Sensibility in the Hand*, 1431–1447. Baltimore: Williams & Wilkins.

Tests

- Froment's sign (lateral pinch). American Society for Surgery of the Hand. 1990. *The Hand: Examination and Diagnosis*, 3rd ed., 121–122. New York: Churchill-Livingstone. (Extension or hyperextension of the metacarpalphalangeal [MCP] joint with hyperflexion of the IP joint.)
- localization of touch. Sensibility testing: Clinical methods by Callahan, A.D. 1990. In *Rehabilitation of the Hand*, 3rd ed., ed. J.M. Hunter et al., 594–610. St Louis MO: Mosby.
- *Moberg Pick-Up Test* by Moberg, E. 1958. Objective methods for determining the functional value of sensibility in the hand. *Journal of Bone and Joint Surgery* 40B:454–476.
- *Moving Two-Point Discrimination Test* by Dellon, A.L. 1978. The moving two-point discrimination test. *Journal of Hand Surgery* 3:474–481.
- *Object Identification Test* by Wynn-Parry, C.B. 1981. *Rehabilitation of the Hand*. London: Butterworths.
- *Sensibility Evaluation Form* by Leveridge, A. 1996. In *Occupational Therapy and Physical Dysfunction: Principles, Skills and Practice,* 4th ed., ed. A. Turner, 591. New York: Churchill Livingstone.
- *Shape-Identification Test*. Omer, G.E. 1983. Report of the committee for evaluation of clincial results in peripheral nerve injury. *Journal of Hand Surgery* 8:754–759.
- *Sollerman Grip Test* by Sollerman, C. and A. Ejeskär. 1995. Sollerman hand function test: A standardized method and its use in tetraplegic patients. *Scandinavian Journal of Plastic Reconstruction Surgery and Hand Surgery* 29:167–173.
- *Stereognosis Test Chart* by Leveridge, A. 1996. In *Occupational Therapy and Physical Dysfunction: Principles, Skills and Practice.* 4th ed., ed. A. Turner, 595. New York: Churchill Livingstone.
- Tinel's sign. The sign is positive when percussion along the route of a nerve elicits pain or hypersensitivity.
- Two-Point Discrimination Test (2PD) using the Disk-Criminator. Moberg, E. 1990. Two-point discrimination—a valuable part of hand surgical rehabilitation in tetraplegia. *Scandinavian Journal of Rehabilitation* 22:127–134.
- *Visual Analogue Scale* (pain). Wewers, M.E. and N.K. Lowe. 1990. A critical review of visual analogue scales in the measurement of clinical phenomena. *Research in Nursing and Health* 13:227–236.

PROBLEMS

Self-Care

- The person may be unable to perform some ADLs because of loss of intrinsics, which reduces the effect of total grasp and normal release patterns.
- The person may experience difficulty in writing with the dominant hand.
- Holding activities in the nondominant hand may be difficult.

Productivity

- The person may be unable to perform some job tasks, such as heavy labor, driving a truck, typing or keypunching, or taking dictation.

Leisure

- The person may be unable to perform some leisure activities, such as playing the piano or other musical instruments requiring finger dexterity and coordination.

Sensorimotor

Ulnar Nerve: Low Lesion (Colditz 1995, 681–683)

- Laceration at the level of the wrist (low ulnar palsy) results in deinnervation of most of the intrinsic muscles of the hand.
- The ulnar border of the transverse metacarpal arch is lost because the ulnar nerve innervates all of the hypothenar muscles: abductor digiti minimi, flexor digit minimi, and the opponens digit minimi.
- Inability to abduct and adduct the fingers, due to loss of dorsal and volar interossei.
- Loss of fine manipulative skills in the hand, due to loss of the interossei.
- Ring and little finger lose function of lumbricales, which results in loss of intrinsic balancing control or force to the normal extrinsics to the two digits.
- The loss of intrinsic control means that the tension of the long flexors is opposed only by the extrinsic extension, which primarily extend the MCP joints.
- There is loss of the prime flexors of the MCP joint because the intrinsic muscles normally flex the MCP joint and extend the IP joint.
- The functional deformity is clawing of the ring and little fingers.
- In the claw hand position, both the lumbricales and interossei are held in a stretched position.
- The functional loss is the inability to open the hand to grasp large objects.
- Pinch is compromised because the adductor of the thumb and deep head of the flexor policis brevis are lost.
- The person demonstrates Froment's sign: hyperextension of the MCP joint with hyperflexion of the IP joint. Deformity is difficult to splint because stabilizing the thumb is difficult without restricting other essential mobility.

Ulnar Palsy: High Lesion (Colditz 1995, 684)

- In addition to involvement of the muscles mentioned in the lower lesion, the profundi of the ring and little fingers and the flexor carpi ulnaris are missing.
- The claw hand is not as obvious because the tension of the profundi and all the intrinsics of the ring and little finger are also absent.
- As the profundi become reinnervated, the claw deformity becomes more apparent.

Median Nerve: Low Lesion (Colditz 1995, 684–686; Kasch 1996, 671)

- Because the median nerve contributes much of the motor function of the thumb and the sensibility to the radial 3-1/2 digits, laceration of median nerve at the wrist level is a serious loss.
- In addition to the above, there is motor loss to the radial portion of the hand.
- The thumb cannot be abducted or extended from the hand because the opponens pollicis and abductor pollicis brevis are lost. The thumb can be moved only across the palm by extrinsic muscles in an adducted position.
- The total extent of the thumb deformity may not be obvious because the median nerve injury may be incomplete or there may be cross-innervation from the ulnar nerve.

- Lumbricales, which move the index and long fingers, are also lost but claw hand deformity is not present because the palmar and dorsal interossei are still present (ulnar nerve).
- Adduction contractures of the thumb occur frequently in the thumb, which decreases the web space.
- The clinical picture shows a flat thenar eminence with no sensation to the volar aspects of the thumb, index, middle, and radial side of the ring finger. If blindfolded, the person uses the ring and little fingers to compensate when feeling or manipulating objects in the hand (Kasch 1996, 671). The appearance of the hand is sometimes called a "monkey hand" because of the flat appearance and lack of opposition (Leveridge 1996, 579).

Median Nerve: High Lesion (Colditz 1995, 686, Kasch 1996, 671)
- High lesions often occur at or near the elbow, which results in the loss of the profundi to the index and long fingers and the superficialis to all fingers, resulting in a loss of all function except gross actions.
- Loss of innervation of the pronator teres and quadratus inactivate active pronation but slight abduction of the arm allows gravity-assisted pronation.
- Clinical signs are ulnar flexion or deviation of the wrist due to loss of the flexor carpi radialis, loss of palmar abduction, and opposition of the thumb (Kasch 1996, 671).

Radial Nerve: High Lesion (Colditz 1995, 686–670)
- High lesion to the radial nerve is more common than to the ulnar or median nerve, especially where the radial nerve spirals around the humerus.
- Injury in the spiral groove is associated with humeral fractures and compression syndrome.
- Sensory loss with the radial nerve causes less functional loss because the sensibility lies over the dorsoradial aspect in the hand, leaving the palmar surface intact (median nerve).
- If the injury is at or below the spiral groove, the triceps are spared, leaving elbow motions intact.
- The wrist and finger extensors and supinator will be lost, resulting in the "drop wrist" position of the hand.
- The primary function loss is inability to stabilize the wrist in extension so that the fingers can flex normally. The loss of wrist and finger extension destroys the reciprocal tenodesis action used in normal grasp-and-release patterns.
- Clinical signs are pronation of the forearm, wrist flexion, and the thumb held in palmar abduction, resulting from the unopposed action of the flexor pollicis brevis and abductor pollicis brevis (Kasch 1996, 671)

Radial Nerve: Low Lesion (Colditz 1995, 690, Kasch 1996, 670–671)
- Posterior interosseous nerve palsy or syndrome. (The radial nerve divides after crossing the elbow, forming two branches. The deep motor is called the *posterior interosseous branch*.)
  1. The clinical picture of the hand is strong radial deviation of the wrist during attempted wrist extension (Colditz 1995, 690). Sensation and wrist extension are normal but finger and thumb extension is lost. There is incomplete extension of the MCP joints of the fingers and thumb. The interossei extend the IP joints of the fingers, but the MCP joints in resting position have about 30 degrees of flexion (Kasch 1996, 671).
  2. Attempts at finger extension will show an intrinsic plus pattern of MCP flexion and interphalangeal extension due to lack of innervation to the extensor digitorum.

3. In partial lesions, isolated absence of finger extension with adjacent normal finger extension may be seen.
4. The extensor carpi radialis, extensor carpi longus, and extensor carpi brevis are not involved.
- The superficial sensory branch is not discussed by Colditz.

Mixed Median and Ulnar Nerve Lesions (Colditz 1995, 690–692)
- The two nerves may be injured at the same time because they both lie on the palmar aspect of the wrist.
- If both are injured, the hand has no intrinsic muscles and, therefore, claw deformity occurs in all four digits.
- No muscles are available to stabilize the thumb.

Cognitive
- Cognitive faculties are not affected directly by the disorder.

Psychosocial
- The person may fear permanent disability and disfigurement.
- The person may fear loss of function if the injury is to dominant hand.
- The person may avoid social situations because of his or her appearance.

TREATMENT/INTERVENTION
Models of treatment are based on biomechanical learning models, such as behavioral or cognitive behavioral and compensatory approaches.

Self-Care
- Provide self-help devices and training as needed to perform self-care activities.
- Promote independence in ADLs.

Productivity
- Determine what hand and upper extremity functions are needed in work settings.
- Make recommendations regarding modifications or adaptations in the work environment that would permit the person to return to productive activities during recovery or as soon as possible.

Leisure
- Explore leisure interests and make suggestions for modifications that would permit the person to enjoy leisure activities during recovery.

Sensorimotor
- A splint can be useful to:
  1. keep denervated muscles from remaining in an overstretched position,
  2. prevent joint contractures,
  3. prevent development of substitution patterns, and
  4. maximize functional use of the hand (Colditz 1995, 679).

Muscle Innervation of the Upper Extremity

Muscles Innervated by the Median Nerve (Cervical vertebrae number 6 through thoracic vertebrae number 1)
Muscular Branches in the Forearm:
- flexor carpi radialis   C6–C7
- pronator teres   C6–C7
- palmaris longus   C6–C7
- flexor digitorum superficialis   C7–C8

Anterior Interosseus Nerve:
- flexor pollicis longus   C8–T1
- flexor digitorum profundus (digits 2, 3) C8–T1
- pronator quadratus   C8–T1

Muscular Branch in the Hand:
- abductor pollicis brevis   C8–T1
- flexor pollicis brevis (superficial)   C8–T1
- opponens pollicis   C8–T1

1st Common Palmar Digital Nerve:
- first lumbrical   C8–T1

2nd Common Palmar Digital Nerve:
- second lumbrical   C8–T1

Muscles Innervated by the Radial Nerve *(Cervical vertebrae 5 through cervical vertebrae 8)*
- brachioradialis   C5–C6
- extensor carpi radialis longus   C6 (with C5 and C7)
- triceps (all three heads)   C7–C8
- anconeous   C7–C8

Deep Branch (of the Radial Nerve)
- supinator   C5–C7
- abductor policis longus   C6–C7
- extensor policis brevis   C6–C7
- extensor carpi radialis brevis   C6–C7
- extensor indicis   C6–C7
- extensor carpi ulnaris   C6–C8
- extensor digiti minimi   C6–C8
- extensor digitorum communis   C6–C8
- extensor policis longus   C6–C8

Muscles Innervated by the Ulnar Nerve *(Cervical vertebrae 8 through thoracic vertebrae 1) (all muscles are innervated by C8–T1)*
- abductor digiti minimi
- adductor pollicis
- dorsal interossei
- flexor carpi ulnaris

continues

continued

- flexor digiti minimi brevis
- flexor digitorum profundus (digits 4, 5)
- flexor pollicis brevis (deep head)
- lumbricales, 3rd and 4th
- opponens digiti minimi
- palmar interossei
- palmaris brevis

Source: Data from H.J. Hislop and J. Montgomery, *Daniels and Worthingham's Muscle Testing*, 6th ed., pp. 413–414, © 1995, W.B. Saunders.

Ulnar Nerve: Low Lesion (Colditz 1995, 681–683)

- The purpose of splinting is to prevent overstretching of the denervated intrinsic muscles of the right and little fingers. Thus, the MCP joints must be prevented from fully extending. The splint must block the MCP joint in slight flexion, which will prevent the claw deformity by forcing the extrinsic extensors to transmit force into the dorsal hood mechanism of the finger. The dorsal block should distribute pressure over the dorsum of each proximal phalanx and should end at the axis of the PIP joint.
- The splint should cover as little of the surface of the palm as possible because two-thirds of the palmar surface has normal sensibility.
- For sample splint, see Colditz (1995, 683). The Capener splint wire splint may also be used.

Ulnar Palsy: High Lesion (Colditz 1995, 684)

- Splinting requirements are the same as for the low lesions.
- The person must be instructed to maintain full passive IP flexion of the ring and little fingers when the profundi are absent.

Median Nerve: Low Lesion (Colditz 1995, 684–686)

- A splint is necessary to prevent the opponens pollicis and abductor pollicis brevis from resting in a stretch position, to maintain the soft-tissue length of the first web space, and to balance the pull force of the adductor pollicus, which is functioning normally. Traditionally, a C-bar-type splint was used but the splint interferes with MCP flexion of the index finger. A night splint is now recommended which holds the index finger extended and thumb in full abduction (Colditz 1995, 685).
- Because motor return usually precedes full sensory return (due to proximal to distal reinnervation pattern), the splint may be discontinued before full sensory recovery has occurred. Covering the palmar surface may be useful to avoid further injury. A thumb splint to position the CMC joint for better opposition may be useful (Colditz 1995, 686).
- During early stages of recovery, visual assistance is necessary to use the fingertips. The positioning splint can be used to place the thumb in slight abduction and opposition to counteract the strong extensor pollicis longus and to avoid overpowering the returning intrinsics (Colditz 1995, 686).

- Activities for gross pinch might include coil or pinch pottery, pastry and bread making, and computer and keyboard games. Activities for fine pinch might include macramé work, pinchpot ceramics, or light dowel and pin solitaire (Leveridge 1996, 587).

Median Nerve: High Lesion (Colditz 1995, 686)

- In adults, splinting should maintain PROM in preparation for tendon transfers because full motor and sensory return does not occur.
- Be aware that the index finger may appear to flex actively but is actually being "carried along" into flexion, due to the common muscle belly of the profundi to the long, ring, and little fingers.
- Colditz states that a buddy splint, in which the index finger is taped to the long finger, is inadequate because it does not provide adequate passive motion; however, a suggested alternative is not provided.

Radial Nerve: High Lesion (Colditz 1995, 686–690)

- Function of the hand with a radial nerve lesion is relatively normal with a splint that harnesses the wrist to allow the finger flexors to function.
- The splint should recreate the natural tenodesis action: finger extension with wrist flexion and wrist extension with finger flexion. Static splinting does not meet the criteria.
- The splint should use a static cord system through an outrigger above the MCP joints to suspend the proximal phalangeal area, which allows full finger flexion but the wrist never drops below neutral. As they tighten, the flexors bring the wrist into a position of extension. Gravity drops the wrist during relaxation but extension of MCP joints is achieved by a blocking force that is transmitted to the loops on the proximal phalangeal area. The intrinsics, acting in concert with the blocking action of the splint, provide finger extension (Colditz 1995, 689).
- The thumb may not be included in the outrigger because the wrist has been harnessed by the splint and because the thumb extensor and abductors lie on the dorsiulnar surface of the forearm; the muscles have been taken off maximum strength. In addition, a thumb outrigger would be cumbersome. Also, the intrinsic muscles can still extend the thumb IP joint in the absence of the extrinsic extensors.
- Colditz cautions against designs for dynamic wrist and finger extension, because the powerful unopposed flexors may overcome the force of the dynamic splint during finger flexion (Colditz 1995, 690).

Radial Nerve: Low Lesion (Colditz 1995, 690)

- The same splint as discussed with high radial nerve injury can be used with low lesions or posterior interosseous palsy.
- If there is a partial injury, a buddy splint may be of value.
- Suggested activities that require muscles to work in groups to develop coordination and strength include rolling pottery into coils for coil pots, rolling out pastry, sanding and polishing wood, games such as shuffleboard or dartboard, and computer games with the Microprocess Upper-Limb Exerciser (MULE) (Leveridge 1996, 585).

Mixed Median and Ulnar Nerve Injuries (Colditz 1995, 690–692)
- The splint must block the MCP joints using a dorsal blocking approach. A firm palmar bar is also needed to provide volar counterforce to prevent MCP hyperextension (Colditz 1995, 691).
- The thumb should be splinted in an abducted position. The palmar bar can be shaped to position the thumb in abduction.
- The splint should be removed to carry out PROM.

Median Nerve Repair (Kasch 1996, 672–673)
- Wrist is immobilized in flexed position for 2–3 weeks.
- Following immobilization, protective stretching of the joints is started.
- Care must be taken not to put excessive traction on the repaired nerve.
- Reducing contractures may take from 4 to 6 weeks.
- Active exercise is used to regain extension.
- A dynamic splint may be used to assist or substitute for weakened muscles during nerve regeneration.
- The person should be taught correct patterns of movement, and substitution patterns should be avoided.
- Make revisions in splints or eliminate splinting as nerve regeneration occurs.
- Change exercises and activities as person gains function.
- Discontinue use of assistive devices as soon as their functions are no longer required.
- Proprioceptive neuromuscular facilitation techniques, such as hold-relax, contract-relax, quick stretch, icing, or neuromuscular electrical stimulation may be useful in increasing muscle strength for muscles graded as fair, or 3, on a manual muscle test.
- When muscles reach the grade of good, or 4, functional activities can be started to continue muscle strengthening.
- Sensory reeducation should be started to maximize the functional level of tactile sensation.

Cognitive
- Instruct the person in use of one-handed activities.
- Instruct the person in safety techniques to avoid injury to skin while sensation is poor.

Psychosocial
- Encourage the person to express fears.
- Encourage the person to maintain or reestablish social activities.

PRECAUTIONS
- Protect denervated skin from injuries caused by pressure, friction, chemical agents, heat, or sharp objects. Insulated mugs, padded oven gloves, and long-handled pots and pans may be useful.
- Avoid shortening and eventual contractures of soft tissues (Leveridge 1996, 581). Watch for sites known to be prone to contractures, such as the first web space of the hand.

- Splints should be checked frequently. Static splints should be removed for daily skin care.
- Avoid overstretching paralyzed muscle by unopposed contractures of antagnostic muscles (Leveridge 1996, 581).
- Be aware of decreased function of intact muscle due to loss of the synergistic function of the paralyzed muscles (Leveridge 1996, 581).

PROGNOSIS AND OUTCOME

Generally, the outcome is good. Reinnervation occurs in most cases. However, return of sensation is usually not as good as motor function.
- The person demonstrates the ability to perform functional activities and ADLs.
- The person is able to perform productive activities.
- The person is able to perform leisure activities.
- The person demonstrates hand functions and strength within normal range for his or her sex, age, and type of work.
- The person demonstrates fine motor coordination and dexterity.
- The person has functional range of motion of the hand and wrist.
- The person has sensation for touch pressure, temperature, and two-point discrimination.

REFERENCES

Colditz, J.C. 1995. Splinting the hand with a peripheral nerve injury. In *Rehabilitation of the Hand*, 4th ed., ed. J.M. Hunter, E.J. Mackin, and A.D. Callahan, 678–692. St. Louis: Mosby.

Kasch, M.C. 1996. Peripheral nerve injuries. In *Occupational Therapy: Practice Skills for Physical Dysfunction*, 4th ed., ed. L.W. Pedretti, 669–673. St. Louis: Mosby.

Leveridge, A.C. 1996. Peripheral nerve lesions. In *Occupational Therapy and Physical Dysfunction: Principles, Skills, and Practice,* ed. A. Turner, M. Foster, S.G. Johnson, 571–598. New York: Churchill Livingstone (Case report).

BIBLIOGRAPHY

Rosén, B. 1996. Recovery of sensory and motor function after nerve repair: A rationale for evaluation. *Journal of Hand Therapy* 9(4):315–327.

Spinal Cord Injuries—Adult

DESCRIPTION

Spinal cord injury results in compression caused by contusion or hemorrhage due to laceration or transection of the spinal cord. Contusion causes rapid edematous swelling with increased intradural pressure that can result in severe dysfunction for several days. Spontaneous improvement follows, but some residual disability may remain. Hemorrhage is usually confined to the cervical central gray matter, resulting in signs of lower motor neuron damage, such as muscle weakness and wasting, fasciculation, and diminished tendon reflexes in the arms, which is usually permanent. Motor weakness is often proximal and accompanied by selective impairment of pain and temperature. Extradural, subdural, or subarachnoid hemorrhage can also result from spinal injury (*Merck Manual* 1999, 1483–1484).

Tetraplegia is defined as partial or complete paralysis of the upper and lower extremities caused by compression or dislocation of the spinal cord, which results in disruption of nerve impulses to and from the brain and spinal nerves. *Tetraplegia* is now the preferred term and replaces the term *quadriplegia*, which was commonly used in the United States. *Paraplegia* remains in use to indicate conditions that affect primarily the lower extremities and, depending on the level of the lesion, some trunk functions.

Spinal cord injuries may also be classified as complete or incomplete. Complete means that all ascending and descending pathways are interrupted and there is a total loss of motor and sensory function below the level of the injury. Incomplete injury means that there is still some degree of voluntary movement and/or sensation present below the level of injury.

The injury may also be referred to as an *upper or lower motor neuron injury*. Upper motor neuron injury means that the reflex arcs are intact below the level of injury but are no longer mediated by the brain. Upper neuron injuries are characterized by a loss of voluntary function below the level of the injury, spastic paralysis, and hyperactive reflexes but not muscle atrophy. Lower motor neuron injuries occur below the level of conus medullaris because they affect the spinal nerves after they exit from the cord. Reflex arcs are lost because the impulses cannot enter the cord synapse. Such injuries are characterized by a loss of voluntary function below the level of the injury, flaccid paralysis, absence of reflexes, and muscle atrophy.

CAUSE

The causes of the most serious injuries are accidents (automobile, diving in shallow water, falls, and gun shots), spinal cord tumors, or birth defects. Less serious injuries may occur from lifting heavy objects or minor falls. Tetraplegia most frequently occurs in adolescents and children.

An acute transverse cord lesion causes immediate flaccid paralysis and loss of all sensation and reflex activity, including the autonomic functions below the level of the injury, due to spinal shock. Flaccid paralysis gradually changes over hours or days to spastic paraplegia or tetraplegia, due to exaggeration of the normal stretch reflexes resulting from loss of descending inhibition. Later, flexor muscle spasms appear, and deep tendon reflexes and autonomic reflexes return (*Merck Manual* 1999, 1484).

Less complete lesions cause partial motor and sensory loss. Voluntary movement becomes uncoordinated. Sensory loss depends on the spinal tracts affected: Posture, vibration, and light touch are lost if the posterior columns are affected; pain, temperature, and light or deep touch are affected if the spinothalamic tracts are affected (*Merck Manual* 1999, 1484).

Syndromes and Specific Injuries to the Spinal Cord

- *Anterior (spinal) cord (column) syndrome*: The syndrome results from a flexion injury in which bone or cartilage causes damage to the anterior spinal artery or anterior aspect of the cord. Paralysis of motor functions occurs. The sensory sensation of pain and temperature sensation are lost, but proprioceptive, two-point discriminative, stereognostic, deep-pressure, and vibratory sensations are preserved because the impulses travel in the posterior column.

Stages in Adjustment to Injury

Stage	Response
Shock	Disbelief at what happened
	Denial that anything serious or bad has actually occurred
Expectancy of Recovery	Hope that the injury is only temporary
	Bargaining as a means of ensuring a fast and complete recovery
Mourning	Recognition that the injury is permanent and that a self-image based on previous abilities has been lost
	Constriction of interests
	Focus on self-depreciating behavior, such as self-pity and expressions of hopelessness or worthlessness
	Depressive behavior, including turning away from the support system of family and friends
Defense	New self-image begins to form
	New behavior is tested and tried out, including angry, aggressive, or acting-out behavior
	Dependence-independence struggle of adolescence is repeated
	Emphasis is placed on the here and now
Adjustment	New self-image is formed
	Goals and plans can be made for the future
	Interest in exploring the quality of life for him- or herself and significant others
	Ability to make decisions and solve problems

Source: Data from A.C. Seidel, Spinal Cord Injury, in *Adult Rehabilitation: A Team Approach for Therapists*, M.K. Logigian, ed., pp. 325–346, © 1982, Little, Brown, & Co.

- *Brown-Séquard's syndrome*: Hemisection of the cord that results in ipsilateral spastic paralysis and loss of postural sense (proprioception) below the lesion and contralateral loss of pain, thermal, touch sense (*Merck Manual* 1999, 1484). The syndrome results when only one side of the cord is damaged, as might occur in a stabbing or gunshot injury.
- *Cauda equina:* Injuries to the cauda equina involve peripheral nerves, rather than the cord itself. Because peripheral nerves possess a better regeneration capability than does the cord, there is a better prognosis for recovery. Patterns of sensory deficits are quite variable and usually asymmetrical, depending on which part of the cauda equina is involved.
- *Central (spinal) cord (column) syndrome*: The syndrome results when more cellular destruction occurs in the center of the cord than in the periphery. There is greater paralysis

and sensory loss in the upper extremities because these nerve tracts are located more centrally in the cord than the nerve tracts for the lower extremities. The syndrome is seen in older people with arthritic changes resulting in a narrowing of the spinal cord or in situations where cervical hyperextension occurs without vertebral fracture, which results in greater compression to the central aspects of the cord than to the periphery.

- *Conus medullaris syndrome*. The injury occurs to the sacral and lumbar nerve roots, which results in areflexic bladder, bowel, and lower limbs.
- *Posterior (spinal) cord (column) syndrome*: The syndrome results from a tumor or infarction that causes damage to the posterior spinal artery and/or posterior aspect of the cord. The motor tracts are mostly unaffected. Pain and temperature remain intact, but there is loss of proprioceptive, two-point discriminative, stereognostic, deep-pressure, and vibratory sensation.
- *Mixed syndrome*: The combination of two or more of the previously mentioned syndromes is called a *mixed syndrome*.

ASSESSMENT

Of special interest are the level of injury and remaining muscle strength. However, all areas of function must be assessed to provide a base level of function and identify interests to increase motivation.

Areas

- daily living skills
- productive history, skills, values, and interests
- leisure skills and interests
- muscle strength (examine the scapula, shoulder, elbow, wrist, and digits grip and pinch strength)
- endurance
- range of motion
- muscle tone (check for spasticity)
- gross motor coordination
- wrist and hand function
- trunk control and posture
- reflexes present and lost
- sensibility (examine light touch, pin prick, joint proprioception, stereognosis, and kinesthesia)
- temperature control
- pain
- problem-solving and decision-making skills
- self-concept
- mood or affect
- social and family support
- communication skills
- architectural barriers
- adaptive driving

Levels of Spinal Cord and Function

C1–C3	Has face and neck muscles innervated by cranial nerves	Can chew, swallow, talk, see, hear, smell, taste, suck, blow, sense motion
C4	Has phrenic nerve to innervate diaphragm, trapezius, and levator scapulae	Can breathe independently and has shoulder girdle elevation
C5	Has teres minor, rhomboids, deltoid, and infraspinatus and supraspinatus. Should have some biceps, brachialis, supraspinatus, and teres major.	Has shoulder external rotation and abduction to 90 degrees, and elbow flexion and supination. There is good control of the glenohumeral joint
C6	Has serratus anterior, pectoralis major and minor, serratus anterior, supinator, subscapularis, and brachioradialis. May have some extensor carpi radialis longus and brevis and pronator teres.	Has shoulder internal rotation, flexion extension, and adduction. May have forearm pronation. May have wrist extension allowing some passive finger flexion
C7	Has triceps, anconeous pronator teres, extensor digitorum, extensor carpi ulnaris, flexor carpi ulnaris, flexor carpi radialis, extensor pollicus longus and brevis, abductor pollicis longus	Has elbow extension, forearm pronation, wrist extension and flexion, thumb extension and abduction, passive finger flexion
C8, T1	Has ulnar wrist flexors and extensors, thumb flexors, extensors, abductors, abductors opposition, and finger intrinsics	Has power grasp, thumb movements, finger abduction and adduction and fine motor coordination

Note: Innervation of upper extremity muscles has some variability. The chart is an overview but will not be an exact pattern for all persons.

Source: Data from C. Formal and J. Smith, Upper Extremity Function in Spinal Cord Injury, *Topics in Spinal Cord Injury Rehabilitation*, © 1996, Vol. 1, No. 4, pp. 1–14.

Instruments

- *Barthel Index* by Mahoney, F.I. and D.W. Barthel. 1985. Functional evaluation: The Barthel Index. *Maryland State Medical Journal* 14:61–65.

- *Functional Independence Measure*, v. 4 by Uniform Data System for Medical Rehabilitation. 1994. Buffalo, NY: State University of New York at Buffalo.
- *Klein-Bell ADL Scale* by Klein, R.M. and B.J. Bell. 1982. Self-care skills: Behavior measurement with the Klein-Bell ADL Scale. *Archives of Physical Medicine and Rehabilitation* 63:335–338.
- manual muscle test by Hislop, H.J. and J. Montgomery. 1995. *Daniels and Worthingham's Muscle Testing: Techniques of Manual Examination*, 6th ed. Philadelphia, WB Saunders.
- passive range of motion evaluation.
- *Quadriplegic Index of Function* by Gresham, G.E., M.L. Labi, S.S. Dittmar, J.T. Hicks, S.Z. Joyce, and M.A. Stehlik. 1986. The quadriplegic index of function (QIF): Sensitivity and reliability demonstrated in a study of thirty quadriplegic patients. *Paraplegia* 24:38–44.
- *Qual-OT* by Robnett, R.H. and J.A. Gliner. 1995. Qual-OT: A quality of life assessment tool. *Occupational Therapy Journal of Research* 15(3);198–214.
- sensory evaluation
- *Sollerman Hand Test* by Sollerman, C. 1984. Assessment of grip function: Evaluation of a new test method. Stockholm, Sweden: MITAB.
- *Standard Neurological Classification of Spinal Cord Injury* by American Spinal Injury Association. 1992. Chicago, IL: The Association.

PROBLEMS

Self-Care
- The person will initially experience difficulty performing simple ADLs without assistance.
- The level of injury will determine, in part, the degree of self-care that the person can achieve.

Productivity
- The person usually will be unable to perform most job tasks requiring physical motor performance, such as lifting, carrying, bending, stooping, climbing, or assembling.
- The person probably will need vocational assessment or reassessment.

Leisure
- The person usually will be unable to perform leisure activities requiring physical motor performance, such as walking, running, jumping, climbing, kicking, throwing, swinging a bat, playing the piano, or playing a stringed or wind instrument.

Sensorimotor
- The person may have total or partial loss of movement of all the muscle groups affected.
- The person may have weakness or complete loss of strength in all muscle groups affected.
- The person usually has spasticity that results from lack of inhibition from higher centers.
- The person usually has decreased cardiovascular fitness due to loss of skeletal muscle support, which leads to less energy reserve.
- The person may have decreased vital capacity.
- The person may experience skin breakdown, pressure sores, or decubitus ulcers in dermatome areas innervated by nerves affected by the lesion.

American Spinal Injury Association (ASIA) Impairment Scale

A = Complete   There is no motor or sensory function preserved in the sacral segments S4–S5

B = Incomplete   Sensory but not motor function is preserved below the neurologic level and extends through the sacral segments S4–S5.

C = Incomplete   Motor function is preserved below the neurologic level, and the majority of key muscles below the neurologic level have a muscle grade less than 3.

D = Incomplete   Motor function is preserved below the neurologic level, and the majority of key muscles below the neurologic level have a muscle grade greater than or equal to 3.

E = Normal   Motor and sensory function is normal.

Source: Data from *Standards for Neurological and Functional Classification of Spinal Cord Injury*, © 1992, American Spinal Injury Association.

- Vital capacity may be decreased, especially for a person who sustained cervical or high thoracic lesion.
- The person may experience orthostatic hypotension, due to lack of muscle tone in the abdomen and lower extremities, leading to pooling of blood in these areas when the body is put in the vertical position and there is resultant decrease in blood pressure (hypotension).
- The person may experience osteoporosis or bone loss due to disuse. Pathological fractures may occur, especially in the supracondylar area of the femur, proximal tibia, distal femur, and neck of the femur. The upper extremities are usually not affected.
- The person may experience heterotopic ossification or ectopic bone that develops in abnormal anatomic locations, usually in the muscles around the hip and knee, but occasionally around the elbow and shoulder. Symptoms are swelling, warmth, and decreased joint range of motion that occur between 1 and 4 months after injury.
- The person usually has loss of the sense of touch and tactile discrimination below the level of the lesion site.
- The person usually has loss of kinesthesia and proprioception in affected areas.
- The person usually has loss of temperature control in the affected areas.
- The person's vision, hearing, taste, and smell are usually not affected because innervation is from cranial, not cervical, nerves.
- The person with C4-C7 tetraplegia may experience shoulder pain, due to scapular immobilization from prolonged bed rest or nerve root compression as a result of original injury.
- The person may report a phantom phenomenon. The typical pattern is flexion at the hip or knee, or both. Visual checking to see that the limb is extended helps the person to define reality from sensation.

Cognitive

- Cognitive faculties are not affected directly by the disorder, although people with high-level spinal cord injuries may also have some injury to the brain that may go undetected unless the therapist notes and reports any observed cognitive disabilities.

Psychosocial
- The person may express feelings of helplessness until the basic ADLs are relearned.
- The person may deny reality and expect to be walking independently in a few months.
- The person may become depressed when reality is accepted.
- The person may express feelings of hopelessness and a wish to die.
- The person may experience loss of loved ones or friends who cannot accept the person's change from physically able to physically challenged.
- The person may experience difficulty in finding new friends and interacting in group situations.

Environment
- The family's lifestyle is altered.
- The family financial resources are stretched.

TREATMENT/INTERVENTION

Treatment models include biomechanical and rehabilitative (compensatory). Biomechanical approaches are used to strengthen innervated muscle groups, and rehabilitative approaches are used to help the individual function as independently as possible.

Self-Care

For additional details, see Garber et al. 1994, 189–225 or Henshaw 1996, 599–624)
- Develop maximal level of independence in all self-care activities, including mobility.
- Assist the person to select assistive devices and orthoses that will be useful to accomplish tasks, and teach the use of self-help devices.
- Evaluate, recommend, and train in the use and care of needed durable medical devices, such as wheelchairs, seating systems, or scooters.
- Teach alternate methods and body positions for performing self-care activities.
- Assist the person and family in planning ahead for independent living.
- Consider the lifestyle of the person before encouraging the person to perform ADLs that require more time and energy to perform than would be expended by a normal person, such as dressing for level C6.
- The person may prefer to use the time and limited energy on productive or leisure activities.
- Eating and drinking: Provide opportunity to practice using assistive eating utensils with molded grips or a universal cuff to accommodate an ordinary spoon or fork. A nonslip mat, a deep-rimmed disk, or a plate guard may be useful initially but can be discontinued as the person's skill improves. A lightweight plastic cup or mug held with both hands can be used for drinking. A double-handle cup is also a possibility. A flexible straw may be preferred to picking up a cup. Antislide material may be useful on the table surface.
- Hair: Style should be easy to maintain by washing and towel drying. Brushes and combs that have rounded or adapted handles can be made with thermoplastic splinting material. Warn the person about the use of styling equipment and hair dryers that burn anesthetic skin. Washing the hair is most easily done in the shower or with a spray attachment in a sink. Filling the basin with water is not recommended because the person might slip forward face first into the basin and be unable to get out.
- Teeth: The toothbrush can be placed in a universal cuff, or a thermoplastic loop hand can be made that allows the hand to be slipped in easily. Electric toothbrushes may be useful for

some but for others will be too heavy and may have the on/off switch in a position that is inaccessible. Such devices are not easily adapted. Pump-action toothpaste dispensers are helpful.

- Makeup: Most applicators can be slipped into a universal cuff, or thermoplastic handles can be made.
- Washing: The basin and counter top should be low enough to support the person's elbows and forearm, and mounted so that there is room for feet and knees under the basin. The faucets should be lever style. Liquid soap or soap-on-a-rope make washing easier.
- Bathing: Some possible items that may be helpful include a rolling shower/commode wheelchair, transfer bench, shower chair with back and suction cup feet, grab bars for support and stability, a hand-held shower nozzle with on/off control in the handle, wash mitt with a Velcro D-ring closure or elastic edge, long-handled bath brush with angled handle, soap-on-a-rope worn around the neck or attached to a bath chair, towels adapted by adding loops to the ends or sewing eyelet holes in the ends.
- Clothing: Clothing that is tight or has back pockets or studs and elastic bands should be avoided. Clothing should not bind, back pockets or studs should be removed, and elastic bands, such as socks or bras, should be loose-fitting so as not to cause pressure marks. Natural fiber clothing is best. Some manmade fabrics may rub or scratch. Shoes should be a size larger to prevent rubbing and allow for some edema.
- Dressing: A technique for a person with paraplegia: The person sits up in bed. Additional pillows may provide support. One leg is bent at the knee and lifted over the other, making sure that the foot does not drag on the bed. Socks can be put on in this position while checking placement of the seams to avoid pressure on the toes. The process is repeated with the other leg. Trousers (slacks or jeans) are put on after the socks to avoid toes being caught in the seams. The process is the same. Trousers are then pulled up as far as possible. Note that underpants are not included. If they are worn, they must not be too tight so that they do not obstruct the leg-bag tubing. The person then lies down and pulls the trousers up by rolling from one side to the other to pull the garment over the buttocks. By sitting up again, shoes can be put on in the same way. For upper torso garments, the person may sit on the bed or transfer to a chair. Many variations are possible, and the person should be encouraged to problem solve. For example, shoes can be sandals, loafers, or sports shoes. Sports shoes may be tied or may use Velcro straps.
- Sitting transfers: Two methods are used. For the "forward-on" transfer, the person places the wheelchair at right angles to the surface, such as a bed, and lifts the legs onto the surface one at a time. The footrests are removed or swung away, and the chair is moved closer. The person moves forward as necessary until the buttocks are on the surface. The process is reversed to get into the chair. For the "legs-down" or side-transfer method, the chair is positioned beside the surface to which the transfer will occur. The foot plates are swung away or removed. The person moves forward on the seat until the feet are flat on the floor. The near side armrest is removed, the far side of the surface is grabbed, and the person lifts the buttocks off the chair and onto the surface. Then the legs are repositioned.
- Reproductive function: Correct information is most important. There is an interval of weeks or months when menstruation ceases but it usually starts again and returns to normal. Thus, a woman's fertility is not affected by the spinal cord injury. She can still bear children. However, there are health risks, such as autonomic dysreflexia, blood clots, problems with respiratory function, and bladder infections that need to be closely monitored. Medications

taken during pregnancy should be carefully evaluated for possible impact on the fetus. Male fertility usually is decreased, due to reduced sperm count. If birth control is desired, options should be carefully evaluated. Birth control pills pose a risk of blood clots, especially when combined with smoking. Diaphragms are difficult to position because of loss of sensation and hand function. Probably the best method is use of a condom by the male partner (Adler 1996, 769–770, Henshaw 1996, 623–624).

- Sexuality: The need for physical and emotional intimacy and the sex drive are not changed by the injury itself. However, there are practical problems. Male erection and ejaculation are often affected by spinal cord injury, although the extent of the problem varies. Body image, lack of sensation, the attitude of partners and society, and personal readiness are important factors. The person needs practical advice on aspects such as the benefits and drawbacks of various body positions and care of the bladder or catheter during intercourse. Also, different approaches to facilitating and maintaining an erection and augmenting the ejaculation should be discussed (Adler 1996, 769–770, Henshaw 1996, 623–624).

Productivity

- Develop maximal level of independence in homemaking skills.
- Develop parenting skills if needed.
- Assist in determining vocational choices based on interests, cognitive abilities, and skill level. Castle (1994, 182–187) found that employment postinjury tended toward administration, clerical, and finance positions.
- Assist in determining changes in the person's work environment needed to permit the person to work safely and effectively.
- Assist in evaluating and selecting an educational institution for continuing the person's education if more education is a goal.
- Evaluate the person's potential for driving a car or van and provide simulated driver training.

Leisure

- Assist the person to develop, explore, or expand leisure activities based on interests, cognitive abilities, and skill level.
- Assist in providing adaptations that may facilitate the person's participation in chosen leisure activities.
- Assist the person in making constructive use of time during acute stage of bed rest or when resting between activities. Equipment that may be useful include:
  1. Bed mirrors mounted to the bed and over-bed frame to enable the person to see the ward or to watch television and others in the room.
  2. Prism glasses that enable the person to see horizontally while looking at the ceiling.
  3. Books on tape, which are available from most public libraries or book stores.
  4. Reading frames or over-the-bed table that tilts to permit reading.
  5. Electric page turners.
  6. Overhead computer mounted for access using a mouth-stick or hand stick in a universal cuff. The person can play games or use word processing software.

Sensorimotor

- Maintain or increase joint range of motion.
- Prevent deformity via active and PROM, splinting, and positioning.

- Strengthen remaining muscle groups through use of enabling and purposeful activities.
- Increase physical endurance via functional activities.
- Provide care for the individual's hands, such as:
  1. Maintain the function position of the hand, including supporting the palmar transverse arch, stabilizing and supporting the thumb in abduction and opposition, and maintaining adequate web space.
  2. Maintain good cosmetic appearance of the hand and prevent contractures.
  3. Maintain good range of movement in all joints of the hand and wrist.
  4. Maintain good wrist extension.
  5. Examples of possible splints include: palmar hand, foot drop, short or long opponents, wrist-driven tenodesis, power-driven tenodesis, and dorsal wrist support.
- Teach compensatory or substitute motions.
- Provide splints to maintain the functional position of the wrist and hand and to assist in substitute motions (flexor hinge).
- Teach conservation of energy in all activities requiring motor activity.
- Assist in teaching wheelchair mobility skills.
- Teach safety using visual inspection and hearing as substitutes for tactile and temperature sensation.
- Teach the importance of visual inspection of skin surfaces to avoid decubitus ulcers.

Cognitive
- It may be useful to increase the person's memory skills so that he or she can remember the location of items because energy reserve is less.

Psychosocial
- Use previous interests to motivate the person to learn and relearn useful skills.
- Encourage a positive outlook through demonstration of possibilities.
- Aid in the adjustment to disability.
- Provide opportunities for social interaction with handicapped and able-bodied persons.
- Teach the person how to instruct nonmedical personnel to assist in pushing a wheelchair safely, using ramps, and transferring from a wheelchair to a chair or bed.

Environment
- Ensure safe and independent home accessibility through evaluation and recommendation for home modification.
- Provide information on architectural requirements for the safe use of a wheelchair in the home and community.
- Encourage family and friends of the individual to learn techniques for managing person.
- Provide psychological support to the family and friends.
- Provide knowledge about community resources and encourage participation in community activities.

PRECAUTIONS
- Always observe skin for redness or indications of skin breakdown.

Types of Splints Worn by Persons with Spinal Cord Injury

Resting pan or paddle splint—worn by patients who have wrist extensors and finger muscles below grade 3 on the Oxford Scale, usually at night.
Wrist extension splint—worn by patients with wrist extensors of grade 3 or below, but who have elbow flexors and need to use their hands.

  Futuro-type wrist splint
  Long opponens splint
  Dorsal cock-up splint
  Spiral splint

Short hand splints—worn to maintain web space, promote a functional hand position, and prevent hyperextension of the MP joints. Patients should have good wrist extension but show an imbalance between the extrinsic and intrinsic finger muscles.

  Short resting pan or paddle splint
  Short opponens splint
  Thumb post splint
  Commercially available MP flexion splint—Bunnell

Tenodesis splints—worn by patients with wrist extensor of above grade 3 with flickers or no movement of the fingers.

  Taping
  Heidleberg splint
  Volar splint

Source: Data from M. Curtin, Development of a Tetraplegic Hand Assessment and Splinting Protocol, *Paraplegia*, © 1994, Vol. 32, No. 3, pp. 159–169.

- Always observe temperature. Overheating is especially harmful. Time in the sun should be kept to a minimum. Body fluids should be maintained at all times.
- Watch for signs of autonomic reflexia, such as pounding headache, anxiety, perspiration, flushing, chills, nasal congestion, paroxysmal hypertension, and bradycardia. Person should be placed in an upright position and any restriction removed, such as abdominal binders or elastic stockings, to reduce blood pressure. Check for obstructions, such as leg bag tubing, and drain bladder.
- Watch for sudden increases in spasticity, which may be a symptom of other medical problems, such as bladder infections, skin breakdown, or fever.

PROGNOSIS AND OUTCOME

At present, totally severed or degenerated nerves in the spinal cord cannot recover—functional damage is permanent. However, animal studies suggest that regeneration of nerves damaged by contusion or transection may be possible. Compressed nerve tissue often recovers its function. Dysfunction remaining after 6 months is likely to be permanent (*Merck Manual* 1999, 1484).

A successful rehabilitation outcome depends on the person's willingness and ability to monitor fluid input and output and skin integrity, and to observe safety rules to reduce disease and accidents. The person's general intelligence and variety of interests increase opportunities for education and work. Social support and leisure interests increase life satisfaction.

Several references provide sample charts of expected functional performance: Adler 1996; 775–777; Adler and Hardy 1998, 600–604; Dolhi 1996, 21–28; Holler 1995, 798–803; Miller 1993, 252–253.

- The person is able to perform self-care activities independently but may have agreed to the use of an attendant to conserve energy and time for productive or leisure activities.
- The person uses self-help devices and equipment to facilitate performance.
- The person is able to perform productive activities, with or without assistive technology.
- The person is able to perform leisure activities. Assistive devices may be used.
- The person demonstrates maximum muscle strength that can be obtained, given the level of the lesion.
- The person demonstrates full range of motion, given the level of the lesion, except where contractures are encouraged because they may facilitate performance of certain activities.
- The person demonstrates the use of substitute and compensatory movements to increase functional performance.
- The person uses hand splints to augment performance, if needed.
- The person is independent in mobility when using powered mobility.
- The person is able to communicate using a variety of communication devices.
- The person is able to control his or her environment using a variety of electronic devices.
- The person understands and uses energy conservation and work-simplification techniques.

REFERENCES

Adler, C. 1996. Spinal cord injury. In *Occupational Therapy: Practice Skills for Physical Dysfunction*, 4th ed., ed. L.W. Pedretti, 765–784. St. Louis: Mosby.

Adler, C. and D.D. Hardy. 1998. Spinal cord injuries. In *Physical Dysfunction: Practice Skills for the Occupational Therapy Assistant*, ed. M.B. Early, 589–607. St. Louis: Mosby.

Beers, M.H., and R. Berkow, eds. 1999. *The Merck Manual of Diagnosis and Therapy,* 17th ed. Whitehouse Station, NJ: Merck Research Laboratories.

Castle, R. 1994. An investigation into the employment and occupation of patients with a spinal cord injury. *Paraplegia* 32:182–187.

Dolhi, C.D. 1996. *Occupational Therapy Practice Guidelines for Adults with Spinal Cord Injury.* Bethesda, MD: American Occupational Therapy Association.

Formal, C. and J. Smith. 1996. Upper extremity function in spinal cord injury. *Topics in Spinal Cord Injury Rehabilitation.* 1(4):1–14.

Garber, S.L., T.L. Gregorio, N. Pumphrey, and P. Lathem. 1994. Self-care strategies for persons living with spinal cord injuries. In *Ways of Living: Self-Care Strategies for Special Needs*, ed. C. Christiansen, 189–226. Rockville, MD: American Occupational Therapy Association.

Henshaw, J. 1996. Spinal cord lesions. In *Occupational Therapy and Physical Dysfunction: Principles, Skills, and Practice*, ed. A. Turner, M. Foster, and S.G. Johnson, 599–624. New York: Churchill Livingstone.

Holler, L.D. 1995. Spinal cord injury. In *Occupational Therapy for Physical Dysfunction*, 4th ed., ed. C.A. Trombly, 795–814. Baltimore: Williams & Wilkins.

Robnett, R.H. and J.A. Gliner. 1995. Qual-OT: A quality of life assessment tool. *Occupational Therapy Journal of Research* 15(3);198–214.
Miller, L.V. 1993. Spinal cord injury. In *Conditions in Occupational Therapy: Effects on Occupational Performance*, R.A. Hansen and B. Atchison, 229–265. Baltimore: Williams & Wilkins.

BIBLIOGRAPHY

Bates, P.S., J.C. Spencer, M.E. Young, and D.H. Rintala. 1993. Assistive technology and the newly disabled adult: Adaptation to wheelchair use. *American Journal of Occupational Therapy* 47(11):1014–1021.
Bell, P. and J. Hinojosa. 1995. Perception of the impact of assistive devices on daily life of three individuals with quadriplegia. *Assistive Technology* 7(2):87–94.
Carroll, S.G. and Meeney, C.F. 1993. Electrical stimulation for restoring independent feeding in a man with quadriplegia. *American Journal of Occupational Therapy* 47(8):739–742.
Colan, B.J. 1995. The other side of FES: Strengthening the arms. *Advance for Occupational Therapists* 11(43):9.
Creighton, C., M. Dijkers, N. Bennet, and K. Brown. 1995. Reasoning and the art of therapy for spinal cord injury. *American Journal of Occupational Therapy* 49(3):311–317.
Cunliffe, M.W. 1993. Adjustable thoracolumbar spinal orthoses: Direct molding using thermoplastic mesh sheet. *British Journal of Occupational Therapy* 56(12):441–446.
Curtin, M. 1993. Powered wheelchairs and tetraplegic patients: Improving the service. *British Journal of Occupational Therapy* 56(6):204–206.
Curtin, M. 1994. Technology for people with tetraplegia, part 1: Accessing computers. *British Journal of Occupational Therapy* 57(10):376–380.
Curtin, M. 1994. Technology for people with tetraplegia, part 2: Environmental control units. *British Journal of Occupational Therapy* 57(11):419–424.
Curtin, M. 1994. Development of a tetraplegic hand assessment and splinting protocol. *Paraplegia* 32(3):159–169.
DiPasquale-Lehnerz, P. 1994. Orthotic intervention for development of hand function with C-6 quadriplegia. *American Journal of Occupational Therapy* 48(2):138–144.
Dyson, M. 1995. Living with halo traction: A survival guide for clients in halo traction. *Australian Occupational Therapy Journal* 42(2):87–89.
Eberhardt, K. 1998. Home modification for persons with spinal cord injury. *OT Practice* 3(10):24–27.
Edmiston, H. 1998. In the driver's seat: OTs meet the challenges of today's health care. *Advance for Occupational Therapy Practitioners* 14(33):27–29 [Reprinted from *Outlook Magazine*, a Washington University School of Medicine publication. Summer, 1998].
Fahlgren, K.J. 1993. Use of assistive devices by persons with quadriplegia: A literature review. *Journal of Occupational Therapy Students* 7(1):55–62.
Fike, M.L., M. Weiner, and S. Parlak. 1993. The young adult with a spinal cord injury. In *Practice Issues in Occupational Therapy: Principles, Skills, and Practice*, ed. S.E. Ryan, 93–102. Thorofare, NJ: Slack.
Fuhrer, M.J., S.L. Garber, D.H. Rintala, R. Clearman, and K.A. Hart. 1993. Pressure ulcers in community-resident persons with spinal cord injury: Prevalence and risk factors. *Archives of Physical Medicine and Rehabilitation* 74(11):1172–1177.
Gadberry, L., and T. Frauenheim-Finke. 1996. *Motivating Life Skill Modules: For Individuals with Spinal Cord Injury*. Bethesda, MD: American Occupational Therapy Association.
Garber, S.L. and P. Lathem. 1995. Adaptive driving: mobility and community integration for persons with spinal cord injury. *Topics in Spinal Cord Injury Rehabilitation*. 1(1):59–65.

Garber, S.L., D.H. Rintala, C.D. Rossi, K.A. Hart, and M.J. Fuhrer. 1996. Reported pressure ulcer prevention and management techniques by persons with spinal cord injury. *Archives of Physical Medicine and Rehabilitation* 77(8):744–748.

Hammell, K.R.W. 1994. Establishing objectives in occupational therapy practice, part 1. *British Journal of Occupational Therapy* 57(1):9–14.

Hammell, K.R.W. 1994. Psychosocial outcome following spinal cord injury. *Paraplegia* 32:771–779.

Hammell, K.R.W. 1995. Spinal cord injury: Quality of life; Occupational therapy: Is there a connection? *British Journal of Occupational Therapy* 58(4):151–157.

Henderson, J.L., S.H. Price, M.E. Brnadstater, and B.R. Mandac. 1994. Efficacy of three measures to relieve pressure in seated persons with spinal cord injury. *Archives of Physical Medicine and Rehabilitation* 75(5):535–539.

Holme, S.A., E.M. Kanny, M.R. Guthrie, and K.L. Johnson. 1997. The use of environmental control units by occupational therapists in spinal cord injury and disease services. *American Journal of Occupational Therapy* 51(1):42–48.

Hodges, C. and L. Bender. 1994. Phantom pain: A critical review of the proposed mechanisms. *British Journal of Occupational Therapy* 57(60):209–212.

Johnson, K. 1998. Bladder and bowel management in SCI: An analysis of six approaches. *Advance for Occupational Therapists* 14(15):22–24.

Kerr, T. 1995. The mom or dad with SCI: Parenting is possible with a little OT help. *Advance for Occupational Therapists* 11(24):15,19.

Klose, K.J., B.M. Needham, D. Schmidt, J.G. Broton, and B.A. Green. 1993. An assessment of the contribution of electromyographic biofeedback as an adjunct therapy in the physical training of spinal cord injured persons. *Archives of Physical Medicine and Rehabilitation* 74(5):453–456.

Kohlmeyer, K.M., J.P. Hill, G.M. Yarkony, and R.J. Jaeger. 1996. Electrical stimulation and biofeedback effect on recovery of tenodesis grasp: a controlled study. *Archives of Physical Medicine and Rehabilitation* 77(7):702–706.

Kohlmeyer, K.M. and C. Rom. 1994. Driver assessment. In *Spinal Cord Injury: Medical Management and Rehabilitation*, ed. G.M. Yarkony, 205–210. Gaithersburg, MD: Aspen Publishers.

Kohlmeyer, K.M. and G.M. Yarkony. 1994. Functional outcome after spinal cord injury rehabilitation. In *Spinal Cord Injury: Medical Management and Rehabilitation*, ed. G.M. Yarkony, 9–14.Gaithersburg, MD: Aspen Publishers.

Kreutz, D., S.J. Taylor, and D.F. Apple. 1995. A wheelchair seating challenge. *Topics in Spinal Cord Injury Rehabilitation* 1(1):37–41.

Lee, B. and T. Nantais. 1996. Use of electronic music as an occupational therapy modality in spinal cord injury rehabilitation: An occupational performance model. *American Journal of Occupational Therapy* 50(5):362–369.

Lightbody, S. 1994. Dynamic pronation splint in high level spinal cord injury: A case study. *Australian Occupational Therapy Journal* 41(2):83–85.

Lynch, S.M. and S.L. Edwards. 1995. Meeting the challenge. *TeamRehab Report* 6(8):24–28.

Marmer, L. 1997. Saving the day for SCI patients. *Advance for Occupational Therapists* 13(12):15, 46.

Marmer, L. 1996. Model treatment systems for SCI target quality of life. *Advance for Occupational Therapists* 12(26):13,46.

Maurer, C., M. Floersheim, and P. Craig. 1998. Fitness training for healthy lifestyle: Working with SCI patients to enhance upper extremity strength. *Rehab Management* 11(2):36, 38–9, 41,43.

McAlonan, S. 1996. Improving sexual rehabilitation services: The patient's perspective. *American Journal of Occupational Therapy* 50(10):826–834.

Pentland, W., A.S. Harvey, and J. Walker. 1998. The relationships between time use and health and well-being in men with spinal cord injury. *Journal of Occupational Science* 5(1):14–25.

Pentland, W., A.S. Harvey, T. Smith, and J. Walker. 1999. The impact of spinal cord injury on men's time use. *Spinal Cord* 37(11):786–792.

Price, G. and S. Lightbody. 1994. A community living skills education programme within spinal cord injury rehabilitation. *Australian Occupational Therapy Journal* 41(1):37–40.

Quigley, M.C. 1995. Impact of spinal cord injury on the life roles of women. *American Journal of Occupational Therapy* 49(8):780–786.

Rodriguez, G.P. and S.L. Garber. 1994. Prospective study of pressure ulcer risk in spinal cord injury patients. *Paraplegia* 32:150–158.

Schlindler, L., G. Robbins, and C. Hamlin. 1994. Functional effect of bilateral tendon transfer on a person with C-5 quadriplegia. *American Journal of Occupational Therapy* 48(8):750–757.

Spencer, J., M.E. Young, D. Rintala, and S. Bates. 1995. Socialization to the culture of a rehabilitation hospital: An ethnographic study. *American Journal of Occupational Therapy* 49(1):53–62.

Sutton, S. 1993. An overview of the management of the C-6 quadriplegic patient's hand: An occupational therapist's perspective. *British Journal of Occupational Therapy* 56(10):376–380.

Taylor, B., M.E. Cupo, and S.J. Sheredos. 1993. Workstation robotics: A pilot study of a desktop vocational assistant robot. *American Journal of Occupational Therapy* 47(11):1009–1013.

Van Deusen, J. 1993. The physically challenged adult—spinal cord injury. In *Body Image and Perceptual Dysfunction in Adults*, ed. J. Van Deusen, 217–222. Philadelphia: WB Saunders.

Watson, A.H., E.M. Kanny, D.M. White, and D.K. Anson. 1995. Use of standardized activities of daily living rating scales in spinal cord injury and disease services. *American Journal of Occupational Therapy* 49(3):229–234.

Spinal Cord Injuries—Child/Adolescent

DESCRIPTION

Spinal cord injury results in abrupt motor paralysis; sensory, bowel, bladder, and sexual dysfunction; temporary cessation of developmental, scholastic, and social milestones; and eventual alteration of development from poor growth in paralyzed extremities, paralytic scoliosis, hip instability, pressure ulcers, pathologic fractures, contractures, and severe spasticity. As if these problems do not pose enough challenges, spinal injury in childhood also can result in underachievement in social, educational, and vocational pursuits; conflict in peer relationships; alteration in leisure activities; financial devastation; family stress; and forced lifestyle changes for the child and his or her family members.

The manifestations and complications of childhood spinal cord injury are magnified by the interaction of injury with growth and development and the reciprocal impact of the injured child and family members. Thus, rehabilitation efforts must accommodate the dynamic nature of growing children by restoring lost abilities and promoting new and unlearned skills. Sensitivity to the developmental needs of children and inclusion of the family are instrumental in defining and realizing rehabilitation and habilitation goals (Mulcahey and Betz 1997, 31).

CAUSE

Causes for spinal cord injury in children and adolescents are motor vehicle accidents (40%), sports injuries (24%), diving accidents (13%), gunshot wounds (8%), falls (8%), transverse myelitis (4%), and spinal cord tumors (3%) (Betz and Mulcahey 1994, 782).

ASSESSMENT

Areas
- daily living skills
- productivity skills, values, and interests
- leisure skills and interests
- muscle tone and spasticity
- hand functions

Instruments
- *Bayley Scales of Infant Development*, 2nd ed. by Bayley, N. 1992. San Antonio, TX: The Psychological Corporation.
- *Common Object Test* by Stroh, K., C. Van Doren, G. Thorpe, and C. Wijman. 1989. Common object test: A functional assessment for quadriplegic patients using an FNS hand system. *Proceedings of the RENSA 12 Annual Conference,* 387–388.
- *Denver II* by Frankenberg, W.K., J. Dodds, P. Archer et al. 1990. Denver, CO: Denver Developmental Materials.
- *Grasp and Release Test* by Stroh-Wuolle K.C., C.L. Van Doren, G.B. Thorpe, M.W. Keith, and P.H. Peckham. 1994. Developmental of a quantitative hand grasp and release test for patients with tetraplegia using a hand neuroprosthesis. *Journal of Hand Surgery* 19A:209–218.
- *Hawaii Early Learning Profile* by Furuno, S., K. O'Reilly, C.M. Hoska et al. 1985. Palo Atlo, CA: Vort Corporation.
- *Peabody Developmental Motor Scales* by Folio, R. and R. Fewell. 1983. Austin, TX: ProEd.
- *Pediatric Evaluation of Disability Inventory* by Haley, S.M., W.J. Coster, L.J. Ludlow et al. 1999. San Antonio, TX: Psychological Corporation/Therapy Skill Builders.
- *Standards for Neurological and Functional Classification of Spinal Cord Injury* by American Spinal Injury Association. 1992. Atlanta, GA: The Association.
- *Vineland Adaptive Behavior Scales*, 2nd ed. by Sparrow, S.S., D. Balla, and D. Cicchetti. 1990. Circle Pines, MN: American Guidance Service.
- *WeeFIM* by Uniform Data System for Medical Rehabilitation. 1991. Buffalo, NY: State University of New York at Buffalo.

PROBLEMS

Self-Care
- The person is likely to experience difficulty performing self care activities.
- The person may need to have modifications to the home to facilitate moving about the rooms.
- The person may require special equipment and assistive devices to perform self-care activities.

Productivity
- The child may underachieve in school.

- Adolescent may underachieve in vocational pursuits.
- The person may need to have modifications made at school to facilitate moving about the building.
- The person may need specialized equipment and assistive devices to perform school work.

Leisure
- The child or adolescent will experience changes in leisure activities.

Sensorimotor
- Child will experience poor growth of paralyzed extremities.
- The person usually will experience paralytic scoliosis or spinal deformity (Betz and Mulcahey 1994, 790).
- The person may have increased muscle tone.
- The person usually has spasticity or excessive reflex activity associated with involuntary movement.
- The person may experience hip instability, dislocation, or subluxation, due to spasticity (Betz and Mulcahey 1994, 791–792).
- The person may have contractures. The most common are flexion and adduction of the hips, equinus of the ankles, adduction-internal rotation of the shoulders, flexion supination contractures of the elbows, and intrinsic minus hands (Betz and Mulcahey 1994, 789).
- The person may develop heterotopic ossification (Betz and Mulcahey 1994, 790).
- The person may have reflex sympathetic dystrophy (see chapter on complex regional pain syndrome).
- The person always experiences osteopenia or osteoporosis. Person may experience pathological fractures as a result of osteopenia (Betz and Mulcahey 1994, 792–793).
- The person may experience posttraumatic syrinx or cysts (Betz and Mulcahey 1994, 793).
- The person may experience pressure sores.
  1. Grade I involves irregular, ill-defined areas of soft tissue swelling and induration with associated erythema overlying a bony prominence.
  2. Grade II involves all soft tissues, presenting with a full-thickness skin ulcer extending to the underlying subcutaneous fat.
  3. Grade III is typical decubitus with necrotic, foul-smelling, infected ulcer limited by deep fascia but involving the fat and undermining the skin.
  4. Grade IV is a sore that has penetrated the deep fascia, causing extensive soft tissue spread with osteomyelitis and septic, dislocated joints (Betz and Mulcahey 1994, 793).
- The person may have a brachial plexus palsy (see chapter on brachial plexus injury).
- The person usually has loss of hand function related to grasp and release.
- The person may experience urinary tract infections (Betz and Mulcahey 1994, 787).
- The person may have respiratory insufficiency (Betz and Mulcahey 1994, 786–787).
- The person may experience deep venous thrombosis (Betz and Mulcahey 1994, 785).
- The person may experience immobilization hypercalcemia (Betz and Mulcahey 1994, 785).
- The person may experience problems in thermal regulation (Betz and Mulcahey 1994, 798).
- The person may have fever of unknown origin (Betz and Mulcahey 1994, 788).
- Adolescents may refuse to wear lower extremity orthoses.

Cognitive
- Spinal cord injury does not directly affect cognitive skills but the person may have experienced a head injury at the same time that the spinal cord injury occurred.

Psychosocial
- The child may experience conflict in peer relations.
- Adolescents may lose friends following their injury because their friends do not know how to relate to a person with a disability.
- Adolescents may experience difficulty reentering the school environment because of inadequate support systems within the schools.

Environment
- The family will experience changes in lifestyle.
- The family may experience financial devastation.
- The family may experience stress.
- The person and family will experience architectural barriers.
- The person and family may experience geographic barriers, especially in regard to transportation.
- The person and family may experience stigmas and preconceptions about what a child or adolescent with a spinal cord injury can be expected to do in the community and at school.

TREATMENT/INTERVENTION

The treatment program must provide rehabilitation services to restore lost abilities or skills and rehabilitation services to promote the development of new skills and abilities that were not previously established (Mulcahey and Betz 1997, 31–32). Models include compensatory or rehabilitation techniques, primarily.

Self-Care (Betz and Mulcahey 1994, 801–803)
- Self-care goals should be established with input from the parents, child, and medical personnel.
- Dressing: A child with paraplegia can dress independently with practice in maintaining balance but those with tetraplegia will have difficulty. Concentrate on what the child is able to do and limit frustration. Adolescents with tetraplegia should be able to dress independently but need to decide how to spend limited energy. Dressing and other self-care activities may be less important tasks to perform independently on a daily basis than going to school and participating in social activities.
- Eating/feeding: For the child with paraplegia, self-feeding should be accomplished according to developmental norms. For an adolescent with tetraplegia, assistive devices may be necessary for independent eating. Some may prefer to have a helper feed them.
- Grooming: Most children and adolescents can manage brushing teeth and hair with assistive devices, if needed.
- Bowel and bladder/catheterization: Every effort should be made to promote independence in bowel and bladder management including, self-catheterization and changing the leg bag.

- Skin care: Skin care and skin checks should be integrated into the parents' routines for young children and all adolescents' routines.
- Applying makeup, deodorant, and perfume: Most adolescents want to be able to perform these tasks. With assistive devices, these tasks can be mastered.
- Bed mobility: The person should learn how to move about in bed, if possible. Adaptations may include changing the height of the bed; stabilizing the bed; adding loops, straps, or bed rails; using an overhead frame with a trapeze or loop; using an electrical elevating head section for respiratory and pressure release; changing the type of mattress or changing to nylon or silk matte sheets to decrease friction.
- Wheelchair mobility: The better the child's mobility is, the better will be his or her independence. Participate with the multidisciplinary team in the selection of the best chair, based on range of motion; strength; endurance; posture; height, width, and depth measurements; balance; and the effect of spasticity on seating posture and sitting balance. Other considerations are the vendor's reputation, availability of repair parts in the home community, availability of new equipment on the market, family acceptance, and number of additional items the chair requires that can get lost or stolen (González-Mueller and Kelly 1996, 483–500).
- Transfers: A child often needs assistance with transfers, regardless of the level of injury, due to problems with balance, immature muscle strength, and back orthosis. Adolescents with paraplegia can transfer independently. Some adolescents with low tetraplegia (C7 or C8) can transfer independently but, more importantly, should know how to instruct others to aid in transfers safely for the other person and the helper(s). Transfer boards and hydraulic pump lifts may be needed, especially for tetraplegia.
- Communication: An adolescent with tetraplegia may learn to write with a felt-tipped pen interwoven between the fingers or through use of assistive technology, such as computer keyboards and voice-activated tape recorders. The ability to use a touch-tone telephone (cord, cordless, or cell phone) is important, especially for emergencies.

Productivity

- Attending school should be a top priority (Chambers and Lasher 1997, 1–3). Education is an important factor in future vocations, as well as an opportunity to reestablish contacts with friends and peers. The school should be evaluated for wheelchair accessibility of the entrances, exits, and bathrooms, and the teacher should be provided with information about educating a child with a disability. Parents should know about the public laws that concern public education for children with disabilities (Kolodner and Ameci 1996, 639–652).
- Adolescents who are of legal age to drive should be consulted about their interest in driving. With modifications and assistive devices, most are able to drive. A major consideration is the financial cost of modifying a car or adapting a van to fit the adolescent's needs. The Office of Vocational Rehabilitation should be consulted as one source of funding to defray the costs.
- Assist the adolescent in considering vocational and career options. Coordinate with vocational counseling and the local or state Office of Vocational Rehabilitation. Massagli et al. (1996) found that adolescents with spinal cord injury had adequate education but may not have adequate vocational counseling and opportunities for paid employment.

Leisure

- For children, use age-appropriate play activities. Play techniques should be incorporated into treatment sessions.
- Adolescents should be educated about community activities available to them.
- Some adolescents may want to participate in wheelchair sports and consider trying out for the ParaOlympics or Special Olympics.

Sensorimotor

- Prevent deformity by maintaining functional range of motion and mobility in all affected joints. During the acute stage, nursing and therapy are responsible but the responsibility should be transferred to the person and family as soon as possible. Positioning during sleeping or rest periods can also help.
- Prevent contractures using passive stretch by therapy personnel, the person (if possible), and family members. Night splints can help but skin integrity must be monitored. Some contractures can be useful, such as contracture of the long finger flexors in a person with C6-level injury, which facilitates the tenodesis action of the wrist.
- Increase muscle strength of remaining muscles using functional activities and play routines. Traditional exercises used in adults, such as weights, wall pulleys, slings, suspension, and forearm skateboards are not usually effective with children (Betz and Mulcahey 1994, 796). Biofeedback, electrical stimulation, and bicycle ergonometry can also be used.
- Assist in return to vertical position by increasing tolerance to vertical sitting and standing. If hypotension occurs, recline person or provide pressure-gradient stocking or abdominal binders.
- Reduce hypertonicity though prolonged stretching, proper positioning, and use of orthoses. The person should recognize his or her reflex patterns of spasticity and learn to avoid the stimuli that elicit the spasticity. Electric stimulation of the antagonistic muscles can temporarily reduce tone through reciprocal innervation but is not recommended for long-term use. Occasionally, spasticity can be used to advantage, such as pinching the calf muscle to initiate flexion to assist in dressing (Betz and Mulcahey 1994, 796).
- Prevent pressure sores by promoting skin care, safety, hygiene, skin checks, and pressure relief. Cushions should be provided in the wheelchair. Instruction to family is important after discharge. Coordinate efforts with nursing staff. At home, an egg crate mattress, sheepskin, or water bed may be helpful but do not take the place of daily skin care and monitoring. Instruction to avoid extreme heat or cold is important, as is avoiding burns from bathing, cigarettes, heating pads, or car heaters (Benner 1996, 285–292; Betz and Mulcahey 1994, 796).
- Provide assistive devices as needed and accepted. Most children choose assistive devices (built-up handles, angled utensils) and compensatory movement patterns over orthoses (Mulcahey 1997a, 49).
- Useful orthotic devices include the universal cuff, wrist-driven flexor hinge orthosis (WFHO), and mobile arm support (MAS), also called *balanced forearm orthosis* (BFO). Orthoses used by children should be cosmetically pleasing, easy to put on and take off, reliable, size- and weight-efficient, effective, and durable; their wear and use must be supported by parents and teachers.

- The universal cuff orthosis is worn in the palm and has a pocket to accommodate small objects, such as pen, pencil, keyboard, stick, or eating utensil. The cuff can be attached to volar- or dorsal-based splints if more support is required for the wrist. It is useful for midcervical injuries when there is no functional hand grasp. Children as young as 3 or 4 can use the universal cuff (Mulcahey 1996, 375–392; Mulcahey 1997a, 49, Overview).
- The WFHO is used for specific tasks, such as writing or catheterization. Mostly adolescents use the WFHO. Acceptance is increased if the WFHO is cosmetically acceptable, can be put on in a timely manner, and can be used to accomplish a specific task or tasks (Mulcahey 1996, 375–392; Mulcahey 1997a, 49–50, Overview).
- The MAS may be used to stabilize the forearm and facilitate shoulder and arm movements. Persons with partial motor preservation at the C5–C6 level are most likely to benefit from the MAS. However, acceptance of the MAS is low because of poor cosmesis, poor portability, and difficulty with setup (Mulcahey 1996, 375–392; Mulcahey, 1997a, 50, Overview).
- Overhead slings may be useful but may not provide the level of proximal stability or arm control necessary to facilitate hand use. The issues of acceptance are the same as those for the MAS, above.
- Person may benefit from tendon transfer. Best candidates are those with C5–C7 injuries. A C5-level injury can gain voluntary elbow and wrist extension. C6–C7 level injuries can regain hand grasp and release. Skills gained may include ability to catheterize without assistance, to perform advanced wheelchair skills, such as negotiating curbs or ramps, and to grasp assistive devices for stance and upright mobility (Mulcahey 1997a, 50, Overview; see also chapter on tendon transfers).
- Adolescents with midcervical injury may benefit from implantation of the Freehand System, which has been shown to improve hand function and increase level of independence in ADL skills (Mulcahey et al. 1997a, 597–607, Implanted; Davis et al. 1998, 220–226). Recent studies have focused on upright mobility (Bonaroti et al. 1999a and 1999b).
- A child with tetraplegia or paraplegia is at greater risk for developing upper extremity pain. Prevention may include stretching, warm-up and cool-down exercises, energy conservation, and avoiding overuse syndrome. For pain management, gentle passive joint range of motion exercise, visual imagery, submotor threshold surface electrical stimulation, and supervised applications of heat may be effective (Lau and McCormack 1996, 653–670; Mulcahey 1997a, 53, Overview).
- Assist in respiratory and cardiovascular function with other team members to provide training in more efficient coordinated breathing patterns, maintaining chest mobility and bronchial hygiene. Group games, such as sipping through straws and blowing bubbles, are helpful.
- Muscle tendon transfers may be done to facilitate function (see chapter on tendon transfers).
- Assist with standing and ambulation. Children with injury at T4 or below can stand and may ambulate with knee-ankle-foot orthosis (KAFO), hip-knee-ankle-foot orthosis (HKAFO), reciprocating gait orthosis (RGO), or hip guidance orthosis (Para walker).
- Functional neuromuscular stimulation (FNS) and functional electrical stimulation (FES) have been used to stimulate nerves, resulting in muscle contraction, but the effects are usually of short term. Implanted systems have been more successful (Smith et al 1996, 16–23).

Cognitive

- The person should be instructed in terms and level appropriate to the age.
- Because no specific damage to cognitive skills is expected, no specific intervention is provided.

Psychosocial

- Therapy personnel should keep in mind that adolescents are primarily interested in autonomy, peer acceptance, and group conformity, which may lead to behavior judged to be noncompliant, poorly motivated, or acting out.
- The adolescent program should focus on social skills, assertiveness training, and exploration of sexuality, body image, social stigmas, peer pressure, substance use, and self-worth (Mulcahey and Betz 1997, 33).
- Provide opportunity for the person to learn to interact with able-bodied peers and with other children and adolescents with disabilities.
- Provide information about substance use and abuse and the risk for a person with a spinal cord injury.

Environment

- Parents need reeducation in parenting a child with a disability, especially with regard to hygiene, nutrition, safety, and medical needs.
- The home may require modification. Of special consideration are accessibility of the entrances, exits, bathroom, and bedroom using a wheelchair (Benner 1996, 573–579).

PRECAUTIONS

- If pain is present, performance of strenuous activities, such as wheelchair sports, body transfers, weight training, and ambulation should be discouraged.
- Watch for signs and symptoms of autonomic dysreflexia, which include pounding headache, vasodilation, flushing, blotching of the skin, and cold sweating above the level of spinal cord lesion. Look for cause of noxious stimuli, such as an overfull bladder due to kink in the drainage tube or other blockage and impacted fecal material in the anus.
- If any orthosis is used, monitor skin integrity very closely (every few hours) when the device is newly applied and regularly thereafter (every time the device is removed or at least daily).
- Avoid hypotension in vertical position. Symptoms include decreased blood pressure, increased pulse, pallor, and dizziness.
- Avoid quick stretching, which may elicit the stretch reflex. Use slow stretching.
- Watch for signs of substance abuse, such as alcohol and drug abuse.

PROGNOSIS/OUTCOMES

Outcome depends on the involvement of the family and child or adolescent in the rehabilitation process and in home and community reintegration. Cooperation of a school system is also important. Spinal cord injury is a lifetime disability. Changes and adjustments will continue to be made.

- The person is able to perform self-care activities independently but may have agreed to the use of an attendant to conserve energy and time for productive or leisure activities.

- The person uses self-help devices and equipment to facilitate performance.
- The person is able to perform productive activities with or without assistive technology.
- The person is able to perform leisure activities. Assistive devices may be used.
- The person demonstrates normal developmental skills and milestones consistent with limitation of function imposed by level of spinal cord injury.
- The person demonstrates maximum muscle strength that can be obtained, given the level of the lesion.
- The person demonstrates full range of motion, given the level of the lesion, except where contractures are encouraged because they may facilitate performance of certain activities.
- The person demonstrates the use of substitute and compensatory movements to increase functional performance.
- The person uses hand splints to augment performance, if needed.
- The person is independent in mobility when using powered mobility.
- The person is able to communicate using a variety of communication devices.
- The person participates in social activities appropriate to chronologic age.

REFERENCES

Benner, L. 1996. Equipment needs and environmental accessibility. In *The Child with a Spinal Cord Injury,* ed. R.R. Betz, M.J. Mulcahey, 573–588. Rosemont, IL: American Academy of Orthopaedic Surgeons.

Betz, R.R. and M.J. Mulcahey. 1994. Spinal cord injury rehabilitation. In *The Pediatric spine: Principles and Practice,* Vol 1., ed. S.L. Weinstein, 781–810. New York: Raven Press.

Bonaroti, D. et al. 1999a. A comparison of FES with KAFO for providing ambulation and upright mobility for a child with a complete thoracic spinal cord injury. *Journal of Spinal Cord Medicine* 22(3):159–166.

Bonaroti, D. et al. 1999b. Comparison of functional electrical stimulation to long leg braces or upright mobility for children with complete thoracic level spinal injuries. *Archives of Physical Medicine and Rehabilitation* 80(9):1047–1057.

Chambers, P. and E. Lasher. 1997. A team approach in returning adolescents with spinal cord injuries to the classroom. *Physical Disabilities Special Interest Section Newsletter* 20(2):1–3.

Davis, S.E., M.J. Mulcahey, B.T. Smith, and R.R. Betz. 1998. Self-reported use of an implanted FES hand system by adolescents with tetraplegia. *Journal of Spinal Cord Medicine* 21(30):220–226.

González-Mueller, I. and M.A. Kelly. 1996. In *The Child with a Spinal Cord Injury,* ed. Betz R.R., M.J. Mulcahey, 483–500. Rosemont, IL: American Academy of Orthopaedic Surgeons.

Kolodner, E.L. and G.M. Ameci. 1996. Disability laws. In *The Child with a Spinal Cord Injury,* ed. R.R. Betz and M.J. Mulcahey, 639–652. Rosemont, IL: American Academy of Orthopaedic Surgeons.

Lau, C. and G. McCormack. 1996. Chronic pain management in pediatric spinal cord injury. In *The Child with a Spinal Cord Injury,* ed. R.R. Betz and M.J. Mulcahey, 653–670. Rosemont, IL: American Academy of Orthopaedic Surgeons.

Massagli, T.L., B.J. Dudgeon, and B.W. Ross. 1996. Education performance and vocation participation after spinal cord injury in childhood. *Archives of Physical Medicine and Rehabilitation* 77(10):995–999.

Mulcahey, M.J. 1996. Upper extremity orthoses and splints. In *The child with a spinal cord injury,* ed. R.R. Betz and M.J. Mulcahey, 375–392. Rosemont, IL: American Academy of Orthopedic Surgeons.

Mulcahey, M.J. and R.R. Betz. 1997. Considerations in the rehabilitation of children with spinal cord injuries. *Topics in Spinal Cord Injury Rehabilitation* 3(2):31–36.

Mulcahey, M.J. 1997a. An overview of the upper extremity in pediatric spinal cord injury. *Topics in Spinal Cord Injury Rehabilitation* 3(2):48–55.

Mulcahey, M.J., R.R. Betz, B.T. Smith, A.A. Weiss, and S.E. Davis. 1997a. Implanted functional electrical stimulation hand system in adolescents with spinal injuries: An evaluation. *Archives of Physical Medicine and Rehabilitation* 78(6):597–607.

BIBLIOGRAPHY

Anderson, C.J., M.J. Mulcahey, and L.C. Vogel. 1997. Menstruation and pediatric spinal cord injury. *Journal of Spinal Cord Medicine* 20(1):56–59.

Benner, L. 1996. Pressure ulcer prevention. In *The Child with a Spinal Cord Injury*, ed. R.R. Betz and M.J. Mulcahey, 285–292. Rosemont, IL: American Academy of Orthopaedic Surgeons.

Dudgeon, B.J., T.L. Massagli, and B.W. Ross. 1997. Educational participation of children with spinal cord injury. *American Journal of Occupational Therapy* 51(7):553–561.

Granger, C.V. and S.L. Braun. 1996. Outcome assessments and measures in pediatrics. In *The Child with a Spinal Cord Injury*, ed. R.R. Betz and M.J. Mulcahey, 285–292. Rosemont, IL: American Academy of Orthopaedic Surgeons.

Kerr, T. 1996. Getting teens with SCI back to school. *Advance for Occupational Therapists* 12(2):12.

Marmer, L. 1996. In touch with kids: How Terry Terrific found out about OT! *Advance for Occupational Therapists* 12(34):4–5.

Mulcahey, M.J., B.T. Smith, R.R. Betz, R.J. Triolo, and P.H. Peckham. 1994. Functional neuromuscular stimulation: Outcomes in young people with tetraplegia. *Journal of the American Paraplegia Society* 17(1):20–35.

Mulcahey, M.J., R.R. Betz, B.T. Smith, and A.A. Weiss. 1995. Outcomes of functional electrical stimulation using a totally implanted stimulator and electrodes in adolescents with tetraplegia. *Journal of Spinal Cord Medicine* 18(4):265–266.

Mulcahey, M.J. 1999. Evaluation of the lower motor neuron integrity of upper extremity muscles in high level spinal cord injury. *Spinal Cord.* 37(8):585–591.

Mulcahey, M.J. 1997b. Unique management needs of pediatric spinal cord injury patients: Rehabilitation. *Journal of Spinal Cord Medicine* 20(1):25–30.

Mulcahey, M.J. 1996. Wheelchairs and seating systems: Evaluation and training. In *The Child with a Spinal Cord Injury*, ed. R.R. Betz and M.J. Mulcahey, 483–500. Rosemont, IL: American Academy of Orthopaedic Surgeons.

Mulcahey, M.J. and R.R. Betz. 1997. Upper and lower extremity applications of functional electrical stimulation: A decade of research with children and adolescents with spinal injuries. *Pediatric Physical Therapy* 9:113–122.

Mulcahey, M.J., B.T. Smith, and R.R. Betz. 1999. Evaluation of the lower motor neuron integrity of upper extremity muscles in high level spinal cord injury. *Spinal Cord* 37(8):585–591.

Mulcahey, M.J., R.R. Betz, S.T. Smith, A.A. Weiss, and S.E. Davis. 1997b. Implanted functional electrical stimulation hand system in adolescents with spinal injuries: An evaluation. *Archives of Physical Medicine and Rehabilitation* (6):597–607.

Mulcahey, M., R. Betz, B. Smith et al. 1994. An upper extremity neuroprosthesis using totally implanted stimulator and implanted electrodes: Evaluation process and candidate selection. *Journal of the American Paraplegia Society* 17:226–264.

Nelson, V.S., L.E. Driver, B. Gretchen, D.F. Hilker, B. Howell, and B.B. Wolfe. 1996. High tetraplegia. In *The Child with a Spinal Cord Injury*, ed. R.R. Betz and M.J. Mulcahey, 773–790. Rosemont, IL: American Academy of Orthopaedic Surgeons.

Rizzo, M., R.R. Betz, M.J. Mulcahey, and B.T. Smith. 1998. Magnetic resonance imaging data in the evaluation of effects of functional electrical stimulation on knee joints of adolescents with spinal cord injury. *Journal of Spinal Cord Medicine* 21(2):124–130.

Sarver, J.J., B.T. Smith, R. Seliktar, M.J. Mulcahey, and R.R. Betz. 1999. A study of shoulder motions as a control source for adolescents with C4 level SCI. *IEEE Transactions in Rehabilitation Engineering* 7(1):27–34.

Smith, B., M.J. Mulcahey, and R. Betz. 1996. Development of an upper extremity FES system for individual with C4 tetraplegia. *IEEE Transactions in Rehabilitation Engineering* 4(4):264–270.

Smith, B., M.J. Mulcahey, and R. Betz. 1995. Development of a FES system for C4 tetraplegia. In *Proceedings of the RESNA Annual Conference*, 366–368. Vancouver, BC, Canada.

Smith, B., M.J. Mulcahey, and R. Betz. 1996. Quantitative comparison of grasp and release abilities with and without functional neuromuscular stimulation in adolescents with tetraplegia. *Paraplegia* 34(1):16–23.

Smith, B.T., R.R. Betz, M.J. Mulcahey, and R.J. Triolo. 1994. Reliability of percutaneous intramuscular electrodes for upper extremity functional neuromuscular stimulation in adolescents with C5 tetraplegia. *Archives of Physical Medicine and Rehabilitation* 75(9):939–945.

Triolo, R.J., R.R. Betz, M.J. Mulcahey, and E.R. Gardner. 1994. Application of functional neuromuscular stimulation to children with spinal cord injuries: Candidate selection for upper and lower extremity research. *Paraplegia* 32(12):824–843.

Part VI

Musculoskeletal System

Arthritic Hand and Wrist

DESCRIPTION
Arthritis causes changes in the structure and function of the hand and wrist.

Hand Deformities Associated with Osteoarthritis
- *Bouchard's node* involves osteophyte formation (node) in the proximal interphalangeal (PIP) joint that changes the look of the hand and may cause changes in the functional use of the fingers.
- *Heberden's node* involves osteophyte formation (node) in the distal interphalangeal (DIP) joint that changes the look of the hand and may cause changes in the functional use of the fingers.
- *Nabebuff Type II deformity of the thumb* involves hyperextension at the interphalangeal joint, flexion at the metacarpophalangeal joint, and subluxation of the carpometacarpal joint that reduces the functional use of the thumb.
- *Trigger finger* is a limitation of all finger movements due to a module on a tendon or narrowing of the tendon sheath that is most apparent in hand grasp functions.
- *Volar subluxation of the wrist or metacarpophalangeal* is loss of the integrity of the joint due to weakened ligaments, which changes the dynamic structure and function of the hand, thereby reducing the effectiveness of hand movements.

Hand Deformities Associated with Rheumatoid Arthritis
- *Boutonniere deformity* results in DIP hyperextension and PIP flexion, which may "lock" the joint, reducing the functional use of the finger.
- *Joint laxity* is caused by instability of the collateral ligaments, which may interfere with the movement and function of the joints.
- *Nabebuff Type I deformity of the thumb* involves hyperextension at the interphalangeal joint and flexion at the metacarpophalangeal joint that reduces the functional use of the thumb.
- *Nabebuff Type II deformity of the thumb* involves hyperextension at the interphalangeal joint, flexion at the metacarpophalangeal joint, and subluxation of the carpometacarpal joint (rare in rheumatoid arthritis) that reduces the functional use of the thumb.
- *Nabebuff Type III deformity of the thumb* involves flexion at the interphalangeal joint, hyperextension at the metacarpophalangeal joint, and subluxation of the carpometacarpal joint that reduces the functional use of the thumb.
- *Swan neck deformity* results in PIP hyperextension and DIP flexion, which "locks" the finger, reducing the functional use of the finger.
- *Ulnar drift or deviation* involves joint changes, especially destruction of and loosening of the radial collateral ligaments, that allow the metacarpophalangeal joints to move medially (anatomic position) or laterally (functional hand position) as a group, thereby reducing the grasp and grip functions of the hand, especially between the thumb and index fingers.

CAUSE
The arthritic hand and wrist disorders are associated with the factors involved in osteoarthritis, rheumatoid arthritis, and other arthritic conditions, including synovitis and tenosyno-

vitis. The stiffening and tightening in the hand may be due to edema, fibrosis, collagen alternation, anatomic changes in joint alignment, and inflammation.

ASSESSMENT

Areas
*   daily living skills: personal and instrumental activities of daily living
*   productivity history, skills, interests, and values
*   leisure skills and interests
*   grip and pinch strength (An average grip strength of 20 pounds and an average pinch strength of 5 to 7 pounds are considered necessary to perform most daily living activities.)
*   muscle strength based on performance of functional activities
*   range of motion: active, passive, and total
*   fine motor skills, coordination, manipulation, and dexterity
*   hand functions
*   joint stability
*   vasomotor changes, such as being red or warm to the touch
*   trophic changes, such as brittle nails, pulp atrophy, and hyperemia
*   pain and swelling
*   sensory registration
*   coping skills

Instruments
*   *Arthritis Hand Function Test* by C. Backman, H. Mackie, and J. Harris, in *Occupational Therapy Journal of Research* 11 (1991): 245–255.
*   *Assessment of Motor and Process Skills* (AMPS), 2nd ed. by A.G. Fisher, Fort Collins, CO: Three Star Press, 1997.
*   *Box and Block Test* by P. Holser and E. Fuchs, in F.S. Cromwell, ed., in Primary prevocational evaluation: Occupational therapists manual for basic skills assessment. Pasadena, CA: Fair Oaks Printing Company, 1965. For adult norms see V. Mathiowetz et al., in Adult norms for the Box and Block Test of manual dexterity, *American Journal of Occupational Therapy* 39, no. 6 (1985): 386–391. Test available from Sammons Preston, Bolingbrook, IL.
*   *Canadian Occupational Performance Measure* (COPM), 2nd ed. by M. Law et al., Ottawa, Canada: Canadian Association of Occupational Therapists, 1994.
*   *Jebsen Hand Function Test* by R.H. Jebsen et al., in *Archives of Physical Medicine and Rehabilitation* 50 (1969): 311–319.
*   *Moberg Pickup Test* by E. Moberg, in *Journal of Bone and Joint Surgery* 40 (1958): 454–459.
*   *Nine Hole Peg Test* by M. Kellor et al., in Hand strength and dexterity: Norms for clinical use, *American Journal of Occupational Therapy* 25, no. 1 (1971): 77–83. For adult norms see V. Mathiowetz et al., in Adult norms for the Nine Hole Peg Test of finger dexterity, *Occupational Therapy Journal of Research* 5, no. 1 (1985): 25–38. Test available from Sammons Preston, Bolingbrook, IL.
*   *Purdue Pegboard Test* by J. Tiffin, Lafayette, IN: Lafayette Instrument Co., 1960.

- *TEMPA* by J. Desrosier et al., in Upper extremity performance test for the elderly (TEMPA): Normative data and correlates with sensorimotor parameters, *Archives of Physical Medicine and Rehabilitation* 76, no. 12 (1995): 1125–1129.
- *Visual Analog Scale* by E.C. Husskinsson, in *Lancet* 2, no. 7889 (1974): 1127–1131.
- dynamometer or sphygmomanometer and pinch meter
- goniometer
- activities of daily living scale
- productive history, skills, and values instruments
- leisure checklist

PROBLEMS

Self-Care
- The person usually has experienced difficulty performing self-care and daily activities because of pain, loss of range of motion, or loss of grip or pinch strength.

Productivity
- The person usually has experienced difficulty performing productive activities in the home or at work due to pain, loss of range of motion, or loss of grip or pinch strength.
- The person may be performing productive activities in a manner that is harmful to the joints.

Leisure
- The person may be performing leisure activities that are harmful to the joints.
- The person may have given up many leisure activities because of pain, loss of range of motion, or loss of grip or pinch strength.

Sensorimotor
- The person may have weak grip and pinch strength below the minimum required to perform daily living activities.
- The person may have limited range of motion.
- The person may have deformities such as ulnar deviation of the wrist, swan neck deformity, boutonniere deformity, nodules, joint subluxation, joint dislocation, and bone spurs.
- The person may have poor manipulative and dexterity skills.
- The person may have instability in joints, such as the carpometacarpal joint of the thumb.
- The person may have muscle atrophy (intrinsics).
- Some joints may become immobile due to the disease process (tightness of the intrinsics), and other joints may be immobilized by the person to reduce pain.
- The person usually has pain.

Cognitive
- Chronic pain may reduce problem-solving skills.
- The person may have cognitive disorders not directly related to the arthritic disorder.

Psychosocial

• The person may report frustration and annoyance at being unable to use the involved finger(s) and hands to accomplish intended actions.
• The person may be concerned about the visual appearance of the hand and being considered disabled.

TREATMENT/INTERVENTION

Major models of treatment are biomechanical, compensatory, environmental modification, and assistive technology.

Self-Care

• Compensatory techniques may be needed to continue function.
• Self-help aids, such as enlarged handles or extended handles, should help improve performance of self-care and daily living activities.

Productivity

• Modifications to the arrangement of the home or work environment may be needed.
• Adapted equipment, such as grippers to open jars, should help productivity.

Leisure

• Explore and develop leisure activities that do not aggravate the disorder.
• The person's favorite leisure activities may be adapted to eliminate or decrease the undesirable aspects of the activity.

Sensorimotor

• Maintain or increase muscle, grip, and pinch strength through the performance of daily living activities and selected exercise and activities as needed.
• Maintain or increase range of motion through the performance of daily living activities and selected exercise and activities as needed.
• Maintain or increase manipulative and dexterity skills.
• Consider splinting to maintain good position or alignment, such as a volar resting splint or ulnar deviation splint, and to provide joint stabilization, such as a thumb splint, wrist stabilization splint, or protective metacarpophalengeal (MP) splint.
• Consider splinting to relieve pain, such as a wrist cock-up splint.

Cognitive

• Instruct the person in joint protection, especially of the hand.
• Instruct the person in energy conservation, pacing, and work simplification to reduce stress on the hands.
• Instruct the person in the progress of the disease, including the role of synovitis and tenosynovitis as related to hand dysfunction and the importance of preventive maintenance.

PRECAUTIONS

- The person should avoid static holding positions of the hands and small, repetitive actions, such as writing by hand or knitting. Activity should be divided into short sessions of about 10 minutes followed by a short break to move the fingers (flex and extend); or the person should avoid the activity by using a device such as a book holder to hold the object.
- The person should avoid placing weight on the radial side of the hand and fingers. The person should use the heel of the palm.
- The person should avoid holding small objects that require a strong grip. Enlarged handles will help.
- The person should avoid pulling him- or herself to a standing position with the hands. Instead, the person should push off with weight on the palms of the hands.
- The person should avoid twisting movements of the hand, wrist, and thumb, such as opening sealed jars.

PROGNOSIS AND OUTCOME

- The person is able to perform self-care and instrumental daily activities independently with self-help devices, if needed.
- The person is able to perform productive activities using adapted equipment or environmental modifications, if needed.
- The person is able to perform leisure activities.
- The person is able to maintain or increase grip and pinch strength.
- The person is able to maintain or increase range of motion in the upper extremity.
- The person is able to use his or her hands for functional activities.
- The person is wearing a splint, if prescribed, for the purpose specified.
- The person demonstrates knowledge of joint protection techniques.
- The person demonstrates knowledge of energy conservation, pacing, and work simplification techniques.

BIBLIOGRAPHY

Adams, R.C. 1995. Patients with arthritis in hands require custom-made splints. *Advance for Occupational Therapists* 11, no. 30: 17, 19.

Agnew, P.J., and F. Maas. 1995. Compliance in wearing wrist working splints in rheumatoid arthritis. *Occupational Therapy Journal of Research* 15, no. 3: 165–180.

Backman, C., and H. Mackie. 1993. Arthritis Hand Function Test: Inter-rater reliability among self-trained raters. *Arthritis Care and Research* 6, no. 1: 10–15.

Backman, C., and H. Mackie. 1996. The Arthritis Hand Function Test. *Physical Disabilities Special Interest Section Newsletter* 19, no. 4: 1–2.

Backman, C., and H. Mackie. 1997. Reliability and validity of the Arthritis Hand Function Test in adults with osteoarthritis. *Occupational Therapy Journal of Research* 17, no. 1: 55–66.

Callinan, N.J., and V. Mathiowetz. 1996. Soft versus hard resting hand splints in rheumatoid arthritis: Pain relief, preference, and compliance. *American Journal of Occupational Therapy* 50, no. 5: 347–353.

Collins, L.F. 1996. Hand therapy for clients with arthritis. *OT Practice* 1, no. 4: 28–29, 31, 33.

Dellhag, B., and S. Burckhardt. 1995. Predictors of hand function in patients with rheumatoid arthritis. *Arthritis Care and Research* 8, no. 1: 16–20.

Desrosier, J. et al. 1995. Upper extremity performance test for the elderly (TEMPA): Normative data and correlates with sensorimotor parameters. *Archives of Physical Medicine and Rehabilitation* 76, no. 12: 1125–1129.

Emerson, S.A. 1993. The rheumatoid hand: Postoperative splint options. *Journal of Hand Therapy* 6, no. 3: 214–215.

Falconer, J.A. 1996. Hand splinting in rheumatoid arthritis: A perspective on current knowledge and directions for research. In *Rehabilitation of persons with rheumatoid arthritis,* ed. R.W. Chang, 103–108. Gaithersburg, MD: Aspen Publishers.

Feinberg, J.R., and C.A. Trombly. 1995. Arthritis. In *Occupational therapy for physical dysfunction,* 4th ed., 815–830. Baltimore: Williams & Wilkins.

Glassman, S. 1998. Managing osteoarthritis of the hand: Balance rest, activity is vital. *Advance for Occupational Therapists* 14, no. 18: 19–20.

Klinger, J.L. 1997. The client with arthritis. In *Meal planning and training: The healthcare professional's guide,* ed. J.L. Klinger, 63–68. Thorofare, NJ: Slack.

Kurtz, P.E. 1977. Conservative treatment of arthritis. In *Hand rehabilitation: A practical guide,* 2nd ed., eds. G.L. Clark et al., 395–400. New York: Churchill Livingstone.

Mann, W.C. et al. 1995. Assistive devices used by home-based elderly persons with arthritis. *American Journal of Occupational Therapy* 49, no. 8: 810–820.

Melvin, J.L. 1994. Self-care strategies for persons with arthritis and connective tissue diseases. In *Ways of living: Self-care strategies for special needs,* ed. C.H. Christiansen, 157–188. Rockville, MD: American Occupational Therapy Association.

Melvin, J.L. 1995. *Osteoarthritis: Caring for Your Hands.* Bethesda, MD: American Occupational Therapy Association.

Phillips, C.A. 1995. Therapist's management of patients with rheumatoid arthritis. In *Rehabilitation of the hand: Surgery and therapy,* 4th ed., eds. J.M. Hunter et al., 1345–1350. St. Louis, MO: Mosby.

Sobel, D., and A.C. Klein. 1993. *Arthritis: What Exercises Work.* New York: St. Martin's Press.

Terrono, A.L. et al. 1995. The rheumatoid thumb. In *Rehabilitation of the hand: Surgery and therapy,* 4th ed., eds. J.M. Hunter et al., 1329–1343. St. Louis, MO: Mosby.

Arthritis—Juvenile Rheumatoid

DESCRIPTION

Juvenile rheumatoid arthritis is a chronic syndrome characterized by nonspecific, usually systemic, inflammation of the peripheral joints that begins before the person reaches 16 years of age. It can be divided into three types: (1) systemic onset (Still's disease) often begins with a high fever and rash and affects multiple joints plus other organ systems, including the spleen, liver, and lymph nodes; (2) pauciarticular onset usually affects only a limited number of joints, such as the knee, hip, ankle, or elbow joints, often asymmetrically, and is accompanied by iridocyclitis, an inflamed condition of the iris and ciliary body of the eye that can lead to blindness if not treated; and (3) polyarticular onset may be abrupt and painful, with symmetrical involvement of the joints, such as hands, wrists, feet, ankles, knees, and sometimes the cervical vertebrae of the spine, plus other symptoms, such as weight loss, low-grade fever, and general malaise.

The systemic type, also called juvenile chronic arthritis, was first described by George F. Still in 1897. The criteria for diagnosis were last revised in 1977 as follows: (1) the disease must be present before the person is 16 years old; (2) true arthritis in one or more joints must be evident for at least six weeks; (3) the arthritic joint must show signs of swelling or limitation of movement, with heat, pain, or tenderness; and (4) the disease must not be attributable to any other known cause (e.g., infection, trauma, or disease such as systemic lupus erythematosus or rheumatic fever) (Bender et al. 1994, 143).

CAUSE

The cause is unknown. Possible causes include genetic disorders, psychological trauma, viruses, histocompatibility antigens, and antigen-antibody immune complexes. The percentage of cases is about 20 percent systemic, 40 percent pauciarticular, and 40 percent polyarticular (Merck 1999, 2402). Some references say 10 percent systemic and 50 percent polyarticular. About equal numbers of boys and girls have the systemic type, which can occur at any time from birth to 16 years. The ratio of polyarticular is 3:1 girls to boys. The onset may be at any age but most commonly is between 1 year and 3 years of age. The ratio of pauciarticular is 5:1 boys to girls, with the onset usually before age 10. Boys with the pauciarticular type are at risk for developing spondyloarthropathy (arthritis of the spine) in later life.

ASSESSMENT

Areas
- daily living skills: personal and instrumental activities of daily living
- productivity history, values, skills, and interests
- play skills
- leisure skills and interests
- developmental milestones
- range of motion, passive and active
- muscle strength, grip strength, and pinch strength
- muscle spasms
- gross motor development, coordination, and skills
- fine motor development, coordination, manipulation, dexterity
- physical endurance
- ambulation and physical mobility
- joint stiffness, inflammation, or swelling
- joint integrity, mobility, and stability (Note laxity, tendon alignment, rheumatoid nodules, crepitation, or subluxation.)
- reflex maturation (Note especially the development of equilibrium and protective and righting reactions.)
- balance and postural control
- posture (Note leg length, position of pelvis, and any deformities.)
- motor planning or praxis
- edema in joints: presence of effusion, synovial thickening, heat, and redness

- pain and child's perception of the pain
- sensory registration
- visual perception
- attention and concentration
- self-concept
- affect or mood
- social skills
- communication skills, especially assertiveness
- architectural or environmental barriers or accessibility
- home safety

Instruments

Instruments Developed by Occupational Therapy Personnel

- *Functional Independence Measure for Children* (WeeFIM) by Uniform Data System for Medical Rehabilitation, Buffalo, NY: State University of New York at Buffalo, 1993.
- *Klein-Bell Activities of Daily Living Scale* by R.M. Klein and B. Bell, Seattle, WA: University of Washington, 1982.
- *Pediatric Evaluation of Disability Inventory* (PEDI) by S. Haley et al., San Antonio, TX: Psychological Corporation-Therapy Skill Builders, 1992.
- *Tufts Assessment of Motor Performance* by B.M. Gang, S.M. Haley, and S.C. Hallenborg, in *American Journal of Physical Medicine and Rehabilitation* 67 (1989): 202–210.

Instruments Developed by Other Professionals and Used by Occupational Therapy Personnel

- *Bruininks-Oseretsky Test of Motor Proficiency* (BOTMP) by R.H. Bruininks, Circle Pines, MN: American Guidance Services, 1978.
- *Childhood Arthritis Health Profile* (CAHP) by L.B. Tucker, in The Childhood Arthritis Health Profile (CAHP): Validity and reliability of the condition-specific scales, *Arthritis and Rheumatism* 38 (1995): S183. (Abstract; questionnaire)
- *Childhood Arthritis Impact Measurement Scale* (CAIMS) by C. Coulton et al., in Assessment of the reliability of the Arthritis Impact Scales for children with juvenile arthritis, *Arthritis and Rheumatism* 30 (1987): 819–824. (Questionnaire)
- *Childhood Health Assessment Questionnaire* (CHAQ) by G. Singh et al., in Measurement of functional status in juvenile rheumatoid arthritis, *Arthritis and Rheumatism* 37 (1990): 1761–1769. (Self-report questionnaire)
- *The Beery-Buktenica Developmental Test of Visual-Motor Integration* (VMI-4), 4th ed. by K.E. Beery and N.A. Buktenica, Parisppany, NJ: Modern Curriculum Press, 1997.
- *Juvenile Arthritis Functional Assessment Report* (JAFAR) by S. Howe et al., in Development of a disability measurement tool for juvenile rheumatoid arthritis: The Juvenile Arthritis Functional Assessment Report for Children and Their Parents, *Arthritis and Rheumatism* 34 (1991): 873–880. (Self-report of parent report questionnaire)
- *Juvenile Arthritis Functional Assessment Scale* (JAFAS) by D.J. Lowell et al., in Development of a disability measurement tool for juvenile rheumatoid arthritis: The Juvenile Arthritis Functional Assessment Scale, *Arthritis and Rheumatism* 32 (1989): 1390–1395. (Rating scale)

- *Juvenile Arthritis Quality of Life Questionnaire* (JAQQ) by C.M. Duffy, L. Arsenault, and K.N.W. Duffy, in Level of agreement between parents and children in rating dysfunction in juvenile rheumatoid arthritis and juvenile spondyloarthritis, *Journal of Rheumatology* 20 (1993): 2134–2139. (Questionnaire)
- *Juvenile Arthritis Self-Report Index* (JASI) by F.V. Wright et al., in Development of a self-report functional status index for juvenile rheumatoid arthritis, *Journal of Rheumatology* 21 (1994): 536–544. (Self-report questionnaire)
- *Mother and Child Rating Scales* by B. Egeland, L. Croufe, and D. Rahe, Minneapolis, MN: Mother-Child Project, University of Minnesota, 1978.
- *Motor-Free Visual Perception Test—Revised* (MVPT-R) by R. Colarusso and D.D. Hamill, Novato, CA: Academic Therapy Publications, 1995.
- *Peabody Developmental Motor Scales* (PDMS) by M.R. Folio and R.R. Fewell, Austin, TX: Pro-Ed, 1983.
- *Test of Visual-Motor Skills—Revised* (TVMS-R) by M.F. Gardner, Hydesville, CA: Psychological and Educational Publications, 1995.
- *Test of Visual-Perceptual Skills (Non-motor)—Revised* (TVPS-R) by M.F. Gardner, Hydesville, CA: Psychological and Educational Publications, 1996.
- *Vineland Adaptive Behavior Scales—Revised* (VABS-R) by S.S. Sparrow, D.A. Balla, and D.V. Cicchetti, Circle Pines, MN: American Guidance Services, 1984.
- dynamometer and pinch meter
- goniometer

PROBLEMS

Self-Care
- The person may be unable to perform certain activities of daily living due to wrist or hand involvement.
- The person may be behind his or her chronological age in developmental skills associated with self-care, especially dressing skills.

Productivity
- The person may have difficulty performing hand and wrist activities, such as holding a pencil or pen.
- The person may have difficulty sitting comfortably for productive activities.

Leisure
- The person may be unable to participate in sports that require standing or walking for long periods of time or running, jumping, or climbing.

Sensorimotor
- The person may have limited joint range of motion.
- The person may have tightness or flexion contractures of hips, knees, or elbows.
- The person may have morning stiffness, inflammation, and swelling of the joints.
- The person may have difficulty walking due to unequal growth in the long bones, instability of the pelvis, scoliosis, or pain.

- The person may fatigue easily and have low endurance.
- The person may have weak hand grasp and weakness in affected joints, especially the hips, neck, quadriceps, wrist extensors, and finger flexors and extensors.
- The person may have ligament (joint) instability, subluxation, or dislocation.
- The person may have developmental delays in gross motor skills, especially in running, hopping, and standing on one leg.
- The person may have developmental delays in fine motor skills.
- The person may have muscle spasms, especially in the wrist flexors and knee extensors.
- The person may have poor posture.
- The person may have underdeveloped equilibrium and protective and righting reactions.
- The person may have loss of sight (pauciarticular form).
- The person frequently has pain in affected joints.

Cognitive
- Cognitive faculties are usually not affected directly by the disorder, but taking notes regarding the person's attending behavior, concentration, and interest in learning will be useful in program management.

Psychosocial
- The person may feel a loss of self-esteem and self-confidence.
- The person may have feelings of being different.
- The person may become depressed.
- The person may become irritable.
- The person may become listless.
- The person may develop a dependency on others.
- The person may express hostility.
- The person may be uncooperative during treatment.

TREATMENT/INTERVENTION

Models of treatment include normal growth and development, prevention, biomechanical, and rehabilitation (compensatory).

Self-Care
- Provide opportunity for mastery of independence in as many self-care activities as possible.
- Recommend or teach adapted techniques as needed to increase functional independence. Examples include wearing loose-fitting clothing and using Velcro and/or elastic thread for fastenings.
- Provide adaptive equipment, such as reachers and elongated handles, to help the person compensate for limited range of motion.
- Provide enlarged handles, lightweight utensils, elastic shoelaces, an electric toothbrush, and button hooks to help the person compensate for weakened grasp or backpacks to reduce the need to grasp.

Productivity
- Provide children with opportunities to develop play skills and promote play development.

- Help people explore vocational interests in view of physical limitations.
- Assist in evaluating and recommending changes in living quarters (home or apartment).
- Assist in reorganizing the person's kitchen to permit easier reach of utensils and food items.
- Help teachers to develop routines that permit the person to change positions and activities every 20 to 30 minutes to decrease static positioning.

Leisure

- Encourage continuous motion activities such as creative dance, bicycle riding, swimming, or walking.
- Explore and assist in developing interests that may be explored during the rest periods required when exacerbations occur.
- Recommend adapted equipment for leisure activities if such equipment will facilitate participation.

Sensorimotor

- Consider splinting the affected joints to prevent flexion contractures and increase function. Resting splints, cock-up splints, ulnar gutter splints, or stabilizing splints may be helpful. If contractures have already occurred, splints can be used to prevent further deforming and promote soft tissue lengthening. Wearing a splint at night can reduce morning stiffness.
- Maintain or increase range of motion using activities such as swimming, riding a tricycle or bicycle, creative dance, and hitting softballs, but be careful about doing activities that force the joints or require resistive motions.
- Increase muscle strength using isometric rather than resistive exercises.
- Increase physical endurance and cardiovascular fitness through such activities as walking, swimming, and cycling.
- Promote reflex maturation through using tilt boards, rocking boards, and large balls and bicycle riding.
- Promote gross motor development through games such as hopscotch, obstacle courses, and kickball.
- Promote fine motor development through activities and games requiring manipulation, various hand grasps, and dexterity, such as playing with pop beads, squeezing and rolling clay, and lacing cards.
- Splints may be useful to decrease pain in inflamed joints.
- Provide sensory stimulation, including tactile, proprioceptive, and vestibular.
- A pain management program may be useful to control pain.

Cognitive

- Instruct the person and his or her family on how to use warm compresses and a paraffin bath, if indicated.
- Instruct the person and his or her family in joint protection and positioning techniques. For example, the person can lie prone for 20 minutes to relax joints and prevent flexion contractures of the knees.
- Instruct the person and his or her family in time management to organize self-care, resting, productivity, and leisure activities.
- Instruct the person and his or her family in energy conservation, pacing, and work simplification.

- Instruct the person and his or her family in a home therapy program and encourage compliance. Videotaping the home program may be useful.

Psychosocial

- Provide the person with opportunities to increase self-concept and self-esteem through creative activities, such as art, crafts, dance, drama, or music.
- Provide opportunities to express feelings and emotions through discussion, role playing, or creative outlets.
- Use behavior modification techniques to achieve cooperation with specific objectives of treatment.
- Encourage the person and family to identify specific roles for the person within the family that are not associated with the sick or disabled role.
- Encourage the person to participate in social activities.

Environment

- Encourage the person and his or her family to participate in a self-help group and use other community resources.
- Assist in teaching the person and family about the disease, its possible causes, and its course.
- Help the family respond constructively to the disease.

PRECAUTIONS

- Watch for signs of deformity.
- Watch for signs of tendon rupture.
- Generally, have the person avoid activities that require placing his or her total body weight on non–weight-bearing joints, such as doing handstands, doing cartwheels, or crutch walking.
- Generally, have the person avoid activities that require repeated pounding of a joint, such as jumping rope, doing jumping jacks, or jogging.
- Generally, contact sports, such as football or boxing, should be avoided, but cycling and swimming may be tolerated.
- Generally, the person should avoid being in static positions for long periods of time. Break routines into short periods of time.
- Aspirin is not used with young children because of the concern about Reye's syndrome.
- Complications and side effects of the systemic type are growth retardation and delayed development of sexual characteristics.
- Complications and side effects of the polyarticular type are growth retardation, delayed development of sexual characteristics, and subcutaneous nodules attached to tendon sheaths.
- A complication of the pauciarticular type is iridocyclitis that develops into functional blindness.

PROGNOSIS AND OUTCOME

Approximately 50 percent to 75 percent of cases recover completely within one to two years from the onset of juvenile rheumatoid arthritis. Persons with polyarticular onset and positive rheumatoid factors have a less favorable prognosis. About 15 percent of those with the polyarticular type have permanent disabilities.

- The person has normal range of motion for his or her age or functional range of motion if permanent disability remains.
- The person has normal muscle strength in all muscle groups or maximum muscle strength given the degree of permanent disability.
- The person has normal endurance and cardiovascular fitness.
- The person has functional mobility, whether by ambulation or powered mobility.
- The person has achieved normal developmental levels for his or her age.
- The person demonstrates knowledge and use of joint protection techniques.
- The person demonstrates knowledge and use of energy conservation, pacing, and work simplification techniques.
- The person demonstrates knowledge of a home program, if needed, including using heat modalities, wearing splints, and taking medications.
- The person is able to perform daily living activities with self-help devices if needed.
- The person is able to perform productive activities.
- The person is able to perform leisure activities.
- The person and his or her family are knowledgeable about community resources.

REFERENCES

Beers, M.H., and R. Berkow, eds. 1999. *The Merck Manual of Diagnosis and Therapy*, 17th ed. Whitehouse Station, NJ: Merck Research Laboratories.

Bender, L. et al. 1994. The effects of juvenile rheumatoid arthritis on functional development: A literature review. *British Journal of Occupational Therapy* 57, no. 4: 143–147.

BIBLIOGRAPHY

Abdel-Moty, A.R. 1997. A chance encounter with arthritis. *Advance for Occupational Therapists* 13, no. 41: 11.

Brown, E.J. et al. 1998. The Glenn Rispler story: A story of JRA. *Advance for Occupational Therapy Practitioners* 14, no. 44: 22–23. (Case report)

Brown, G.T. 1996. A review of functional assessment measures for pediatric clients with juvenile rheumatoid arthritis. *Occupational Therapy International* 3, no. 4: 284–299.

Dorries, T. 1996. "I thought the doctor must be crazy. . . ." *Advance for Occupational Therapists* 12, no. 43: 13, 17. (Case report)

Dunn, W. 1993. Grip strength of children aged 3 to 7 years using a modified sphygmomanometer: Comparison of typical children with rheumatic disorders. *American Journal of Occupational Therapy* 47, no. 5: 421–428.

Goodman, S. 1998. A closer look at the many faces of JRA. *Advance for Occupational Therapy Practitioners* 14, no. 44: 24–26, 30.

Hackett, J. et al. 1996. Physiotherapy and occupational therapy for juvenile chronic arthritis: Custom and practice in five centres in the UK, USA, and Canada. *British Journal of Rheumatology* 35, no. 7: 695–699.

Hafner, R. et al. 1998. Rehabilitation in children with juvenile chronic arthritis. *Bailliere's Clinical Rheumatology* 12, no. 2: 329–361.

Liburd, N.L. 1996. Meeting the classroom needs of kids with arthritis. *Advance for Occupational Therapists* 12, no. 43: 12, 16.

Reichley, M.L. 1995. Aquatic program offers kids with JRA relief, fun. *Advance for Occupational Therapists* 11, no. 37: 16.

Spraul, G., and G. Koenning. 1994. A descriptive study of foot problems in children with juvenile rheumatoid arthritis. *Arthritis Care and Research* 7, no. 3: 144–150.

Tomcheck, S.D. 1999. The musculoskeletal system: Juvenile rheumatoid arthritis. In *Pediatric therapy: A systems approach*, eds. S.M. Porr and E.B. Rainville, 230–236. Philadelphia: F.A. Davis.

Arthritis—Osteoarthritis

DESCRIPTION

Osteoarthritis is a progressive disorder characterized by altered hyaline cartilage, loss of articular cartilage, and hypertrophy of bone, producing osteophytes. Osteoarthritis is the most common articular disorder (Merck 1999, 449). It is also called degenerative joint disease or hypertrophic osteoarthritis.

CAUSE

Osteoarthritis appears to be the result of a complex system of interacting mechanical, biological, biochemical, and enzymatic feedback loops. Factors include congenital joint abnormalities; genetic defects; infections; metabolic, endocrine, and neuropathic diseases; diseases of the hyaline cartilage, such as rheumatoid arthritis or gout; acute trauma, such as a fracture; and chronic trauma that may occur in certain occupations. Traditionally, osteoarthritis has been divided into two broad groups, primary or idiopathic and secondary, which is due to a known cause. Onset usually occurs when the person is in his or her twenties and thirties but is almost universal by age 70. Both men and women are affected, but loss of hand function is greatest in women.

ASSESSMENT

Areas

- daily living skills: personal and instrumental activities of daily living
- productivity history, skills, and interests
- leisure skills and interests
- range of motion
- muscle strength, including grip and pinch strength
- hand functions
- fine motor coordination, manipulation, and dexterity
- functional mobility, especially walking
- work tolerance, especially bending, lifting, and carrying

- physical endurance
- pain and swelling
- self-concept
- architectural or environmental barriers
- home safety

Instruments

Instruments Developed by Occupational Therapy Personnel

- *Kenny Self-Care Evaluation* by I.A. Iversen et al., Minneapolis, MN: Sister Kenny Institute Abbort-Northwestern Hospital, 1973.
- *Smith Hand Function Evaluation* by H.B. Smith, in *American Journal of Occupational Therapy* 27 (1973): 244–251.
- occupational history
- leisure checklist
- goniometer
- manual muscle test, dynamometer, and pinch meter

Instruments Developed by Other Professionals and Used by Occupational Therapy Personnel

- *Arthritis Evaluation Checklist* by W. Buckner, in Arthritic diseases, *Occupational therapy: Practice skills for physical dysfunction,* 4th ed., ed. L.W. Pedretti, 441–442, St. Louis, MO: Mosby, 1996.
- *Functional Independence Measure,* 4th ed. by Uniform Data System for Medical Rehabilitation, Buffalo, NY: Research Foundation, State University of New York at Buffalo, 1993.
- *Stanford Health Assessment Questionnaire* by J.F. Fries, in Measurement of patient outcome in arthritis, *Arthritis and Rheumatology* 23 (1980): 137–145.
- *Visual Analogue Scales* by E.C. Huskisson, J. Jones, and P.J. Scot, in *Rheumatology and Rehabilitation* 15 (1976): 185–187.

PROBLEMS

Self-Care

- Performance of self-care and daily living activities may become more difficult, especially in the morning, due to stiffness.

Productivity

- Performance of some job tasks may become impossible or very difficult.
- The person may not be able to continue in his or her present job.

Leisure

- The person may find that engaging in rigorous sports causes excessive pain.
- Activities that require static holding may also become painful.

Sensorimotor

- The person usually has limited range of motion. In the hand, the joints that are most commonly involved are the distal interphalangeal joints and the trapeziometacarpal joint of the thumb. The proximal interphalangeal joints may be involved, but the metacarpal phalangeal joints are involved only rarely. In the wrist, loss of motion is greatest in wrist flexion.

- The person may experience morning stiffness following inactivity, but improvement occurs with exercise. Stiffness also occurs after 15 to 30 minutes of static positioning.
- The person may develop flexion contractures.
- The person's joints may be enlarged and deformed.
- Heberden's or Bouchard's nodes (bone overgrowths) may be present on the fingers.
- The person may experience muscle spasm, and muscle inhibition may occur.
- The person may experience crepitation upon movement.
- The person may have muscle weakness and disuse atrophy.
- The person may lack endurance and become easily fatigued, especially if pain is present.
- The person may have inflammation of the joint.
- The person usually has pain upon movement of certain joints, especially in certain motions or exercises.
- The person may experience aching during cold weather.
- The person's body image (sense of self) may be altered.

Cognitive

- Cognitive faculties are not affected directly by the disorder, but cognitive disorders may be present due to other causes.

Psychosocial

- The person may complain of feeling old because of movement limitations.
- The person may feel less able to cope.
- The person may experience loss of self-concept.
- The person may become emotionally and physically dependent on others.
- The person may become demanding.

TREATMENT/INTERVENTION

The model of treatment is based on the biomechanical model (to maintain joint mobility and muscle strength) or the compensatory model (to enable the person to cope with everyday living). Assistive devices and environmental modification may also be needed.

Self-Care

- Increase or maintain the person's ability to perform activities of daily living with less trauma to the joints.
- Provide self-help devices to assist in performing activities of daily living, such as built-up handles, elongated handles, or reachers. Alternate techniques, such as using both hands to lift, should also be considered.
- Suggest modifications of furniture, such as elevated chairs, high beds, sofas with firm padding, and armrests, to assist in getting up.
- Suggest wearing loose-fitting clothing with front openings to make dressing and undressing easier.

Productivity

- Encourage the person to participate in productive activities, including volunteer activities, paid employment, home management, and classes or senior citizen meetings.
- Provide assistance in dealing with barriers to participation in the home and in the workplace.

Leisure

- Encourage the person to continue exploring old interests and develop new ones.
- Suggest modifications that may help the person to continue participating in leisure activities.

Sensorimotor

- Maintain or increase functional range of motion. Immersing hands in warm water or using paraffin wax treatments before doing range of motion exercises may be useful. Stiffness may be helped by use of pressure gradient or cotton stretch gloves.
- Consider using splints to prevent flexion contractures of the fingers (finger gutter splint) and provide thumb stability at the carpometacarpal joint for better pinch grasp (thumb post splint). Other commonly used splints are the wrist cock-up splint and the volar resting hand splint.
- Mild graded physical activities and exercises can improve movement patterns and reduce stiffness. Aerobic exercise under water is now considered useful in maintaining musculoskeletal function.
- Increase muscle strength, especially around the affected joints, to increase stability.
- Reduce joint stress and practice correct joint use for lifting, or suggest alternate methods for accomplishing a task.
- Maintain mobility, especially in walking, by encouraging the person to take daily walks.
- A pain management program may be useful.
- Body image may improve along with the person's ability to move.
- Splints, especially for the hand and neck, may reduce pain.

Cognitive

- Instruct the person in energy conservation, pacing, and work simplification.
- Instruct the person in joint protection.
- Instruct the person in home safety and reduction of architectural barriers.

Psychosocial

- Increase self-concept and sense of mastery.
- Provide training in relaxation techniques to reduce muscle tension and pain.
- Encourage the person to continue social activities.

PRECAUTIONS

- The person should not be encouraged to overdo any activity.
- If splints are provided, check for redness or discomfort.
- Discourage the person from sleeping prone, using more than one pillow, or using other unusual sleeping positions. Recommend a cervical pillow instead.

PROGNOSIS AND OUTCOME

Osteoarthritis is a slowly progressive disorder. Management depends on the person's willingness to avoid activities and situations that tend to accelerate the progression and to learn to live within the limitations of the disorder.

- The person has maintained functional range of motion, using splints if necessary.
- The person has maintained hand functions, pinch, and grasp, using splints if necessary.
- The person demonstrates knowledge and use of joint protection techniques.
- The person demonstrates knowledge and use of energy conservation and work simplification techniques.
- The person continues to walk independently.
- The person is able to perform daily living activities, using self-help devices if needed.
- The person is able to perform productive activities, using splints or other adaptations, if needed.
- The person is able to perform leisure activities.
- The person has a modified living environment to promote safety, mobility, and functional performance of self-care and home management activities.

REFERENCE

Beers, M.H., and R. Berkow, eds. 1999. *The Merck Manual of Diagnosis and Therapy*, 17th ed. Whitehouse Station, NJ: Merck Research Laboratories.

BIBLIOGRAPHY

Barton, R., and J. Feinberg. 1998. The role of occupational therapy. In *Osteoarthritis*, eds. K.D. Brant et al., 315–324. Oxford, England: Oxford University Press.

Block, J.A., and T.J. Schnitzer. 1997. Therapeutic approaches to osteoarthritis. *Hospital Practice* (office ed.) 32, no. 2: 159–164.

Coppard, B.M. et al. 1998. Working with elders who have orthopedic conditions: Arthritis. In *Occupational therapy with elders: Strategies for the COTA*, eds. H. Lohman et al., 250, 252–256. St. Louis, MO: Mosby.

Feinberg, J.R., and C.A. Trombly. 1995. Arthritis—osteoarthritis (degenerative joint disease). In *Occupational therapy for physical dysfunction*, 4th ed., ed. C.A. Trombly, 827–830. Baltimore: Williams & Wilkins.

Gecht, M.R. et al. 1996. A survey of exercise belief and exercise habits among people with arthritis. *Arthritis Care and Research* 9, no. 2: 82–88.

Gunaydin, I. et al. 1996. Therapeutic approaches of German and Turkish physicians to rheumatoid arthritis and to osteoarthritis of the knee. *Clinical Rheumatology* 15, no. 1: 55–58.

Hayes, K.W. 1994. An examination of Cyriax's passive motion tests with patients having osteoarthritis of the knee. *Physical Therapy* 74, no. 8: 697–709.

Hochberg, M.C. et al. 1995. Guidelines for the medical management of osteoarthritis: Part I: Osteoarthritis of the hip. *Arthritis and Rheumatology* 38, no. 11: 1535–1540.

Hochberg, M.C. et al. 1995. Guidelines for the medical management of osteoarthritis: Part II: Osteoarthritis of the knee. *Arthritis and Rheumatology* 38, no. 11: 1541–1546.

James, J. 1996. Osteoarthritis. In *Occupational therapy and physical dysfunction: Principles, skills, and practice*, eds. A. Turner et al., 731–746. New York: Churchill Livingstone.

Mann, W.C. et al. 1995. Assistive devices used by home-based elderly persons with arthritis. *American Journal of Occupational Therapy* 49, no. 8: 810–820.

Marmer, L. 1995. The arthritis epidemic and the workplace. *Advance for Occupational Therapists* 11, no. 34: 17, 22.

Marmer, L. 1995. Preparing for the arthritis epidemic. *Advance for Occupational Therapists* 11, no. 34: 12–13, 54.

McLaughlin, C., and T. Kerr. 1996. ACR publishes first guidelines for osteoarthritis treatment. *Advance for Occupational Therapists* 12, no. 4: 20.

Murphy, J. 1995. Dancing away arthritis pain. *Advance for Occupational Therapists* 11, no. 42: 20.

Spenser, E.A. 1998. Arthritis. In *Willard and Spackman's occupational therapy*, 9th ed., eds. M.E. Neistadt and E.B. Crepeau, 689–690. Philadelphia: Lippincott-Raven.

Stahl, C. 1995. Coping with the pain of arthritis. *Advance for Occupational Therapists* 11, no. 4: 14.

Steib, P. 1997. New research promises hope for RA and osteoarthritis sufferers. *OT Week* 11, no. 47: 5.

Arthritis—Rheumatoid

DESCRIPTION

Rheumatoid arthritis is a chronic syndrome characterized by nonspecific, usually symmetric inflammation of the peripheral joints, potentially resulting in progressive destruction of articular and periarticular structures, with or without generalized manifestations (Merck 1999, 416). The onset is usually insidious, with progressive joint involvement, but may be abrupt, with simultaneous inflammation in multiple joints. Tenderness in nearly all inflamed joints is the most sensitive physical finding. Symmetrical involvement of the small hand joints (especially proximal interphalangeal and metacarpophalangeal), foot joints (metatarsophalangeal), wrists, elbows, and ankles is typical, but initially manifestations may occur in any joint.

CAUSE

The cause is unknown. Multiple factors may be involved, including autoimmune reactions and environmental factors. A genetic predisposition has been identified, and in the white population, localization to a pentapeptide is known. The disorder is two to three times more common in women than in men. Onset usually occurs between age 25 and 50 but may occur at any age.

ASSESSMENT

Areas
- daily living skills: personal and instrumental activities of daily living
- productivity skills and interests
- leisure skills and interests
- range of motion, active and passive

- grip and pinch strength
- muscle strength
- hand deformities (See section on arthritis in the hand and wrist.)
- hand functions
- physical endurance and fitness
- sensory functions
- memory
- goal-directed behavior and motivation
- self-concept
- coping skills
- interpersonal and social skills
- communication skills
- support structure

Instruments

- *Robinson Bashall Functional Assessment* by H.S. Robinson and D.A. Bashall, in Functional assessment in rheumatoid arthritis, *Canadian Journal of Occupational Therapy* 29 (1962): 123–138; or L. McCloy and L. Jongbloed, Robinson Bashall functional assessment for arthritis patients: Reliability and validity, *Archives of Physical Medicine and Rehabilitation* 68, no. 8 (1987): 486–489.
- *Stanford Health Assessment Questionnaire,* in F. Wolfe et al., in The clinical value of the Stanford Health Assessment Questionnaire Functional Disability Index in patients with rheumatoid arthritis, *Journal of Rheumatology* 15, no. 10 (1988): 1480–1488.
- manual muscle test
- goniometer
- dynamometer and pinch meter

PROBLEMS

Self-Care
- The person may be unable to perform various activities of daily living because of motor limitations, especially those related to bending, reaching, lifting, and carrying.

Productivity
- The person may be unable to perform some job tasks when pain and swelling intensify, especially those related to bending, reaching, lifting, or carrying.

Leisure
- The disorder limits the variety of leisure pursuits in which the person can participate.

Sensorimotor
- The person may have limited or decreased range of motion of the major joints.
- The person may have joint deformities, especially in the hand and wrist.
- The person may have muscle weakness in major muscle groups.
- The person may have swelling in the major joints.

- The person may have stiffness in the morning.
- The person may complain of frequently feeling fatigued.
- The person may experience pain and tenderness in the joints.

Cognitive
- Cognitive faculties are not directly affected by arthritis. Indirect changes may occur through reduction in activity or inactivity.

Psychosocial
- The person may have feelings of hopelessness and helplessness.
- The person may have a poor self-concept.
- The person may have anxiety.
- The person may become depressed.
- The person may exhibit manipulative behavior.

TREATMENT/INTERVENTION

Self-Care
- Provide self-help devices, if needed, and instruction in how to use them.

Productivity
- Suggest modifications or adaptations in the workplace that will help the person to perform job tasks.
- Suggest modifications or adaptations in the home that will improve safety and help the person perform household tasks.

Leisure
- Explore interests and develop leisure activities based on interests and physical abilities.
- Suggest possible modification of existing activities that might make continued participation possible.

Sensorimotor
- Maintain or increase joint range of motion and mobility.
- Consider splints, such as a resting splint, to maintain wrist extension of the hand.
- Consider night leg splints to maintain knee extension.
- Maintain or increase muscle strength.
- Maintain or improve positioning. Consider a splint to prevent ulnar deviation deformity of the hand and wrist.
- Maintain or improve endurance.
- Maintain or improve functional ability.
- Prevent or correct joint deformity through use of joint protection principles.
- Decrease the person's response to pain.

Cognitive
- Teach the person safe limits of activity to avoid overexertion.

- Teach the person energy conservation and work simplification.
- Teach the person joint protection.
- Develop problem-solving skills to enable the person to modify daily activities, protect joints, and conserve energy.

Psychosocial
- Promote acceptance of chronic disability.
- Teach stress management techniques.
- Promote social activities.

PRECAUTIONS
- Persons with arthritis often do not comply with treatment and management regimes. Increased compliance can be obtained by using good learning or teaching techniques, sharing expectations about treatment and management, encouraging personal assumption of responsibility, and maintaining a relaxed, friendly atmosphere to encourage communication.
- Observe hand functions for signs of carpal tunnel syndrome.

PROGNOSIS AND OUTCOME
The prognosis varies and cannot be predicted early in the course of the disease.
- The amount of joint inflammation has decreased.
- Range of motion has been maintained or increased.
- Muscle strength and tone have been maintained or increased.
- The person demonstrates an understanding of joint protection.
- The person demonstrates knowledge of work simplification and energy conservation.
- The person demonstrates knowledge of proper body positioning techniques during work, rest, and play.
- The person has been provided with a hand splint and wears the splint as prescribed, if needed.
- The person has been provided with adapted aids and equipment and uses the devices, if needed.
- The person can describe the problems of living with arthritis and the resources available to assist in coping with the disabilities to minimize handicaps.
- The person demonstrates coping skills to decrease the stresses of living with a chronic disability.
- The person maintains social relations and support.
- The person is able to perform activities of daily living within the limits of his or her disability.
- The person is able to perform productive activities within the limits of his or her disability.
- The person is able to perform leisure activities that are of interest and provide satisfaction within the limits of his or her disability.

REFERENCE

Beers, M.H., and R. Berkow, eds. 1999. *The Merck Manual of Diagnosis and Therapy*, 17th ed. Whitehouse Station, NJ: Merck Research Laboratories.

BIBLIOGRAPHY

Bakheit, A.M.O. et al. 1995. A comparison between the Stanford Health Assessment Questionnaire and the Barthel Index in patients with rheumatoid arthritis. *British Journal of Occupational Therapy* 58, no. 6: 253–254.

Bates, C.D. 1993. Rheumatoid arthritis. In *Conditions in occupational therapy: Effects on occupational performance*, eds. R.A. Hansen and B. Atchinson, 306–334. Baltimore: Williams & Wilkins.

Breines, E. 1996. Don't overlook some handcrafts for your rheumatoid patients. *Advance for Occupational Therapists* 12, no. 37: 5.

Buckner, W. 1998. Arthritic diseases. In *Physical dysfunction practice skills for the occupational therapy assistant*, ed. M.B. Early, 433–455. St. Louis, MO: Mosby.

Dalgas, M. et al. 1994. Disability issues in rheumatoid arthritis. *Physical Medicine and Rehabilitation Clinics of North America* 5, no. 4: 859–866.

Driessen, M-J et al. 1997. Occupational therapy for patients with chronic diseases: CVA, rheumatoid arthritis, and progressive diseases of the central nervous system. *Disability and Rehabilitation* 19, no. 5: 198–204.

Feinberg, J.R., and C.A. Trombly. 1995. Arthritis—Rheumatoid arthritis. In *Occupational therapy for physical dysfunction*, 4th ed., ed. C.A. Trombly, 815–827. Baltimore: Williams & Wilkins.

Hammond, A. 1994. Joint protection behavior in patients with rheumatoid arthritis following an education program: A pilot study. *Arthritis Care and Research* 7, no. 1: 5–9.

Hammond, A. 1996. Functional and health assessments used in rheumatology occupational therapy: A review and United Kingdom survey. *British Journal of Occupational Therapy* 59, no. 6: 254–259.

Hammond, A. 1996. Rheumatoid arthritis. In *Occupational therapy and physical dysfunction: Principles, skills, and practice*, eds. A. Turner et al., 747–766. New York: Churchill Livingstone.

Hammond, A. 1997. Joint protection education: What are we doing? *British Journal of Occupational Therapy* 60, no. 9: 401–406.

Hittle, J.M. et al. 1996. Rheumatoid arthritis. In *Occupational therapy: Practice skills for physical dysfunction*, 4th ed., ed. L.W. Pedretti, 639–660. St. Louis, MO: Mosby.

Joe, B.E. 1995. OAS exhibit forges links between art, disability, and OT. *OT Week* 9, no. 3: 12.

Jones, R.A., and S.K. Blackman. 1993. The young adult with rheumatoid arthritis. In *Practice issues in occupational therapy: Intraprofessional team building*, ed. S.E. Ryan, 111–118. Thorofare, NJ: Slack.

Katz, P.P. 1995. The impact of rheumatoid arthritis on life activities. *Arthritis Care and Research* 8, no. 4: 272–278.

Kjeken, I. et al. 1995. Use of commercially produced elastic wrist orthoses in chronic arthritis: A controlled study. *Arthritis Care and Research* 8, no. 2: 108–113.

Kornblau, B. 1996. Facing up to arthritis: A hidden disability: ADA and workplace issues. *Advance for Occupational Therapists* 12, no. 44: 11.

Kornblau, B. 1996. Maintaining intimacy when arthritis strikes. *Advance for Occupational Therapists* 12, no. 44: 54.

Kraaimaat, F.W. et al. 1995. The effect of cognitive behavior therapy in patients with rheumatoid arthritis. *Behavior Research Therapy* 33, no. 5: 487–495.

MacKinnon, J. et al. 1994. Pain and functional limitations in individuals with rheumatoid arthritis. *International Journal of Rehabilitation Research* 17: 49–59.

MacKinnon, J. et al. 1998. Occupation as a mediator of depression in people with rheumatoid arthritis. *Journal of Occupational Science* 5, no. 2: 82–92.

Morrow, S. 1995. Physical and occupational therapy for arthritis. *Arthritis Today* 9, no. 2: 47–51.

Noreau, L. et al. 1995. Effects of a modified dance-based exercise on cardiorespiratory fitness, psychological state and health status on persons with rheumatoid arthritis. *American Journal of Physical Medicine and Rehabilitation* 74, no. 1: 19–27.

Pagnotta, A. et al. 1998. The effect of a static wrist orthosis on hand function in individuals with rheumatoid arthritis. *Journal of Rheumatology* 25, no. 5: 879–885.

Parker, J.C., and G.E. Wright. 1995. The implications of depression for pain and disability in rheumatoid arthritis. *Arthritis Care and Research* 8, no. 4: 279–283.

Penrose, D. 1993. Rheumatoid arthritis. In *Occupational therapy for orthopaedic conditions*, ed. D. Penrose, 1–27. London: Chapman & Hall.

Sanford, M.K. et al. 1996. Effectiveness of computer-assisted interactive videodisc instruction in teaching rheumatology to physical and occupational therapy students. *Journal of Allied Health* 25, no. 2: 141–148.

Sharma, S. et al. 1994. Evaluation of the Jebson Hand Function Test for use in patients with rheumatoid arthritis. *Arthritis Care and Research* 7, no. 1: 16–19. (Note: The name of the test is misspelled in the article. Jebson should be Jebsen.)

Spenser, E.A. 1998. Arthritis. In *Willard and Spackman's occupational therapy*, 9th ed., eds. M.E. Neistadt and E.B. Crepeau, 689–690. Philadelphia: Lippincott-Raven.

Stern, E.B. et al. 1996. Finger dexterity and hand function: Effect of three commercial wrist extensor orthoses on patients with rheumatoid arthritis. *Arthritis Care and Research* 9, no. 3: 197–205.

Stern, E.B. et al. 1996. Immediate and short-term effects of three commercial wrist extensor orthoses on grip strength and function in patients with rheumatoid arthritis. *Arthritis Care and Research* 9, no. 1: 42–50.

Stern, E.B. et al. 1997. Commercial wrist extensor orthoses: A descriptive study of use and preference in patients with rheumatoid arthritis. *Arthritis Care and Research* 10, no. 1: 27–35.

Sweeney, G.M. et al. 1994. Choosing lever taps for people with rheumatoid arthritis. *British Journal of Occupational Therapy* 57, no. 7: 263–265.

Van Deusen, J. 1993. The physically challenged adult. In *Body image and perceptual dysfunction in adults*, ed. J. Van Deusen, 222–228. Philadelphia: W.B. Saunders.

Dupuytren's Contracture

DESCRIPTION

Dupuytren's contracture is a progressive contracture of the palmar fascial bands that produces flexion deformities of the fingers. The disorder usually begins as a tender nodule in the palm (most often at the third or fourth fingers) followed by formation of a superficial pretendinous cord, which leads to contracture of the metacarpophalangeal and interphalangeal joints of the fingers. The nodule may initially cause discomfort but becomes painless as it matures. Eventually the contracture worsens, and the hand becomes arched (Merck 1999, 491).

CAUSE

The cause is unknown. Repeated microtrauma may be involved. A low-grade inflammatory fibrosis is present in the palmar fascia and surrounds the adjacent digital flexor tendon sheaths. There is some familial association, but genetic origin is not established. Men of Northern European descent are affected much more often than women. The incidence increases after age 40 and has been associated with chronic invalidism, alcoholism, epilepsy, pulmonary tuberculosis, diabetes mellitus, and liver disease. It may be a late sequela to the shoulder-hand syndrome or reflex sympathetic dystrophy syndrome following myocardial infarction or other causes of shoulder immobility. The condition usually appears spontaneously and may have a slow or rapid progression. The ulnar side of the hand is most often affected.

ASSESSMENT

Areas
- daily living skills: personal and instrumental activities of daily living
- hand functions: grasp, grip, and pinch
- range of motion: active and passive
- edema
- pain
- postoperative wound and skin care

Instruments
No specific assessments are reported. The following assessment categories may be helpful:
- activities of daily living test
- hand function test
- range of motion test
- edema assessment
- pain assessment

PROBLEMS

Self-Care
- The person has difficulty performing tasks that involve having the fingers in an extended position, such as putting on gloves.
- The person may report that the contractured fingers get in the way of performing activities with the hands, such as tucking in a shirttail.

Productivity
- The person has difficulty performing work tasks that require extension of the fingers in preparation for a grasp, such as a hook or cylindrical hand grasp.
- The person may have difficulty keyboarding because the contracture prevents fingers from being positioned on the keyboard and moving into new positions to strike specific keys.
- The person may report that the contractured fingers get in the way of using the hand for some tasks such as dusting or cleaning countertops.

Leisure
- The person may report difficulty performing leisure activities that require finger extension in preparation for a grasp, such as holding a tennis racket or catching a football.

Sensorimotor
- The person is unable to fully flex or extend fingers and hands due to the contracture.
- Grasp functions that involve the full hand and fingers are impaired.
- Sensation is not involved per se, but lack of ability to position the hand may reduce the opportunity to receive sensory input from the involved fingers and hand.

Cognitive
- No cognitive functions are involved.

Psychosocial
- The person may report frustration and annoyance at being unable to use the involved finger(s) and hand(s) to accomplish intended actions.
- The person may be concerned about the visual appearance of the hand and being considered disabled.

TREATMENT/INTERVENTION

Surgery is considered the best approach and is usually recommended when the metacarpophalangeal joint contracts to 30 degrees, producing functional restrictions in the use of the hand. Some surgeons suggest surgery for any amount of proximal interphalangeal joint contracture because of the greater likelihood of permanent damage to the capsular ligament structure.

Self-Care
- Begin with light activities of daily living during the early postoperative phase (about two weeks after surgery).
- Observe and listen to the person's report of his or her ability to perform daily life tasks. Provide information and techniques for handling temporary problems caused by the healing process.

Sensorimotor
- Maintain the range of motion of uninvolved joints and digits.
- Control postoperative edema using elevation, retrograde massage, and gloves. If the open-palm technique was used in surgery, gauze compression wraps may be used until the wound is closed.
- Promote wound health, especially for those who had open-palm technique surgery, with use of a whirlpool. The hand should be positioned horizontally in the whirlpool.
- Increase active and passive range of motion in both flexion and extension of the involved finger(s). The person should have a home exercise program that includes joint range of motion and tendon gliding exercises.
- Control and guide scar formation by making a molded splint from splint materials to place on the palm after the wound has closed. The splint may be worn for up to six months or more.
- Other techniques for scar management include static and dynamic prolonged stretching, deep friction massage, compressive inserts, ultrasound, or iontophoresis (an electric modality that transmits medication such as potassium iodide into the dermis).

- If hypersensitivity occurs, use desensitizing techniques to prevent dysfunction.
- Provide a volar or dorsal forearm removable extension splint to maintain the wrist in a neutral position and the involved digits in extension. The splint is worn all the time during the first two weeks, except for therapy and hygiene. After two weeks, the splint is worn at night for about three months.
- Provide light strengthening exercises, progressing to heavier resistance as the wound heals, edema is controlled, and pressure to the area is tolerated. Strengthening is usually introduced four to six weeks after surgery, depending on the integrity of the wound.

Cognitive
- Inform the person about the therapy protocol.
- Provide instructions for wearing and caring for the splint.
- Provide instructions for a home exercise program.

PRECAUTIONS
- Nonoperative treatment such as splinting has not been effective in preventing the contracture from occurring.
- Watch for signs of diseased fascia postoperatively and report any signs to the surgeon.
- Watch for signs of intraoperative complications involving the neurovascular bundles.
- Check to see if concomitant surgical procedures such as capsulectomy might have been performed. When these procedures have been done, the rate of healing and therapy methods can change.
- Check if a skin graft was done to close the operative site.
- Watch for signs of hematoma, skin necrosis, infection, stiffness, pain, reflex sympathetic dystrophy, and recurrence of disease.
- Avoid applying tension to the palmar skin flaps; the tension can interfere with the healing of the tissue.

PROGNOSIS AND OUTCOME
- The person is able to perform daily living tasks independently.
- The person is able to perform work-related tasks and routines.
- The person is able to perform leisure activities.
- The person is able to fully extend all digits on the involved hand and place the hand flat on a flat surface.
- The person has full active and passive movement of the involved hand for functional hand grasp and release.

REFERENCE

Beers, M.H., and R. Berkow, eds. 1999. *The Merck Manual of Diagnosis and Therapy*, 17th ed. Whitehouse Station, NJ: Merck Research Laboratories.

BIBLIOGRAPHY

Eckhaus, D. 1997. Dupuytren's disease. In *Hand rehabilitation: A practical guide*, 2nd ed., eds. G.L. Clark et al., 37–46. New York: Churchill Livingstone.

Garfield, G., and K. Helsher. 1996. Dupuytren's disease: Surgical techniques and treatment. *Physical Disabilities Special Interest Section Newsletter* 19, no. 2: 3–4.

Fibromyalgia Syndrome

DESCRIPTION

Fibromyalgia syndrome is a group of common nonarticular disorders characterized by achy pain, tenderness and stiffness of muscles, areas of tendon insertions, and adjacent soft tissue structures. Fibromyalgia indicates pain in fibrous tissues, muscles, tendons, ligaments, and other sites. Any fibromuscular tissues may be involved, but those of the occiput, neck (neck pain or spasm), shoulders, thorax (pleurodynia), low back (lumbago), and thighs (aches and charley horses) are especially affected (Merck 1999, 481). Some people are misdiagnosed because physicians are not familiar with the disorder or believe it does not exist. Other names for fibromyalgia syndrome include myofascial pain syndrome, fibrositis, and fibromyositis.

Specific diagnosis criteria set by the American College of Rheumatology are (1) widespread pain or tenderness in the trunk and limb muscles present at least three months and (2) excessive tenderness in 11 of 18 tender points located in the neck, shoulder girdle, elbow, hip, and knee (Decker 1983, 1029–1032). Tender points are normal areas in the muscles that are tender to pressure in everyone but are especially tender in people with fibromyalgia syndrome. Some people also have trigger points on the back that can cause pain throughout a specific region or in a separate location.

CAUSE

The cause is unknown. It is unclear whether the condition has a viral, immunologic, genetic, or allergenic basis. There may be a disruption of neurohormone metabolism or serotonin in the central nervous system. Males and females of all ages are affected, but it is most common among females between the ages of 20 and 60.

ASSESSMENT

Areas

- daily living skills: personal and instrumental activities of daily living
- productivity
- leisure

- sleep patterns
- pain

Instruments
- *Fibromyalgia Impact Questionnaire* by C.S. Burckhardt, S.R. Clark, and R.M. Bennett, in *Journal of Rheumatology* 18 (1991): 728–733.
- activity configuration
- analogue pain scale

PROBLEMS

Self-Care
- The person may complain of indigestion, functional bowel disorder or irritable bowel syndrome, irritable bladder syndrome, and urinary frequency.
- The person may have difficulty falling asleep, wake up in the middle of the night, or feel exhausted or unrested after adequate sleep. Stage IV non-REM sleep is often missing.
- The person usually complains of fatigue.

Sensorimotor
- The person may have diffuse aching, stiffness, tenderness, or pain in muscles of back and all four extremities.
- The person may have pain in intrinsic hand muscles where the tendons connect to the bone, called noninflammatory enthesopathy.
- The person may have tingling, numbness, or a burning sensation, often in odd patterns.
- The person may have hypersensitivity to touch, sound, light, smells, or chemical fumes.
- The person may have headaches.
- The person may have temperature sensitivity.
- The person may have subjective or objective swelling of the hands, feet, or face.
- The person may have skin rashes and skin sensitivity.
- The person may complain of malaise and generally not feeling well.
- The person may have changes in vision, hearing, and balance.

Cognitive
- The person may have memory problems such as diminished reading retention, short-term memory lapse, problems with misnaming items, and word-finding problems.

Psychosocial
- The person may experience depression and anxiety.
- The person may become irritable and have a negative mood.

TREATMENT/INTERVENTION

Treatment is aimed at changing the chemistry of the person's brain through exercise, sleep, nutrition, relaxation training, and cognitive therapy.

Self-Care
- Encourage the person to keep a log of symptoms.
- Assist the person in changing sleep behavior so the person feels rested five out of seven mornings without medication.
- Encourage the person to have a healthy lifestyle, including good nutrition.
- Improve general fitness by participating in a low-impact aerobics class or doing a 20-minute to 30-minute stretching program.
- The person may find that a hot bath or shower and massage reduce the pain.
- Encourage the person to learn self-accupressure and self-massage.

Sensorimotor
- Encourage the person to get more exercise (e.g., walking, swimming, yoga, t'ai chi, qigong, stationary cycling).
- Help the person learn deep breathing exercises to facilitate relaxation.
- Support splints may be helpful in reducing pain.
- Encourage proper positioning to decrease pain.

Cognitive
- Teach the person about the condition and help the person to discuss symptoms and problems.
- Help the person to focus on how to make his or her body healthier, stronger, and less sensitive.
- Teach time management and planning and pacing activities to increase the person's sense of control and to reduce stress.

Psychosocial
- Teach stress management through relaxation training, stress management training, visualization, and meditation.
- Encourage the person to participate in a support group.
- Teach the person coping skills.

PRECAUTIONS

- Using exercise machines and weight lifting are not recommended because the focus is on strengthening, not lengthening, the muscles.
- Jogging and running are not recommended because of the repetitive jarring and static position of the shoulder.
- Competitive exercises and sports are not recommended because they may cause the person to overdo, thus increasing pain and fatigue.

PROGNOSIS AND OUTCOME

Some people do recover from fibromyalgia and its symptoms.
- The person is able to perform daily activities without pain or muscle tenderness.

- The person demonstrates participation in a regular exercise program.
- The person demonstrates coping skills designed to reduce stress.

REFERENCES

Beers, M.H., and R. Berkow, eds. 1999. *The Merck Manual of Diagnosis and Therapy*, 17th ed. Whitehouse Station, NJ: Merck Research Laboratories.
Decker, J.L. 1983. American Rheumatism Association nomenclature and classification of arthritis and rheumatism. *Arthritis and Rheumatism* 26, no. 8: 1029–1032.

BIBLIOGRAPHY

Kerr, T. 1996. A whole-person approach to fibromyalgia treatment. *Advance for Occupational Therapists* 12, no. 28: 17, 46.
Melvin, J.L. 1996. *Fibromyalgia Syndrome: Getting Healthy*. Bethesda, MD: America Occupational Therapy Association.
Thiers, N. 1994. Fighting the pain of fibromyalgia. *OT Week* 8, no. 38: 22–23.

Muscular Dystrophies

DESCRIPTION

Muscular dystrophies are a group of inherited, progressive muscle disorders that are distinguished clinically by selective distribution of weakness (Merck 1999, 1499).

Becker muscular dystrophy is an X-linked recessive disorder characterized by progressive proximal muscle weakness. It is a less severe form of Duchenne dystrophy.

Duchenne dystrophy is an X-linked recessive disorder characterized by progressive proximal muscle weakness with destruction and regeneration of muscle fibers and replacement by connective tissue. Symptoms typically start in boys between the ages of 3 and 7 and include a waddling gait, toe walking, lordosis, frequent falls, and difficulty in standing up and climbing stairs.

Facioscapulohumeral (Landouzy-Dejerine) muscular dystrophy is an autosomal dominant disorder characterized by weakness of the facial muscles and shoulder girdle. It usually begins between ages 7 and 20 years.

Limb-girdle muscular dystrophy is characterized by weakness that develops in a limb girdle and proximal limb distribution. It usually begins in the teens or early adulthood.

On its website (www.mda.org), the Muscular Dystrophy Association (MDA) lists nine types of myopathies, including muscular dystrophy. In the *Merck Manual,* only four are listed as muscular dystrophies (Merck 1999, 1499). The other five listed by MDA are myotonic, congenital, oculopharyngeal, distal, and Emery-Dreifuss muscular dystrophy.

CAUSE

Becker muscular dystrophy is due to a mutation at the Xp21 locus. Dystrophin is reduced in quantity or in molecular weight. Many persons with Becker muscular dystrophy survive into their thirties and forties.

Stages of Duchenne Muscular Dystrophy and Treatment

1. Diagnostic period (ages 3 to 4 years): The purpose of treatment is primarily patient and family education about age-appropriate activities.
2. Early childhood (ages 5 to 7 years): The purpose of treatment is to assist the child with early problems in gross motor and upper extremity activities related to play, self-care, and school.
3. Childhood-ambulatory (ages 7 to 12 years): The purpose of treatment is to keep the child mainstreamed in school and the community and independent in home activities, with self-help aids as needed and lifts, ramps, or other architectural modifications designed primarily to aid mobility.
4. Late childhood-nonambulatory (ages 13 to 18 years): The purpose of treatment is to maintain range of motion and use of the upper extremities with assistive devices, such as balanced forearm orthosis, feeding aids, reachers, adaptive clothing, and lapboards. Assist the multidisciplinary team with lower limb stretching and respiratory care.
5. Young adulthood (19 years and older): The purpose of treatment is to maintain as much function as possible and assist with social interaction and educational or vocational planning. Maximum use of adaptive technology is needed.

Source: Adapted with permission from I.M. Siegel, Occupational Therapy, in *Muscle and Its Diseases: An Outline Primer of Basic Science*, pp. 278–284, © 1986, W.B. Saunders Company.

Duchenne dystrophy is caused by a mutation at the Xp21 locus that results in the absence of dystrophin, a protein found inside the muscle cell membrane. It affects 1 in 3,000 live male births. Death because of respiratory complications usually occurs by the age of 20.

Facioscapulohumeral muscular dystrophy is caused by a gene located on chromosome 4q35, but the genetic defect has not been identified.

Limb-girdle muscular dystrophy has been identified on several chromosomal loci with several different substances involved, including beta-sarcoglycan, gamma-sarcoglycan, calpain, and alpha-sarcoglycan. Genes 2q, 4q, 5q, 13q, 15q, and 17q have all been implicated. All but 5q occur in recessive inheritance.

ASSESSMENT

Areas
- daily living skills: personal and instrumental activities of daily living
- productivity skills
- play and leisure skills
- muscle strength

- endurance
- functional range of motion
- gross motor developmental and milestone attainment
- fine motor development, coordination, manipulation, and dexterity
- balance and postural control
- visual perception
- visual motor integration
- self-concept
- social roles
- assistive technology
- environmental modifications

Instruments

Instruments Developed by Occupational Therapy Personnel

- *Miller Assessment for Preschoolers* (MAP) by L.A. Miller, San Antonio, TX: The Psychological Corporation, 1988.
- *School Assessment of Motor and Process Skills* (SAMPS) by A. Fisher, K. Bryze, and L. Magalhaes, Fort Collins, CO: Occupational Therapy Department, Colorado State University, 1998.
- *Wee Functional Independence Measure* (WeeFIM) by Uniform Data Systems, Buffalo, NY: Uniform Data Systems, 1993.

Instruments Developed by Other Professionals and Used by Occupational Therapy Personnel

- *Battelle Developmental Inventory* by J. Newborg et al., Itasca, IL: Riverside Publication Co., 1988.
- *The Beery-Buktenica Developmental Test of Visual-Motor Integration* (VMI-4), 4th ed. by K.E. Beery and N.A. Buktenica, Parsippany, NJ: Modern Curriculum Press, 1997.
- *Bruininks-Oseretsky Test of Motor Proficiency* (BOTMP) by R. Bruininks, Circle Pines, MN: American Guidance Services, 1978.
- *Developmental Profile II* (DPII) by G.D. Alpren, T.J. Boll, and M.S. Shearer, Los Angeles: Western Psychological Services, 1984.
- *Motor-Free Visual Perception Test—Revised* (MVPT-R) by R. Colarusso and D.D. Hammill, Novato, CA: Academic Therapy Publications, 1995.
- *Peabody Developmental Motor Scales* by M.R. Folio and R.R. Fewell, Austin, TX: Pro-Ed, 1983.
- *Test of Visual-Perceptual Skills–Revised* (TVPS-R) by M.F. Gardner, Hydesville, CA: Psychological and Education Publications, 1996.
- *Vineland Adaptive Behavior Scales–Revised* by S.S. Sparrow, D.A. Balla, and D.V. Cicchetti, Circle Pines, MN: American Guidance Services, 1984.

PROBLEMS

Self-Care

- The person loses the ability to perform self-care skills as hand muscle function is lost.

- The person loses functional independence as functional skills are lost.

Productivity
- As the disorder progresses, the person may become unable to attend school and need home schooling.
- As the disorder progresses, the person may be unable to continue working or will need modifications in the workplace environment.

Leisure
- The person loses the ability to participate in certain activities as gross and fine motor skills are lost.
- The person is unable to play some games or participate in some activities with other children because of weakness and loss of function.
- Teenagers or adults may not be able to continue some leisure activities because of loss of motor skills.

Sensorimotor
- The person has a waddling gait due to an attempt to broaden the base of support.
- The person may walk on his or her toes.
- The person's posture is lordotic and may include scoliosis due to muscle imbalance.
- The person may fall frequently due to unsteady gait and muscle weakness.
- The person may have difficulty getting to a standing position and do so by "climbing" his or her legs (Gower's sign).
- The person usually has weakness in the proximal muscles, starting with the pelvis and then the shoulders.
- The person may have difficulty climbing stairs.
- The person may be reluctant to run.
- The person may appear to have enlargement of the calf muscles and sometimes of the forearm and thigh muscles.
- The person may have decreased range of motion.
- The person may have decreased endurance and physical tolerance.
- The person may have decreased mobility, leading to wheelchair dependence.
- Respiratory muscles usually become progressively weaker, leading to decreased pulmonary function.
- The person may develop flexion contractures or have other deformities that occur as muscles become weaker.
- The person may have a tendency toward obesity, especially as endurance decreases.
- The person is unable to keep up with peers whose development is continuing.
- Sensory faculties are not usually involved as a direct consequence of the disorder.

Cognitive
- Persons with Becker muscular dystrophy or Duchenne dystrophy may have mild, nonprogressive intellectual impairment that affects verbal ability. Other forms of muscular dystrophy are not associated with any specific cognitive impairment. However, cognitive impairment may be present as a result of other disorders or dementia.

Psychosocial

- The person may become depressed and lose motivation as the skill gap between him- or herself and his or her peers increases.
- The person may feel that he or she has no control over life or the environment.
- The person may have a poor self-concept, low self-esteem, and a poor sense of mastery.
- The person may lack self-identity and body image.
- The person may have poor coping skills.
- The person may fear dying.
- The person may fear becoming helpless.
- The person may lack motivation.
- Dependence on others increases as the disability increases.
- The person may become demanding.
- The person may lose role identification in the family as the disability increases.

TREATMENT/INTERVENTION

Treatment models include maintenance, prevention, compensatory, and environmental adaptation. A developmental model may be especially useful for the early stages of Duchenne dystrophy or Becker muscular dystrophy. Usually, a team approach is used. The age of the individual may change the specific task, but the objectives remain the same whether the person is a child, teenager, or adult.

Self-Care

- Provide assistive devices or environmental adaptations to help the person continue to handle self-care independently. Low-tech devices might include a reacher; elastic shoelaces; a sock aid for lower extremity dressing; and button hooks, zipper pulls, elastic waistband pants, and shirts that can be pulled over the head easily for upper extremity dressing. A table placed at axilla height may enable the person to continue feeding him- or herself.
- Provide an environmental control unit for household functions such as answering the door or telephone and turning on and off lights, the television, the VCR, or the CD player.
- As function is lost, consider a seating system that can be used on an outdoor and indoor base.

Productivity

- Provide upper extremity support such as computer access for academic or work performance. Keyboarding instead of writing by hand may be helpful. Taping lectures or meetings rather than taking notes may be helpful. Overhead slings or mobile arm supports may also be helpful.
- Facilitate the person's continuing participation in all school and work activities. Encourage the person to use assistive devices and technology, to adapt tasks (e.g., to use less heavy equipment), or to serve as time- or scorekeeper, referee, or recorder of data in gym class.
- If changing classes or moving about the workplace is a problem, encourage the person to allow a little more time for walking in the hallway or to enlist the help of another student or coworker.

- A wheelchair may be necessary at school or work to facilitate movement between classes or meeting rooms and to the lunchroom or auditorium. A scooter can be used if the person's postural control is sufficient.
- Help the family and the person identify productive activities that the individual can perform within the family structure.
- Help the person explore vocational interests and develop occupational skills.

Leisure
- Assist the person in exploring and identifying leisure interests that are within his or her physical limits.
- Explore how technology might help the person participate in leisure activities.
- Suggest modifications of activities that would permit the person to continue participating in chosen interests.

Sensorimotor
- Maintain gross motor skills, especially ambulation, and neuromuscular status for as long as possible through activities and exercises.
- Maintain positioning and postural control. Environmental adaptations such as a chair with foot- and armrests may be needed.
- Prevent deformities and contractures by providing or arranging for daily passive and active range of motion exercises, correct positioning during all activities, and splinting or bracing, if needed.
- Maintain endurance through activities and games.
- Maintain the person's muscle strength, especially in the hips, through activities and games that require kicking, climbing, pushing, and pulling.
- Maintain muscle tone through walking exercises.
- Maintain grip strength and finger dexterity.
- Maintain upper extremity mobility and range of motion through activities and games requiring throwing, tossing, catching, and reaching. A deltoid aid or overhead slings may be useful when shoulder girdle muscles weaken.
- Consider splinting the person's ankle to maintain dorsiflexion when the person becomes wheelchair dependent.
- Assist in maintaining the strength of respiratory muscles through activities and games requiring blowing or taking deep breaths, such as swimming.
- Assist the medical team in selecting powered mobility equipment when walking is no longer feasible.

Cognitive
- Learning tasks may need to be divided into shorter sessions to allow for rest periods.
- Instruct the person and his or her family members on energy conservation, pacing, and work simplification.
- Assist the dietician or nutritionist in instructing the family about diet and preparation of nutritious, nonfattening meals.

Psychosocial
- Help the person to use assistive technology to regain some control over his or her life and environment.
- Increase the person's self-concept (mastery) through the use of selected craft or game activities.
- Encourage the person to express his or her feelings, including feelings of hopelessness and helplessness and fear of dying.
- Encourage the person to engage in family and social activities that are within his or her safe limits.
- Help the family or support group to adjust role expectations as the person's performance permits.

Environmental
- Provide the person's parents with information about how the disease progresses.
- Encourage family members to participate in support groups such as the local chapter of the Muscular Dystrophy Association or a group for parents with exceptional children.
- Help family members to locate and use local resources for information, educational assistance, and leisure activities.
- Confer with family members about modifications to the home that may make caring for the person easier (e.g., installing a wheelchair ramp, having hardwood or linoleum floors rather than area carpets to reduce trips and falls, widening doors to bedrooms and bathrooms, creating a downstairs bedroom to eliminate the need to climb stairs, adding grab rails for the toilet or using a free-standing commode, and installing a shower chair and having the person shower instead of bathing).
- Talk with family members about time management so that the person is able to participate in meaningful activities but gets adequate rest between activities.
- Recommend a pressure-diffusing mattress at home so family members do not have to turn the person in the bed every two hours.
- Instruct the family members in the purpose, correct use, and maintenance of all assistive technology (e.g., a seating system, specialized computer programs, and a hoist).

PRECAUTIONS
- Remember that the diagnosis and its implications will probably shock parents and that they will need support to learn to handle the situation.
- Encourage parents, teachers, and caregivers not to overprotect or "baby" the person.
- The person will tire easily, especially as weakness increases. Activities need to be alternated with rest periods.
- Observe respiratory function, which can be compromised as muscle weakness increases. Avoid exposure to respiratory infections. Report signs of respiratory distress (coughing, choking, or difficulty breathing) to the physician and caregivers promptly.
- Watch for signs of pressure sores that result from the person's inability to turn over or change position.
- There is a tendency to gain weight as mobility decreases. Work with family members and a dietician to keep the person's weight as normal as possible, which will improve health status and make transfer activities easier.

PROGNOSIS/OUTCOME

The progression of muscular dystrophy cannot be stopped or reversed. The person with Duchenne dystrophy or Becker muscular dystrophy will die usually from respiratory difficulties. Other types of muscular dystrophy are more chronic disabling conditions.

- The person will maintain independence in self-care and mobility for as long as possible with the help of assistive devices and home modifications.
- The person will continue attending school or going to work for as long as possible with the help of assistive devices and environmental modifications.
- The person will continue to participate in leisure activities. The type of activity may change as motor functions are lost.
- The person will move using a seating system when or if ambulation is no longer possible.
- The person demonstrates functional range of motion of the upper extremities independently or with the use of mobile arm supports.
- The person has a positive self-concept.
- The person demonstrates stress management techniques.
- The person will continue to have designated roles in the family.

REFERENCE

Beers, M.H., and R. Berkow, eds. 1999. *The Merck Manual of Diagnosis and Therapy*, 17th ed. Whitehouse Station, NJ: Merck Research Laboratories.

BIBLIOGRAPHY

McCormack, G.L. et al. 1998. Motor unit dysfunction—myopathic disorders. In *Physical dysfunction: Practice skills for the occupational therapy assistant*, ed. M.B. Early, 563–564. St. Louis, MO: Mosby.

McCormak, G.L., and L.W. Pedretti. 1996. Motor unit dysfunction—myopathic disorders. In *Occupational therapy: Practice skills for physical dysfunction*, 4th ed., ed. L.W. Pedretti, 757. St. Louis, MO: CV Mosby.

Newman, E.M. et al. 1995. Degenerative diseases—muscular dystrophies. In *Occupational therapy for physical dysfunction*, 4th ed., ed. C.A. Trombly, 742–743. Baltimore: Williams & Wilkins.

Tomchek, S.D. 1999. The musculoskeletal system—muscular dystrophy. In *Pediatric therapy: A systems approach*, eds. S.M. Porr and E.B. Rainville, 207–215. Philadelphia: F.A. Davis.

Wagner, W.B. et al. 1993. Assessment of hand function in Duchenne Muscular Dystrophy. *Archives of Physical Medicine and Rehabilitation* 74, no. 8: 801–804.

Wilsdom, J. 1996. Muscular dystrophy. In *Occupational therapy and physical dysfunction: Principles, skills, and practice*, eds. A. Turner et al., 513–533. New York: Churchill Livingstone.

Myasthenia Gravis

DESCRIPTION

Myasthenia gravis is characterized by episodic muscle weakness caused by loss or dysfunction of acetylcholine receptors at the neuromuscular junction (Merck 1999, 1497). It is a chronic, progressive, degenerative disorder of striated muscles that leads to weakness in the voluntary muscles. Neonatal myasthenia is a syndrome of generalized muscle weakness that affects infants born to women with myasthenia gravis because antibodies passively cross the placenta. Symptoms resolve after the antibody titers decline. Congenital myasthenia is a rare autosomal recessive disorder of neuromuscular transmission that begins in childhood. This disease is not due to autoimmunity. Ocular myasthenia gravis is a subclass of the generalized disease involving only extraocular muscles.

CAUSE

Adult onset myasthenia gravis appears to be an autoimmune disorder. Two possible explanations exist: (1) immunoglobulin G autoantibodies block acetylcholine receptors on the postsynaptic membrane at the myoneurojunction or (2) there is a defect in the resynthesis of acetylcholine on the presynaptic membrane. The disorder occurs more frequently in 20- to 30-year-old women than in men of the same age. After the age of 40, the frequency is about the same. Surgical removal of the thymus gland (thymectomy) helps some patients, although the reasons for the improvement are not well understood. Plasmapheresis (blood filtering) has also been used in addition to pharmacologic agents. Remissions and exacerbations occur.

ASSESSMENT

Areas

- daily living skills, especially swallowing, and other personal and instrumental activities of daily living
- productivity skills
- leisure interests and skills
- muscle strength (Note that muscle testing adds to fatigue. Testing just a few muscles at a time may be necessary.)
- fatigue
- oral-motor skills
- range of motion
- physical endurance
- fine motor skills, dexterity, and manipulation
- ocular motor skills (tracking, scanning)
- balance and equilibrium reactions
- soft tissue integrity
- visual-motor skills

- mood or affect
- life roles

Instruments

No tests have been identified in the literature as developed by occupational therapists. The following types of tests may be useful:
- activities of daily living scale
- occupational history
- leisure checklist
- manual muscle test (include facial muscles)
- goniometer

PROBLEMS

Self-Care

- Note potential difficulties with chewing and swallowing during meals.
- The person may have difficulty with overhead arm raising during dressing.
- The person may experience fine motor impairment in performing buttoning, writing, and typing activities.
- The person may have difficulty with mobility due to diplopia or lack of oculomotor control.

Productivity

- The person may be unable to perform many homemaking tasks because of fatigue.
- Job tasks that require physical exertion or fine motor performance may become impossible to continue or need to be curtailed.
- If balance and posture are involved, the person may be unable to move about the community safely.
- The person may be too tired to perform work tasks.

Leisure

- The person may be too tired to enjoy leisure interests.

Sensorimotor

- The person may have muscle fatigue and weakness, especially after exertion or at the end of the day.
- There may be difficulties associated with the person's extraocular muscles: diplopia (double vision), ptosis (drooping eyelids), and decreased oculomotor control.
- There may be facial problems: the person looks tired, his or her jaw may be open, and his or her smiles may look more like snarls.
- Chewing tires the person.
- The person may drool or have difficulty managing saliva.
- The person's voice may become a whisper.
- The person's head may fall forward because of weak neck muscles.
- It may be difficult for the person to reach overhead.

- Fine motor activities of the hand may be impaired, and hand muscles may fatigue quickly.
- The person may have respiratory insufficiency because intercostals and the diaphragm are involved.
- The person may have low physical endurance and tire easily.
- Kinesthesia and proprioception may be affected in the upper extremities and hands.
- Generally, there is little atrophy of the muscles and rarely any pain.

Cognitive
- Cognitive faculties are not affected directly by the disorder.

Psychosocial
- The person may express feelings of hopelessness or helplessness.
- The person may become depressed.
- The person may express anger at being unable to do what others can do easily.
- The person may try to deny to others that anything is wrong.
- The person may make excuses to avoid social situations.
- The person may be unable to perform many life roles or role functions.

TREATMENT/INTERVENTION

The model of treatment is usually compensatory. Quality of life should also be a major concern.

Self-Care
- Provide self-help aids that will help the person perform activities of daily living. If the person is bedridden, arm supports or electronic devices that can control the environment may be useful (e.g., communication devices and devices that turn on or off the radio or television).
- Teach the person to cut pieces of meat into small bites, take small bites, and drink plenty of liquid to aid swallowing.
- Help the person to plan and prepare meals that contain soft foods that are easy to swallow.
- The person should use energy conservation, pacing, and work simplification techniques.

Productivity
- If the person cannot continue performing his or her present job, help the person consider other job options.
- Recommend modifications in job tasks or workplaces that could permit the person to continue in his or her present job.

Leisure
- Recommend modifications of leisure activities that might help the person continue doing his or her favorite activities.
- Help the person develop an interest in new leisure activities that are within the person's physical capacity.

Sensorimotor
- Increase muscle strength and endurance through gentle, nonresistive activities and games.
- Maintain range of motion.
- Use overhead slings or mobile arm supports if upper extremity muscles are too weak to permit hand function. If the person is bedridden, electronic aids may be needed.

Cognitive
- Assist in teaching the person about the disease and its management.
- Help the person determine what tasks need to be done, decide when during the day or week the tasks should be done, and develop a time management program.
- Teach the person energy conservation, pacing, and work simplification techniques.
- Teach the person to examine his or her home for architectural barriers and how to use grab bars or railings to increase safety.

Psychosocial
- Provide stress management training.
- Encourage the person to continue social activities but modify plans to permit rest breaks or shorten the length of the outing.
- Consider expanding home communication systems such as a voice-activated telephone or intercom to permit easier communication with the family and community agencies.

Environment
- Recommend modifications in the home to increase efficiency, such as using electronic communication devices, reducing architectural barriers, and increasing safety.

PRECAUTIONS
- The person must avoid overexertion. Watch the person for signs of fatigue by observing the face and eyes.
- Observe the person for changes in respiration. Encourage relaxation. If a respiratory crisis occurs, seek medical assistance immediately.
- Do not use strenuous or resistive activities.
- Do not use activities that aggravate respiratory problems.
- Note any changes in appearance (e.g., ptosis, drooping facial muscles, skin breakdown, or changes in breathing or swallowing) to the person's physician.
- The person should avoid emotional distress whenever possible.
- The person should avoid extremes in heat and cold.
- All infections should be monitored by the physician.

PROGNOSIS AND OUTCOME
This disease is progressive. The person may become bedridden. Death usually occurs due to respiratory failure.
- The person is able to perform daily living tasks with self-help devices, if needed.
- The person is able to perform productive activities with assistive technology as needed.

- The person is able to perform his or her chosen leisure activities.
- The person maintains muscle strength consistent with the stage of the disease.
- The person maintains range of motion consistent with the stage of the disease.
- The person maintains hand function and use of upper extremities consistent with the stage of the disease.
- The person uses assistive devices, if needed, to perform activities.
- The person is able to develop a time management plan.
- The person demonstrates knowledge of energy conservation, pacing, and work simplification.
- The person demonstrates knowledge of safety procedures.

REFERENCE

Beers, M.H., and R. Berkow, eds. 1999. *The Merck Manual of Diagnosis and Therapy*, 17th ed. Whitehouse Station, NJ: Merck Research Laboratories.

BIBLIOGRAPHY

McCormack, G.L. et al. Motor unit dysfunction—myasthenia gravis. In *Physical dysfunction: Practice skills for the occupational therapy assistant,* ed. M.B. Early, 563. St. Louis, MO: Mosby.
McCormak, G.L., and L.W. Pedretti. 1996. Myasthenia gravis. In *Occupational therapy: Practice skills for physical dysfunction*, 4th ed., ed. L.W. Pedretti, 756–757. St. Louis, MO: Mosby.
Pulaski, K.H. 1998. Myasthenia gravis. In *Willard and Spackman's occupational therapy*, 9th ed., eds. M.E. Neistadt and E.B. Crepeau, 678–679. Philadelphia: Williams & Wilkins.

Osteoporosis

DESCRIPTION

Osteoporosis is a metabolic bone disorder in which the rate of bone resorption accelerates while the rate of bone formation slows down, causing a loss of bone mass. Bones affected by the disease lose calcium and phosphate salts and thus become porous, brittle, and vulnerable to fracture. The disorder causes a generalized and progressive diminution of bone density (bone mass per unit volume), resulting in skeletal weakness, although the ratio of mineral to organic elements is unchanged (Merck 1999, 469).

CAUSE

The cause of primary osteoporosis is unknown. Types of primary osteoporosis include involutional (type 1, ages 50 to 70, and type 2, age 70 or greater), idiopathic, and juvenile osteoporosis. Risk factors include inadequate intake of calcium, declining gonadal adrenal function, estrogen deficiency, and a sedentary lifestyle. The causes of secondary osteoporosis are related to alcoholism, immobilization, hyperthyroidism, lactose intolerance, malnutrition, malabsorption, osteogenesis imperfecta, Sudeck's atrophy, or prolonged therapy with steroids or heparin. Caucasian women 50 years or older who are postmenopausal with inadequate dietary calcium intake, small bone structure, and a sedentary lifestyle are most frequently affected.

ASSESSMENT

Areas
- daily living skills: personal and instrumental activities of daily living
- productivity history, skills, interests, and values
- leisure skills and interests
- muscle strength
- range of motion
- balance and postural control
- learning skills
- self-concept
- coping skills
- social skills
- home safety
- architectural and environmental barriers

Instruments
No specific, named assessment instruments were identified from the references. The following may be useful:
- activities of daily living scale
- occupational history
- leisure checklist
- manual muscle test
- goniometer
- roles and role performance test
- depression test

PROBLEMS

Self-Care
- The person may experience difficulty performing some activities of daily living because of changes in skeletal function such as functional reach.
- The person may have difficulty finding clothing that fits properly due to kyphosis and lordosis.
- The person may have difficulty with bathing and washing, dressing, and transfers due to decreased range of motion.
- The person may have difficulty with toileting and continence.
- The person may have sleep disturbance due to reduced inspiratory function.
- The person may have limited positioning options due to kyphosis and lordosis.

- The person may have increased fatigue due to lack of restful sleep.

Productivity
- The person may have difficulty performing home management activities that require an upright position and weight bearing.
- The person may be unable to lift or carry heavy loads due to pain or risk of fracture.
- The person may have reduced sitting and standing tolerance.

Leisure
- The person may have only a few interests that can be done primarily in a sitting or reclining position rather than an upright position and that do not involve weight bearing.

Sensorimotor
- The person usually has dorsal kyphosis in the thoracic region.
- The person usually has lordosis in the cervical region.
- The person usually has loss of height.
- The person usually has decreased bone strength.
- The person may have marked changes in posture and increased anterior flexion.
- The person is at risk for vertebral crush fractures at T-8 or below as a result of back flexion, heavy lifting, or weak back extensor muscles.
- The person is at risk for hip fractures at the femoral neck and intratrochanteric and subcapital sites usually associated with falling.
- The person is at risk for wrist fractures usually associated with falling.
- The person may have decreased neuromuscular stability.
- The person may have decreased postural control and balance.
- The person may have reduced range of lumbar extension.
- The person may have reduced inspiratory function due to severe kyphosis.
- The person may have pain in the lower back that radiates around the trunk.
- The person may need a back support.

Cognitive
- Cognitive faculties are not affected directly by the disease.

Psychosocial
- The person may feel and act old because of changes in appearance.
- The person may withdraw from social contacts.
- The person may avoid certain situations for fear of falling or fractures.
- The person may become dependent on others due to decreased ability to perform tasks.

TREATMENT/INTERVENTION

Treatment models in occupational therapy include the Canadian Model of Occupational Performance.

Principles of Energy Conservation for Osteoporosis

- Set priorities and do those tasks that are most important or necessary.
- Distribute tasks over a period of time instead of trying to complete them all in one short time period.
- Take frequent rest breaks, several times a day, so that rest and activity are balanced.
- Sit instead of standing whenever possible.
- Use relaxation techniques to reduce stress and anxiety.
- Continue to lead a balanced lifestyle, taking time for leisure and spiritual enrichment.
- Work more slowly to save energy instead of rushing through tasks or work assignments.
- Pace activity at a comfortable rhythm.
- Do the portion of a task or job that is enjoyable and let someone else do the rest.

Source: Reprinted with permission from R. Barton and J. Feinberg, The Role of Occupational Therapy, in *Osteoarthritis*, pp. 315–324, K.D. Brant et al., eds. © 1998, Oxford University Press.

Self-Care
- Provide self-help devices that will facilitate safe performance of activities of daily living, such as long-handled items, reachers, seats for toilet and bath, and remote control devices for lighting.

Productivity
- Explore with the person home management activities that can satisfy the need for more physical activity (and can be performed safely), such as cleaning, washing, folding sheets, and hanging up garments.

Leisure
- Explore with the person possible leisure interests that can satisfy the need for more physical activity, such as shopping, visiting art galleries or museums, and going on garden tours or nature walks.

Sensorimotor
- Provide graded activities to exercise joints, especially hyperextension of the back by raising arms overhead.
- Encourage good positioning in performing any activity.
- Encourage weight-bearing activities, such as walking and social dancing, that can maintain or increase muscle strength around the hip joint.
- Decrease pain by promoting better posture and increased level of physical activity.
- Provide activities to promote the use of protective reflexes in a safe environment.

Principles of Joint Protection for Osteoporosis

- Distribute stress evenly over joints and keep weight distribution equal.
- Place stress on larger joints, usually more proximal to the trunk, or over surface area that is not a joint.
- Use joints in their most mechanically effective position, in the midrange of arc of motion.
- Avoid static holding positions for extended periods of time; alternate with movement.
- Eliminate excess weight when lifting objects, or completely avoid lifting.
- Use adaptive equipment as a form of joint protection.
- Avoid twisting movements with the hand, wrist, and thumb.
- Raise seats to eliminate stress to lower extremity joints.
- Avoid doing repetitive activities for extended periods of time; alternate with rest breaks.

Source: Reprinted with permission from R. Barton and J. Feinberg, The Role of Occupational Therapy, in *Osteoarthritis*, pp. 315–324, K.D. Brant et al, eds. Copyright © 1998, Oxford University Press.

Cognitive

- Instruct the person in safety procedures, including the use of grab bars and handrails, the elimination of floor hazards, such as rugs or cords, and the value of good lighting and contrast.
- Instruct the person in basic body mechanics, especially proper lifting and carrying, to avoid back strain.
- Instruct the person in selecting furniture that will provide good support for the back and neck as well as solid armrests to facilitate sitting and standing.
- Instruct the person in energy conservation and work simplification. Emphasize task analysis for safety.
- The person may benefit from a discussion of an activity schedule that provides for alternate cycles of activity and rest.

Psychosocial

- The person may find that increased physical activity reduces the feeling of being old.
- Use creative crafts, music, drama, or dance to improve the person's self-concept.
- If withdrawal has occurred, encourage the person to reestablish or make new contacts with community members who may also need more physical activity.

PRECAUTIONS

- Fractures of the hip and radius may occur from minor falls. Insist on safety measures.
- The person should not sleep in the fetal position.

PROGNOSIS AND OUTCOME

- The person is able to use self-help devices to perform activities that would otherwise lead to back strain or excess body flexion.
- The person maintains postural control and balance.
- The person maintains or increases the level of physical activities associated with weight bearing.
- The person demonstrates knowledge of safety issues and takes actions to reduce hazards.
- The person is able to adjust cycles of activity and rest to increase physical activity but not pain.

REFERENCE

Beers, M.H., and R. Berkow, eds. 1999. *The Merck Manual of Diagnosis and Therapy*, 17th ed. Whitehouse Station, NJ: Merck Research Laboratories.

BIBLIOGRAPHY

Grant, D., and K. Lundon. 1999. The Canadian Model of Occupational Performance applied to females with osteoporosis. *Canadian Journal of Occupational Therapy* 66, no. 1: 3–13.
Kalu, N. 1996. Osteoporosis: What the research shows. *Advance for Occupational Therapists* 12, no. 23: 19, 50.

Part VII

Systemic Disorders

Chronic Fatigue Syndrome

DESCRIPTION

Chronic fatigue syndrome (CFS) is characterized by long-standing, relapsing, severe fatigue without substantial muscle weakness and without proven psychological or physical causes (Merck 1999, 2481). The fatigue impairs daily function and is often made worse by exertion, exercise, headache, sore throat, and other stress. Other symptoms are enlarged, painful lymph nodes, sore throat, arthralgia, abdominal and muscle pain, low-grade fever, and difficulty concentrating and sleeping. The illness is observed primarily among adults between the ages of 20 and 40. Females outnumber males by a ratio of 2:1. To meet the case definition of the Centers for Disease Control and Prevention, the patient must fulfill 2 major criteria and either 8 of 11 symptom criteria or 6 of the symptom criteria and 2 of 3 physical criteria. Other names include epidemic neuromyasthenia, yuppie flu, post-viral fatigue syndrome, chronic Epstein-Barr syndrome, chronic fatigue immune dysfunction syndrome, myalgic encephalo-myelitis, and Royal Free disease. CFS was first formally described in 1988.

CAUSE

There is controversy about what causes CFS. Researchers suspect the HHV-6 or other herpes virus, enterovirus, or retrovirus. Rising levels of antibodies to the Epstein-Barr virus, once thought to implicate Epstein-Barr virus infections as a cause, now are considered a result of the disease. The illness is also thought to be associated with a reaction to viral illness that is complicated by a dysfunctional immune response along with other factors such as gender, age, genetic disposition, prior illness, stress, and environment.

ASSESSMENT

Areas

- daily living skills: personal and instrumental activities of daily living
- productivity skills, interests, and values
- leisure interests and skills
- muscle strength
- joint range of motion
- grasp strength
- endurance
- physical fitness
- coordination and dexterity
- lifting and carrying
- functional capacity
- attention span
- memory: short- and long-term
- reasoning: concrete and abstract

**Centers for Disease Control and Prevention
1994 Criteria for Diagnosing CFS**

1. New onset of self-reported persistent or relapsing, debilitating fatigue in a person who has no previous history of similar symptoms, which has lasted for 6 months or longer, is disabling, affects physical and mental function, and:
   a. Is characterized by fatigue as the principal symptom
   b. Is of new or definite onset (has not been lifelong)
   c. Is not the result of ongoing exertion
   d. Is not substantially alleviated by rest
   e. Results in substantial reduction in previous levels of occupation, educational, social, or personal activities.

2. Other clinical conditions that may produce similar symptoms, including pre-existing psychiatric diseases, must be excluded by thorough evaluation, based on history, physical examination, and appropriate laboratory findings.

3. Four or more of the following symptoms must be concurrently present for 6 or more months:
   a. Impaired concentration or memory
   b. Sore throat
   c. Tender cervical or axillary lymph nodes
   d. Muscle pain
   e. Multijoint pain without joint swelling or redness
   f. Headaches of a new type, pattern, or severity
   g. Unrefreshing sleep
   h. Post-exertional malaise lasting more than 24 hours.

- judgment and safety
- roles and role performance
- coping skills

Instruments

Instruments Developed by Occupational Therapy Personnel

- *Activity Record* by N. Pollock et al., *Canadian Journal of Occupational Therapy* 57, no. 2 (1990): 77–81.
- *Functional Capacity Evaluation Battery* by D.M. Barrows, in Functional capacity evaluations of persons with chronic fatigue immune dysfunction syndrome, *American Journal of Occupational Therapy* 49, no. 4 (1995): 327–337.
- *Occupational Case Analysis and Interview Rating Scale* (OCAIRS) by K. Kaplan and G. Kielhofner, Thorofare, NJ: Slack, 1989.

Instruments Developed by Other Professionals and Used by Occupational Therapy Personnel
- *Fatigue Severity Scale* by L.B. Krupp et al., in The Fatigue Severity Scale: Applications to patients with multiple sclerosis and systemic lupus erythematosus, *Archives of Neurology* 46 (1989): 1121–1123.
- *Human Activity Profile* by A.J. Fix and M.S. Daughton, Odessa, FL: Psychological Assessment Resources, 1988.
- *Nottingham Health Profile* by S. Hunt and S.P. McKenna, Manchester, England: Galen Research and Consultancy, 1991.

PROBLEMS

Self-Care
- The person may be too tired to perform personal self-care.
- The person may have difficulty sleeping.

Productivity
- The person may be unable to work a regular workday because of fatigue.
- The person may be unable to complete regular homemaking tasks because of fatigue.

Leisure
- The person may discontinue leisure interests because of fatigue.

Sensorimotor
- The person may complain of feeling weak.
- The person may become deconditioned due to inactivity.

Cognitive
- The person may have difficulty maintaining attention and concentration.

Psychosocial
- The person may be depressed and discouraged.
- The person may express feelings of failure at being unable to manage daily life.
- The person may have loss of self-esteem.
- The person may feel isolated and alone, especially if the diagnosis has taken many weeks or months to establish.
- The person may feel that health professionals lack understanding, are unsympathetic, and are unsupportive.
- The person may stop socializing with friends because of fatigue.

TREATMENT/INTERVENTION
Models of treatment developed by occupational therapists include the Model of Human Occupation and the Canadian Occupational Performance Model or client-centered approach.

Other models include the bio-psycho-social (medical) model and the cognitive behavior therapy (medical-psychology) model.

Self-Care
- Discuss healthy eating habits with the person and consider including a nutritionist or dietician in the discussions.
- Help the person develop a schedule of action and rest (relaxation).

Productivity
- The person may need to reduce work hours or find a job with flexible work hours.

Leisure
- Discuss which of the person's leisure interests can be adapted to his or her available level of energy and aid in relaxation of both mind and body.

Sensorimotor
- Use a graded activity program with small increments to increase endurance using activities agreed upon with the client.
- Reduce sensory overload, especially during periods of relaxation.

Cognitive
- Instruct the person in energy conservation, pacing, and work simplification.
- Instruct the person in time management techniques.
- Instruct the person in lifestyle management, including maintaining a balance of rest and activity.
- Instruct the person in stress management and relaxation techniques.

Psychosocial
- Develop a trusting relationship with the person, if possible. If the person distrusts health care personnel, a group approach may be best.
- Help the person regain control of his or her life by challenging the "I can't" statements such as "I can't work anymore." Suggest new statements such as "I can work, but I must adjust how I do it."
- Use of group approaches encourages the development of a new social network of mutual support that acknowledges difficulties and provides relief and bonding.
- A group approach should be structured and based on problem solving but not be dogmatic or prescriptive. A group can cover topics such as energy conservation, work simplification, lifestyle management, and stress management.
- Group member support and feedback may increase an individual's motivation and morale.
- Explore with the person which roles and role performances are important and which could be changed. Family members should also be consulted.
- Increase use of alternative coping skills through individual or group tasks.
- Help the person and family examine habits and routines that relate to fatigue to determine if certain changes might improve the person's performance.

PRECAUTION

- The person should avoid the "weekend warrior" approach in which the person does as much as possible and then "crashes" in exhaustion (also called the "peaks and troughs" approach). This approach prolongs the disorder and creates a vicious cycle.

PROGNOSIS AND OUTCOME

- The person is able to perform daily living tasks with rest breaks as needed.
- The person is able to perform productive tasks using modifications as needed.
- The person is able to participate in leisure interests.
- The person demonstrates knowledge of energy conservation, pacing, and work simplification.
- The person demonstrates knowledge of time and stress management techniques.
- The person is able to plan and eat a balanced diet.
- The person is able to socialize with friends and participate in social situations.

REFERENCE

Beers, M.H., and R. Berkow, eds. 1999. *The Merck Manual of Diagnosis and Therapy*, 17th ed. Whitehouse Station, NJ: Merck Research Laboratories.

BIBLIOGRAPHY

Barrows, D.M. 1995. Functional capacity evaluations of persons with chronic fatigue immune dysfunction syndrome. *American Journal of Occupational Therapy* 49, no. 4: 327–337.

Cox, D. 1998. Chronic fatigue syndrome—an occupational therapy programme. *Occupational Therapy International* 6, no. 1: 52–64.

Cox, D.L. et al. 1996. Focus on research: Chronic fatigue syndrome. *British Journal of Occupational Therapy* 59, no. 2: 87–90.

Kerr, T. 1996. CFS cause still eluding medical science. *Advance for Occupational Therapists* 12, no. 9: 19.

Packer, T.L. et al. 1997. Fatigue and activity patterns of people with chronic fatigue syndrome. *Occupational Therapy Journal of Research* 17, no. 3: 186–199.

Pembertson, S. et al. 1994. Chronic fatigue syndrome: A way forward. *British Journal of Occupational Therapy* 57, no. 10: 381–383.

Diabetes Mellitus

DESCRIPTION

Diabetes mellitus (DM) is a syndrome characterized by hyperglycemia resulting from absolute or relative impairment in insulin secretion and/or insulin reaction (Merck 1999, 165). There are two major types, Type I DM and Type II DM.

Type I DM is usually diagnosed in childhood, adolescence, or young adulthood (before age 30). It is characterized by hyperglycemia and a propensity to develop diabetic ketoacidosis. The pancreas produces little or no insulin, and thus the person is dependent on insulin being added to the system.

Type II DM is characterized clinically by hyperglycemia and insulin resistance, but diabetic ketoacidosis is rare. The person is not dependent on insulin being added and often can be treated with diet, exercise, and oral drugs. Type II DM is associated with obesity, hypertension, hyperlipidemia, and coronary artery disease (the syndrome of insulin resistance).

Complications associated with poorly controlled diabetes are related to macrovascular disease such as atherosclerosis, which in turn leads to coronary artery disease, claudication, skin breakdown, and infections. Diabetic polyneuropathy causes a number of problems. The most common occurs as a distal, symmetric, predominantly sensory disorder that causes numbness, tingling, and paresthesia. In severe cases, foot ulcers and joint problems may occur. Another type is mononeuropathy, which affects the third, fourth, or sixth cranial nerves in particular (vision), but other nerves may be involved as a result of nerve infarction. Autonomic neuropathy causes postural hypotension, disorder sweating, impotence and retrograde ejaculation in men, impaired bladder function, delayed gastric emptying, esophageal dysfunction, and constipation or diarrhea (including nocturnal diarrhea). Diabetic nephropathy develops in about one-third of Type I DM cases but less frequently in Type II DM. End-stage renal disease can result.

In addition, diabetes may be a primary or secondary diagnosis.

CAUSE

In Type I DM, about 80 percent of cases have a genetically susceptible, immune-mediated, selective destruction of the insulin-secreting beta cells. However, environmental factors do affect the appearance of Type I DM. Viruses such as congenital rubella, mumps, and Coxsackie B may incite the development of autoimmune beta-cell destruction. Other environmental factors are geography and exposure to cow's milk.

Type II DM, which is actually a heterogeneous group of disorders, does not have the same genetic link, but genetics do play a role in the postreceptor defects. Onset is usually after age 30.

ASSESSMENT

Areas
- daily living skills: personal and instrumental activities of daily living
- productivity history, skills, interests, and values
- leisure interests and skills
- muscle strength by groups of muscles
- fine motor skills, manipulation, dexterity, and eye-hand coordination
- grip and pinch strength
- balance and postural control
- sensory registration and modulation, especially vision

- sensory processing (tactile, pain, proprioceptive, vibration) of the feet, hands, and limbs
- perception skills, especially visual
- self-concept
- role behavior

Instruments

No specific instruments developed by occupational therapists were identified in the literature. The following types of instruments may be useful:
- daily living scale
- occupational history
- leisure checklist
- dynamometers and pinch meters
- two-point discrimination tool, such as a Disk-Criminator or Boley gauge
- balance beam and tilt board test

PROBLEMS

Self-Care

- The person may need to learn to administer insulin, whether orally or by injections.
- The person may have difficulty using glucose monitoring equipment.

Productivity

- The person may be unable to perform productive activities due to fatigue.

Leisure

- The person may have stopped participating in his or her favorite leisure activities due to fatigue.

Sensorimotor

- The person may have general weakness and loss of weight.
- The person usually has decreased endurance and physical tolerance and fatigues easily.
- The person may have loss of reflexes or reactions.
- The person may have muscle aches and pains.
- The person may have specific muscle weaknesses, such as in the intrinsics of the foot (diabetic neuropathy).
- The person may have flexion contractures in the hand.
- The person may have limited grasp and release in the hand.
- The person may have impaired circulation associated with diabetes, which may cause myocardial or cerebral infarction or result in amputation of a leg.
- The person may have renal disease associated with diabetes.
- The person may have loss of vision and other eye changes (diabetic retinopathy, diabetic retinitis, or diabetic cataract).
- The person may have loss of the sense of touch.
- The person may experience paresthesia, hyperesthesia, or hypesthesia.
- The person may lose vibration and position sense.

- The person may have decreased sensitivity to pain in the extremities but experience chronic pain in other body parts.
- The person may have decreased temperature sensation.

Cognitive
- Cognitive faculties are not affected directly by the disorder but may be present due to other disorders such as a stroke, the aging process, and Alzheimer's.

Psychosocial
- The person may fear being dependent on insulin.
- The person may feel loss of control of life and purpose.
- The person may have anxiety about living with diet restrictions.
- The person may become depressed or angry (Why me? Why am I being punished?).
- The person may become irritable.
- The person may be easily discouraged.
- The person may worry about the future.
- The person may have decreased social activities due to fatigue or diet restrictions.

TREATMENT/INTERVENTION
Models of treatment do not appear to be well established but include aspects of compensation/substitution, biomechanical modes, and the model of human occupation.

Self-Care
- Provide adapted equipment, if necessary, to facilitate performance of self-care activities.
- Encourage the person to maintain independence in activities of daily living.
- Recommend or design alternate equipment or methods for the person to self-administer insulin safely using the correct dose and monitor glucose levels.

Productivity
- Explore possible needs for modifications in the work or home environment to conserve energy and simplify work tasks.
- If the current job situation is dangerous to the person's health, explore alternative vocational interests.
- Encourage the person to participate in home management tasks.

Leisure
- Help the person to determine which leisure interests must be modified or discontinued.
- Help the person to explore new interests to replace those that cannot continue to be pursued.
- Provide information on available community programs and resources.

Sensorimotor
- Increase muscle strength through the use of specific activities.
- Increase endurance and physical tolerance through the use of functional activities.
- Provide a home program to maintain movement of feet and ankles and decrease edema, such as picking up small objects with the toes or rolling a bottle back and forth with the feet.

- Biofeedback may be helpful in increasing circulation, maintaining temperature in the extremities, decreasing heart rate and blood pressure, and maintaining or increasing muscle contraction.
- Serial casting may be used to prevent contractures and increase joint mobility during or after ulcer healing of the foot.
- Maintain sensory awareness, especially in the feet, through the use of foot activities and games or biofeedback.
- If sensory loss has occurred, provide an opportunity to practice compensatory skills using remaining sensory systems as backups or substitutes.
- If visual loss is suspected, provide a screening test for functional problems and review the person's living environment so that safety hazards may be eliminated.
- If the person has low vision, see the section on low vision or Cate et al. (1995).

COGNITIVE
- Instruct the person on energy conservation and work simplification.
- If sensory loss has occurred, instruct the person on safety requirements necessary to avoid injury.
- Instruct the person in time management to organize cycles of rest and activity.
- Assist in instructing the person to modify his or her diet according to recommended guidelines, including changing recipes and planning meal menus.
- Assist in instructing the person about the secondary complications of diabetes, such as decreased tactile awareness (routine visual inspection, especially of the feet, is necessary), circulation impairment (shoes designed to protect against pressure should be worn), and visual problems (relationship of increased systolic pressure to retinal aneurysms).
- Instruct the person on the relationship of exercise to blood sugar level.

Psychosocial
- Maintain or increase the person's self-concept and sense of mastery.
- Maintain or increase the person's self-identity and sense of responsibility.
- Increase the person's coping skills, helping him or her adjust to life with a disability.
- Provide instruction and practice in relaxation techniques to reduce stress.
- Encourage the person to maintain dyadic relationships.
- Support group interaction, including a support group for persons with diabetes and their family members.
- Assist the family to adjust roles and functions to maintain the person's active participation in the family unit.

PRECAUTIONS
- Observe the person for symptoms of insulin shock.
- Observe safety rules.

PROGNOSIS AND OUTCOME
- The person has sufficient strength and endurance to perform activities of daily living.

Ways To Improve Coping Skills

- Change your job to meet your changing health needs.
- Change your personal schedule to better meet your health needs.
- Decide what is more and less important in your daily life and relationships.
- Refuse to be overwhelmed by too much information. Put things aside for later.
- Use humor to let off steam.
- Put some distance between yourself and the illness at times.
- Rely on faith and spirituality.
- Get enough recreation and leisure activity.
- Release emotions by doing, talking, crying, singing, and playing sports.
- Get enough social support.
- Get counseling.

Source: Adapted with permission from R. Krinsky, The Link between Depression, Diabetes, *Advance for Occupational Therapists*, Vol. 12, No. 49, p. 18, © 1996.

- The person demonstrates the use of good energy conservation and work simplification techniques during functional activities.
- The person demonstrates time management skills in regulating physical activities according to rest and activity cycles based on insulin and diet considerations.
- The person demonstrates knowledge regarding skin care to prevent skin breakdown.
- The person has learned compensatory skills for any sensory loss and can perform activities safely.
- The person has learned coping skills to live within the restrictions of the disease without becoming handicapped.

REFERENCES

Beers, M.H., and R. Berkon, eds. 1999. *The Merck Manual of Diagnosis and Therapy*, 17th ed. Whitehouse Station, NJ: Merck Research Laboratories.
Cate, Y. et al. 1995. Occupational therapy and the person with diabetes and vision impairment (review). *American Journal of Occupational Therapy* 49, no. 9: 905–911.

BIBLIOGRAPHY

Copley-Nigro, J. 1997. Ralph and talking glucose monitor. *Advance for Occupational Therapists* 13, no. 24: 42.
Krinsky, R. 1996. The link between depression, diabetes. *Advance for Occupational Therapists* 12, no. 49: 18.

Systemic Sclerosis

DESCRIPTION

Systemic sclerosis is a chronic disease characterized by diffuse fibrosis; degenerative changes; and vascular abnormalities in the skin (scleroderma), articular structures, and internal organs (especially the esophagus, gastrointestinal tract, lung, heart, and kidney; Merck 1999, 421). The disease varies in degree of severity and rate of progression. The localized form of scleroderma occurs as circumscribed patches (morphea) or linear sclerosis of the integument and immediate subjacent tissues without system involvement. The subtype sclerodactyly is confined to the hands for many years. A major variant of the limited cutaneous scleroderma is the CREST syndrome (calcinosis, Raynaud's phenomenon, esophageal dysfunction, sclerodactyly, and telangiectasia).

Mixed connective tissue disease or diffuse cutaneous systemic sclerosis combines features of scleroderma with clinical and serologic features of systemic lupus erythematosus, polymyositis, or rheumatoid arthritis. The mixed or diffuse form may progress to total body involvement within one year. Symptoms may subside for many months, but the course of the disease is not reversed. Death usually occurs because of visceral involvement.

Associated conditions that affect the hand are Raynaud's phenomenon, digital ischemic ulcers, telangiectasia, calcium deposits, resorption, and tendon friction rubs.

CAUSE

The cause is unknown. The ratio of women with the disease to men with the disease is about 4:1. Diagnosis usually occurs between the ages of 30 and 50. The disorder is rare in children and the elderly. Involvement usually is symmetrical, beginning in the hands and progressing proximally to the arms, neck, and face, followed by involvement of the trunk and lower extremities. As the disorder progresses, the skin, musculoskeletal system, gastrointestinal tract, cardiorespiratory system, and renal system become involved.

ASSESSMENT

Areas

- daily living skills: personal and instrumental activities of daily living
- productivity history, skills, interests, and values
- leisure skills and interests
- range of motion, active and passive
- hand prehension functions
- fine motor skills, manipulation, dexterity, and bilateral coordination
- physical endurance
- functional mobility
- affect or mood
- social skills
- social roles

Instruments

- *Health Assessment Questionnaire,* Disability Index portion by J.F. Fries et al., in Measurement of patient outcomes in arthritis, *Arthritis and Rheumatism* 23 (1980): 137–145.
- activities of daily living
- occupational history
- leisure checklist
- goniometer or tracing digit and thumb abduction on a piece of paper
- dynamometer and pinch meter
- dexterity and coordination tests

PROBLEMS

Self-Care

- The person usually has increasing difficulty performing activities of daily living, especially those requiring range of motion or reaching, such as dressing, grooming, housekeeping, and cleaning.
- The person may regurgitate food.
- The person's mouth opening (oral aperture) has usually decreased in size, which may restrict oral hygiene, dental care, and the ability to chew solid food.
- The person may experience dry mouth (sicca syndrome), which interferes with chewing and swallowing.

Productivity

- The person may become increasingly unable to perform certain job tasks due to limited range of motion, limited endurance, or pain.
- The person may be unable to continue working in a specific job because he or she cannot perform the required job tasks.

Leisure

- The person may find that certain leisure activities are difficult to continue due to limited range of motion, endurance, or pain.

Sensorimotor

- The person may have decreased range of motion and loss of joint mobility.
- The person may have decreased physical endurance.
- The person may have stiffness and swelling of the joints, especially in the hands and feet.
- Flexion contractures of the wrists and elbows may occur.
- Claw hand deformity may occur (metacarpophalangeal joints in extension, proximal interphalangeal joints in flexion, and adduction of the thumb, which results in loss of opposition).
- The person may have myopathy, including muscle weakness and wasting.
- The person may have resorption of fingertips.
- The person may have hypopigmentation.

- The person may develop ulcers on the fingertips and dorsum of the knuckles due to repeated ischemic attacks related to vasospasms.
- The person may lose normal hand prehension functions and fine motor skills due to bony resorption, which results in shortening of the fingers (resorption), sores on the fingers, or calcium deposits that occur subcutaneously or intracutaneously.
- The person may have episodic vasospasms of the peripheral arteries that result in balancing and cyanosis of the hands (loss of temperature control) during spasms and erythema following spasm (Raynaud's phenomena). The disorder may also affect the toes, earlobes, tip of the nose, and tongue.
- The person may have polyarthralgia (pain in multiple joints).
- The person may have changes in body image.
- The person may have pain and paresthesia.
- The person's skin may become puffy, swollen, and edematous. Thickening may occur, then atrophy and deformity.
- The person's hands may become hypersensitive. The person may respond by keeping his or her hands in a protected or guarded position (elbows and wrists flexed in front of the body) that affects posture and balance.

Cognitive
- Cognitive faculties are not directly affected.

Psychosocial
- The person may have a fear of or difficulty adjusting to what others think about his or her changing body.
- The person may have a fear of dying.
- The person may have a fear of or difficulty adjusting to becoming increasingly helpless.
- The person may have a fear of or difficulty adjusting to facial and upper extremity disfigurement.
- The person may withdraw from social situations.
- The person may experience difficulty speaking clearly if his or her mouth, lips, and respiratory system are involved.
- The person may experience changes in roles and role performance.

TREATMENT/INTERVENTION
- Models of treatment are based on biomechanical and rehabilitation models.

Self-Care
- Encourage the person to maintain independence in self-care activities. Choosing clothing without buttons or with Velcro and loafers or shoes with elastic ties is useful. Clothing that is a size too large is easier to get on and off than more tightly fitting clothing.
- Recommend self-help devices and provide training in their use if needed. Commonly used devices have built-up handles, extended handles, and parts that can make small pinching motions. If ulcers or calcium deposits limit functional ability, pressure on sensitive areas may be relieved by using padding on utensils or using strap loops, faucet turners, button hooks, and pencil holders.

- For hypomotility, reflux esophagitis (regurgitation), and dysphagia, suggest sitting very erect during meals, using relaxation techniques before eating, eating smaller and more frequent meals, remaining erect for 15 to 20 minutes after eating, sleeping with the head elevated eight inches above the body, and using antacids.
- Recommend joint protection, energy conservation, pacing, and work simplification techniques.

Productivity

- Make recommendations for modifications in the work setting that might enable the person to continue working.
- Provide opportunities for exploring other interests and career options if the person cannot safely or effectively continue in his or her present job.
- Make recommendations for modifications in the home that might enable the person to function more independently and contribute to home management.
- Recommend homemaking devices that reduce the degree of general strength and endurance that is needed (e.g., jar openers, electric can openers, suctioned cutting boards, and ergonomically designed knives).

Leisure

- Encourage the person to identify new interests and explore leisure activities that can be pursued within the limitations of the disability.

Sensorimotor

- Maintain range of motion and joint mobility as long as possible to avoid contractures. Exercises should be done frequently and beyond the point of initial resistance. Special attention should be paid to maintaining metacarpophalangeal (MCP) joint flexion, proximal interphalangeal (PIP) joint extension, thumb abduction (to maintain web space and opposition), and wrist extension. (Claw hand deformity limits these motions.) Encourage the individual to make a fist, emphasizing flexion of the MCP joints. The heel of one hand can be used to press the fingers of the other hand flat down against a table, or place the hands and fingers flat against each other in a "prayer" position.
- If contractures are developing, pressure points can also be used. The first point is the pulp of the index finger on the volar surface of the middle phalanx of a contracted finger. The second point is the pulp of the third finger on the volar surface of the proximal phalanx of the contracted finger. The third point is the thumb against the dorsum of the contracted PIP joint. The thumb pushes against the joint while the index and middle fingers apply counterpressure to try to straighten the joint (Poole 1996, 581).
- Finger and hand range of motion and stretching exercises can be done while using rubber bands, by putting rolls made from facial tissue between the fingers, by clasping and unclasping the hands, and by making and unmaking a fist.
- Maintain hand prehension functions through exercises and use of alternate or variant grasp patterns (Poole 1994, 46–54).
- Maintain facial mobility (oral aperture, lip closure, and temporomandibular joint excursion) through exercises. Massage with a warm washcloth or use of a vibrator may facilitate performance of the exercises. For facial contractures of the temporomandibular joints, three exercises are recommended: exaggerated facial movements, manual stretching, and oral

augmentation. Exaggerated facial movements include pursing the lips, puffing out the cheeks, and exaggerated smiling. Manual stretching is done by placing the right thumb in the corner of the left side of mouth and vice versa with the left thumb. The thumbs are then used to stretch the mouth laterally. Oral augmentation involves the insertion of a stack of tongue depressors or similar items between the molar teeth. Additional depressors can be added if more jaw opening is attained.

- Exercises to maintain motion of the chest consist of retracting the shoulders and fully flexing and abducting the shoulders. Good posture is also important.
- Consider providing hand splints if the person is unable to carry out range of motion exercises. MCP flexion and PIP extension may be maintained by using a dynamic volar wrist splint with dynamic finger flexion slings added and using rubber bands to apply tension. The person wears a splint for 15 to 30 minutes while performing daily activities. A splint with a C-bar may be used to maintain web space. This splint may be worn at night. Watch for signs of edema, decreased circulation, and skin changes. Static splints that restrict joint motion should be used with caution unless the person has carpal tunnel syndrome or a ruptured tendon.
- Single joints may be wrapped with Coban tape or Co-wrap.
- Dynamic splints have been found to be unsuccessful in increasing range of motion in the hand (Poole 1996, 584).
- Maintain physical endurance and conditioning for as long as possible. Swimming in a very warm pool is a good aerobic exercise. Use a skin lotion with lanolin to counteract the drying effects of chlorine.
- Slow the process of contracture development and prevent contractures due to poor positioning, disuse, or inadequate range of motion exercise.
- Maintain or increase strength. For the proximal muscles in the pelvic and shoulder girdle, resistance can be provided with elastic material such as a theraband, theratubing, and a dental dam. For hand strengthening, exercise putty is available in several grades of resistance.
- Wearing gloves or mittens for hands and socks for feet may decrease temperature loss.
- Biofeedback may be useful to control symptoms, relieve pain, and improve function.
- Pain control may be accomplished through use of heat modalities, such as paraffin bath, hot packs, hydrotherapy, or fluidotherapy. Occupational therapy personnel should use only heat modalities that they have been properly trained to use.

Cognitive

- Instruct the person about symptoms, progression of the disorder, and treatments that are effective and ineffective.
- Instruct the person on joint protection and the best postures for activities requiring standing, sitting, and lying down.
- Instruct the person on time management, energy conservation, pacing, and work simplification.
- Provide the person with an objective system for checking range of motion to permit self-monitoring of the progress of the disorder, such as templates of the hands and fingers drawn during the most recent visit (Melvin 1995, 1391).
- Provide a home program of daily exercises. Check to ensure that the person understands how the exercise is to be performed and why the exercise is important (to maintain range of

motion and joint mobility). Pay special attention to metacarpophalangeal flexion, followed by thumb abduction and opposition, and finger proximal interphalangeal extension.
- Instruct the person on how to measure range of motion using templates of the hand and/or drawings of the hand on paper, which can be compared to a template showing desired range of motion in abduction and extension of the digits.

Psychosocial
- Permit the person to voice fears about changing body image, possible disfigurement, death and dying, and the reaction of family and friends.
- Assist in providing counseling to the person and family or friends regarding the need for physical and emotional support.
- Provide training in stress management and relaxation techniques. Deep breathing is especially useful since it reinforces breathing exercises. Biofeedback may be useful to develop relaxation skills.
- Encourage the person to continue socialization.
- Encourage the person to seek social support from family and friends.
- Encourage the person and family to participate in a self-help group if available and use other community resources as needed.

PRECAUTIONS
- Provide information on the need to avoid or limit contact with household detergents because of their drying effect on the skin. The person should use gloves and/or lanolin lotions.
- Provide information on the need to avoid or limit contact with cold air or tobacco because of their effect on vasoconstriction, especially if the person has Raynaud's phenomenon.
- Provide information on the need to avoid or limit contact with abrasives that may irritate the skin and lead to infection.
- Watch for signs of carpal tunnel syndrome or ruptured tendons, which may occur due to dorsal or volar wrist tenosynovitis.
- Caution the person on the use of heating pads or heat modalities. The person is subject to burns because the vascular system is compromised.
- Avoid exercises that utilize lifting of books to strengthen muscles, which may cause a paper cut injury.

PROGNOSIS AND OUTCOME
There is no cure. Various drugs can treat some symptoms but not the disease itself. The prognosis varies. The person may have remission and lead a relatively healthy life or may become chronically ill and have multiple systemic involvement.
- The person is able to maintain range of motion and joint mobility, especially in the hands, upper extremities, and oral musculature.
- The person demonstrates the use of joint protection techniques in the performance of all daily activities.
- The person demonstrates the use of energy conservation and work simplification techniques.

- The person demonstrates the use of coping strategies or stress management techniques to reduce stress.
- The person maintains social interaction with family and friends.
- The person has the social support of family and friends.
- The person performs daily living activities independently, using self-help devices as needed.
- The person performs productive activities.
- The person performs leisure activities.

REFERENCES

Beers, M.H., and R. Berkow, eds. 1999. *The Merck Manual of Diagnosis and Therapy*, 17th ed. Whitehouse Station, NJ: Merck Research Laboratories.

Melvin, J.L. 1995. Scleroderma (systemic sclerosis): Treatment of the hand. In *Rehabilitation of the hand: Surgery and therapy,* 4th ed., eds. J.M. Hunter et al., 1385–1400. St. Louis, MO: Mosby.

Poole, J.L. 1994. Grasp pattern variations seen in the scleroderma hand. *American Journal of Occupational Therapy* 48, no. 1: 46–54.

Poole, J.L. 1996. Occupational and physical therapy. In *Systemic sclerosis,* eds. P.J. Clements and D.E. Furst, 581–590. Baltimore: Williams & Wilkins.

BIBLIOGRAPHY

Carr, S. et al. 1997. Use of continuous passive motion to increase hand range of motion in a woman with scleroderma: A single subject study. *Physiotherapy Canada* 49, no. 4: 292–296.

Marmer, L. 1993. Systemic sclerosis: Outwitting a baffling disorder. *Advance for Occupational Therapists* 9, no. 17: 13.

Melvin, J.L. 1994. *Scleroderma: Caring for your hands and face.* Bethesda, MD: American Occupational Therapy Association.

Poole, J.L. et al. 1995. Concurrent validity of the Health Assessment Questionnaire Disability Index in scleroderma. *Arthritis Care and Research* 8, no. 3: 189–193.

Part VIII

Immunologic and Infectious Diseases

Human Immunodeficiency Virus and Acquired Immunodeficiency Syndrome—Adult

DESCRIPTION

Human immunodeficiency virus (HIV) infection results in a wide range of clinical manifestations, varying from asymptomatic carrier status to severely debilitating and fatal disorders related to defective cell-mediated immunity. The human retrovirus that has had the greatest social and medical impact is HIV-1, which was identified in 1984 as the cause of a widespread epidemic of severe immunosuppression called acquired immunodeficiency syndrome (AIDS). AIDS is a secondary immunodeficiency syndrome disorder of cell-mediated immunity characterized by opportunistic infections, malignancies, neurologic dysfunction, and a variety of other syndromes (Merck 1999, 1312). AIDS was formally recognized in 1981 and was identified as an epidemic in 1985. Mean survival rate for women has been significantly shorter than for men, but newer combined drug treatments have greatly increased life expectancy.

HIV infection has the following stages:

1. Acute infection: This is the body's initial short-lived flulike response to the virus. (Note: Not all persons report this stage.)
2. Asymptomatic disease: HIV continues to replicate in the body and affect the immune system, but not enough to cause signs and symptoms.
3. Symptomatic: HIV has done enough damage to the immune system to cause signs and symptoms.
4. Advanced HIV disease or AIDS: The immune system is severely compromised.

CAUSE

The cause of infection is the HIV retrovirus, which appears in two major forms, HIV-1 and HIV-2. Other names include the human T-lymphotrophic virus type, the lymphadenopathy-associated virus, and the AIDS-associated retrovirus. Transmission of HIV requires contact with body fluids containing infected cells with lymphocytes or plasma (e.g., blood, semen, vaginal secretions, breast milk, saliva, or wound exudates). Secondary disorders include opportunistic infections such as Pneumocystis carinii pneumonia, Candida albicans, Cryptococcus neoformans, Toxoplasma gondii, cytomegalovirus, Mycobacterium avium-intracellular complex, or Mycobacterium tuberculosis and malignancies such as Karposi's sarcoma. Additional disorders caused by the AIDS virus include segmental demyelination, mononeuritis multiplex, polyneuropathy, ganglioneuronitis, and radiculopathy. The groups most affected are sexually active homosexual and bisexual men, intravenous drug users, hemophiliacs infected by blood transfusions, and Haitians, but increasing numbers of women and their infants are infected from the women's relationships with HIV-positive bisexual men and drug users.

Not all HIV infections lead to AIDS. AIDS requires the presence of HIV infection and CD4+ (helper-T cells) counts below 200/ml.

ASSESSMENT

Note: Because the status of people with HIV and AIDS can change quickly, frequent reassessment is recommended.

Areas

- daily living tasks: personal and instrumental activities of daily living
- productivity: homemaking and work-related tasks
- community management
- medication schedule
- accustomed life roles
- leisure and avocational interests and skills
- balance and gait
- coordination
- muscle tone
- muscle strength
- activity tolerance
- sensation/pain
- visual perception
- motor planning
- reality orientation
- memory
- organizational skills
- safety awareness
- judgment
- oral and written communication
- coping mechanisms
- social support system
- home and community safety

Instruments

- *Pizzi Assessment of Productive Living for Adults with HIV Infection and AIDS* (PAPL) by M. Pizzi, Silver Spring, MD: Positive Images and Wellness, 1991.
- activities of daily living scale
- work capacities evaluation
- occupational history
- leisure checklist
- manual muscle test
- dexterity and coordination test

PROBLEMS

Most of the problems seen by occupational therapy personnel are related to neuropathologic aspects of HIV infection, specifically the central nervous system, the peripheral nervous system, and the autonomic nervous system.

Self-Care

- The person may have difficulty performing or be unable to perform daily living tasks.
- The person may lose his or her appetite and interest in food and not eat regularly.
- The person may have disturbed sleep patterns.
- The person may experience difficulty in basic communication.
- The person may be unable to hold onto and use effectively self-care "tools" (e.g., forks, hairbrushes) because of changes (hypo- or hypersensitivity) in both somatic and visual senses.
- The person may have dysphagia due to oral candidiasis (yeast infection) or neurologic manifestations.

Productivity

- The person may have difficulty with or be unable to perform work-related tasks.
- The person may have difficulty with or be unable to perform homemaking tasks.

Leisure

- The person may be unable to continue participating in some leisure activities.

Sensorimotor

- The person usually has loss of physical endurance.
- The person may have a fever.
- The person may complain of fatigue, especially with lymphadenopathy.
- The person may complain of general malaise, especially with lymphadenopathy.
- The person may lose weight, especially with lymphadenopathy, because the nutrients are used by the metabolism of the virus itself.
- The person may experience diarrhea, which further reduces nutrients available.
- The person may have progressive loss of muscle strength.
- The person may experience gait ataxia.
- The person may have tremors.
- The person may have release of primitive reflex patterns.
- The person may experience changes in or loss of postural control related to loss of weight.
- The person may experience loss of coordination.
- The person may experience shortness of breath.
- The person may have hemiplegia due to a cerebrovascular disorder. (See the section on hemiplegia.)
- The person may demonstrate diminished ankle and knee reflexes.
- The person may have autonomic changes such as tachycardia, abnormal blood pressure readings in response to isometric exercise, and positional changes (sit to stand, tilting).
- The person may have pain related to changes in posture.
- The person may experience loss of sensation: temperature, vibration, and proprioception.

Conventional Stages of Mourning

- shock or alarm
- denial or realization, often accompanied by self-isolation
- anger, guilt, fear
- search for health, new lifestyle, healthier living
- altruism or identity with loss
- sadness or feeling of loss
- continued depression and/or anxiety, pathological grief
- acceptance
- resignation

Source: Adapted with permission from L. Cusack and L. Phillips, HIV Disease and AIDS, in *Occupational Therapy and Physical Dysfunction: Principles, Skills, and Practice*, A. Turner, M. Foster, and S.G. Johnson, eds., p. 833, © 1996, Churchill Livingstone.

- The person may be hypersensitive to touch.
- The person may experience loss of vision as a result of cytomegalovirus retinitis.
- The person may have loss of visual perceptual skills.

Cognitive
- The person may experience signs of dementia, including confusion and loss of problem-solving skills.
- The person with cognitive deficits may be unable to live independently due to poor judgment about safety.

Psychosocial
- The person may express shock at the diagnosis and go through the conventional stages of mourning. The person may also fear death.
- The person may express anxiety related to uncertainty about the following issues:
  1. his or her prognosis and course of illness
  2. the effectiveness and side effects of medication and treatment
  3. his or her relationship with a partner or family member, that person's ability and willingness to cope, and possible rejection from that person
  4. the reaction of others (coworkers and friends) and possible loss of friendships
  5. the loss of cognitive, physical, social, and occupational abilities
  6. the risk of getting infections from others
  7. the risk of infecting others with HIV
  8. finances
- The person may become depressed because of
  1. feelings of helplessness in the face of changing circumstances
  2. the perception that the virus and illness are in control of the person as opposed to the person in control of him- or herself
  3. feelings of hopelessness because of gloomy prognosis and possibly because of pain, discomfort, and disfigurement

4. poorer quality of life
5. self-blame for past "sins" and "indiscretions"
6. reduced social and sexual acceptance and increased sense of isolation
- The person may express anger about
  1. participating in a high-risk lifestyle and activities in the past
  2. his or her inability to defeat the virus
  3. new restrictions on his or her lifestyle that were not freely chosen
- The person may express guilt about being homosexual, being bisexual, being a drug user, or having been "found out" because of the illness.
- The person may be obsessed, preoccupied, or immobilized by
  1. a search for an explanation of how he or she acquired the virus
  2. a search for new diagnostic evidence in his or her body
  3. fads related to health, drug combinations, and diets
  4. the inevitability of decline and death
- The person may have loss of self-esteem and self-worth.
- The person's personality may change.
- The person may have mood disorders of the manic type.
- The person may have a thought disorder in the schizophrenia family of disorders.
- The person's life roles and relationships may be significantly altered.
- The person may have a loss of coping skills, especially if the person has been a perfectionist with high standards and rigid schedules.
- The person may experience loss of friends or rejection by his or her partner or family members.

Environment
- The person may be unable to negotiate his or her surroundings due to loss of endurance, sensory disturbances, fatigue, and shortness of breath.
- The person could lose his or her home because he or she is unable to produce income to pay the mortgage or rent.
- The person may not have the money to participate in many pleasurable leisure activities, such as eating out or going to the movies.

TREATMENT/INTERVENTION

Treatment is usually provided by a multidisciplinary team. Models of treatment in occupational therapy are based on neurodevelopmental (child), biomechanical, cognitive-learning, compensatory or rehabilitation, model of human occupation, balance of occupation, and human occupation (called personal adaptation through occupation) models. Alternative medicine has also been used, including therapeutic touch, myofascial release, craniosacral therapy, imagery, visualization, progressive relations, Chinese traditional medicine, and prayer.

Because the problems vary depending on both the individual and the course of the disease, the suggested treatment and management techniques are a composite of ideas rather than a single approach.

**Types of Disorders Seen in Occupational Therapy
as a Result of HIV/AIDS Infections**

- central nervous system: dementia, spinal cord dysfunction, stroke, gait disturbances, restricted mobility, changes in muscle tone
- peripheral nervous system:
  1. sensory: paresthesia; decreased temperature, vibration, and proprioceptive sensitivity; decreased ankle and knee reflexes; hyperesthesia; balance impairment
  2. motor: progressive muscle weakness, paralysis, decreased deep tendon reflexes, possible deformities, loss of range of motion and coordination
- autonomic nervous system: tachycardia, abnormal blood pressure, myelopathy, and peripheral sensory neuropathies

Note: Some disorders result from both central nervous system and peripheral nervous system disorders.
Source: Data from Neurological Rehabilitation, 1996, *Willard & Spackman's Occupational Therapy*, 1998.

Self-Care

- Assist the person in maintaining skills needed to perform activities of daily living.
- Provide self-care retraining if the person has stopped doing a skill that is within his or her capacity.
- Recommend use of energy conservation, pacing, and work simplification techniques.
- Provide training in community management skills.
- Recommend compensatory techniques and/or adaptive equipment as needed.

Productivity

- Encourage the person to maintain productive activities at work and at home for as long as possible.
- Suggest modifications of the work or home environment that will permit the person to continue to perform productive tasks.
- Explore with the person alternate work situations that require skills the person is able to perform and permit more flexibility for rest breaks (e.g., flexible hours, working from home).

Leisure

- Encourage the person to continue or increase participation in leisure activities, especially if work alternatives are available or desired.
- Assist the person in exploring and developing new leisure interests to replace those that cannot be continued.

Considerations While Conducting Interviews

Do
- Allow enough time to complete the interview.
- Ensure privacy during the interview.
- Respect confidentiality after the interview.
- Let the person talk.
- Listen to what the person says.
- Observe and report nonverbal cues such as facial expression.
- Gauge the need for information on an individual basis.
- Permit the person to discuss painful topics.
- Permit silence during the interview.
- Use humor sparingly, unless rapport has been established and the person enjoys the humor.

Don't
- Rush the interview process or the interviewee's answers.
- Assume you know what is troubling the person.
- Give false reassurance.
- Overload the person with information.
- Feel obligated to keep talking all the time.
- Withhold information.
- Tell lies.
- Criticize or make judgments.
- Give dirct advice about psychological matters.

Sensorimotor
- Maintain or improve the person's physical endurance, but be aware when changes in routine are necessary to compensate for reduced endurance.
- Maintain or improve muscle strength, but be aware when to compensate for reduced strength.
- Maintain or improve functional range of motion.
- Maintain normal muscle tone.
- Maintain functional mobility, including use of ambulation aids.
- Maintain hand grip functions, but if weakness or lack of proprioception occur, provide alternative strategies such as elastic shoelaces or Velcro fasteners to eliminate the need for shoe tying or safety checks for sharp objects to avoid injury to the skin.
- Provide techniques for pain management, including relaxation techniques or complementary therapies such as aromatherapy or massage.
- Provide sensory stimulation for an adequate sensory diet, especially if the person is unable to leave the living quarters or is confined primarily to one room.
- If loss of vision or low vision has occurred, examine the living environment to make sure there is adequate lighting and color contrast. For instance, mark temperature controls, dials,

and knobs of stoves, microwave ovens, and washing machines with brightly colored tape, or get a telephone with large numbers. Mark edges of steps with tape that contrasts and install banisters. For reading tasks, magnifying glasses or sheets are available. (See also the section on low vision.)

- If proprioception has been lost, review the environment to make sure it is safe for walking, checking for uneven surfaces or quick changes in surface characteristics, and adequate lighting.

Cognitive
- Maintain or improve short- and long-term memory.
- Maintain or improve problem-solving and decision-making skills.
- Maintain or improve judgment of safety and risks.
- Stress goal-directed actions within the person's ability to perform.
- Instruct the person on energy conservation, pacing, and work simplification.
- Instruct the person on time management techniques.
- Assist in instructing the person about the secondary complications that may occur, such as neurologic changes, tumors, infections, and weight loss.
- Encourage the person to define and engage in purposeful and meaningful occupations.
- Assist the person in developing and following an activity schedule that provides for periods of activity and relaxation.
- Stress the importance of maintaining the immune system through good body mechanics, proper nutrition, and an adequate exercise program.
- Provide instruction about safety issues associated with protecting the person from opportunistic infections and other diseases.
- If cerebral toxoplasmosis or cryptococcal meningitis have occurred, compensation for memory loss may be necessary. The person may need an appointment book, memory lists, or a schedule board. A diary can help the person keep track of what has occurred, especially if multiple agencies are involved in providing care.

Psychosocial
- Maintain or increase the person's self-concept and sense of mastery using tasks or routines that the person feels are important.
- Assist the person in regaining a sense of control by allowing the person to select the occupation or task that will be the focus of each day's session.
- Maintain or increase the person's sense of identity and responsibility by helping the person continue in his or her established routine with modifications for current impairments and functional limitations.
- Help the person learn to adjust to and cope with life with a chronic disability.
- Address issues that the person finds depressing or that create anxiety.
- Steer the person away from obsessive thoughts, perfectionist goals, and rigid schedules.
- Provide instruction and practice in relaxation techniques to reduce stress.
- Help the person and his or her partner or family to review social and occupational roles, role tasks, and role relationships to permit the person to maintain active participation for as long as possible.

- Encourage the person to maintain a dyadic relationship with his or her partner.
- Encourage the person to maintain relationships with family and friends but be aware that the person may be mourning the loss of social contacts with some people who are unable to accept the person's illness or lifestyle. The person also may have lost friends to HIV and AIDS infections or complications.
- Reminiscence may be useful during the final stage of the illness. A memory book composed of photographs and other memorabilia may provide closure for the person and a chance to review his or her accomplishments.

Environment

- Provide the person's partner, family, and friends with information about AIDS and the course of treatment.
- Encourage the person's partner and others to attend group sessions on living with AIDS.
- Discuss with the person, his or her partner, and his or her family available community resources, including statutory and voluntary agencies.
- Consider with the person and family if environmental control devices might be useful (e.g., an intercom system or switches that allow the door to be opened remotely and appliances to be turned on and off remotely).
- Encourage the person to participate in a self-help group.

PRECAUTIONS

- Protect the person from communicable diseases. The therapist should wear a mask if he or she has cold or flu symptoms.
- Occupational therapy personnel should follow universal precautions, including using gloves if they will be exposed to body fluids, washing hands before and after working with the person, and being alert when using sharp objects to avoid pricking or puncturing themselves.
- Occupational therapy personnel must follow isolation procedures if they are posted on the person's room door.
- If a therapy pool is used, be sure the pool is properly maintained and disinfected.
- The person's house, apartment, or room should be cleaned regularly with bleach.
- Detergent and bleach should be used for cleaning laundry.
- Food preparation surfaces should be cleaned frequently.
- Check for pressure sores. Change to pressure-relieving cushions and mattresses, if needed.
- All treatment/intervention should be provided in a nonjudgmental manner that conveys acceptance of the person and is free of discrimination.

PROGNOSIS AND OUTCOME

The outcome of persons with full-blown AIDS is poor. Most persons die of opportunistic infections within two years or less. Persons with HIV infection who take combined drug therapy (drug cocktail) are surviving much longer: years, not months. Maximum survival is not yet known. As a result of the increased survival rate, expectations have changed and people with HIV are being taught to live with a chronic disease.

- The person demonstrates knowledge of how to maintain physical fitness and endurance as long as possible.
- The person demonstrates knowledge of work simplification, pacing, and energy conservation techniques.
- The person demonstrates knowledge of stress management techniques, including relaxation.
- The person demonstrates a positive self-concept.
- The person is able to maintain independence in daily living skills using self-help devices as needed.
- The person is able to maintain productive activities at work and at home.
- The person has a variety of leisure activities.

REFERENCE

Beers, M.H., and R. Berkow, eds. 1999. *The Merck Manual of Diagnosis and Therapy*, 17th ed. Whitehouse Station, NJ: Merck Research Laboratories.

BIBLIOGRAPHY

Balogun, J.A. et al. 1998. The effect of professional education on the knowledge and attitudes of physical therapist and occupational therapist students about acquired immunodeficiency syndrome. *Physical Therapy* 78, no. 10: 1073–1082.

Bedell, G., and M. Kaplan. 1996. Providing services for persons with HIV/AIDS and their caregivers (position paper). *American Journal of Occupational Therapy* 50, no. 10: 853–854.

Burkhardt, A., and L. Joachim. 1996. Acquired immune deficiency syndrome (AIDS). In *A therapist's guide to oncology: Medical issues affecting management*, eds. A. Burkhardt and L. Joachim, 163–168. San Antonio, TX: Therapy Skill Builders. (Case reports)

Cusack, L., and L. Phillips. 1996. HIV disease and AIDS. In *Occupational therapy and physical dysfunction: Principles, skills, and practice*, eds. A. Turner et al., 829–850. New York: Churchill Livingstone. (Case report)

Dunn, M., and J. Giacone. 1993. Occupational therapy and AIDS on an acute care hospital unit. *Occupational Therapy Forum* 8, no. 10: 4–5, 8–10.

Herzberg, G.L. 1996. Positive parenting. . .an OT finds an unexpected setting for her skills: An agency that serves mothers with HIV or AIDS. *OT Practice* 1, no. 12: 21–26.

Katzman, E. 1996. Adults with AIDS: Taking the long view. *OT Week* 10, no. 13: 18–19.

Krinsky, R. 1996. New York hospital audience reviews AIDS tape. *Advance for Occupational Therapists* 12, no. 23: 17.

Lang, C. 1993. Experience of community physiotherapy for people with HIV infection. *British Journal of Occupational Therapy* 56, no. 6: 213–216.

LeCocq, L. et al. 1995. The role of rehabilitation after human immunodeficiency virus (HIV) infection. In *Neurological rehabilitation*, 3rd ed., ed. D.A. Umphred, 556–570. St. Louis, MO: Mosby. (Case reports)

Marcil, W.M. 1993. The adult with AIDS. In *Practice issues in occupational therapy: Intraprofessional team building*, ed. S.E. Ryan, 129–136. Thorofare, NJ: Slack. (Case report)

Marmer, L. 1995. Making the choice to accept HIV. *Advance for Occupational Therapists* 11, no. 28: 11.

Marmer, L. 1995. Rehab is the biggest change in AIDS treatment. *Advance for Occupational Therapists* 11, no. 46: 16.

McNelis, D.N., and T. McNelis. 1994. AIDS and the person with mental retardation: Critical issues for practice. *Developmental Disabilities Special Interest Section Newsletter* 17, no. 1: 5–6.

Meyers, R.A.M. 1995. AIDS and occupational therapy: One therapist's journey. *Occupational Therapy Forum* 1, no. 13: 4–5, 11.

Newman, E.M. et al. 1995. Acquired immune deficiency syndrome. In *Occupational therapy for physical dysfunction*, 4th ed., ed. C.A. Trombly, 735–741. Baltimore: Williams & Wilkins. (Case reports)

Pizzi, M. 1993. HIV infections and AIDS: An update for occupational therapists. *Physical Disabilities Special Interest Section Newsletter* 16, no. 3: 2–4.

Pizzi, M. 1998. HIV infection and AIDS. In *Physical dysfunction: Practice skills for the occupational therapy assistant*, ed. M.B. Early, 530–538. St. Louis, MO: Mosby. (Case report)

Pizzi, M., and A. Burkhardt. 1998. HIV infection and AIDS. In *Willard and Spackman's occupational therapy*, 9th ed., eds. M.E. Neistadt and E.B. Crepeau, 705–710. Philadelphia: Lippincott-Raven.

Schlinder, V.P., and S. Ferguson. 1995. An education program on acquired immunodeficiency syndrome for patients with mental illness. *American Journal of Occupational Therapy* 49, no. 4: 359–361.

Shaw, A. 1996. Prepare yourself to treat people with AIDS. *Journal of Occupational Therapy Students* 10, no 1: 17–20.

Snyder, C. 1993. AIDS: Awareness, assistance, and acceptance. *Journal of Occupational Therapy Students* 7, no. 1: 49–54.

Thiers, N. 1993. Helping people hold on. *OT Week* 7, no. 34: 40–43.

Turner, A. 1996. Introduction to AIDS and cancer. In *Occupational therapy and physical dysfunction: Principles, skills, and practice*, eds. A. Turner et al., 819–828. New York: Churchill Livingstone.

Wolf, M. 1995. HIV/AIDS means disability. *Advance for Directors in Rehabilitation* 4, no. 10: 12–17.

Human Immunodeficiency Virus and Acquired Immunodeficiency Syndrome—Child

DESCRIPTION

This section focuses on children below age 13. For teenagers, see the preceding section.

Human immunodeficiency virus (HIV-1) is a retrovirus that can lead to progressive immunologic deterioration and associated opportunistic infections and malignancies. The end stage is acquired immunodeficiency syndrome (AIDS) (Merck 1999, 2345).

In the United States, AIDS probably occurred in children almost as early as it did in adults (first described in 1981 but occurring since the mid-1970s). Two percent of the total cases of HIV and AIDS are in children. Infants and children at highest risk for HIV infection and AIDS are those born to women who use drugs or are sexual partners of drug users or bisexual men. Boys with hemophilia who received clotting factor concentrates before the mid-1980s are also at high risk, and children who received a blood transfusion before 1985 had a significant risk of having been infected (Merck 1999, 2345). The clinical course is highly variable. The Centers for Disease Control and Prevention uses categories for classifying HIV infection depending on the clinical condition (MMWR, 1–19):

- Category N, nonsymptomatic: The child has no signs or symptoms of HIV infection or only one listed in category A.
- Category A, mildly symptomatic: The child has two or more of the following items but none of the items in category B or C: dermatitis, hepatomegaly, lymphadenopathy, parotitis, recurrent or resistant upper respiratory tract infection, sinusitis, otitis media, or splenomegaly.
- Category B, moderately symptomatic: The child has signs and symptoms listed in categories A and B but none in category C. Examples are anemia, bacterial meningitis, cardiomyopathy, cytomegalovirus infection, hepatitis, herpes zoster, leiomyosarcoma, mycobacterium tuberculosis, nephropathy, nocardiosis, persistent fever, or toxoplasmosis.
- Category C, severely symptomatic: The child has serious bacterial infections that are multiple or recurrent. Examples are candidiasis; coccidioidomycosis, disseminated; cryptococcosis, extrapulmonary; encephalopathy; Kaposi's sarcoma; lymphoma; Pneumocystis carinii pneumonia; salmonella septicemia; or wasting syndrome (loss of weight, body tissue, and function).

CAUSE

Infection is caused by a cytopathic human retrovirus (HIV-1 and HIV-2). Congenital or perinatal transmission, called vertical transmission, accounts for 90 percent of the cases in children under 13 years of age. Cesarean section appears to reduce the risk, as does drug therapy for AIDS during pregnancy. Blood transfusion or contaminated blood products, hemophilia, and cases of unknown causes complete the remaining 10 percent. Black children are twice as likely to be infected (52 percent), as Hispanics (26 percent) or whites (22 percent). The risk of infection from an infected mother ranges from 13 percent to 39 percent. Testing for AIDS in children is not definitive until about 18 months.

ASSESSMENT

Areas
- daily living tasks: personal and instrumental activities of daily living
- productivity: play skills, educational skills
- leisure interests and skills
- developmental milestones
- reflex development
- regulatory functions
- gross motor development: coordination of the two sides of the body
- fine motor skills: dexterity, manipulation, eye-hand coordination
- sensory registration and modulation
- attention span
- coping skills
- interpersonal skills

Instruments
Therapists should know that children with HIV and AIDS are known to perform poorly on timed tests since they tend to work slowly and have limited endurance. Such problems should

be noted in test analysis and interpretation.
• interview with caregivers regarding medication schedules and other care issues

Instruments Developed by Occupational Therapy Personnel
• *Evaluation Tool of Children's Handwriting* (ETCH) by S. Amundesn, Homer, AL: OT Kids, 1995.
• *FirstSTEp Screening Test for Evaluating Preschoolers* by L.A. Miller, San Antonio, TX: The Psychological Corporation, 1993.
• *Pediatric Evaluation of Disability Index* (PEDI) by S. Haley et al., San Antonio, TX: Psychological Corporation-Therapy Skill Builders, 1992.

Instruments Developed by Other Professionals and Used by Occupational Therapy Personnel
• *Bayley Scales of Infant Development—Revised* (BSID-R) by N. Bayley, San Antonio, TX: The Psychological Corporation, 1992.
• *Bruininks-Oseretsky Test of Motor Proficiency* (BOTMP) by R. Bruininks, Circle Pines, MN: American Guidance Services, 1978.
• *Denver II* by W.K. Frankenburg et al., Denver, CO: Denver Developmental Materials, 1990.
• *The Berry-Buktenica Developmental Test of Visual-Motor Integration* (VMI-4), 4th ed. by K.E. Beery and N.A. Buktenica, Parsippany, NJ: Modern Curriculum Press, 1997.
• *Holistic Feeding Observation Form* by D.K. Lowman and S.M. Murphy, in *The Educator's Guide to Feeding Children with Disabilities,* Baltimore: Paul H. Brookes, 1998. Adapted version appears in S.M. Porr and E.B. Rainville, eds., *Pediatric Therapy: A Systems Approach,* Philadelphia: F.A. Davis, 1999.
• *Peabody Developmental Motor Scales* by M.R. Folio and R.R. Fewell, Austin, TX: Pro-Ed, 1983.

PROBLEMS

Self-Care
• The child may be delayed in the development of self-care skills.
• The child may become easily fatigued.
• The child may have oral thrush, poor appetite, and decreased respiratory function, which may cause difficulties in feeding, eating, and swallowing. The child may be on a special diet of soft, bland foods.
• The child may have regulatory dysfunction, especially related to eating and respiration.
• The child may lack functional speech or communication skills.

Productivity
• The child may be delayed in the development of play skills.
• The child may have difficulty functioning in school because of fatigue.

Leisure
• The child may not develop leisure interests.

Sensorimotor
- The child may have developmental delays in sensorimotor milestone skills and loss of developmental milestones.
- The child may show classic signs of failure to thrive. (See section on failure to thrive.)
- The child may have progressive encephalopathy that occurs when HIV or related infections develop in the central nervous system.
- The child may have static encephalopathy occurring from perinatal factors associated with cerebral palsy.
- The child may have an opportunistic infection in the central nervous system that has a progressive effect.
- The child may exhibit hyper- or hyporesponsiveness to various sensations in the environment.
- The child may have abnormal muscle tone: hyper- or hypotonic.
- The child may have delays in gross motor skills, especially motor coordination in running and playing sports.
- The child may have persistence of primitive reflexes.
- The child may perform poorly on timed tasks.
- The child may experience pain regularly or intermittently.

Cognitive
- The child may have developmental delays in cognitive milestone skills.

Psychosocial
- The child may have developmental delays in psychosocial milestone skills.
- The child may be difficult to console due to regulatory dysfunction.
- The child may be easily frustrated.
- The child may become irritable at the slightest provocation.
- The child may show signs of depression.

Environment
- The child may be prevented from participating in some community programs because community members are fearful of having their children associate with children with HIV or AIDS.
- One or both parents may also have HIV or AIDS, which will alter parent-child relations. If one parent or both parents have died, the child may be living with relatives or foster parents.

TREATMENT/INTERVENTION

Treatment of HIV and AIDS in children is usually conducted by a team, with the hospital staff, the family, and community members working together to handle a wide range of issues. Usually, the focus of intervention is on habilitation and remediation. Practice models used in occupational therapy include neurodevelopment treatment to address the postural tone, balance, motor control, and coordination; sensory integrative therapy to provide sensory modulation and sensory regulation; and the biomechanical approach to improve strength and endurance and provide positioning equipment. Other techniques include motor control techniques, learning approaches, cognitive-behavioral approaches, and assistive technology.

Self-Care
- Provide opportunity to develop self-care skills, including eating and dressing.
- Improve oral motor functions, including desensitizing perioral area and addressing dysphagia.
- Provide adapted equipment and techniques to foster self-care skills (e.g., adapted spoons and drinking cups, Velcro fasteners for buttons, finger rings on zippers).
- Assist speech pathologist in development of functional speech or communication system.

Productivity and Leisure
- Assist the child in school tasks such as positioning.
- Provide an opportunity to develop play skills, especially exploratory play skills.

Sensorimotor
- Work toward increasing sensorimotor skills and achieving developmental milestones such as sitting and walking.
- Positioning, seating, and mobility equipment may be needed (e.g., suitable chairs, tables, lapboards, wheelchairs, strollers, walkers).
- Orthotic devices such as hand splints and ankle-foot orthoses may be needed.
- Increase range of motion.
- Increase endurance.

Cognitive
- Increase orientation to task and attention span.
- Increase short- and long-term memory.
- Increase organization in task performance.

Psychosocial
- Role playing stressful situations during therapy may allow the child to express feelings and reduce fears, anxieties, and grief.
- Help the child learn new coping strategies to deal with situations occurring in the child's life.
- Provide an opportunity for social interaction with other children and with adults who are not associated with medical care.
- Provide the child with opportunities to take control of him- or herself and master the environment.

Environment
- Instruct caregivers and teachers in energy conservation, work simplification, time management, and adaptive strategies and equipment.
- Use environmental cues to assist the child in learning his or her daily routine.
- Provide the child with context-specific feedback, reinforcement, and encouragement in learning tasks and skills needed to function at home, in school, and in the community.

PRECAUTIONS

- Occupational therapy personnel should know and follow infectious disease guidelines (universal precautions) when handling blood or body secretions containing visible blood when working with children with HIV and AIDS. The universal precautions were developed by the Centers for Disease Control and Prevention and the Food and Drug Administration.
- Occupational therapy personnel should be aware that responses to drug therapy may vary from hour to hour and from day to day. The child's responses may change suddenly.
- Watch for signs and symptoms of opportunistic infections and report them to the physician immediately.
- Encourage the child to be as active as possible but to be mindful of limitations caused by the disease process. Redirect interests as loss of function occurs.
- Because of the stigma attached to HIV and AIDS, the therapist should take extra precautions to safeguard the child's confidentiality. Only those who need to know should be told of the diagnosis.
- Occupational therapy personnel should be nonjudgmental in working with families of children with HIV and AIDS. The focus should be on helping the child, not on the lifestyle decisions made by the parents before the child was born.

PROGNOSIS AND OUTCOME

There is no cure for HIV infection or AIDS at this time. Some children with HIV and AIDS are surviving past 10 years of age, and better treatment is improving life expectancy. Still, many children with HIV and AIDS do not survive childhood. In general, the earlier the symptoms appear, the worse the prognosis.

- The child is able to perform self-care skills that are appropriate for his or her chronological age or expected functional level.
- The child demonstrates age-appropriate play skills.
- The child is able to participate in school at the expected grade level for his or her chronological age or expected functional level.
- The child attains expected developmental milestones for his or her chronological age.
- The child demonstrates effective coping skills.
- The child demonstrates skills in interacting with other children and adults.
- The child demonstrates the ability to use adapted equipment and devices.
- Parents or caregivers demonstrate effective management skills.

REFERENCES

Beers, M.H., and R. Berkow, eds. 1999. *The Merck Manual of Diagnosis and Therapy*, 17th ed. Whitehouse Station, NJ: Merck Research Laboratories.
Centers for Disease Control and Prevention. 1994. Revised classification system for HIV infection in children less than 13 years of age; official authorized addendum: HIV infection codes and official guidelines for coding and reporting ICD-9-CM. *MMWR* 43, no RR-12: 1–19.

BIBLIOGRAPHY

Hinojosa, J. et al. 1993. Immune system dysfunction: Children with HIV or AIDS and their families. In *Willard and Spackman's occupational therapy*, 8th ed., eds. H.L. Hopkins and H.D. Smith, 618–621. Philadelphia: J.B. Lippincott.

Joe, B.E. 1996. How AIDS affects our children. *OT Week* 10, no. 4: 14–16.

Kelly, L. 1994. Developmental patterns in Zimbabwean children with HIV+ serology: A guide to planning a service delivery model. *British Journal of Occupational Therapy* 57, no. 4: 121–123.

Krinsky, R. 1995. What's best for women, kids with AIDS? *Advance for Occupational Therapists* 11, no. 28: 10.

Parks, R.A. 1994. HIV-positive infants. In *Working with substance-exposed children: Strategies for professionals*, ed. C.H. Puttkammer, 25–34. Tucson, AZ: Therapy Skill Builders.

Parks, R.A. 1994. Occupational therapy with children who are HIV positive. *Developmental Disabilities Special Interest Section Newsletter* 17, no. 1: 5–6.

Porr, S.M. 1999. Chronic illness, terminal illness, and closure—AIDS: The clinical picture. In *Pediatric therapy: A systems approach*, eds. S.M. Porr and E.B. Rainville, 565–583. Philadelphia: F.A. Davis.

Rogers, L.A. 1994. Developmental and functional status of children with HIV or AIDS. *Physical and Occupational Therapy in Pediatrics* 14, no. 2: 67–77. (Bibliography)

Sherwen, L.N. 1994. Pediatric HIV infection: Implications for provision of care. *Developmental Disabilities Special Interest Section Newsletter* 17, no. 1: 1–4.

Lymphedema

DESCRIPTION

The disorder is characterized by an accumulation of excessive lymph fluid and swelling of subcutaneous tissues. Lymphedema may be primary or secondary. The primary type can be present from birth (congenital lymphedema) or may occur during puberty (Lymphedema praecox) or, less frequently, later in life (lymphedema tarda). Secondary lymphedema occurs with infection and malignant disease (Merck 1999, 1798). This section is concerned with secondary lymphedema associated with surgical treatment of breast cancer (not discussed in Merck).

CAUSE

The causes of lymphedema are obstruction, destruction, or hypoplasia of the lymph vessels. Secondary lymphedema is due to poor tissue fluid drainage resulting from surgical removal, trauma and damage to, or radiation of any part of the lymphatic system, usually to treat malignancies such as breast or cervical cancer in women and prostate cancer in men. In third-world countries, the cause may be parasitic infections. Inadequate tissue fluid drainage results in the buildup of proteins and stagnant fluid in the tissue, which can lead to chronic low-grade inflammation, elevated skin temperature, increase in limb girth, decrease in tissue healing ability, and high susceptibility to infection or cellulitis (Weatherly 1996, 17).

ASSESSMENT

Areas

- daily living skills: personal and instrumental activities of daily living
- productivity skills, interests, and values
- leisure interests and skills
- edema
- pain and discomfort
- depression

Instruments

- *Lymphedema Evaluation Form* by A. Burkhardt and L. Joachim, in *A Therapist's Guide to Oncology: Medical Issues Affecting Management,* San Antonio, TX: Therapy Skill Builders, 1996.

PROBLEMS

Self-Care

- The person may have difficulty with activities of daily living such as dressing and bathing.

Productivity

- The person may experience difficulty performing homemaking tasks such as preparing meals and cleaning the house.
- The person may find employment difficult to maintain due to lack of endurance, pain, or appearance.

Leisure

- The person may discontinue or reduce participation in leisure interests due to difficulty in movement, pain or discomfort, or lack of strength and endurance.

Sensorimotor

- The person may have decreased range of motion.
- The person may have decreased strength and endurance.
- The person may have difficulty walking due to pain or due to increased weight of the limb, which changes the dynamics of balance.
- The person may experience isolated pain with movement or palpation or a generalized pain and discomfort throughout the extremity.
- The person may experience episodes of infection called cellulitis.

Cognitive

- Cognition is not directly affected by the disorder.

Psychosocial

- The person may not want to appear in public because the limb looks ugly or unsightly.

- The person may become depressed, especially if treatment is not successful.
- The person may have limited social support from family and friends.

TREATMENT/INTERVENTION

Several treatment approaches have been described. One is the manual lymphatic drainage (MLD) method developed by Albert LeDuc, PhD, a professor at the University of Brussels in Belgium. The technique is designed to reroute lymph around blocked, damaged, or absent lymph node sites. This rerouting is accomplished by hands-on massage, bandaging with nonelastic bandages, an exercise and skin care program, and a sequential gradient compression pump set at no more than 40 mgH.

Second is the method developed in 1932 by Dr. Emil Vodder and his wife, Estrid, a Danish couple living in France. In 1971, a Dr. Vodder School was founded in Austria, and in 1993 a Dr. Vodder School of North America was established in Canada.

Third is the taping method developed by Kenzo Kase, D.C., a Japanese sports trainer educated in an American school of chiropractic medicine. He developed a tape called kinesiotape or Kinesio Tex Tape. The tape is elastic enough to permit active range of motion. Originally, the tape was used only on sports injuries, but it has recently been used for other pathological conditions. Fascial release techniques may also be used.

Self-Care

- Improve the person's ability to perform self-care tasks by decreasing the swelling.
- Determine if adaptive equipment or assistive devices may be helpful in performing self-care tasks. Recommend those that appear most useful.

Productivity

- Improve the person's ability to perform homemaking tasks.
- If the person is employed or wants to work, encourage the person to continue working or seek work.

Leisure

- Improve or increase the person's participation in leisure activities.

Sensorimotor

- LeDuc's massage is designed to reach the tissue depth without affecting the muscle by rolling or laying on the skin to help stretch it so the small lymphatics open and absorb more protein-filled lymphatic fluid from the affected areas. After the massage, the affected limb is wrapped in nonelastic bandages to provide a counterforce for resistive exercise.
- LeDuc exercises for the upper extremity include shoulder abduction and elbow flexion and extension. Proprioceptive neuromuscular facilitation exercises may also be used. For the lower extremity, foot or hip flexion and extension exercises may be used.
- In the LeDuc method, the skin is washed with a mild soap. A hypoallergenic, fragrance-free moisturizing lotion may be used to keep the skin in good condition.
- In the LeDuc method, a compression pump is used for no more than one hour a day. The pump is set at a maximum of 40 mgH.

- The traditional American model uses custom-fit compression garments and a compression pump set as high as 100 mgH for up to eight hours. This model is no longer recommended.
- Vodder massage requires a firm touch to make small, heavy circles in the skin.
- The Vodder method uses low-stretch elastic bandages that are wrapped in a four-layer technique designed to increase tissue pressure in the edematous region and speed up reabsorption.
- Kinesiotape seems to help encourage the lymph to drain through alternate pathways. Because the tape is elastic, it can be stretched over the fascia, creating a rippling effect on the superficial skin where the lymph starts. It also decreases the interstial pressure of the epidermis to open up the system (Kerr 1998, 26–27).

Cognitive
- Instruct the person in good skin care techniques.
- Instruct the person in daily management of the lymphedema.
- Instruct the person on methods to prevent bacterial and fungal infections.

Psychosocial
- Massage helps in stress reduction.

PRECAUTIONS
- Occupational therapy personnel using the Vodder massage method should watch for signs and symptoms of hand and finger overuse injuries, including cumulative trauma syndrome, in themselves.
- Manual lymph drainage techniques are contraindicated for people with active cancer, people receiving radiation therapy, people on chemotherapy with low platelet counts, people with active infections, people with deep vein thrombosis, and people with congestive heart failure.
- Resting the affected limb is counterproductive because the drainage stops. However, a person may have been told to rest the limb by a physician unfamiliar with the mechanics of lymphedema. Education is essential.
- The person should avoid stings or bites from insects, injections or shots, burns, blood pressure monitoring in the affected arm, and situations that might result in cuts.
- Repetitive resistive exercise should not be used since it may increase the production of lymphatic fluid in the involved limb.
- Being overweight may contribute to a poorer outcome.

PROGNOSIS AND OUTCOME
- The size of the affected limb decreases, becoming more normal again. Note: Complete reduction of edema is not always attained or maintained.
- The person is able to perform all self-care routines.
- The person is able to perform homemaking tasks.
- The person is able to perform work tasks.
- The person is able to engage in leisure pursuits.

- The person reports less pain and discomfort.
- The person participates in social situations.

REFERENCES

Beers, M.H., and R. Berkow, eds. 1999. *The Merck Manual of Diagnosis and Therapy*, 17th ed. Whitehouse Station, NJ: Merck Research Laboratories.
Kerr, A. 1998. Try catching lymphedema 'on tape.' *Advance for Occupational Therapy Practitioners* 14, no. 42: 26–27.
Weatherly, K. 1996. Bringing lymphedema treatment home. *Advance for Directors in Rehabilitation* 5, no. 9: 17, 19, 21.

BIBLIOGRAPHY

Berg, T. 1998. Out of the dark: Lymphedema gets its deserved recognition, treatment, and reimbursement. *Rehab Management* 11, no. 5: 28, 30–31.
Chin, M. 1996. MLD certification worth obtaining, says Washington OTR. *Advance for Occupational Therapists* 12, no. 17: 4.
Colan, B.J. 1995. Education important in treating women with lymphedema. *Advance for Occupational Therapists* 11, no. 22: 16.
Dennis, B. 1993. Acquired lymphedema: A chart review of nine women's responses to intervention. *American Journal of Occupational Therapy* 47, no. 10: 891–899.
Kerr, T. 1996. Lymphedema center takes holistic approach to treatment. *Advance for Occupational Therapists* 12, no. 15: 19, 21.

Neoplasms/Cancer

DESCRIPTION

A neoplasm or cancer is a cellular structure that has lost normal controls. The result may be unregulated growth, lack of differentiation, invasion into surrounding tissue, and metastasis to other sites in the body. Cancer (malignancy) can develop in any tissue of any organ at any age (Merck 1999, 973). There are some 200 types of cancers. Some can be treated, and some are still resistant to known treatments.

Cancerous tumors can be divided into two groups: benign or malignant. Benign tumors are composed of normal cells that resemble the host tissue. Usually benign tumors grow slowly, are encapsulated, and do not move to other sites (metastasize). Benign tumors often can be surgically removed. However, benign tumors can kill or paralyze if they grow in places where surgery or radiation is not possible or if they compress vital tissue (e.g., tissue in the brain or spinal cord). Malignant tumors are fast-growing cells that are abnormal to the host area and that spread, if left untreated, via the lymphatic and circulatory systems.

Cancer tumors can also be divided into low-grade and high-grade tumors. Low-grade tumors tend to grow more slowly than high-grade tumors, and the cell structures are more uniform and consistent, like more benign tumors. However, low-grade tumors can be

---

Stages of Tumors: The TNM System

- T: the size, site, and depth of the primary tumor's invasion, depending on the type of tumor, using a scale that ranges from T1 (minimal) to T5 (maximal)
- N: the lymph node spread, using a scale that ranges from N0 (no spread) to N5 (wide spread)
- M: the presence of distant metastases, using a scale that ranges from M0 (no metastasis) to M5 (metastases to multiple sites)

Examples: T1, N0, M0 means a person has a detectable tumor that has not spread. T1, N2, M2 means the person has a detectable tumor that has begun to spread through the lymph nodes.

---

malignant (as in prostate cancer). In general, low-grade tumors are responsive to current treatment. In contrast, high-grade tumors tend to grow rapidly, to metastasize to other organs, and to be resistant to current treatment (as in inflammatory breast cancer).

Standard therapies for neoplasms or cancer are surgery, radiotherapy, chemotherapy, and transplantation.

CAUSE

Known causes include mutations in genes such as oncogenes and tumor suppressor genes, chromosomal abnormalities, viruses, parasites, chemicals (including occupational, lifestyle, and drug carcinogens), ultraviolet radiation, ionizing radiation, and chronic skin irritation. Immunologic disorders can predispose a person to neoplastic disease. Age is a significant factor in the incidence and mortality of cancer. Certain cancers are associated with children, such as acute lymphoblastic leukemia; others are associated with young adults, such as Hodgkin's disease; while still others are associated with older people, such as cancer of the prostate, stomach, and colon. The most common cancer sites are prostate, breast, lung, colon and rectum, bladder, and uterus.

ASSESSMENT

Areas
- daily living skills
- productivity history, skills, interests, and values
- work or physical capacities evaluation
- leisure interests and skills
- range of motion
- muscle strength
- postural control and balance
- fine motor skills, manipulation, dexterity, and coordination

---

Stages of Tumors: The Roman Numeral System

- Stage I: The tumor is localized to one region (usually occurs in the early stage of the disease process).
- Stage II: The tumor is in one region with one metastasis site to an adjacent region of the body.
- Stage III: The tumor is in one organ and one metastasis to another organ of the body.
- Stage IV: There are multiple sites of metastases.

Source: Reprinted with permission from A. Burkhardt, Oncology, in *Physical Dysfunction: Practice Skills for the Occupational Therapy Assistant*, M.B. Early, ed., p. 520, © 1998, Mosby-Year Book, Inc.

- sensory registration and processing
- cognition
- perceptual skills: acuity and visual perception
- self-concept
- coping skills
- social skills
- communication skills
- architectural and environmental barriers
- home safety

Instruments

Instruments Developed by Occupational Therapy Personnel

- *Canadian Occupational Performance Measure*, 2nd ed. by M. Law et al., Ottawa, Canada: Canadian Association of Occupational Therapists, 1994.
- *Chessington Occupational Therapy Neurological Assessment Battery* (COTNAB) by R. Tyerman et al., Nottingham, England: Nottingham Rehab., 1986.
- *Structured Observational Test of Function* by A. Laver, Windsor, Berkshire, England: NFER-Nelson, 1995.

Instruments Developed by Other Professionals and Used by Occupational Therapy Personnel

- *Barthel Index* by F.I. Mahoney and D.W. Barthel, *Maryland State Medical Journal* 14 (1965): 61–65.
- *Pressure-Relieving Cushion Assessment* by Merton and Sutton NHS Trust Wheelchair Service, in J. Cooper, *Occupational Therapy in Oncology and Palliative Care,* San Diego, CA. Singular Publishing Group, 1997.
- *Pressure Sore Prevention Manual* by J.A. Waterlow, in J. Cooper, *Occupational Therapy in Oncology and Palliative Care,* San Diego, CA. Singular Publishing Group, 1997.

PROBLEMS

Self-Care

- The person may be unable to perform certain activities of daily living, depending on the type of cancer, cognitive status, level of fatigue, and resulting disability.
- The person may have dysphagia, which may be severe.
- The person may be anorexic.
- The person may complain of a sore and dry mouth.
- The person may experience nausea and vomiting as a side effect to chemotherapy or radiation.
- The person may have urinary retention or frequency.
- The person may have diarrhea or constipation.
- The person may experience alopecia (hair loss) due to chemotherapy.
- The person may have insomnia or other problems with sleep, rest, and relaxation.

Productivity

- The person may be unable to continue productive tasks, depending on the type of cancer, cognitive status, functional status, level of fatigue, and resulting disability.

Leisure

- The person may be unable to continue leisure activities that he or she once enjoyed.

Sensorimotor

- The person may lose muscle strength.
- The person may lose range of motion.
- The person may lose joint mobility due to onset of adhesive capsulitis.
- The person may have instability of the trunk or limbs.
- The person may have loss or impairment of hand or upper extremity function.
- The person may have low physical tolerance and fatigue easily.
- The person may experience upper extremity dysfunction due to side effects of chemotherapy, radiotherapy, tumor growth, metastases, surgery, or spinal cord compression.
- The person may experience lymphedema due to obstruction of the lymphatics (see section on lymphedema).
- The person may experience peripheral neuropathy such as paresthesias, hyperesthesias, and loss of proprioception.
- The person may have dyspnea or shortness of breath.
- The person may experience a variety of types of pain or a single, intense type of pain.
- The person may lose one or more sensory systems, depending on the type of cancer. Loss of visual acuity may occur due to cytomegalovirus (CMV) infection following bone marrow transplant.
- The person may complain of an altered sense of smell.
- The person may have an altered body image.

Cognitive

- If the tumor is in the brain, cognitive functions may be adversely affected.
- Drug therapy may cause some cognitive dysfunction, such as mental confusion.

Psychosocial
- The person may express fear of pain, suffering, and dying.
- The person may fear loss of ability to function independently and to have control over his or her life.
- The person may be depressed and express a sense of despair.
- The person may suffer loss of self-esteem.
- The person may feel hopeless and helpless.
- The person may express feelings of anger (Why me?).
- The person may become tense and overanxious.
- The person may become highly defensive or deny anything is wrong.
- The person may lose social support as friends find excuses for not visiting a person with cancer or a person who is dying.

TREATMENT/INTERVENTION
The approach to treatment and management must be individualized to the needs of the person, to the specific disease state, and to the degree of disability. The focus of intervention is prevention, restoration, adaptation, support, or palliation, compensation, and learning/acquisition. Occupational therapy models of treatment include occupational behavior, the human occupations model, and the model of human occupation.

Self-Care
- Maintain or increase the person's ability to independently perform personal activities of daily living (dressing, eating, hygiene) and instrumental skills (writing, cooking, driving).
- Provide adaptive equipment and train the person in its use, if needed. Adapted devices for eating or grooming and installation of grab bars and non-skid materials may be useful.
- Make recommendations regarding seating needs and mobility systems such as a wheelchair or scooter.

Productivity
- Maintain participation in productive activities as long as possible, including participation in work for pay, volunteer duties, or student life.
- Make recommendations for modifications of the work environment to provide easier access, promote task performance, and increase safety.
- Retrain the person to perform homemaking tasks.

Leisure
- Explore leisure interests and encourage the development or expansion of leisure activities that are within the person's physical and psychosocial abilities.

Sensorimotor
- Help the person to maintain as much physical strength as possible through organization of rest and activity cycles.
- Maintain or increase range of motion through activities selected to promote the use of joints.

- Provide orthotic devices, such as splints and other positioning support as needed, to reduce deformity and promote function.
- Maintain or increase muscle strength through the use of graded activities.
- Provide pre- and postprosthesis training, if needed. (See the section on amputations.)
- If pain is present, help the person to reduce his or her responses to pain.
- The use of therapeutic touch may promote relaxation or promote a sense of caring.
- Provide sensory stimulation to the vestibular, tactile, proprioceptive, and visual senses to facilitate maintenance of sensorimotor integration.

Cognitive

- Teach the person about work simplification and energy conservation.
- Teach the person about safety in the home and workplace to reduce the possibility of added injury.
- Assist in explaining the possible side effects of treatment from surgery, chemotherapy, or radiation therapy.
- Teach the person and family about the disease.
- Provide cognitive and perceptual retraining, if it is needed.

Psychosocial

- Maintain or improve the person's quality of life, including his or her present lifestyle, past experiences, hope for the future, and ambitions.
- Provide stress management training, including training in relaxation techniques.
- Doing craft activities may help a person maintain self-esteem. Crafts should be chosen based on the person's age, level of function, stage of illness, and degree of disability.
- Listening to music may promote relaxation or arousal by changing respiration, pulse rate, or blood pressure.
- Using humor may help change a person's outlook on the situation and help that person interact with others.
- Maintain the person's sense of dignity, and respect the person's sense of privacy.
- Assist the person in expressing his or her spiritual side, if that is important to the person.
- Maintain or improve the person's social support system.
- Provide training in the use of alternative communication systems, especially if the ability to talk is impaired or lost.

Environment

- Help the family to provide caregiving, cope with problems, and set realistic goals.
- Provide education for caregivers regarding work simplification and energy conservation.
- Make recommendations about modifications of the living environment that may increase the ability of the person to function independently or make caregiving easier, including eliminating architectural barriers and making provisions for safety. Examples include installing a ramp for access to the house, widening the door for easier wheelchair access to the bathroom, changing the height of countertops, improving heating or air conditioning systems, adapting lighting controls to make them easier to use, or removing carpeting and installing linoleum or wood flooring to improve wheelchair access.

PRECAUTIONS
- Be alert to possible side effects of medication and radiation treatments, such as nausea and vomiting.
- Occupational therapy personnel should be aware that working with persons who are very sick or dying is stressful and take steps to relieve or counteract the effects of stress on a regular schedule.
- If the person has had a bone marrow transplant, watch for signs or symptoms of opportunistic infections.

PROGNOSIS AND OUTCOME
- The person can demonstrate knowledge of his or her health status and disabilities, if any.
- The person performs self-care activities independently with self-help devices, if needed.
- The person performs productive activities within the range of his or her health status.
- The person performs leisure activities that require active participation.
- The person can demonstrate knowledge of community support services.
- Family and friends encourage the person to perform as independently as possible within his or her health status.

REFERENCE
Beers, M.H., and R. Berkow, eds. 1999. *The Merck Manual of Diagnosis and Therapy*, 17th ed. Whitehouse Station, NJ: Merck Research Laboratories.

BIBLIOGRAPHY
Beresford, S. 1996. Cancer. In *Occupational therapy and physical dysfunction: Principles, skills, and practice*, eds. A. Turner et al., 851–870. New York: Churchill Livingstone. (Case report)
Berg, J. 1997. A wellness model for cancer recovery. *OT Week* 11, no. 23: 16–17.
Black, T.J. 1993. OT and "cancervive" patients. *Occupational Therapy Forum* 7, no. 2: 4–5.
Burkhardt, A. 1998. Oncology. In *Physical dysfunction: Practice skills for the occupational therapy assistant*, ed. M.B. Early, 519–529. St. Louis, MO: Mosby.
Burkhardt, A., and L. Joachim. 1996. *A Therapist's Guide to Oncology: Medical Issues Affecting Management*. San Antonio, TX: Therapy Skill Builders. (Case reports)
Cook, A., and A. Burkhardt. 1994. The effect of cancer diagnosis and treatment on hand function. *American Journal of Occupational Therapy* 48, no. 9: 836–839.
Cooper, J. 1997. *Occupational Therapy in Oncology and Palliative Care*. San Diego, CA. Singular Publishing Group.
Dawson, S., and J. Barker. 1995. Hospice and palliative care: A Delphi survey of occupational therapists' roles and training needs. *Australian Occupational Therapy Journal* 42, no. 3: 119–127.
Guidelines recommended aggressive treatment for cancer pain. *OT Week* 8, no. 15: 10.
Joannidis, S. 1997. Cancer rehab: Learning to treat the whole patient. *OT Week* 11, no. 35: 68.
Kerr, T. 1998. A window of hope. *Advance for Occupational Therapists* 14, no. 7: 28–29.
Klinger, J.L. 1997. The client who has cancer. In *Meal preparation and training: The healthcare professional's guide*, ed. J.L. Klinger, 129–134. Thorofare, NJ: Slack.
Kumiega, K. 1995. Occupational therapy for patients undergoing chemotherapy. *Physical Disabilities Special Interest Section Newsletter* 18, no. 3: 2–3.

Kumiega, K. 1997. *Windows to cancer rehabilitation: An occupational therapy treatment guide.* Bisbee, AZ: Imaginart.

Marmer, L. 1996. Researching the effect of occupation on pain level. *Advance for Occupational Therapists* 12, no. 40: 18, 50.

Mostert, E. et al. 1996. Claiming the illness experience: Using narrative to enhance theoretical understanding. *Australian Occupational Therapy Journal* 43, no. 3/4: 125–132.

Penfold, S.L. 1996. The role of the occupational therapist in oncology. *Cancer Treatment Review* 22, no. 1: 75–81.

Pizzi, M., and A. Burkhardt. 1998. Cancer. In *Willard and Spackman's occupational therapy*, 9th ed., eds. M.E. Neistadt and E.B. Crepeau, 711–715. Philadelphia: Lippincott-Raven Publishers.

Ratki, S. 1997. The road to recovery—and beyond. *OT Week* 11, no. 35: 20–21. (Case report)

Van Deusen, J. 1993. Mastectomy and body image. In *Body image and perceptual dysfunction in adults*, ed. J. Van Deusen, 191–205. Philadelphia: W.B. Saunders.

Part IX

Skin Disorders

Burns—Adult

DESCRIPTION

Burns are tissue injuries that result in protein denaturation, burn wound edema, and loss of intravascular fluid volume due to increased vascular permeability. Burns are classified as first, second, or third degree. First-degree burns are red, very sensitive to touch, and usually moist. The surface skin will blanch markedly and widely to light pressure; no blisters develop. Second-degree burns are more likely to produce blisters. The bases of the blisters may be erythematous or whitish with a fibrous exudate; they are sensitive to touch and may blanch to pressure. Third-degree burns usually do not produce blisters. The burn's surface may be white and pliable; black, charred, and leathery; or bright red because of fixed hemoglobin in the subdermal region. Pale third-degree burns may be mistaken for normal skin, but the subdermal vessels do not blanch to pressure. Third-degree burns are generally anesthetic or hypoesthetic (Merck 1999, 2434). Some people also list a fourth-degree burn which generally means all soft tissue, including muscle, has been burned and bone may be seen. The incidence of burns is estimated at 1.25 million per year in the United States, of which approximately 51,000 require hospitalization and 5,500 die in spite of continuing improvement in burn care rehabilitation (Brigham and McLoughlin 1996, 95).

CAUSE

The causes include thermal (heat or cold), radiation, chemical (acids or alkalis), or electrical contact.

Thermal burns may be due to any external heat source capable of raising the temperature of skin and deeper tissues to a level that causes cell death and protein coagulation or charring. The most common causes are flame, scalding liquids, and hot objects such as hot metal, or gases such as steam contacting the skin.

Radiation burns are most commonly due to prolonged exposure to the sun's ultraviolet radiation (sunburn) but may be due to prolonged or intense exposure to sources of ultraviolet radiation such as tanning beds, to X-ray, or to other radiation.

Chemical burns may be due to strong acids or alkalis, phenols, cresols, mustard gas, or phosphorus. All of the agents produce necrosis, which may extend slowly for several hours.

Electrical burns result from the generation of heat, which may reach 5000 degrees Celsius (9032 degrees Fahrenheit). Because most of the resistance to electric current occurs where the conductor contacts the skin, electrical burns usually affect the skin and tissues immediately underneath; they may be of almost any size and depth. Electrical injury, particularly from alternating currents, may cause immediate respiratory paralysis, ventricular fibrillation, or both (Merck 1999, 2434).

ASSESSMENT

Severity is measured by the percentage of total body surface area (TBSA) burned.
* small: 15 percent TBSA

Methods for Calculating the Percent of Body Burned

Wallace's Rule of Nines (for an adult):
- head and neck: 9 percent (4.5 percent anterior or face, 4.5 percent posterior)
- trunk: anterior 18 percent, posterior 18 percent
- arms: 9 percent one (4.5 percent anterior, 4.5 percent posterior), 18 percent both
- legs: 18 percent one (9 percent anterior, 9 percent posterior), 36 percent both
- genitalia and perineum: 1 percent

Percentage of Body

	0 years	1 year	5 years	10 years	15 years	Adult
half of head	9.5	8.5	6.5	5.5	4.5	3.5
half of one thigh	2.75	3.25	4	4.25	4.5	4.75
half of one lower leg	2.5	2.5	2.75	3	3.25	3.5

Measurements that do not change with age:
- arm: 2 percent anterior, 2 percent posterior
- forearm: 1.5 percent anterior, 1.5 percent posterior
- hand: 1.5 percent anterior, 1.5 percent posterior
- trunk: 13 percent anterior, 13 percent posterior
- buttocks: 2.5 percent each
- genitalia: 1 percent
- feet: 1.75 percent anterior, 1.75 percent posterior

- moderate: 15 percent to 49 percent TBSA
- large: 50 percent to 69 percent TBSA
- massive: more than 70 percent TBSA

Depth is measured by the number of layers of skin burned.
- First-degree burns involve the superficial or partial-thickness epidermis, causing burns that are red, that are very sensitive to touch, that blanch to light pressure, and that are usually moist, but there are no blisters.
- Second-degree burns involve deep partial thickness of the epidermis and varying depths of the dermis, causing the wound to be sensitive to touch. The wound may also blanch to pressure and blister.
- Third-degree burns involve the full thickness of the epidermis, the dermis, and varying degrees of subcutaneous tissues, tendons, or muscles. The surface may be white and pliable

---

Classification by Depth of Injury

- Superficial partial-thickness burns involve the epidermis and may involve the upper dermis. Burns are characterized by edema, blister formation, pain, and erythema (redness). Skin will heal spontaneously by reepithelialization, with good functional ability and appearance. Deformity and disability are rarely a problem.
- Deep partial-thickness burns involve damage to the epidermis and dermis. They may heal spontaneously, but with decreased function and poor appearance. The person may develop contractures and hypertrophic scarring that can result in major deformity and disability.
- Full-thickness burns involve loss of the epidermis and most or all of the dermis. The burned area does not heal spontaneously, and grafting is required for closure. Development of contractures and hypertrophic scarring can result in major deformity and disability.

---

or black, charred, and leathery. Subdermal vessels do not blanch to pressure, and generally the wound is anesthetic or hypoesthetic. Hairs may be pulled from their follicles easily.

Areas
- daily living skills: personal and instrumental activities of daily living
- productivity history, skills, interests, and values
- leisure skills and interests
- burned areas, including type, percentage, depth, and location
- skin and scar condition as healing occurs
- range of motion, active and passive
- muscle strength
- hand dominance
- edema
- pain
- mobility and ambulation
- sensory registration, modulation, and processing
- affect or mood
- self-concept
- coping skills
- role responsibilities
- spiritual and cultural values
- home and work environments

Instruments
No instruments developed by occupational therapists for this disorder were identified in the literature. The following types of instruments may be useful:

- activities of daily living scale
- occupational history
- job analysis interview
- leisure checklist
- goniometer (not during acute phase)
- manual muscle test (not during acute phase)
- sensory testing (not during acute phase)
- pain questionnaire
- role performance interview
- home environment

PROBLEMS

Self-Care
- The site and degree of injury usually determine the degree of loss of performance of activities of daily living. Burns to the hands and arms result in greater loss of skills than do burns elsewhere.
- The person tends to assume a guarding position of flexion and adduction, which makes putting on garments difficult since most dressing activities require extension.

Productivity
- The person usually will be unable to work for several months and may be unable to return to his or her former occupation.
- The person may lose skills or require modification to perform skills necessary for productivity and need retraining or work hardening.

Leisure
- If the lower limbs are injured, sports activities may be limited.
- If the hands are injured, the person may be unable to perform fine motor skills.

Sensorimotor
- The person may have limitations in range of motion.
- The person may have muscle weakness and disuse atrophy.
- The person may experience loss of hand strength and upper extremity skill.
- The person may have contractures.
- The person may have faulty posture.
- The person may have deformities.
  1. in the face: mouth microstomia, closure of the nares, and loss of ear cartilage
  2. in the neck: flexion and lateral scar banding
  3. in the shoulder: elevation, protraction, adduction, and internal rotation
  4. in the elbow: flexion with forearm pronation
  5. in the trunk: scoliosis and kyphosis
  6. in the hip: flexion and adduction
  7. in the knee: flexion or hyperextension
  8. in the ankle: equinovarus, foot plantar flexion, and inversion

9. in the foot, equinovarus or foot plantar flexion and inversion and metatarsophalangeal hyperextension
- The person usually has severe physical pain and discomfort.
- The person usually experiences deconditioning due to prolonged bed rest in areas of the body that are not burned.
- The person experiences loss of energy level due to increased metabolic demands of the healing process.
- The person may have loss of sensory registration and processing in tactile, proprioceptive, temperature, and pressure senses.

Cognitive
- Cognitive faculties are not affected directly, but the experience of trauma, pain, and discomfort limits the person's attention span and ability to concentrate.
- The person may become disoriented and unresponsive due to drug therapy or prolonged isolation.

Psychosocial
- The person may fear permanent physical deformity, disfigurement, and permanent change in body image.
- The person may fear chronic pain.
- The person may express feelings of being overwhelmed by the trauma.
- The person may express feelings of inadequacy and physical helplessness.
- The person may express feelings of frustration at being inactive and dependent for so long.
- The person may express anger or hostility at his or her employer for permitting the burn-related situation to occur.
- The person may feel that the injury is a punishment for misdeeds or express feelings of guilt.
- The person may have loss of self-esteem and self-confidence.
- The person may become dependent or regress.
- The person may become depressed and express a sense of loss or despair.
- The person may become irritable.
- The person may have limited or no verbal communication ability if his or her face is burned or the person is intubated.
- The person may withdraw from social situations and feel rejected.
- The person may lose interests, values, and motivation.
- The person usually experiences loss or disruption of familiar role performance and role identity, at least temporarily. The new role of patient is acquired and may be experienced for several months. Resumption of role performance may be limited to self-care.
- The person may experience post-traumatic stress disorder (see section on this disorder).

TREATMENT/INTERVENTION
Models are based on biomechanical, compensatory/rehabilitation, learning (cognitive/behavioral), and phenomenologic concepts and principles. Specific models in occupational therapy include the model of human occupation and the client-centered approach.

Stages of Wound Healing

- The inflammation stage, which lasts 1 day to 5 days.
- The migration and proliferation stage, which begins at 5 days postinjury and may last up to 14 days.
- The matrix formation and remodeling stage, which lasts about two months, when 70 percent of tensile strength is attained.

Self-Care

- Facilitate performance of activities of daily living by providing the opportunity to perform, which may include positioning such as sitting or using special equipment.
- Provide self-care devices and instruction if needed temporarily, such as built-up handles to compensate for lack of grasp. Do not use extension handles for the elbow; encourage use of normal elbow range of motion. Remove specialized devices as soon as possible to encourage normal movement performance of self-care and activities of daily living.
- Encourage the person to participate in all self-care and activities of daily living and remind other staff to build in some participation to foster independence and learning about wound healing.
- Task performance may need to be divided into small steps that are easily followed to overcome the person's sense of helplessness and dependence.
- Make recommendations and suggestions to the person and his or her family about clothing modifications that may be needed to accommodate functional limitations (e.g., garments that are easy to put on, alternate fasteners, and appropriate clothing for sensitive skin).

Productivity

- Help the person to prepare for a return to productive activities as stages of recovery permit.
- Explore the need for environmental changes that might permit an earlier return to productive tasks.
- If the person must work outside in the heat, suggest working in shaded areas; wearing light-colored, lightweight, nonrestrictive clothing; wearing a cap or hat with a brim; bringing a battery-operated fan; using a spray bottle of water; wearing sunglasses; and drinking lots of fluid.
- Stress the importance of keeping vehicles in good running order, using a mobile phone, and keeping emergency supplies available such as blankets, warm clothing, flashlights, and snacks.
- If the person is exposed to cold temperatures inside or outside while at work, he or she should use insulated, waterproof boots; safety shoes; an insulated jacket with a hood; and multiple layers of clothing that are wind-resistant. The person should avoid taking vasodilating or vasoconstricting drugs.
- Provide practice in the physical tasks required for the person's job (e.g., reaching, lifting, stooping, pulling, pushing, handling, and manipulating).

Leisure
- Help the person to explore leisure interests that are within his or her functional capacity at various stages of recovery.

Sensorimotor

Therapeutic Positioning
- Edema control and reduction should be accomplished through elevation of the limbs and head above the heart at about 30 degrees
- Maintain normal muscle length during rest using extension and abduction patterns.
- Facilitate wound coverage after skin grafts.
- Limit the degree of scar contracture.
- Help the person to learn methods for reducing the impact of skin tightness on function.
- Reduce stress on suture lines when a skin flap graft is performed.
- Maintain graft placement; avoid positions that can contribute to graft shifting.

Specific Deformities
- General rule: Position the body segments opposite to anticipated deformity.
- Mouth: Use mouth spreader or incorporate mouth spreader with face mask.
- Eye: Use face mask.
- Nose: Use nasal obturators.
- Ear: Use no pillows and avoid pressure to the ear helix.
- Neck: Position the neck in a neutral position or in slight extension using a neck splint made from foam, wastusi, or thermoplastic or a clear plastic conformer. Do not use a pillow.
- Shoulder, supine: Use a small roll between scapulae, abduction troughs, or small wedges. Keep shoulders abducted to 90 degrees and in forward flexion at 45 degrees.
- Shoulder, prone: Use a short mattress below the head, a separate foam piece for the head, axilla pads, a foam positioner, and an airplane splint.
- Elbow: Use an arm conformer in extension and supination, use a three-point extension splint, and elevate.
- Hand, dorsal: Position in wrist extension, metacarpophalangeal flexion, and proximal interphalangeal and distal interphalangeal extension with a volar splint and the arm elevated above the heart.
- Hand, volar: Position the hand in full digit and palmar extension with an extension splint.
- Trunk: Align with shoulders and hips in bed and in sitting position.
- Hip: Place in neutral (extension) position or up to 15 degrees abduction, use form positioner between lower extremity, and avoid prolonged sitting if burns are across anterior pelvis.
- Knee: Place in extended position, with knee extension splint, but with no pillows under knees or heels.
- Knee hyperextension: Use an extension splint such as a conformer, three point immobilizer or knee immobilizer and elevate lower extremities while sitting.
- Ankle: Position in dorsiflexion using a footboard, the back of the bed at the end of the mattress, or a foot splint that incorporates ankles (ankle-foot orthosis type).
- Foot: Place in neutral position with a footboard or splint.

Skin Grafting Terms

- autograft: surgical transplantation of a person's own skin from an un-burned area (the donor site)
- allograft: viable skin from another person, usually a cadaver donor, that is used as temporary coverage
- xenograft or heterograft: skin from an animal from another species, such as a pig
- split-thickness graft (STSG): removal of various layers of skin from the donor site and application to the graft recipient site
- sheet STSG: a skin graft used as it was removed from the donor site
- mesh STSG: a skin graft perforated evenly by a machine to stretch or enlarge the skin available for grafting
- cultured epidermal autograft: the person's skin grown in the laboratory so that it may cover a larger surface area
- full-thickness skin graft: blood supply is moved along with skin from the donor site to the recipient site
- microvascular skin flap autograft: blood supply is moved along with skin by cutting three sides, turning the flap, and suturing over the burned area

---

Acute Care or Pregrafting Stage

- General goals are to prevent contracture and deformity by maintaining range of motion, muscle function, and strength.
- Provide positioning devices as needed, such as
  1. foam head donut to prevent neck flexion contracture
  2. foam ear protector to prevent pressure on ear that is burned
  3. arm trough to maintain abduction of shoulder
  4. footboard to keep ankle in neutral or dorsiflexed position
- Provide orthotic devices and splints as needed, such as
  1. neck conformer or soft cervical collar to prevent contractures of neck tissue
  2. axillary or airplane splint to maintain shoulder abduction
  3. elbow conformer or three-point extension splint to maintain elbow extension
  4. cock-up splint to maintain wrist extension with or without C-bar to maintain web space
  5. abductor wedge to maintain hip abduction
  6. knee conformer or three-point extension splint to maintain knee extension
  7. foot drop splint to maintain ankle in neutral position
- Encourage active range of motion when changing positioning device, splint, or bandage.
- Use of continuous passive motion may help prevent contractures and decrease deformity.
- Maintain or increase muscle strength in affected and unaffected areas through activities that provide graded, progressive-resistive exercise.
- Simple adaptive devices may be used temporarily (e.g., overhead mirrors, prism glasses for reading supine in bed, or universal cuffs). Extended handles should be used only if the person is restricted from using joints necessary to reach objects.

- Bedside activities, such as pegboard or other upper extremity exercises, can be performed while wearing cuff weights to promote flexibility and strength if burns are primarily to lower extremities.
- Encourage normal posture to avoid guarding positions (usually flexion and adduction).

Grafting Stage

- Additional positioning devices or splints may be needed, depending on the graft site, to prevent movement that might damage or destroy the capillary bed and thus the graft.
- Limited movement of the graft site area may be permitted after the fourth day.

Postoperative or Postgrafting Stage

- Minimize scarring by applying pressure to the person's skin through the use of pressure garments.
- Provide sensory stimuli according to the person's needs to prevent environmental deprivation.

Rehabilitation Inpatient or Outpatient Stage (with or without Grafting)

- Provide range of motion exercises involving multiple joints to maintain flexibility. Be aware that a person with burns does not like to move because of pain and deconditioning, so movement is likely to be very slow, labored, robotlike, and lacking in fluidity and spontaneity.
- Stretching exercises can be combined with other activities. The shoulder and elbows can be stretched while the person uses a vibrator to reduce back itch, reaches for an overhead bar added to a walker, combs his or her hair, or reaches overhead to punch a balloon after a set number of revolutions on the stationary bicycle. Or arms may be elevated while the person eats, with feet tucked under a chair to stretch knee flexion and ankle dorsiflexion during a meal.
- Continuous passive motion may be useful as an adjunct to the regular exercise regimen. Other exercise equipment may include grippers, hand manipulation boards, pipe trees, reciprocal pulleys, stationary bicycles, the BTE (Baltimore Therapeutic Equipment) work simulator, work evaluation system technology (WEST), the Valpar whole body exerciser, and musical or computer keyboards.
- Provide stretching exercises to reduce tightness in the soft tissue, tendons, ligaments, blood vessels, and nerves around the joints. A person can also use free weights (using the Delorem method), electronically controlled dynamometers, or a bicycle ergometer. In the Delorem method, the maximum load or weight a person can lift through the entire range of motion for 10 repetitions is established. Then a program is designed so the person completes 10 repetitions of a weight 50 percent of maximal load, progressing to 10 more repetitions using a weight 75 percent of maximal load, and finally 10 repetitions at 100 percent of maximal load. Rest periods are from two minutes to four minutes between progressions with more weight.
- Increase muscle strength to counteract prolonged immobilization.
- Increase endurance to counteract deconditioning.
- Decrease hypersensitivity to touch.

Splinting

For comprehensive information on splinting, see Daugherty and Carr-Collins (1994) and Ott and colleagues (1996).

- The use of splints for burns varies from one burn center to another. Splints used to be worn most of the time, except for during baths or changes of dressings. Now wearing time is less.
- The primary splint for burns is designed to permit the claw hand (flexion of the wrist, hyperextension of the metacarpophalangeal joints, and flexion of the interphalangeal joints). The wrist is in 30 degrees to 35 degrees extension, the metacarpophalangeal joints are flexed to between 50 degrees and 70 degrees, and the interphalangeal joints are extended, with the thumb in abduction. The splint is held with gauge or elastic wrap. Wrapping should be applied distal to proximal to assist venous return. Straps are not used because of infection control concerns and the possibility of distal edema.
- Splints used during the acute stage are usually conformer splints with total body contact. Most are designed to maintain extension except for the ankle dorsiflexion splint and the airplane splint for maintaining the shoulder at about 90 degrees of abduction.
- Static splints used during wound maturation should avoid restricting functional movement as much as possible.
- Dynamic splints are designed to assist in regaining function or to provide slow, dynamic stretching to contracting tissues.
- Dynamic splints should avoid exerting ligamentous stress, friction, or joint compression as much as possible.
- Use commercially available splints with caution because fit is critical and adjustments may need to be made frequently.
- Splinting materials may include clear or transparent plastic for the face or opaque materials for other parts of the body. Usually the splint material is made of a low-temperature thermoplastic material.

Plaster Casts

- Plaster casts can be used to correct positions or stretch and soften contractures.
- A serial fall-out or drop-out cast can be used to block flexion positioning at night during sleep by limiting the amount of flexion permitted before the cast stops the flexion movement.
- Plaster casts offer conformity to body surface at minimum cost.

Pressure Wraps and Garments

- Pressure garments are used primarily for scar management.
- Pressure should be applied perpendicularly to approximate capillary pressure. It is believed that wounds mature more rapidly, with fewer scars, when deprived of circulation and oxygen.
- Elastic wrap supports prevent dependent edema under grafts on dependent extremities.
- Wraps can be changed to cotton or rubber tubes or custom-made garments when the skin can tolerate a shear force.
- Vascular supports control edema, minimize vascular and lymphatic pooling, and condition new skin for the shear force demands of the pressure garments.

- Pressure garments should conform to the body as closely as possible, but inserts and overlays will be needed to account for body contours, bony prominences, and postural adjustments made by the person. Inserts may be made from orthopaedic felt, Plastazote (finger webs, hand dorsum, axillary webs), Aliplast (thumb webs, shoe inserts), Aquaplast (face contours, finger webs), silicone gel (hands, face, areas of limited friction), silastic elastomer (hands, face, chest), prosthetic foam (chest), or adhesive-based closed cell foam (concave areas). Maceration of skin or friction should be avoided.
- Pressure garments can be used to assist in skin desensitization and sensory reeducation.

Cognitive

- Provide instruction to the person about the recovery process from burns and what to expect at various stages of recovery. The person should understand the purpose of a specific treatment, such as a surgery; the potential outcomes if the individual remains in treatment; the consequences for discontinuing treatment; the length of time for recovery; and how to assess scar maturation.
- The person may need information and instructions repeated on several occasions over a period of time before the instructions are fully understood.
- If the person was burned with hot water or liquid, instruct the person on how to safely test water temperatures, how to set the thermostat of the hot water heater below 120 degrees Fahrenheit, and how to cook using safety procedures.
- Instruct the person in skin and scar care, including caring for wounds, moisturizing and lubricating skin, and putting on vascular support or compression garments. New skin must be protected against shear and friction forces to avoid breakdown.
- Recommend that the person wear a hat with a wide brim to avoid sun exposure, especially if the neck or face was burned.
- Help the person understand that his or her circulatory system may have been changed permanently and that sweat glands may be absent, so exposure to heat and cold may be a problem. Also explain that injured skin is very sensitive to temperature extremes.

Psychosocial

- Use craft or game activities to enhance self-esteem and provide purposeful activity. Generally, avoid skin irritants or hazardous tools. While the person is in bed or confined to his or her room, avoid dirty or messy activities or ones that require many parts. Consider working with ceramic tiles, painting, doing needlework, leather lacing, playing board games, and doing puzzles.
- Instruct the person in techniques for coping with pain and managing stress.
- Provide a communication board for the person who is intubated and cannot talk.
- Using job-related tasks or tasks that require movements similar to those required on the job may increase the person's self-confidence and self-worth.
- Provide an opportunity for a discussion of sexuality and burn victims.

Environment

- The burn team should maintain a schedule to help the person with temporal awareness.
- Educate the person and his or her family about the course of treatment and what to expect regarding response to pain, length of hospitalization, immobilization, appearance of wounds at various stages, and goals.

- Provide education and training in nutrition, exercise, pain management, and wound changes. Help the person return to performance self-care tasks independently.
- Prepare the family for discharge well in advance of the discharge date.
- Encourage the family to participate in a support group.
- Provide the family with information about community resources such as burn camps and burn recovery groups.

PRECAUTIONS

- Do not permit the person to assume a fetal or protective position, such as adduction and flexion of the upper extremities, adduction of thumb, flexion of the hips and knees, plantar flexion of the ankles, or resting the neck and head on a pillow in an upright position when there are trunk burns. These positions contribute to development of contractures and limit function. Positioning should be in extension patterns.
- Watch for signs of infection. Splints can be a source of microorganisms. Whenever splints are removed from the person, they should be cleaned with a disinfecting agent, such as a quaternary ammonia solution.
- Watch for signs of skin breakdown or failure of grafts, such as blisters.
- Be aware that new skin is very fragile and sensitive and must be protected from friction.
- Watch for signs of heterotopic ossification (calcium deposits in a joint, such as the elbow).
- Watch for signs of peripheral nerve injury from compression.
- Watch for signs of hypertrophic scarring.
- Watch for signs of contracture formation.
- Watch for increase in edema and changes in skin color suggesting poor venous return of fluid, which may be due to noncompliance.
- Before starting exercise, use a lubricant to reduce the chance of skin rupture from dryness and scar rigidity.
- During exercise, monitor pulse rate, blood pressure, and respiration.
- Caution the person about unprotected sun exposure to avoid blotchy and variable tanning.
- Caution the person about temperature extremes. The person should stay in areas where the temperature is above 70 degrees Fahrenheit.

PROGNOSIS AND OUTCOME

The prognosis for first-degree burns is very good to excellent. Recovery occurs in 1 day to 14 days, and hospitalization is not required. There should be no problems in healing, although some changes may occur in pigmentation, or the color of the skin. Second-degree burn recovery takes 21 days or more and usually occurs in a hospital. Pigment changes are probable, and skin will have reduced durability. Other changes include scarring, changes in sensation, reducing sweating capacity, loss of temperature control, and dependent edema, which may be temporary. Third-degree burn recovery is highly variable and always requires hospitalization. In addition to the changes listed for second-degree burns, sweating potential will be further decreased, more sensory loss occurs, hair does not grow on graft sites, and finger- and toenails may be lost. Fourth-degree burn recovery is highly variable, with permanent changes in functional performance. In addition, amputation, reconstructive surgery, and prosthetic use may be necessary.

- The person demonstrates the maximum level of independence in performance of self-care activities, such as bathing, grooming, eating, toileting, and dressing.
- The person is able to control pain to permit maximum function in performing daily tasks.
- The person is able to perform productive activities, such as homemaking, attending school, or working at a vocation.
- The person is able to perform leisure, recreational, or avocational activities at home or in the community.
- The person has recovered, as much as possible, preburn status for active range of motion, strength, endurance, and coordination.
- The person demonstrates knowledge of how to prevent and ability to prevent decreased joint and skin mobility and avoid joint deterioration through stretching exercises.
- Edema is controlled by elevated positioning and external vascular supports.
- The person uses protective interventions for sensory, vascular, and pigment changes.
- The person is able to explain and demonstrate use of any assistive technology that helps the person perform daily tasks at home, at work, or in the community.
- The person demonstrates knowledge of and ability to perform techniques of skin conditioning, including caring for wounds, moisturizing skin, putting on and removing vascular supports, and protecting of wounds, grafts, and donor sites.
- The person is able to control skin sensitivity to permit maximum function in performing daily tasks.
- Deformities are eliminated or minimized.
- Hypertrophic scarring is reduced as much as possible and does not interfere with performance of daily tasks.
- The person copes constructively with symptoms of stress and changes in body appearance.
- The person is able to demonstrate role performance in the home and community.

REFERENCES

Beers, M.H., and R. Berkow, eds. 1999. *The Merck Manual of Diagnosis and Therapy*, 17th ed. Whitehouse Station, NJ: Merck Research Laboratories.

Brigham, P.A., and E. McLoughlin. 1996. *Journal of Burn Care and Rehabilitation* 17, no. 2: 95–107.

Daugherty, M.B., and J.A. Carr-Collins. 1994. Splinting techniques for the burn patient. In *Burn care and rehabilitation: Principles and practice,* eds. R.L. Richard and M.J. Staley, 242–323. Philadelphia: F.A. Davis. (Case report)

Ott, S. et al. 1996. Treating deformities via positioning and splinting, using skeletal suspension and traction, and with prosthetics and orthotics. In *Total burn care*, ed. D.N. Herndon, 455–470. London: W.B. Saunders.

BIBLIOGRAPHY

Adams, R.C. 1995. Treating patients with burns at home. *Advance for Occupational Therapists* 11, no. 20: 10, 16.

Alvarado, M.I. 1996. Burns. In *Occupational therapy for physical dysfunction*, 4th ed., ed. C.A. Trombly, 831–848. Baltimore: Williams & Wilkins.

Androwick, J. et al. 1995. OT intervention for people with burns. *Advance for Occupational Therapists* 11, no. 20: 18, 54. Also in *Advance for Rehabilitation* 4, no. 3: 23–24, 57.

Apfel, L.M. et al. 1994. Approaches to positioning the burn patient. In *Burn care and rehabilitation: Principles and practice*, eds. R.L. Richard and M.J. Staley, 221–241. Philadelphia: F.A. Davis. (Case report)

Barone, C.M. et al. 1994. Evaluation of treatment modalities in perioral electrical burns. *Journal of Burn Care and Rehabilitation* 15, no. 4: 335–340.

Baruch, L.D. 1993. More information about burn treatment. *OT Week* 7, no. 15: 17. (Bibliography)

Baruch, L.D. 1993. UVA therapists meet the challenge of scar management. *OT Week* 7, no. 15: 14–17.

Biggs, K.S. et al. 1998. Determining the current roles of physical and occupational therapists in burn care. *Journal of Burn Care and Rehabilitation* 19, no. 5: 442–449.

Carter, Y.M. et al. 1999. Incidence of the concrete scalp deformity associated with deep scalp donor sites and management with the unna cap. *Journal of Burn Care and Rehabilitation* 20, no. 2: 141–144.

Chiburis, L. et al. 1997. Ethics and rehabilitation of the patient with severe burns. *Journal of Burn Care and Rehabilitation* 18, no. 5: 443–446.

Church, P.M., and R. Cooper. 1996. Burns. In *Occupational therapy and physical dysfunction: Principles, skills, and practice*, eds. A. Turner et al., 691–708. New York: Churchill Livingstone. (Case report)

Colan, B.J. 1996. No place to hide: Treating patients with facial burns. *Advance for Occupational Therapists* 12, no. 47: 18. Also in *Advance for Physical Therapists,* November 18, 15.

Crowe, J.M. et al. 1998. Reliability of photographic analysis in determining change in scar appearance. *Journal of Burn Care Rehabilitation* 19, no. 2: 183–186.

Fletchall, S., and W.L. Hickerson. 1995. Quality burn rehabilitation: Cost-effective approach. *Journal of Burn Care and Rehabilitation* 16, no. 5: S39–S42.

Fletchall, S., and W.L. Hickerson. 1997. Managed health care: Therapist responsibilities. *Journal of Burn Care and Rehabilitation* 18, no. 1, part 1: 61–63.

Fraulin, F.O.G. et al. 1996. Assessment of cosmetic and functional results of conservative versus surgical management of facial burns. *Journal of Burn Care and Rehabilitation* 17, no. 1: 19–29.

Giele, H.P. et al. 1995. Early use of pressure masks to avoid facial contracture during the pregrafting phase. *Journal of Burn Care and Rehabilitation* 16, no. 6: 641–645.

Gill, R. 1993. Special room encourages patient activity. *OT Week* 7, no. 31: 18–19.

Gripp, C.L. et al. 1995. Use of burn intensive care unit gymnasium as an adjunct to therapy. *Journal of Burn Care and Rehabilitation* 16, no. 2, part 1: 160–161.

Haley, R. 1993. Massachusetts OTs find diversity on burn unit. *OT Week* 7, no. 15: 18–19.

Johnson, J. et al. 1994. Compliance with pressure garment use in burn rehabilitation. *Journal of Burn Care and Rehabilitation* 15, no. 2: 181–188.

Jordan, C.L. et al. 1994. Self-care strategies following severe burns. In *Ways of living: Self-care strategies for special needs,* ed. C. Christiansen, 305–332. Rockville, MD: American Occupational Therapy Association. (Case reports)

Jordan, C.L., and R.R. Allely. 1996. Burns and burn rehabilitation. In *Occupational therapy: Practice skills for physical dysfunction*, 4th ed., ed. L.W. Pedretti, 613–638. St. Louis, MO: CV Mosby. (Case report)

Kerr, T. 1995. The ups and downs of the burn unit. *Advance for Occupational Therapists* 11, no. 20: 9, 54.

Leman, C.J., and N. Ricks. 1994. Discharge planning and follow-up burn care. In *Burn care and rehabilitation: Principles and practice*, eds. R.L. Richard and M.J. Staley, 447–472. Philadelphia: F.A. Davis.

Reichley, M.L. 1995. New technology improves burn care rehabilitation. *Advance for Occupational Therapists* 11, no. 20: 3, 16.

Ridgway, C.L., and G.D. Warden. 1995. Evaluation of vertical mouth stretching orthosis: Two case reports. *Journal of Burn Care and Rehabilitation* 16, no. 1: 74–78.

Rivers, E.A. 1998. Burns. In *Physical dysfunction: Practice skills for the occupational therapy assistant*, ed. M.B. Early, 622–637. St. Louis, MO: Mosby.

Rivers, E.A., and C.L. Jordan. 1998. Skin system disorders: Burns. In *Willard and Spackman's occupational therapy*, 9th ed., eds. M.E. Neistadt and E.B. Crepeau, 741–755. Philadelphia: J.B. Lippincott.

Rock, K., and M. Costigan. 1996. The use of the edema bar for the treatment of burn patients. *American Journal of Occupational Therapy* 50, no. 5: 386–388.

Sanford, S., and D. Gore. 1996. Unna's boot dressings facilitate outpatient skin grafting of hands. *Journal of Burn Care and Rehabilitation* 17, no. 4: 323–326.

Serghiou, M., and M. Staley. 1998. Proceedings of the physical and occupational therapy special interest group meeting. *Journal of Burn Care and Rehabilitation* 19, no. 2: 147–150.

Stahl, C. 1995. Burn care in the home setting. *Advance for Occupational Therapists* 11, no. 3: 22.

Staley, M., and M. Serghiou. 1998. Casting guidelines, tips, and techniques: Proceedings from the 1997 American Burn Association PT/OT casting workshop. *Journal of Burn Care and Rehabilitation* 19, no. 3: 254–260.

Summer, G.J. et al. 1999. The unna "cap" as a scalp donor site dressing. *Journal of Burn Care and Rehabilitation* 20, no. 2: 183–188.

Van Deusen, J., and D. Harlow. 1993. The physically challenged adult—burns. In *Body image and perceptual dysfunction in adults*, ed. J. Van Deusen, 207–217. Philadelphia: W.B. Saunders.

Zeller, J. et al. 1993. Patients with burns are successful in work hardening programs. *Journal of Burn Care and Rehabilitation* 14, no. 2, part 1: 189–196.

Burns—Child

DESCRIPTION

Burns in children are defined as tissue injury to the layers of skin and in some cases the soft tissue structure under the skin, resulting in protein denaturation, burn wound edema, and loss of intravascular fluid volume due to increased vascular permeability. Systemic effects, such as hypovolemic shock, infection, or respiratory tract injury, pose a greater threat to life than does the injury to the skin and soft tissue directly.

CAUSE

The most common sources of burns in children are fire and hot water. Other sources are electrical burns that occur from biting an electrical cord, sunburn, various caustic chemicals, or radiation. Young children ages one to three are likely to be burned by hot water, while children older than three are more likely to be burned by fire in their clothing or their home.

ASSESSMENT

Areas
- daily living skills
- play skills
- academic skills
- leisure interests

- developmental profile
- range of motion
- muscle strength
- fine motor skills, manipulation, dexterity, and bilateral coordination
- sensory registration and processing
- self-concept
- coping skills
- communication skills

Instruments

No specific instruments developed by occupational therapists for this disorder were identified in the literature. The following types of instruments may be useful:
- activities of daily living scale
- play history
- leisure checklist
- developmental tests (Note: It may be necessary to interview parents or caregivers if the child is severely burned.)
- goniometer
- manual muscle test
- dexterity and coordination tests

PROBLEMS

Self-Care

- The child may lose the ability to perform self-care skills or fall behind in the development of self-care activities.

Productivity

- The child may lose play skills or fall behind in play skill development.
- The child may fall behind in academic skills.

Leisure

- The child may be unable to participate in favorite leisure activities.

Sensorimotor

- The child usually has limited range of motion.
- The child usually has loss of muscle strength.
- The child may have loss of dexterity and coordination.
- The child may have contractures.
- The child may have deformities.
- The child may have hypertrophic scar formation.
- The child may have a distorted body image.
- The child usually has pain.

Cognitive
- The child may have difficulty concentrating on tasks due to pain and/or pain medication.

Psychosocial
- The child may fear dying.
- The child may have anxiety about what is happening.
- The child may have guilt that the burns are his or her fault or are a punishment.
- The child may be angry and irritable.
- The child may become depressed, listless, or apathetic.
- The child may have low self-esteem.
- The child may suffer loss and separation from his or her family.
- The child may have loss of verbal communication if intubated or if a microstomia splint is used.

TREATMENT/INTERVENTION

Self-Care
- Provide adapted self-care equipment as needed, such as built-up handles, one-handed devices, prism glasses, reachers, large hook handles, nonslip devices or material, long straws, or long handles.

Productivity
- Provide opportunities to maintain or develop play skills.
- Assist in promoting academic development by providing suggestions for adapted devices or equipment.

Leisure
- Promote participation in leisure activities using adapted devices or techniques if needed.

Sensorimotor
- Assist in positioning of body parts through the use of splints to prevent contractures and deformities. Common splints include (1) anterior neck conformer for neck, (2) pan splint for hands, (3) axillary splint for shoulders, (4) bivalve splint for elbow or knee, or (5) posterior knee splint. Less common is the transparent face mask and microstomia splint to maintain the size of the mouth.
- Provide exercises for the burned hand to avoid possible damage to the extension mechanisms: tabletop (metacarpophalangeal flexion, proximal and distal interphalangeal extension), and curl (metacarpophalangeal extension, proximal and distal interphalangeal flexion).
- Provide pressure garments to reduce scar hypertrophy.

Cognitive
- Provide instructions to family members on the care of burns and progress of rehabilitation.

- Assist the physician in providing factual information on the prognosis and outcome of the burn sites.

Psychosocial
- Provide opportunities for self-expression, such as storytelling, simple craft projects, or games.
- Provide instruction in stress management techniques, including relaxation training.
- Provide a communication board if needed to facilitate communication.

PRECAUTIONS

- Watch for signs of infection. Clean splints with approved solution.
- Watch for skin breakdown or graft site failure.
- Watch for heterotopic ossification.
- Watch for peripheral nerve injury from compression, which may occur from a splint.
- Watch for hypertrophic scarring.
- Watch for contractures.

PROGNOSIS AND OUTCOME

- The child is able to perform self-care activities independently, using self-help devices if needed.
- The child demonstrates age-appropriate play skills.
- The child is able to maintain or improve academic skills, with adapted devices or equipment if needed.
- The child is able to participate in leisure activities.
- The child maintains or improves developmental profile to his or her chronologic age.
- The child maintains or improves muscle strength in muscle groups affected by burns.
- The child maintains or improves range of motion in joints affected by burns.
- The child maintains or improves fine motor dexterity and bilateral coordination.
- The child maintains or improves sensory registration and processing of sensory information.
- The child demonstrates positive self-concept and self-esteem.
- The child demonstrates coping techniques.

BIBLIOGRAPHY

de Linde, L.G. 1994. Rehabilitation of the child with burns. In *Pediatric physical therapy*, ed. J.S. Tecklin, 208–248. Philadelphia: J.B. Lippincott.
Dorga, D. et al. 1999. The physical, functional, and developmental outcome of pediatric burn survivors from 1–12 months postinjury. *Journal of Burn Care and Rehabilitation* 20, no. 2: 171–178.
Gibbons, M. et al. 1994. Experience with silastic gel sheeting in pediatric scarring. *Journal of Burn Care and Rehabilitation* 15, no. 1: 69–73.

Greenhalgh, D.G. et al. 1993. The early release of axillary contractures in pediatric patients with burns. *Journal of Burn Care and Rehabilitation* 14, no. 1: 39–42.

Grigsby de Linde, L. 1997. Healing burns in children. *Advance for Directors in Rehabilitation* 6, no. 5: 37–38, 41.

Hoffman, B.E., and K. Cozean. 1993. The adolescent with burns. In *Practice issues in occupational therapy: Intraprofessional team building*, ed. S.E. Ryan, 81–90. Thorofare, NJ: Slack.

Nakamura, D.Y. et al. 1998. The Unna 'sleeve': An effective postoperative dressing for pediatric arm burns. *Journal of Burn Care and Rehabilitation* 19, no. 4: 349–351.

Porr, S.M. 1999. Children as burn patients. In *Pediatric therapy: A systems approach*, eds. S.M. Porr and E.B. Rainville, 507–524. Philadelphia: F.A. Davis.

Raible, R. 1995. Old techniques, new hopes. *OT Week* 9, no. 13: 16–17.

Reeves, S.U. et al. 1994. Management of the pediatric burn patient. In *Burn care and rehabilitation: Principles and practice*, eds. R.L. Richard and M.J. Staley, 499–530. Philadelphia: F.A. Davis.

Roberts, L. et al. 1993. Longitudinal hand grip and pinch strength recovery in the child with burns. *Journal of Burn Care and Rehabilitation* 14, no. 1: 99–101.

Schwanholt, C.A. et al. 1993. A comparison of full-thickness versus split-thickness autograft for the coverage of deep palm burns in the very young pediatric patient. *Journal of Burn Care and Rehabilitation* 14, no. 1: 29–33.

Schwanholt, C.A. et al. 1994. A prospective study of burn scar maturation in pediatrics: Does age matter? *Journal of Burn Care and Rehabilitation* 15, no. 5: 416–420.

Wavrek, B.B. 1996. Hospital services—burn unit. In *Occupational therapy for children*, 3rd ed., eds. J. Case-Smith et al., 750–752. St. Louis, MO: Mosby.

Thermal Injuries—Hands

DESCRIPTION

This section discusses burns to wrists, hands, fingers, and thumbs. See the section on burns in adults for more description.

CAUSE

Causes include thermal, radiation, chemical, or electrical. Cold injuries are classified into two major groups: freezing (frostbite) and nonfreezing (chilblains and immersion injury). Frostbite is the result of crystallization of the water in cell tissue due to exposure to temperatures below freezing. Peripheral vasoconstriction occurs because heat is channeled to the body core. Three factors contribute to frostbite: conditions that facilitate heat loss, such as wet clothing, exposed skin, immobility, fever, injury, hyperventilation, overexercise, and alcohol; mechanical or physical restriction of the peripheral circulation, such as tight boots or gloves, peripheral vascular disease, blood vessel injury, fracture or crush injury, or vasoconstriction due to drug action; and conditions that decrease the ability of the person to cope with cold, such as fatigue, emaciation, dehydration, poor caloric intake, underlying systemic disease, previous frostbite, and mental disorders. Chilblains occur when the person is exposed repeatedly to a dry, nonfreezing cold environment without adequate protection. Immersion

> ### Classification of Cold Injury Involving the Hand
>
> - First degree: After rewarming, the skin becomes mottled, cyanotic, red, hot, and dry. The person may complain of a burning sensation and aching.
> - Second degree: Hyperemia, edema, and burning pain develop after rewarming. The person may not respond to light touch, and his or her sense of position may be absent. Clear blisters appear within 6 hours to 12 hours and subsequently dry to form eschars.
> - Third degree: Necrosis of skin and subcutaneous tissue occurs. Vesicles which form are small, hemorrhagic, and violaceous. Anesthesia is present early and is followed by severe pain of a burning, aching, or throbbing type. Eschars separate late, exposing granulation tissue.
> - Fourth degree: There is necrosis of all skin, soft tissue, and bone. Upon rewarming, the skin appears deep red, mottled, or cyanotic. The area is anesthetic, and there is no edema or vesicle formation. There is a progression to dry gangrene and mummification.
>
> *Source:* Data from Brown, Hamlet, McDowell, and Sudekump, pp. 1297–1298.

injuries result from exposure to a wet, nonfreezing cold environment (Brown et al. 1995, 1295–1296).

ASSESSMENT

Areas
- hand function
- edema
- active and passive range of motion
- two-point discrimination
- grip strength
- wound status: open or closed
- sensation: hypersensitivity, hyposensitivity
- sensory registration and processing: touch, proprioception

Instruments
- *EVAL Hand Evaluation System* by Greenleaf Medical Systems, Palo Alto, CA. (Computerized evaluation system)
- *Vancouver Burn Scar Assessment* by the Occupational Therapy Department, Vancouver General Hospital, Vancouver, British Columbia, Canada, 1990.
- dynamometer and pinch meter
- goniometer
- two-point discrimination wheel

- tape measure and ruler
- Tinel's sign

PROBLEMS

Self-Care
- Loss of hand function interferes with performance of daily living skills.

Sensorimotor
- The person may have deformities such as the claw hand with metacarpophalangeal hypertension, proximal interphalangeal and distal interphalangeal flexion, thumb interphalangeal flexion and adduction, and flattened palmar arch. With palmar burns, there may be proximal interphalangeal and distal interphalangeal flexion; with burns to the thumb, there may be interphalangeal flexion and adduction.
- Chronic conditions after frostbite include excessive sweating, pain, coldness in the extremities, numbness, abnormal skin color, joint stiffness, contractures, and osteoporosis.
- Chilblains lead to edema, a cyanotic rubor, and vestibular dermatitis. Repeated exposure leads to an itching and burning sensation. The skin becomes erythematous and vesiculated. Ulcers may develop.
- Immersion injuries produce peripheral vasoconstriction, followed by ischemia, with compromise of endothelial cell function. Loss of intravascular fluid produces peripheral edema and vascular sludging. Thrombosis can occur during rewarming.
- The person has edema, possibly persistent edema.
- The person may have reduced range of motion.
- The person may lose hand functions.
- The person may have damage to the anatomical structures of the hand and wrist.
- The person may have hypertrophic scarring.
- The person may have soft tissue contractions.
- There may be obstacles to treatment such as poor positioning or improper mobilization, which may be caused by the client, the caregiver, or other health professionals.
- Obstacles to recovery include inappropriate positioning, poor-fitting splints, prolonged immobilization, and delayed initiation of active range of motion and participation in functional activities.

Cognitive
- Cognitive functions are not usually a problem in burn or terminal injuries of the hand.

Psychosocial
- The person may be noncompliant with the recommended treatment regimen.

TREATMENT/INTERVENTION

The team approach is commonly used. Good communication between physicians and therapists is essential for effective outcomes. The occupational therapy model of treatment is biomechanical. A treatment protocol for the evaluation and treatment of burned hands appears in the article by Torres-Gray et al. (1996, 165–168).

Self-Care
- Use feeding and grooming tasks to help the person maintain use of his or her hands and prevent the pattern of protecting the burned hand.

Productivity
- After hand therapy has reached a plateau, referral to a work hardening program may be helpful in continuing the gains made in hand functions.

Sensorimotor
- Promote early positioning and splinting, which is generally done by placing the joint in the opposite direction of the anticipated deformity and maintaining the length of the ligaments.
- Promote early mobilization to decrease problems with prolonged immobilization using short, frequent periods of light and repetitive active range of motion exercises.
- Maintain or restore hand motions and functions.
- For partially exposed tendons (buttonhole), active range of motion exercises include isolated tendon gliding exercises such as hook fisting (interphalangeal joint flexion with metacarpophalangeal joint extension), tabletop (metacarpophalangeal flexion with interphalangeal joint extension), partial fist (metacarpophalangeal and proximal interphalangeal flexion with distal interphalangeal extension), and composite fisting (metacarpophalangeal and interphalangeal joint flexion). A resting hand, radial, or ulnar gutter splint may be used. See the Torres-Gray et al. (1996, 165–168) protocol for additional recommendations.
- Prevent deformities or deficits such as soft tissue contractures and adhesions through positioning, active and active-assisted, or passive range of motion exercises or splinting.
- Most common deformities are thumb web-space contractures, proximal interphalangeal joint flexion contractures, and fifth-digit boutonniere deformities, whether "true" boutonniere, with damage to the extensor apparatus, or "pseudo," involving hyperextension of the proximal interphalangeal joint.
- Prevent thumb web-space contractures by early positioning and exercise to avoid loss of cylindrical grasp and opposition with fingers.
- Prevent proximal interphalangeal flexion contracture by using joint mobilization, passive stretching, active exercise, or casting or splinting with a finger gutter or hand-based splint.
- Prevent "true" boutonniere deformity using immobilization of the proximal interphalangeal joint with a splint or surgical fixation with Kirschner wire placement.
- Prevent "pseudo" boutonniere by use of serial casting or static progressive splinting to restore metacarpophalangeal joint flexion and proximal interphalangeal and distal interphalangeal joint extension.
- Prevent specific hand deformities.
  1. claw hand: resting hand splint, metacarpophalangeal at 75 degrees flexion, proximal interphalangeal and distal interphalangeal at 0 degrees, thumb in radial or palmar abduction, wrist at 30 degrees extension
  2. palmar burns: dorsal hand splint, proximal interphalangeal, distal interphalangeal, and metacarpophalangeal at 0 degrees
  3. thumb burns: thumb splint, thumb in radial adduction, wrist at 30 degree extension

- Control edema through elevation and positioning of the hand to avoid the dependent position. Splinting may provide better positioning but must be monitored daily to adjust for fluctuations in edema. After a few days, a resting hand splint may be used to maintain a position of zero degrees to 20 degrees of wrist extension, 50 degrees to 70 degrees of metacarpophalangeal flexion, and full proximal interphalangeal and distal interphalangeal extension. Note: Richard and colleagues (1994) suggest that there is little agreement about the best splinting position for the wrist, metacarpophalangeal, distal interphalangeal, or proximal interphalangeal joints.
- After graft surgery, more aggressive intervention is recommended, including range of motion to a normal limit and increased strength and functional activities.
- Joint mobilization techniques may be applied to relieve joint tightness and stiffness.
- Splinting may be switched from a static splint to a static-progressive or dynamic splint.
- Continuous passive motion can be useful in a home program because the unit is portable and the range can be set to avoid over- or underexercising.
- Prevent hypertrophic scar formation using pressure garments.
- Pressure garments, such as gloves, for the dorsum of the hand can be effective but are generally not effective for the palm. Other products such as silicone gel, sheeting, or other silicone-based products can be used in combination with or independent of compression products.

Cognitive

- Use of educational videos and printed or written information about the importance of following treatment procedures can increase compliance.

Psychosocial

- Provide psychological support.
- Promote compliance with the treatment program.
- Encourage the person to have contact with other burn survivors.

PRECAUTIONS

- During the acute stage, be alert for exposed tendons. Be careful with active-assisted exercises, passive range of motion exercises, or pressure on the dorsal hand from edema because too much pressure can cause a rupture or other damage to the extensor tendon mechanism. Isolated range of motion exercises are strongly recommended.
- Paraffin baths should be used cautiously if the person has open wounds or is sensitive to heat. Options include painting the paraffin on the hand or dipping strips of gauze in the wax and then applying the strips to the hand.
- No heat modality should be applied directly to open wounds or those that are sensitive to heat.
- Identify the type of contracture for proper treatment: a scar band contracture involves skin only; more advanced contractures may include muscle contracture or fibrosis or both. Therapy is effective with skin-only contractures, but surgery is needed for advanced contractures.

PROGNOSIS AND OUTCOME

- The person is able to perform daily living tasks and routines.
- The person is able to perform productive tasks.
- The person is able to engage in leisure interests.
- The person has functional range of motion.
- The person has functional hand skills.

REFERENCES

Brown, F.E. et al. 1995. Acute care and rehabilitation of the hand after cold injury. In *Rehabilitation of the hand: Surgery and therapy*, 4th ed., eds. J.M. Hunter et al., 1295–1303. St. Louis, MO: Mosby.
Richard, R. et al. 1994. The wide variety of designs for dorsal hand burn splints. *Journal of Burn Care and Rehabilitation* 15: 275–280.
Torres-Gray, D. et al. 1996. Rehabilitation of the burned hand: Questionnaire results. *Journal of Burn Care and Rehabilitation* 17, no. 2: 161–168.

BIBLIOGRAPHY

DeLinde, L.G., and W.K. Miles. 1995. Remodeling of scar tissue in the burned hand. In *Rehabilitation of the hand: Surgery and therapy*, 4th ed., eds. J.M. Hunter et al., 1267–1294. St. Louis, MO: Mosby.
Harvey, K.D. et al. 1996. Computer-assisted evaluation of hand and arm function after thermal injury. *Journal of Burn Care and Rehabilitation* 17, no. 2: 176–180.
Matsumura, H. et al. 1999. The use of the Millard "crane" flap for deep hand burns with exposed tendons and joints. *Journal of Burn Care and Rehabilitation* 20, no. 4: 316–319.
Murphy, J. 1996. The tricky art of treating hand burns. *Advance for Occupational Therapists* 12, no. 4: 17.
Nuchtern, J.G. et al. 1995. Treatment of fourth-degree hand burns. *Journal of Burn Care and Rehabilitation* 16, no. 1: 36–42.

Part X

Cognitive-
Perceptual
Disorders

Agnosia

DESCRIPTION

Agnosia is a rare neuropsychological deficit in which a person cannot identify an object despite the capacity to identify its tactile or visual elements (Merck 1999, 1382). The word "gnosia" means knowledge, so the loose translation of agnosia is "not to know" what objects (or persons) are. The following are types of agnosia (Laver and Unsworth 1999):

* alexia—an acquired inability to comprehend written language
* anosognosia—lack of awareness, or denial, of a paretic extremity as belonging to the person; or lack of insight concerning, or denial of, paralysis
* astereognosis—inability to recognize objects by touch alone (with vision occluded) despite intact sensory abilities
* vauditory agnosia—inability to distinguish between sounds or to recognize familiar sounds
* color perception disturbances
    — achronmatopsia—difficulty recognizing or matching colors or sorting different shades of the same color
    — color agnosia—inability to associate objects with particular colors
* finger agnosia—inability to identify correctly which finger has been touched
* prosopagnosia—inability to recognize familiar faces despite intact sensory abilities
* simultanagnosia—difficulty recognizing the elements of a visual array
* tactile agnosia—see astereognosis
* visual object agnosia—inability to recognize objects by looking at them despite intact vision

CAUSE

Agnosia is caused by the impairment or loss of information processing and interpretation skills previously stored in the secondary projection association cortex area and related to objects' tactile or visual (or other sensory system) characteristics. If the primary project areas had been lost or impaired, the person would have lost the sensory modality itself.

ASSESSMENT

Areas

* daily living skills—activities of daily living (ADLs), instrumental ADLs (IADLs)
* productivity skills, values, history, interests
* leisure skills and interests
* gross motor skills
* fine motor skills—dexterity, manipulation, eye-hand coordination
* visual perception—form discrimination, prosopagnosia, color recognition, reading skills
* tactile perception—stereognosis
* auditory perception—noises, spoken word, music
* body image and scheme

- taste perception
- perception of temperature—hot or cold
- cognition—awareness, alertness, attention, concentration, memory skills
- problem-solving and decision-making skills
- judgment of safety
- roles and role behaviors
- social skills

Instruments

Note: Laver and Unsworth (1999, 340–341) provide a useful set of interview questions for understanding a client's agnosia. These questions have been adapted in the box, "Interview Quesions for Undertanding Agnosia."

Instruments Developed by Occupational Therapy Personnel

- *Arnadottir OT-ADL Neurobehavioral Evaluation* (A-ONE) by G. Arnadottir, in *The Brain and Behavior: Assessing Cortical Dysfunction through Activities of Daily Living* (ADL). St. Louis, MO: CV Mosby, 1990.
- *Assessment of Motor and Process Skills*, 2nd ed., by A. Fisher, Ft. Collins, CO: Three Star Press, 1997.
- *Chessington Occupational Therapy Neurological Assessment Battery* (COTNAB) by R. Tyerman et al., Nottingham, England: Nottingham Rehab., 1986.
- *Loewenstein Occupational Therapy Cognitive Assessment* (LOTCA) by M. Itzkovich et al., Pequanock, NJ: Maddak, 1990.
- *Kitchen Task Assessment* (KTA) by C.M. Baum and D.F. Edwards, *American Journal of Occupational Therapy* 47, no. 5 (1993): 431–436.
- *Rabideau Kitchen Assessment,* revised by M.E. Neistadt, *Occupational Therapy Journal of Research* 12, no. 4 (1992): 242–255.
- *Rivermead Perceptual Assessment Battery* (RPAB) by S. Whiting et al., Windsor, Berkshire, England: NFER-Nelson, 1985. (Distributed in the United States by Western Psychological Services, Los Angeles.)
- *Sensory Integration and Praxis Tests* by A.J. Ayres, Los Angeles: Western Psychological Services, 1989.
- *Structured Observational Test of Function* by A.J. Laver and G.E. Powell, Windsor, Berkshire, England: NFER-Nelson, 1995.

Instruments Developed by Other Professionals and Used by Occupational Therapy Personnel

- *Cognitive Competency Test* by P.I. Wang and K.E. Ennis, in Competency assessment in clinical populations: An introduction to the Cognitive Competency Test, *Clinical neuropsychology of intervention,* eds. B. Uzzel and E. Gross, Boston: Marinus Nijhoff Publishing, 1986.
- *Ishihara Color Plates* by Kanehura & Company, Tokyo: 1977.
- *Memory and Behavior Problems Checklist* by S.H. Zarit, N.K. Orr, and J.M. Zarit, in *The hidden victims of Alzheimer's disease: Families under stress,* New York: New York University Press, 1985.

Interview Questions for Understanding Agnosia

1. Can you describe to me what you can see, feel, hear, or taste?
2. When you look at an object and try to identify what you are seeing, what are you thinking?
3. Look at this object (use a familiar object) and tell me all your thoughts out loud as you try to identify it.
4. Are you able to remember what a particular object should look like or what color an object should be?
5. Are you able to identify the weight, size, and shape of an object?
6. Can you remember objects that have the same weight, shape, and size?
7. When you recognize an object and can match it to a picture or memory of other similar objects in your head, can you find the name or word for the object and speak it out loud?
8. How do you know the object is a (cup or other familiar object)?
9. Why did you think it was a spoon instead of a fork? (Or a cup instead of a plate?)
10. Can you recognize faces of people you know?
11. Can you recognize your own face in the mirror?
12. How do you try to recognize common objects?
13. What do you see on the page when you try to read?
14. How do you approach a page or sentence when you try to read?
15. Do you try to break down the sentence and focus on one word or letter at a time?

Source: Data from A. Laver and C. Unsworth, Evaluation and Intervention with Simple Perceptual Impairment (Agnosias), in C. Unsworth, ed., *Cognitive and Perceptual Dysfunction: A Clinical Reasoning Approach to Evaluation and Intervention*, pp. 340–341, © 1999, F.A. Davis Company

---

- *Test of Facial Recognition* by A.L. Benton and M.W. Van Allen, in Impairment of facial recognition in patients with cerebral disease, *Cortex* 4 (1968): 344–358.
- *Zarit Caregiver Burden Survey* by S.H. Zarit, P.A. Todd, and J.M. Zarit, in Relatives of the impaired elderly: Correlates of feelings of burden, *Gerontologist* 20 (1986): 649–655.

PROBLEMS

Self-Care

- The person may have difficulty with some self-care activities, such as buttoning or fastening.
- The person may have difficulty recognizing self-care objects and combining them for use; for example, identifying the toothbrush and toothpaste, and getting the toothpaste on the toothbrush.
- The person may complain that some foods do not taste right.

- The person may be unable to participate or perform instrumental ADLs such as meal preparation, writing checks, paying for purchases, or locating items in the store because of difficulty recognizing and responding to objects and persons in the environment.
- The person may be unable to drive because of inability to make sense of road signs.

Productivity

- The person may be unable to perform job duties because of failure to recognize and respond correctly to objects or persons in the work environment.
- The person may be unable to perform homemaking duties because of failure to recognize and respond correctly to objects or persons in the home environment.

Leisure

The person may be unable to participate in favorite leisure activities because of difficulty recognizing and responding correctly or normally to objects or persons associated with the leisure activity.

Sensorimotor

- The person may have difficulty discerning the lines, depth, color, or angles of an object.
- The person may have difficulty integrating relationships between objects, overall form, and possible movement.
- The person may be unable to differentiate colors, which may all seem to be shades of gray.
- The person may be unable to differentiate different tastes.

Cognitive

- The person may have difficulty drawing on past memories and associations.
- The person may have difficulty telling or showing how an object is used, described, or identified.

Psychosocial

The person may be unable to perform roles or role behaviors because of inability to recognize and respond correctly or at the expected level of performance to objects or persons in normal context.

TREATMENT/INTERVENTION

The primary models of treatment are based on remediation of deficits and compensatory strategies.

Self-Care

- Have the person practice recognition of self-care objects in the normal context and environment.
- Have the person plan a meal, shop for and buy the ingredients, prepare the meal, and eat it with utensils.
- The Easy Street Environments (Habitat Inc., 6031 S. Maple Ave., Tempe, AZ 85283; phone 800–733–8442) can be used for realistic home and community settings for self-care, meal

preparation, home management, negotiating streets and sidewalks, shopping for groceries and clothes, banking, going to a movie, and so on.

- Photographs or drawings of objects with labels may be helpful if the person does not have aphasia as well as agnosia.
- Matching words on the shopping list to words on the package label may facilitate shopping tasks (e.g., "tomato soup"). Also, describing the object in advance may aid in recognition on the store shelf.

Productivity

Use objects the patient encountered in the workplace in treatment situations. For example, if the person used carpentry tools at work, select a hammer and screwdriver for object recognition. For a more complex task, have the person identify different types of hammers and screwdrivers.

Leisure

Objects used in favorite leisure activities (for example, small gardening tools) can be used for matching and discrimination tasks. Be aware of safety considerations such as sharp points or edges.

Sensorimotor

- Multiple sensory input may be helpful; for example, seeing and touching an object while listening to the noise it makes.
- Use task grading to increase the level of difficulty; for example, change the environmental context in which an object is viewed from a normal context to a contrived context.
- Increase the complexity of the task as the person improves by increasing the number of objects presented for recognition, from a single object to multiple objects.
- Increase the complexity of the task by varying the client's level of familiarity with the objects, from common self-related objects to unfamiliar or unconventional objects.
- Increase the complexity by altering the spatial arrangement from the usual left-to-right view with well-spaced placement to an unusual view with a scattered, crowded arrangement.
- For form discrimination, begin with matching the same objects present in the same view using familiar, everyday objects placed in a contextual setting. Increase the task demand to matching the same object in different views. Next, have the person match objects that are different but have the same function, such as drinking cups of different shapes, materials, and sizes. Next, have the person differentiate between drinking and eating objects. Finally, have the person identify a variety of objects related to drinking and eating in a context not associated with either activity.
- An open box with mirrors on the bottom and three sides may help the person examine the object from all angles and build up memory units of what the object looks like from different angles.
- Little information about intervention for achromatopsia is available. Grieve (1993) reports that color, shape, and depth (hue) are processed separately, suggesting they should be remediated separately.
  - — For hue, start by having the person discriminate between light and dark shades on color cards. Gradually increase the number of color cards, and have the person sequence them from lightest to darkest color.

— For colors, ask the person if he or she remembers the color of an object such as a stop sign. Present the person with three color cards and see if he or she can pick out the color red. A color chart with the names of colors printed on them may be useful.

— For shape, ask person to sort different objects of the same color, but of different shape.

- For tactile agnosia, begin by having the person discriminate among different sizes and weights of familiar objects, first using vision and then with vision occluded. The person is instructed to hold two objects, one in each hand simultaneously or one after another in the same hand, and identify which is larger, smaller, heavier, or lighter. Objects should initially be as different as possible and gradually become more similar. Next, objects can be placed on the table and identified by touch and vision (no holding) and then by touch only. Again, start with objects that are quite different and gradually decrease the differences.

- For tactile agnosia of texture, begin by having the person match textures on a texture board—such as sandpaper, silk, wood, metal, plastic—first with vision and then with vision occluded. Next, have the person describe the texture in terms of rough, smooth, soft, or hard. Have the person name everyday objects such as a cup, spoon, pen, soap, and book, starting with those that are obviously three-dimensional. Then add flatter objects, such as a key, paper clip, or coin. Finally, place objects in a container with rice or beans and ask the person to find the objects one at a time and name them.

Cognitive

- Use cue grading, from easy to difficult:
  — Repetition cues involve asking the person to "look again."
  — Analysis cues involve asking the person to describe the attributes such as size, shape, weight, or color of the object that was misidentified.
  — Perceptual cues involve directing the person to attend to a critical feature of the object, which may involve repositioning the object so that the critical feature is in the center of vision and pointing to the feature and directing the person to "look here."
  — Semantic cues involve providing the person with a choice of several categories, such as "is it food, a tool, or clothing?"
- Asking the person to keep a journal about daily tasks attempted and relative success or failure can help with writing and reading skills. The journal can be handwritten or kept on a computer. At each session, the person and the therapist review successes and difficulties, and adjust the treatment program to work on difficult items that the person wants to master.

Psychosocial

Items for matching and discrimination can be selected from a valued role such as meal preparer. Common kitchen utensils can be used.

PRECAUTIONS

- Be aware of safety considerations. A person with tactile agnosia may not deal appropriately with sharp edges or points. A person with temperature agnosia may not respond to water hot enough to scald or burn.
- Agnosia should be differentiated from homonomous hemianopia and visual neglect.

PROGNOSIS/OUTCOME

- The person is able to perform self-care and IADLs using remedial techniques or compensatory strategies.
- The person is able to perform a job to his or her satisfaction.
- The person is able to engage in leisure occupations that are enjoyable and satisfying.
- The person is able to use remedial techniques or compensatory strategies to perform tasks requiring sensory processing of information in one or more of the sensory systems.
- The person is able to use problem-solving and decision-making strategies to achieve desired results.
- The person is able to judge personal safety.
- The person is able to perform role tasks and behaviors.

REFERENCES

Beers, M.H., and R. Berkow, eds. 1999. *The Merck Manual of Diagnosis and Therapy,* 17th ed. Whitehouse Station, NJ: Merck Research Laboratories.
Grieve, J.I. 1993. Visual perceptual deficits and agnosia. In *Neuropsychology for occupational therapists,* ed. J.I. Grieve, 96–104. Oxford: Blackwell Scientific Publications.
Laver, A., and C. Unsworth. 1999. Evaluation and intervention with simple perceptual impairment (agnosias). In *Cognitive and perceptual dysfunction: A clinical reasoning approach to evaluation and intervention,* ed. C. Unsworth, 299–356. Philadelphia: F.A. Davis.

BIBLIOGRAPHY

Zoltan, B. 1996. Agnosia. In *Vision, perception, and cognition: A manual for the evaluation and treatment of the neurologically impaired adult,* 3rd ed., ed. B. Zoltan, 53–72. Thorofare, NJ: Slack.

Apraxia

DESCRIPTION

Apraxia, as discussed here, refers to adult-onset apraxia. Developmental apraxia is covered separately. Apraxia is the inability to execute or perform purposeful, previously learned motor acts despite physical ability and willingness. Typically, the person cannot follow a motor command, although he or she understands the words, and cannot recall how to perform learned complex acts despite the fact that he or she may perform the component movements (Merck 1999, 1382). Apraxia is a disorder of skilled movement that cannot be adequately accounted for by incoordination, sensory loss, visual spatial problems, language comprehension difficulties, or cognitive problems alone (Golisz and Tolgia 1998, 272). Apraxia is common in many metabolic and structural diseases that affect the brain diffusely, particularly those that impair frontal lobe function (Merck 1999, 1382). The association areas of the brain are also thought to be involved.

Apraxia may include *temporal* errors, such as those involving rate of movement, temporal coordination of the subcomponents of the movement, or problems and delays in initiating movements; *spatial* errors in orientation and targeting; *postural* errors in hand-arm position; *action* errors, such as clumsiness or augmentation of motor behavior; *sequential* errors such as omissions, faulty sequential organization, or perseveration; *object* errors, such as object misuse, object substitutions, or body part used as an object; *added movement* errors, such as movement of head during limb gesture or other extraneous movements not related to purposeful movement; and *lack of movement* errors, such as failing to move as necessary for the task (Landry and Spaulding 1999, 56). Errors typical of problems in ideomotor (production) apraxia are categorized as content, temporal, spatial, and other (Butler 1999, 266–268). Content errors include perseverative movements, movements related to the target but not correct, and movements nonrelated to the target. Temporal errors are related to sequencing, timing, occurrence, and delay. Spatial errors are called internal configuration for limb only, amplitude, external configuration or orientation for limb only, body-art-as-object for limb only, movement, extraneous, and place of articulation. Other errors are no response, unrecognizable response, or verbalization instead of movement. Errors typical of problems in ideational (conceptual) apraxia are elements occurring in the wrong order, sections of the sequence omitted or performed out of order, two or more elements blended together, action remains incomplete, action overshoots what is necessary, objects are used inappropriately, movements are made in the wrong plane or direction, perseveration occurs, and many abortive runs at the task are made before succeeding or giving up (Zoltan 1996, 56). Poole et al. (1997) found that children and adults make the same errors, which suggests that developmental apraxia and adult-onset apraxia are the same disorder.

Subtypes of apraxia may include any of the following, depending on the author's point of view regarding apraxia.
- akinesia or dyskinesia—a behavioral state of diminished motor and psychic spontaneity
- constructional apraxia—impairment in producing designs in two or three dimensions by copying, drawing, or constructing, whether upon verbal command, imitation, actual object use, or spontaneously (Zoltan 1996, 59)
- developmental apraxia or dyspraxia—difficulty with gross and fine motor skills in children (see section on Developmental Dyspraxia)
- dressing apraxia—difficulty organizing the sequence of actions necessary to put on one's clothes because of a disorder in body scheme and/or spatial relations (Zoltan 1996, 67)
- ideational or conceptual apraxia—a disorder in the performance of purposeful movement resulting from loss of the concept of movement. The person cannot carry out activities using objects and tools automatically or on command (Grieve 1993, 115). The problem is one of conceptualization rather than production and execution.
- ideomotor or production apraxia—a disorder in the planning, timing, and spatial organization of purposeful movement. The person cannot carry out what is intended, even though the idea is understood (Grieve 1993, 115). The problem is one of production and execution, not conceptualization, such as reaching for a glass of water to take a drink.
- kinetic apraxia—inability to coordinate a limb or part of limb, such as the wrist and fingers. May be a component of ideomotor apraxia.
- motor apraxia—a disorder of movement in the performance of purposeful activities, with the presence of normal muscle tone, normal sensation, and good comprehension (Grieve 1993, 114)

- oral-motor or buccofacial apraxia—difficulty in forming and organizing intelligible words, although the musculature required to do so remains intact. This differs from dysarthria, in which the muscles are affected and the speech is slurred (Zoltan 1996, 59). This disorder is usually treated by a speech pathologist, although occupational therapy personnel can assist in treatment.
- sequential or sequencing apraxia—difficulty organizing the sequence of actions necessary to perform a task such as getting dressed

CAUSE

There is little agreement about the underlying mechanisms that cause apraxia. Theories include a disconnection syndrome, conceptual disorder, spatial disorder, conceptual-production disorder, and movement disorder (Landry and Spaulding 1999, 54). In some cases, a lesion in the postrolandic neural pathway appears to be the cause, but it is unclear whether a lesion or some other disturbance in the brain is the causative factor, as different types of apraxia are attributed to different areas of the brain. Ideational and ideomotor apraxia are associated more often with left-side lesions while constructional apraxia is associated more with right-side lesions.

ASSESSMENT

Areas

(Rule out problems caused by spasticity, ataxia, or paresis.)
- daily living skills, ADLs, and IADLs
- occupational history, interests, skills, and values
- leisure interests and skills
- muscle tone
- range of motion
- coordination—reciprocal, bilateral, and visual motor
- gross motor skills
- fine motor skills, manipulation, and dexterity
- postural control and balance
- functional mobility
- sensory registration
- sensory sensibility or processing
- perceptual skills
- attending behavior
- imitation of movement
- expressive and receptive language
- social skills

Instruments

Assessment of apraxia currently uses six basic formats: (1) *actual performance* of motor actions and tasks; (2) *pictures* of actions and tasks are presented and the person must state what is being done and/or sequence the pictures in the correct order; (3) *gesture production* (person uses gestures to indicate how the task would be performed but the actual task is not done); (4) *gesture comprehension* (person watches a videotape of a gesture being panto-mimed, such as use of a hammer, and then selects a picture of the object, the hammer); (5) *gesture identification* (person watches a gesture, such as use of a hammer, and then selects the object that goes with the gesture, a nail); and (6) *gesture discrimination* (person watches a video and discriminates between well-performed and poorly performed pantomimed acts).

Instruments Developed by Occupational Therapy Personnel

- *Assessment of Motor and Process Skills* (AMPS), 2nd ed., by A. Fisher, Ft. Collins, CO: Three Star Press, 1997.
- *Cambridge Apraxia Battery* by C. Fraser and A. Turton, *British Journal of Occupational Therapy* 49, no. 8 (1986): 248–252.
- *Loewenstein Occupational Therapy Cognitive Assessment* (LOTCA) by M. Itzkovich et al., Pequanock, NJ: Maddak, 1990.
- *Matchstick Designs* by M.E. Gregory and J.A. Aitkin, in Assessment of parietal lobe function in hemiplegia, *Occupational Therapy* 34 (1971): 9–17.
- *Parquetry Block Test* by M.E. Neistadt, in Using research literature to develop a perceptual retraining treatment protocol, *American Journal of Occupational Therapy* 48, no. 1 (1994): 62–72.
- *Praxis (Motor Planning)* by L.W. Pedretti, B. Zoltan, and C.J. Wheatley, in *Occupational therapy: Practice skills for physical dysfunction,* ed. L.W. Pedretti, 237, St. Louis: Mosby, 1996.
- *Praxis Test* by B. Zoltan et al., in *Perceptual Motor Evaluation for Head Injured and Other Neurologically Impaired Adults,* San Jose, CA: Santa Clara Valley Medical Center, 1983.
- *Rivermead Perceptual Assessment Battery* (PRAB) by S Whiting et al., Windsor, Berkshire, England: NFER Nelson, 1985. (Distributed in the United States by Western Psychological Services, Los Angeles.)
- *Sensory Integration and Praxis Tests* by A.J. Ayres, Los Angeles: Western Psychological Services, 1989.
- *Solet Test for Apraxia* by J.M. Solet, available from the author, 5 Channing Road, Newton Center, MA 02159.
- *Test for Apraxia* by B. Longs-Christopher, in Life's a maze: Treating patients with apraxia, *Occupational Therapy Forum* 8, no. 8 (1993): 4–5, 8–9.

Instruments Developed by Other Professionals and Used by Occupational Therapy Personnel

- *Bender-Gestalt Test—Its Quantification and Validity for Adults* by G.K. Pascal and B. Suttell, New York: Grune & Stratton, 1951.
- *Benton Visual Retention Test* by A.B. Sivan, San Antonio, TX: Psychological Corporation, 1992.
- *Boston Diagnostic Aphasia Examination* (Parietal Lobe Tests) by H. Goodglass and E. Kaplan, in *Assessment of aphasia and related disorders,* Philadelphia: Lea & Febiger, 1972.
- *Constructional Praxis Tests* by A. Benton, in *Tests of three-dimensional block construction,* New York: Oxford University Press, 1973

- *Copying Designs* by E.J. Lorenze and R. Cancro, in Dysfunction in visual perception with hemiplegia: Its relation to activities of daily living, *Archives of Physical Medicine* 43 (1962): 514–517.
- *DeRenzi, Pieczuro, and Vignol Test of Apraxia* by E. DeRenzi, A. Pieczuro, and L.A. Vignol, in Ideational apraxia: A quantitative study, *Neuropsychologia* 6 (1966): 41–52.
- *Deuel's Test of Manual Apraxia* by R.K. Deuel, C. Feely, and C. Bonskowski, in Manual apraxia in learning disabled children (abstract), *Annals of Neurology* 16 (1984): 388, and R.K. Deuel et al., in Constructional apraxia in Alzheimer's disease: Contributions to functional loss, *Physical and Occupational Therapy in Geriatrics* 9, no. 3/4 (1991): 53–68.
- *Florida Apraxia Screening Test* (FAST) by L.G. Rothi and K.M. Heilman, in Ideomotor apraxia: Gestural discrimination, comprehension and memory, *Neuropsychological studies in apraxia and related disorders,* ed. E.A. Roy, 65–74, Amsterdam: Elsevier, 1985. (Printed in Butler, 262–265.)
- *Goodglass Test of Apraxia* by H. Goodglass and E. Kaplan, in *Assessment of aphasia and related disorders*, Philadelphia: Lea & Febiger, 1972. (Reproduced in Quintana, 213.)
- *Ideational Apraxia Test* by E. DeRenzi and F. Lucchelli, in Ideational apraxia, *Brain* 111 (1988): 1173–1185. (Scoring sheet appears in Butler, 269.)
- *Ideomotor Apraxia Test* by E. DeRenzi, M. Fabrizia, and P. Nichelli, in Imitating gestures: A quantitative approach to ideomotor apraxia, *Archives of Neurology* 37 (1980): 6–10.
- *Kohs Block Test* by S.C. Kohs, in Intelligence measurement: A psychological and statistical study based on the block design test. New York: Macmillan, 1923.
- *Rey-Osterreith Complex Figure* by J. Meyers and K. Meyers, Odessa, FL: Psychological Assessment Resources, Inc., 1995.
- *Test of Oral and Limb Apraxia* (TOLA) by N. Helm-Estabrooks, Chicago: Riverside Publishing, 1992.
- *Test of Visual-Motor Skills—Revised* (TVMS-R) by M.F. Gardner, Hydesville, CA: Psychological and Educational Publications, 1996.
- *Test of Three-Dimensional Construction Praxis* by A.L. Benton and M.L. Fogel, *Archives of Neurology* 7 (1962):347–354.

PROBLEMS

Self-Care

The person usually has some difficulty performing activities of daily living, such as dressing, grooming, or writing.

Productivity

The person may be unable to perform some job tasks, especially those that require use of both hands simultaneously.

Leisure

The person may be unable to do some leisure activities that require highly skilled, coordinated movements.

Sensorimotor

- The person has difficulty planning or carrying out motor movements.
- The person may appear clumsy, especially when performing a series of movements (ideomotor).
- The person may appear uncoordinated, especially when trying to perform a task that requires the use of both sides of the body at the same time (ideational).
- The person may have difficulty with manipulation and dexterity (kinetic apraxia).
- The person may have loss of range of motion, including contractures resulting from disuse.
- The person may have muscle weakness or atrophy resulting from disuse.
- The person may have sparing of some movements that are performed in isolation.
- The person may have decreased sensory registration.
- The person may have loss of sensory sensitivity.
- The person may have associated perceptual disorders, such as visual or auditory perceptual dysfunction, dyskinesia, agraphia, astereognosis, or tactile defensiveness.
- A person with left cardiovascular accident (CVA) may perform less well on gesture comprehension and praxis production (York and Cermak 1995).
- A person with right CVA may perform less well on gesture discrimination and visual perception (York and Cermak 1995).

Cognitive

- The person may have decreased or poor visualization skills.
- The person may have decreased ability to imitate.

Psychosocial

- The person may have low self-esteem and self-confidence.
- The person may have difficulty making and keeping friends because of odd behavior (clumsy and uncoordinated).
- The person may not be permitted to assume certain roles within the family because of clumsiness.
- The person may have expressive or receptive aphasia, or both.

TREATMENT/INTERVENTION

Effective techniques for addressing apraxia have not been established. Multiple approaches are currently suggested. The model of treatment most often mentioned in occupational therapy is based on sensory integration and the Affolter approach.

Self-Care

- Use environmental cues and knowledge of the person's previous habits to evoke self-care skills. For example, if the person brushed his or her teeth in the morning upon rising, take the person to the bathroom sink where toothbrush and toothpaste have been placed. Placing a familiar object in the person's hand may also be helpful in evoking the desired movement (ideational apraxia).
- Practice performing functional activities in the context in which the person would normally perform them.

- Use functional (occupational) tasks rather than remedial activities for best carryover.

Productivity
- The work situation may require modification to eliminate or reduce the need for praxis skills that the person cannot perform reliably.
- The person may need to explore interests, career goals, and vocational choices that do not require praxis skills that he or she cannot perform.

Leisure
   Explore with the person leisure interests and activities that are within his or her ability to perform.

Sensorimotor
- Improve gross motor skills through guided practice.
- Provide opportunity for repetition of successful performance.
- Maintain or increase range of motion (ideational apraxia).
- Prevent atrophy by facilitating whatever movements are possible (ideational apraxia).
- Use developmental sequence of postural reflexes to evoke movements (ideomotor apraxia).
- Have the person perform a movement using the noninvolved side first, then try to copy or imitate the movement on the involved side (kinetic apraxia).
- The use of parquetry block assembly in puzzles graded from simple to complex may be helpful for persons with constructional apraxia (remedial approach) (Neistadt 1994).
- Provide sensory input through the tactile and touch systems using deep pressure, neutral warmth, discrimination of objects in other media such as sand, a variety of textures on the skin, and alternating passive touch and active tactile activities.
- Provide sensory input through the kinesthetic and proprioceptive systems using movement of body parts and resistance to movement.
- Provide proprioceptive, tactile, and kinesthetic input before and during the task, such as taking the person's leg through the required motion to propel a wheelchair before requesting the person try the motion (remedial approach to ideomotor apraxia).
- Provide sensory input through the vestibular system using rocking, swinging, turning, jumping, forward and backward acceleration, and deceleration.
- Provide sensory input through the visual system using familiar objects when possible (kinetic apraxia) to assist the haptic sense. Begin with models or actual objects and progress to drawings or schematic representations as improvement occurs (constructional apraxia).
- Provide sensory input through the auditory system using familiar sounds or music when possible.
- Provide sensory input through the gustatory and olfactory senses.
- Combine sensory input, such as tactile and vision, when possible.
- The use of sensorimotor techniques—including tapping, icing, brushing, rubbing, kneading, and vibration—may be helpful with ideomotor apraxia (see "Treatment" section on inhibitory and facilitation techniques).

Cognitive
- Instructions should be clear and concise, and should reflect the desired results.

- Use appropriate methods of providing instruction. For example, for total body apraxia, the command "Get up" is more inclusive of the desired result than breaking the process into steps of scooting toward the edge of the chair, pushing down, and leaning forward.
- Instructions using different and multisensory cues (contextual, auditory, visual, and tactile) provide multiple sources of information.
- Provide therapeutic guiding and modeling by showing the desired movement rather than using verbal or pictorial instruction (Affolter approach). For example, place your hand over the hand of the person and guide the person to comb the hair or brush the teeth.
- Use visualization techniques or imagining with eyes closed before actual task performance.
- Teach compensatory strategies, such as goal-oriented verbal strategies, which involve breaking down tasks into their component parts, then performing each part in sequence while talking oneself through the process.
- Keep verbal commands to a minimum and encourage subcortical performance. Instead of telling the person to "Lock your brakes," say "There's something on your brakes" (adaptive approach) (Zoltan 1996).
- Help the person develop effective personal strategies.
- For constructional apraxia, use backward chaining techniques; for example, start by having the person do only the last step, such as tightening the bow, then have the person pull the loop through and tighten the bow. Keep adding steps in reverse order until the person is performing all the steps.

Psychosocial

- Provide support for the person when he or she becomes frustrated. Let the person know you recognize that he or she is not being uncooperative and that the task is difficult to perform.
- Provide opportunities for success.

Environment

- Instruct the family and caregivers in techniques that are found to be effective for the person.
- Inform the family and caregivers about possible safety issues.

PRECAUTIONS

Performance varies with the type and method of test administration. Drawings or photographs produce different results than three-dimensional models, and the time permitted for performance is important for older persons.

PROGNOSIS AND OUTCOME

The prognosis and outcome vary depending on the type of apraxia and the causative factors. In degenerative disorders, the prognosis is poor, but in other disorders, such as head injury, the prognosis may be good. Therefore, the outcomes listed below are examples of possible outcomes rather than typically expected outcomes. Outcome statements should be selected on the basis of expectation for the individual.

- The person is able to plan, organize, and execute a motor act requiring motor planning with which the person is unfamiliar.

- The person is able to perform a motor act requiring motor planning in a smooth (not jerky) and coordinated (using two sides of the body together) manner.
- The person's resting muscle tone is within normal limits with no evidence of hyper- or hypotonicity.
- The person's muscle tone is balanced between flexion and extension, not biased toward flexion or extension.
- The person can perform motor acts requiring motor planning through the range of motion, not within a narrow arc of motion.
- The person is able to perform motor acts requiring motor planning and bilateral or reciprocal coordination.
- The person can perform motor acts requiring motor planning and execution through the use of postural control and balance reactions in a variety of body positions.
- The person is able to perform motor acts requiring motor planning and execution of constructional or assembly tasks.
- The person can perform motor acts requiring motor planning and execution of a prescribed series of sequential or ordered tasks.
- The person is able to perform motor acts requiring motor planning and execution of rapidly alternating movement of body parts, such as the hand, wrist, tongue, or mouth.

REFERENCES

Beers, M.H., and R. Berkow, eds. 1999. *The Merck Manual of Diagnosis and Therapy,* 17th ed. Whitehouse Station, NJ: Merck Research Laboratories.
Butler, J.A. 1999. Evaluation and intervention with apraxia. In *Cognitive and perceptual dysfunction: A clinical reasoning approach to evaluation and intervention,* ed. C. Unsworth, 257–298. Philadelphia: F.A. Davis.
Golisz, K.M., and J.P. Toglia. 1998. Evaluation of perception and cognition. In *Willard and Spackman's occupational therapy,* 9th ed., eds. M.E. Neistadt and E.B. Crepeau, 260–281. Philadelphia: Lippincott-Raven.
Grieve J.I. 1993. The apraxias. In *Neuropsychology for occupational therapists: Assessment of perception and cognition,* ed. J.I. Grieve, 114–122. Oxford: Blackwell Scientific Publications.
Landry, J., and S. Spaulding. 1999. Assessment and intervention with clients with apraxia: Contributions from the literature. *Canadian Journal of Occupational Therapy* 66, no. 1:52–61.
Neistadt, M.E. 1994. Using research literature to develop a perceptual retraining treatment protocol. *American Journal of Occupational Therapy* 48, no. 1:62–72.
Poole, J.L., et al. 1997. The mechanisms for adult onset-apraxia and developmental dyspraxia: An examination and comparison of error patterns. *American Journal of Occupational Therapy* 51, no. 5:339–346.
Quintana, L.A. 1995. Evaluation of perception and cognition—apraxia and constructional apraxia. In *Occupational therapy for physical dysfunctions,* 4th ed., ed. C. Trombly, 211–216. Baltimore, MD: Williams & Wilkins.
York, C.D., and S.A. Cermak. 1995. Visual perception and praxis in adults after stroke. *American Journal of Occupational Therapy* 49, no. 6:543–550.
Zoltan, B. 1996. Apraxia. In *Vision, perception and cognition: A manual for the evaluation and treatment of the neurologically impaired adult,* ed. B. Zoltan, 53–70. Thorofare, NJ: Slack.

BIBLIOGRAPHY

Kohlmeyer, K. 1998. Motor planning. In *Willard and Spackman's occupational therapy*, 9th ed., eds. M.E. Neistadt and E.B. Crepeau, 272–275. Philadelphia: Lippincott-Raven.

Longs-Christopher, B. 1993. Life's a maze: Treating patients with apraxia. *Occupational Therapy Forum* 8, no. 8:4–5, 8–9.

Pedretti, L.W., B. Zoltan, and C.J. Wheatley. 1996. Praxis. In *Occupational therapy: Practice skills for physical dysfunction*, 4th ed., ed. L.W. Pedretti, 235–238. St Louis: Mosby.

Toglia, J.P. 1998. Motor planning: Specific skills training: Limb apraxia. In *Willard and Spackman's occupational therapy*, 9th ed., eds. M.E. Neistadt and E.B. Crepau, 445–446. Philadelphia: Lippincott-Raven.

Van Heugten C.M., et al. 1998. Outcome of strategy training in stroke patients with apraxia: A phase II study. *Clinical Rehabilitation* 12, no. 4:294–303.

Cognition Disorders—Attention, Orientation, and Concentration

DESCRIPTION

Cognition disorders or cognitive dysfunction are difficulties in information processing due to brain damage, which alters a person's experiences and responses to stimuli and interferes with the performance of everyday living tasks. Cognition disorders include problems in attention, orientation, and concentration; problems in short-term and long-term memory, storage and retrieval, and learning approaches; and executive functions such as problem solving, decision making, planning, organizing, reasoning, concept formation, goal formation and selection, and error detection. The deficits may be global, specific, or both, and they affect the brain, especially the cerebral hemispheres, although lower-level structures are involved in some skills. Treatment to remediate problems in cognition had been studied sporadically for many years in persons with strokes, but renewed interest began in 1966 when Ben-Yishay was asked by the Israeli government to develop a program for soldiers with head injuries suffered during the 1967 war (see sections on Memory Disorders and Dementia).

Cognitive disorders are most commonly seen in brain injury and cerebral vascular accidents. They are also seen in neurodegenerative disorders such as multiple sclerosis and Alzheimer's disease. Mental health disorders often have cognitive disorders as well, especially schizophrenia.

Disorders of attention may include insufficient alertness, inability to selectively attend to relevant information and inhibit irrelevant information, inability to sustain attention over a period of time, and response perseveration due to the inability to shift attention (Duchek and Abreu 1997, 291). Deficits in attention and memory present an obstacle to learning and impede the person's ability to interact effectively with the environment (Toglia 1993). Because these deficits are silent and not directly observable, they are easily overlooked.

- Alternating concentration—capacity to move flexibly between tasks and respond appropriately to the demands of each task (Unsworth 1999, 129).

- Alertness—the ability to respond to environmental stimuli beyond the level of reflex reactions (Mosey 1993, 25). Alertness refers to both the physical and mental level of arousal that is necessary to respond (Duchek and Abreu 1997, 290).
- Allocation of attention—the division or recruitment of attention to certain tasks. (See attentional capacity.)
- Arousal—involves the capacity to maintain a state of wakefulness (Unsworth 1999, 127).
- Attention—the ability to focus on an activity involving internal stimuli (thoughts) and external stimuli, such as information, tasks, and events. It includes elements such as concentration, selective attention, and attentional flexibility (Mosey 1993, 26).
- Attentional capacity—refers to the cognitive resources available for allocation for any given cognitive task (Duchek and Abreu 1997, 290).
- Attentional flexibility—involves the ability to shift one's focus from one set of stimuli to another (Mosey 1993, 26). Also called alternating attention, switching attention, mental flexibility, and disengagement.
- Automatic processing—involves activating a learned, organized sequence of behavior (Toglia 1993, 15).
- Concentration—the process of sustaining attention to and persisting in an activity (also referred to as attention span) (Mosey 1993, 26).
- Controlled processing—use of conscious effect and attentional capacity to perform a task. Usually the capacity for controlled processing is limited, slow, and serial in nature (Toglia 1993, 16). Also called supervisory attentional system.
- Divided concentration or attention—capacity to respond simultaneously to two or more tasks (Unsworth 1999, 129).
- Divided concentration deficit, also called divided attention deficit—difficulty responding simultaneously to two or more tasks (based on Unsworth 1999, 129).
- Focused attention—the capacity to concentrate on relevant information while engaged in occupations or maintain a consistent response during a continuous activity (Unsworth 1999, 128).
- Focused attention deficit (FAD)—difficulty concentrating on relevant information (based on Unsworth 1999, 128).
- Mental tracking—refers to the ability to attend to several pieces of information simultaneously (Toglia 1993, 12). Also called divided attention.
- Orientation—the ability to locate oneself in one's environment with reference to knowing time, place, and person (Mosey 1993, 25).
- Habituation—the ability to inhibit or ignore stimuli that are no longer relevant (Toglia 1993, 10).
- Phasic arousal—refers to a specific level of alertness resulting from some kind of warning signal and depends on the functioning of appropriate brain structures such as the ascending reticular formation (Duchek and Abreu 1997, 290). Also called orienting reflex.
- Selective attention—the process of identifying and focusing on relevant stimuli to the exclusion of other, competing stimuli (Mosey 1993, 26).
- Sustained concentration—see focused attention.
- Tonic arousal—refers to a general level of wakefulness or generalized readiness of the nervous system to respond, which depends on physiological indices (Duchek and Abreu 1997, 290; Toglia 1993, 10).
- Vigilance—ability to sustain attention over extended periods of time (Haase 1997, 336).

CAUSE

Cognition disorders may be due to developmental delay, an affective disorder, or organic impairment. These problems are frequently seen in adults with mental retardation, schizophrenia, bipolar disorders, head injuries, and cerebrovascular disorders. Divided attention deficit (DAD) is believed to result from speed limitations when trying to consciously process material (Unsworth 1999, 131). Focused attention deficit (FAD) is assumed to occur when automatic processing tendencies conflict with responses demanded in a task (Unsworth 1999, 131). Some problems in cognition in normal aging may be due to a deficit in inhibitory control (Duchek and Abreu 1997, 291).

ASSESSMENT

Areas

- daily living skills—activities of daily living and instrumental ADLs
- productive skills, values, history, and interests
- leisure skills and interests
- alertness—environmental responsiveness
- arousal—state of consciousness
- awareness or level of consciousness
- orientation—temporal, personal, environmental, situational, and left-right
- attention or concentration—span or length of attention, and distractibility
- speed of information processing
- goal formation (cognitive set) and persistence toward goal
- sensory acuity and discrimination—tactile, visual, and auditory
- memory functions—immediate, delayed, and remote
- learning and fund of information
- problem solving
- decision making
- cause and effect
- organization of tasks and sequencing
- judgment of safety
- insight—especially awareness of disability
- abstraction
- concept formation and categorization
- motivation or goal-directed behavior
- frustration tolerance and coping behavior
- behavioral control

Instruments

Instruments Developed by Occupational Therapy Personnel

- *Assessment of Motor and Process Skills* (AMPS), 2nd ed., by A. Fisher, Ft. Collins, CO: Three Star Press, 1997.
- *Awareness Screen* by B. Abreu, in *Occupational therapy: Enabling function and well-being,* 2nd ed., eds. C. Christiansen and C. Baum, 301, Thorofare, NJ: Slack, 1996.

- *Canadian Occupational Performance Measure* (COPM), 2nd ed., by M. Law et al., Ottawa, Ontario, Canada: Canadian Association of Occupational Therapists, 1994.
- *Chessington Occupational Therapy Neurological Assessment Battery* (COTNAB) by R. Tyerman et al., Nottingham, England: Nottingham Rehab., 1986.
- *Dynamic Interactional Assessment* by J. Toglia, in Approaches to cognitive assessment of the brain-injured adult: Traditional methods and dynamic investigation, *Occupational Therapy Practice* 1, no. 1 (1989): 36–57.
- *Loewenstein Occupational Therapy Cognitive Assessment* (LOTCA) by M. Itzkovich et al., Pequanock, NJ: Maddak, 1990.
- *Test of Orientation for Rehabilitation Patients* (TORP) by J. Deitz et al., San Antonio, TX: Psychological Corporation/Therapy Skill Builders, 1993.

Instruments Developed by Other Professionals and Used by Occupational Therapy Personnel
- *Army Individual Test Battery—Trail-making Test* by the United States Army, Washington, D.C.: Adjutant General's Office, 1944.
- *Knox's Cube Test* by M.H. Stone and B.D. Wright, Wood Dale, IL: Stoelting Company, 1980.
- *Mental Status Examination—Random Letter Test* by R.L. Strub and F.W. Black, in *The mental status examination in neurology*, 2nd ed., Philadelphia: F.A. Davis, 1985.
- *Paced Auditory Serial Attention Test* (PASAT) by D. Gronwall, *Perceptual and Motor Skills* 44 (1977): 367–373.
- *Stroop Test* by J.R. Stroop, in Studies of inference in serial verbal reactions, *Journal of Experimental Psychology* 18 (1935): 643–662.
- *Symbol Digit Modalities Test* by A. Smith, Los Angeles: Western Psychological Services, 1982.
- *Test of Everyday Attention* (TEA) by I. Robertson et al., Bury St. Edmunds: Thames Valley Test Company, 1994. (Available in the United States from Northern Speech Services, 117 Elm Street, P.O. Box 1247, Gaylord, MI 49735.)
- *Visual Search Attention Test* by M.R. Trenerry et al., Odessa, FL: Psychological Assessment Resources, 1990.

PROBLEMS

Self-Care
- The person may have difficulty performing self-care routines without prompting.
- The person may have mental lethargy: closes eyes frequently and has difficulty staying awake.

Productivity
The person may have difficulty performing complex routines, such as driving, shopping, preparing meals, and serving.

Leisure
- The person may have difficulty performing the complex coordination skills required in some sports.

Cognitive-Perceptual Disorders

- The person may have difficulty with the attention and concentration required in many table games.

Sensorimotor
- The person may have difficulty with the execution or imitation of simple motor acts on command. Responses are slow or sluggish.
- The person may have difficulty combining or integrating sensory or perceptual information with motor skills; for example, seeing a red light and stopping on the curb or seeing an elevator door open and moving into the elevator.
- The person may have difficulty with motor impersistence.
- The person's performance may show inconsistencies or dramatic fluctuations in task performance.
- The person may be unable to perform more than one action at a time; for example, holding a bag of groceries while unlocking the door with a key, or stirring and pouring at the same time.
- The person may have specific deficits in the registration of sensory input, especially in the auditory, visual, proprioceptive, or tactile modalities; for example, diminished responsiveness to external stimuli or hypersensitivity.
- The person may have difficulty discriminating essential from nonessential (foreground-background) information.
- The person may have difficulty integrating cross-modal information, such as tactile-kinesthetic, tactile-visual, or auditory-visual input.
- The person may make more errors as the task or situation changes.

Cognitive
- The person has difficulty with orientation to the task.
  1. The person may not orient eyes, head, or body toward a new stimulus in the environment.
  2. The person may be easily distracted by stimuli unrelated to the task.
  3. The person may be easily distracted by stimuli inherent in the task, such as the sound of an electric appliance.
  4. The person may have difficulty tuning out competing background environmental stimuli such as a radio, the sound of an air conditioner, or a conversation in the next room.
  5. The person may become distracted by irrelevant thoughts or ideas.
  6. The person may overfocus (fixate, perserverate) on irrelevant details such as the design on the side of a bowl.
  7. The person may become stuck on one aspect of the task or situation and be unable to move to the next step.
  8. The person may be slow to orient him- or herself to a new set or task.
  9. The person may become hyperaroused and unable to inhibit orienting reflex.
- The person may have difficulty maintaining attention and concentration (or freedom from distraction) in performing
  1. psychomotor tasks
  2. organizing, assembling, and sequencing routines
  3. reasoning and learning activities
  4. following directions or other structured interaction

5. unstructured situations
6. modulation of response to stimuli (disinhibition, hyperresponsiveness)
*   The person may have difficulty with attention and memory; for example, problems with
    1. time span (immediate, short-term, and remote). Examples are shortened attention span, decrement of performance observed over time, or slowness in performing serial tasks that require moving from one step to the next sequentially.
    2. retention of content (simple instructions, basic routines of daily life, simple assignments or chores or commitments, and resolutions and promises to significant others)
    3. learning, assimilating, and retaining new information at mastered criterion level
*   The person may have difficulty with the use of language; for example,
    1. poor quality of speech production, such as dysarthria and verbal or oral apraxia
    2. difficulty with use of speech, such as word substitution, anomia, or grammatical errors
    3. difficulty with written communication
*   The person's ability to initiate and achieve goal-directed behavior is decreased.
*   The person may make impulsive responses.

Psychosocial
*   The person may lack initiative or be unable to induce even simple acts, routines, or communications without the help of others.
*   The person may lack the ability to maintain or sustain an act or routine independently without prodding or reminding by others.
*   The person may manifest behavioral lag, delay of response, or slowed-down rhythm.
*   The person may manifest reduced rate of behavioral performance and/or increased passivity.
*   The person may exhibit flat affect, lack of emotion.
*   The person may become increasingly irritable or agitated as the number or complexity of stimuli increase.
*   The person may show irritability with any change in the usual or expected environment, situation, or routine.
*   The person may lack ability to vary behavioral responses because of rigidity of thinking.
*   The person may show poor coping skills when unexpected or unfamiliar situations occur. The person functions in a low-level, stimulus-bound, stereotypical behavior manner.

TREATMENT/INTERVENTION

Models of treatment for cognitive disorders are grouped into four major areas: (1) general stimulation, (2) substitution and transfer techniques, (3) behavioral approach, and (4) systemic approach. Models in occupational therapy include cognitive disabilities (Allen 1992), quadraphonic approach (Abreu 1999), retraining approach, model of human occupation, neurofunctional approach, remedial, dynamic interactional model (Toglia 1993), rehabilitative/compensatory model, and group-work model.

Self-Care
Self-care activities can be used at level 1 because they are performed at an automatic level (see section on Coma and Stupor—Glasgow Coma Scale).

Productivity

Productive activities can be used at level 2 to provide structured activities, such as sorting, matching, and counting; and at level 3 to provide integrated activities, such as planning and organizing work activities, or solving a problem in the work environment (see section on Coma and Stupor—Rancho Los Amigos Cognitive Functioning Scale).

Leisure

Leisure activities can be used at all three levels. Simple, noncompetitive games can be used at level 1. Games with rules and simple crafts can be used at level 2. Games requiring strategy, craft projects requiring planning, and community outings requiring organization can be used at level 3.

Sensorimotor

See sections on apraxia, head injuries, sensory disorders, and sensory integration.

Cognitive

- Cueing methods approach—addresses all dimensions of attention simultaneously
  - vary the task: number of stimuli, number of steps, familiarity of the task
  - vary the environment: familiar, unfamiliar
- Hierarchical approach—present tasks at lower level and progress to higher level
  - alertness (lowest level)
  - sustained attention
  - selective attention
  - attentional flexibility
  - mental tracking (highest level)
- Task category approach (Toglia 1993)
  - attentional flexibility tasks: involves dealing with repeated changes in task or stimuli
    1. follow one change such as copying a sequence of letters: *bbbbbddddd*
    2. alternate between two different sequences or responses such as copying an alternating sequence of letters: *bdbdbdbdbdbd*
    3. generate alternate response or ideas such as figuring out how many combinations of coins would equal 85 cents
  - detect/react tasks: emphasizes ability to detect changes quickly with the environment or task
    1. detect one gross change in environment, such as the telephone ringing
    2. detect changes, such as changes from one commercial to another on television
    3. detect according to rules; for example, pricking the red balloons but not the blue ones
    4. detect with increasing amounts of stimuli with speed; for example, canceling the letter *C* quickly on a page of letters
  - section tasks: involves choosing relevant stimuli while ignoring other stimuli
    1. find one target out of X number (2, 5, 8, 17) of distractors; for example, locating the word *home* in a paragraph
    2. select multiple targets from numerous stimuli (number is unspecified); for example, identifying all the "tails up" nickels from a group of mixed denomination coins

3. select essential information from irrelevant stimuli; for example, selecting the main idea from a paragraph
4. inhibit competing stimuli; for example, attending only to the color blue no matter what color the word says
— mental tracking: emphasizes ability to internally hold onto several pieces of information at once
    1. keep track of rules, facts, stimuli during the course of a task such as repeating a telephone number
    2. keep track of two or more stimuli simultaneously; for example, talking on the telephone while writing a message
— sustaining tasks: emphasizes ability to maintain attention to same task, location, or stimuli over time
    1. repetitive task where the response remains the same, such as putting away dishes
    2. increased selection with repetitive task; for example, putting dishes of one design on the shelves but leaving dishes of another design on the counter
    3. sustain attention and keep track in a task with changing stimuli; for example, #2 task, but keep track of the number of dishes put on the shelf
- General teaching methods approach
    — anchoring: provide the person with a cue as to where to begin a task, such as a red line or star
    — compensatory: teach an alternate response (usually already available in the behavior repertoire) to a given cognitive demand
    — control of stimulus complexity: control the environmental situation to limit or increase the number or amount of stimulus input
    — elaboration: provide visual images or verbal mediation to help the person pursue a task
    — error prevention: start by giving the person a task that is virtually error proof; then slowly add complexity and opportunity for error
    — frequent feedback: use tangible feedback scores, percentages, time, and checklists that show the person his or her level of accuracy and improvement
    — gradual increase in task complexity: start with simple tasks that are subsequently graded with additional requirements of frequency, duration, and difficulty
    — limit sensory stimulation: avoid distractors such as radio, TV, CD or tape player, or clutter, and modalities that require processing and attention to two or more senses
    — repetitive practice: use concrete, familiar, easy-to-learn tasks, activities, and materials that are related to the person's living environment and that can be repeated easily; then use the same or similar materials in different situations
    — response pacing: have the person talk aloud or talk through the steps or sequence of a response
    — saturation cueing: give the person increasingly more information on successive trials to the point that success is virtually assured, then incrementally remove the cues (fading out) so the person learns to perform a task with less and less cueing
    — self-evaluation: have the individual review his or her own performance
    — strategies for information processing: teach organized or methodical approaches using cues, written suggestions, or other compensatory techniques
    — substitution: teach a new set of responses to a given cognitive demand

- — visual cues: use visual as opposed to auditory instructions, such as written directions, cue sheets, and samples of end products
- Teaching modalities
  - — activities of daily living: practice performing daily living tasks that are repetitive and can be repeated easily, such as brushing teeth, getting dressed, and eating
  - — computer programs: practice specific skills (educational programs) or planning strategies (games)
  - — games and crafts: practice planning strategies
  - — group activities: practice decision making, problem solving, and awareness of others
  - — gross and fine motor activities: practice responding to environmental or interpersonal demands
  - — instrumental activities of daily living: practice tasks frequently done around the house or community, such as laundry, meal preparation, cleaning, shopping, writing checks, answering the telephone
  - — survival skills: reading and obeying street signs, making change, writing checks, reading bus or train schedules
- Levels or phases of treatment
  1. Stimulation—activities that require detecting and responding appropriately to the environment (sensory registration and motor response); responses should be at the automatic level (lower brain function) with little or no processing required.
  2. Structure—activities that require discrimination, simple analysis, and manipulation of information from the environment; responses require moderate processing capacity.
  3. Integration—activities that require planning, organization, and problem solving in thoughts, emotions, and ideas; responses require maximum effort, concentration, and analysis.

Psychosocial

See sections on head injuries and schizophrenia.

PRECAUTIONS

- Studies using computer-assisted cognitive retraining have not been shown to be superior to standard cognitive rehabilitation approaches.
- Persons who are confused or disoriented should be supervised at all times. Do not leave them unattended.
- If an activity is not working, do not pursue the activity; change focus.
- Avoid continuous stimulation, such as playing the radio or TV continuously, to reduce habituation.

PROGNOSIS AND OUTCOME

- The person will be able to generalize learning to improve performance of everyday tasks.
- The person can demonstrate or articulate cognitive strategies (organized sets of rules) used to process information and organize a plan to approach the problem or situation.

REFERENCES

Abreu, B.C. 1999. Evaluation and intervention with memory and learning impairments. In *Cognitive and perceptual dysfunction: A clinical reasoning approach to evaluation and intervention,* ed. C. Unsworth, 163–207. Philadelphia: F.A. Davis.

Allen, C.K. 1992. Cognitive disabilities. In *Cognitive rehabilitation: Models for intervention in occupational therapy,* ed. N. Katz, 1–21. Boston, MA: Andover Medical Publishers.

Ducheck, J.M., and B.C. Abreu. 1997. Meeting the challenges of cognitive disabilities. In *Occupational therapy: Enabling function and well-being,* eds. C. Christiansen and C. Baum, 288–311. Thorofare, NJ: Slack, Inc.

Haase, B. 1997. Cognition. In *Assessments in occupational therapy and physical therapy,* eds. J. Van Deusen and D. Brunt, 333–356. Philadelphia: W.B. Saunders.

Mosey, A.C. 1993. Working taxonomies. In *AOTA self-study series: Cognitive rehabilitation,* ed. C.B. Royeen, 23–35. Bethesda, MD: American Occupational Therapy Association.

Toglia, J. 1993. Attention and memory. In *AOTA self-study series: Cognitive rehabilitation,* ed. C.B. Royeen, no. 4. Bethesda, MD: American Occupational Therapy Association.

Unsworth, C. 1999. Evaluation and intervention with concentration impairment. In *Cognitive and perceptual dysfunction: A clinical reasoning approach to evaluation and intervention,* ed. C. Unsworth, 125–161. Philadelphia: F.A. Davis.

BIBLIOGRAPHY

Allen, C.K. 1993. Creating a need-satisfying, safe environment: Management and maintenance approaches. In *AOTA self-study series: Cognitive rehabilitation,* ed. C.B. Royeen, no. 11. Bethesda, MD: American Occupational Therapy Association.

Allen, C.K., J. Goldberg, and J. Tryssenaar. 1995. Treating attentional impairment. *Canadian Journal of Occupational Therapy* 62, no. 1:49–51.

Allen, C.K., and T. Blue. 1998. Cognitive disabilities model: How to make clinical judgments. In *Cognition and occupation in rehabilitation: Cognitive models for intervention in occupational therapy,* ed. N. Katz, 225–280. Bethesda, MD: American Occupational Therapy Association.

Allen, C.K., S.C. Robertson, and C.A. Earhart. 1993. *A Study Guide for Occupational Therapy Treatment Goals for the Physically and Cognitively Disabled.* Rockville, MD: American Occupational Therapy Association.

Brown, C., et al. 1993. Effectiveness of cognitive rehabilitation for improving attention in patients with schizophrenia. *Occupational Therapy Journal of Research* 13, no. 2:71–86.

Golisz, K.M., and J.P. Toglia. 1998. Evaluation of perception and cognition. In *Willard and Spackman's occupational therapy,* 9th ed., eds. M.E. Neistadt and E.B. Crepeau, 260–281. Philadelphia: Lippincott-Raven.

Hobson, S.J.G. 1999. Using a client-centered approach with persons with cognitive impairment. In *Client-centred practice in occupational therapy: A guide to implementation,* ed. T. Sumsion, 51–60. Edinburgh, Scotland: Churchill Livingstone.

Katz, N. 1994. Cognitive rehabilitation: Models for intervention and research on cognition in occupational therapy. *Occupational Therapy International* 1, no. 1:49–63.

Larson, A., et al. 1995. Computer-assisted cognitive rehabilitation for adults with traumatic brain damage: Four case studies. *Occupational Therapy International* 2, no. 3:166–189.

Levy, L.L. 1992. The use of the cognitive disability frame of reference in rehabilitation of cognitively disabled older adults. In *Cognitive rehabilitation: Models for intervention in occupational therapy,* ed. N. Katz, 22–50. Boston: Andover Medical Publishers.

Levy, L.L. 1998. The cognitive disabilities model in rehabilitation of older adults with dementia. In *Cognition and occupation in rehabilitation: Cognitive models for intervention in occupational therapy,* ed. N. Katz, 195–222. Bethesda, MD: American Occupational Therapy Association.

Mann, W.C., et al. 1996. Use of assistive devices for bathing by elderly who are not institutionalized. *Occupational Therapy Journal of Research* 16, no. 4:261–286.

Neistadt, M.E., et al. 1993. An analysis of a board game as a treatment activity. *American Journal of Occupational Therapy* 47, no. 2:154–160.

Quintana, L.A. 1995. Evaluation of perception and cognition. In *Occupational therapy for physical dysfunctions*, 4th ed., ed. C. Trombly, 201–223. Baltimore, MD: Williams & Wilkins.

Quintana, L.A. 1995. Remediating cognitive impairments. In *Occupational therapy for physical dysfunctions*, 4th ed., ed. C. Trombly, 539–548. Baltimore, MD: Williams & Wilkins.

Shimelman, A., and J. Hinojosa. 1995. Gross motor activity and attention in three adults with brain injury. *American Journal of Occupational Therapy* 49, no. 10:973–979.

Stahl, C. 1995. Cognitive rehab: The silent side of work hardening. *Advance for Occupational Therapists* 11, no. 11:15, 54.

Sorensen, L.V. 1995. The O.T. treatment of patients with cognitive disorders in Denmark. *World Federation of Occupational Therapists Bulletin* 32:33–35.

Stone, E.L. 1998. Use of the cognitive disability frame of reference in a short-stay private psychiatric hospital. In *Cognitive rehabilitation: Models for intervention in occupational therapy*, ed. N. Katz, 51–76. Boston: Andover Medical Publishers.

Unsworth, C. 1999. Introduction to cognitive and perceptual dysfunction: Theoretical approaches to therapy. In *Cognitive and perceptual dysfunction: A clinical reasoning approach to evaluation and intervention*, ed. C. Unsworth, 1–41. Philadelphia: F.A. Davis.

Wheatley, C.J. 1994. Cognitive rehabilitation service provision: Results of a survey of practitioners. *American Journal of Occupational Therapy* 48, no. 2:163–166.

Wheatley, C.J. 1996. Evaluation and treatment of cognitive dysfunction. In *Occupational therapy: Practice skills for physical dysfunction*, 4th ed., ed. L.W. Pedretti, 241–252. St. Louis: Mosby.

Wheatley, C.J. 1998. Treatment of cognitive dysfunction. In *Physical dysfunction: Practice skills for the occupational therapy assistant*, ed. M.B. Early, 395–397. St. Louis: Mosby.

Zoltan, B. 1996. Orientation, attention, and memory. In *Vision, perception, and cognition: A manual for the evaluation and treatment of the neurologically impaired adult*, 3rd ed., ed. B. Zoltan, 121–147. Thorofare, NJ: Slack Inc.

Cognition Disorders— Memory and Learning Disorders

DESCRIPTION

Memory disorders are defined as partial or total inability to encode (process), store, or retrieve (recall) information. Encoding determines which stimuli are noticed or attended to and which ones are selected for storage. Storage concerns the saving of information. Retrieval concerns the recall of information from a memory store.

Problems with memory may include loss of strategic search skills of remote episodic memory, deficits in working memory and the speed of information processing, dissociation in performance on explicit and implicit memory tasks, difficulty performing routine tasks, forgetting to perform daily activities, deficits in retaining the contents of working memory, loss of long-term memory, lack of insight into the nature of one's disability, and so on.

Although dementia involves a memory dysfunction, the permanent loss of memory skills is not the focus of this section. (See Dementia—Alzheimer's Type and Dementia—Other.)
The following terminology is related to memory:

- anterograde amnesia—loss of or decreased memory of events after a traumatic situation
- cued recall—ability to recall information when provided with cues
- declarative memory—knowledge of factual information
- emotional memory—memory of all types of affect
- episodic memory—memory of one's personal history
- explicit memory—memory that involves the deliberate and conscious retrieval of information such as would be required on a recall or recognition test
- free recall—ability to recall information when no specific retrieval cues are provided.
- immediate memory—memory held consciously for less than one minute
- implicit memory—a facilitation in performance as a result of previous experience with the task, even though there may be no conscious recollection of the task
- long-term memory—memory held for more than a few minutes
- metamemory—knowledge one has about one's own memory (Toglia 1993, 23)
- motor memory—memory of movements
- posttraumatic amnesia—decreased memory function (storing and retrieving information), confusion, and disorientation in the period following trauma
- procedural memory—knowledge of the necessary procedures to perform some activity
- prospective memory—remembering to carry out some action in the future
- recent memory—memory held for several hours or months (overlaps with the concept of long-term memory)
- recognition—ability to recognize previously presented information
- remote memory—memory held for many years, including back to childhood
- retrograde amnesia—loss of memory of events prior to a traumatic situation
- retrospective memory—remembering information or events that occurred in the past (overlaps with episodic memory)
- semantic memory—personal knowledge of the physical environment or world through linguistic concepts
- sensory memory—memory of sensory information (may be specific to a single sensory system, such as auditory, olfactory, or taste)
- short-term memory—memory held for more than a minute
- temporal memory—memory of the timing of events, their duration and sequence
- verbal memory—memory of words and sentences
- visuospatial memory—memory of objects, spatial relationships, and configurations
- working memory—includes the active representations and executive processes necessary to perform a task, routine, or occupation

CAUSE
The causes of memory disorders can be divided into four types:
1. supratentorial mass lesions, including epidural and subdural hematoma, cerebral infarct or hemorrhage, brain tumor or abscess

2. subtentorial lesions, including brainstem infarct, tumor, hemorrhage, trauma, cerebellar hemorrhage
3. diffuse and metabolic cerebral disorders, such as trauma, epilepsy, postepileptic states, infection, toxins, subarachnoid hemorrhage
4. psychiatric disorders, such as malingering, hysteria, catatonia

ASSESSMENT

Areas

*   daily living skills—activities of daily living and instrumental ADLs
*   productive skills, values, history, and interests
*   leisure skills and interests
*   awareness or level of consciousness
*   orientation—temporal, personal, environmental, situational, and left-right
*   attention or concentration—arousal, span or length of attention, and distractibility
*   sensory acuity and discrimination—tactile, visual, and auditory
*   memory functions—immediate, delayed, and remote
*   learning and fund of information
*   problem solving
*   decision making
*   cause and effect
*   organization of tasks and sequencing
*   judgment of safety
*   insight—especially awareness of disability
*   abstraction
*   concept formation and categorization
*   motivation or goal-directed behavior
*   frustration tolerance and coping behavior
*   behavioral control

Instruments

Instruments Developed by Occupational Therapy Personnel

*   *Assessment of Motor and Process Skills* (AMPS), 2nd ed., by A. Fisher, Ft. Collins, CO: Three Star Press, 1997.
*   *Cognitive Performance Test* by T. Burns, in *Occupational Therapy Treatment Goals for the Physically and Cognitively Disabled,* eds. C.K. Allen, C.A. Earhart, and T. Blue, 46–50, 69–80, Bethesda, MD: American Occupational Therapy Association, 1992.
*   *Contextual Memory Test* by J.P. Toglia, San Antonio, TX: Psychological Corporation/ Therapy Skill Builders, 1993.
*   *Functional Behavior Profile* by C.M. Baum et al., The *Gerontologist* 33, no. 3 (1993): 403–408.
*   *Kitchen Task Assessment* (KTA) by C.M. Baum and D.F. Edwards, *American Journal of Occupational Therapy* 47, no. 5 (1993): 431–436.

- *Rabideau Kitchen Assessment,* revised by M.E. Neistadt, *Occupational Therapy Journal of Research* 12, no. 4 (1992): 242–255.
- *Routine Task Inventory—2* by C.K. Allen, in *Occupational Therapy Treatment Goals for the Physically and Cognitively Disabled,* eds. C.K. Allen, C.A. Earhart, and T. Blue, Bethesda, MD: American Occupational Therapy Association (1992): 31–40, 54–68.

Instruments Developed by Other Professionals and Used by Occupational Therapy Personnel

- *Autobiographical Memory Interview* by M. Kopelman, B. Wilson, and A.D. Baddeley, Bury St. Edmunds, England: Thames Valley Test Co. (Available in the United States from Northern Speech Services, 117 Elm Street, P.O. Box 1247, Gaylord, MI 49735.)
- *Everyday Memory Questionnaire* by A. Sunderland and J. Harris, in Failures in everyday life following severe head injury, *Journal of Clinical Neuropsychology* 6 (1984): 127–142.
- *Hopkins Verbal Learning Test* by J. Brandt, *Clinical Neuropsychologist* 5 (1991): 125–143.
- *Recognition Memory Test* by E.K. Warrington, United Kingdom: NFER-Neklson, 1984.
- *Rivermead Behavioral Memory Test* (RBMT) by B. Wilson, J. Cockburn, and A.D. Baddeley, Bury St. Edmunds, England: Thames Valley Test Company. (Available in the United States from Northern Speech Services, 117 Elm Street, P.O. Box 1247, Gaylord, MI 49735.)
- *Serial Digit Learning Test* by A.L. Benton, Odessa, FL: Psychological Assessment Resources, 1994.
- *Subjective Memory Questionnaire* (SMQ) by J. Bennett-Levy and G. Powell, *British Journal of Social and Clinical Psychology* 19 (1980): 177–188.

PROBLEMS

Self-Care

If loss of remote memory is involved, the person may not remember how to perform basic activities of daily living.

Productivity

- The person may be able to perform some job tasks if remote memory is intact.
- The person may be unable to perform new job tasks because he or she is unable to learn them.

Leisure

- The person may be able to enjoy leisure activities learned many years ago.
- The person may be unable to enjoy new leisure activities because he or she is unable to learn how to do them.

Sensorimotor

- Motor problems—such as reduced range of motion, muscle weakness, and contractures—may exist, depending on the brain disorder.

- Sensory problems—such as loss of vision, hearing, touch, proprioception, taste, or smell—may exist, depending on the brain disorder.

Cognitive
- The person may have loss of immediate memory covering the past few seconds.
- The person may have loss of intermediate (short-term or primary) memory covering the period from a few seconds to a few days.
- The person may have loss of recent (long-term or secondary) memory covering a period from hours to months.
- The person may have loss of remote (very long) memory covering events back to early childhood.
- The person may have retrograde amnesia for the period of time immediately preceding concussion or traumatic head injury.
- The person may have anterograde or posttraumatic amnesia for the time period following concussion or severe head trauma.
- The person may confabulate to fill in memory gaps (Korsakoff's syndrome).
- The person may be unable to learn any new tasks but may be able to carry out complex tasks learned before the illness or injury.
- The person may have lost episodic memory or memory of personal history, such as what clothes he or she wore yesterday.
- The person may have lost semantic memory, which includes linguistic concepts such as colors, sizes, and shapes.
- The person may have lost verbal memory, which includes words and sentences.
- The person may have lost visuospatial memory and be unable to recognize faces, familiar objects, or surroundings.
- The person may have lost motor memory and be unable to remember how to do the movements of a once-familiar task, such as typing, putting on clothes, or setting a table.
- The person may have lost temporal memory and be unable to remember when events occur, how long an event usually lasts, or the sequence of tasks within an event, such as going to a football game.
- The person may have lost sensory memory and be unable to remember common sounds, such as a bell or whistle, and be unable to remember common smells, such as perfume.
- The person may have lost emotional memory and be unable to remember what affect is appropriate for joy, anger, or sadness.

Psychosocial
- The person may become angry or frustrated if he or she is aware of the decreased memory ability.
- The person may lose self-confidence because he or she is aware of memory failures.
- The person may become depressed.
- The person may not recognize family or friends.
- The person may be unable to carry on a conversation because he or she has forgotten many of the subjects used to initiate and maintain a conversation.

TREATMENT/INTERVENTION

Models of treatment are based on retraining the memory, if possible, by improving encoding, increasing attention, and aiding retrieval, or by adaptive techniques designed to compensate for the loss of memory functions.

Self-Care

Behavior modification techniques have been used successfully to help people relearn tasks with fixed sequences of steps, such as washing and dressing. The techniques include (1) social praise to positively reinforce desired behaviors; (2) time-out-on-the-spot (TOOTS), ignoring the client so that no reinforcement follows an undesired behavior; (3) verbal mediation to control behavior through self-instruction and self-regulation.

Productivity

- Job tasks with repetitive motor sequences, visual cues, or step-by-step instruction may help the person function in a job situation.
- A notebook, chalkboard, or computer schedule may provide reminders of tasks to be performed.

Leisure

Activities learned long ago (in remote memory) may be remembered better and thus be useful leisure activities and skills.

Sensorimotor

- Motor routines can assist memory; for example, always putting the checkbook in the same place on the desk or putting the egg slicer in the same drawer each time.
- Visual imagery may be useful. The person consolidates information by making a mental picture of the information to be remembered.
- Sensory contextual modifiers can be used:
  — Auditory: give verbal repetition or use verbal cues such as questions or probes
  — Visual: give visual cue with nonverbal feedback, use pictorial representations, provide written cues, or increase illumination, contrast, or brightness
- Postural readiness can be guided by cueing the person to position eyes, head/neck, limbs, hands, hips, or feet a certain way.

Cognitive

- Storage devices may be helpful as external memory aids, including lists, schedules, notebooks, calculators, diaries, and computers. Training in the use of memory aids is necessary; for example, reminding the person to look at the list.
- Computers can be used to provide practice in memory tasks.
- Games, such as remembering objects on a tray and Twenty Questions, may be used in groups.
- A person with left-hemisphere problems may find visual cues more useful, while a person with right-hemisphere problems may find linguistic cues more helpful.
- First letter mnemonics may be helpful to remember a list of items, for example, "mice" for milk, ice cream, cheese, and eggs.

- PQRST is a memory rehearsal system in which Preview stands for skimming the material for general content. Questions are then asked about the content. The person Reads to answer the questions. He or she then States, rehearses, or repeats the information read and finally Tests him- or herself by answering the questions.
- Semantic elaboration is a memory technique in which a person makes up a simple story about information to be remembered, such as "Tom needs a clean suit to go to the Pilgrims' Ball" for "Go pick up Tom's suit at Pilgrim Cleaners."
- Modify the amount of contextual information provided by (1) giving a cue to initiate; (2) giving one-step instructions; (3) reducing the number of steps in the task; (4) shortening the task.
- Modify the complexity by simplifying the information: (1) use concrete explanations; (2) provide a demonstration; (3) use familiar tasks; (4) use items/objects the person relates to; (5) increase the spacing between items or objects presented (nonscattered); (6) decrease spatial relation traits or position of objects (all in same position).
- Modify or change the pace or speed and consistency with which information in presented by (1) giving a slow presentation; (2) giving a fast presentation; (3) giving a predictable or stable presentation; (4) giving a random or unpredictable presentation.
- Modify or change the interval of time the person is given in which to respond to (1) 15 seconds; (2) 30 seconds; (3) 1 minute.
- Modify the information given to the person to perform safely: (1) explain safety measures; (2) explain preventive measures; (3) explain dangerous consequences; (4) explain emergency procedures; (5) repeat preventive measures.
- Modify cues provided to increase person's awareness of impairment, dysfunction, restriction, and/or personal or social disadvantage: (1) give general cues that a problem exists; (2) give specific cues when an error happens or a problem exists; (3) give gentle confrontation about the undetected problem; (4) give the answer or solution.
- Modify cues regarding error detection and correction: (1) cue for error detection; (2) cue for how to correct the error; (3) encourage the person to self-cue for error detection; (4) encourage the person to self-cue for error correction.
- Modify the type and structure of verbal corrective feedback given: (1) give knowledge of performance [KP] feedback, which includes corrective information about a component or part of a task, test, or movement; (2) give knowledge of results based on feedback [KF], which includes corrective information about the total or whole task, test, or movement goal; (3) give positive feedback such as approval, assurance, or reinforcement; (4) give negative feedback such as disapproval or negative reinforcement; (5) give private feedback in a confidential or private environment; (6) give public feedback in a group situation or community environment.
- Modify the information provided to help a person in organizational strategy toward a task or situation: (1) provide guidelines about where to start and end; (2) provide guidelines about where to look for information or objects; (3) provide guidelines about what to say; (4) provide rules and guidelines for behavior; (5) provide guidance for reorganizing information; (6) encourage the person to initiate a strategy.
- Modify the information provided to person during the activity phase in which the person's functioning breaks down and the therapist offers feedback that might occur (1) before or during the preparatory state; (2) at the initiation stage; (3) at the middle stage; (4) at the end; (5) after completion of the activity.

Psychosocial

- Increase self-confidence and decrease depression by providing opportunities for success.
- Family or friends may help the person by providing cues regarding the memory assistive devices; for example, asking if the person has checked the daily schedule board to determine the next task to be done.
- Modify the references made to the person's needs, values, interests, or preferences: (1) connect the current task with the person's interests or preferences; (2) connect the task with the person's hobbies; (3) refer to the person's needs or goals; (4) refer to the person's values; (5) use a personally relevant task; (6) use a task that is concrete to the person.
- Modify the therapy set by (1) explaining the goal or purpose of the task; (2) explaining the goal or purpose of the therapy; (3) explaining the role of the therapist
- Modify the social milieu or environment: (1) seat the person near a friend; (2) ask the person to help another; (3) ask a client-helper to work with the person; (4) ask a question to elicit an interaction.
- Modify the therapist's use of self: (1) give expressive touch; (2) use gentle humor; (3) move closer to the person; (4) actively listen to the person's concerns; (5) use encouraging words or gestures; (6) offer the power of choice.
- Modify the verbal tone of voice used with the person: (1) use a "therapy voice" or formal therapeutic language; (2) use a directive voice that implies interpersonal control and command; (3) use a sympathetic voice—calm, confident, yet gentle; (4) use a modulated voice—speak slower, louder, or use shorter sentences.
- Modify the therapist's expectation of the person's success or failure: (1) therapist anticipates task failure; (2) therapist anticipates task success; (3) no anticipation.

PRECAUTIONS

- Do not confuse decreased attention span or poor concentration with memory disorders. Attention span and concentration affect performance but not the actual memory.
- Persons with brain injuries have difficulty using internal strategies that require learning. External strategies may be more successful, especially during the early stages of recovery.

PROGNOSIS AND OUTCOME

The literature is mixed regarding improvement of memory in general or for specific types of memory.
- The person is able to perform self-care and daily living activities with or without memory aids.
- The person is able to perform productive activities with or without memory aids.
- The person is able to perform leisure activities with or without memory aids.

REFERENCE

Toglia, J. 1993. Attention and memory. In *AOTA self-study series: Cognitive rehabilitation,* ed. C.B. Royeen, no. 4. Bethesda, MD: American Occupational Therapy Association.

BIBLIOGRAPHY

Bourgeois, M.D. 1993. Using memory aids to stimulate conversation and reinforce accurate memories. *Gerontology Special Interest Section Newsletter* 16, no. 4:1–3.

Cunninghis, R.N. 1994. A new look at reality and memory techniques. *Occupational Therapy Forum* 9, no. 4:4–5, 10.

Donnelly, S. 1994. Behavioral modification in retraining showering and dressing skills for a person with severe memory loss. *Australian Occupational Therapy Journal* 41, no. 4:177–182.

Farber, S.D, and B.C. Abreu. 1993. Understanding the brain and learning theories related to cognitive function and rehabilitation. In *AOTA self-study series: Cognitive rehabilitation,* ed. C.B. Royeen, no. 2. Bethesda, MD: American Occupational Therapy Association.

Golisz, K.M., and J.P. Toglia. 1998. Evaluation of perception and cognition. In *Willard and Spackman's occupational therapy,* 9th ed., eds. M.E. Neistadt and E.B. Crepeau, 260–281. Philadelphia: Lippincott-Raven.

Grieve, J.I. 1993. Memory. In *Neuropsychology for occupational therapists: Assessment of perception and cognition,* ed. J.I. Grieve, 71–82. Oxford: Blackwell Scientific Publications.

Grieve, J.I. 1993. Memory problems. In *Neuropsychology for occupational therapists: Assessment of perception and cognition,* ed. J.I. Grieve, 132–142. Oxford: Blackwell Scientific Publications.

Haase, B. 1997. Cognition. In *Assessments in occupational therapy and physical therapy,* eds., J. Van Deusen and. D. Brunt, 333–356. Philadelphia: W.B. Saunders.

Kohlmeyer, K. 1998. Memory. In *Willard and Spackman's occupational therapy,* 9th ed., eds. M.E. Neistadt and E.B. Crepeau, 275–276. Philadelphia: Lippincott-Raven.

Krinsky, R. 1995. How to tell if forgetfulness is serious. *Advance for Occupational Therapists* 11, no. 6:24.

Marmer, L. 1996. Mental fitness also takes "exercise." *Advance for Occupational Therapists* 12, no. 39:19.

Painter, J. 1993. Cognitive impairment in the elderly. *Physical and Occupational Therapy in Geriatrics* 11, no. 3:27–42.

So, Y.P., J. Toglia, and M.V. Donohue. 1997. A study of memory functioning in chronic schizophrenic patients. *Occupational Therapy in Mental Health* 13, no. 2:1–23.

Wheatley, C.J. 1996. Evaluation and treatment of cognitive dysfunction. In *Occupational therapy: Practice skills for physical dysfunction,* 4th ed., ed. L.W. Pedretti, 241–252. St. Louis: Mosby.

Wheatley, C.J. 1998. Treatment of cognitive dysfunction. In *Physical dysfunction: Practice skills for the occupational therapy assistant,* ed. M.B. Early, 395–397. St. Louis: Mosby.

Zoltan, B. 1996. Orientation, attention, and memory. In *Vision, perception, and cognition: A manual for the evaluation and treatment of the neurologically impaired adult,* 3rd ed., ed. B. Zoltan, 133–147. Thorofare, NJ: Slack.

Cognitive Disabilities— Executive Functions

DESCRIPTION

Executive functions are a broad band of skills that allow a person to engage in independent, purposeful, and self-directed behavior (Golisz and Toglia 1998, 276). As a group of capacities and mental processes, they are considered higher level cortical capacities (Unsworth 1999). Executive functions provide the self-regulating and control functions that direct and organize behavior (Zoltan 1996, 149). Executive functions include the ability to organize and carry out specific occupations, including the ability to make decisions, organize, sequence, problem solve, generalize, and demonstrate judgment (Haase 1997, 339). Persons with poor executive function are often impulsive, display tangential conversations, have perseveration problems, and are socially inappropriate (Zoltan 1996, 149).

Cognitive disability may be regarded as maladaptation to environmental demands because of difficulties with acquisition, application, and transfer of knowledge (Birnboim 1995, 61).

Loss of executive function, especially metacognition, results in a decrease in the use of efficient processing strategies to select, discriminate, organize, and structure incoming information, as well as a reduced ability to access previous knowledge and to apply knowledge and skills flexibly to a variety of situations (Birnboim 1995, 61).

Terminology
- Abstract thinking—enables a person to see relationships among objects, events, or ideas; to discriminate relevant from irrelevant detail; and to recognize absurdities (Wheatley 1996, 248)
- Acquisition—the ability to learn (and remember) new tasks or routines in order to adapt to environmental demands (Birnboim 1995, 61)
- Anticipation awareness—the ability to anticipate that a problem is going to happen because of some deficit (Zoltan 1996, 152)
- Application—the ability to use what is learned spontaneously in the same context (Birnboim 1995, 61)
- Concept formation—the ability to define objects, compare and differentiate, establish logical relationships, and categorize (Zoltan 1996, 168)
- Convergent thinking—enables a person to arrive at a central idea (Wheatley 1996, 248)
- Cue—subjective or objective information or data provided or received by the client designed to assist the client in gathering information to a difficulty (reworded from Unsworth 1999, 476)
- Decision making—the process of making choices about preferred courses of action (Unsworth 1999, 476)
- Deductive reasoning—the ability to arrive at a conclusion (Wheatley 1996, 248)
- Divergent thinking—generating alternatives (Wheatley 1996, 248)
- Emergent awareness—the ability to recognize a problem when it is occurring (Zoltan 1996, 152)
- Generalization—taking information learned in one situation and applying it to another situation that is similar but different in some manner (Haase 1997, 339)
- High road transfer—requires planned cognitive effort and "mindful" abstraction of transferable principles, rules, labels, or concepts, resulting in a skilled performance (Birnboim 1995, 62)
- Incentive learning—understanding that the use of a particular strategy in everyday life will result in getting something in return (Zoltan 1996, 150)
- Inductive reasoning—enables a person to draw generalizations from specific experiences (Wheatley 1996, 248)

- Initiation of activity—ability to start a task or activity
- Insight—conscious and unconscious knowledge of one's behavior and recognition of one's symptoms (Haase 1997, 340)
- Intellectual awareness—the cognitive capacity of the client to understand to some degree that a particular function is diminished from premorbid levels (Zoltan 1996, 152)
- Judgment—the ability to anticipate consequences and use reason (Haase 1997, 339) or the capacity to make realistic decisions based on environmental information (Unsworth 1999, 479)
- Low road transfer—well-rehearsed knowledge that is applied automatically in somewhat novel contexts, resulting in a trained performance (Birnboim 1995, 62)
- Mental or cognitive flexibility—the ability to shift attentional sets from one subject or task to another
- Metacognition—knowledge about knowledge: knowing "how" we think and awareness of our limitations; includes the ability to evaluate the difficulty of a task, to plan, to choose the right strategies, to anticipate the results, and to monitor the process (Birnboim 1995, 61)
- Mindfulness—a motivational factor that determines the amount of effort and control that are invested in a cognitive operation and is essential in abstraction (Birnboim 1995, 62)
- Novice performer—one who learns new tasks and routines to acquire cognitive knowledge
- Organization—the ability to sequence and plan the steps of an occupation (Haase 1997, 339)
- Planning—the ability to efficiently organize the steps or elements of the behavior or task and to look ahead, anticipate consequences, weigh and make choices, conceive of alternatives, sustain attention, and sequence the task (Golisz and Toglia 1998)
- Problem solving—the ability to recognize an error, generate solutions, select the proper solution, implement a solution, and assess the effectiveness of a solution (Haase 1997, 339)
- Purposeful action—the translation of an intention or plan into the activity; the carrying out of plans, which requires the ability to initiate, switch, and stop sequences (flexibility as well as self-regulation) (Golisz and Toglia 1998)
- Self-awareness, decreased—inability to recognize deficits or problem circumstances caused by neurological injury (Zoltan 1996, 152)
- Self-regulation—includes initiation, shifting to and from different activities, and problem solving (Haase 1997, 340)
- Stimulus-bound behavior—the person impulsively begins a task before instructed or is unable to draw his or her attention away from a task when necessary (Wheatley 1996, 247)
- Skilled performer—has metacognitive knowledge, has practice in multicontext situations, and can do high road transfer of training (Birnhoim 1995, 61).
- Strategy learning—the acquisition and development of compensatory behaviors, memory techniques, and problem-solving methods (Zoltan 1996, 150)
- Trained performer—a person who has extensively practiced routines and has the ability to do low road transfer (Birnboim 1995, 61)
- Transfer of training—the ability to use learned strategies in different situations (Birnboim 1995, 61)
- Volition—capacity to formulate an intention or goal and initiate action (Golisz and Toglia 1998)

CAUSE

Impaired executive function has been associated with damage to frontal lobe and subcortical limbic system (Zoltan 1996, 149).

ASSESSMENT

Areas
- daily living skills—activities of daily living and instrumental ADLs
- productive skills, values, history, and interests
- leisure skills and interests
- awareness or level of consciousness
- orientation—temporal, personal, environmental, situational, and left-right
- attention or concentration—arousal, span or length of attention, and distractibility
- sensory acuity and discrimination—tactile, visual, and auditory
- memory functions—immediate, delayed, and remote
- learning and fund of information
- problem solving
- decision making
- cause and effect
- organization of tasks and sequencing
- judgment of safety
- insight—especially awareness of disability
- mental flexibility
- abstraction
- concept formation and categorization
- motivation or goal-directed behavior
- frustration tolerance and coping behavior
- behavioral control

Instruments
Instruments Developed by Occupational Therapy Personnel
- *Allen Cognitive Level Screening Test* by C.K. Allen, Colchester, CT: S&S Worldwide, 1996.
- *Allen Cognitive Level Test—Problem Solving* by N. Josman and N. Katz, *American Journal of Occupational Therapy* 45, no. 4 (1991): 331–338.
- *Assessment of Motor and Process Skills* (AMPS), 2nd ed., by A. Fisher, Ft. Collins, CO: Three Star Press, 1997.
- *Bay Area Functional Performance Evaluation*, 2nd ed., by S.L. Williams and J. Bloomer, Palo Alto, CA: Consulting Psychologists Press, 1987.
- *Block Design* by B. Zoltan, in Visual, visual-perceptual, and perceptual-motor deficits in brain injured adults: Evaluation, treatment and functional implication, *Rehabilitation Clinics of North America* 3, no. 2 (1992): 337–355.
- *Cognitive Assessment of Minnesota* by R. Rustad et al., San Antonio, TX: Psychological Corporation/Therapy Skill Builders, 1993.

- *Cognitive Performance Test* by T. Burns, in *Occupational therapy treatment goals for the physically and cognitively disabled,* eds. C.K. Allen, C.A. Earhart, and T. Blue, 46–50, 69–80, Bethesda, MD: American Occupational Therapy Association, 1992.
- *Dynamic Interactional Assessment* by J.P. Toglia, in Generalization of treatment: A multicontextual approach to cognitive perceptual impairment in the brain-injured adult, *American Journal of Occupational Therapy* 45, no. 6 (1991): 505–516.
- *Loewenstein Occupational Therapy Cognitive Assessment* (LOTCA) by M. Itzkovich et al., Pequanock, NJ: Maddak, 1990.
- *Modification of ADL* by M.E. Neistadt, in Assessing learning capabilities during cognitive and perceptual evaluations for adults with traumatic brain injury, *Occupational Therapy in Health Care* 9, no. 1 (1995): 3–16.
- *Toglia Category Assessment* by J. Toglia, San Antonio, TX: Psychological Corporation/ Therapy Skill Builders, 1994.

Instruments Developed by Other Professionals and Used by Occupational Therapy Personnel

- *Cognitive Behavior Rating Scales* by J.M. Williams, Odessa, FL: Psychological Assessment Resources, 1987.
- *Concept Formation and Abstractions* by A.L. Christenson, *Luria's Neuropsychological Investigation,* New York: Spectrum Publications, 1975.
- *Executive Function—Route-Finding Task* by T.M. Boyd and S.W. Sautter, in Route-finding: A measure of everyday executive functioning in the head-injured adult, *Applied Cognitive Psychology* 7 (1993): 171–181.
- *Mini-Mental State Examination* (MMSE) by M.F. Folstein, S.E. Folstein, and P.R. McHugh, in Mini-mental state: A practical method for grading the cognitive state of patients for the clinician, *Journal of Psychiatric Research* 12 (1975): 189–198.
- *Minnesota Paper Formboard—Revised* by R. Likert and W.H. Quasha, San Antonio, TX: The Psychological Corporation, 1970.
- *Neurobehavioral Cognitive Status Examination* by R. Kierman et al., *Annals of Internal Medicine* 107 (1987): 481–485.
- *Odd-Even Cross-Out* by J.F. Craine, in The retraining of frontal lobe dysfunction, *Cognitive rehabilitation: Conceptualization and intervention,* ed. L.E. Trexler, New York: Plenum Press, 1982.
- *Profile of Executive Control System* by D. Branswell et al., Puyallup, WA: Association for Neuropsychological Research and Development, 1992.
- *Raven's Progressive Matrices* by J.C. Raven, J.H. Court, and J. Raven, London: Oxford Psychologists Press, 1988.
- *Rey-Osterrieth Complex Figure* by J. Meyers and K. Meyers, Odessa, FL: Psychological Assessment Resources, 1995.
- *Self-Awareness Questionnaire* by P.G. Gasquoine and T.A. Gibbons, in Lack of awareness of impairment in institutionalized, severely and chronically disabled survivors of traumatic brain injury: A preliminary investigation, *Journal of Head Trauma Rehabilitation* 9, no. 4 (1994): 16–24.
- *Short Category Test* by L. Wetzel and T. Boll, Los Angeles: Western Psychological Services, 1987.

- *Test of Nonverbal Intelligence* by L. Brown, R.J. Sherbenou, and S.K. Johnsen, Austin, TX: Pro-Ed, 1982.
- *Wisconsin Card-Sorting Test* by R.K. Heaton et al., Odessa, FL: Psychological Assessment Resources, 1993.

PROBLEMS

Self-care
- The person may have difficulty performing self-care tasks without physical assistance and/or cueing.
- The person may be unable to perform instrumental ADLs without physical assistance and/or cueing.

Productivity
- The person may be unable to work because of difficulty initiating, terminating, or judging, and lack of problem-solving or decision-making skills.
- The person may be unable to perform homemaking tasks without physical assistance and/or cueing.
- The person may be unable to drive or walk safely because of problems with judgment and insight.

Leisure
The person may be unable to participate in favorite sports because of difficulty following the rules, inability to use judgment of safety, or lack of insight into disability.

Sensorimotor
- The person may overestimate his or her ability in gross and fine motor skills.
- The person may overestimate his or her ability to process sensory input.

Cognitive
- The person may have problems in thinking, such as difficulty
  1. articulating thoughts
  2. comprehending the main idea
  3. weighing alternatives
  4. planning a course of action
  5. arriving at conclusions
  6. drawing inferences
  7. thinking in symbolic terms; for example, thinking abstractly or using abstract reasoning
- The person may have difficulty in problem solving; for example,
  1. carrying out routine self-care and household chores
  2. carrying out basic adaptive behaviors, such as making a phone call, asking for directions, or using public transportation
  3. using convergent reasoning; that is, formulating the problem, determining the objective sought, and considering the relevant factors

4. using divergent reasoning; that is considering alternatives systematically and choosing a strategy
5. using executive abilities; that is, formulating a plan, prioritizing the details, executing the plan, monitoring the performance, and verifying the solution obtained against the original plan
- The person may have difficulty with judgment, such as
  1. appropriateness in manner of dress, use of verbal and nonverbal expression or gestures, awareness of what "fits" the occasion
  2. propriety concerning privacy, invasion of privacy, friendliness or chumminess
  3. overestimating his or her ability to perform a task correctly and safely
- The person may have difficulty understanding roles, such as
  1. family roles: wife, husband, child, parent
  2. work roles: employee, volunteer, student
  3. social or community roles: traveler, shopper, customer, theatergoer
- The person may have disruption in planning skills, volition, quality control of performance, and self-regulation.
- The person may not recognize errors.
- The person may have generated appropriate solutions to wrong information.
- Attention to safety in relation to judgment may be impaired.
- The person may have decreased insight into his or her deficits.
- The person may get into situations that his or her cognitive skills cannot handle.
- The person may have poor decision-making skills.
- The person may make poor choices of goals.

Psychological
- The person may not apply enough motivation to get a task completed, especially if the individual overestimates his or her ability to complete the task.
- The person may not be able to cope with social situations or use good judgment.

TREATMENT/INTERVENTION

Treatment models are based on remedial and adaptive approaches.

Cognitive
- Treatment of imitation deficit (Zoltan 1996, 151)
  — Remedial approach
    1. Provide incentive training by first identifying the person's needs and interests to determine the most appropriate incentives. Make the incentive available regularly. Create a learning environment in which the value of the incentive will be sufficient to elicit the desired behavior. Use teaching strategies and repetition until behavior is habitual. Change incentive learning to a token economy so the person receives rewards such as money, praise, a movie, and so on for using learned strategies in a proper context.
    2. Provide sensory input combined with verbal cueing to initiate the task.

3. The Affolter approach (physically guiding the person through the necessary movements) may be helpful in initiating the activity.
— Adaptive approach
1. Provide starting signals to begin an activity.
2. Provide step-by-step instruction using either an audiocassette with verbal instructions or a notebook with written instructions.
3. Help the person develop insight into and awareness of his or her problem(s) so he or she can begin to develop an internal cueing system to initiate tasks without having to rely on someone else.
• Treatment of decreased awareness (Zoltan 1996, 155–157)
— Remedial approach
1. Intellectual awareness
   a. The person must have a minimal amount of intellectual awareness for the remedial approach to be appropriate.
   b. Assuming a minimal amount of intellectual awareness, provide immediate, objective, and concrete feedback to the person during task performance or situation.
   c. Have the person make a list of his or her strengths and weaknesses and show it to the therapist.
2. Emergent awareness
   a. Provide feedback during and after the task to the person that is consistent, understandable, and direct.
   b. Have the person do a self-rating scale about the specific problem. Family or therapist can also do a rating and then compare the two so the person can see what others think. Questions might include what happened, how did I feel, what did I do, how could I have behaved differently, how could I have avoided the situation, how can I handle the situation better next time?
3. Anticipatory awareness
   a. Help the person plan ahead and anticipate how deficits could affect performance and what to do about the situation or task.
   b. As the person becomes more aware, the therapist can fade out cues and the person can provide him- or herself with more cues.
   c. Videotaping, audiotaping, roleplaying, and group sessions may be useful devices to increase the person's awareness, especially concerning social situations.
   d. Rewards should be given for anticipating a problem correctly as well as for responding correctly.
— Adaptive approach
1. Intellectual awareness
   a. Provide education to the person and the family regarding the individual's decreased awareness and how it will affect function.
   b. Provide external cues as needed and make necessary environmental modification to ensure safety.
2. Emergent awareness—compensatory strategies must address the specific situation: for example, provide an auditory tape on how to dress or a checklist of household cleaning tasks.

3. Anticipatory awareness—when the person recognizes that a problem may occur, help him or her develop a strategy for solving it, such as notebook to refer to for helpful hints or instructions.
- Treatment for planning and organization (Zoltan 1996, 158–160)
  — Remedial approach
    1. Help the person focus on the organizational structure of information; for example, major points of a discussion can be prefaced by a number or, in written material, a bold heading can be used that can be incorporated into a personal outline.
    2. Have the person verbalize the entire plan of action in sequence before performing it, verbalize each step as it is performed, and summarize the plan upon completion. As the person's performance improves, verbal prompts can be faded out.
    3. Have the person estimate the degree of difficulty he or she will experience doing a task, then recall difficulties, if any, after performing the task. See how closely the estimation matched the results.
    4. Have the person use a question-and-answer approach to a task; for example, What do I need to do to begin this task? I need to. . . . What do I do next? I . . . . What do I need to do now? I need to. . . . The person may write ideas or thought processes down before beginning the task and have the therapist or a family member review the plan.
    5. Use question technique in a variety of tasks and settings; for example, searching for an object (What are we looking for?); developing a tentative plan (Where do you think it might be?); developing a comprehensive plan (How can we find it?); considering a time frame (How much time do we have to look?); and predicting success (Do you think we can find it?).
  — Adaptive approach
    1. Provide reminders; for example, an appointment calendar or a daily "to do" list along with information necessary to complete the tasks.
    2. Identify times of day when the person performs best and try to use these times for therapy; recommend that the person do important tasks at these times.
    3. Have the person prioritize tasks and prepare instructions to complete the tasks.
    4. Educate the family or caregiver about the planning and organization deficit and how to compensate at home and in the community.
- Treatment for problem solving (Zoltan 1996, 163–165)
  — Remedial approach
    1. Focus on improving the skills necessary to solve a problem; for example, acknowledging that a problem exists (situation needs action); formulating the problem (verbalize or write down the problem); analyzing the conditions of the problem (how hard is the problem to solve?); formulating a strategy or plan of action (examine ways to solve the problem); identifying relevant tactics (what information is needed?); deciding on a plan (develop steps); executing the plan (perform steps); comparing results to the problem (did the plan work?); revising the plan if necessary (determine where errors occurred and redevelop steps); determining the level of satisfaction with the outcome (evaluate the results).
    2. Use problem-solving worksheets; for example, locating a hair salon in the Yellow Pages and planning how to get to it. The therapist should have a copy of the written instructions for the practice task, a pencil, a copy of the Yellow Pages, an Answer

Key, a therapist observation sheet, a self-assessment quiz, and a stopwatch (if timing is important). Other tasks might be locating a doughnut shop, finding a shop that sells fishing gear, buying water softener, getting a plumber, or getting a picture framed.
    3. Have the person practice "chaining" the activities of problem solving, especially the identification of external and internal cues. Rehearse the solution before actually doing it. Have the person label the steps in the problem-solving process using his or her own words.
    4. Provide a variety of situations in which to practice skills, alternating among worksheets, games, and functional activities.
— Adaptive approach
    1. Monitor performance and provide adaptive solutions as needed; for example, providing more external cues to a situation (more pictures, more written directions, more diagrams, more audiotaped reminders) to decrease inappropriate strategies and instructing the person to check for errors before proceeding
    2. Identify the areas of occupational task performance that are most affected and provide step-by-step instructions for those tasks.
    3. Teach the person to ask for help when he or she is unable to solve a problem, using role planning and guided experience in the community.
    4. Have the person verbalize the strategies that are being used to solve a problem; identify faulty strategies, suggest more effective strategies, and provide the opportunity to practice the new strategies.
• Treatment for mental flexibility and abstraction (Zoltan 1996, 168–169)
— Remedial approach
    1. Have the person perform tasks that require changing mental focus from one kind of mental task to another; for example, changing from picture instructions to written instructions to verbal instruction; or from watching a game to participating in the game; or following a conversation in a group situation.
    2. Use computer software programs designed to increased mental flexibility.
— Adaptive approach
    1. Ask the person to perform a task with several steps; for example, fixing a breakfast that includes a hot drink and cereal with milk. Observe whether the person can shift and organize behavior as needed.
    2. Have the person sort different types of laundry that are stored differently; for example, towels are folded and put in a drawer, T-shirts are hung in the closet.
    3. Memory aids, such as written or audiotaped instructions, can be used to help the person in changing his or her mental approach to a task; for example, reminding the person that glasses and coffee cups go in the right cabinet from the dishwasher; dishes go in the left cabinet; eating utensils go in the left drawer.
    4. If the person has difficulty with mental flexibility, provide more concrete support, such as putting pictures of glasses, dishes, and eating utensils on the cabinets and drawer and encouraging visual scanning.
    5. Teach the person and the family how lack of mental flexibility and abstraction affect everyday life.
• Treatment of generalization and transfer (Zoltan 1996, 170–171)
— Remedial approach

1. Help the person recognize new situations and provide opportunities to generalize techniques; for example, finding groceries in different grocery stores. Help the person identify the parts of the situation that are the same and those that are different: same list of groceries; different location in the store.
2. Help the person focus on the mental operations, not the external environment, because the latter often changes.
3. Use simulation, then provide real-life situations or have the person report on performance in a real-life situation; for example, you can simulate the person's work environment, then have the person return to the actual work setting and report on successes and problems.
4. More complex tasks require more similarity to transfer; simple tasks can be carried out in a greater variety of situations. Therapists should consider the complexity of the task before considering where and how the task should be practiced and performed.
   — Adaptive approach
     1. Target the processing strategies and behaviors that are most needed by the person.
     2. Begin with near transfer tasks: those that transfer easily.
- Treatment of metacognition (Birnboim 1995)
  — Teach procedures of new strategies first by modeling and later by transferring responsibility to the learner. Begin by introducing the modality.
  — Provide extensive training of these procedures for achieving low road transfer. Encourage the person to master the modality.
  — Analyze (done by both the therapist and the client) the metacognitive strategies the person has for better understanding and to facilitate awareness and motivation. Help the person analyze and identify the metacognitive strategies necessary to master the modality.
  — Provide explicit learning and training of high road transfer to various life situations. Transfer the skills to daily life.
- Teaching modalities
  — Make use of computer games, such as PFB (Pico, Fermi, Bagels), a number guessing game which has multiple levels of difficulty.

PRECAUTIONS
- Monitor the person carefully during initial training in executive functions. Person can still have lapses in self control and self regulation.
- The person may become impulsive in the middle of a task, especially if the task is too difficult or the person is tired.
- The person may display inappropriate social behavior.
- The person may display poor judgment of personal safety.
- The person may perseverate and have difficulty solving problems in spite of training.

PROGNOSIS/OUTCOME
- The person is able to make decisions that meet the demands of the situation and carry out task or tasks based on those decisions.

- The person is able to organize and sequence a series of steps to complete a task or tasks.
- The person is able to correctly identify that a problem exists, solve the problem, and apply the solution to the situation in which the problem arose.
- The person is able to generalize learning of knowlege and skills gained in one situation and apply that learning to another similar situation.
- The person is able to exercise judgment as to what constitutes an appropriate response in various situations and act based on that judgment. Appropriateness may be in terms of a social situation or personal safety.

REFERENCES

Birnboim, S. 1995. A metacognition approach to cognitive rehabilitation. *British Journal of Occupational Therapy* 58, no. 2:61–64.

Golisz, K.M., and J.P. Toglia. 1998. Evaluation of perception and cognition—Executive functions, organization, and problem solving. In *Willard and Spackman's occupational therapy*, 9th ed., eds. M.E. Neistadt and E.B. Crepeau, 276–279. Philadelphia: Lippincott-Raven.

Haase, B. 1997. Cognition. In *Assessments in occupational therapy and physical therapy,* eds. J. Van Deusen and D. Brunt, 333–356. Philadelphia: W.B. Saunders.

Unsworth, C. 1999. Glossary of terms. In *Cognitive and perceptual dysfunction: A clinical reasoning approach to evaluation and intervention,* ed. C. Unsworth, 473–484. Philadelphia: F.A. Davis.

Wheatley, C.J. 1996. Evaluation and treatment of cognitive dysfunction. In *Occupational therapy: practice skills for physical dysfunction*, 4th ed., ed. L.W. Pedretti, 241–252. St. Louis: Mosby.

Zoltan, B. 1996. Executive functions. In *Vision, perception and cognition: A manual for the evaluation and treatment of the neurologically impaired adult,* 3rd. ed., ed. B. Zoltan, 149–176. Thorofare, NJ: Slack, Inc.

BIBLIOGRAPHY

Abreu, B., et al. 1993. Occupational performance and the functional approach. In *AOTA self-study series: Cognitive rehabilitation,* ed. C.B. Royeen, no. 9. Bethesda, MD: American Occupational Therapy Association.

Bruce, M.A.G. 1993. Cognitive rehabilitation: Intelligence, insight, and knowledge. In *AOTA self-study series: Cognitive rehabilitation,* ed. C.B. Royeen, no. 5. Bethesda, MD: American Occupational Therapy Association.

Duran, L., and A.G. Fisher. 1999. Evaluation and intervention with executive functions impairment. In *Cognitive and perceptual dysfunction: A clinical reasoning approach to evaluation and intervention,* ed. C. Unsworth, 209–255. Philadelphia: F.A. Davis.

Katz, N., and A. Hartman-Maeir. 1998. Metacognition: The relationships of awareness and executive functions to occupational performance. In *Cognition and occupation in rehabilitation: Cognitive models for intervention in occupational therapy,* ed. N. Katz, 323–342. Bethesda, MD: American Occupational Therapy Association.

Neistadt, M.E., et al. 1993. An analysis of a board game as a treatment activity. *American Journal of Occupational Therapy* 47, no. 2:154–160.

Wheatley, C.J. 1998. Treatment of cognitive dysfunction. In *Physical dysfunction: Practice skills for the occupational therapy assistant,* ed. M.B. Early, 395–397. St. Louis: Mosby.

Zemke, R. 1993. Task skills, problem solving, and social interaction. In *AOTA self-study series: Cognitive rehabilitation,* ed. C.B. Royeen, no. 6. Bethesda, MD: American Occupational Therapy Association.

Dementia—Alzheimer's Type

DESCRIPTION

Dementia of the Alzheimer's type is a progressive, inexorable loss of cognitive function associated with an excessive number of senile plaques in the cerebral cortex and subcortical gray matter, which also contain beta-amyloid and neurofibrillary tangles consisting of tau protein (Merck 1999, 1395–1396). The DSM-IV requires the following criteria for a diagnosis of dementia of the Alzheimer's type: (1) the development of multiple cognitive deficits manifested by other memory impairment and one or more of the following cognitive disturbances: aphasia, apraxia, agnosia, or disturbance in executive functioning such as planning, organizing, sequencing, or abstracting; (2) the cognitive deficits cause significant impairment in social or occupational functioning and represent a significant decline from a previous level of functioning; (3) the course is characterized by gradual onset and continuing cognitive decline; (4) the cognitive deficits do not occur exclusively during the course of a delirium; and (5) the cognitive deficits are not caused by central nervous system disorders, systemic conditions, substance-induced conditions, or other mental illness. Two types are recognized: early onset, which occurs before age 65, and late onset, which occurs after age 65 (American Psychiatric Association 1994, 142–143).

Alzheimer's disease is a diagnosis by exclusion; that is, all other possible reasons must be ruled out before the diagnosis of Alzheimer's disease or senile dementia of the Alzheimer's type (SDAT) is applied. The diagnosis cannot be confirmed during a lifetime with current technology but may be confirmed by pathological examination of brain tissue after death. The prevalence is between 2 percent and 4 percent of the population over age 65; the prevalence increases after age 75.

The disorder is named for Alois Alzheimer, a German neurologist who first described the condition in 1907.

CAUSE

The cause is unknown but may be a combination of any of the following: deficiency in neurotransmitter acetylcholine, especially in the frontal and temporal lobes; presence of the protein amyloid, which causes destruction of blood vessels and brain neurons; environmental factors; slow-acting virus; exogenous toxins such as aluminum; head trauma earlier in life; or genetic immunologic factors. The early onset type of the disease runs in families in about 15 percent to 20 percent of cases. Genes located on chromosomes 1, 14, 19, and 21 are known to influence initiation and progression. Persons with trisomy 21 type Down syndrome have a high incidence of early Alzheimer's disease. Thus, autosomal dominant genetic patterns are involved in early onset Alzheimer's, but the factors involved in the late onset type are less clear. Females are more often diagnosed with late onset Alzheimer's, but this may be due to their longer average lifespan than to a specific factor. All racial, ethnic, and socioeconomic groups are equally affected. The course of the disease may run from 5 to 25 years.

DSM-IV Diagnostic Criteria for Dementia of the Alzheimer's Type

A. The development of multiple cognitive deficits manifested by both
   1. memory impairment (impaired ability to learn new information or recall previously learned information)
   2. one or more of the following cognitive disturbances:
      a. aphasia (language disturbance)
      b. apraxia (impaired ability to carry out motor activities despite intact motor function)
      c. agnosia (failure to recognize or identify objects despite intact sensory function)
      d. disturbance in executive functioning (i.e., planning, organization, sequencing, abstracting)
B. The cognitive deficits in Criteria A1 and A2 each cause significant impairment in social or occupational functioning and represent a significant decline from a previous level of functioning.
C. The course is characterized by gradual onset and continuing cognitive decline.
D. The cognitive deficits in Criteria A1 and A2 are not due to any of the following:
   1. other central nervous system conditions that cause progressive deficits in memory and cognition (e.g., cerebrovascular disease, Parkinson's disease, Huntington's disease, subdural hematoma, normal-pressure hydrocephalus, brain tumor)
   2. systemic conditions that are known to cause dementia (e.g., hypothyroidism, vitamin B12 or folic acid deficiency, niacin deficiency, hypercalcemia, neurosyphilis, HIV infection)
   3. substance-induced conditions
E. The deficits do not occur exclusively during the course of a delirium.
F. The disturbance is not better accounted for by another Axis I disorder.

Source: Reprinted with permission from the *Diagnostic and Statistical Manual of Mental Disorders, Fourth Edition.* Copyright © 1994, American Psychiatric Association.

ASSESSMENT

Areas
- daily living skills—self-care and instrumental ADLs
- productivity history, skills, interests, and values
- leisure skills and interests
- gross motor skills and coordination
- fine motor skills—manipulation, dexterity, and bilateral coordination

- postural control and balance
- mobility
- motor planning or praxis
- sensory registration
- sensory processing
- perceptual skills
- attending behavior
- attention span
- memory—short-term vs. long-term
- orientation
- executive skills—planning, organizing, executing actions and activities
- conceptualization or abstract reasoning
- learning skills
- mood or affect changes
- judgment of safety
- communication skills
- social interaction skills
- home safety

Instruments
Instruments Developed by Occupational Therapy Personnel
- *Activities of Daily Living (ADL) Situational Test* by E. Skula and T. Sunderland, in Direct assessment of activities of daily living in Alzheimer's disease: A controlled study, *Journal of American Geriatrics Society* 36, no. 2 (1988): 97–103.
- *Allen Cognitive Level Screening Test* by C.K. Allen, Colchester, CT: S&S Worldwide. 1996.
- *Assessment of Motor and Process Skills* (AMPS), 2nd ed., by A. Fisher, Ft. Collins, CO: Three Star Press, 1997.
- *Cognitive Performance Test* by T. Burns, J.A. Mortimer, and P. Merchak, in Cognitive performance test: A new approach to functional assessment in Alzheimer's disease, *Journal of Geriatric Psychiatry and Neurology* 7 (1994): 46–54.
- *Functional Performance Measure* by A. Carswell et al., in Functional performance measure for persons with Alzheimer's disease: Reliability and validity, *Canadian Journal of Occupational Therapy* 60, no. 3 (1995): 62–69.
- *Kingston Geriatric Cognitive Battery* by R.W. Hopkins, P. Dixon-Medora, and L. Krefting, in Kingston Geriatric Cognitive Battery, *Occupational Therapy Journal of Research* 13, no. 4 (1993): 241–252.
- *Kitchen Task Assessment* (KTA) by C.M. Baum and D.F. Edwards, *American Journal of Occupational Therapy* 47, no. 5 (1993): 431–436.
- *Right-Left Discrimination,* subtest of the *Southern California Sensory Integration Test* by A.J. Ayres, Los Angeles, CA: Western Psychological Services, 1972.
- *Routine Task Inventory-2* by C.K. Allen, D.A. Earhart, and T. Blue, *Occupational Therapy Treatment Goals for Physically and Cognitively Disabled,* 63–72, Bethesda, MD: American Occupational Therapy Association, 1992.

Instruments Developed by Other Professionals and Used by Occupational Therapy Personnel

- *Alzheimer's Disease Assessment Scale* by W.G. Rosen et al., in A new rating scale for Alzheimer's Disease, *American Journal of Psychiatry* 141 (1984): 1356–1364.
- *Blessed Dementia Scale*, short form by R. Katzman et al., in Validation of a short orientation-memory-concentration test of cognitive impairment, *American Journal of Psychiatry* 140 (1993): 734–739.
- *Clinical Dementia Rating* (CDR) by L. Berg, in Clinical dementia rating (CDR), *Psychopharmacology Bulletin* 24 (1988): 637–639.
- *FROMAJE* by L. Libow, in A rapidly administered, easily remembered mental status evaluation: FROMAJE, *The care of geriatric medicine,* eds. L. Libow and F.T. Sherman, 85–91, St Louis: CV Mosby, 1981.
- *Global Deterioration Scale* by B. Reisberg et al., *American Journal of Psychiatry* 139, no. 9 (1982): 1136–1139.
- *Map-Reading Test* by J. Semmes et al., in Spatial orientation in man after cerebral injury: I. Analysis by locus of lesions, *Journal of Psychology* 39 (1955): 227–243.
- *Mini-Mental State Examination* (MMSE) by M.F. Folstein, S.E. Folstein, and P.R. McHugh, in Mini-mental state: A practical method for grading the cognitive state of patients for the clinician, *Journal of Psychiatric Research* 12 (1975): 189–198.
- *Road-Map Test* by D. Alexander, H.T. Walker, and J. Money, in Studies in direction sense: I. Turner's Syndrome, *Archives of General Psychiatry* 10 (1964): 337–339.
- *Worry Scale* by E. LaBarge, in A preliminary scale to measure the degree of worry among mildly demented Alzheimer's disease patients, *Physical and Occupational Therapy in Geriatrics* 11, no. 3 (1993): 43–57.

Other assessments to measure motor system: range of motion, coordination, equilibrium, muscle tone, gait, posture, and movement speed and rhythm.

PROBLEMS

Clinical features can be divided into four stages:
1. Initial or early stage: The person has difficulty with short-term memory, lacks concentration, and experiences mood changes. The person may deny difficulty and try to cover by confabulating.
2. Middle stage: The person has difficulty with orientation and shows marked loss of memory regarding recent events, although remote events are preserved. The person gets lost easily, and problems with hygiene, dressing, eating, and speech appear. Aphasia, apraxia, and agnosia become more apparent.
3. Late stage: The person is unable to recognize close family members. Severe language deficits emerge, and disorientation is severe. Catastrophic reaction may occur and the person needs 24-hour supervision.
4. Final or terminal stage: The person is completely dependent in all aspects of daily living, is apathetic and unresponsive except for facial grimacing, has no meaningful language or memory, does not interact with the environment, and has poor motor function.

Self-Care
- The person may experience loss of self-care skills, especially those requiring fine motor hand skills and complex motor planning.
- The person may have sleep disturbances.

Productivity
- The person may have loss of productive skills because of memory loss and other cognitive impairments.
- The person may lose his or her job or be forced to take early retirement.

Leisure
- The person may lose interest in activities that used to be important leisure pursuits.
- The person may lose motor coordination, which may limit participation in some leisure pursuits.

Sensorimotor
- The person usually has increasing loss of gross motor skills and coordination.
- The person usually has increasing loss of balance and equilibrium reactions.
- The person usually has increasing loss of fine motor skills, manipulation, dexterity, and bilateral coordination.
- The person may have gait disturbances such as stumbling, wide-based gait, or shuffling feet.
- In advanced or terminal stages, the person may have contractures.
- Positioning may be an issue in advanced or terminal stages.
- The person may have increasing loss of sensory awareness and registration.
- The person may have increasing loss of sensory processing.
- The person may have reduced ability to monitor (inhibit) incoming stimuli, which leads to overstimulation.
- The person usually has apraxia and thus has difficulty with motor planning activities. An example is difficulty with dressing, because the person is unable to execute the movements necessary to don the clothes.
- The person may have increasing loss of spatial relations and spatial visualization and thus may become lost or disoriented even in familiar situations.
- The person usually has agnosia and is unable to remember familiar objects or persons. An example is inability to recognize a son or daughter.
- The person may lose binocular vision or visual accommodation, which affects depth perception.
- The person may wander around or pace without apparent sense of purpose or direction.

Cognitive
- The person usually has increasing memory loss, which begins with recent events (short-term memory) and increases to include remote events (long-term memory). Initial sign.
- The person usually has increasing forgetfulness and disorientation. Initial sign.
- The person usually has increasing difficulty learning and remembering new information.
- The person usually has increasing inability to concentrate. Initial sign.

- The person usually has increasing loss of abstract thinking skills.
- The person usually has anomia or difficulty remembering the names of things.
- The person usually has loss of judgment about personal safety.
- The person may experience loss of the sense of time passing. For example, the person may accuse a caregiver of being gone for many hours when actually the caregiver was out of the room for only a minute or two.
- The person may experience the sundowning effect; that is, symptoms become worse at night.

Psychosocial
- The person may become restless, especially at night.
- The person may become increasingly irritable and may become combative or aggressive if unable to cope.
- The person may experience paranoid thinking, because memory loss does not permit the person to remember what actually happened. For example, the person may accuse someone of taking an object when actually the person put the object somewhere and now does not remember where.
- The person may experience delusions.
- The person usually becomes increasingly disoriented to time, place, or person.
- The person may become easily frustrated while performing what should be easy tasks.
- The person may experience mood and affect changes, especially apathy or lability.
- The person may appear depressed. It is important to differentiate depression, a treatable problem, from changes in mood and affect that are signs of Alzheimer's disease.
- The person usually has loss of spontaneity.
- The person may be hypochondriacal.
- The person may have a catastrophic reaction or may overreact to seemingly inconsequential things or even to something the caretaker cannot identify.
- The person usually experiences decreased ability to write or speak as a result of aphasia.
- The person may blame others for personal problems; for example, accusing others of stealing items that have been misplaced or were discarded many years ago.
- The person may withdraw from social situations or become very agitated.

TREATMENT/INTERVENTION
   Models of treatment include reminiscent therapy and validation therapy. Models of treatment in occupational therapy include the cognitive disability model, person-environment fit models (Edwards and Baum 1996), and model of human occupation.
- Early stage: Enable the person to maintain as much independence as possible and teach caregivers how to cope with the stress of dealing with a person who has Alzheimer's.
- Middle stage: Encourage physical fitness, facilitate socialization and communication, and promote adjustment to the environment.
- Advanced stage: Maximize the quality of life, promote awareness of self and others, maintain overall fitness, and increase sensory stimulation.
- Terminal stage: Prevent or decrease contractures and make the person comfortable.

Self-Care
- Encourage the person to maintain independent performance of daily living activities as long as possible. Select activities within the person's physical and mental capacity.
- Provide assistive devices and instruct the person in the use of the devices if his or her use will prolong independent or semi-independent performance.
- Structure the environment and cue the person to help him or her participate in self-care activities for a longer period of time.
- Instruct the caregiver (family member or home health aide) on helping the person perform the daily living activities that the individual can no longer perform independently in a satisfactory or safe manner.
- Grade self-care activities using environmental modification and task simplification as the person's capacities decline. For example, serve the person one food at a time on a plate or in a bowl and provide the appropriate utensil. Keep other food out of view. When one food is finished, serve the next food.
- Increase physical comfort to promote relaxation and sleep.

Productivity
- Encourage the person to participate in productive activities (work, homemaking, volunteering) as long as possible; that is, as long as the person performs at a satisfactory level or meets an acceptable standard set by an employer or other person charged with establishing and maintaining these criteria.
- Modify (simplify or redesign) productive tasks if such changes will permit the individual to continue productive activity at a level of performance that is satisfactory or meets an acceptable standard.

Leisure
- Maintain the person's leisure interests as long as possible by offering opportunities to engage in favorite activities.
- Modify leisure activities within the scope of the person's interests if original activities are no longer possible or practical.

Sensorimotor
- Encourage exercise and participation in activities to maintain mobility and general fitness.
- Use more gross motor or large motor activities when fine motor activities become difficult or impossible. Examples are walking groups, bowling, a rhythm band, musical chairs games, balloon volleyball, or exercise groups.
- Consider splints to prevent contractures.
- Stimulate sensory systems regularly to maintain contact with the environment, but avoid overstimulation, which may cause agitation, confusion, and catastrophic reaction.
- Maintain balance and equilibrium reactions as long as possible to reduce possible falls and injuries. Examples are the use of vestibular boards, large balls or inflatables, swings, seesaws, or merry-go-rounds.
- Rhythmic activities such as walking and dancing may be used to advantage.

Cognitive

- Maintain current level of attention and memory for as long as possible.
- Provide structure and predictability. Be consistent in approach and use clear, concise instructions. Use the person's habitual skills when possible to facilitate performance.
- Teach compensatory memory techniques, such as writing down a daily schedule and keeping a notebook of important personal information.
- In conjunction with sensory stimulation, have the person name the type of stimulation and review a past experience with the same or similar sensory input.
- To reduce confusion and anxiety, use simple one- or two-step commands when providing instructions.

Psychosocial

- Orient the person to the environment through reality orientation sessions, including the name, place, date, day, and weather. Use memory aids if the person can read. A life story book may help the person connect with reality and can become a source of self-expression and pride.
- Promote self-esteem and self-worth by praising the person for maintaining self-care skills (dressing and grooming), for completing a task as requested, or for engaging in a leisure activity.
- Reduce anxiety by providing a structured, organized, and scheduled environment, telling the person what is going to happen in advance and what behavior is expected of him or her (e.g., wash hands before sitting at the table for lunch).
- Increase opportunities for and participation in socialization activities through such programs as pet therapy, sing-a-longs, field trips, show-and-tell sessions, parties, and entertainment.
- Promote vocalization and interaction skills through such activities as word games, object identification games, remember-when games, or name that tune. Modify according to the person's ability level.
- In group activities, assign one task or part of the process to each member so each can contribute. Active involvement and human contact can decrease behavioral problems.

Environment

- Keep the physical and temporal environments as consistent, free of ambiguity, familiar, and dependable as possible. Avoid clutter, excess noise, or too much activity and allow for optimal cue-finding. Signs, photos, or line drawings can be used to help identify rooms or objects.
- Contrasting colors and textures can be used to help a person distinguish figures from backgrounds or to camouflage safety hazards; for example, disguising doors to decrease wandering.
- Educate the family and caregiver(s) about managing the person with Alzheimer's: offer tips for facilitating care; encourage caregivers to help without doing for the person during early stages; and tell them what to expect as the disease progresses.
- Provide the family and caregiver(s) with emotional support, stress reduction, environmental adaptation, and assistance with problem solving, including opportunities to talk about specific problems and get suggestions for handling difficult situations.

- Recommend that the family and caregiver(s) join a local support group or Internet chat group for persons dealing with Alzheimer's disease.
- Provide the family with information about community resources, including day care and respite care.

PRECAUTIONS

- The person can become lost even in familiar environments. Do not leave him or her unattended.
- Avoid giving false expectations of the person's ability to perform cognitive tasks.
- Avoid overstimulating the person, and provide a quiet space if overstimulation occurs. Keep track of what tends to upset the person and try to avoid those situations.
- Avoid arguing with the person if he or she is not telling the truth. Redirect the person to an activity.
- Be aware that the person may be unable to modify his or her behavior. Do not argue with the person or engage in behaviors that are known to upset him or her.
- Watch for changes in sensory acuity that affect safety, such as decreased depth perception, decreased response to warning sounds, or decreased sense of tactile perception and touch to heat.
- In the advanced stage, avoid stairs or climbing when possible because of balance and gait problems.
- In the terminal stage, avoid the use of sharp objects, especially feeding utensils, to reduce the possibility of injury.
- In the terminal stage, if splints are used, check the person's skin frequently for changes in circulation, as the person may be unaware of or not able to report sensory changes him- or herself.

PROGNOSIS AND OUTCOME

Progressive loss of cognitive functions generally occurs. The physical body may remain in relatively good health for years after the cognitive functions are lost. Outcomes apply to early stages of the disorder. In advanced and terminal stages, loss of skills is unavoidable.

- The person demonstrates the ability to perform self-care and instrumental activities of daily living with modifications, such as a memory aid.
- The person demonstrates the ability to perform productive activities with modifications.
- The person demonstrates the ability to perform leisure activities with or without modifications.
- The person maintains or improves gross motor skills, including rolling, sitting, standing, and walking.
- The person maintains or improves fine motor skills, including dexterity and bilateral coordination.
- The person maintains or improves postural control and balance, including use of protective and equilibrium reactions.
- The person maintains or improves functional mobility.
- The person maintains or improves sensory registration and processing.
- The person maintains or improves perceptual skills, especially vision.

- The person maintains or improves attending behavior and attention span.
- The person maintains or improves memory skills.
- The person maintains or improves learning skills.
- The person maintains or improves orientation to person, place, and time.
- The person maintains or improves communication skills.

REFERENCES

American Psychiatric Association. 1994. *Diagnostic and Statistical Manual of Mental Disorders: DSM-IV,* 4th ed. Washington, DC: American Psychiatric Association. Task Force on DSM-IV.

Beers, M.H., and R. Berkow, eds. 1999. *The Merck Manual of Diagnosis and Therapy,* 17th ed. Whitehouse Station, NJ: Merck Research Laboratories.

Edwards D.F., and C.M. Baum. 1996. Functional performance of inner city African-American older persons with dementia. *Topics in Geriatric Rehabilitation* 12, no. 2:17–27.

BIBLIOGRAPHY

American Occupational Therapy Association. 1994. Statement: Occupational therapy services for persons with Alzheimer's disease and other dementias. *American Journal of Occupational Therapy* 48 no. 11:1029–1031.

Aspinall, G. 1996. Alzheimer's disease: Taking up a label. In *Occupational therapy in short-term psychiatry,* 3rd ed., ed. M. Willson, 55–56. New York: Churchill Livingstone.

Atchison, P. 1994. Helping people with Alzheimer's preserve independence. *OT Week* 8, no. 5:16–17.

Atchison, P. 1996. Alzheimer's disease. In *Occupational therapy: Practice skills for physical dysfunction,* 4th ed., ed. L.W. Pedretti, 851–856. St. Louis: Mosby.

Baum, C., and D.F. Edwards. 1993. Cognitive performance in senile dementia of the Alzheimer's type: The Kitchen Task Assessment. *American Journal of Occupational Therapy* 47, no. 5:431–436.

Ber, P. 1998. Degenerative diseases of the central nervous system—Alzheimer's disease. In *Physical dysfunction: Practice skills for the occupational therapy assistant,* ed. M.B. Early, 486–490. St. Louis: Mosby.

Benzing, P. 1994. The place to be: The development and implementation of an Alzheimer's day-care/respite program as a level in fieldwork experience for occupational therapy students. *Educational Gerontology* 20, no. 3:251–263.

Borell, L., et al. 1994. Occupational therapy in a day hospital for patients with dementia. *Occupational Therapy Journal of Research* 14, no. 4:219–238.

Borell, L., L, Ronnberg, and P.O. Sandman. 1995. The ability to use familiar objects among patients with Alzheimer's disease. *Occupational Therapy Journal of Research* 15, no. 2:111–121.

Bowlby, C. 1993. *Therapeutic activities with persons disabled by Alzheimer's disease and related disorders.* Gaithersburg, MD: Aspen Publishers.

Brown, I., and C.F. Epstein. 1993. The elderly with Alzheimer's disease. In *Practice issues in occupational therapy: Intraprofessional team building,* ed. S.E. Ryan, 153–160. Thorofare, NJ: Slack, Inc.

Burns, T., J.A. Mortimer, and P. Merchak. 1994. Cognitive Performance Test: A new approach to functional assessment in Alzheimer's disease. *Journal of Geriatric Psychiatry and Neurology* 7:46–54.

Canadian Occupational Therapy Association. 1998. *Living at Home with Alzheimer's Disease and Related Dementias: A Manual of Resources, References and Information.* Ottawa, Ontario: The Association.

Carswell, A., et al. 1995. The Functional Performance Measure for persons with Alzheimer's disease: Reliability and validity. *Canadian Journal of Occupational Therapy* 62, no. 2:62–69.

Carswell, A., and R. Eastwood. 1993. Activities of daily living, cognitive impairment and social function in community residents with Alzheimer's disease. *Canadian Journal of Occupational Therapy* 60, no. 3:130–136.

Casby, J.A., and M.B. Holm. 1994. The effect of music on repetitive disruptive vocalization of persons with dementia. *American Journal of Occupational Therapy* 48, no. 10:883–889.

Corcoran, M.A. 1994. Management decisions made by caregiver spouses of persons with Alzheimer's disease. *American Journal of Occupational Therapy* 48, no. 1:38–45.

Corcoran, M.A. 1997. *Occupational therapy practice guidelines for individuals with Alzheimer's disease.* Bethesda, MD: American Occupational Therapy Association.

Corcoran, M.A., and L.N. Gitlin. 1996. Managing eating difficulties related to dementia: A case comparison. *Topics in Geriatric Rehabilitation* 12, no. 2:63–69.

Devine, M.R. 1998. Reintroducing "Jack" to himself: A student learns the lesions of OT. *Advance for Occupational Therapy Practitioners* 14, no. 30:19–20

Gagnon, D. 1996. A review of reality orientation (RO), validation therapy (VT), and reminiscence therapy (RT) with the Alzheimer's client. *Physical and Occupational Therapy in Geriatrics* 14, no. 2:61–77.

Glickstein, J. 1996. Alzheimer's diagnosis doesn't mean "do not treat." *Advance for Occupational Therapists* 12, no. 34:15, 50.

Hellen, C.R. 1998. *Alzheimer's disease: Activity-focused care,* 2nd ed. Boston: Butterworth-Heinemann.

Hellen, C.R. 1998. Working with elders who have dementia and Alzheimer's disease. In *Occupational therapy with elders: Strategies for the COTA,* eds. H. Lohman, R.L. Padilla, and S. Byers-Connon, 224–234. St. Louis: Mosby.

Hopkins, R.W., P. Dixon-Medora, and L. Krefting. 1993. The Kingston Geriatric Cognitive Battery. *Occupational Therapy Journal of Research* 13, no. 4:241–252.

Kerr, T. 1995. Creating caregiver coalitions for Alzheimer's patients. *Advance for Occupational Therapists* 11, no. 45:18.

Kerr, T. 1995. Unusual new approach to Alzheimer's care. *Advance for Occupational Therapists* 11, no. 30:11, 50.

Liu, L., L. Gauthier, and S. Gauthier. 1996. Personal and extrapersonal orientation in persons with Alzheimer's disease: Reliability and validity of three assessments. *Canadian Journal of Occupational Therapy* 63, no. 3:162–172.

Lonergan, S.E. 1996. Benevolent touch: Use for persons with Alzheimer's disease and related dementias. *Mental Health Special Interest Section Newsletter* 19, no. 4:3, 6.

Mann, W.C., et al. 1996. Changes over one year in assistive device use and home modifications by home-based older persons with Alzheimer's disease. *Topics in Geriatric Rehabilitation* 12, no. 2:9–16.

Nieman, D., and M. Silver. 1997. Safe homes for people with Alzheimer's. *Advance for Occupational Therapists* 13, no. 42:21.

Paulanka, B.J., and L.S. Griffin. 1993. Behavioral responses of memory impaired clients to selected nursing interventions. *Physical and Occupational Therapy in Geriatrics* 12, no. 1:65–78.

Thiers, N. 1993. Meeting the needs of the elderly. *OT Week* 7, no. 16:14–15

Ward, J.D. 1998. Alzheimer's disease and other dementias. In *Willard and Spackman's occupational therapy,* 9th ed., eds. M.E. Neistadt and E.B. Crepeau, 717–720. Philadelphia: Lippincott-Raven.

Dementia—Other

DESCRIPTION

Dementia is a structurally caused permanent or progressive decline in several dimensions of intellectual function that interferes substantially with the individual's normal social or economic activity. There are two types: static or fixed dementia and progressive dementia. The essential feature of a dementia is the development of multiple cognitive deficits that include memory impairment and at least one of the following cognitive disturbances: aphasia, apraxia, agnosia, or a disturbance in executive functioning (American Psychiatric Association 1994, 134).

The DSM-IV lists 11 types of dementia, including dementia of the Alzheimer's type (see separate chapter), vascular dementia (also called multi-infarct dementia), dementia due to HIV disease, dementia due to head trauma, dementia due to Parkinson's disease (see separate chapter), dementia due to Huntington's disease (see separate chapter), dementia due to Pick's disease, dementia due to Creutzfeldt-Jakob disease, dementia due to other general medical conditions, substance-induced persisting dementia, and dementia due to multiple etiologies (American Psychiatric Association 1994, 133).

CAUSE

The cause of static dementia usually is a single major injury, such as severe head trauma, cardiac arrest, or cerebral hemorrhage. The causes of progressive dementia include all of the disorders listed below. In most cases, the dementia occurs because there is actual loss of tissue. These causes can be grouped into three categories: (1) metabolic or toxic, (2) structural, and (3) infectious. Metabolic or toxic causes include anoxia; vitamin B12 deficiency; chronic drug-alcohol-nutritional abuse; hypercalcemia associated with hyperparathyroidism; hypoglycemia; hypothyroidism; hepatic, respiratory, or uremic organ system failure; pellagra; and possibly folic acid deficiency. Structural causes include Alzheimer's disease, amyotrophic lateral sclerosis, brain trauma, brain tumor, cerebellar degeneration, communicating hydrocephalus, Huntington's disease, irradiation to frontal lobes, multiple sclerosis, normal-pressure hydrocephalus, Parkinson's disease, Pick's disease, progressive multifocal leukoencephalopathy, progressive supranuclear palsy, surgery, vascular disease, and Wilson's disease. Infectious causes include bacterial endocarditis, some brain tumors, Creutzfeldt-Jakob disease, Gerstmann-Sträusler-Scheinker disease, HIV-related disorders, neurosyphilis, tuberculosis and fungal meningitis, and viral encephalitis (Merck 1999, 1393).

ASSESSMENT

Areas

- daily living skills: note changes in the person's ability to perform self-care skills, manage finances, and balance a checkbook

---

Level of Dementia and Environmental Strategies

Mild stage with memory difficulties or impairment and minimal deficits in social interaction and task performance—use object-based modification such as removing clutter and unnecessary clothing, assistive devices, and home alterations.

Moderate stage with increase in disturbing behaviors and decrease in independent performance of daily routines—use task simplification such as setting up a daily routine, limiting number of items presented at a time to one, and using verbal or tactile cues.

Severe stage with loss of orientation skills and further increase in behavioral symptoms—use environmental modification such as painting a room in soft colors or placing an aquarium in the room to increase comfort and a sense of calm.

Source: Data from N.L. Gitlin and M.A. Corcoran, Managing Dementia at Home: The Role of Home Environment Modifications, *Topics in Geriatric Rehabilitation*, Vol. 12, No. 2, pp. 28–39, © 1996, Aspen Publishers, Inc.

- productivity history, work tasks, skills, and interests
- home management
- leisure skills and interests
- balance of activity
- sensorimotor skills: range of motion, functional range of motion, muscle tone, balance, posture, strength, quality of movement, fine motor coordination, manipulation, dexterity
- functional mobility skills
- motor planning skills
- agnosia: note the person's inability to recognize deficits in his or her own abilities and behaviors (anosognosia), failure to recognize objects by feel alone (stereognosis), failure to recognize faces (prosopagnosia), disorientation in personal space (autotopagnosia)
- visual motor integration: note the person's ability to copy figures or draw simple objects, such as a clock
- orientation skills: note response to unfamiliar surroundings
- memory: note changes in recent memory; also note visual, auditory, topographical (location), episodic (personal events/history), semantic (general learned knowledge), procedural (series of actions), and prospective (future events)
- judgment
- problem solving
- mental flexibility
- personality changes: note paranoid ideation
- emotions, mood, or affect: note signs of depression, emotional outbursts, uncontrolled crying or laughing, perseverative behaviors (repetitive, meaningless actions such as rubbing)

- inflexibility to change
- communication skills: note changes in handwriting
- social support networks
- accessibility and safety in the home
- appropriateness of living situation for stage of disease
- community mobility
- community safety

Note: depression, distress, and coping skills of the primary caregiver should also be assessed.

Instruments

Instruments Developed by Occupational Therapy Personnel

- *Allen Cognitive Level Test* by C.K. Allen, Colchester, CT: S&S Worldwide, 1996.
- *Assessment of Motor and Process Skills* (AMPS), 2nd ed., by A. Fisher, Fort Collins, CO: Three Star Press, 1997.
- *Cognitive Performance Test* by T. Burns, J.A. Mortimer, and P. Merchak, in Cognitive performance test: A new approach to functional assessment in Alzheimer's disease, *Journal of Geriatric Psychiatry and Neurology* 7, no. 1 (1994): 46–54.
- *Contextual Memory Test* by J.P. Toglia, San Antonio, TX: Psychological Corporation/ Therapy Skill Builders, 1993.
- *Descriptive Home Evaluation* by H. Davidson, Rehabilitation Institute, Kansas City, MO, in Assessing environmental factors, *Occupational therapy: Overcoming human occupation deficits,* eds. C. Christiansen and C. Baum, 444, Thorofare, NJ: Slack, Inc., 1991.
- *Functional Behavior Profile* by C.M. Baum, D.F. Edwards, and N. Morrow-Howell, in Identification and measurement of productive behaviors in senile dementia of the Alzheimer type, *Gerontologist* 33, no. 3 (1993): 403–408.
- *Interest Checklist* by J. Matsutsuyu, The interest checklist, *American Journal of Occupational Therapy* 23, no. 4 (1969): 323–328.
- *Kitchen Task Assessment* (KTA) by C.M. Baum and D.F. Edwards, *American Journal of Occupational Therapy* 47, no. 5 (1993): 431–436.
- *Klein-Bell ADL Scales* by R. Klein and B. Bell, Seattle, WA: Health Sciences Center for Educational Resources, 1982.
- *Kohlman Evaluation of Living Skills,* 3rd ed., by L.K. Thomason, Rockville, MD: American Occupational Therapy Association, 1992.
- *Milwaukee Evaluation of Daily Living Skills* by C.A. Leonardelli, Thorofare, NJ: Slack, Inc., 1988.
- *Performance Assessment of Self-Care Skills* (PASS) by J.C. Rogers et al., in Stability and change in functional assessment of patients with geropsychiatric disorders, *American Journal of Occupational Therapy* 48, no. 4 (1994): 355–360.
- *Routine Task Inventory-2* by C.K. Allen, D.A. Earhart, and T. Blue, *Occupational Therapy Treatment Goals for Physically and Cognitively Disabled,* 63–72, Bethesda, MD: American Occupational Therapy Association, 1992.
- *Test of Orientation for Rehabilitation Patients* (TORP) by J. Deitz et al., San Antonio, TX: Therapy Skill Builders/Psychological Corporation, 1986.

Instruments Developed by Other Professionals and Used by Occupational Therapy Personnel

*   *Barthel Self-Care Index* by F. Mahoney and D. Barthel, in Functional evaluations: The Barthel index, *Maryland State Medical Journal* 14 (1965): 61–65.
*   *Benton Visual Retention Test*, 5th ed., by A.B. Sivan, San Antonio, TX: The Psychological Corporation, 1992.
*   *Boston Aphasia Evaluation* by H. Goodglass and E. Kaplan, in *The assessment of aphasia and related disorders,* Philadelphia: Lea & Febiger, 1983.
*   *Brighton Clinic Adaptive Behaviour Scale* by R.T. Wood and P.G. Britton, *Clinical psychology with the elderly,* Beckenham, England: Croom Helm, 1984.
*   *Center for Epidemiological Studies—Depression Scale* (CES-D Scale) by L.S. Radloff and L. Teri, in Use of the Center for Epidemiological Studies—Depression Scale with older adults, *Clinics in Gerontology* 5, no. 12 (1986): 119–136.
*   *Clinical Dementia Rating* (CDR) by L. Berg, in Clinical dementia rating (CDR), *Psychopharmacology Bulletin* 24 (1988): 637–639.
*   *Deuel's Test of Manual Apraxia* by R.K. Deuel, C. Feely, and C. Bonskowski, in Manual apraxia in learning disabled children (abstract), *Annals of Neurology* 16 (1984): 388, and R.K. Deuel et al., in Constructional apraxia in Alzheimer's disease: Contributions to functional loss, *Physical and Occupational Therapy in Geriatrics* 9, no. 3/4 (1991): 53–68.
*   *Functional Independence Measure* (FIM) by Uniform Data System for Medical Research, Buffalo, NY: State University of New York at Buffalo, 1990.
*   *Global Deterioration Scale* (GDS) by B. Reisberg, in *Assessment in Geriatric Psychopharmacology*, eds. S.H. Ferris, T. Crook, and R. Bartus, New Canaan, CT: Mark Powlex, 1983, 19–35.
*   *Hamilton Depression Rating Scale* (HAMD) by M. Hamilton, in A rating for depression, *Journal of Neurology, Neurosurgery, and Psychiatry* 23 (1960): 56–62.
*   *Index of ADL* by S. Katz et al., in The index of ADL: A standardized measure of biological and psychosocial function, *JAMA* 195 (1963): 914–919.
*   *Learning Efficiency Test* by R.E. Webster, Novato, CA: Academic Therapy Publications, 1992.
*   *London Psycho-Geriatric Rating Scale* by D.L. Hersch, V.A. Kral, and R.B. Ralmer, in Clinical value of the London Psycho-Geriatric Rating Scale, *Journal of the American Geriatric Society* 26 (1978): 348–354.
*   *Mental Status Questionnaire* (MSQ) by R. Kahn et al., in Brief objective measures for the determination of mental status in the aged, *American Journal of Psychiatry* (117) 1960: 326–328.
*   *Memory and Behavior Problems Checklist* by S.H. Zarit, N.K. Orr, and J.M. Zarit, in *The hidden victims of Alzheimer's disease: Families under stress,* New York: New York University Press, 1985.
*   *Mini-Mental Status Examination* (MMSE) by M.F. Folstein, S.E. Folstein, and P.R. McHugh, in Mini-mental state: A practical method for grading the cognitive state of patients for the clinician, *Journal of Psychiatric Research* 12 (1975): 189–198.
*   *Older Americans Resource and Services Multidimensional Functional Assessment* by Duke University Center for the Study on Aging, in *Multidimensional Functional Assessment: The OARS Methodology*, 2nd ed., Durham, NC: Duke University Press, 1978.

- *Revised Memory and Behavior Problems Checklist* by L. Teri et al., in Assessment of behavioral problems in dementia, *Psychology and Aging* 7 (1992): 622–631.
- *Revised Ways of Coping Checklist* by P.P. Vitaliano, *Manual for the Revised Ways of Coping Checklist,* Seattle, WA: Stress and Coping Project, University of Washington, 1993.
- *Rivermead Behavioral Memory Test* by B. Wilson, J. Cockburn, and A. Baddeley, Suffolk, England: Thames Valley Test, 1985.
- *Sandoz Clinical Assessment Geriatric Scale,* by H.B. Hamot, R.J. Patin, and M.J. Singer, in Factor structure of the Sandoz Clinical Assessment Geriatric (SCAG) scale, *Psychopharmacology Bulletin* 20 (1984): 142–150.
- *Trail Making Test* (A&B), U.S. Army Individual Test Battery, Washington, D.C.: War Department, Adjutant General's Office, 1944.
- *Zarit Burden Interview* by S.H. Zarit, N.K. Orr, and J.M. Zarit, in *The hidden victims of Alzheimer's disease: Families under stress*, 84, New York: New York University Press, 1985.
- *Zung Depression Status Inventory* by W.W.K. Zung, in A self-rating depression scale, *Archives of General Psychiatry* 12 (1965): 63–70.

PROBLEMS

Note: Dementia is a variable condition that can be exhibited in numerous groups of symptoms; therefore, there is no "typical" pattern of problems. Both the type and severity of symptoms vary because of the many and sometimes multiple causes of dementia.

Self-Care

- The person's habits of self-care usually deteriorate.
- In the later stages of dementia, the person may be unable to perform self-care activities.

Productivity

- The person may be unable to perform productive occupations.
- The person may neglect job tasks unless he or she is supervised.
- The person may require supervision to perform any productive occupation.

Leisure

- The person may lose interest in leisure activities.
- The person may be unable to perform activities previously enjoyed.

Sensorimotor

- The person may have apraxia or difficulty performing motor activities even though the sensory motor function is intact and the person understands the requirements of the task.
- Limb rigidity may be present.
- Flexed posture may occur.
- The person may have agnosia or difficulty recognizing familiar objects in spite of intact sensory capacities.
- The person may be apraxic and have difficulty with motor planning.
- The person may have spatial or topographic disorientation and thus get lost easily even in familiar surroundings.

Types of Presenile Dementias

In addition to Alzheimer's disease, Parkinson's disease, and Huntington's disease, the following disorders may be seen:

Binswanger disease—progressive arteriosclerotic disorder marked by unsteady gait, urinary incontinence, memory and emotional disorders, convulsions and hallucinations, typically appearing in ages 50s and 60s.

Joseph disease—a neurological disorder characterized by progressive unsteady gait, spasticity and rigidity of the lower limbs, impaired vision, slow speech and dystonia of the head, face, trunk and extremities.

Hallervorden-Spatz syndrome (HSS)—marked by muscle tone disorders, involuntary movements and progressive dementia, with early symptoms appearing in childhood and adolescence.

Olivopontocerebellar atrophy (OPCA)—a chronic progressive ataxia characterized by progressive cerebellar atrophy with ataxic disorders of the trunk and limbs, equilibrium and gait disorders, tremors and dysphagia.

Seitelberger syndrome—a ganglioside storage disorder characterized by petit or grand mal seizures and cyclonic jerks, blindness, incoordination and tremors. Most patients die between ages 4 and 8 years.

Creutsfeldt-Jakob—classified as a "slow virus" characterized in the early stages by failing memory, changes in behavior, lack of coordination, or visual disturbances. Mental deterioration becomes more pronounced as the disease progresses, and involuntary movements appear. The person may become blind, develop weakness in the arms or legs and ultimately lapse into a coma.

Pick's disease—characterized by slowly progressive deterioration of social skills and changes in personality leading to impairment to intellect, memory loss, lack of spontaneity, difficulty in thinking or concentrating, speech disturbances, loss of moral judgment and progressive dementia.

Source: Data from C. Stahl, Presenile Dementias are Rare Disorders, *Advance for Occupational Therapists*, Vol. 12, No. 34, p. 14, © 1996, Merion Publications, Inc.

Cognitive

- Familiar tasks may be performed well but learning new skills is very difficult.
- The person is distractible and his or her attention span is short.
- The person's ability for conceptual thinking is decreased.
- The person may have poverty of thought.
- The person's recent memory impairment increases, beginning with problems recalling recent events or remembering names (registration of information).
- The person's remote memory may be spared in fixed dementia but becomes involved in progressive dementia. Problems are due to difficulty with retention and recall.

- The person may have acute episodes of severe confusion, especially in response to a stressful situation.
- The person may confabulate (recite imaginary events to fill in for gaps in memory).
- The person may have difficulty with executive functions or metacognition.
- The person may have aphasia (impairment of language), including receptive aphasia (inability to understand spoken or written language) and expressive aphasia (impairment in use of verbal and written language).

Psychosocial
- The person may become depressed.
- The person may become anxious or restless.
- The person may show signs of paranoia.
- The person's insight usually is impaired.
- The person's judgment usually is impaired.
- The person's affect may be exaggerated and then become blunted or flat.
- The person's initiative usually decreases.
- Changes in the person's personality structure may occur.
- The person may have acute episodes of severe emotional disturbance, especially in response to a stressful situation.
- The person may be aware of decreasing abilities and suffer loss of self-esteem.
- The person may lose social interaction skills.
- The person may demonstrate echolalia (parroting words or phrases said by others).
- The person may demonstrate palilalia (repeating part or all of a sentence while speaking).
- The person may speak nonsensical sentences or include jargon (a string of nonsense words) in a sentence.
- The person may become mute.
- The caregiver may report being anxious, having sleeping problems, or feeling depressed.

TREATMENT/INTERVENTION

Models of treatment include the medical model, family-oriented approach, stress theory, ecologic-behavioral, competence-environmental press, and disablement model. Models of treatment in occupational therapy include the Five Stage Model, reactivating model (Bach et al. 1995), model of human occupation.

Self-Care
- Develop and maintain a routine of daily living tasks.
- Printing a schedule of the tasks may be helpful. Pictures or photographs may help.
- Printing a sequence of steps to perform routine tasks, such as brushing teeth or putting on clothes, may be helpful. Use line drawings or simple pictures if the person no longer comprehends printed text.
- Imitation of gestures or verbal or tactile cues can be used to accomplish some self-care activities.
- If the person wears inappropriate clothing, the caregiver may select clothing and put it out for the person or hand the items to the person one at a time in the correct order.

- Expect difficulty in learning any new routines in the later stages of the disorder. Anticipate needed changes early, when learning is still possible.

Productivity

- Provide constant or frequent supervision if the person is helping with household activities or volunteering services.
- Alert the family that even activities that have been done many times by the person may be performed poorly because of memory lapses and inattention. For example, baking cookies: The person may have baked cookies successfully for 50 years but now leaves out some critical ingredients. Suggest doing the activity together so that the person can be monitored.

Leisure

If reading is a favorite activity of the person, be aware that his or her comprehension is decreasing. Short stories may work better than novels, and more photos and less text may be better. Talking books may aid comprehension.

Sensorimotor

- Plan activities that are within the person's level of function.
- Emphasize gross motor rather than fine motor activities.
- Use familiar rather than novel movements.
- Provide sensory stimuli, including nightlights, a radio, or television; avoid sensory deprivation but do not overstimulate the person.
- Maintain familiar settings when possible to help with spatial orientation.
- Minimize distractions, such as the background noise of a radio or television during a treatment session. Reduce visual distractions too, if possible.
- Be aware of sensory deficits. Make sure that persons who need glasses are wearing them, and that hearing aids are functioning.
- Use visual cues such as pictures, labels, or name cards to facilitate recognition and reminiscing.

Cognitive

- Improve the person's quality of life by providing opportunities for him or her to engage in purposeful activity.
- Keep explanations brief and simple. Use short, simple, and concrete statements that are literal and direct.
- Give one instruction at a time and repeat it if necessary. Break complex activities into simple, easy-to-follow steps.
- Ask questions that can be answered with yes or no to reduce the problem of trying to organize ideas for a response.
- Use calendars and clocks to help orient the person to time.
- Call the person by name or touch the person and establish eye contact to get his or her attention before giving instructions.
- Expect poor recall of the treatment program. Review any instructions that must be followed from one treatment session to the next.
- Compile a photo album of the person's family members and other significant images, such as homes or businesses, to use as a memory aid and point of discussion.

- Anticipate poor independent practice of exercises or activities at home. The caregiver will need to monitor exercises in a home program.
- Anticipate denial of the disability. The person may be unaware of his or her limitations.

Psychosocial

- Increase social interactions to decrease social isolation.
- Plan activities within the person's level of function.
- Include the person in any discussion about his or her condition with caregivers. Do not speak as if the person were not aware of what is happening.
- Be aware that the person may comprehend nonverbal gestures much longer than verbal language. Monitor your facial expressions and tone of voice to project positive signals.
- To promote group interaction, compile a photo album that includes the photographs and names of group members.
- Anticipate the need to interpret what the person says. Rephrase the message and ask for confirmation rather than ignoring a rambling sentence.

Environment

- Provide activities that are culturally appropriate and meaningful to the person or group. Example: For a group of African Americans, Baum et al. (1996) found that good group activities included singing gospel music, Bible discussions, storytelling groups on holiday traditions, fashion shows, exercise sessions, and competitive games such as pool and bingo.
- Clearly label physical structures, with unique symbols if possible. Numbers or names should appear on doors. Arrows can help with directions.
- Increase lighting to promote safety, especially in hallways and entrances.
- Physical objects can be modified to improve performance and increase safety; for example, unplugging or disabling dangerous appliances, removing clutter, removing unnecessary objects from the living environment, placing the bed next to a wall (the person sleeps next to the wall, the caregiver away from wall, so the caregiver will wake up if the person gets out of bed).
- Tasks can be simplified to minimize the complexity of the environment and its demands on task performance. Examples include verbal coaching or written and tactile cueing by caregivers.
- Assistive devices—such as grab bars, safety locks, commodes, tub benches, shower seats, detachable shower hoses, stair glides, and monitoring systems—can be helpful.
- Environmental modification is expensive, but it may be necessary; for example, adding alarms to bathroom doors and outside doors that sound if the door is opened, widening doors, reconstructing rooms, or installing ramps or stair rails to improve safety.
- Gitlin, Corcoran, and Leinmiller-Eckhardt (1995) suggest that occupational therapists can use four ethnographic principles in working with caregivers: (1) informant (provide knowledge); (2) emic (uncover personal meaning); (3) reflexivity (facilitate hypothesis development, test and question); interpretation (analyze and implement treatment).
- Increase the caregiver's sense of efficacy through increased problem-solving and coping skills by increasing his or her knowledge of available resources, such as support group, and by educating the caregiver about management techniques for dealing with the person who has dementia.

- Permit caregivers to express emotions and frustrations in one-on-one sessions or in a support group, but avoid focusing only on negative aspects, which may promote feelings of hopelessness, helplessness, and despair. Include the strategy of counting one's blessings for the positive feelings and experiences of the caregiver with the person who has dementia.
- Focus the caregiver away from blaming others, or wishful thinking that directs responsibility away from the caregiver.
- Provide information on community resources such as respite care, so the caregiver can take a break from the 24-hour-per-day care requirements and run errands.

PRECAUTIONS

- The person should not be left unattended.
- Lock up, restrict access to, or remove hazardous items such as electrical appliances and tools, knives, medications (including vitamin pills), car keys, cleaning fluids, and guns. Use child-proof doorknobs and locks on cabinets.
- Cover burners on the stove or remove the knobs.
- Install nightlights in hallways and bathrooms to provide illumination for night trips to the bathroom. Increase light in all locations where the person carries out activities in the home.
- Install locks on all doors that lead outside and install alarms to alert the caregiver to the person's location.
- Have the person wear an identification bracelet in case he or she gets lost and cannot tell anyone who she is or where he belongs.
- Avoid teasing the person, as he or she may not comprehend the intent or meaning.
- Avoid high-level humor, such as plays on words; the person may not understand and may think someone is making fun of him or her.
- Avoid being overly optimistic about his or her condition. State the facts to family and caregivers.
- Avoid situations in which the caregiver perceives a problem as someone's else's doing. Encourage the caregiver to take action and try to resolve problems.

PROGNOSIS

The prognosis is not good. The person's course usually continues downhill until death, which may occur within a few years or after many years. However, intervention can teach the individual and the family or other caregivers how to compensate for the person's loss of cognitive skills to reduce the impact of the decline.

- The person is able to perform motor skills consistent with the stage of the disorder.
- The person is aware and registers sensory input in all major senses consistent with the stage of the disorder.
- The person is able to remember and to orient him- or herself using assistive devices or techniques consistent with the stage of the disorder.
- The person has maintained social skills consistent with the stage of the disorder.
- The person is able to perform daily living skills using assistive devices or techniques, as needed, in a supervised environment consistent with the stage of the disorder.
- The person is able to perform productive activities consistent with the stage of the disorder.
- The person is able to perform leisure activities consistent with the stage of the disorder.

Activities in Reactivating Occupational Therapy Program

- Animals and plants
- Birds and insects
- Cities and countryside
- Clothes—textiles and materials
- Colors
- Cooking with eggs
- Different professions
- Food and drink—preparing a meal
- Foreign countries
- Gardens—flowers, fruits, vegetables
- Holidays—Christmas, Easter
- Learning and playing group games
- Leisure activities
- Music—listening, performing
- My family
- My hometown
- Seasons—calendars and timetables, associations such as poems or songs
- Sun, moon, and stars
- Weather reports

Source: Bach et al., Reactivating occupational therapy, a method to improve cognition performance in geriatric patients, *Age and Aging*, Vol. 24, p. 223, reproduced by permission of Oxford University Press, 1995.

- The person's living environment has been modified to provide maximum opportunity for independence consistent with safety considerations.
- The person and the caregiver demonstrate knowledge of community resources, such as mobile meal programs, self-help groups, and respite care.

REFERENCES

American Psychiatric Association. 1994. *Diagnostic and Statistical Manual of Mental Disorders: DSM-IV,* 4th ed. Washington, DC: American Psychiatric Association. Task Force on DSM-IV.

Bach, D., et al. 1995. Reactivating occupational therapy: A method to improve cognitive performance in geriatric patients. *Age and Aging* 24:222–226.

Baum, C.M., et al. 1996. An activity program for cognitively impaired low-income inner city residents. *Topics in Geriatric Rehabilitation* 12, no. 2:54–62.

Beers, M.H., and R. Berkow, eds. 1999. *The Merck Manual of Diagnosis and Therapy,* 17th ed. Whitehouse Station, NJ: Merck Research Laboratories.

Gitlin, L.N., M. Corcoran, and S. Leinmiller-Eckhardt. 1995. Understanding the family perspective: An ethnographic framework for providing occupational therapy in the home. *American Journal of Occupational Therapy* 49, no. 8:802–809.

BIBLIOGRAPHY

American Occupational Therapy Association. 1996. Occupational therapy services for persons with Alzheimer's disease and other dementias. In *Reference Manual of the Official Documents of the American Occupational Therapy Association, 297–302.* Bethesda, MD: American Occupational Therapy Association.

Batt-Leiba, M.I., et al. 1998. Implications of coping strategies for spousal caregivers of elders with dementia. *Topics in Geriatric Rehabilitation* 14, no. 1:54–63.

Butin, D.N., et al. 1996. COPE (caregiver options for practical experiences): An activity group for caregivers with relatives with dementia. In *ROTE: The role of occupational therapy with the elderly,* 2nd ed., eds. K.O. Larsen et al., 597–609. Bethesda, MD: American Occupational Therapy Association.

Cartwright, D.L., H.M. Madill, and S. Dennis. 1996. Cognitive impairment and functional performance of patients admitted to a geriatric assessment and rehabilitation center. *Physical and Occupational Therapy in Geriatrics* 14, no. 3:1–21.

Decker, M.R. 1996. Evaluating the client with dementia. *Mental Health Special Interest Section Newsletter* 19, no. 4:1–2.

Elliot, S.J. 1997. Collaboration of treatment to enhance functioning of persons with dementia: A case study. *Gerontology Special Interest Section Newsletter* 20, no. 2:1–2.

Gitlin, L.N., and Corcoran, M.A. 1996. Managing dementia at home: The role of home environment modifications. *Topics in Geriatric Rehabilitation* 12, no. 2:28–39.

Glogoski-Williams, C., D. Foti, and M. Covalt. 1998. Dementia. In *Psychosocial occupational therapy: A clinical practice,* eds. E. Cara and A. MacRae, 199–226. Albany, NY: Delmar.

Gregory, S. 1996. Memory maintenance groups in the community. *British Journal of Occupational Therapy* 59, no. 1:25–26.

Hasselkus, B.R. 1994. Occupational programming in a day hospital for patients with dementia (commentary). *Occupational Therapy Journal of Research* 14, no. 4:239–243.

Josephsson, S., et al. 1995. Effectiveness of an intervention to improve occupational performance in dementia. *Occupational Therapy Journal of Research* 15, no. 1:36–49.

Josephsson, S., et al. 1993. Supporting everyday activities in dementia: An intervention study. *International Journal of Geriatric Psychiatry* 8:395–400.

Levy, L.L. 1998. The cognitive disabilities model in rehabilitation of older adults with dementia. In *Cognition and occupation in rehabilitation: Cognitive models for intervention in occupational therapy,* ed. N. Katz, 195–221. Bethesda, MD: American Occupational Therapy Association.

Law, P., G. Coffey, and R. Zamora. 1995. Caring for clients with dementia. *OT Week* 9, no. 42:18–19.

Maddox, M., and T. Burns. 1997. Positive approaches to dementia care in the home. *Geriatrics* 52, suppl. 2:S54–58.

Nygard, L., et al. 1994. Comparing motor and process ability of persons with suspected dementia in home and clinic settings. *American Journal of Occupational Therapy* 48, no. 8:689–696.

Robichaud, L., R. Herbert, and J. Desrosiers. 1994. Efficacy of a sensory integration program on behaviors of inpatients with dementia. *American Journal of Occupational Therapy* 48, no. 4:355–360.

Rogers, J.C., et al. 1994. Stability and change in functional assessment of patients with geropsychiatric disorders. *American Journal of Occupational Therapy* 48, no. 10:914–918.

Ross, M. 1994. Attempts to study Ross's five-stage group program are welcome (letter; comment). *American Journal of Occupational Therapy* 48, no. 11:1112.

Sainty, M. 1993. Dementia: The marriage relationship and the concept of relief. *British Journal of Occupational Therapy* 56, no. 7:238–242.

Stahl, C. 1996. Presenile dementias are rare disorders. *Advance for Occupational Therapists* 12, no. 34:14.

Walsh, P.G., et al. 1995. The effects of a "pets as therapy" dog on persons with dementia in a psychiatric ward. *Australian Occupational Therapy Journal* 42, no. 4:161–166.

Part XI

Mental Disorders

Anxiety Disorders

DESCRIPTION

Anxiety disorders are a group of disorders in which anxiety or anxiousness are central features. Anxiety is defined as apprehension of danger and dread accompanied by restlessness, tension, tachycardia, and dyspnea unattached to a clearly identifiable situation (Stedman 1995). The DSM-IV delineates five broad categories of anxiety disorders: panic disorders (two types), phobic disorders (three types), obsessive-compulsive disorder (one type), posttraumatic stress disorders (one type), and anxiety states (four types). Panic disorders usually begin in late adolescence or early adulthood. Phobic disorders usually begin early in life and are common in children and younger adults. Obsessive-compulsive disorder is common throughout life including children, adults, and the aged. Posttraumatic stress disorders (PTSDs) usually occur as a reaction to natural disasters, sexual abuse, violent crime, or war experiences and thus are associated with childhood and young adults. (See section on PTSD.) General and specific anxiety states are most common in older adults. Anxiety disorders are reported as Axis I disorders on the multiaxial assessment scale.

CAUSE

The causes of anxiety disorders depend on which theory of psychodynamics is consulted.

ASSESSMENT

Areas

- daily living skills
- productivity values, tasks, and skills
- leisure interests and skills
- problem-solving skills
- time management
- role performance and skills
- social skills

Instruments

Instruments Developed by Occupational Therapy Personnel

- *Activity Configuration* by V.B. Levitt, in Anxiety disorders, *Psychosocial occupational therapy: A clinical practice,* eds. E. Cara and A. MacRae, 383, Albany, NY: Delmar, 1998.
- *Role Checklist,* 2nd ed., by F. Oakley, Bethesda, MD: Occupational Therapy Service, National Institutes of Health, 1988.
- *Self-Assessment of Activities* by V.B. Levitt, in Anxiety disorders, *Psychosocial occupational therapy: A clinical practice,* eds. E. Cara and A. MacRae, 382, Albany, NY: Delmar, 1998.

Instrument Developed by Other Professionals and Used by Occupational Therapy Personnel

- *Function Questionnaire,* adapted from the Fear Questionnaire by B. Taylor and B. Arnow, in *The nature and treatment of anxiety disorders,* New York: Free Press, 1988.

PROBLEMS

Self-Care

- The person may experience increased cardiovascular symptoms such as heart rate, tachycardia, chest pain, and pressure.
- The person may experience gastrointestinal symptoms such as diarrhea, constipation, nausea, vomiting, gas, cramps, or loss of appetite, or may eat excessive amounts of food.
- The person may experience respiratory symptoms such as dyspnea (shortness of breath) or choking sensation.
- The person may experience a more frequent and urgent need to urinate.
- The person may experience sexual dysfunction such as loss of libido, premature ejaculation, or amenorrhea.
- The person may experience automatic symptoms such as sweating, flushing, dry mouth, dizziness, and fainting.
- The person may complain that he or she is unable to perform certain self-care skills or that certain tasks must be performed in a ritualistic way.
- The person may have sleep disturbances that leave him or her too fatigued to participate in therapy sessions.

Productivity

- The person may complain that he or she is unable to perform certain productivity skills or that certain tasks must be performed in a ritualistic way. For example, the person may be chronically late or unable to maintain a normal work schedule, or work may be inaccurate.
- The person may not perform important tasks related to homemaking or parenting, such as meal preparation or getting the children ready for school.

Leisure

The person may give up leisure interests and activities because of difficulty in performing certain aspects or tasks of the activity.

Sensorimotor

- The person may demonstrate restlessness and an inability to stay seated or attentive.
- The person may experience muscle tension sufficient to cause pain in the neck and headache.

Cognitive

- The person may be confused.
- The person may have poor memory.
- The person may be easily distractible with poor concentration.
- The person may have thought blocking.

- The person may have loss of perspective or cognitive distortion, including catastrophic thinking and negative self-evaluation.
- The person may have obsessive thoughts.
- The person may have fears of loss of control, going crazy, injury, death, and not coping.
- The person may have poor problem-solving abilities.
- The person may look preoccupied.

Psychosocial

- The person may complain of feeling uneasy or off balance.
- The person may complain of feeling overwhelmed.
- The person may feel a sense of impending doom.
- The person may feel helpless and out of control.
- The person may feel that he or she is going insane.
- The person may have feelings of depersonalization (unreality).
- The person may have feelings of derealization (feeling detached from one's surroundings).
- The person may become overactive, restless, or agitated.
- The person may become immobile and withdrawn.
- The person may be excessively worried about loved ones, personal health, and impending catastrophes.
- The person may become irritable when others are nearby and, in a health care setting, may refuse to participate in treatment sessions.

TREATMENT/INTERVENTION

Self-Care, Productivity, and Leisure

- Functional behavior training—carry out a behavioral training program that deals directly with improving functioning or performance by decreasing symptoms associated with that daily activity.
- Graded activity and activity analysis—help the person identify target behavior and then break the behavior into smaller, more manageable units.

Sensorimotor

- Relaxation training—including breathing exercises, progressive muscle relaxation, visualization, and autogenic training. The purpose is to diminish arousal state, increase feelings of well-being, and prevent anxiety attacks. The program begins with external directions, but the goal is to teach the client self-directed use of the technique.
- Breathing exercises—the person learns to self-monitor breathing by placing the hands on the abdomen and watching the hands rise on inhalation and fall with exhalation as the person slows and deepens his or her breathing rate. The technique should be introduced slowly to avoid lightheadedness from increased oxygen consumption. Imagery may be used to help the person focus on breathing.
- Progressive muscle relaxation—teach a person to slowly, methodically, and progressively tighten and release voluntary muscle groups to control states of tension and relaxation.

- Visualization—the person is directed to close the eyes and picture the self in a pleasant scene. The technique can be combined with breathing exercises, and the addition of soothing music may help evoke images. Some people can learn to do this themselves, but others will need verbal guidance. The technique should not be used with persons who have perceptual distortions (hallucinations) or thought disorders (delusions).
- Autogenic training—a method of teaching the person to relax through self-directed verbal commands, developed by Schultz and Luthe (1969).
- Alexander technique—teaches "use" and "misuse" of the body while carrying out an action or posture (Gelb 1981).
- Mitchell technique—based on the principles of reciprocal inhibition relating to voluntary movement, so that agonist muscle groups move the body part into a more relaxed position (Mitchell 1977).

Cognitive

- Education/lifestyle alterations—instructing the person about external environmental influences on internal feelings; for example, increased caffeine intake or side effects of over-the-counter drug, which might increase anxiety, and regular exercise and a balanced diet, which might decrease anxiety.
- Rational/cognitive approaches—helping the person replace negative statements about him- or herself with more positive statements. This technique is usually most successful when the statements are written down.
- Time management—the person learns how to organize time and increase productive activity using a graphic or written format. Help the person prioritize activities according to their importance.

Psychosocial

- Assertiveness training and social skills training can be used to identify irrational beliefs and fears about social situations and to practice through role-playing in a controlled environment.
- Expressive activities, including journal writing and structured craft and art activities, provide for physical and emotional outlet and release.
- Journal and diary writing provide a symbolic act of writing down concerns and feelings that may help the individual become better able to understand and cope with feelings.
- Structured crafts provide limits through repetition, true boundaries, and predictable outcome. Examples are mosaics, plastic "stained glass," and presketched coloring canvases or sheets.
- Expressive activities offer a release of tension through physical activity such as ripping paper or cloth, using a stippling brush for painting, or drawing with felt pens on a large paper canvas.

Environment

Community mobility and reentry to learn how to locate, make contact, and participate in community resources that are related to the person's interests.

PRECAUTIONS

Visualization and guided imagery techniques should not be used with persons who are experiencing visual hallucinations or delusions, because the technique may increase the intensity of those symptoms.

PROGNOSIS AND OUTCOME

- The person is able to perform daily activities in a manner that controls or does not elicit anxiety.
- The person is able to perform homemaking tasks and go to work and perform work tasks by controlling the effects of anxiety.
- The person participates in leisure activities of choice.
- The person is able to plan a daily schedule that allows all necessary tasks to be completed.
- The person is able to attend and concentrate on a task for the time necessary to complete it.
- The person can demonstrate self-management techniques, such as relaxation exercises, for the control of anxiety symptoms.
- The person is able to participate in social situations without having panic attacks.
- The person is able to go out into the neighborhood and community, for example, to the grocery store, church, or a movie theater.

REFERENCES

American Psychiatric Association. 1994. *Diagnostic and Statistical Manual of Mental Disorders: DSM-IV*, 4th ed. Washington, DC: American Psychiatric Association. Task Force on DSM-IV.

Gelb, M. 1981. *Body Learning*. London: Aurum Press.

Mitchell, L. 1977. *Simple Relaxation*. London: John Murray.

Schultz, J.M., and W. Luthe. 1969. *Autogenic Therapy, Vol. 1. Autogenic Methods*. New York: Grune & Stratton.

Stedman's Medical Dictionary. 1995. Baltimore, MD: Williams & Wilkins.

BIBLIOGRAPHY

Bonder, B.R. 1995. Anxiety disorders. In *Psychopathology and function*, 2nd ed., ed. B.R. Bonder, 129–142. Thorofare, NJ: Slack.

Drake, L.M., and P.L. Barnett. 1998. Working with elders who have psychiatric conditions—Anxiety. In *Occupational therapy with elders: Strategies for the COTA*, eds. L. Lohman, R.L. Padilla, and S. Byers-Connon, 239–240. St. Louis: Mosby.

Keable, D. 1997. *The management of anxiety: A guide for therapists*, 2nd ed. New York: Churchill Livingstone.

Levitt, V.B. 1998. Anxiety disorders. In *Psychosocial occupational therapy: A clinical practice*, eds. E. Cara and A. MacRae, 139–404. Albany, NY: Delmar.

Marmer, L. 1995. Anxiety disorders can wreak havoc on ADL. *Advance for Occupational Therapists* 11, no. 32: 19.

Morgan-Brown, M. 1997. An association of the asymmetrical tonic neck reflex (ATNR) and agoraphobia and panic attacks. *British Journal of Occupational Therapy* 60, no. 5: 223–225.

Depression and Manic (Mood) Disorders

DESCRIPTION

Mood disorders are a group of heterogeneous, typically recurrent illnesses including unipolar (depressive) and bipolar (manic-depressive) disorders that are characterized by pervasive mood disturbance, psychomotor dysfunction, and vegetative symptoms (Merck 1999, 1525). Mood disorders used to be classified as affective disorders.

Depression, in a clinical sense, is a psychopathologic state in which the disturbance of mood or affect is characterized by agitation, weight loss, guilt, insomnia, decreased activity, and an inability to experience pleasure. The state may be part of a bipolar disorder in which depression alternates with mania, or the condition may be unipolar, in which depression is the major disorder. Many terms and expressions are used to describe episodes of depression: the blues; melancholia; dysthymia; unipolar disorder; bipolar II disorder; endogenous, involutional, and reactive.

Mania is characterized by expansiveness, elation, agitation, hyperexcitability, hyperactivity, and increased speed of thought and speech (flight of ideas); it can be seen in manic bipolar disorder (Dorland 1988, 978). Mania may also be described as hypomania or bipolar I disorder.

Mood disorders, including depression, are classified as Axis I disorders on the multiaxial assessment scale. If the mood disorder is caused by a general medical condition, that condition should be listed with the mood disorder on Axis I and specifically named and listed on Axis III.

CAUSE

The cause may be singular or multiple, depending on the theory. Psychoanalytic theories view depression as a result of the loss of a loved object. Behavioral theories that emphasize reinforcement view depression as the result of negative person-environment interaction. Behavioral theories that emphasize cognition view depression as the result of negative cognitive patterns of thinking. Biochemical theories focus on depression as the result of decreased neurotransmitter amines at the synaptic junction. Sociologic theories focus on life roles, the stresses related to these roles, and the individual's ability to cope with stress. Existential theories view depression as an inability to find meaning in life. About one in four persons experiences some form of affective disturbance in his or her lifetime. Women are affected more frequently than men. Bipolar disorders usually begin in the person's teens, 20s, or 30s. Unipolar forms occur throughout the person's lifespan.

ASSESSMENT

Areas

- daily living skills
- productivity history, skills, and interests

- leisure skills and interests
- postural control and balance
- posture during gross motor activities
- physical fitness and endurance
- fine motor skills, manipulation, dexterity, and bilateral coordination
- perceptual skills
- attending behavior
- attention span and concentration
- understanding and following direction
- memory
- problem solving and decision making
- conceptualization
- categorization
- organizational skills—time and materials
- ability to abstract
- mood or affect
- self-concept
- independence or dependence
- goals and values
- communication skills
- social roles

Instruments

Instruments Developed by Occupational Therapy Personnel

- *Adolescent Role Assessment* by M. Black, *American Journal of Occupational Therapy* 30 (1976): 73–79.
- *Allen Cognitive Level Test* by C.K. Allen, in *Occupational therapy for psychiatric diseases: Measurement and management of cognitive disabilities*, ed. C.K. Allen, 108–113, Boston: Little, Brown & Co, 1985.
- *Canadian Occupational Performance Measure* (COPM), 2nd ed., by M. Law et al., Ottawa, Ontario, Canada: Canadian Association of Occupational Therapists, 1994.
- *The Interest Checklist* by J. Matsutsuyu, in The interest checklist, *American Journal of Occupational Therapy* 23, no. 4 (1969): 323–328.
- *Kohlman Evaluation of Living Skills*, 3rd ed., by L. Kohlman-Thomson, Rockville, MD: American Occupational Therapy Association, 1992.
- *Milwaukee Evaluation of Daily Living Skills* by C.A. Leonardelli, Thorofare, NJ: Slack, 1988.
- *Occupational Case Analysis Interview and Rating Scale* by K.L. Kaplan and G. Kielhofner, Thorofare, NJ: Slack, 1989.
- *Occupational Questionnaire* by N. Riopel, G. Kielhofner, and J. Watts, in The relationship between volition, activity patterns, and life satisfaction in the elderly, *American Journal of Occupational Therapy* 40, no. 4 (1986): 278–283.
- *Performance Assessment of Self-Care Skills*, rev 3.1 (PASS) by J. Rogers and M.B. Holm, WPIC #1237, 3811 O'Hara Street, Pittsburgh, PA 15213.

- *Scorable Self-Care Evaluation*, rev. ed., by M. Peters and N. Clark, Thorofare, NJ: Slack, 1993.

Instruments Developed by Other Professionals and Used by Occupational Therapy Personnel

- *Beck Anxiety Inventory* by A.T. Beck, N. Epstein, and G. Brown, in An inventory for measuring clinical anxiety, *Journal of Clinical Psychology* 56 (1988): 892–897.
- *Beck Depression Inventory*, rev., by A. Beck, in Internal consistencies of the original and revised Beck Depression Inventory, *Journal of Clinical Psychology* 40, no. 6 (1984): 1365–1367.
- *Burns Depression Checklist* by D. Burns, *The feeling good handbook: The new mood therapy,* New York: Plume/Penguin, 1989.
- *Dysfunctional Attitudes Scale* by D. Burns, *Feeling good: The new mood therapy,* 241–255, New York: Signet Penguin, 1980.
- *Future Time Perspective Inventory* by L.K. Heimberg, in The measurement of future time perspective, *Dissertation Abstracts International* (University Microfilms No. 63–7346), 1963.
- *Internal-External Locus of Control Scale* by J.B. Rotter, in Generalized expectancies for internal versus external control of reinforcement, *Psychological Monographs* 80 (1966): 1–28.
- *Multidimensional Observation Scale for Elderly Subjects* (MOSES) by E. Helmes, R.G. Caspo, and J.A. Short, *Journal of Gerontology* 42 (1987): 395–405.
- *Older Americans Resource and Services Multidimensional Functional Assessment* by Duke University Center for the Study on Aging, in *Multidimensional Functional Assessment: The OARS Methodology*, 2nd ed., Durham, NC: Duke University Press, 1978.
- *Pleasant Events Schedule III* by D.J. MacPhillamy and P.M. Lewinsohn, in The pleasant events schedule: Studies on reliability, validity, and scale intercorrelation, *Journal of Consulting and Clinical Psychology* 50 (1982): 363–380.
- *Self-Esteem Scale* by M. Rosenberg, in *Society and the adolescent self-image,* Princeton, NJ: Princeton University Press, 1965.
- *Social Readjustment Rating Scale* by T.H. Homes and R.H. Rahe, *Journal of Psychosomatic Research* 11 (1967): 216.

PROBLEMS

Self-Care
Depression

- The person is usually disinterested in most activities of daily living.
- The person may refuse to eat, become anorexic, or lose weight.
- The person may have insomnia and awaken early in the morning.

Mania

- The person may go on a buying spree and buy many things that are not needed or are very expensive. The person may reach the spending limit on all credit cards owned and be overdrawn at the bank.
- The person may make foolish investments.
- The person may engage in sexual indiscretions because of increased sexual desire.
- The person has a decreased need for sleep and may stay up for many hours or sleep only two or three hours a night.

Productivity

Depression

The person may be unable to perform job tasks.

Mania

- The person may complete work tasks in record time.
- The person may accomplish many tasks much more quickly than normal (which may irritate coworkers who object to a person who appears to be a "brown noser").

Leisure

Depression

The person may lose interest in leisure activities he or she used to enjoy.

Mania

The person is interested in many activities.

Sensorimotor

Depression

- The person may exhibit psychomotor retardation (difficulty initiating the action of moving the body or parts of the body).
- The person may have psychomotor agitation with restlessness and wringing of the hands.
- The person may lack physical endurance and may tire easily.
- The person may have hallucinations; auditory and visual hallucinations are the most common, but occasionally tactile or olfactory hallucinations occur as well.

Mania

- The person may have psychomotor acceleration and move very quickly.
- The person may give the impression of physical fitness but may actually be losing weight from increased activity and inattention to proper dietary habits.
- The person may have fleeting auditory or visual hallucinations.

Cognitive

Depression

- The person may have difficulty attending to a task.
- The person may express recurrent thoughts of death and suicide.

- The person may have difficulty making decisions and solving problems.
- The person may have difficulty finding activities of interest.

Mania
- The person is interested in new activities but does not complete existing tasks.
- The person has a short attention span and is very distractable.

Psychosocial

Depression
- The person may have a poor self-concept or be self-denigrating.
- The person may express feelings of helplessness and hopelessness.
- The person may be preoccupied with feelings of guilt.
- The person may be unable to feel or express emotions.
- The person may express fear of going insane or losing his or her mind.
- The person may be irritable.
- The person may appear agitated.
- The person may lack self-confidence.
- The person may be dependent.
- The person may express feelings of worthlessness.
- The person may cry for no apparent reason or say that he or she doesn't feel any emotion.
- The person may become socially withdrawn.
- The person may not speak at all or may speak with great effort.

Mania
- The person may demonstrate inflated self-esteem and boast of skills or accomplishments.
- The person may be elated, irritable, or hostile.
- The person may have racing thoughts or clang associations.
- The person may increase his or her involvement with others in ways that are inappropriate, and thus other people may be alienated by the person's intrusive and meddlesome behavior.
- The person may have delusions of exceptional talent or physical fitness.
- The person may have delusions of wealth, aristocratic ancestry, or other grandiose identity.
- The person may not take responsibility for the consequences of his or her behavior.

TREATMENT/INTERVENTION

General models of treatment include cognitive therapy. Models of treatment in occupational therapy include the model of human occupation.

Self-Care (Both Depression and Mania)
- Express expectations that the person will perform activities of daily living.
- Help the person reestablish normal routines: structured planning of daily occupations, making and following simple behavioral lists.
- Provide instruction in daily living skills, such as money management, locating living quarters, shopping, or preparing meals.

Productivity (Both Depression and Mania)
- Encourage the person to participate in home-management tasks. The family can be encouraged to assign specific tasks for the person to perform.
- If the person is working, explore career goals and interests.
- If the person is retired, explore the possibility of volunteer activities.

Leisure (Both Depression and Mania)
Encourage the person to explore interests and develop enjoyable leisure activities.

Sensorimotor
Depression
- Increase the person's energy through participation in activities, including recreation.
- Maintain or increase sensory stimulation through participation in activities.

Mania
Encourage the person to help in appraising and reflecting on the amount of energy expended in constructive, goal-directed activities and occupations as opposed to non-goal-directed activities.

Cognitive
Depression
- Initially limit choices and gradually provide opportunities to make more choices, solve problems, and make decisions, for example, in the selection of color, type of activity, or amount of time devoted to an activity.
- Provide opportunities to successfully accomplish short-term, simple, concrete activities.
- Set realistic, step-by-step goals and create behavioral "to do" lists.
- Engage the person in recognizing, monitoring, and changing thoughts.
- Help the person perform reality testing and question unrealistic beliefs.
- Provide instruction in time management and activity scheduling.
- Provide learning groups that discuss subjects such as problems of depression, growing old, and managing emotions.

Mania
- Provide opportunities for the person to engage in concrete, short-term activities during initial treatment sessions.
- Provide clear expectations for expected behavior and end products.
- Refocus the person on goal-directed action when he or she becomes distracted.
- Encourage the person to help in goal setting and planning, and in anticipating the consequences of actions by monitoring behavior during activities.

Psychosocial
Depression
- Engage the person in activities that he or she values.
- Provide opportunities for the person to engage in more than one activity.

- Increase self-concept (self-mastery, sense of competence, self-confidence) through creative activities—such as art, crafts, drama, dance, or music—that can result in task accomplishment.
- Provide training in stress reduction, including discussion about life stresses, assertion, and relaxation training.
- Relate present activities to immediate feelings and goals to increase concept of purposeful activity and goal-directed behavior.
- Provide opportunities to develop social skills and participate in group activities through structured task groups, discussion groups, or informal work-related groups.
- Encourage interpersonal relationships through group activities. Encourage the person to join a group in the community.
- Increase communication skills, verbal and nonverbal, through practice in group situations, role playing, discussion, and review.
- Provide limits that are consistent, direct, presented frequently, and understandable.

Mania
- Provide honest, realistic appraisals of behavior, finished products, or outcomes of activities and occupations.
- Encourage the person to appraise and reflect upon his or her behavior and finished products.
- Engage the person in activities that focus on self-exploration, such as recognizing and dealing with emotions and self-expression through creative media and expanding coping styles.

Environment
Mania
- Provide a structured environment that is as free of distractions as possible.
- Begin with short-term projects and activities and work toward longer term projects and activities.

PRECAUTIONS
- Watch the person to prevent self-inflicted injuries and suicide attempts.
- Watch for signs of overmedication, such as tremor and loss of visual acuity.
- In older persons it is important to determine whether cognitive dysfunction is due to depression (which is reversible) or dementia (which may not be reversible).
- Therapy personnel should remind physicians that low energy, apathy, and lack of motivation (which may be signs of depression) should alert the physician to refer the person to occupational therapy, rather than assume that the person is unlikely to benefit from therapy and thus not refer him or her.
- A person with depression who is discharged home is more likely to function as a disabled person than a person in a hospital, even though he or she has had therapy services.

PROGNOSIS AND OUTCOME
Between episodes of depression or mania, there is full recovery of function.

- The person is able to perform activities of daily living and functional skills independently.
- The person is able to perform productive activities while setting realistic goals, conserving energy, and setting limits.
- The person assumes responsibility for performing leisure activities.
- The person is able to test reality and control his or her mood and activity level independently.
- The person is able to perform cognitive activities, including using judgment for personal safety, decision making, problem solving, and time management.
- The person is able to function in one-to-one and group situations.
- The person is able to resume his or her previous level of participation in the community.

REFERENCES

Beers, M.H., and R. Berkow, eds. 1999. *The Merck Manual of Diagnosis and Therapy*, 17th ed. Whitehouse Station, NJ: Merck Research Laboratories.

Dorland, W.A. 1988. *Dorland's Illustrated Medical Dictionary*, Philadelphia: W.B. Saunders.

BIBLIOGRAPHY

Adams, R.C. 1996. Geriatric rehab: Treat depression to improve function. *Advance for Occupational Therapists* 12, no. 49: 19.

Brollier, C., N. Hamrick, and B. Jacobson. 1994. Aerobic exercise: A potential occupational therapy modality for adolescents with depression. *Occupational Therapy in Mental Health* 12, no. 4: 19–29.

Cara, E. 1998. Mood disorders. In *Psychosocial occupational therapy: A clinical practice,* eds. E. Cara and A. MacRae, 285–312. Albany: Delmar.

Cracknell, E. 1995. A small achievable task. *British Journal of Occupational Therapy* 58, no. 8: 343–344.

Doe, J. 1995. Depression: A personal account. *Mental Health Special Interest Section Newsletter* 18, no. 3: 3–4.

Drake, L.M., and P.L. Barnett. 1998. Working with elders who have psychiatric conditions—Depression. In *Occupational therapy with elders: Strategies for the COTA,* eds. H. Lohman, R.L. Padilla, and S. Byers-Connon, 236–239. St. Louis: Mosby.

Engel, J.M. 1995. Evaluation and treatment of persons with major depressive disorder. *Mental Health Special Interest Section Newsletter* 18, no. 3: 1–3.

Engel, J.M. 1995. Bipolar disorders: The "Moody Blues." *Mental Health Special Interest Section Newsletter* 18, no. 4: 1–3.

Florey, L. 1993. The adolescent with depression. In *Practice issues in occupational therapy: Intraprofessional team building,* ed. S.E. Ryan, 65–70. Thorofare, NJ: Slack.

Gilbert, J., and J. Strong. 1994. Dysfunctional attitudes in patients with depression: A study of patients admitted to a private psychiatric hospital. *British Journal of Occupational Therapy* 57, no. 1: 15–19.

Henry, A.D., and W.J. Foster. 1996. Predictors of functional outcome among adolescents and young adults with psychotic disorders. *American Journal of Occupational Therapy* 50, no. 3: 171–181.

Katz, N. 1993. Cognitive performance and psychomotor retardation in depression: A pilot study. *Israel Journal of Occupational Therapy* 2, no. 2: E43–E52.

Neville-Jan, A. 1994. The relationship of volition to adaptive occupational behavior among individuals with varying degrees of depression. Presented at the AOTF research symposium, American Occupational Therapy Association Conference. *Occupational Therapy in Mental Health* 12, no. 4: 1–18.

Rogers, J.C., et al. 1994. Stability and change in functional assessment of patients with geropsychiatric disorders. *American Journal of Occupational Therapy* 48, no. 10: 914–918.

Stahl, C. 1995. Electroconvulsive therapy: Saving lives or keeping psychiatrists in business? *Advance for Occupational Therapists* 11, no. 17: 12–13.

Stevens-Ratchford, R.G. 1993. The effect of life review reminiscence activities on depression and self-esteem in older adults (review). *American Journal of Occupational Therapy* 47, no. 5: 413–420.

Waters, D. 1995. Recovering from a depressive episode using the Canadian Occupational Performance Measure. *Canadian Journal of Occupational Therapy* 62, no. 5: 278–282.

Zisselman, M.N., et al. 1995. A pet therapy intervention with geriatric psychiatry inpatients. *American Journal of Occupational Therapy* 50, no. 1: 47–51.

Dissociative Disorders—Dissociative Identity Disorder

DESCRIPTION

The criteria for the diagnosis of dissociative identity disorder (DID), formerly called multiple personality disorder (MPD), are (1) the presence of two or more distinct identities or personality states, each with its own relatively enduring pattern of perceiving, relating to, and thinking about the environment and self; (2) at least two of these identities or personality states recurrently take control of the person's behavior; (3) inability to recall important personal information that is too extensive to be explained by ordinary forgetfulness; (4) the disturbance is not due to the direct physiologic effects of a substance such as blackouts or chaotic behavior during alcohol intoxication or a general medical condition such as complex partial seizures (American Psychiatric Association 1994, 487). The diagnosis is controversial. Some psychiatrists do not believe the diagnosis exists.

All dissociative disorders, including DID, are classified as Axis I disorders on the multiaxial assessment scale.

CAUSE

The causative factors are assumed to be related to extreme psychosocial stress, shock, or trauma, or physical, emotional, or sexual abuse occurring early in childhood. The reaction is dissociation or splitting, an intrapsychic defense process in which one or more mental processes separates from the normal consciousness and functions as a whole within itself.

ASSESSMENT

Definitions

- *personality*: an entity with a firm, persistent sense of self, having a range of functions, emotions, and history
- *birth personality*: personality or identity developed just after birth, which at some point splits off the first new personality in order to help the body survive severe stress

---

**Greaves Suggestive Signs of Multiple Personality
Disorder or Dissociative Identity Disorder**

- Person reports time loss or time distortion.
- Observers report changes in the person's behavior.
- Person reports being told of disremembered behavior.
- Personalities can be elicited by hypnosis.
- Person uses "we" when referring to self.
- Person discovers objects in his or her possession that he or she cannot explain.
- Person reports severe headaches.
- Person reports hearing internal voices that are separate from the self.

Source: Data from G. Greaves, Multiple Personality: 165 Years after Mary Reynolds, *Journal of Nervous and Mental Disorders*, Vol. 168, p. 577–596, © 1980.

- *presenting personality*: the personality seeking treatment
- *host personality*: the personality that maintains executive control of the body
- *anesthetic personality*: the personality that is impervious to pain; it is developed to endure abuse
- *alter*: a generic term used to denote a fragment or personality
- *fragment*: an entity with limited function, emotion, and history
- *splitting*: creating a new personality
- *switching*: changing from one personality to another
- *fusion/integration*: the unification of personalities into one functional individual

Areas

Note: Different alters usually have different abilities and skills. These abilities and skills may or may not be transferred to the fused or integrated personality. Some abilities and skills that are performed well by one or more alters may have to be learned as new skills by the fused or integrated personality.

- memory
- problem-solving skills
- generalization of learning
- integration of learning
- synthesis of learning
- self-concept
- coping skills
- goals and values
- social skills
- communication skills
- daily living skills
- productive history, skills, and interests
- leisure interests and skills

Instruments

- *Allen Cognitive Level Test* by C.K. Allen, in *Occupational therapy for psychiatric diseases: Measurement and management of cognitive disabilities*, ed. C.K. Allen, 108–113, Boston: Little, Brown & Co, 1985.
- *Comprehensive Occupational Therapy Evaluation* by S.J. Brayman et al., *American Journal of Occupational Therapy* 30, no. 2 (1976): 94–100.
- *Interdependence Activity Scale* by P.L. Denton, in Occupational therapy for inpatients and outpatients with multiple personality disorder, *Expressive and functional therapies in the treatment of multiple personality disorder,* ed. E.S. Fluft, 245–257, Springfield, IL: Charles C Thomas, 1993.
- *Interest Checklist* by J. Matsutsuyu, in The interest checklist, *American Journal of Occupational Therapy* 23, no. 4 (1969): 323–328.
- *Occupational Case Analysis Interview and Rating Scale* by K.L. Kaplan and G. Kielhofner, Thorofare, NJ: Slack, 1989.
- *Role Checklist*, 2nd ed., by F. Oakley, Bethesda, MD: Occupational Therapy Service, National Institutes of Health, 1988.
- *Routine Task Inventory-2* by C.K. Allen, D.A. Earhart, and T. Blue, *Occupational Therapy Treatment Goals for Physically and Cognitively Disabled,* 63–72, Bethesda, MD: American Occupational Therapy Association, 1992.

PROBLEMS

Self-Care

- The degree to which activities of daily living are performed may depend on which alter (personality) is in charge at a particular time.
- The person may report that strange or unwanted items, such as items of clothing or food, sometimes are purchased because an alter (personality) wanted the item, although the host personality was unaware of the alter's existence or desire.

Productivity

- The degree to which the person can perform work tasks may depend on a personality being in charge when the self is at the work setting or getting ready to report to work.
- The person may have been fired from a job for not showing up for work because one or more alters (personalities) was in charge of the body and did not view the job as important.

Leisure

The alters (personalities) may have different leisure interests.

Sensorimotor

- The person may have headaches that the presenting personality cannot initially explain.
- The auditory sense is most commonly involved because the personalities talk to or about the other personalities at various times.

Cognitive

- The person is unable to account for certain time periods. The presenting personality has no memory of the time period or of events that occurred during that time.
- Certain times and events are distorted by the person as being either much longer or much shorter than actual occurrence.
- The person cannot explain the discovery of some objects in his or her possession.
- The person cannot explain how he or she got to a certain place.

Psychosocial

- The person usually is fearful of being "found out"; that is, that he or she was sexually or physically abused.
- The person may use compulsivity as an external structure to deal with an inner sense of disorganization.
- The person may be fearful of new adventures and any type of risk taking.
- The person may use a high level of activity, bordering on mania, and impulsive "springing into action" as a means of keeping busy to avoid uncomfortable thoughts.
- The person may report hearing voices that are separate from the self.
- In stressful situations, various alters (personalities) come out to deal with the situation and then retreat.
- The person may be suicidal or homicidal in an attempt to solve the original trigger event.
- The person may have been told by others that his or her personality sometimes changes dramatically.

TREATMENT/INTERVENTION

Models of treatment are based on D.A.R.E. (Frye 1994), the synthesis approach, the sensorimotor approach (Waid 1993), human occupation, and cognitive disabilities.

Self-Care

- Include self-care activities in the time-management program.
- Provide instruction in activities of daily living that may not have been learned.

Productivity

- Explore work interests and work capacities.
- Provide basic work skill training, if needed.

Leisure

Explore leisure interests and provide opportunities to try them out.

Sensorimotor

- The person may find physical activities—including exercises, physical fitness routines, and physically demanding sports—useful to provide structure and gain control.
- A sensorimotor program approach can be used in treatment, which incorporates a number of ideas presented in this section (see Waid 1993).

Cognitive

- Encourage all the personalities to learn about multiple personality disorder and how the disorder works.
- Set limits or rules that the alters (personalities) will support to discourage alters from breaking the rules.
- Provide learning situations that emphasize the importance of consistent behavior in a normal group situation.
- Provide an opportunity to plan and carry out goal-directed activities independently and in groups.
- Use projects made in occupational therapy as concrete representations to alters of their intrapersonal coexistence.
- Provide time-management training. It may be necessary to start with time awareness by having the person write down how long various tasks take to increase knowledge for planning an activity schedule.

Psychosocial

- The person must learn normal coping skills and adaptive strategies instead of splitting, especially in handling anger and rage. Opportunities to practice handling emotions need to be provided.
- Task-oriented activities provide different levels of structure and organization to which different alters (personalities) can be assigned and encouraged to achieve a higher level of organization or to facilitate the attainment of a higher level skill by the host personality.
- Task-oriented activities may permit other personalities to emerge that should be observed, evaluated, and reported to the case manager. In particular, nonverbal personalities may present, as the occupational therapy clinic may provide more opportunities for nonverbal behavior, such as drawing and painting.
- Gradually increase the opportunities for making choices to increase the person's sense of control over the environment.
- Activity analysis can be used to provide structure and external focus to counteract the internal chaos and disorganization.
- Different personalities may be assigned to different social group situations to encourage further development of social and communication skills.
- The person may find the use of constructively destructive tasks useful in dealing with anger and frustration; for example, kneading bread, wedging clay, sawing, sanding, cutting and sewing cloth, gardening, remodeling or refinishing the home, and splitting wood.
- Help the person identify comforting activities such as taking a warm bath, going for a walk, listening to music, eating specific foods, taking time alone to draw or write, or doing repetitive needlework such as cross-stitch.
- The D.A.R.E. model includes four stages: (1) denial, reflecting the person's discovery of a well-established defense system designed to protect him or her from "knowing" about past physical or sexual abuse; (2) awarenesss, which slowly erodes the denial and is graphically and painfully "trauma-rich," as the person learns of past events; (3) resolution, which involves working through the feelings the awareness brings to the present; and (4) emergence, when evidence begins to appear of cooperative and collective functioning as the person envisions a "unified self"—scarred but whole. During denial the person needs small,

controlled, structured tasks; boundaries; repetition; and short-term projects. During awareness the person needs constructive-destructive and physical outlets that are socially acceptable. During resolution the person needs opportunities to make choices; plan; take control over his or her own stress; practice logical, not emotional, decision making; complete tasks that are started; and work on "taking apart and putting back together" tasks. During emergence the person needs to give of him- or herself, analyze layers of an activity, be playful, and enjoy changes (Frye 1994).
- The person may be able to continue functioning in the primary roles of his or her life with minimum difficulty except for periods of acute stress.

PRECAUTIONS
- Occupational therapy personnel who themselves were abused as children should consider professional care if they choose to work with clients who have DID.
- Occupational therapy personnel may experience secondary posttraumatic stress syndrome as a result of working with persons with DID.
- Occupational therapy personnel should be aware that one or more alters may want to harm the body or harm others.
- Occupational therapy personnel should be aware that keeping track of clock time, location, and purposeful task can be derailed by one or more alters taking control of the body. Clients may be late, become lost, or fail to complete tasks as a result of alters switching.

PROGNOSIS AND OUTCOME
- The person is able to function as an integrated whole without splitting or switching.
- The person demonstrates normal coping skills.
- The person performs daily living activities independently.
- The person performs productive activities on a regular basis.
- The person performs leisure activities.

REFERENCES

American Psychiatric Association. 1994. *Diagnostic and Statistical Manual of Mental Disorders: DSM-IV,* 4th ed. Washington, DC: American Psychiatric Association. Task Force on DSM-IV.

Frye, B. 1994. D.A.R.E. to function: A purposeful story of multiple personality disorder recovery. *Occupational Therapy Forum* 9, no. 13: 4–5, 8–9.

Waid, K.M. 1993. An occupational therapy perspective in the treatment of multiple personality disorder. *American Journal of Occupational Therapy* 47, no. 10: 872–876.

BIBLIOGRAPHY

Dawson, P.L. 1993. Occupational therapy for inpatients and outpatients with multiple personality disorder. In *Expressive and functional therapies in the treatment of multiple personality disorder,* ed. E.S. Kluft, 245–248. Springfield, IL: Charles C Thomas.

Greaves, G. 1980. Multiple personality: 165 years after Mary Reynolds. *Journal of Nervous and Mental Disorders* 168: 577–596.

Santschi, H.S. 1993. Occupational therapy treatment of multiple personality disorder. In *Expressive and functional therapies in the treatment of multiple personality disorder,* ed. E.S. Kluft, 231–244. Springfield, IL: Charles C Thomas.

Skinner, S.T. 1993. Multiple personality in acute care psychiatry: Occupational therapy assessment. In *Expressive and functional therapies in the treatment of multiple personality disorder,* ed. E.S. Kluft, 219–230. Springfield, IL: Charles C Thomas.

Stahl, C. 1995. DSM-IV reclassifies MPD as dissociative identity disorder. *Advance for Occupational Therapists* 11, no. 32: 14.

Vergeer, G., and E. Cara. 1996. Dissociative disorders. In *Psychosocial occupational therapy: A clinical practice,* eds., E. Cara and A. MacRae, 405–434. Albany: Delmar.

Eating Disorders—Anorexia Nervosa

DESCRIPTION

The essential features of anorexia nervosa are the refusal to maintain a minimally normal body weight, intense fear of gaining weight, and exhibition of a significant disturbance in the perception of the shape or size of the body. In addition, postmenarcheal females are amenorrheic (American Psychiatric Association 1994, 539). Complications include cardiac arrhythmias, sterility, and osteoporosis. The death rate may be as high as 20 percent.

Anorexia nervosa is classified as an Axis I disorder on the multiaxial assessment scale.

CAUSE

The cause is unclear, although many explanations appear, including psychological issues, cognitive distortions, dysfunctional families, social pressure, learned behavior, faulty behavior, and physiologic disturbances (Lim and Agnew 1994). Emphasis on the desirability of being thin pervades Western society, and obesity is considered unattractive, unhealthy, and undesirable (Merck 1999, 1595). The history of the person may suggest a model child. The disorder is more common among sisters and mothers of those with the disorder than among the general population. Onset usually occurs in early to late adolescence, but onset in the 20s also occurs. The disorder is predominant among females (95 percent). In males, the onset usually presents in preadolescence or immature adolescent boys.

ASSESSMENT

Areas

- daily living skills
- productivity in school, home, and job, including history, skills, values, and interests
- leisure skills and interests
- motor activity level, especially hyperactivity
- body scheme or body image

Diagnostic Criteria for Anorexia Nervosa

A. Refusal to maintain body weight at or above a minimally normal weight for age and height (e.g., weight loss leading to maintenance of body weight less than 85 percent of that expected; or failure to make expected weight gain during period growth, leading to body weight less than 85 percent of that expected).
B. Intense fear of gaining weight or becoming fat, even though underweight.
C. Disturbance in the way in which one's body weight or shape is experienced, undue influence of body weight or shape on self-evaluation, or denial of the seriousness of the current low body weight.
D. In postmenarcheal females, amenorrhea, that is, the absence of at least three consecutive menstrual cycles.

Type:

*   **Restricting type**: During the current episode of anorexia nervosa, the person is not regularly engaged in binge-eating or purging behavior (self-induced vomiting or the misuse of laxatives, diuretics, or enemas).
*   **Binge-eating/purging type**: During the current episode of anorexia nervosa, the person has regularly engaged in binge-eating or purging behavior (self-induced vomiting or the misuse of laxatives, diuretics, or enemas).

Source: Reprinted with permission from the *Diagnostic and Statistical Manual of Mental Disorders, Fourth Edition.* Copyright © 1994, American Psychiatric Association.

---

*   problem solving or decision making
*   goals and values
*   reality testing
*   affect or mood
*   self-concept and self-esteem
*   social skills
*   social roles

Instruments

Instruments Developed by Occupational Therapy Personnel

*   *Occupational Therapy Assessment Protocol* by B. Bridgett, in Occupational therapy evaluation for patients with eating disorders, *Occupational Therapy for Mental Health* 12, no. 2 (1993): 79–89.
*   *Interest Checklist* by J. Matsutsuyu, in The interest checklist, *American Journal of Occupational Therapy* 23, no. 4 (1969): 323–328.

- *Occupational Questionnaire* by N. Riopel, G. Kielhofner, and J. Watts, in The relationship between volition, activity patterns, and life satisfaction in the elderly, *American Journal of Occupational Therapy* 40, no. 4 (1986): 278–283.
- *Role Checklist*, 2nd ed., by F. Oakley, Bethesda, MD: Occupational Therapy Service, National Institutes of Health, 1988.
- *Role Activity Performance Scale* by M.A. Good-Ellis et al., in Developing a role activity performance scale, *American Journal of Occupational Therapy* 41, no. 4 (1987): 323–341.

Instruments Developed by Other Professionals and Used by Occupational Therapy Personnel

- *Bruininks-Oseretsky Test of Motor Proficiency* (BOTMP) by R. Bruininks, Circle Pines, MN: American Guidance Services, 1978.
- *Internal-External Locus of Control Scale* by J.B. Rotter, in Generalized expectancies for internal versus external control of reinforcement, *Psychological Monographs* 80 (1966): 1–28.
- *Leisure Satisfaction Questionnaire* by J.G. Beard and M.G. Ragheb, in Measuring leisure satisfaction, *Journal of Leisure Research* 12 (1980): 20–33.
- *Life Attitude Profile* by G.T. Reker and E.J. Peacock, in The life attitude profile: A multidimensional instruction for assessing attitudes toward life, *Journal of Behavioral Science* 13 (1981): 264–273.
- *Reid Ware Factor Internal External Scale* by D.W. Reid and E.E. Ware, in Multidimensionality of internal versus external control, *Canadian Journal of Behavioral Science* 5 (1973): 264–271.

PROBLEMS

Self-Care

- The person may avoid performing some daily living activities, such as grooming.
- The person usually has periods of fasting when all food is refused.
- The person usually has been abusive to the body through starvation, vomiting, excessive exercise, overactivity, and/or lack of sleep.
- The person may have bulimic episodes (eating binges), often followed by vomiting.
- The person may hoard, conceal, crumble, or throw away food.
- The person may prepare an elaborate meal for others but limit him- or herself to eating low-calorie foods.
- The person may have no menstrual cycles.
- The person may complain of being cold when the weather is mild or of being in pain when the weather is cold.
- The person's skin may appear dark and dirty even though personal cleanliness is rarely, if ever, a problem.
- The hair on the person's head may be thinning, while fine, downy hair may cover normally hairless parts of the body.
- The person is dysfunctional in individual pursuit of engagement in meaningful occupation.

Productivity

- The person may fail to perform home-management tasks or may perform them irregularly.
- Although the person may have a good record of productivity, he or she does not derive meaning or satisfaction from performance or achievement.
- The person may express little interest in a discussion of career goals or vocational choice.

Leisure

The person neglects previously enjoyed activities; instead, leisure time may be characterized by boredom, restlessness, and aimlessness.

Sensorimotor

- Body weight is 15 percent or more below that expected for a person of this age and height.
- The person has increased motor activity and frequently overexercises to "keep the calories off" or stands in preference to sitting for such activities as reading and watching television.
- The person has a distorted body image or schema of the actual body size and shape and lacks an awareness of the real self. The body is usually seen as fatter and larger than it is; the degree of distortion varies with the person and stage of intervention.
- The person may misinterpret or fail to interpret internal and external stimuli, including the way hunger, tiredness, temperature, and pain are experienced or denied.
- The person may have atrophy of muscles and muscle weakness if the illness is of long duration.
- The person may be much shorter than normal due to failure to grow and may thus appear younger than he or she is.

Cognitive

- The person may have a short attention span.
- The person may appear alert but aloof.
- The person may use the need to study school subjects as a tool to avoid confronting problems.
- Cognitive skills are diminished but may be used as devices for avoidance behavior.
- The person may base cognitive decisions on incorrect information about nutrition, digestion, and metabolism.
- The person may have great difficulty making decisions; for example, making choices from restaurant menus.
- The person may have difficulty establishing and maintaining an appropriate balance of work, play, and social activities. Time spent on preparing and eating food may be out of balance with other activities.
- The person may have difficulty accepting new ideas for fear of losing control.
- The person may be unable to describe his or her assets or strengths.
- The person may be able to state that he or she feels increasingly "out of control."
- The person may set unrealistically high standards of performance (usually perfection or no errors), which dooms the person to failure, thus reinforcing feelings of inadequacy.

Psychosocial

- Anorexics demonstrate some type A behavioral patterns (Folts, Tigges, and Jackson 1993).

- The person has intense fear of gaining weight or becoming fat, even though he or she is underweight.
- The person's reality testing and belief systems may be distorted and not based on reality or fact.
- The person usually denies or minimizes the severity of the illness and his or her emaciated body. The person may be uninterested in or resistant to therapy because "nothing is wrong."
- The person is dysfunctional in his or her attitudes and habits related to eating and weight control.
- The person tends to be perfectionistic and set high standards of performance, although the specific occupational goal may be unclear.
- The person may have compulsive or ritualistic behavior, such as cutting food into minute pieces, putting food in bowls, eating with teaspoons, heavily spicing food, rearranging food so it appears to take up less space, and drawing meals out over long periods of time.
- Phobic behavior may be present so that certain foods, such as sweets, are viewed as "bad" or "forbidden."
- Anxiety behavior may occur if the person has to handle certain foods, such as meats or fats.
- The person usually does not feel competent or have feelings of mastery even though he or she may have a list of accomplishments. The person feels helpless against forces outside his or her control, such as family and social areas.
- The person may have difficulty managing stress and tension and using coping mechanisms effectively.
- The person may have delayed psychosexual development and a fear of sexuality.
- The person may misinterpret emotional and social cues.
- The person may have difficulty enjoying him- or herself or having fun doing activities that others enjoy.
- The person is struggling for a sense of identity, competence, and effectiveness.
- The person may undervalue him- or herself (poor self-concept) in spite of obvious abilities.
- The person may have an underlying sense of inability and helplessness to change anything. The person may report feeling devalued.
- The person's feelings or beliefs about pleasure may be distorted.
- The person may describe a childhood as one of constantly trying to live up to the expectations of his or her family.
- The person may have a limited repertoire of roles, and they may be below the person's chronologic age.
- The person may have pressured, defiant speech.
- The person may demonstrate explosive anger.
- The person may have a low frustration tolerance.
- The person's behavior may be described as "obstinate," "manipulative," "deceitful," and "stubborn."
- The person may have poorly developed social skills, especially in group situations that involve food and eating.
- The person tends to be lonely and withdrawn.

Environment
- The family may undermine or undervalue efforts of the person at achievement and success.

- The family may have very close relationships between family members without defined boundaries that allow each person to function as an individual.
- The family may be overprotective and may shelter the person from risk-taking experiences that would allow feelings of achievement to occur.
- The family may rescue the person from any experience that might result in failure.
- The family may avoid direct confrontation, which prevents the development of successful negotiating skills and the ability to compromise.
- The family may set strict limits that discourage individuality and personal freedom.

TREATMENT/INTERVENTION

Intervention is usually initiated and maintained as part of the team management approach. General models of treatment include cognitive behavioral and psychoanalytic models. Occupational therapy models include the occupational behavior model, and the model of human occupation. Other models described in the literature are the medical model, behavior model, developmental model, and family therapy approach.

Self-Care

- Provide opportunities to practice shopping for food, preparing it, and eating it in a controlled setting, then slowly releasing control as the person is able to gain responsibility for his or her actions and channel anxiety associated with food into more acceptable activities.
- Therapy personnel may accompany the person to shop for new clothes after some weight has been regained to help the person to realistically respond to being "fat" in public. An alternative approach could be sewing new clothes.
- Beauty and makeup sessions may be useful to help in developing a new, positive image.
- The person may be asked to keep an eating record that is discussed in a stress management group. The daily record may include when the person eats, amount eaten, hunger level, and stress before and after eating.

Productivity

- Help the person explore possible career options to promote a positive self-concept.
- Encourage the person to continue schoolwork and education, but as part of a balanced program of self-care, productive, and leisure activities.

Leisure

- Explore with the person new interests to substitute for food behaviors that must be given up.
- Encourage the person to find interests that permit relaxation, fun, humor, and variety.

Sensorimotor

- Encourage daily participation in a physical fitness program to improve muscle tone, strength, and cardiopulmonary conditioning, but change the type of exercise and promote moderation. Yoga exercises and other relaxation techniques may be useful.
- Increase the person's awareness of his or her physical body and perceptual body image by providing sensory stimulation such as proprioceptive, tactile, and visual information. Videotaping and use of a mirror may be useful in confronting the person with a realistic appraisal of his or her body image and its relationship to the illness.

Cognitive

- Instruct the person in concepts of time and activity management to create a balance of self-care, productivity, and leisure.
- Instruct the person in the role of food in metabolism and the adverse effects of abnormal eating behavior.
- Values clarification exercises may be useful in helping the person determine personal likes and dislikes.
- Time frames and schedules (activity configurations) may be useful in helping the person learn to balance work and play activities.
- Encourage the person to set goals but keep them flexible. Micro-goals are those covering the next 15–60 minutes, mini-goals cover from one day to one month, short-range goals cover from one month to one year, and medium-range goals cover the next five years and usually are educational goals.
- The person should engage in controlled risk taking without the fear of feeling rebuked for it.

Psychosocial

- Encourage awareness of emotional and social needs.
- Provide opportunities for mastery, control, and self-expression through creative crafts, art activities, games, dance, and drama.
- Facilitate psychological, physical, and social competence by helping the person to achieve maximum function at all levels.
- Provide training in relaxation techniques to reduce anxiety and deal with stress.
- A contract may be useful to help the person set objectives or goals and work toward them.
- Assertiveness training may be useful to encourage the person to understand and control aggressive behavior and to validate feelings.
- Stress management activities may be useful in developing alternative means of coping with tension and stress to replace the destructive eating behaviors. The person needs to learn how to channel stress constructively into creative outlets, and to learn the appropriate use of exercise and relaxation techniques.
- Therapy personnel should establish a trusting relationship that accepts the person and permits discussion of feelings and opinions.
- Help the person improve his or her interpersonal skills, especially insight into how others see the individual, to permit a realistic comparison between self-perception and the perception of others.
- Encourage the person to participate in social situations that include food and practice eating with others, such as dining at a restaurant.
- Folts, Tigges, and Jackson (1993) list the following social skills to be taught: initiating a conversion, continuing a conversation, terminating a conversation, making a request, requesting assistance, following direction, active listening, giving directions, giving compliments, empathic assertion, criticizing, expressing anger, expressing feelings, admitting a mistake, accepting criticism, reacting to another's anger, responding to nonverbal communication, dealing with mixed messages, bargaining, assertiveness, problem solving, and decision making.

Environment

Family members need to be instructed not to focus on eating behavior and to refrain from arguments, yelling, threatening, punishment, or other negative behavior at mealtimes.

PRECAUTIONS
- Monitor cardiac performance for arrhythmias, such as ventricular fibrillation associated with hypokalemia.
- Watch for signs of depression and possible suicide attempts.
- The variety of models and treatment approaches suggests that the disorder is not well understood. Therapists should be aware of changing viewpoints in working with such persons.
- Do not get into power struggles with the person.

PROGNOSIS AND OUTCOME
- The person is able to maintain body weight at an established level.
- The person correctly describes his or her body.
- The person demonstrates improved ability to express feelings and thoughts.
- The person participates in social group activities.
- The person is able to prepare and eat food in a group setting.
- The person demonstrates knowledge of his or her skills and assets.
- The person has increased the number of leisure skills performed.

REFERENCES

American Psychiatric Association. 1994. *Diagnostic and Statistical Manual of Mental Disorders: DSM-IV,* 4th ed. Washington, DC: American Psychiatric Association. Task Force on DSM-IV.
Beers, M.H., and R. Berkow, eds. 1999. *The Merck Manual of Diagnosis and Therapy,* 17th ed. Whitehouse Station, NJ: Merck Research Laboratories.
Folts, D.J., K. Tigges, and G. Jackson. 1993. Occupational therapy treatment of anorexia nervosa. In *The eating disorders,* eds. A.J. Giannini and A.E. Slaby, 227–242. New York: Springer-Verlag.
Lim, P.Y., and P. Agnew. 1994. Occupational therapy with eating disorders: A study on treatment approaches. *British Journal of Occupational Therapy* 57, no. 8: 309–314.

BIBLIOGRAPHY

Bowers, W.A., and A.E. Andersen. 1994. Inpatient treatment of anorexia nervosa: Review and recommendations. *Harvard Review of Psychiatry* 2, no. 4: 193–203.
Bridgett, B. 1993. Occupational therapy evaluation for patients with eating disorders. *Occupational Therapy in Mental Health* 12, no. 2: 79–89.
Henderson, S. 1998. Frames of reference utilized in the rehabilitation of individuals with eating disorders. *Canadian Journal of Occupational Therapy* 66, no. 1: 43–51.
Martin, J.E. 1998. Occupational therapy in the treatment of eating disorders. In *Eating disorders, food and occupational therapy,* ed. J.E. Martin, 183–208. London, England: Whurr Publications Ltd.

Van Deusen, J. 1991. Anorexia nervosa. In *Body image and perceptual dysfunction in adults,* ed. J. Van Deusen, 149–172. Philadelphia: W.B. Saunders.
Ward, J.D. 1998. Eating disorders. In *Willard and Spackman's occupational therapy*, 9th ed., eds. M.E. Neistadt and E.B. Crepeau, 728–732. Philadelphia: Lippincott-Raven.

Eating Disorders—Bulimia Nervosa

DESCRIPTION

The essential features of bulimia nervosa are binge eating and inappropriate compensatory methods to prevent weight gain. In addition, the self-evaluation of individuals with bulimia is excessively influenced by body shape and weight. To qualify for the diagnosis, the binge eating and inappropriate compensatory behaviors must occur, on average, at least twice a week for three months (American Psychiatric Association 1994, 545).

Bulimia nervosa is classified as an Axis I disorder on the multiaxial assessment scale.

CAUSE

Mood swings, disturbed family dynamics, impulsivity, lack of internal control, high anxiety, and low self-esteem are predisposing factors, but the exact etiology is unknown. Both men and women are affected, but the typical person is a woman in her 20s.

ASSESSMENT

Areas

- gross motor skills
- fine motor coordination, manipulation, and dexterity
- attention span
- ability to follow directions
- problem-solving and decision-making skills
- goals and values awareness
- self-concept and self-esteem
- group interaction skills
- daily living skills
- productivity history, skills, and interests
- leisure interests and skills

Instruments

Instruments Developed by Occupational Therapy Personnel

- *Occupational History* by L. Moorhead, in The occupational history, *American Journal of Occupational Therapy* 23, no. 4 (1969): 329–338.

Diagnostic Criteria for Bulimia Nervosa

A. Recurrent episodes of binge eating. An episode of binge eating is characterized by both of the following:
   1. Eating, in a discrete period of time (e.g., within any 2-hour period), an amount of food that is definitely larger than most people would eat during a similar period of time and under similar circumstances.
   2. A sense of lack of control over eating during the episode (a feeling that one cannot stop eating or control what or how much one is eating).
B. Recurrent inappropriate compensatory behavior in order to prevent weight gain, such as self-induced vomiting; misuse of laxatives, diuretics, enemas, or other medications; fasting; or excessive exercise.
C. The binge eating and inappropriate compensatory behaviors both occur, on average, at least twice a week for three months.
D. Self-evaluation is unduly influenced by body shape and weight.
E. The disturbance does not occur exclusively during episodes of anorexia nervosa.
- **Purging type**: During the current episode of bulimia nervosa, the person has regularly engaged in self-induced vomiting or the misuse of laxatives, diuretics, or enemas.
- **Nonpurging type**: During the current episode of bulimia nervosa, the person has used other inappropriate compensatory behaviors, such as fasting or excessive exercise, but has not regularly engaged in self-induced vomiting or the misuse of laxatives, diuretics, or enemas.

Source: Reprinted with permission from the *Diagnostic and Statistical Manual of Mental Disorders, Fourth Edition.* Copyright © 1994, American Psychiatric Association.

- *Occupational Therapy Assessment Protocol* by B. Bridgett, in Occupational therapy evaluation for patients with eating disorders, *Occupational Therapy for Mental Health* 12, no. 2 (1993): 79–89.

PROBLEMS

Self-Care
- The person has a history of recurrent episodes of binge eating in which large amounts of food are consumed, followed by periods of eating little food. Normal eating becomes uncommon.
- The person uses eating to deal not only with hunger but also with frustration, emptiness, tension, boredom, anxiety, and self-sedation.
- The person may eat so rapidly that the food is hardly chewed or tasted.
- The person may engage in self-induced vomiting.

- The person may use laxatives or diuretics excessively.
- The person may attempt strict dieting or fasting.
- The person may have frequent weight fluctuations as a result of alternating episodes of gorging and fasting.
- The person may also abuse drugs and alcohol.
- The person may be obsessed with personal hygiene, which is carried out methodically and meticulously.
- The person may have physical side effects such as tooth decay and sore throats from vomiting and abdominal pain from excessive use of laxatives.
- The person may lack independence in several self-care areas.

Productivity
- The person may have poorly developed vocational interests or may consider only those related to food, fitness, modeling, dance, or caregiver occupations.
- The person may have difficulty accepting supervision and following directions.
- The person may have a history of underproductivity and excessive absences from school or work.

Leisure

  The person may have few leisure interests other than food: eating, bingeing, or dieting.

Sensorimotor
- The person may engage in vigorous exercise to prevent weight gain.
- The person may have distortion of body scheme.
- The person may have swelling around the ankles due to retention of fluids.
- The person may have puffiness around the eyes due to retention of fluids.
- The person may have calluses on the dominant index finger as a result of using the finger to induce vomiting.

Cognitive
- The person may have difficulty concentrating on a task.
- The person manages time more by food than any other way.
- The person usually has difficulty planning ahead and has unrealistic goals.
- The person is susceptible to dichotomous thinking; for example, "If I'm not thin, then I must be fat as a cow."

Psychosocial
- The person may describe feelings of being misunderstood in terms of the illness.
- The person usually does not deny or minimize symptoms.
- The person feels a lack of control over eating behavior, especially during binges.
- The person is overconcerned with body shape and weight and usually has a distorted body image.
- The person may express feelings of being foolish, ridiculous, pathetic, damaged, or worthless.
- The person may have an extreme fear of being overweight; after years of trying to keep the weight under control, he or she discovered purging.

- The person may feel that his or her life is dominated by conflicts about eating.
- The person has poor reality testing as evidenced by life-threatening behaviors, such as starvation, use of laxatives, and induced vomiting.
- The person may exhibit suicidal behavior by slashing wrists or overdosing.
- The person may describe feelings of sadness or depression.
- The person usually has low self-esteem and a feeling of being a failure or of being rejected.
- The person usually is a perfectionist and an overachiever.
- The person may compulsively overexercise.
- The person may have an extroverted personality.
- The person may avoid interpersonal situations, when possible, to reduce the chances of being found out.
- The person may engage only in social activities that he or she can control.
- The person may be fearful of sustained closeness or intimacy.
- The person may have a history of stealing food because the binge behavior exceeds the income available.

Environment

Episodes of bingeing may occur at the same time of day, every day. Evenings are most common.

TREATMENT/INTERVENTION

Models of treatment have been based on cognitive behavior therapy (cognitive restructuring), medical model, behavioral model, psychoanalytic model, family therapy model, developmental model, and psychoeducation. Occupational therapy models include occupational behavior and the model of human occupation.

Self-Care

- Increase independence skills in self-care and daily living based on problem areas identified in the original assessment.
- Interrupt the binge-purge cycle and improve the person's ability to monitor eating behavior. A cooking class is useful to correct misinformation about food, such as caloric value and what constitutes nutritionally balanced meals. Planning meals in advance and shopping only for the food needed for the planned meals may be helpful to control binge eating. Later in treatment, ordering and eating at a restaurant may be useful to help the person practice self-control. Keeping a diary of food intake provides a reference for discussion of nutritional values in various foods.
- The person may need to shop for new clothes when weight has been stabilized because his or her existing wardrobe does not fit. Practice in making decisions about and planning a wardrobe for work activities as well as leisure activities can be stressed.

Productivity

- Increase skills in independent living, such as money management or living in an apartment.
- Provide work adjustment programs that develop work habits and skills.
- The person may need assistance in looking for job opportunities and developing interview techniques, and practice in completing an application form.

Leisure

- Provide opportunities to explore and develop leisure skills and activities. In later stages of treatment, the person should be encouraged to use community resources, rather than the hospital, for leisure activities, to practice independence skills.
- Leisure activities should be directed away from food and eating interests.

Sensorimotor

Provide movement and exercise experiences emphasizing body toning, general strengthening, and general fitness while discouraging excessive exercise.

Cognitive

- Instruct the person about body weight regulation, including caloric intake, homeostasis, and eating a balanced diet.
- Help the person organize an activity schedule with specific tasks, especially during times of the day or week when binge eating is most likely to occur.
- Instruct the person in stress-management techniques, including the use of exercise, yoga, and other relaxation techniques.
- Videotapes may be useful in discussing disturbances of body image. Reading materials may provide factual information about the disorder and its effects on a person's life, which can facilitate discussion with the therapist or in group therapy.
- Provide information about the complications and course of the illness if it is not corrected.
- Increase problem-solving skills to anticipate problems and develop strategies for handling the problems before the situations get out of the person's control.
- Teach time-management skills that include a balance of work and leisure activities.

Psychosocial

- Help the person set graded goals related to eating and select rewards for not bingeing.
- Increase the person's sense of competency, achievement, and self-esteem through activities that will provide a sense of mastery, such as leatherwork or ceramics. Art, drama, or music may also be useful.
- Encourage the person to verbalize feelings. Role-playing may be a useful technique.
- Correct dysfunctional thinking patterns or faulty constructions of reality, such as overgeneralization, all-or-nothing reasoning, superstition, or attaching too much significance to specific events. Keeping a diary of dysfunctional thoughts and participating in group discussions may help the person identify these kinds of thoughts.
- Identify and help the person evaluate automatic (ritualistic, obsessive) thoughts or images by examining the advantages, disadvantages, or logical inconsistencies of such thoughts.
- Increase the person's coping skills and alternative strategies to bingeing and purging by identifying what triggers the bingeing, teaching relaxation techniques, and providing assertiveness training.
- Increase the person's self-control and decrease impulsive behavior.
- Create a group situation in which beliefs and values can be identified and examined.
- Provide opportunities for the person to be assertive and enjoy creativity within a safe group setting, such as role-playing, drama, or dance.
- Encourage the person to participate in group activities outside the treatment situation.

PRECAUTIONS
- Watch for signs of relapse into binge eating.
- Follow-up programs are important to maintain short-term gains.

PROGNOSIS AND OUTCOME
- The person is able to express, verbally and nonverbally, a positive sense of self.
- The person is able to set goals and perform activities without resorting to binge eating behaviors.
- The person is able to eat regular, normal meals independently, without supervision.
- The person is able to express opinions and accept feedback without withdrawing or becoming hostile.
- The person has increased skills toward independence or achieved independence in self-care activities.
- The person has increased skills in home management and career choice.
- The person demonstrates regular performance of leisure skills.

REFERENCE
American Psychiatric Association. 1994. *Diagnostic and Statistical Manual of Mental Disorders: DSM-IV,* 4th ed. Washington, DC: American Psychiatric Association. Task Force on DSM-IV.

BIBLIOGRAPHY
Bridgett, B. 1993. Occupational therapy evaluation for patients with eating disorders. *Occupational Therapy in Mental Health* 12, no. 2: 79–89.
Folts, D.J., and A.J. Giannini. 1993. Occupational therapy treatment of bulimia nervosa. In *The eating disorders,* eds. A.J. Giannini and A.E. Slaby, 243–254. New York: Springer-Verlag.
Lin, P.Y., and P. Agnew. 1994. Occupational therapy with eating disorders: a study on treatment approaches. *British Journal of Occupational Therapy* 57, no. 8: 309–314.
Martin, J.E. 1998. Occupational therapy in bulimia nervosa. In *Eating disorders, food and occupational therapy,* ed. J.E. Martin, 209–222. London, England: Whurr Publications Ltd.
Ward, J.D. 1998. Eating disorders. In *Willard and Spackman's occupational therapy*, 9th ed., eds. M.E. Neistadt and E.B. Crepeau, 728–732. Philadelphia: Lippincott-Raven.

Emotionally Disturbed Children and Adolescents

DESCRIPTION
The definition of this disorder includes a broad group of potential diagnoses. The common factor in the description of emotionally disturbed children and adolescents is the label applied

by educational institutions to children who (1) are under 19 years of age and (2) have emotional or behavioral problems that are difficult or impossible for teachers to handle in regular classrooms. Actual diagnoses may include mood disorders, depressive disorders, bipolar disorders, disruptive behavior disorders, anxiety disorders, eating disorders, personality disorders, pervasive developmental disorders, schizophrenia, and others. (See specific sections for descriptions of attention deficit disorder and autism.)

The term "emotional disturbance" is defined by the Individual Disabilities Education Act (IDEA) of 1997 as an inability to learn that cannot be explained by intellectual, sensory, or health factors; an inability to build or maintain satisfactory interpersonal relationships with peers and teachers; inappropriate types of behavior or feelings under normal circumstances; a general pervasive mood of unhappiness or depression; and a tendency to develop physical symptoms or fears associated with personal or school problems (IDEA, 1977, 34 CFR, Sec 300.7).

"Emotional disturbance" is not a term used in the DSM-IV; therefore, there is no specific axis for the disorder. The axis would be based on the psychiatric disorder given the child, not the educational term.

CAUSE

The causative factors may be singular or multiple but generally can be organized into four areas: (1) primary, such as a neurologic disorder; (2) predisposing, such as failure to learn adaptive behavior; (3) precipitating, such as an unstable home life; and (4) reinforcing, such as being rewarded by a parent or sibling for stealing or selling drugs.

ASSESSMENT

Areas
- muscle tone
- range of motion
- reflex development, especially continuing existence of primitive reflexes
- physical endurance
- motor skills, including gross and fine skills
- developmental milestones—delayed or normal achievement
- sensation—normal, hypersensitive, or hyposensitive
- sensory integrative skills, including visual, tactile, proprioceptive, auditory, and vestibular
- cognitive skills, including intellectual and memory
- behavior patterns, including type, frequency, and location
- temperament, including locus of control, autonomy, motivation, affect, and expectancy
- emotional function, including fear, hostility, aggression, and withdrawal
- family dynamics, including parent-child interactions, appearance, attitudes, and concerns
- environmental influences, including home, school, parents, and peers
- role history
- daily living skills
- play history and skills and/or productivity history, skills, and interests
- leisure interests and skills

Instruments

Instruments Developed by Occupational Therapy Personnel

- *Assessment of Communication and Interaction Skills* by M. Salamy, S. Simon, and G. Kielhofner, Bethesda, MD: American Occupational Therapy Association, 1993.
- *Assessment of Motor and Process Skills* (AMPS), 2nd ed., by A. Fisher, Fort Collins, CO: Three Star Press, 1997.
- *Comprehensive Occupational Therapy Evaluation* by S.J. Brayman and T. Kirby, *American Journal of Occupational Therapy* 30, no. 2 (1976): 94–100.
- *Erhardt Developmental Prehension Assessment,* rev., by R. Erhardt, San Antonio, TX: Therapy Skill Builders, 1982.
- *FirstSTEP Screening Test for Evaluating Preschoolers* by L.J. Miller, San Antonio, TX: The Psychological Corporation, 1993.
- *Interest Checklist* by J. Matsutsuya, *American Journal of Occupational Therapy* 23, no. 4 (1969): 323–328.
- *Knox Preschool Play Scale* by S. Knox, in Development and current use of the Knox Preschool Play Scale, *Play: A clinical focus in occupational therapy for children,* eds. D. Parham and L. Fazio, 35–51, St. Louis: Mosby, 1996.
- *Occupational Performance History Interview* by G. Kielhofner, A. Henry, and D. Walens, Rockville, MD: American Occupational Therapy Association, 1989. (See pages 480–483 in Porr and Rainville for suggested questions for adolescents.)
- *Occupational Questionnaire* by N. Riopel, G. Kielhofner, and J. Watts, in The relationship between volition, activity patterns, and life satisfaction in the elderly, *American Journal of Occupational Therapy* 40, no. 4 (1986): 278–283.
- *Role Checklist*, 2nd ed., by F. Oakley, Bethesda, MD: Occupational Therapy Service, National Institutes of Health, 1988.
- *Self-Assessment of Occupational Function—Children's Version* by C. Curtin and K. Baron, Chicago: Department of Occupational Therapy, University of Illinois, 1990.

Instruments Developed by Other Professionals and Used by Occupational Therapy Personnel

- *The Beery-Buktenica Developmental Test of Visual-Motor Integration* (VMI-4), 4th ed., by K.E. Beery and N.A. Buktenica, Parsippany, NJ: Modern Curriculum Press, 1997.
- *Goodenough-Harris Drawing Test* by D.B. Harris, San Antonio, TX: The Psychological Corporation, 1963.
- *Kinetic Self-Image Test* by R.M. Abramson, in Developmental and diagnostic assessment, *The evaluation and care of severely disturbed children,* ed. L. Hoffman, 37–44, New York: SP Medical & Scientific Books, 1982.
- *Test of Visual-Perceptual Skills-Revised* (TVPS-R) by M.F. Gardner, Hydesville, CA: Psychological and Educational Publications, 1996.
- *Vineland Adaptive Behavior Scales—Revised* (VABS-R) by S.S. Sparrow, P.A. Balla, and D.V. Cicchetti, Circle Pines, MN: American Guidance Services, 1984.

PROBLEMS

This section describes a group of childhood disorders that have specific names according to some classification schemes, such as conduct disorders, school phobia, childhood schizophrenia, and others. The problems are a composite from the literature in occupational therapy.

Self-Care

The child or adolescent may not have learned self-care skills.

Productivity

- The child or adolescent's play skills may be delayed.
- Academic skills usually are below the child or adolescent's chronologic age.

Leisure

The child or adolescent may have few leisure interests.

Sensorimotor

- The child or adolescent may have poor fine motor skills.
- The child or adolescent may show developmental delay in gross motor skills.
- The child or adolescent may have impaired postural control and balance.
- The child or adolescent may have injuries from physical abuse that result in loss of muscle strength or range of motion.
- The child or adolescent may have poor motor planning skills.
- The child or adolescent may have had limited tactile stimulation or be tactilely defensive.
- The child or adolescent may have difficulty with visual scanning and tracking.
- The child or adolescent may have poor perception of spatial relationships.
- The child or adolescent may have poor stereognosis.
- The child or adolescent may be hyper- or hyporesponsive to vestibular stimulation.

Cognitive

- The child or adolescent may have poor attending behavior.
- The child or adolescent may have difficulty following directions.
- The child or adolescent may have difficulty with problem solving and decision making.
- The child or adolescent may have poor time-management skills.

Psychosocial

- The child or adolescent may have a poor self-concept.
- The child or adolescent may have had inadequate or faulty discipline.
- The child or adolescent may have suffered continued stress.
- The child or adolescent may have poor impulse control.
- The child or adolescent may have been overprotected.
- The child or adolescent may lack goal-directed behaviors or skills.
- The child or adolescent may have had faulty (verbal abuse) or little communication with adults.
- The child or adolescent may lack social skills.
- The child or adolescent may lack group interaction skills.

TREATMENT/INTERVENTION

Models of treatment vary and may include developmental, neurodevelopmental, behavioral, neurobehavioral, educational, cognitive, psychodynamic, milieu, and family therapy. Models of practice in occupational therapy include the model of human occupation.

Self-Care
- Develop grooming and etiquette habits.
- Practice performing activities of daily living without reminders.

Productivity
- Practice working in groups of increasing size.
- Practice taking directions, suggestions, and corrections from a supervisor.

Leisure

Explore the child or adolescent's interests and provide opportunities for participation in these activities.

Sensorimotor
- Increase or improve the child or adolescent's gross motor skills.
- Increase or improve fine motor skills.
- Increase or improve coordination (eye-hand, eye-foot, two sides of the body).
- Improve balance reactions.
- Increase or improve visual motor skills (scanning, tracking).
- Increase or improve visual perception skills.
- Normalize response to tactile and vestibular stimuli. (See sections on tactile defensiveness and gravitational insecurity if needed.)
- Consider whether deficits in sensory input—such as hearing loss, amblyopia, or color blindness—may be contributing to the emotional problems.

Cognitive
- Teach the child or adolescent to pay attention to and follow directions.
- Plan and perform a series of steps leading to task completion.
- Practice problem-solving techniques, including alternative solutions to problems.
- Have the child or adolescent practice critiquing (evaluating) his or her own work, including positive and negative aspects.
- Help the child or adolescent learn time orientation (past, present, and future) by reviewing a sequence of activities during a day, week, month, and year.
- Help the child or adolescent plan and review daily routines.

Psychosocial
- Increase the child or adolescent's self-mastery, self-awareness, and sense of competence by completing tasks and practicing in activities such as crafts, cooking, cooperative action games, board games, and role-playing exercises.
- Have the child or adolescent accept responsibility for his or her own actions by acknowledging his or her behavior and accepting the consequences.
- Help the child or adolescent develop internal control by expressing feelings in words rather than actions.
- Help the child or adolescent practice channeling anger and aggression into socially acceptable activities.

- Demonstrate goal-directed behavior by stating or writing a goal, methods for achieving the goal, progress in achieving the goal, and the reward for completing the goal.
- Have the child or adolescent practice changing behavior based on suggestions from adults or peers.
- Teach the child or adolescent to respect the rights of others by sharing space and materials.
- Have the child or adolescent practice expressing ideas and feelings in a group situation.
- Have the child or adolescent practice praising others for expressing good ideas, controlling behavior, or performing good work.
- Increase adaptive and coping strategies using meal planning and preparation, newspaper production, theatrical productions, or furniture refinishing.
- Have the child or adolescent practice new roles and increasing responsibility within old roles.
- Increase social interaction skills through practice in following the rules of a game, rules for driving a vehicle, and observing safety precautions. For differences in play skills, including peer relationships, rules and games, and play interests between younger and older children, see Florey and Green (1997, 130).
- Increase skills in peer interaction and relationships with adults using group tasks such as role playing or planning a group project.
- Increase communication skills between peers and adults using tasks such as crafts and cooking.

Environment

Encourage participation in youth groups such as Cub Scouts, Girl Scouts, or other youth organizations.

PRECAUTIONS
- Watch for signs of side effects of medication.
- Be aware of changes in the environment that may alter the child's behavior.

PROGNOSIS AND OUTCOME
- The child or adolescent demonstrates increased ability to concentrate on a task.
- The child or adolescent demonstrates problem-solving skills.
- The child or adolescent is able to remember and follow directions.
- The child or adolescent demonstrates improved and positive self-concept.
- The child or adolescent demonstrates judgment regarding safety of self and others.
- The child or adolescent is able to participate in a group setting.
- The child or adolescent performs self-care activities independently or with verbal or visual assistance only.
- The child or adolescent is attending and learning academic skills in a classroom setting or home program.
- The adolescent participates in vocational exploration or a work skill training program.
- The child or adolescent demonstrates increased play and leisure interests.
- The child or adolescent demonstrates improved leisure interests and skills.

REFERENCES

Florey, L., and S. Greene. 1997. Play in middle childhood: A focus on children with behavioral and emotional disorders. In *Play in occupational therapy for children,* eds. L.D. Parham and L. Fazio, 126–143. St. Louis: Mosby.
Individuals with Disabilities Education Act (IDEA) Amendments, 34 CFR, § 300.7 (1977).

BIBLIOGRAPHY

Bonder, B.R. 1995. Disorders of infancy, childhood, and adolescence. In *Psychopathology and function,* 2nd ed., ed. B.R. Bonder, 19–44. Thorofare, NJ: Slack.
Borg, B., and M.A. Bruce. 1995. Aggressive behavior. In *Occupational therapy stories: Psychosocial interaction in practice,* eds. B. Borg and M.A. Bruce, 55–61. Thorofare, NJ: Slack.
Davidson, D.A. 1996. Programs and services for children with psychosocial dysfunction. In *Occupational therapy for children,* 3rd ed., eds. J. Case-Smith, A.S. Allen, and P.N. Pratt, 796–807. St. Louis: Mosby.
Fahl, M.A. 1997. Determining the relevant causative factors in children with emotional disturbance in community-based treatment. *Mental Health Special Interest Section Quarterly* 20, no. 4: 1–4.
Florey, L. 1993. The child with a conduct disorder. In *Practice issues in occupational therapy: Intraprofessional team building,* ed. S.E. Ryan, 57–62. Thorofare, NJ: Slack.
Joe, B.E. 1993. Conference 93 preview: Recognizing and treating children with SED in the classroom. *OT Week* 7, no. 16: 28.
Lambert, W.L., and B.J. Rodrigues. 1998. Disorders of children and adolescents. In *Psychosocial occupational therapy: A clinical practice,* eds. E. Cara and A. MacRae, 161–198. Albany, NY: Delmar.
Lougher, L. 1997. Child and adolescent mental health services. In *Occupational therapy and mental health,* 2nd ed., ed. J. Creek, 377–398. New York: Churchill Livingstone.
Simons, D.F. 1999. The psychological system in adolescence. In *Pediatric therapy: A systems approach,* eds. S.M. Porr and E.B. Rainville, 424–506. Philadelphia: F.A. Davis.

Forensic Psychiatry

DESCRIPTION

Forensic psychiatry includes a group of disorders that have as their common denominator a person who has entered the criminal justice system because of aggressive, dangerous, or socially unacceptable behavior. Among the typical diagnoses are personality disorders, such as antisocial personalities; major psychiatric disorders, such as schizophrenia; anxiety disorders, such as compulsive behavior; and substance abuse, including alcohol and drugs. Mental retardation and learning disabilities may also be present.

Generally, forensic occupational therapy deals with three groups of people: (1) those who have severe psychoses or addictions that do not respond to current therapies sufficiently to consider release; (2) those who need rehabilitation to the status of mental competence so they can stand trial; and (3) those who can be rehabilitated for release back into the community. Therapy programs need to be developed for each group. Such services usually are located in specialized forensic psychiatric units, which may be located at a hospital, prison, or jail. Other services may include functioning as an expert witness, providing aftercare, or offering community services.

Forensic psychiatry is a term related to place and type of employment setting, not a clinically diagnosed disorder. Therefore, there is no specific axis classification. The axis classification would depend on the psychiatric disorder given each individual in the forensic setting.

CAUSE

The causes include a variety of etiologic factors, such as inherited disorders, congenital disorders, family interaction disturbances, and social deprivation. The etiology may also be a combination of factors triggered by a specific stressful situation.

ASSESSMENT

Areas
- self-care activities
- productivity, including history, skills, aptitudes, and interests
- leisure activities, including skills and interests
- academic learning skills
- time management
- problem-solving skills
- coping skills, adaptive strategies
- interaction skills, including peer and authority relationships

Instruments
Instruments Developed by Occupational Therapy Personnel
- *Allen Cognitive Level Screening Test* by C.K. Allen, Colchester, CT: S&S Worldwide, 1996.
- *Bay Area Functional Performance Evaluation,* 2nd ed., by S.L. Williams and J. Bloomer. Palo Alto, CA: Consulting Psychologists Press, 1987.
- *Client Satisfaction Survey* by C. Lloyd, in *Forensic psychiatry for health professions,* 96–97, London: Chapman & Hall, 1995.
- *Forensic Activities of Daily Living Questionnaire* by C. Lloyd, in *Forensic psychiatry for health professions,* 73–76, London: Chapman & Hall, 1995.
- *Interest Checklist* by J. Matsutsuya, *American Journal of Occupational Therapy* 23, no. 4 (1969): 323–328.
- *Occupational Case Analysis Interview and Rating Scale* by K.L. Kaplan and G. Kielhofner, Thorofare, NJ: Slack, 1989.
- *Role Checklist*, 2nd ed., by F. Oakley, Bethesda, MD: Occupational Therapy Service, National Institutes of Health, 1988.
- *Self-Assessment of Occupational Functioning* by K. Baron and C. Curtin, Chicago: Department of Occupational Therapy, University of Illinois, 1990.

Instruments Developed by Other Professionals and Used by Occupational Therapy Personnel

- *New Scale of Interrogative Suggestibility* by G. Gudjonsson, *Personality and Individual Differences* 4 (1984): 303.
- *Competency Screening Test* by P. Lipsitt, D. Lelos, and A. McGarry, in Competency to stand trial: A screening instrument, *American Journal of Psychiatry* 128 (1971): 105.
- *Coping Responses Inventory* by R.H. Moos, Odessa, FL: Psychological Assessment Resources, 1976.
- *Interdisciplinary Fitness Interview* by S. Galding, R. Roesch, and J. Schreiber, in Assessment and conceptualization of competency to stand trial: Preliminary data on the interdisciplinary fitness interview, *Law and Human Behavior* 8 (1984): 321.
- *Rogers Criminal Responsibility Assessment Scales* by B. Rogers, Odessa, FL: Psychological Assessment Resources, 1984.

PROBLEMS

Self-Care
- The person may be unable to perform functional skills, such as meal preparation and paying bills.
- The person may lack community skills, such as how to shop for food, locate affordable housing, or read a bus schedule.

Productivity
- The person may lack job-seeking skills.
- The person may lack the knowledge or skills necessary to keep a job.
- The person may lack home-management skills.

Leisure
The person may lack leisure interests and skills.

Sensorimotor
- The person may experience deconditioning from inactivity in a restricted living situation.
- The person may have problems in sensory integration.

Cognitive
- The person may lack decision-making and problem-solving skills.
- The person may have learning disorder patterns, such as dyslexia, poor bilateral integration, or hyperactivity.
- The person may lack basic education skills, such as reading, arithmetic, and writing, or be functionally illiterate.
- The person may lack time-management skills.

Psychosocial
- The person may be unable to manage affection in a socially acceptable manner.

- The person may have feelings of inadequacy and inferiority (a poor self-concept and lack of self-esteem).
- The person may lack feeling for and recognition of responsibilities.
- The person may lack adequate coping skills or adaptive behavior.
- The person may lack the social skills necessary to carry on a social conversation.
- The person may lack interpersonal skills related to caring and sharing.
- The person may lack role skills other than criminal.

TREATMENT/INTERVENTION
Models of treatment include behavioral therapy, motivational change, and social skills training. Major program models are based on increasing occupational adaptation, sense of competency in occupational behavior, human occupation, personal adaptation through occupation, cognitive disability, activities therapy, sensory integration, and activities health.

Self-Care
- Provide opportunities to learn about self-care and maintenance activities such as dressing for a job interview and work situation.
- Provide instruction in instrumental activities of daily living such as cooking and nutrition, budgeting, shopping, doing laundry, basic cleaning, and finding living accommodations.
- Provide skills in food preparation using a hot plate or microwave oven that might be available in an efficiency apartment or local fast food restaurant.

Productivity
- Provide work-skills training, including work readiness, work habits, and job practice.
- Provide job survival skills, including human relations skills, worker characteristics, resume writing, practicing employment interviews, and completing job applications.
- Provide vocational information and discussion related to employment resources, assessing the job market, contacting prospective employers, and coping with stress on the job.

Leisure
- Provide group sessions to explore and develop leisure interests.
- Provide opportunities to practice leisure skills such as games, art, crafts, creative writing, reading poetry, drama, and so on.

Sensorimotor
- Provide programs designed to maintain general physical fitness and conditioning.
- Sensory integration programs may be helpful to those identified as having problems in bilateral integration, dyspraxia, or gravitational security.

Cognitive
- Teach the person to recognize and break the cycle of criminal behavior.
- Teach the person alternative behaviors to suppress, control, manage, or stop the criminal behavior pattern.
- Provide situations for individual and group decision making and problem solving through the use of craft projects, games, or task groups.

- Provide tasks and activities that require basic reading, arithmetic, and writing, such as reading the directions to heat a frozen food dinner, adding up the costs of groceries, or writing a letter.
- Teach time management through a daily schedule, organizing the steps in a project, or discussions about the health and social values of balancing work, rest, and play.

Psychosocial

- Encourage the person to accept responsibility for his or her behavior and to establish an internal locus of control.
- Encourage the person to express feelings of guilt related to acts of criminal behavior.
- Improve the person's self-concept through completion of tasks, such as craft projects, playing board games, musical activities, or drama.
- Have the person participate in victim empathy therapy to enable him or her to view the crime from the point of view of the victims.
- Provide instruction in stress management techniques, such as relaxation training.
- Provide insight-oriented groups through the use of psychodrama, simulated games, or goal-oriented group tasks.
- Help the person experience positive interpersonal relationships that are satisfying, pleasurable, and nonthreatening through the use of sports or musical activities or discussion groups based on viewing films or television programs.
- Provide group situations through discussion, role playing, and task groups to explore different role behaviors, such as leader, follower, supervisor, employee, parent, or child.

Environment

- While the person is in the institution, occupational therapy personnel must provide a safe environment to try out behaviors in an activity-based situation.
- Provide information about resources in the community that may be helpful when the person is released.
- Provide instruction in time management and scheduling in the community as opposed to in the institution.

PRECAUTIONS

- Occupational therapy personnel must understand the basics of the legal system to understand the rules of sentencing and the rights of prisoners.
- Occupational therapy personnel must understand the need for security and how to handle dangerous clients who may harm themselves or others.
- All equipment and most supplies should be checked before and after therapy sessions to determine lost and potential misuse.
- Occupational therapy personnel should be aware of possible suicide risks and take necessary precautions.
- Occupational therapy personnel should be prepared to recognize malingering to avoid prosecution, continue a drug habit, or ease the frustration and boredom associated with incarceration.

PROGNOSIS AND OUTCOME

- The person can demonstrate skills in self-care.
- The person can demonstrate skills in locating and maintaining employment.
- The person can demonstrate skills in homemaking and home management.
- The person can demonstrate leisure skills.
- The person can demonstrate effective problem-solving techniques.
- The person can demonstrate skills in behavioral control.
- The person can demonstrate coping or adaptive strategies for dealing with stressful situations.
- The person can demonstrate social interaction skills that are acceptable to other members of a group.
- The person can demonstrate role performance that is socially accepted, such as worker, volunteer, student, homemaker, club member, recreational sport team member, and so on.

BIBLIOGRAPHY

Busuttil, J. 1997. Forensic occupational therapy in Malta: A historical overview. *WFOT Bulletin* 36: 25–26.

Chacksfield, J. 1997. Forensic occupational therapy: Is it a developing specialism? *British Journal of Therapy and Rehabilitation* 4, no. 7: 371–374.

Chacksfield, J. 1997. Occupational therapy and forensic addictive behaviors. *British Journal of Therapy and Rehabilitation* 4, no. 7: 381–386.

Colpaert, A., Y. Cattier, and C. Valentin. 1997. Experiences of creative workshops in a Belgian prison. *WFOT Bulletin* 36: 20–24.

Crawford, M., and J. Mee. 1994. The role of occupational therapy in the rehabilitation of the mentally disordered offender. *British Journal of Occupational Therapy* 57, no. 1: 26–28.

Dressler, J., and F. Snively. 1998. Occupational therapy in the criminal justice system. In *Psychosocial occupational therapy: A clinical practice,* eds. E. Cara and A. MacRae, 527–552. Albany: Delmar.

Flood, B. 1993. Implications for occupational therapy services following the Reed Report. *British Journal of Occupational Therapy* 56, no. 8: 293–294.

Flood, B. 1997. An introduction to occupational therapy in forensic psychiatry. *British Journal of Therapy and Rehabilitation* 4, no. 7: 375–376, 378–380.

Forward, M.J., C. Lloyd, and J. Trevan-Hawke. 1999. The OT in the forensic psychiatric setting. *British Journal of Therapy and Rehabilitation* 6, no. 9: 442–446.

Garner, R. 1995. Prevocational training within a secure environment: A programme designed to enable the forensic patient to prepare for mainstream opportunities. *British Journal of Occupational Therapy* 58, no. 1: 2–6.

Idringa, R. 1997. Occupational therapy, forensics and the care and treatment of addicts. *WFOT Bulletin* 36: 16–19.

Joe, B.E. 1997. Rehab's ultimate challenge. *OT Week* 11, no. 26: 20.

Kerr, T. 1997. Holiday activities: Good rehab for violent offenders. *Advance for Occupational Therapists* 13, no. 49: 21.

Lloyd, C. 1995. Trends in forensic psychiatry. *British Journal of Occupational Therapy* 58, no. 5: 209–213.

Lloyd, C. 1995. *Forensic Psychiatry for Health Professionals.* London, England: Chapman & Hall.

Marmer, L. 1997. Occupation-centered therapy: How to make a lasting difference in mental health. *Advance for Occupational Therapists* 13, no. 39: 13, 46.

Rogowski, A. 1997. Forensic psychiatry. In *Occupational therapy and mental health*, 2nd ed., ed. J. Creek, 459–480. New York: Churchill Livingstone.

Stancliff, B.L. 1997. Emerging practice areas: Going where no OT has gone before; Forensic OT: Filling a void; OT on the "inside." *OT Practice* 2, no. 7: 16–20.

Taylor, E.A., et al. 1997. Forensic practice for occupational therapists—the Alberta Experience. *WFOT Bulletin* 36: 6–10.

Whiteford, G. 1997. Occupational deprivation and incarceration. *Journal of Occupational Science: Australia* 4, no. 3: 126–130.

Homelessness—Adult

DESCRIPTION

Homeless describes a person who lacks a permanent home and address. Other terms include vagrant, vagabond, panhandler, hobo, or bum. Homelessness is not necessarily a mental health disorder itself, but because of associated problems often related to psychiatric disorders, the mental health section seemed to be the best location for this condition.

Homelessness is a sociocultural term, not a psychiatric disorder; therefore, no axis classification can be assigned. A person who is homeless may have a psychiatric disorder, in which case the axis classification is determined by that disorder.

CAUSE

There are many causes of homelessness. Mental illness, substance abuse, head injury, Alzheimer's, or other conditions may disable the person so that he or she is unable to earn money to pay rent or keep a residence in satisfactory enough condition to avoid eviction. Domestic violence is another cause of homelessness, especially for a mother who does not have the resources to find a safe place to live or the skills to get a job. Social policy may cause homelessness if urban redevelopment substantially reduces the number of available low-income housing units.

ASSESSMENT

Areas

- self-care skills, including activities of daily living (ADLs) and instrumental ADLs
- productivity skills, including values and skills
- leisure skills and interests
- problem-solving and decision-making skills
- time-management skills
- coping and adaptive strategies
- roles and role behavior, former and present
- social interaction skills
- social support system

Instruments

- *Kohlman Evaluation of Living Skills*, 3rd ed., by L. Kohlman-Thomson, Rockville, MD: American Occupational Therapy Association, 1992.

PROBLEMS

Self-Care

- The person may depend on others for instrumental ADLs.
- The person may be picked up by the police for lack of hygiene.

Productivity

The person is usually unemployed.

Leisure

The person may be performing few or no leisure activities.

Sensorimotor

No specific information is reported.

Cognitive

- The person may lack knowledge about parenting and normal child development.
- The person may have memory loss or dementia.

Psychosocial

- The person may be abusing substances or be chemically dependent on alcohol and recreational drugs.
- The person may have a chronic mental illness such as schizophrenia.
- The person may feel a lack of control over his or her life and/or feel that other family members are in control. As a result, the person may feel that any action will have little or no impact on being homeless.
- The person may blame others for the homelessness.
- The person may have experienced physical, sexual, and/or emotional abuse, as either the abuser or the person who was abused.
- The person may have experienced violence or abusive relationships in the former home.
- The person may lack trust in others as a result of experiences such as abuse. The person may also be distrustful of health care workers.
- The person may have street-smart skills—including manipulative behavior—that are not acceptable in other situations.
- The person may be an ex-prisoner or have family members in prison.
- The person may be withdrawn or depressed.
- The person may fail to take prescribed medications to control behavioral symptoms.
- The person may experience social isolation.
- The person may have loss of self-esteem.

- The person may express feelings of hopelessness and helplessness.
- The person may show low levels of interest and motivation.
- The person usually has lost roles and role identities held before he or she became homeless.
- The person may have little or no family or social support. Often the person has alienated family and friends by his or her behavior toward them.

Environment
- The person may come from a dysfunctional family that provides little or no social support.
- Lack of coordination and cooperation may exist among agencies that offer services to homeless persons.
- There may be no central location for services.
- Legal issues may exist, such as divorce, child custody, or criminal behavior.

TREATMENT/INTERVENTION
Models of occupational therapy include the model of human occupation.

Self-Care
Increase independence in instrumental ADLs such as budgeting, transportation, and household management.

Productivity
Provide opportunities to engage in productive tasks, starting with crafts or tasks that need to be done about the shelter.

Leisure
Help the person explore the community and available resources, including music and art, through field trips, lectures, and discussion.

Sensorimotor
The person may need to increase his or her endurance and physical fitness.

Cognitive
Help the person recognize that his or her former life was unmanageable and a new plan needs to be made.

Psychosocial
- The "tough love" approach may be helpful.
- A 12-step recovery program may provide the structure the person needs to "start over."
- Built-in child care is essential for programs that deal with women.
- The person needs opportunities to increase his or her self-esteem and sense of self-worth.
- Provide opportunities for the person to increase social interaction skills.

Environment
- Provide troubleshooting, information, and resources to help the professionals in charge of the program.

- Provide a program in the community that matches persons who need homes with persons who need physical and social help (Collins, 1997).
- Work on specific activities that will help the person reintegrate into the community, such as finding suitable housing, using public transportation, and using community resources.

PRECAUTIONS
Clients may not be taking medication and could become violent.

PROGNOSIS AND OUTCOME
- The person demonstrates skills and performs self-care activities.
- The person demonstrates skills in instrumental ADLs.
- The person demonstrates productivity skills such as volunteering, finding a job, resuming studies, or parenting.
- The person demonstrates leisure skills by participating in a chosen activity.
- The person demonstrates coping skills and adaptive strategies.
- The person demonstrates knowledge of and skill in using community resources.

REFERENCE
Collins, L.F. 1997. Connecting the community: Shared housing in New Orleans. *OT Practice* 2, no. 4: 40–43, 45–47.

BIBLIOGRAPHY
Barth, T. 1994. Occupational therapy interventions at a shelter for homeless, addicted adults with mental illness. *Mental Health Special Interest Section Newsletter* 17, no. 1: 7–8.

Borg, B., and M.A. Bruce. 1997. Reengagement. In *Occupational therapy stories: Psychosocial interaction in practice,* eds. B. Borg and M.A. Bruce, 111–116. Thorofare, NJ: Slack.

Heubner, J.E., and J. Tryssenaar. 1996. Development of an occupational therapy practice perspective in a homeless shelter: A fieldwork experience. *Canadian Journal of Occupational Therapy* 63, no. 1: 24–32.

Kavanagh, J., and J. Fares. 1995. Using the model of human occupation with homeless mentally ill clients. *British Journal of Occupational Therapy* 58, no. 10: 419–422.

Kerr, T. 1997. Student program gets homeless back on their feet. *Advance for Occupational Therapists* 13, no. 18: 12.

Stahl, C. 1997. Research project tests impact of PTSD on homeless women. *Advance for Occupational Therapists* 13, no. 30: 11.

Stancliff, B.L. 1997. Emerging practice areas: Going where no OT has gone before—Homeless program benefits from OT skills. *OT Practice* 2, no. 7: 22–23.

Personality Disorders

DESCRIPTION

The major feature of a personality disorder is an enduring pattern of inner experience and behavior that deviates markedly from the expectations of the individual's culture and is manifested in at least two of the following areas: affectivity, cognition, impulse control, and interpersonal functioning. Personality disorders are coded on Axis II on the multiaxial assessment scale. The enduring pattern is inflexible and pervasive across a broad range of personal and social situations, is stable and of long duration, and leads to clinically significant distress or impairment in social, occupational, or other areas of functioning. Other mental disorders, substance abuse, medical conditions, and problems associated with acculturation must be ruled out. There are 10 specific types of personality disorders that can be grouped into three major clusters according to the DSM-IV (American Psychiatric Association 1994, 629–630).

Cluster A

Individuals with these disorders often appear odd or eccentric.
- **Paranoid** personality disorder is a pattern of distrust and suspiciousness in which others' motives are interpreted as malevolent.
- **Schizoid** personality disorder is a pattern of detachment from social relationships and a restricted range of emotional expression.
- **Schizotypal** personality disorder is a pattern of acute discomfort in close relationships, cognitive or perceptual distortions, and eccentricities of behavior.

Cluster B

Individuals with these disorders often appear dramatic, emotional, or erratic.
- **Antisocial** personality disorder is a pattern of disregard for and violation of the rights of others.
- **Borderline** personality disorder is a pattern of instability in interpersonal relationships, self-image, and affects, and marked impulsivity.
- **Histrionic** personality disorder is a pattern of excessive emotionality and attention seeking.
- **Narcissistic** personality disorder is a pattern of grandiosity, need for admiration, and lack of empathy.

Cluster C

Individuals with these disorders often appear anxious or fearful.
- **Avoidant** personality disorder is a pattern of social inhibition, feelings of inadequacy, and hypersensitivity to negative evaluation.
- **Dependent** personality disorder is a pattern of submissive and clinging behavior related to an excessive need to be taken care of.
- **Obsessive-compulsive** personality disorder is a pattern of preoccupation with orderliness, perfectionism, and control.

CAUSE

The cause of personality disorders is unknown but is associated with early childhood experiences; the disorder must be traced back at least to adolescence or early adulthood as part of the diagnostic criteria. The disorders in Cluster A are more common in men, while those in Clusters B and C are more common in women. Individuals rarely seek help; they are usually referred by family members or social agencies because of the difficulties their maladaptive behavior causes others.

ASSESSMENT

Areas

- daily living skills, including activities of daily living (ADLs) and instrumental ADLs
- productivity history, values, and skills
- leisure skills and interests
- level of arousal or awareness
- orientation to person, place, and time
- recognition
- attending behavior
- attention span
- memory
- concept formation
- comprehension
- generalization and integration of learning
- problem-solving and decision-making skills
- judgment of safety
- time management
- self-concept and self-esteem
- self-identity or role identity
- coping skills
- self-control
- social interaction skills or conduct
- language and communication skills
- group interaction skills
- social support

Instruments

- *Allen Diagnostic Module* by C. Allen, C.A. Earhart, and T. Blue, in *Understanding cognitive performance modes,* Colchester, CT: S&S Worldwide, 1996.
- *Occupational Performance History Interview* by G. Kielhofner and A. Henry, Bethesda, MD: American Occupational Therapy Association, 1995.

PROBLEMS

Self-Care

- The ability to perform basic ADLs is not a problem, but motivation may be.
- The person may encounter difficulties with instrumental ADLs because of behavioral patterns that are not accepted in society.

Productivity

- The person usually has a poor work history; for example, being fired from several jobs, many changes in the type of job held, or a history of underemployment in relation to his or her education and skill level. The person may also have a marginal school record.
- The person usually has poorly defined vocational goals.
- The person may experience difficulty in job situations with coworkers because of his or her inappropriate expression of emotions.
- The person may experience job-related conflict with supervisors regarding dependence/independence problems.
- The person may be unable to meet the standards of performance expected at work, especially unwritten standards.
- The person may lack motivation to help with home-management tasks.
- The person tends to be unclear about career choices.
- The person may express dissatisfaction with work situations and sees work activities as meaningless.
- The person may have poor work habits accompanied by avoidance and procrastination.

Leisure

- The person may lack the ability to gain satisfaction from recreational or leisure pursuits because of rigid, narrow interests; fearful behavior; or fear of closeness to others.
- The person may experience difficulty engaging in group leisure activities, such as sports, because of a low tolerance for frustration and the need to maintain control.
- The person may select certain leisure activities to permit spontaneity, a sense of achievement, and relief from inner turmoil that cannot be obtained in any other way.
- The person's leisure interests may be poorly defined.

Sensorimotor

- The person may complain of vague somatic symptoms.
- The person may have brief episodes of delusions or hallucinatory experiences.

Cognitive

- The person may have a short attention span and poor concentration.
- The person may have poor comprehension or understanding of situations and the possible consequences of personal actions.
- The person may have difficulty planning long-term goals and tends to be impulsive.
- The person may have difficulty integrating learned skills into useful patterns of behavior.
- The person usually has difficulty with problem-solving and decision-making tasks. He or she tends to select from a very narrow list of possible choices.

- The person tends to take extreme views: The world is either black or white. This is called *dichotomous thinking* or *splitting.*
- The person's judgment may be impaired concerning his or her personal safety.
- The person's memory skills may be underdeveloped.
- The person's time-management skills usually are poor.

Psychosocial
- The person may have a poor self-concept, including a poor sense of mastery.
- The person usually lacks a sense of responsibility for individual actions.
- The person may exhibit impulsive behavior that is potentially self-damaging.
- The person may have difficulty distinguishing his or her own needs from others' needs.
- The person's coping skills are limited. The person does not tolerate frustration or anxiety, has poor impulse control, and does not sublimate his or her drives into socially acceptable channels.
- The person usually has low motivation to change his or her behavior.
- The person may have suicidal ideation.
- The person may have a charming personality in casual relations but lacks the ability to engage in sustained interdependent relationships.
- The person may have difficulty relating to authority figures.
- The person may have difficulty cooperating with a group to perform tasks unless the task is performed according to his or her personal specifications.
- The person may have difficulty maintaining relationships within the family.
- The person's moods may shift among depression, irritability, and anxiety.
- The person lacks control of anger and may display a temper or get into physical fights.
- The person makes recurrent suicidal threats or gestures or exhibits self-mutilating behavior.
- The person's self-image is unstable and may vacillate between dependency and self-assertion.
- The person has chronic feelings of emptiness or boredom.
- The person may be unsure about his or her sexual orientation.
- The person is uncertain about which values to adopt.
- The person may have unrealistic expectations for perfection.
- A splitting of feelings into good and bad with no integration may have led to identity diffusion.
- The person has a pattern of unstable interpersonal relationships characterized by alternating between extremes of overidealization and devaluation.
- The person tries to avoid real or imagined abandonment and hates to be alone.
- The person has difficulty deciding what type of friends to have and maintaining friendships.
- The person may manipulate others through self-destructive behavior.

TREATMENT/INTERVENTION

Treatment models have been based on biophysical, neuropsychiatric, psychodynamic, behavioral, cognitive, interpersonal, biopsychosocial or evolutionary, and neurobiological or temperament theories. Models in occupational therapy include the model of human occupation. Bonder (1995) suggests that the underlying issues in personality disorders are similar

Functional Deficits of Persons with Personality Disorders

Antisocial	Work, leisure, social, instrumental ADL (especially financial)
Avoidant	Social, possibly work and leisure
Borderline	Work, leisure, social, ADL, instrumental ADL
Dependent	Social, possibly work and leisure
Histrionic	Work, leisure, social
Obsessive-compulsive	Social, possibly work and leisure
Paranoid	Work, leisure, social
Schizoid	Work, leisure, social
Schizotypal	Work, leisure, social, ADL, instrumental ADL

Source: Data from B.R. Bonder, *Psychopathology and Function*, 2nd ed., pp. 123–142, © 1995, Slack.

from the standpoint of occupational therapy. These issues are (1) inaccurate perceptions of self and others, (2) inadequate social skills, (3) poorly developed personal values and goals, and (4) poor self-esteem.

Self-Care

- Help the person increase skills in self-care and daily living, such as cooking, meal planning, shopping, and personal finance. The person may need assistance in shopping for suitable clothes for a productive role.
- Praise the person for completing self-care activities or performing other ADLs that he or she has tended not to perform in the past.

Productivity

- Help the person to explore vocational interests, including simulated or temporary job responsibilities.
- Help the person to learn and perform life-management and home-management skills.
- Supervised work activities may be useful in helping the person learn to continue performing while experiencing conflicting feelings.
- The work setting should provide a consistent set of demands within a given time period to permit the development of work cycles that can be discussed later in a group or individual session.
- The work activities should permit exploration and curiosity about how the work is done, such as how leather is carved or how clay becomes a solid object.
- Encourage the person to sort out productive from unproductive work habits.
- Help the person explore vocational interests and identify career goals.
- Increase the person's skills in home management.

Leisure

- Help the person explore leisure interests and learn about community resources.

- Help the person select leisure activities that will provide a creative outlet for his or her feelings.
- Encourage exploration of activities that are fun to do and support the person's recognition of having fun.

Sensorimotor

Persons diagnosed with one of the Cluster A disorders may respond to sensory-integrative and sensorimotor interventions because of a neurologic component to their disorder.

Cognitive

- Persons diagnosed with one of the Cluster B disorders may respond to behavioral learning strategies because of deficits in early learning experiences.
- Provide activities to improve reality testing and the person's understanding of the consequences of his or her actions.
- Provide graded tasks that require anywhere from few decisions or choices to many possibilities in order to improve the person's ability to solve problems and make decisions.
- Help the person to develop time-management skills by requiring him or her to organize and follow a schedule.
- Assist the person in making a realistic self-appraisal in which both strengths and weaknesses are addressed. Success with this objective may be limited because of the enduring pattern of behavior.

Psychosocial

- Persons diagnosed with one of the Cluster C disorders may be amenable to social skills training, as this is the predominant deficit in these individuals.
- Maintain or improve the person's self-concept through the use of craft or game activities.
- Help the person rechannel his or her behavior into more socially accepted activities.
- Use group activities as a basis for providing instruction and giving feedback on communication skills and for confronting the person on the effects of his or her social behavior on others.
- Provide an outlet for mixed feelings through the use of creative media.
- Provide opportunities for the person to select an activity, to encourage self-awareness.
- Encourage mastery of the task activities to reinforce the concepts of rewarding, pleasurable, self-actualizing experiences with objects in the environment.
- Permit the objects created to be used as projections for the person's vacillating feeling states.
- Confront defensive behavior and inaccurate perceptions of self and others in group situations.
- Provide opportunities for cooperative behavior in a group setting by using tasks that require two or more persons to get the job done within the time frame.
- Contracting (behavior therapy) may be useful to encourage the person to demonstrate responsible behavior, control actions, and make decisions.

PRECAUTIONS

- A person with a personality disorder often tries to bend or break the rules. The management team must agree on the rules and consistently follow through on carrying out the rules and

their assigned consequences. Otherwise, the person may spend most of his or her time looking for ways to divide the staff or undermine authority and will spend little time learning better self-management behaviors.
- A person with a personality disorder may be skilled at "uproar games" or "let's you and him fight." These games distract attention from the self and circumvent efforts to change the person's behavior patterns.

PROGNOSIS AND OUTCOME

The prognosis is guarded. People with personality disorders usually require long-term therapy to make modest gains.
- The person is able to perform daily living activities independently.
- The person demonstrates improved performance of work skills, work tolerance, and work habits and attitudes.
- The person is able to select and perform productive activities.
- The person demonstrates skill in performing home-management tasks.
- The person is able to select and perform leisure activities.
- The person demonstrates socially approved behaviors in group settings.
- The person is able to maintain a productive role or situation.
- The person demonstrates the ability to plan a daily calendar of activities and follow the schedule.

REFERENCES

American Psychiatric Association. 1994. *Diagnostic and Statistical Manual of Mental Disorders: DSM-IV,* 4th ed. Washington, DC: American Psychiatric Association. Task Force on DSM-IV.
Bonder, B.R. 1995. Personality disorders. In *Psychopathology and function*, 2nd ed., ed. B.R. Bonder, 123–124. Thorofare, NJ: Slack.

BIBLIOGRAPHY

Cara, E. 1998. Personality disorders. In *Psychosocial occupational therapy: A clinical practice,* eds. E. Cara and A. MacRae, 435–459. Albany, NY: Delmar.
Ward, J.D. 1998. Borderline personality disorder. In *Willard and Spackman's occupational therapy*, 9th ed., eds. M.E. Neistadt and E.B. Crepeau, 732–735. Philadelphia: Lippincott-Raven.

Post-Traumatic Stress Disorder

DESCRIPTION

The essential feature of posttraumatic stress disorder (PTSD) is the development of characteristic symptoms following exposure to an extreme traumatic stressor involving direct personal experience of an event. The event may involve actual or threatened death or serious injury; a threat to the physical integrity of another person; or learning about unexpected or violent death, serious harm, or threat of death or injury experienced by a family member or other close associate. In adults, the person's response to the event includes intense fear, helplessness, or horror. In children, the response must involve disorganization or agitated behavior. The characteristic symptoms of PTSD include persistent reexperiencing of the traumatic event, persistent avoidance of stimuli associated with the trauma, numbing of general responsiveness, and persistent symptoms of increased arousal. To be clinically significant, the distress or impairment must interfere with social, occupational, or other important areas of functioning (American Psychiatric Association 1994, 424). Persons seen in occupational therapy may have experienced sexual abuse, a natural or man-made disaster, or military combat.

PTSD is a subtype of anxiety disorder. The axis classification is Axis I on the multiaxial assessment scale.

CAUSE

The disorder occurs in response to situations or events that are extremely distressing, such as natural or man-made disasters, physical or sexual abuse, violent crime or accident, or acts of war. Some examples are destruction of a person's home or community by a fire, flood, bombing, tornado, hurricane, earthquake, or other disaster. Other examples are witnessing a violent crime such as murder, torture, or abuse, or witnessing an automobile or airplane crash. Survivors of war—whether military or civilian—are also candidates for PTSD.

ASSESSMENT

Areas
- daily living skills, including activities of daily living (ADLs) and instrumental ADLs
- productivity values and skills
- leisure interests
- time-management skills
- self-image
- social roles and role behavior
- social support system

Instruments
- *Barth Time Construction* by T. Barth, New York: Health Related Consulting Services, 1985.
- *Bay Area Functional Performance Evaluation*, 2nd ed., by S.L. Williams and J. Bloomer, Palo Alto, CA: Consulting Psychologists Press, 1987.
- *Canadian Occupational Performance Measure* (COPM), 2nd ed., by M. Law et al., Ottawa, Ontario, Canada: Canadian Association of Occupational Therapists, 1994.
- *Comprehensive Occupational Therapy Evaluation* by S.J. Brayman, et al., *American Journal of Occupational Therapy* 30, no. 2 (1976): 94–100.
- *Kohlman Evaluation of Living Skills,* 3rd ed., by L. Kohlman-Thomson, Rockville, MD: American Occupational Therapy Association, 1992.

Victims of Disasters At Risk for Post-Traumatic Stress Disorder

- Primary-level victims—the actual survivors of a particular disaster or persons exposed directly to the traumatic events.
- Secondary-level victims—relatives, friends, colleagues, and neighbors of the primary-level victims.
- Third-level victims—individual emergency and support workers involved in rescue, recovery, transport, and care of primary victims, such as police, firefighters, ambulance paramedics, doctors, nurses, and all health care professionals exposed to trauma cases.
- Fourth-level victims—individuals who are part of the immediate community involved in the disaster, including those affected by the total disruption and breakdown of the normal community services such as might occur in a plane crash, tornado, or earthquake.
- Fifth-level victims—"media victims" who suffer emotional and psychological problems as a result of viewing horrific scenes of a disaster on television.
- Sixth-level victims—individuals who would have, except by chance or fate, been primary victims themselves (missed the plane that crashed) or persons who see themselves as being partly responsible for the trauma because they persuaded others to take a course that made them primary victims (suggested person take a vacation and the plane crashed).

Source: Data from B.W. Roberts, Trauma Following Major Disasters: The Role of the Occupational Therapist, *British Journal of Occupational Therapy*, Vol. 58, No. 5, pp. 204–208, © 1995.

- *Role Checklist*, 2nd ed., by F. Oakley, Bethesda, MD: Occupational Therapy Service, National Institutes of Health, 1988.

PROBLEMS

Self-Care
- The person may experience sleep disturbances, including insomnia and nightmares.
- The person may experience difficulty performing some instrumental ADL tasks, such as shopping, driving, or paying bills.
- The person may be homeless and living in a temporary shelter or on the streets.

Productivity
- The person may be unable to work because of flashbacks.
- The person may be using unsafe techniques in a work situation.

Leisure

The person may have lost the skills and the opportunity to engage in leisure activities.

Sensorimotor

- The person may have symptoms of increased anxiety and distress, such as high heart rate, flushed face, or sweating while engaged in or performing certain activities.
- The person may have an exaggerated startle response to noises that are the same as or similar to those associated with the original traumatic situation; for example, an air raid siren. Or the person might respond to a particular odor or to certain visual images in pictures or on videotapes.

Cognitive

- The person may experience intrusive and distressing thoughts.
- The person may try to avoid situations that are the same as or similar to the trauma situation.

Psychosocial

- The person usually tries to avoid situations that might evoke the memory of the trauma.
- The person may have flashbacks to traumatic events.
- The person may have feelings of detachment or unreality when a memory of the trauma surfaces.
- The person, especially a woman or child, may have experienced verbal, physical, or sexual abuse.
- The person may feel guilt or shame for surviving a traumatic situation when others did not.
- The person may feel stigmatized by the events that led to PTSD.
- The person may feel frustrated and angry at what happened and at whoever is perceived to be responsible for the disaster.
- The person may have learned a sense of helplessness, hopelessness, and powerlessness.
- The person may question his or her faith or religion. How could God let this happen?
- The person may become socially withdrawn and isolated, avoiding contact with others.
- The person may lose coping skills.
- The person may lack social support.

TREATMENT/INTERVENTION

The primary model of treatment in psychology is a behavioral therapy using repeated exposure to the trauma-related stimuli to desensitize and extinguish the response. In occupational therapy, models of practice include object relations (Froehlich 1992), approaches emphasizing therapeutic rituals and emotional catharsis (Short-DeGraff and Engelmann 1992), and the model of human occupation.

Self-Care

Practice can be used to enable the person to perform independently where withdrawal or isolation have reduced his or her involvement in instrumental ADL tasks such as shopping, doing errands in the community, or driving.

Productivity

Work simulation tasks can be useful in extinguishing responses in cases in which the PTSD is related to work situations.

Sensorimotor

- Help the person learn to use breathing exercises to counteract the physiologic symptoms of PTSD.
- To help identify feelings and reactions, use music that is related to the trauma; for example, war songs.
- Pictures, videotapes, or patriotic colors may be useful in helping the person identify feelings and responses to certain situations.

Cognitive

- Teach the person stress management techniques, including relaxation techniques.
- Systematic desensitization to threatening stimuli is the treatment of choice by psychologists. Occupational therapy personnel can provide simulated or real environments in which desensitization can occur in a controlled environment.
- Facilitate discussions of values and interests to help the person understand personal causation in activity and interpersonal choices.
- Creative writing may allow the person to express feelings.

Psychosocial

- Help the person learn to use mental imagery to counteract flashbacks.
- Creative and expressive media such as art or ceramics can be helpful in allowing the person to express feelings, thoughts, and experiences related to the trauma.
- Help the person increase his or her self-esteem by participating in meaningful activities that provide a successful result.
- Support and encourage the performance of role behaviors and tasks that encompass daily habits.

Environment

Teach the person about community resources.

PRECAUTIONS

Occupational therapy personnel should be aware that some clients may be a danger to themselves and possibly to others.

PROGNOSIS AND OUTCOME

- The person demonstrates the ability to perform instrumental ADLs.
- The person demonstrates the ability to get and keep a job for at least one year.
- The person is able to express feelings, including enjoyment and fun, while performing a leisure activity.
- The person is able to discuss the trauma and the accompanying feelings.

- The person demonstrates social interaction skills.
- The person performs roles and tasks in a socially acceptable manner.

REFERENCES

American Psychiatric Association. 1994. *Diagnostic and Statistical Manual of Mental Disorders: DSM-IV,* 4th ed. Washington, DC: American Psychiatric Association. Task Force on DSM-IV.
Froelich, J. 1992. Occupational therapy interventions with survivors of sexual abuse. *Occupational Therapy in Health Care* 8, no. 2–3: 1–25.
Short-DeGraff, M.A., and T. Engelmann. 1992. Activities for the treatment of combat-related post-traumatic stress disorder. *Occupational Therapy in Health Care* 8, no. 2–3: 27–47.

BIBLIOGRAPHY

Phillips, M.E., S. Bruehl, and R.N. Harden. 1997. Work-related post-traumatic stress disorder: Use of exposure therapy in work-simulation activities. *American Journal of Occupational Therapy* 51, no. 8: 696–700.
Roberts, B.W. 1995. Trauma following major disasters: The role of the occupational therapist. *British Journal of Occupational Therapy* 58, no. 5: 204–208.
Stahl, C. 1997. Research project tests impact of PTSD on homeless women. *Advance for Occupational Therapists* 13, no. 30: 11.

Schizophrenia and Other Psychotic Disorders

DESCRIPTION

The characteristic signs and symptoms of schizophrenia are two or more of the following: delusions; hallucinations; disorganized speech; grossly disorganized or catatonic behavior; or negative symptoms such as affective flattening, alogia, or avolition that have been present for a significant portion of time during a one-month period with some signs of the disorder persisting for at least six months. These signs and symptoms are associated with marked social or occupational dysfunction (American Psychiatric Association 1994, 285).

Schizophrenia is an Axis I disorder on the multiaxial assessment scale.

The following terminology associated with schizophrenia and other psychotic disorders is based on DSM-IV and other sources.

- *alogia*—an impoverishment in thinking that is inferred from observing speech and language behavior
- *avolition*—an inability to initiate and persist in goal-directed activities
- *delusion*—a false belief based on incorrect inference about external reality that is firmly sustained despite what almost everyone else believes and despite what constitutes incontrovertible and obvious proof or evidence to the contrary

- *hallucination*—a sensory perception that has the compelling sense of reality of a true perception but that occurs without external stimulation of the relevant sensory organ
- *negative symptoms*—loss of normal function, including poverty of speech; blunting of emotional affect; avolition (loss of will, energy, and drive); anhedonia (loss of ability to experience pleasures); and diminished interpersonal skills (Andreasen 1987)
- *positive symptoms*—distortions of normal functions and perceptions, including delusions, hallucinations, disorganized speech, and disorganized behavior (Andreasen 1987)

CAUSE

The cause is unknown. Current thinking suggests that the disorder is caused by a complex interaction of inherited and environmental factors, including disturbances of brain circuitry and chemical imbalances in the brain.

ASSESSMENT

Areas
- daily living skills
- productivity history, skills, interests, and values
- leisure interests and skills
- postural control and balance
- gross movement patterns
- stereotypical behaviors
- sensory awareness and discrimination
- judgment of personal safety
- problem-solving and decision-making skills
- reality testing
- orientation to time, place, and person
- self-concept
- coping skills and adaptive strategies
- social skills
- social support system

Instruments
Instruments Developed by Occupational Therapy Personnel
- *Activity Configuration* by S. Cynkin and A.M. Robinson, in *Occupational therapy and activities health: Toward health through activities,* Boston: Little, Brown & Co., 1990.
- *Allen Cognitive Level Test-90* by C.K. Allen, C.A. Earhardt, and T. Blue, in *Treatment goals for the physically and cognitively disabled,* Rockville, MD: American Occupational Therapy Association, 1992.
- *Allen Diagnostic Module* by C.A. Earhardt, C.K. Allen, and T. Blue, Colchester, CT: S&S Worldwide, 1993.
- *Assessment of Motor and Process Skills* (AMPS), 2nd ed., by A. Fisher, Fort Collins, CO: Three Star Press, 1997.

- *Bay Area Functional Performance Evaluation* (BAFPE), 2nd ed., by S.L. Williams and J. Bloomer, Palo Alto, CA: Consulting Psychologists Press, 1987.
- *Contextual Memory Test* by J.P. Toglia, San Antonio, TX: Psychological Corporation/ Therapy Skill Builders, 1993.
- *Kohlman Evaluation of Living Skills* (KELS), 3rd ed., by L. Kolhman-Thomson, Rockville, MD: American Occupational Therapy Association, 1992.
- *Milwaukee Evaluation of Daily Living Skills* by C.A. Leonardelli, Thorofare, NJ: Slack, 1988.
- *Occupational Performance History Interview* by G. Kielhofner, A. Henry, and D. Walens, Bethesda, MD: American Occupational Therapy Association, 1995.
- *Role Checklist*, 2nd ed., by F. Oakley, Bethesda, MD: Occupational Therapy Service, National Institutes of Health, 1988.
- *Routine Task Inventory-2* by C.K. Allen, D.A. Earhart, and T. Blue, *Occupational Therapy Treatment Goals for Physically and Cognitively Disabled,* 63–72, Bethesda, MD: American Occupational Therapy Association, 1992.
- *Schroeder Block Campbell Adult Psychiatric Sensory Integration Evaluation* by C.V. Schroeder et al., Kailua, HA: Schroeder Publishing & Consulting, 1979.
- *Scorable Self-Care Evaluation*, rev. ed., by M. Peters and N. Clark, Thorofare, NJ: Slack, 1993.
- *Stress Inventory* by F. Stein and S. Nikolic, in Teaching stress management techniques to a schizophrenic patient, *American Journal of Occupational Therapy* 43, no. 3 (1989): 162–169.
- *Toglia Category Assessment* by J.P. Toglia, Pequannock, NJ: Maddak, 1994.

Instruments Developed by Other Professionals and Used by Occupational Therapy Personnel

- *Motor-Free Visual Perception Test–Revised* (MVPT-R) by R. Colarusso and D.D. Hamill, Novato, CA: Academic Therapy Press, 1996.
- *Scale for the Assessment of Negative Symptoms* by N. Andreason, Iowa City, IA: University of Iowa, 1981.
- *Wisconsin Card-Sorting Test* by R.K. Heaton et al., Odessa, FL: Psychological Assessment Resources, 1993.

PROBLEMS

Self-Care
- The person may be indifferent to performing activities of daily living (ADLs), especially dressing and grooming.
- The person may have difficulty with instrumental ADLs, such as using public transportation, financial management, meal planning, shopping, or using a telephone book to locate a phone number.

Productivity
- The person may be unable to perform job tasks consistently.
- The person may not have developed work skills consistent with any work situation.

Leisure

The person usually has few leisure interests.

Sensorimotor

- The person may exhibit catatonia, stupor, or immobility.
- The person may have poorly developed gross motor skills, including lack of fluid body movement.
- The person may exhibit repetitive movement patterns, such as rocking or pacing.
- Auditory hallucinations are most common, but visual, tactile, gustatory, or olfactory hallucinations may also occur.
- The person may have perceptual deficits such as difficulty with figure-ground or topographical orientation.
- The person may have sensory integrative dysfunction.
- The person may show signs of tardive dyskinesia, such as a neck jerk or pill-rolling motion of the fingers.
- The person may be slow to process information in the sensory motor system.

Cognitive

- The person may have difficulty sustaining an arousal level sufficient to permit focused attention.
- The person may be easily distracted.
- The person may have difficulty detecting relevant stimuli when they are embedded in irrelevant "noise."
- The person may have difficulty with concept formation.
- The person may be inefficient in organizing information into short-term memory.
- The person may have difficulty organizing thoughts in a goal-directed manner.
- The person may have difficulty following a time schedule, especially if the schedule is not written.
- The person may have difficulty starting and finishing a task.
- The person may have difficulty following directions.
- The person may have difficulty with problem solving and decision making.
- The person may have difficulty using judgment and safety skills.
- The person may have difficulty generalizing information from one situation to another.

Psychosocial

- The person may have blunted or flat affect.
- The person's emotions may alternate from depression to excitement, anxiety, elation, or sadness.
- Delusions of persecution or religious ideas are common, but other themes also occur.
- The person may become aggressive toward others.
- The person may have a poorly defined or inaccurate self-concept.
- The person may demonstrate abnormal overresponse to stress.
- The person may have decreased coping skills and adaptive strategies.
- The person may demonstrate limited role performance.
- The person may have poor verbal and nonverbal communication skills.

- The person may have limited social interaction skills.
- The person usually has difficulty maintaining social relations.

TREATMENT/INTERVENTION

Models of treatment in schizophrenia include behavior modification, social skills training such as psychiatric rehabilitation, and cognitive rehabilitation. Models in occupational therapy include the model of human occupation (MOHO, schizophrenia), cognitive disabilities, dynamic interactional model, perceptual cognitive rehabilitation (Abreu), and sensory integration for adults.

Self-Care

- Encourage attention to personal hygiene, including bathing, grooming, and dressing.
- Establish a reward system, such as verbal praise, for improving and maintaining personal appearance.
- Increase functional skills in independent living such as meal preparation, shopping, money management, using public transportation, and driving safely.

Productivity

- Help the person improve his or her work habits and skills.
- Provide opportunities for the person to try out different jobs through supervised practice or job coaching.
- Provide opportunities for the person to develop job acquisition skills, including locating a potential job, interviewing, and learning the requirements for performing the job.

Leisure

- Provide opportunities to explore leisure interests.
- Provide opportunities to practice recreational pursuits.

Sensorimotor

- Increase the person's gross motor coordination.
- Increase motor planning ability.
- Decrease body rigidity.
- Increase the person's balance and equilibrium.
- Increase body awareness.
- Provide more direct visual sensory stimulation and less auditory stimulation, and reduce auditory and visual clutter.
- Increase perceptual skills in topographic orientation using maps and planned trips.

Cognitive

- Help the person learn to regulate arousal and alertness.
- Increase problem-solving ability.
- Encourage independent decision making.
- Increase knowledge of community resources.
- Provide opportunities to practice time-management skills.

- Teach the person to use judgment skills and safety awareness.
- Provide assertiveness training.

Psychosocial

- Decrease the person's depressed behavior.
- Decrease inappropriate expressions of anger.
- Provide reality orientation training.
- Provide values clarification exercises.
- Increase coping skills and adaptive strategies.
- Increase self-esteem and positive self-image through individual accomplishment with expressive activities such as drawing, painting, or pottery.
- Provide opportunities for graded, structured verbalization.
- Provide one-on-one contact for individuals who are withdrawn or are too psychotic to benefit from a group approach.
- Provide opportunities for working cooperatively in a group setting.
- Provide opportunities for practicing appropriate behavior in the community.
- Use role playing to increase social skills.

PRECAUTIONS

- The variety of symptoms and levels of function or dysfunction in schizophrenia suggest that any single treatment approach will not be successful for all cases. Multiple approaches may be needed for different clients functioning at different levels and for any one client at a particular point in the course of the disorder.
- Schizophrenia is a life-long process. Relapses occur frequently in some cases.
- Occupational therapy personnel should be aware that persons with schizophrenia may be suicide risks because of misperceptions about their environment. Persons with paranoid symptoms may strike out at others if they perceive a situation to be threatening.

PROGNOSIS AND OUTCOME

- The person can perform self-care skills and function independently in the community.
- The person is able to perform productivity tasks in a worker role.
- The person is able to take responsibility for and control of his or her life.
- The person is able to interpret his or her environment correctly and react appropriately.
- The person is able to solve problems and make decisions independently.
- The person can express emotions in socially approved ways.
- The person can plan and follow a time schedule.
- The person is oriented to reality.

REFERENCES

American Psychiatric Association. 1994. *Diagnostic and Statistical Manual of Mental Disorders: DSM-IV*, 4th ed. Washington, DC: American Psychiatric Association. Task Force on DSM-IV.

Andreasen, N.C. 1987. The diagnosis of schizophrenia. *Schizophrenia Bulletin* 13: 9–22.

BIBLIOGRAPHY

Barnett, P.L. 1993. The young adult with schizophrenia. In *Practice issues in occupational therapy: Intraprofessional team building,* ed. S.E. Ryan, 103–110. Thorofare, NJ: Slack.

Barrows, C. 1996. Clinical interpretation of predictors of functional outcome among adolescents and young adults with psychotic disorders (comment). *American Journal of Occupational Therapy* 50, no. 3: 182–183.

Benetton, M.J. 1995. A case study applying a psychodynamic approach to occupational therapy. *Occupational Therapy International* 2, no. 3: 220–228.

Bonder, B.R. 1995. Schizophrenia, paranoid disorders, and other psychoses. In *Psychopathology and function,* 2nd ed., ed. B.R. Bonder, 77–92. Thorofare, NJ: Slack.

Brown. C., et al. 1993. Effectiveness of cognitive rehabilitation for improving attention in patients with schizophrenia. *Occupational Therapy Journal of Research* 13, no. 2: 71–86.

Fine, S. 1993. Neurobehavioral perspectives on schizophrenia. In *Body image and perceptual dysfunction in adults,* ed. J. Van Duesen, 83–115. Philadelphia: W.B. Saunders.

Fine, S. 1994. Reframing rehabilitation: Putting skill acquisition and the mental health system into proper perspective. In *Cognitive technology in psychiatric rehabilitation,* ed. W.D. Spaulding, 87–113. Lincoln, NE: University of Nebraska Press.

Hemphill-Pearson, B.J., and M. Hunter. 1997. Holism in mental health practice. *Occupational Therapy in Mental Health* 13, no. 2: 35–49.

Henry, A.D., and W.J. Foster. 1996. Predictors of functional outcome among adolescents and young adults with psychotic disorders. *American Journal of Occupational Therapy* 50, no. 3: 171–181.

Hirsh, I.G. 1993. At Harper Hospital, client's treatment is work. *OT Week* 7, no. 30: 16–17.

Josman, N. 1996. The dynamic interactional model in schizophrenia. In *Cognition and occupation in rehabilitation: Cognitive models for intervention in occupational therapy,* ed. N. Katz, 151–164. Bethesda, MD: American Occupational Therapy Association.

Kannenberg, K.R. 1997. *Occupational therapy practice guidelines for adults with schizophrenia.* Bethesda, MD: American Occupational Therapy Association.

Kautzmann, L.N. 1996. Schizophrenia. Parts 1 and 2. *Mental Health Special Interest Section Newsletter* 19, no. 1: 1–3; 19, no. 2: 1–4.

Liberman, R.P., et al. 1998. Skills training versus psychosocial occupational therapy for persons with persistent schizophrenia. *American Journal of Psychiatry* 155, no. 8: 1087–1091.

MacRae, A. 1997. The model of functional deficits associated with hallucinations. *American Journal of Occupational Therapy* 51, no. 1: 57–63.

MacRae, A. 1998. Schizophrenia. In *Psychosocial occupational therapy: A clinical practice,* eds. E. Cara and A. MacRae, 261–284. Albany, NY: Delmar.

Marmer, L. 1996. OTs need to help MH clients live independently. *Advance for Occupational Therapists* 12, no. 30: 14.

Niemcyk, M., P.A. Smith, and L. Knis. 1997. Occupations for schizophrenia: On the road to room maintenance. *Advance for Occupational Therapists* 13, no. 39: 17–18.

Penny, N.H., K.T. Mueser, and C.T. North. 1995. The Allen Cognitive Level Test and social competence in adult psychiatric patients. *American Journal of Occupational Therapy* 49, no. 5: 420–427.

Salo-Chydenius, S. 1996. Changing helplessness to coping: An exploratory study of social skills training with individuals with long-term mental illness. *Occupational Therapy International* 3, no. 3: 174–189.

Suto, M., and G. Frank. 1994. Future time perspective and daily occupations of persons with chronic schizophrenia in a board and care home. *American Journal of Occupational Therapy* 48, no. 1: 7–18.

Teske, Y.R. 1993. Schizophrenia. In *Conditions in occupational therapy: Effects on occupational performance,* eds. R.A. Hansen and B. Atchison, 98–121. Baltimore: Williams & Wilkins.

Tryssenaar, J., and J. Goldberg. 1994. Improving attention in a person with schizophrenia. *Canadian Journal of Occupational Therapy* 61, no. 4: 198–205.
Ward, J.D. 1998. Schizophrenia. In *Willard and Spackman's occupational therapy*, 9th ed., eds. M.E. Neistadt and E.B. Crepeau, 735–739. Philadelphia: Lippincott-Raven.

Self-Injurious Behavior

DESCRIPTION

Self-injurious behavior is a broad term that encompasses any self-inflected behavior that causes physical damage to the person (Lissy 1997). Stereotyped behavior may result in self-injury or interfere with more purposeful behavior. The behavior is repetitive and chronic, with occurrences ranging from a few times per month to several hundred times per hour; it can last for months or years.

Self-injurious behavior is a psychological, not a psychiatric, term. The behavior is not listed as a psychiatric disorder; therefore, there is no axis classification.

CAUSE

Self-injurious behavior occurs frequently in persons with mental retardation and mental disorders. It is more common in females than males, at a ratio of about 3 to 1. The suggested causes are (1) learned behavior that is reinforced by caretakers who provide attention when stopping the behavior, (2) learned avoidance behavior to escape aversive stimulus, (3) self-stimulation to provide additional somatosensory input, (4) organic deficits or abnormal physiologic response systems, and (5) psychodynamic attempts to establish ego boundaries and body reality.

ASSESSMENT

Areas

- daily living skills
- play skills
- gross motor skills
- fine motor skills
- mobility skills
- hand functions
- sensory registration—hypo- or hyperresponsiveness to tactile, auditory, and visual stimuli in particular
- sensory processing—discrimination
- attending behavior
- communication skills
- interaction skills
- stereotypical behaviors

Instruments

Instruments Developed by Occupational Therapy Personnel

- *Sensory Integration and Praxis Tests* by A.J. Ayres, Los Angeles: Western Psychological Services, 1989.
- *Tactile-Vestibular Behavioral Checklist* by J. Brocklehurst-Woods, in *American Journal of Occupational Therapy* 44, no. 6 (1990): 538.

Instruments Developed by Other Professionals and Used by Occupational Therapy Personnel

- *Bruininks-Oseretsky Test of Motor Proficiency* (BOTMP) by R.H. Bruininks, Circle Pines, MN: American Guidance Services, 1978.
- *Motivation Assessment Scale* (MAS) by V.M. Durand and D.B. Crimmins, in Identifying the variables maintaining self-injurious behavior, *Journal of Autism and Developmental Disorders* 18, no. 1 (1988): 99–117.

PROBLEMS

Self-Care

The person smears saliva, food, or excrement on his or her face, hands, or other parts of the body.

Productivity

Behaviors do not have a productive objective, goal, or purpose, and they frequently interfere with such activities.

Leisure

The person usually has few, if any, leisure interests.

Sensorimotor

- Rocking: When sitting, the person usually sways the body in a back and forth repetitive pattern, but when standing, the movement is more often side to side as weight is transferred from one foot to the other.
- Head banging or hitting: The person repeatedly bangs or hits his or her head on some hard surface, such as a wall or the back of a chair.
- Rotating the head clockwise or counterclockwise.
- Pinching or squeezing a body part between the thumb and fingers.
- Scratching the skin with the fingernails.
- Pulling a body part away from the body, usually with the hands.
- Sucking a body part with the tongue, mouth, and lips, causing inflammation and swelling.
- Eye rubbing: The person repeatedly rubs his or her eyes.
- Eye poking or hitting: The person repeatedly pokes or hits his or her eye.
- Waving a hand or moving fingers through the visual field.
- Patting or touching the face on the cheeks with the fingers.
- Hitting the chin or forehead with a closed fist.

- Putting one or more fingers in the mouth.

Cognitive

These behaviors do not appear to require cognitive thinking, memory, or problem solving.

Psychosocial

- The person does not exercise judgment for personal safety.
- Some behaviors may have a communication or attention-getting objective.

TREATMENT/INTERVENTION

Treatment by psychologists is based on behavioral or operant conditioning techniques. Treatment in occupational therapy is based primarily on sensory integration and general techniques of inhibition and relaxation based on the concept that slow, repetitive activity sends inhibitory impulses to the bulbar section of the brain (reticular area), which results in total body inhibition.

Self-Care

Self-care activities are not used in direct treatment but may be initiated after the self-stimulation behavior slows or stops.

Productivity

Productivity activities are not used in direct treatment but may be initiated after the self-stimulation behavior slows or stops.

Leisure

Leisure and play activities are not used in direct treatment but may be initiated after the self-stimulation behavior slows or stops.

Sensorimotor

- Motor skills are not used in treatment, although the person may be permitted to play with toys or other objects between sessions of sensory stimulation.
- Vestibular stimulation (linear): Use slow, repetitive rocking in a net hammock or a rocking chair on a rocker board, on a platform swing, or in the inverted position over a large therapy ball. Movements may be anterior-posterior, lateral, or up and down. Positions may include prone, supine, or sitting. A rate of 40 rocking movements per minute has been used, but maximally effective rates have not been established. A metronome may be helpful to maintain the rate of movement. Length of stimulation using 1-minute to 15-minute intervals has been successful, but maximally effective lengths of stimulation have not been established. A total length of treatment session of 20 to 50 minutes has been used, but maximally effective lengths of treatment have not been established.
- Vestibular stimulation (angular): Use slow, repetitive turning or spinning in a hammock, or in a wheelchair or other surface that can be turned.
- Firm, deep, tactile stimulation: Brushing, using a nonabrasive surgical scrub brush. Stimulation may also be supplied through vibration. Vibration is supplied by a cylindrical,

battery-operated vibrator; hands-on massage applied to hands, neck, arms, shoulders, or temples; rolling a large bolster over legs, back, and shoulder; rolling up in a blanket; or using two mats to form a sandwich through which pressure may be applied.
- Other tactile stimulation: The person locates objects in a medium such as plastic foam beads, or receives tactile stimuli from a feather duster, lotion, powder, a clothes brush, a dish mop, a terrycloth towel, and a vegetable brush.
- Slow, continuous stroking: The person is placed in a prone position without clothing on his or her back so that the skin is exposed. The therapist places the index and middle fingers on either side of the spinal column on the posterior primary rami, starting at the neck and stroking slowly to the coccyx. As one hand reaches the coccyx, the other hand begins at the neck to provide continual stimulation. Three-minute lengths have been used successfully.
- Other inhibitory (dampening) stimuli, including dimmed lighting and soft music.

Cognitive
The person may be encouraged to make choices in the specific sensory activity.

Psychosocial
- The therapist or other staff member or caregiver may hold a child in the lap while rocking in a rocking chair.
- Two people can share a platform swing, push a ball back and forth, or push and pull on each other's arms while seated on a mat.

PRECAUTIONS
- Vestibular stimulation may be contraindicated for some persons with seizure disorders, especially if the person is photosensitive. Sources of light may need to be blocked or dimmed.
- Do not use slow, continuous stroking on persons with hair growth on the back that forms swirls or irregular patterns, because the stroking will stimulate rather than inhibit behavior.
- Observe for extrapyramidal side effects if the person is given neuroleptic medication.

PROGNOSIS AND OUTCOME
- The person has decreased self-injury or self-stimulatory activity.
- The person has increased attention span to external sources of stimuli.

REFERENCE

Lissy, S.S. 1997. Sensory stimulation as treatment for self-injurious behavior in severe or profound mental retardation. *Developmental Disabilities Special Interest Section Quarterly* 20, no. 1: 1–4.

BIBLIOGRAPHY

Gorman, P.A. 1997. Case study: Self-injury and gate dysfunction in dual diagnosis. *OT Practice* 2, no. 3: 49–52.

Kelm, K., and R. Pawley. 1998. Good vibrations: A vibrating seat and back calms a boy's destructive behavior. *TeamRehab Report* 9, no. 9: 37–38, 40.

Reisman, J. 1993. Using a sensory integrative approach to treat self-injurious behavior in an adult with profound mental retardation. *American Journal of Occupational Therapy* 47, no. 5: 403–411.

Substance-Related Disorders

DESCRIPTION

Substance-related disorders become a problem when the person is unable or unwilling to modify behavior to avoid adverse life events; for example, driving after consuming too much alcohol, being arrested for possession of a controlled substance, or missing school or work because of a hangover. Drug abuse, alcohol abuse, and alcoholism are maladaptive patterns of substance use leading to clinically significant impairment or distress, as manifested by one or more of the following problems occurring in a one-year period: (1) failure to fulfill major role obligations at work, school, or home, for example, repeated absences or poor work performance related to alcohol; alcohol-related absences, suspensions, or expulsions from school; neglect of children or household; (2) recurrent substance use in situations that can be physically hazardous, for example, driving an automobile or operating a machine when impaired by alcohol; (3) recurrent alcohol-related legal problems such as arrests for alcohol-related disorderly conduct; or (4) continued alcohol use despite having persistent or recurrent social or interpersonal problems caused or exacerbated by the effects of alcohol, for example, arguments with one's spouse or physical fights (American Psychiatric Association 1994, 182).

Substance intoxication is the development of a reversible substance-specific syndrome resulting from recent ingestion of or exposure to a substance, which leads to significant maladaptive behavior or psychological changes associated with intoxication, such as belligerence, mood lability, cognitive impairment, impaired judgment, or impaired social or occupational function due to the direct physiologic effects of the substance on the central nervous system and develops during or shortly after the exposure to the substance (American Psychiatric Association 1994, 183).

Alcohol intoxication is defined as recent ingestion of alcohol that leads to significant maladaptive behavior or psychological changes, such as inappropriate sexual or aggressive behavior, mood lability, impaired judgment, or impaired social or occupational function and includes one or more of the following signs: slurred speech, incoordination, unsteady gait, nystagmus, impairment in attention or memory, or stupor or coma (American Psychiatric Association 1994, 197).

Alcohol withdrawal is the cessation or reduction in alcohol use that has been heavy and prolonged. It includes two or more of the following: autonomic hyperactivity; increased hand tremor; insomnia; nausea or vomiting; transient visual, tactile, or auditory hallucinations or illusions; psychomotor agitation; anxiety; or grand mal seizures. In addition, the symptoms must cause clinically significant distress or impairment in social, occupational, or other important areas of functioning (American Psychiatric Association 1994, 198–199).

Substance withdrawal is the development of a substance-specific maladaptive behavioral change, with physiologic and cognitive concomitants, that is due to the cessation of or reduction in heavy and prolonged substance use. It leads to a substance-specific syndrome causing clinically significant distress or impairment in social, occupational, or other important areas of functioning (American Psychiatric Association 1994, 184–185).

Terminology used in DSM-IV:

- *substance abuse*—a maladaptive pattern of substance use, leading to clinically significant impairment or distress, as manifested by recurrent and significant adverse consequences related to the repeated use of substances
- *substance dependence*—a maladaptive pattern of repeated self-administration that usually results in tolerance, withdrawal, and compulsive behavior that the person continues to engage in despite significant substance-related problems, such as reduction in important social, occupational, or recreational activities
- *substance intoxication*—development of a reversible substance-specific syndrome resulting from the recent ingestion of or exposure to a substance, leading to clinically significant maladaptive behavioral or psychological changes associated with intoxication, such as belligerence, mood lability, cognitive impairment, impaired judgment, or impaired social or occupational function due to the direct physiologic effects of the substance on the central nervous system
- *tolerance*—a need for greatly increased amounts of the substance to achieve intoxication (or the desired effect) or a markedly diminished effect with continued use of the same amount of the substance
- *withdrawal*—a maladaptive behavioral change, with physiologic and cognitive concomitants, that occurs when blood or tissue concentrations of a substance decline in an individual who had maintained prolonged heavy use of the substance

CAUSE

The cause is not well understood, but three factors usually exist: (1) an addictive substance, (2) a predisposing condition, and (3) the personality or disposition of the user. General factors are related to the culture, socioeconomic class, and psychology of the individual and the availability of the substance. Specific factors include peer pressure, emotional distress, and perception of the inability to change the situation. Frequent personality traits include the following:

1. schizoid qualities (isolation, loneliness, shyness)
2. depression
3. dependency
4. hostile and self-destructive impulsivity
5. sexual immaturity

A family history of drinking increases the risk, but genetic and inherited factors have not been established. The ratio of men to women is 4:1. About 1 in 10 persons experiences some problem with alcoholism (Merck 1999, 1581).

ASSESSMENT

Areas
- daily living skills

- productivity history, values, skills, and interests
- leisure values, skills, and interests
- physical fitness and endurance
- physical appearance
- fine motor coordination, manipulation, dexterity
- sensory registration and processing
- attending behavior, concentration
- orientation
- ability to follow instructions
- organizational skills
- problem solving and decision making
- learning skills
- time-management skills
- judgment and safety awareness
- mood or affect
- self-concept
- self-control
- social interaction skills
- communication skills
- role behavior

Instruments

Instruments Developed by Other Professionals and Used by Occupational Therapy Personnel

- *The Beery-Buktenica Developmental Test of Visual-Motor Integration* (VMI-4), 4th ed., by K.E. Beery and N.A. Buktenica, Parsippany, NJ: Modern Curriculum Press, 1997.
- *Neurobehavioral Cognitive Status Examination* by R. Kierman et al., *Annals of Internal Medicine* 107 (1987): 481–485.
- *Quick Neurological Screening Test-II* by M. Mutti, H.M. Sterling, and N.V. Spalding, Novato, CA: Academic Therapy Publications, 1998.
- *Test of Visual-Perceptual Skills—Revised* (TVPS-R) by M. Gardner, Hydesville, CA: Psychological and Educational Publications, 1996.
- *Therapeutic Factor Questionnaire* by L. Lowett and J. Lovett, in Group therapeutic factors on an alcohol inpatient unit, *British Journal of Psychiatry* 159 (1991): 365–370.

PROBLEMS

Self-Care

- The person may neglect to perform certain daily living skills.
- The person may lack skills in performing instrumental activities of daily living, such as money management, meal planning and preparation, or shopping.

Productivity

- The person usually has an irregular job history or is unemployed.

- The person may have a history of irregular school attendance.
- The person may have an unrealistic perception of his or her job skills.
- The person may be late for work often because of difficulty planning tasks in a time sequence.
- The person may have difficulty organizing and performing job duties.

Leisure

The person may have few leisure interests except alcohol and drugs.

Sensorimotor

- The person may have poor physical fitness and low physical endurance.
- The person may have a peripheral neuropathy.
- The person may have reduced range of motion, especially in the upper extremities.
- The person may have impairments in balance and posture.
- The person may have poor muscle tone as a result of inactivity.
- The person may have impaired coordination and dexterity.
- The person may have slower than normal reaction time.
- The person may have pain, especially in the lower back.
- The person may have sensory changes associated with peripheral neuropathy.

Cognitive

- The person may have cognitive disorders associated with brain damage.
- The person may have difficulty following instructions.
- The person may have impaired judgment regarding personal safety.
- The person may have poor time-management skills, leading to an imbalance among self-care, productivity, and leisure activities.
- Personal goals may be poorly defined and goal-oriented behavior lacking.

Psychosocial

- The person may have a poor self-concept and low self-esteem.
- The person may show signs of immaturity compared with chronologic age.
- The person may show signs of depression.
- The person may be dependent on others.
- The person may show hostility or self-destructive impulsivity.
- The person may be suicidal.
- Personal values and beliefs may be poorly defined.
- The person may have schizoid qualities (isolation, loneliness, shyness, withdrawal).
- The person may tend to be a perfectionist.
- The person may have immature or impaired social interaction skills.

TREATMENT/INTERVENTION

Models of treatment include cognitive-behavioral therapy, the disease model, and the psychodynamic/psychoanalytic model. Models used in occupational therapy include personal adaptation through occupation, the Moyers model (Moyers 1997), and sensory integration.

Self-Care
- Increase the person's skills in organizing and managing daily life tasks, including grooming, dressing, and other self-care routines.
- Increase the person's life skills in meal planning, shopping, meal preparation, using public transportation, doing laundry, managing money in a checking account, and arranging living accommodations.

Productivity
- Provide training in job-finding skills.
- Increase the person's skills in organizing and completing work tasks, such as organizing a workspace, pacing the work activities, trying new ideas, making decisions, and organizing a project into manageable steps.
- Increase the person's ability to follow verbal and written directions.
- Increase the person's skills in managing the home, such as cleaning, dusting, and organizing the home and preparing meals.
- If necessary, help the person explore career options, write a resume, apply for a job, complete an application form, and interview for a job.
- Encourage the person to explore volunteer work, continuing education courses, or study groups.

Leisure
- Help the person explore and develop a variety of leisure activities and skills.
- Encourage the person to use leisure skills and tasks to replace time devoted to alcohol and drinking activities.

Sensorimotor
- Help the person increase his or her range of motion through performance of tasks in the environment and selected exercises.
- Encourage participation in a group exercise program to increase physical tolerance, endurance, fitness, and muscle tone. Exercises may include stretching, bending, twisting, jogging in place, and jumping jacks.
- Increase the person's standing balance and postural reactions.
- Improve coordination and dexterity through activities requiring imitation of simple and complex movements, including crossing the midline.
- Improve fine motor coordination, manipulation, and dexterity through the use of craft projects requiring fine motor skills.
- Encourage regular participation in recreational activities and exercise to increase physical fitness.

Cognitive
- Increase the person's awareness of his or her strengths and weaknesses through participation in arts and crafts activities, creative writing, psychodrama, and group discussion.
- Increase the person's ability to concentrate and his or her attention span through the use of arts and crafts projects.

- Provide opportunities for the person to learn to follow verbal and written instructions through the use of leisure or work activities.
- Provide opportunities to practice problem-solving and decision-making skills through the use of leisure or work activities.
- Provide instruction in organizing an activity schedule and learning time-management skills that include planning for leisure time.
- Provide question-and-answer sessions on the effects of drug withdrawal on physical and psychological health, including how to cope with the craving.
- Provide time-management training and daily scheduling to organize a drug-free lifestyle.
- Teach the person about community resources.
- Provide opportunities to set obtainable short- and long-term goals and identify the steps needed to achieve the goals using behavior-modification techniques.
- Help the person sort out priorities through group discussion.
- Provide instruction in relaxation training as a stress-management technique.

Psychosocial
- Provide the opportunity to learn to deal with frustration and develop frustration tolerance by increasing coping skills and the use of adaptive strategies in actual or real learning situations.
- Encourage the person to control impulsive behavior through practice in handling frustration and anger.
- Increase the person's self-esteem and sense of mastery by using short-term projects in which success is relatively ensured.
- Increase the person's ability to channel anger and aggression into acceptable activities, such as crafts that include destruction (sawing wood), hammering, and drilling.
- Increase the person's self-confidence through experience in dealing with problems arising in completing craft or other activity tasks.
- Increase the person's sense of autonomy and independence by giving him or her opportunities to perform activities without direct supervision.
- Increase self-esteem and self-concept through the use of creative activities, such as art, crafts, drama, music, or dance.
- Provide group-oriented tasks that can be used as a basis for group discussion regarding attitudes, feelings, emotions, and reactions, especially regarding authority figures.
- The use of drama therapy and role playing may be helpful in providing opportunities for the person to try out different roles and alternative behaviors. Sessions may be videotaped to help in analysis.
- Special groups may be organized to concentrate on specific problems, such as women's issues or marital issues.
- Increase the person's social interaction skills, such as meeting new people, expressing ideas, maintaining relationships. Discuss the role of physical appearance in social relationships.
- Encourage the person to participate in support or self-help groups, such as Alcoholics Anonymous.
- Encourage the person to share feelings and experiences in group discussion, role playing, or psychodrama.
- Increase social relationships, including group cooperation.

- Help the person learn new behavior patterns that are socially acceptable through the performance of a variety of activities in group situations.
- Encourage socially acceptable behavior by rewarding such behavior and using the topic in group discussion.

Environment
Increase the person's skill in functioning in the community.

PRECAUTIONS
- Observe the person for relapses in drinking behavior or drug abuse.
- Note shortness of breath, increased sweating, or dizziness, especially during exercises, which may indicate a need for referral to a physician for further analysis of health status.
- Program modifications may be necessary if the person has a history of hypertension, seizures, back pain, or other physical injury.

PROGNOSIS AND OUTCOME
- The person performs self-care and daily living activities regularly.
- The person performs instrumental activities of daily living independently.
- The person is able to plan a budget and manage money using checking, savings, or credit accounts.
- The person performs productive activities on a regular schedule.
- The person is able to obtain and hold a job.
- The person is able to manage a home independently or in cooperation with others.
- The person has identified leisure interests in which he or she participates on a regular basis.
- The person demonstrates self-control.
- The person is able to initiate a goal and follow through to completion.
- The person participates in social activities.
- The person demonstrates the ability to organize and follow a drug-free lifestyle.
- The person is able to solve problems and make decisions without the use of drugs or other unacceptable social behavior.
- The person is able to set goals and plan and execute a program to meet goals without the use of drugs.
- The person is able to participate in group activities without the use of drugs.
- The person is knowledgeable about community resources, such as self-help groups.

REFERENCES

American Psychiatric Association. 1994. *Diagnostic and Statistical Manual of Mental Disorders: DSM-IV,* 4th ed. Washington, DC: American Psychiatric Association. Task Force on DSM-IV.
Beers, M.H., and R. Berkow, eds. 1999. *The Merck Manual of Diagnosis and Therapy,* 17th ed. Whitehouse Station, NJ: Merck Research Laboratories.
Moyers, P.A. 1997. Occupational meanings and spirituality: The quest for sobriety. *American Journal of Occupational Therapy* 51, no. 3: 207–214.

BIBLIOGRAPHY

Barth, T. 1994. Occupational therapy intervention at a shelter for homeless, addicted adults with mental illness. *Mental Health Special Interest Section Newsletter* 17, no. 1: 7–8.

Booth, P.G., and C.J. Mulligan. 1994. Alcohol teaching within occupational therapy courses: A case for larger measures. *British Journal of Occupational Therapy* 57, no. 9: 354–356.

Buijsse, N., W. Caan, and S.F. Davis. 1999. Occupational therapy in the treatment of addictive behaviors. *British Journal of Therapy and Rehabilitation* 6, no. 6: 300–307.

Harrison, T.S., and P. Precin. 1996. Cognitive impairments in clients with dual diagnosis (chronic psychotic disorders and substance abuse): Considerations for treatment. *Occupational Therapy International* 3, no. 2: 122–141.

Kerr, T. 1996. If you can play it straight you can "play it sober." *Advance for Occupational Therapists* 12, no. 1: 19.

Kerr, T. 1996. Beating substance abuse: Get a fresh start in the privacy of your home. *Advance for Occupational Therapists* 11, no. 1: 12, 50.

Kerr, T. 1995. Using OT skills to help children of substance abusers. *Advance for Occupational Therapists* 11, no. 8: 12.

Marmer, L. 1996. OTs need to help MH clients live independently. *Advance for Occupational Therapists* 12, no. 30: 14.

Marmer, L. 1995. Ceramics shop critical stepping stone for recovering alcoholics. *Advance for Occupational Therapists* 11, no. 13: 16, 62.

Ogilvie, S.S., S.E. Blair, and A.L. Paul. 1995. Survey of patients on an alcohol in-patient unit in relation to group therapeutic factors. *Occupational Therapy International* 2, no. 4: 257–277.

Riley, K., R. Ramsey, and E. Cara. 1998. Substance abuse and occupational therapy. In *Psychosocial occupational therapy: A clinical practice,* eds. E. Cara and A. MacRae, 227–260. Albany, NY: Delmar.

Rotert, D.A. 1993. The adolescent with chemical dependency. In *Practice issues in occupational therapy: Intraprofessional team building,* ed. S. Ryan, 71–80. Thorofare, NJ: Slack.

Steib, G. 1995. Recognizing the signs. *OT Week* 9, no. 44: 18–19.

Stoffel, V.C. 1994. Occupational therapists' roles in treating substance abuse. *Hospital Community Psychiatry* 45, no. 1: 21–22.

Stoffel, V., and P. Moyers. 1997. *Occupational therapy practice guidelines for substance use disorders.* Bethesda, MD: American Occupational Therapy Association.

Stratton, J., and D. Gailfus. 1998. A new approach to substance abuse treatment: Adolescents and adults with ADHD. *Journal of Substance Abuse Treatment* 15, no. 2: 89–94.

Van Deusen, J. 1993. Alcohol abuse. In *Body image and perceptual dysfunction in adults,* ed. J. Van Deusen, 65–81. Philadelphia: W.B. Saunders.

Ward, J.D. 1998. Substance abuse. In *Willard and Spackman's occupational therapy*, 9th ed., eds. M.E. Neistadt and E.B. Crepeau, 724–732. Philadelphia: Lippincott-Raven.

Appendix A

Evaluating Hand Injuries

ORDER OF RECOVERY OF SENSATION

1. protective sensation (response to deep pressure and pinprick)
2. moving touch or tactile sensation
3. static light touch
4. discriminative touch (Dellon 1981, 115–122).

SPECIFIC HAND TESTS

Note: There are many tests for evaluating the sensibility of the hand. The tests below are the more commonly mentioned tests.

Testing for Static or Moving Two-Point Discrimination

Test instrument is the (Mackinnon-Dellon) Disk Criminator, which is applied on a longitudinal axis of the digit. The pressure applied should not blanch the skin. Support the person's hand on a table surface and occlude his or her vision. Seven out of 10 correct responses are required for each zone of the hand tested. Begin testing at 5 mm distance between the two points. Randomly touch with one or two points. The person states whether he or she feels one or two points on the skin. Discontinue test if the person cannot discriminate at 15 mm between the stimulus points.

Ratings

1. normal—less than 6 mm
2. fair—6 to 10 mm
3. poor—11 to 15 mm
4. protective—one point perceived
5. anesthetic—no point perceived

Source: Data from American Society for Surgery of the Hand, *The Hand: Examination and Diagnosis*, 3rd ed., 121, © 1990, Churchill Livingstone.

Testing for Light Touch and Deep Pressure
(Semmes-Weinstein Pressure Aesthesiometer)

Testing begins with the monofilament marked 2.83, which is applied perpendicularly to the skin in the center of a selected zone of the hand until the monofilament bows (bends). Vision is occluded. Each monofilament is applied for 1 to 1.5 seconds. Filaments marked 1.65 through 4.08 are applied three times. A positive response (person perceives the stimulus) must be recorded two out of three times to record a positive result in that zone of the hand. If the person cannot detect the stimulus in the range 1.65 to 4.08, continue with filaments marked 4.17 to 6.65, but apply only once. Stop when the person is able to detect the pressure.

Ratings

Green	Normal	1.65–2.83
Blue	Diminished light touch	3.22–3.61
Purple	Diminished protective sensation	3.84–4.31
Red	Loss of protective sensation	4.56–6.65
	Untestable	>6.65

Source: Data from D.S. Martin and E.D. Collins, *Manual of Acute Hand Injuries*, p. 614, © 1998, Mosby Year-Book Publishers.

Interpretation of the Semmes-Weinstein Monofilaments (minikit)

0 = untestable
1 (filament marking 6.65) = loss of deep protective sensation
2 (filament marking 4.56) = loss of protective sensation
3 (filament marking 4.31) = diminished protective sensation
4 (filament marking 3.61) = diminished perception of light touch
5 (filament marking 2.83) = normal perception of touch and pressure

Source: Data from B. Rosén, Recovery of Sensory and Motor Function after Nerve Repair: A Rationale for Evaluation, *Journal of Hand Therapy*, Vol. 9, No. 4, p. 316, © 1996.

Testing for Localization of Stimulus

Use a monofilament from the Semmes-Weinstein series that can be detected in all zones of the hand. Apply the stimulus perpendicular to the skin in the center of a selected zone of the hand until the monofilament bows (bends). Vision is occluded. Then ask the person to open his or her eyes and point to the exact spot touched by the monofilament stimulus. Use a grid worksheet marked with zones and subdivided into approximately equal square areas. If the person responds correctly, circle the dot; if incorrectly, draw an arrow from the dot in the zone stimulated to the point the person indicated was touched (Rosén 1996, 317).

Moberg Pick-Up Test

Small common objects are placed on a table surface (car key, 1" paper clip, 1" safety pin, 1" screw, 3/8" diameter wing nut, 3/8" hexagon nut, a nickel, a dime). The person is asked to pick them up. Examiner notes the time required and the type of prehension employed. With vision occluded, the person will tend not to use sensory surfaces with poor sensibility (Callahan 1984, 25).

Subtest 1—Person picks up objects with the involved hand, eyes opened, and places them in a box.

Subtest 2—Person picks up objects with the noninvolved hand, eyes opened, and places them in a box.

Subtest 3—Person picks up objects with the involved hand, eyes closed, and places them in a box.

Subtest 4—Person picks up objects with the noninvolved hand, eyes closed, and places them in a box.

Vibration

Equipment includes tuning forks at 30 cycles per second (cps or Middle C on the piano) or Hertz (Hz) and 256 cps (A above Middle C on the piano). The tuning fork is applied either by the pronged or the stem end. Dellon (1981, 115–122) prefers the prong end because it has greater amplitude and is more suitable to test the fingertip pulp in persons with altered vibratory threshold. Vibration is scored as more sensation, less, or the same, as compared with the contralateral hand. Bio-Thesiometers and Vibration IIs are commercial instruments that can vary the amplitude but fix the frequency (Martin and Collins 1998, 615).

REFERENCES

Callahan, A. 1984. Nerve injuries in the upper extremities. In *Manual on management of specific hand problems*, eds. M.H. Malick and M.C. Kasch, 25. Pittsburgh: American Rehabilitation Educational Network.

Dellon, A.O. 1981. *Evaluation of sensibility and re-education of the sensation in the hand*, 115–122. Baltimore: Williams & Wilkins.

Martin, D.S., and E.D. Collins. 1998. *Manual of acute hand injuries*, 615. St. Louis: Mosby.

Rosén, B. 1996. Recovery of sensory and motor function after nerve repair: A rationale for evaluation. *Journal of Hand Therapy* 9(4): 317.

Appendix B

Technique References

ENERGY CONSERVATION, PACING, AND WORK SIMPLIFICATION
- Use good body mechanics and muscles that use the least energy.
  a. Use both hands and arms whenever possible (symmetrical vs. asymmetrical).
  b. Use hip and shoulder muscles for lifting tasks (weight-bearing muscles).
- Sit rather than stand whenever possible, or alternate sitting and standing.
- Keep frequently used items within easy reach to avoid stretching and straining, including bending, reaching, stooping, and twisting.
- Let your fingers do the walking: shop by telephone if possible.
- Tell vendors to deliver: let the Post Office or other delivery service bring items to the house.
- Let the laws of physics (gravity and momentum) help reduce workload.
  a. Slide rather than lift or carry objects.
  b. Toss instead of place unbreakable items; toss item into wastebasket rather than putting the item into the wastebasket.
- Use proper work heights according to the job task and the individual. Jobs requiring hand activity require a higher work surface than those requiring arm motion.
- Plan ahead to eliminate wasted motion and time.
  a. Plan activities and assemble needed items before starting. Use a cart, wagon, or basket to keep items assembled.
  b. Reschedule tasks so they can be done less frequently, such as shopping for groceries less often and at times that are less busy at the store.
- Avoid doing unnecessary tasks.
  a. Delegate some tasks to other family members.
  b. Let the grocery clerks carry the bags.
- Schedule rest breaks as well as activities.
- Let power tools, such as electric can openers, do the work when possible.

BIBLIOGRAPHY

Early, M.E. 1998. *Physical dysfunction: Practice skills for the occupational therapy assistant*, 448. St. Louis: Mosby.

Gilbert, D.W. 1965. Energy expenditures for the disabled homemaker: Review of studies. *American Journal of Occupational Therapy* 19: 321–328 (classic article).

Neistadt, M.E., and E.B. Crepeau, eds. 1998. *Willard and Spackman's occupational therapy*, 9th ed., 499–500, 698. Philadelphia: J.B. Lippincott.

Trombly, C.A., ed. 1996. *Occupational therapy for physical dysfunction*, 4th ed., 304, 319–320. Baltimore: Williams & Wilkins.

Turner, A., M. Foster, and S.E. Johnson. 1996. *Occupational therapy and physical dysfunction: Principles, skills, and practice*, 4th ed., 758–759. New York: Churchill Livingstone.

INHIBITION AND FACILITATION TECHNIQUES

I. Categories of Inhibition Techniques

General characteristics of inhibiting or damping techniques to the central nervous system are slow and repetitive movements and activities that send inhibitory impulses to the bulbar section of the brain in the reticular formation. Some techniques can be used in combination with others.

- *Inversion*—By turning the person upside down so that the head is lower than the rest of body, the carotid sinus produces a calming and inhibiting effect on all the stretch reflexes except those facilitated by the labyrinthine reflex. Do not invert person with shunts and use caution with persons who have tracheostomies to be sure the airway is clear and with persons with abdominal feeding tubes to be sure the tube does not cause discomfort.
- *Joint Compression*—The therapist uses one hand to stabilize the shoulder while placing the other hand on the flexed elbow. Force is applied up through the humerus into the shoulder. Gradually and slowly, the therapist rotates the elbow in large radius circles, increasing the amount of flexion and abduction. Joint compression that is less than the person's body weight is inhibitory to all muscles around the joint being compressed.
- *Mobilization of Proximal Joints*—Mobilization of the shoulder girdle and pelvis assists in reducing abnormal muscle tone. Techniques include separation of movement of the upper and lower trunk, elongating the trunk musculature, increasing movement of the shoulder, and increasing anterior pelvic tilt.
- *Neutral Warmth*—Wrap the person's total body in a cotton blanket for 10 to 20 minutes. Avoid extremes of temperature, which may relax initially but may result in rebound later, causing the person to tighten up or experience pain.
- *Pressure on the Insertion of a Muscle*—To relax a tight muscle group, apply pressure on the insertion of the muscle. In the hand, wrist flexors can be relaxed by placing a hand cone in the hand.
- *Reciprocal Inhibition*—Contraction of the agonist muscle causes the motor neurons that supply the antagonist to be inhibited. For example, contraction of the triceps causes the motor neurons in the biceps to be inhibited and thus more relaxed.
- *Reflex-Inhibiting Postures*—Reflex-inhibiting postures are movement patterns that inhibit abnormal postural reactions and thus facilitate voluntary movements. Generally, a reflex-inhibiting posture is based on the use of one or more key points of control, which are the

neck, shoulder, and pelvic girdle. Key points of control usually are proximal body units that tend to influence the rest of the particular posture. For example, to inhibit or counteract an abnormal flexion pattern of the upper extremity, the neck and spine are extended, the shoulder is externally rotated, the elbow is extended, the forearm is supinated, and the thumb is abducted.

- *Selected Sensory Stimuli*—Auditory stimuli that have a regular rhythm less than the heart rate are inhibitory. Dimmed lights or natural indirect light tends to be inhibiting. Perfume or pleasant odors tend to have a calming effect. Warm fluids inhibit hyperactive swallowing.
- *Slow Rocking*—Rhythmic slow rocking in a rocking chair or over a large-diameter ball in a forward and backward position is inhibitory. If a ball is used, the therapists should stabilize the person at the pelvis to reduce any fear of falling.
- *Slow Rolling*—The therapist places one hand on the person's shoulder and the other hand on the person's pelvis. The person is slowly rolled from supine to side-lying and back to supine for several minutes.
- *Slow Stroking*—Slow stroking is done to the posterior primary rami located on either side of the spinal cord. When the person is prone, the therapist places the index finger on one side and the middle finger on the other side of the spinal cord, starting at the neck or occiput. Applying light but firm touch, the therapist moves slowly through the coccyx. Before the therapist lifts the first hand, he or she begins to move the second hand at the neck and slowly down the back. Slow stroking should be applied directly to the skin, not through clothing. Slow stroking should not be used on any person with swirls or irregular hair patterns on the back because the movement of the hairs will stimulate rather than calm the person.
- *Weight Bearing and Cocontraction*—Weight bearing through the lower extremities and pelvis can reduce spasticity. In the upper extremities, cocontraction can assist in restoring the normal agonist and antagonist relationship and muscle tone.

II. Facilitating Techniques

General characteristics of facilitating techniques are rapid, irregular rhythms in a movement or activity.

- *Brushing* is accomplished by using a rotary mixer into which a soft camel-hair brush has been inserted. The brushing is applied to the dermatomal representation of the muscle to be facilitated, which usually is the skin area over the muscle belly. The stimulus is applied 10 to 15 seconds per area. It is assumed that the exteroceptors, probably C fibers, are stimulated.
- *Icing* is accomplished by wrapping an ice cube in a towel or cloth and rubbing it with pressure over the belly muscle to be facilitated. Usually, three quick swipes are applied in a distal to proximal direction and then the skin is dried. Chewing ice is useful for facilitating swallowing and tongue movement. Do not ice the forehead, anterior midline of the trunk, or posterior trunk because blood pressure may be increased.
- *Pressure* (tapping, rubbing, quick stretching) applied to the muscle belly as a quick stretch facilitates the movement produced by the muscle being stretched. Do not apply pressure or quick stretch to a spastic muscle.
- *Joint Approximation or Compression* (pressing the joint together) applied with more than body weight facilitates extensor patterns and cocontraction patterns. Do not use if the person has a fracture of any bones whose joints are being compressed.
- *Joint Traction* (pulling the joint apart) facilitates flexor patterns. Do not use if the person has a fracture of any bones involved with the joints to which traction is being applied.

- *Resistance* is most effective when applied in a pattern of apply, hold, release, apply, hold, release, rather than in a steady pull. The apply, hold, release pattern permits the muscle fibers to adjust rather than fatigue under the steady pull. The amount of resistance applied must be adjusted according to the person (adult or child), particular pattern (static or movement), or position (finger flexion or elbow flexion). Application of strong, steady, static resistance will result in cocontraction. Less resistance is needed for movement patterns.
- *Postural Change* (changes in posture) can be used to increase or decrease muscle tone through the response to gravity. Generally, positions that cause the person to work against gravity increase muscle tone.
- *Sensory Stimuli* (fast, loud, irregular rhythms) are stimulating; bright colors (red, yellow, orange) are stimulating; salty and oily fluids, thin mucus that facilitates swallowing, and noxious odors have a stimulating effect.
- *Successive Induction* is based on the concept that a muscle will contract more strongly if its contraction is preceded by a contraction of the antagonist—in other words, alternate contraction of agonist and antagonist. For example, if the wrist flexors are weak, first give maximum resistance to the wrist extensors, then give resistance to wrist flexors.
- *Vestibular Stimulation* (fast rolling, spinning, tilting, and swinging) can be used to increase muscle tone. Always watch the person for emotional reactions and sympathetic nervous system response. If the person becomes fearful or becomes pale or flushed, reduce the rate of stimulation. Generally, spinning should not be used with persons who are prone to seizures or who have seizure disorders.
- *Vibration* is applied through a battery-operated vibrator. The reaction is immediate but wears off in about three minutes. Vibration is assumed to stimulate proprioceptors and arouse the reticular system, which activates the cortex. Vibration should not be used with persons prone to seizures or who have seizure disorders.

BIBLIOGRAPHY

McCormack, G.L. 1996. The Rood approach to treatment of neuromuscular dysfunction. In *Occupational therapy: Practice skills for physical dysfunction*, 4th ed., ed. L.W. Pedretti, 377–399. St. Louis: Mosby.
Trombly, C.A., L. Levit, and B.J. Meyers. 1996. Remediating motor control and performance through traditional therapeutic approaches. In *Occupational therapy for physical dysfunction*, 4th ed., ed. C.A. Trombly, 433–498. Baltimore: Williams & Wilkins.

JOINT PROTECTION

- Maintain joint in correct position and avoid positions of deformity.
- Maintain body in correct posture and avoid positions that lead to injury.
- Use stronger, larger joints and the biggest muscles to lift and carry. Use shoulders instead of hands. Use palms of hands instead of fingers.
- Use each joint in the most stable anatomic and functional position. Stand with both feet on the floor in flat shoes with toes pointed ahead. Bend hips and knees, but keep back straight when picking up objects.
- Distribute load over two or more joints. Lift small objects, such as bowls and pans, with two hands.

- Avoid sustaining the same position for long periods of time, such as holding a pencil. Use a built-up or enlarged-diameter pencil.
- Avoid static positions for long periods of time, such as standing and sitting.
- Plan alternate periods of activities and rest.
- Stop before becoming fatigued. Bad habits creep in more easily when a person is tired and not concentrating.
- Divide work into light and heavy tasks. Alternate and take frequent rest breaks.
- Reduce effort needed to do the job.
- Avoid tight grasp.
- Avoid pressure against the radial side of each finger (thumb side).
- Avoid strong and constant pressure against the pad of the thumb.

BIBLIOGRAPHY

Hittle, J.H., L.W. Pedretti, and M.C. Kasch. 1996. Rheumatoid arthritis. In *Occupational therapy: Practice skills for physical dysfunction*, 4th ed., ed. L.W. Pedretti, 644–645. St. Louis: Mosby.
Trombly, C.A. 1996. Arthritis. In *Occupational therapy for physical dysfunction*, 4th ed., ed. C.A. Trombly, 821–826. Baltimore: Williams & Wilkins.

For additional resources, see the resource bibliography on Media, Modalities, and Techniques in Appendix G.

MUSCLE TONE

Hypotonia

The person has diminished or lost deep tendon reflexes, has less than normal resilience or resistance to movement (limbs feel heavy when moved), has muscles that feel flabby and soft when palpated, and may have instability or laxity of joints and weakened or lost reflexive or voluntary motion.

Severe Hypotonia

The person exhibits an inability to resist gravity, lack of cocontraction at proximal joints for stability, weakness, and limited voluntary movements. For passive movement, there is joint hyperextensibility, no resistance to movement imposed by examiner, and full or excessive passive range of motion.

Moderate Hypotonia

The person exhibits decreased tone, primarily in axial muscles and proximal muscles of the extremities, which interferes with the rate of development and length of time a posture can be sustained. For passive movement, there is mild resistance to movement when imposed by an examiner in distal parts of extremities only, and joint hyperextensibility at elbows and knees.

Mild Hypotonia

A decreased tone interferes with axial muscle cocontraction and delays initiation of movement against gravity and speed of adjustment to postural change. For passive movement, there is mild resistance in proximal as well as distal segments, and a full passive range of motion.

Normal Tone

The person exhibits quick and immediate postural adjustment during movement. The ability to use muscles in synergistic and reciprocal patterns for stability and mobility depends on task of the movement. For passive movement, body parts resist displacement, momentarily maintain new posture when placed in space, and can rapidly follow changing movements improved by examiner.

Hypertonicity

The person has hyperactive deep tendon reflexes; has resistance to passive motion or quick stretch of a joint when motion is against the involved muscle's action; has movements that are linked into total body patterns that prevent isolated joint motion, reduce the variability of active joint motion, and decrease relative consistency of strength and joint range; has isolated joint motions that are slow, weak, inefficient, and uncoordinated, especially in reciprocal movements; has inability to produce stabilizing and mobilizing components for skilled motor performance; and, when conscious effort is used, the effort reinforces hypertonus and abnormal movement patterns.

Mild Hypertonus

The increased tone causes delay in postural adjustment, poor coordination, and slowness of movement. For passive movement, there is resistance to change of posture in part or throughout the range, and poor ability to accommodate to passive movements.

Moderate Hypertonus

An increased tone limits speed, coordination, a variety of movement patterns, and active range of motion. For passive movement, there is resistance to change of posture throughout the range, and limited passive range of motion at some joints.

Severe Hypertonus

A severe stiffness of muscles in stereotyped patterns limits the active range of motion. There is little or no ability to move against gravity, and very limited patterns of movement. The passive range of motion is limited. The person is unable to overcome resistance of muscle to complete the full range of motion.

Intermittent Tone

The person exhibits an occasional and unpredictable resistance to postural changes alternating with normal adjustment and may have difficulty initiating active movement or sustaining posture. For passive movement, there is an unpredictable resistance to imposed movements alternating with a complete absence of resistance.

BIBLIOGRAPHY

Wilson, J.M. 1984. Cerebral palsy. In *Pediatric neurologic physical therapy*, ed. S.K. Campbell, 363. New York: Churchill Livingstone (Clinics in Physical Therapy, vol. 5); and Ryerson, S., and K. Levit. 1997. *Functional movement reeducation*. New York: Churchill Livingstone.

CATEGORIES OF REFLEXES

Primitive or Primary Reflexes

These reflexes are involuntary responses, usually present at birth, that affect posture and movement. Generally, these reflexes are gradually suppressed or they integrate as higher control centers mature. All are assumed to be mediated at the brainstem level. The most commonly discussed reflexes are:

1. Moro Response or Reflex

a. This response is elicited by extending the infant's head backward, which results in an extension of the head, neck, and arms followed by a flexion or "embrace" posture.
b. The Moro should integrate between three to five months of age.
c. If the Moro remains active, it decreases sitting balance, as the neck extension is transferred to the spine, resulting in the person slipping forward out of a chair.
d. The Moro can be inhibited by keeping the head and neck in neutral or slight anterior flexion and keeping the hips and legs flexed.

2. Asymmetrical Tonic Neck Reflex (ATNR)

a. The ATNR is elicited by turning the head to one side. The face limb is extended while the skull limb is flexed in the so-called fencer's position The lower limbs may follow a similar pattern.
b. The ATNR should integrate between three to five months, except when the infant is asleep.
c. Initially, the ATNR is useful in helping the infant look at his or her hand and experience eye-hand coordination, but if the ATNR remains active, it interferes with bringing the hands together at the midline of the body for such activities as eating or using both hands. Also structural changes such as scoliosis and hip subluxation may occur due to the asymmetrical posture.
d. The ATNR may be inhibited by positioning the person with the head in the midline in any of the following positions: side-lying, supine with legs flexed at about 100 degrees over a bolster, prone with arms extended over a bolster, sitting with legs extended at 160 to 180 degrees in front of the body.

3. Tonic Labyrinthine Reflex, Supine (TLR, supine)

a. The TLR, supine, is elicited when the labyrinth (and head) are in the supine position, which results in extension of the neck and legs, retraction of the shoulders, and variable positions of the arms.
b. The TLR, supine, usually integrates between one to three months, permitting lifting of the head or head righting.
c. If the TLR, supine, remains active, it is difficult for the person to lift his or her head from the supporting surface.
d. The TLR, supine, can be inhibited by flexing the head, neck, and legs. Generally, it is best to avoid this position, when possible, by using the side-lying position.

4. Tonic Labyrinthine Reflex, Prone (TLR, prone)

a. The TLR, prone, is elicited when the labyrinth (and head) is in the prone position, which results in flexion of the neck, arms, and legs.

b. The TLR, prone, usually integrates between one to three months, permitting lifting of the head or head righting.

c. If the TLR, prone, remains active, it is difficult for the person to lift his or her head from the supporting surface.

d. The TLR, prone, can be inhibited by placing a bolster under the shoulder and a pillow or small wedge under the legs, or by placing under the person a wedge long enough to accommodate the length of the body from the shoulders to the thighs. The shoulders should be positioned at the high end of the bolster and the arms permitted to extend to the floor. A wedge may be placed between the legs to keep them in abduction.

5. Symmetrical Tonic Neck Reflex, Extension (STNR, extension)

a. The STNR, extension, is elicited when the head and neck are extended in the horizontal plane (all-fours position), which results in extension of the arms and flexion of the legs.

b. The STNR, extension, usually integrates between the fourth and sixth months.

c. If the response is obligatory, it will interfere with creeping on all fours, kneeling, and half-kneeling, which are needed to get to standing.

d. The STNR, extension, can be inhibited by keeping the head in a neutral position when the person is on all fours, kneeling, or half-kneeling.

6. Symmetrical Tonic Neck Reflex, Flexion (STNR, flexion)

a. STNR, flexion, is elicited when the head and neck are flexed in the horizontal plane (all-fours position), which results in flexion of the arms and extension of the legs.

b. The STNR, flexion, usually integrates between the fourth and sixth months.

c. If the response is obligatory, it will interfere with creeping on all fours, kneeling, and half-kneeling, which are needed to get to a standing position.

d. The STNR, flexion, can be inhibited by keeping the head in a neutral position when the person is on all fours, kneeling, or half-kneeling.

7. Positive Supporting Reflex

a. The positive supporting reflex is elicited by touching the soles of the feet to a hard surface, which results in extension of the legs so they straighten out to support the body's weight.

b. The positive supporting reflex usually integrates between six to nine months.

c. Abnormally strong influences of the positive supporting reflex will result in crossing or scissoring of the legs. If the reflex remains, walking will not be possible.

d. The positive supporting reflex can be inhibited by placing body weight or greater on the heels of the foot before touching the soles.

Automatic Reflexes

These reflexes are not present at birth but evolve during the first two years of life and remain active throughout the lifespan in the normal individual.

1. Righting Reflexes

These reflexes assist in maintaining the position of the head, trunk, arms, and legs in proper relationship to one another and to gravity by supplying information regarding the position of the body in relationship to the up/down, right/left, straight/rotated position of the body parts. These reflexes are assumed to be mediated at the midbrain level.

   a. Labyrinthine Head-Righting Reflex
- This reflex is responsible for keeping the head in an upright or vertical posture regardless of the position of the rest of the body.
- The reflex begins to develop at about four to six weeks and matures through the third month.
- This reflex facilitates head control as the person's body moves in space and permits the person to lift the head from prone and supine positions.
- The reflex can be stimulated by occluding the person's vision and holding the person in space in various positions. Usually this reflex is not treated directly because people do not like their vision occluded. Because the optical righting reflex usually develops at the same time, therapy is directed toward promoting the optical righting reflex and indirectly promoting the head-righting reflex.

   b. Optical Righting Reflex
- The optical righting reflex uses vision to right the head.
- The reflex develops between four and six weeks and matures throughout the third month.
- It assists in orienting the head to the vertical position by righting the head and body in relation to space.

   c. Body Righting Acting on the Head
- This reflex acts to right the head in relation to the body.
- The reflex develops during the first two months and matures by eight months.
- It facilitates head control in relation to the body in all positions of the body—supine, prone, sitting, on hands and knees, and standing.

   d. Neck Righting Acting on the Body (derotation righting)
- This reflex acts to turn the body in the direction the head is turning, starting with the rotation of the shoulders, then the trunk, and then the pelvis.
- The reflex develops between four and six months. It can be inhibited by age five.
- This reflex facilitates rolling from supine to prone and prone to supine.

   e. Body Righting Acting on the Body (derotation righting)
- If the head and neck are rotated to one side, the shoulder, thorax, abdomen, hips, and legs will tend to rotate in the same direction in sequential order. The sequence may be started from the legs and hips and move up toward the neck and head.
- The reflex starts about four to six months and becomes mature at eight to 10 months. It can be inhibited by the age of five.
- The reflex facilitates attainment of the sitting position, getting to the all-fours position, and attaining the standing position.

2. Protective or Propping Reflexes/Reactions/Responses

   a. These reflexes are activated by rapid changes in body position to break a fall.
   b. The subtypes and age of onset are:

- Downward (sometimes called Parachute)—occurs at about four months.
- Posterior (also called Backward)—occurs at about 10 months.
- Lateral (also called Sideward)—occurs at about eight months.
- Forward (sometimes called Parachute)—occurs at about seven to nine months.

c. The reflexes are needed to protect the person in upright positions, including when sitting, kneeling, and standing.

- Downward—The legs and arms externally rotate and abduct. The feet dorsiflex in preparation for landing. If the hips internally rotate and adduct, and the feet plantar flex, the person has increased muscle tone, which is abnormal. Also, if the response is asymmetrical, brain injury may have occurred on one side of the brain, or there may be muscle weakness or peripheral nerve injury.
- Posterior—The arms extend backward at the shoulder, elbow, and wrist and the fingers are extended and abducted to break the fall. An alternate response may be one arm extended with trunk rotation. If the response is asymmetrical, brain injury may have occurred on one side of the brain, or there may be muscle weakness or peripheral nerve injury.
- Lateral—The person abducts an arm on the side opposite from the force, with abduction at the shoulder, extension of the elbow and wrist, and abduction and extension of the fingers to break the fall. Asymmetrical response may indicate brain injury, muscle weakness, or peripheral nerve injury.
- Forward—The person flexes and abducts his or her shoulder, extends elbow and wrist, and extends and abducts fingers to break the fall. Asymmetrical response may indicate brain injury, muscle weakness, or peripheral nerve injury.

d. Protective reflexes can be facilitated by pushing the person off balance in the sitting, kneeling, or standing positions in any of the four directions: downward, posterior, lateral, or forward. *Note*: The therapist should be prepared to catch the person if the reflex does not function or should create an environment in which it is safe to fall, such as with the use of mats.

3. Equilibrium or Tilting Reflexes/Reactions/Responses

These reflexes are activated when there is a mild change in the position of the body. Equilibrium reflexes differ from protective reflexes in that they develop in all body positions, including prone, supine, sitting, and standing positions. The proficiency increases from initial appearance at about four months in the prone position, eight months in the sitting position, and one year in the standing position. These reflexes are assumed to be mediated at the cortex level.

a. Equilibrium reflexes are activated by subtle or slow changes in the posture or position of the body.

b. The types and age of development are:

- Prone—onset about six months and persists throughout life
- Supine—onset about seven to eight months and persists throughout life
- Sitting—onset about seven to eight months and persists throughout life

- All Fours—onset about nine to 12 months and persists throughout life
- Standing—onset about 12 to 21 months and persists throughout life
c. Equilibrium reflexes modify the righting (labyrinthine) reflexes. Asymmetrical responses suggest unilateral brain injury or muscle weakness.
    - Prone—The person's trunk is curved away from the tilt, with the concavity of the spine upward toward the tilt; the upper arm and leg may be slightly abducted.
    - Supine—The person's trunk is curved away from the tilt, with the concavity of the spine upward toward the tilt; the upper arm and leg may be slightly abducted.
    - Sitting, Lateral Tilt—The body remains in an upright position flexed against the tilt, with the concavity of the spine upward, neck flexed laterally, and the head slightly rotated with the face toward the upper side. The arm and leg on the upper side are abducted, while those on the lower side are adducted and extended.
    - Sitting, Forward (Anterior) Tilt—The body remains in an upright position with the spine extended and the limbs retracted.
    - Sitting, Backward (Posterior) Tilt—The body remains in an upright position with the spine flexed and the limbs slightly extended and abducted.
    - All Fours, Lateral Tilt—The body is flexed against the tilt with the concavity of the spine upward. The head is slightly rotated so that the face is turned toward the upper side. The arm and leg on the upper side flex while the arm and leg on the lower side extend and abduct.
    - All Fours, Anterior Tilt—The body remains in an upright position with the trunk moving posterior while the head and arms extend and the legs flex.
    - All Fours, Posterior Tilt—The body remains in an upright position with the trunk moving anterior while the head and elbows flex and the shoulders and hips extend.
    - Standing, Lateral Tilt—The body is flexed against the tilt with the concavity of the spine upward. The upper arm is abducted while the upper leg is flexed. The lower leg is extended to act as a strong brace.
    - Standing, Anterior Tilt—The body remains in an upright position with the spine extended, displacing the body backward; the arms are extended at the shoulder but flexed at the elbows.
    - Standing, Posterior Tilt—The body remains in an upright position with the spine flexed, displacing the trunk forward; the arms are flexed at the shoulders but extended at the elbows while the legs are extended.
d. The equilibrium reflexes can be facilitated using a tilt board, large ball, rolls, bolsters, or t-stool (sitting surface is mounted on one peg in the center). The person should be slowly tilted in the direction desired. The therapist should be prepared to catch the person if the reflex does not function.

BIBLIOGRAPHY

Johnston, R.B. 1976. Motor function: normal development and cerebral palsy. In *Developmental disorders: Assessment, treatment, education*, eds. R.B. Johnston and P.R. Magrab, 15–55. Baltimore: University Park Press; and Stuberg, W. 1994. *The Milani-Comparetti Motor Development Screening Test*, 3rd ed. Rev. Omaha, NE: Meyer Rehabilitation Institute, University of Nebraska Medical Center.

FUNCTIONAL SIGNIFICANCE OF POSTURAL REFLEXES

Activity (reflex, reaction)	Assist	Interfere
Early Prone		
Head up	Head righting	Tonic labyrinthine, supine, and prone
		Asymmetrical tonic neck
		Symmetrical tonic neck
Early Supine		
Head lift	Head righting	Tonic labyrinthine, supine, and prone
		Asymmetrical tonic neck
Reach		Tonic labyrinthine, supine, and prone
		Asymmetrical tonic neck
Rolling Over	Head righting	Tonic labyrinthine, supine, and prone
	Derotation	Asymmetrical tonic neck
Sitting		
Come to sit	Head righting	Asymmetrical tonic neck
	Derotation	Tonic labyrinthine, supine, and prone
Stable sitting	Protective	Asymmetrical tonic neck
	Equilibrium	Symmetrical tonic neck, flexed and extended
		Tonic labyrinthine, supine and prone
		Moro
Crawling		
Reciprocal crawl	Equilibrium	Symmetrical tonic neck, flexed and extended
		Tonic labyrinthine, supine and prone
		Positive supporting
Standing		
Pull to stand	Positive support	Positive supporting
		Asymmetrical tonic neck
Stable stand	Positive support	Positive supporting
	Protective	Tonic labyrinthine, supine and prone
	Equilibrium	
Ambulating		
Cruise	Equilibrium	Positive supporting
Walk	Protective	Positive supporting
	Equilibrium	Tonic labyrinthine, supine and prone
		Asymmetrical tonic neck
		Moro
Crossing		
Midline		Tonic labyrinthine, supine and prone
		Asymmetrical tonic neck
		Symmetrical tonic neck, flexed and extended
Derotation		Tonic labyrinthine, supine and prone
		Asymmetrical tonic neck
		Neonatal neck righting (log rolling)

Source: Data from R.B. Johnston and P.R. Magrab, *Developmental Disorders: Assessment, Treatment, Education*, © 1976, University Park Press.

RELAXATION

Simple Techniques

1. *Deep Breathing*. Deep breath is taken through the nose or mouth, held briefly, released slowly, and then another breath is taken. Counting the number of breaths taken focuses attention on breathing.
2. *Fist Tightening*. A deep breath is taken while clenching the fists, position is held for a count of three, breath is released, and fists are unclenched. Action is repeated.
3. *Stretching*. Person stands on toes, raises arms overhead (reaches for the sky or ceiling), and takes a deep breath. Position is held and then person goes limp while exhaling. Action is repeated. Technique can be done while sitting by having person extend legs and point toes. Arm position is the same.
4. *Shoulder Shrug*. Shoulders are lifted toward the ears, held for five seconds, slowly brought down, held in position, and relaxed.

Progressive Relaxation

Beginning with either the top or bottom of the body, a group of muscles is tightened while taking a deep breath and then relaxed while breath is released. The routine may be altered to begin with a group of muscles that are causing discomfort. In either case, the routine progresses through groups of muscles until attention has been paid to all parts of the body. The procedure is called a script and may be done while sitting, standing, or lying down. The person may memorize the script, have it tape recorded, or have it read. Total length of time may be a few minutes to half an hour.

Imagery

The person begins by visualizing a peaceful scene or fantasizing being in a peaceful setting. Some people may need to write their script while others may prefer to tape record it. Eventually, the script is memorized. For persons who need ideas to get started, some examples may be useful, such as lying on the sand at a favorite beach, floating like a balloon looking down at the earth, sitting by a brook in the woods, listening to the birds sing on an early spring morning, resting on a soft cloud gazing at the blue sky, or fishing in a lake on a lazy afternoon. The procedure then follows a theme from progressive relaxation.

Visualization

The person focuses on getting rid of or plucking the tension or pain from a tense or painful part of the body and sending it away. Technique is similar to imagery, except for the localization of the problem. For example, the person might visualize plucking the pain from a knee joint, putting it in a brook, and watching it bubble away, or taking the tension from a headache, putting it on a balloon, and watching it sail away.

Meditation

The person selects a word, object, or body part on which to focus or center. The person then centers or concentrates on the selected target while sitting and breathing deeply and regularly. A quiet environment is usually helpful when learning the technique.

Self-Hypnosis

To prepare for self-hypnosis, the person is told by the therapist to concentrate on an object or on breathing. When a state of hypnosis has been achieved, a suggestion is given to the person, such as "Picture yourself floating on a soft cloud and begin to relax." After practicing several times, the person will be able to self-recall the image and begin relaxing without help from another person.

Biofeedback

The person practices a relaxation technique as described above but observes the relaxation response in muscles through an audiovisual response from the biofeedback machine. Usually, training begins in a clinic by a trained therapist, but after the person has learned the technique, the training may be used at home. The therapist then monitors the person's progress in using the technique.

BIBLIOGRAPHY

Keable, D. 1997. *The management of anxiety: A guide for therapists*, 2nd ed. New York: Churchill Livingstone; and Stein, F., and S.K. Cutler. 1998. Stress management, biofeedback, and relaxation training. In *Psychosocial occupational therapy: A holistic approach*, eds. F. Stein and S.K. Cutler, 375–418. San Diego: Singular Publishing Group.

See also the resource bibliography on Relaxation Techniques and Stress Management in Appendix G.

SELF-CARE TECHNIQUES

Bathing and Toileting

- Use long-handled sponge or brush to soap body (range of motion).
- Use reacher to hold toilet paper for wiping (range of motion).
- Use a tub, shower bench, or webbed plastic lawn chair to permit sitting in tub or shower (energy conservation).
- Put nonskid safety strips or rubber bathmat on tub or shower floor to avoid slipping (safety).
- Consider installing grab bars to assist in climbing in and out of the tub or shower (safety).
- Use a long shower spray hose to make rinsing easier (range of motion).
- Use a terrycloth robe to soak up water on body; pat the body dry (energy conservation).
- Install a grab bar on the wall or floor next to the toilet to assist in sitting and standing (safety).
- Use an electric toothbrush or Water-Pik instead of a manual toothbrush (energy conservation).
- Use a device that holds the dental floss rather than using fingers (fine motor).
- Use the heel of the hand to squeeze the toothpaste tube instead of fingers (fine motor).

BIBLIOGRAPHY

Christiansen, C., ed. 1994. *Ways of living: Self-care strategies for special needs*. Bethesda, MD: American Occupational Therapy Association.
Foti, D., and L.W. Pedretti. 1996. Activities of daily living. In *Occupational therapy: Practice skills for physical dysfunction*, 4th ed., ed. L.W. Pedretti, 463–499. St. Louis: Mosby.

Trombly, C.A. 1996. Retraining basic and instrumental activities of daily living. In *Occupational therapy for physical dysfunction*, 4th. ed., ed. C.A. Trombly, 289–318. Baltimore: Williams & Wilkins.

For additional resources, see the resource bibliography on Media, Modalities, and Techniques in Appendix G.

Cooking/Meal Preparation

- Microwave ovens save time and energy, can be placed at a convenient height, and are safer than traditional ovens to use because the food heats rather than the container (energy conservation, range of motion, safety).
- Avoid lifting heavy pans of food and water. Either remove the food first by ladling the contents out or use a fry basket inside the pot so the food is separate from the water (energy conservation, safety).
- Use lightweight cooking utensils, bowls, and dishes. Avoid cast-iron skillets and heavy ceramic bowls (joint protection).
- Use a jar opener that grips the lid, permitting the use of both hands to turn the jar itself (joint protection).
- Use an electric can opener rather than a manual one (energy conservation, one-handed).
- Select appliances with controls that are easy to operate—that is, their location is easy to reach and the action is easy to engage or stop (safety, range of motion, energy conservation).
- Organize canned goods within easy reach and place labels so they can be easily read (range of motion, energy conservation).
- Plan meals that are easy to fix and easy to clean up. Consider frozen meals, one-pot meals, ready mixes, and convenience foods (energy conservation).
- Serve foods in the same containers in which they were prepared (energy conservation).
- Use throwaway utensils, paper plates, and cups to reduce dishwashing (energy conservation).
- Use a dishwasher that is easy to load rather than manually washing dishes (energy conservation).
- Cook a double portion and freeze the extra portion for easier preparation of a meal on a day that will be busier than most (energy conservation).
- Use pans with nonstick surfaces or spray with nonstick product to reduce clean-up time (energy conservation).
- Line containers with aluminum foil or put aluminum foil on a cookie sheet to prevent sticking to the surface to reduce clean-up time (energy conservation).
- Use a hook (cup holder hook on the end of a dowel or bent coat hanger) to pull out a hot oven shelf (safety).
- Use mitt pot holders so palms can be used to lift pans and bowls instead of fingers (joint protection).
- Place heavy containers, such as flour and sugar, where they do not need to be lifted to get small quantities, or buy smaller quantities (joint protection).
- Place bowls on a nonskid surface (wet washrag, wet terrycloth towel, certain types of plastic mats) so that both hands can be used to stir (joint protection).
- Use a food processor for recipes that require foods to be chopped, sliced, or grated.
- Use a spray to rinse dishes and pour water into cooking pans immediately after use to avoid food drying to the surface before cleaning (energy conservation).

BIBLIOGRAPHY

Foti, D., and L.W. Pedretti. 1996. Activities of daily living. In *Occupational therapy: Practice skills for physical dysfunction*, 4th ed., ed. L.W. Pedretti, 463–499. St. Louis: Mosby.

Klinger, J.L. 1997. *Meal preparation and training: The health care professional's guide*. Thorofare, NJ: Slack.

Klinger, J.L. 1997. *Mealtime manual for people with disabilities and the aging*. Thorofare, NJ: Slack.

Park, S. 1998. Enhancing performance of instrumental activities of daily living. In *Stoke rehabilitation: A function based approach*, eds. G. Gillen and A. Burkhardt, 353–384. St. Louis: Mosby.

Stewart, C. Retraining housekeeping and child care skills. In *Occupational therapy for physical dysfunction*, 4th ed., ed. C.A. Trombly, 319–328. Baltimore: Williams & Wilkins.

For additional resources, see the resource bibliography on Media, Modalities, and Techniques in Appendix G.

Dressing: Clothing, Shoes

- Sew Velcro on clothing to replace small buttons. Sew the button on the top side (fine motor manipulation).
- Sew elasticized thread on button cuffs to provide give for fingers to slide through (fine motor).
- Buy clothes that are easy to put on (range of motion). Get front fasteners and elastic bands that slip over hips.
- Buy clothes that are easy to care for (energy conservation).
- Lower the rod in the closet for easier reach (range of motion).
- Use long-handled shoe horn to assist in putting on shoes (range of motion).
- Use elastic shoelaces that can remain tied (fine motor).
- Place large rings, thread, or leather loops on zipper tabs to facilitate zipping (fine motor).
- Fasten bra in front and then turn it around and pull in place, or get front-closure bras (range of motion).
- Use reacher or dressing stick to assist with pulling up pants, straightening skirts, or getting clothes slightly out of reach (range of motion).
- Use powder on legs before putting on pantyhose to reduce friction (fine motor).
- Buy low heels—no higher than 1 inch (safety).
- Cushion plantar surface with shoe inserts (safety).
- Look for shoes with soft upper material that gives or stretches to relieve pressure (safety).

BIBLIOGRAPHY

Christiansen, C., ed. 1994. *Ways of living: Self-care strategies for special needs*. Bethesda, MD: American Occupational Therapy Association.

Foti, D., and L.W. Pedretti. 1996. Activities of daily living. In *Occupational therapy: Practice skills for physical dysfunction*, 4th ed., ed. L.W. Pedretti, 463–499. St. Louis: Mosby.

Trombly, C.A. 1996. Retraining basic and instrumental activities of daily living. In *Occupational therapy for physical dysfunction*, 4th ed., ed. C.A. Trombly, 289–318. Baltimore: Williams & Wilkins.

See also the resource bibliography on Clothing Adaptations and Activities of Daily Living (ADL) in Appendix G.

Driving

- If possible, buy or lease a car with doors that are easy to open and close, seats that are adjustable, and storage space that is easy to reach (fine motor, grasp manipulation, and range of motion).
- Reduce low back strain by using a cushion designed to fit the curve of the back (joint protection).
- Attach loops to inside door handles so that forearm can be used to assist door closing instead of hand (joint protection).
- Attach auxiliary or wide-angle mirrors to allow for increased visibility when neck motion is limited (range of motion).
- Get a handicapped sticker to permit parking closer to stores (energy conservation).
- Drive and shop when energy level is highest, such as when medication effect is at a peak (energy conservation).
- Shop with family or friends who can carry purchases (joint protection).
- Avoid peak shopping and traffic hours that will lengthen time standing in line or moving through traffic (energy conservation).
- Shop by telephone or mail when possible (energy conservation).
- Keep shopping trips short by planning what and where to buy. Call ahead to make sure items are available, if unsure (energy conservation).
- If tired after shopping for groceries, bring perishable items in first. Other items can wait until later after a nap (energy conservation).

BIBLIOGRAPHY

Lillie, S.M. 1996. Driving with a physical dysfunction. In *Occupational therapy: Practice skills for physical dysfunction*, 3rd ed., ed. L.W. Pedretti, 499–506. St. Louis: Mosby.
Pierce, S.L. 1998. Driving. In *Stroke rehabilitation: A function-based approach*, eds. G. Gillen and A. Burkhardt, 385–406. St. Louis: Mosby.

For additional resources, see the resource bibliography on Media, Modalities, and Techniques in Appendix G.

Eating/Feeding

- Enlarge or build up handles for easier grasp (fine motor, grasp manipulation). Foam curlers, washrags secured with tape, or commercial designs may be used. Applies to forks, knives, spoons, spatulas, or any device with a handle.
- Extend or lengthen the handle for restricted range of motion (range of motion).
- Rocker knife or spooks (spoon and fork combined) may be used by persons with only one functioning hand (one-handed).
- Small-diameter glasses, such as juice glasses, may be useful for persons with limited grasp (fine motor, grasp manipulation).
- Use nonbreakable items (safety).
- Use a friction or nonskid surface (Dycem, suction cup, or wet washrag) for persons using one hand or who have uncontrolled movements (one-handed; tremor, spastic or athetoid movements).

- Use cups with handles large enough to insert fingers for persons with poor grasp (fine motor, grasp manipulation).
- Use a plate guard for persons using one hand or who have uncontrolled movements to keep food on plate and aid in getting food on eating utensil (one-handed; tremor, spastic or athetoid movements).
- Use long straw for persons with limited range of motion (range of motion).
- Use sandwich holders for persons with uncontrolled movements or high level paralysis (tremor, spastic, or athetoid movement; paralyzed).
- Use a utensil cuff for person with limited or no grasp (fine motor, grasp manipulation).
- Use swivel utensils that stay level regardless of the position of the hand, wrist, or forearm for persons with restricted motions (range of motion).
- Use bent handles for persons with limited motion patterns (range of motion). May be combined with extended and enlarged handles.

BIBLIOGRAPHY

Christiansen, C., ed. 1994. *Ways of living: Self-care strategies for special needs*. Bethesda, MD: American Occupational Therapy Association.

Foti, D., and L.W. Pedretti. 1996. Activities of daily living. In *Occupational therapy: Practice skills for physical dysfunction*, 4th ed., ed. L.W. Pedretti, 463–499. St. Louis: Mosby.

Klein, M.D., and S.E. Morris. 1999. *Mealtime participation guide*. San Antonio, TX: Therapy Skill Builders.

Trombly, C.A. 1996. Retraining basic and instrumental activities of daily living. In *Occupational therapy for physical dysfunction*, 4th ed., ed. C.A. Trombly, 289–318. Baltimore: Williams & Wilkins.

For additional resources, see the resource bibliography on Media, Modalities, and Techniques in Appendix G.

Grooming

- Sit on a stool to apply makeup or to shave. Prop elbows on the countertop, if possible (energy conservation).
- Allow enough time to groom "in phase" to permit short rest breaks (energy conservation).
- Use long-handled attachments with combs or brushes to reduce need to reach arms over shoulder height (range of motion, energy conservation).
- Enlarge handles on makeup items, combs, brushes, toothbrush with foam curlers to make grasp easier (fine motor, grasp manipulation).
- Squeeze toothpaste using the palm of the hand on a flat surface rather than with fingers (fine motor, grasp manipulation).
- Take short showers or baths using warm, not hot, water when getting ready to go out. Save longer showers or baths for bedtime (energy conservation).

BIBLIOGRAPHY

Christiansen, C., ed. 1994. *Ways of living: Self-care strategies for special needs*. Bethesda, MD: American Occupational Therapy Association.

Foti, D., and L.W. Pedretti. 1996. Activities of daily living. In *Occupational therapy: Practice skills for physical dysfunction*, 4th ed., ed. L.W. Pedretti, 463–499. St. Louis: Mosby.

Trombly, C.A. 1996. Retraining basic and instrumental activities of daily living. In *Occupational therapy for physical dysfunction*, 4th ed., ed. C.A. Trombly, 289–318. Baltimore: Williams & Wilkins.

For additional resources, see the resource bibliography on Media, Modalities, and Techniques in Appendix G.

Housekeeping

- Keep cleaning supplies in each area where they will be needed to reduce walking with loads, or put cleaning supplies in easy-to-reach containers and place on a movable cart that can be wheeled about the house (energy conservation).
- Use a short stool to sit on to clean low-level surfaces, such as the tub, toilet bowl, or floor (energy conservation).
- Use long-handled tools or create extended handles for sponges, dustpans, mops, or small brooms to reduce the need for stretching and bending (energy conservation, range of motion).
- Use an ironing board that can be adjusted to permit sitting while ironing (energy conservation). Better yet, buy clothes that require little, if any, ironing.
- Use a front-loading washing machine, if possible. Clothes can be dumped out when wet and heavy rather than lifted (joint protection).
- Arrange to shop for groceries with someone who can carry them from the car into the house, or check to see if delivery service is available and affordable. Volunteers may be available to shop (energy conservation, joint protection).
- For light switches on lamps, buy enlarged knobs or a device that allows lamps to be turned on and off by touching them (fine motor, grasp manipulation).
- Casters on furniture make moving it easier when vacuuming (joint protection).

BIBLIOGRAPHY

Foti, D., and L.W. Pedretti. 1996. Activities of daily living. In *Occupational therapy: Practice skills for physical dysfunction*, 4th ed., ed. L.W. Pedretti, 463–499. St. Louis: C.V. Mosby.

Park, S. 1998. Enhancing performance of instrumental activities of daily living. In *Stroke rehabilitation: A function-based approach*, eds. G. Gillen and A. Burkhardt, 353–384. St. Louis: Mosby.

Stewart, C. Retraining housekeeping and child care skills. In *Occupational therapy for physical dysfunction*, 4th ed., ed. C.A. Trombly, 319–328. Baltimore: Williams & Wilkins.

For additional resources, see the resource bibliography on Media, Modalities, and Techniques in Appendix G.

Appendix C

Assessments Developed Entirely or in Part by Occupational Therapy Personnel

Note: This list is an attempt to document assessment instruments authored in total by occupational therapy personnel or authored by a group of professionals of which at least one was an occupational therapist or assistant. The task has been difficult because occupational therapy personnel do not consistently document assessment instruments correctly in the literature, which makes identification of authorship an uncertain art. Errors may have occurred, but the intent is honest: to document the contribution of occupational therapy personnel in the development of assessment instruments. Information on errors is welcome.

The list below is in alphabetical order by title and includes information about the source and development of the assessment instrument as well as articles in which the instrument was part of the research methodology. Because some instruments have more than one name, cross references have been provided.

A Factor Analytically Derived Scale. See Occupational Therapy Trait Rating Scale (OTTRS).

A-One

Árnadóttir, G. 1989. An introduction to the concepts and background of the Arnadottir OT-ADL Neurobehavioral Evaluation (A-ONE). *Bulletin of the World Federation of Occupational Therapists.* 20: 36–43.

Árnadóttir, G. 1990. *The brain and behavior: Assessing cortical dysfunction through activities of daily living.* Philadelphia: Mosby. Form and instructions included.

Árnadóttir, G. 1999. Evaluation and intervention with complex perceptual impairment. In *Cognitive and perceptual dysfunction: A clinical reasoning approach to evaluation and intervention*, ed. C. Unsworth, 393–454. Philadelphia: F.A. Davis. Form included.

The author is indebted to Lee Ann Klombies and Megan Zook for their contribution to the development of this list as part of their professional project in the Master's of Occupational Therapy program at the School of Occupational Therapy, Texas Woman's University—Houston Campus.

Impact of neurobehavior deficits on activities of daily living. In *Stroke rehabilitation: A function-based approach*, eds. G. Gillen and A. Burkhardt, 285–333. St. Louis: Mosby, 1998.

Rogers, J.C., and M.C. Holm. 1998. Árnadóttir OT-ADL Neurobehavioral Evaluation (A-ONE). In *Willard and Spackman's occupational therapy*, 9th ed., eds. M.E. Neistadt and E.B. Crepeau, 203–204. Philadelphia: J.B. Lippincott.

Ropiak, J.A. 1996. The benefits of collaboration: Clinicians, educators, and students joining forces in research. *Journal of Occupational Therapy Students* (October): 19–20.

Rubio, K.B. 1995. The Árnadóttir OT-ADL Neurobehavioral Evaluation (A-ONE). *Physical Disabilities Special Interest Section Newsletter* 18(2): 1–2.

Rubio, K.B., and J. Van Deusen. 1995. Relation of perceptual and body image dysfunction to activities of daily living of persons after stroke. *American Journal of Occupational Therapy* 49(6): 551–556.

Unsworth, C. 1999. The Árnadóttir Occupational Therapy Neurobehavioral Evaluation (A-ONE). In *Cognitive and perceptual dysfunction: A clinical reasoning approach to evaluation and intervention*, ed. C. Unsworth, 85–88. Philadelphia: F.A. Davis.

Achievement Record

Livingston, D.M. 1950. Achievement recording for the cerebral palsied. *American Journal of Occupational Therapy* 6(2): 66–74. Form included.

Activities of Daily Living Assessment

Activities of Daily Living Assessment, Time-Oriented Record. In *Occupational therapy for children*, eds. P.N. Clark and A.S. Allen, 510–523. St. Louis: Mosby, 1985. Form included.

Children's Hospital at Stanford Occupational Therapy. 1978. Activities of Daily Living Assessment, Time-Oriented Record. In *Pediatric assessment of self-care activities*, ed. I.L. Coley, 123–131. St. Louis: Mosby. Form included.

Activities of Daily Living Checklist

Backman, C. 1998. Functional assessment. In *Rheumatologic rehabilitation series: Assessment and management*, Vol. 1, eds. J. Melvin and G. Jensen, 181–191. Bethesda, MD: American Occupational Therapy Association. Form included.

Activities of Daily Living Rating Scale

Dinnerstein, A.J., M. Lowenthal, and M. Dexter. 1965. Evaluation of rating scale of ability in activities of daily living. *Archives of Physical Medicine and Rehabilitation* 46(8): 579–584.

Activities of Daily Living Scale (modified from Northwick Park and Rivermead)

Ebrahim, S., F. Nouri, and D. Barer. 1985. Measuring disability after a stroke. *Journal of Epidemiology and Community Health* 39(1): 86–89.

Activities of Daily Living Screening and Assessment

Melvin, J.L. 1989. *Rheumatic disease in the adult and child: Occupational therapy and rehabilitation*, 2nd ed. Philadelphia: F.A. Davis.

Activities of Daily Living Situational Test. See ADL Situational Test.

Activities of Daily Living Test

Zimmerman, M.E. 1963. Occupational therapy in the ADL program. In *Occupational Therapy*, 3rd ed., eds. H.S. Willard and C.S. Spackman, 320–357. Philadelphia: J.B. Lippincott.

Activity Assessment (in geriatrics)

Crepeau, E.L. 1986. *Activity programming for the elderly*, 39. Boston: Little, Brown.

The process of activity assessment in geriatrics. *Topics in Geriatric Rehabilitation* 1986; (4): 31–44.

Activity Configuration

Hemphill, B.J., ed. 1982. *Evaluative process in psychiatric occupational therapy*, 364. Thorofare, NJ: Slack. Adapted form.

Hopkins, H.L., and H.D. Smith. 1978. Activity configuration chart. In *Willard and Spackman's occupational therapy*, 5th ed., 156–157. Philadelphia: J.B. Lippincott.

Watanabe, S. 1969. Activities configuration: Social adaptation "Making it." In *Regional Institute on the Evaluation Process*. Final Report No. RSA-123-T-68. New York: American Occupational Therapy Association. Adapted from a form developed by Richard Spahn, Austin-Riggs Foundation. Paper presented at the March 1965 meeting of the American Orthopsychiatric Society.

Watanabe, S. 1971. Activity configuration chart. In *Occupational Therapy*, 4th ed., eds. H.S. Willard and C.S. Spackman, 88–89. Philadelphia: J.B. Lippincott.

Activity Configuration

Mosey, A. 1993. *Activities therapy*, 102. New York: Raven Press. Form included.

Activity Laboratory

Fidler, G.S. 1982. The activity laboratory: A structure for observing and assessing perceptual, integrative, and behavioral strategies. In *Evaluative process in psychiatric occupational therapy*, ed. B.J. Hemphill, 195–207, 379–389. Thorofare, NJ: Slack.

Activity Patterns and Leisure Concepts Among the Elderly

Gregory, M.D. 1983. Occupational behavior and life satisfaction among retirees. *American Journal of Occupational Therapy* 35(8): 548–553. Form included. See modified edition.

Nystrom, E. 1974. Activity patterns and leisure concepts among the elderly. *American Journal of Occupational Therapy* 28(6): 337–345.

Activity Questionnaire. See National Institutes of Health Activity Record.

Activity Record. See National Institutes of Health Activity Record.

ADL Situational Test

Skurla, E., J.C. Rogers, and T. Sunderland. 1988. Direct assessment of activities of daily living in Alzheimer's disease: A controlled study. *Journal of the American Geriatrics Society* 36(2): 97–103.

Adolescent Feminine and Occupational Development Questionnaire

Pezzuti, L. 1979. An exploration of adolescent feminine and occupational behavior development. *American Journal of Occupational Therapy* 33(2): 84–91.

Adolescent Leisure Interest Profile (ALIP)

Henry, A.D. 1998. Development of a measure of adolescent leisure interests. *American Journal of Occupational Therapy* 52(7): 531–539.

Adolescent Role Assessment

Black, M. 1976. Adolescent role assessment. *American Journal of Occupational Therapy* 30(2): 73–79. Form included.

Black, M. 1982. Adolescent role assessment. In *The evaluative process in psychiatric occupational therapy*, ed. B.J. Hemphill, 49–53, 333–338. Thorofare, NJ: Slack.

Henry, A.D. 1998. Adolescent role assessment. In *Willard and Spackman's occupational therapy*, 9th ed., eds. M.E. Neistadt and E.B. Crepeau, 163. Philadelphia: J.B. Lippincott.

Adult Psychiatric Sensory Integration Evaluation. See Schroeder Block Campbell Adult Psychiatric Sensory Integration Evaluation.

Adult Skills Evaluation Survey (ASES) for Persons with Mental Retardation

Herrick, J.T., and H.E. Lowe. 1984. Adult Skills Evaluation Survey (ASES) for persons with mental retardation. *Occupational Therapy in Health Care* 1(2): 71–77.

Lowe, H.E. 1990. *Adult Skills Evaluation Survey for persons with mental retardation.* 770 North Fair Oaks Avenue, Pasadena, CA 91103. Published by author.

Affective Self-Report Checklist

Boyer, J., W. Colman, L. Levy, and B. Manoly. 1989. Affective responses to activities: A comparative study. *American Journal of Occupational Therapy* 43(2): 81–87.

Alderson-McGall Hand Function Questionnaire

Alderson, M., and D. McGall. 1999. The Alderson-McGall Hand Function Questionnaire for patients with carpal tunnel syndrome: A pilot evaluation of a future outcome measure. *Journal of Hand Therapy* 12(4): 313–322.

Allen Cognitive Level Screen (ACLS)

Allen, C.K. 1996. *Allen Cognitive Level Screen (ACLS) Test Manual.* S&S, P.O. Box 513, Colchester, CT 06414-0513. Published by S&S.

Allen, C.K., and T. Blue. 1998. Cognitive disabilities model: How to make clinical judgments. In *Cognition and occupation in rehabilitation: Cognitive models for intervention in occupational therapy,* ed. N. Katz, 225–279. Bethesda, MD: American Occupational Therapy Association.

Earhart, C.A., and C.K. Allen. 1988. *Cognitive disabilities: Expanded activity analysis,* 10–15. 3660 Cartwright Street, Pasadena, CA 91107 (author) or S&S, P.O. Box 513, Colchester, CT 06414-0513.

Mayer, M.A. 1988. Analysis of information processing and cognitive disability theory. *American Journal of Occupational Therapy* 42(3): 176–183.

Allen Cognitive Level Test (ACL-O)

Allen, C.K. *Allen Cognitive Level Test,* S&S, P.O. Box 513, Colchester, CT 06414-0513; or AliMed, Inc., 297 High Street, Dedham, MA 02026-9135.

Allen, C.K. 1982. Independence through activity: The practice of occupational therapy. *American Journal of Occupational Therapy* 36(22): 731–739.

Allen, C.K. 1985. *Occupational therapy for psychiatric diseases: Measurement and management of cognitive disabilities.* Boston: Little, Brown.

Allen, C.K. 1988. Occupational therapy: Functional assessment of the severity of mental disorders. *Hospital and Community Psychiatry* 39(2): 140–142.

Allen, C.K., and T. Blue. 1998. Cognitive disabilities model: How to make clinical judgments. In *Cognition and occupation in rehabilitation: Cognitive models for intervention in occupational therapy,* ed. N. Katz, 225–279. Bethesda, MD: American Occupational Therapy Association.

Allen, C.K., C.A. Earhart, and T. Blue. 1996. *Understanding cognitive performance models.* S&S, P.O. Box 513, Colchester, CT 06414-0513.

Burns, T., J.A. Mortimer, and P. Merchak. 1994. Cognitive Performance Test: A new approach to functional assessment in Alzheimer's disease. *Journal of Geriatric Psychiatry and Neurology* 7(1): 46–54.

David, S.K., and W.T. Riley. 1990. The relationship of the Allen Cognitive Level Test to cognitive abilities and psychopathology. *American Journal of Occupational Therapy* 44(6): 493–497.

Felder, R., K. James, C. Crown, S. Lemon, and M. Reveal. 1994. Dexterity testing as a predictor of oral care ability. *Journal of the American Geriatric Society* 42(10): 1081–1086.

Henry A.D., K. Moore, M. Quinlivan, and M. Triggs. 1998. The relationship of the Allen Cognitive Level Test to diagnosis and disposition among psychiatric inpatients. *American Journal of Occupational Therapy* 52(8): 638–643.

Keller, S., and R. Hayes. 1998. The relationship between the Allen Cognitive Level Test and the Life Skills Profile. *American Journal of Occupational Therapy* 52(10): 851–856.

Penny, N.H., K.T. Mueser, and C.T. North. 1995. The Allen Cognitive Level Test and social competence in adult psychiatric patients. *American Journal of Occupational Therapy* 49(5): 420–427.

Richert, G.A., and M.B. Merryman. 1987. The vocational continuum: A model for providing vocational services in a partial hospitalization program. *Occupational Therapy in Mental Health* 7(3): 1–20.

Shapiro, M.E. 1991. Application of the Allen Cognitive Level Test in assessing cognitive level functioning of emotionally disturbed boys. *American Journal of Occupational Therapy* 46(6): 514–520.

Unsworth, C. 1999. Allen Cognitive Level Test (ACL). In *Cognitive and perceptual dysfunction: A clinical reasoning approach to evaluation and intervention*, ed. C. Unsworth, 86–87, 91–92. Philadelphia: F.A. Davis.

Velligan, D.I., C.C. Bow-Thomas, R. Mahurin, A. Miller, A. Dassori, and F. Erdely. 1998. Concurrent and predictive validity of the Allen Cognitive Levels Assessment. *Psychiatry Research* 80(3): 287–298.

Velligan, D.I., J.E. True, R.S. Lefton, T.C. Moore, and C.V. Flores. 1995. Validity of the Allen Cognitive Levels Assessment: A tri-ethnic comparison. *Psychiatry Research* 56(2): 101–109.

Allen Cognitive Level Test —Problem Solving

Josman, N., and N. Katz. 1991. A problem-solving version of the Allen Cognitive Level Test. *American Journal of Occupational Therapy* 45(4): 331–338.

Allen Cognitive Level Test—Revised (ACL-R)

Allen, C.K., K. Kehrberg, and T. Burns. 1992. Evaluation instruments, Part 1: Allen Cognitive Levels (ACL). In *Occupational therapy treatment goals for the physically and cognitively disabled*, eds. C.K. Allen, C.A. Earhart, and T. Blue, 31–34, 51–53. Bethesda, MD: American Occupational Therapy Association.

Davidhizar, R., R. Cosgray, J. Smith, and R. Fawley. 1991. Comparison of three rating scales used with psychiatric patients. *Perspectives in Psychiatric Care* 27(3): 19–25.

Robertson, S. 1988. *Mental health FOCUS: Skills for assessment and treatment*, 3-18 to 3-33. Rockville, MD: American Occupational Therapy Association.

Allen Cognitive Levels—Expanded. See Allen Cognitive Level Test—Revised.

Allen Diagnostic Module (ADM)

Allen, C.K., and A. Reyner. 1995, 1996, 1997. *How to start using the Allen Diagnostic Module*. S&S, P.O. Box 513, Colchester, CT 06415-0513.

Earhart, C., C.K. Allen, and T. Blue. 1993. *Allen Diagnostic Module instruction manual*. S&S, P.O. Box 513, Colchester, CT 06415-0513, or AliMed, Inc., 297 High Street, Dedham, MA 02026-9135.

Roitman, D.M., and N. Katz. 1996. Predictive validity of the Large Allen Cognitive Levels Test (LACL) using the Allen Diagnostic Module (ADM) in an aged, nondisabled population. *Physical and Occupational Therapy in Geriatrics* 14(4): 43–59.

Allen Lacing Test. See Allen Cognitive Level Test.

Allen Lower-Level Cognitive Test

Ross, M. 1997. *Integrative group therapy mobilizing coping abilities with the five-stage group*, 169–170. Bethesda, MD: American Occupational Therapy Association.

Alzheimer Home Assessment

Painter, J. 1996. Home environment considerations for people with Alzheimer's disease. *Occupational Therapy in Health Care* 10(3): 45–63. Form included.

Tullis, A., and M. Nicol. 1999. A systematic review of the evidence for the value of functional assessment of older people with dementia. *British Journal of Occupational Therapy* 62(12): 554–563.

Apfel Hand Function Test

Apfel, E. 1990. Preliminary development of a standardized hand function test. *Journal of Hand Therapy* 3(4): 191–194.

Apraxia Assessment Technique

Sirkanojo, M. 1979. Evaluation of an apraxia assessment technique—Finland. *Bulletin of the World Federation of Occupational Therapists* 3(1): 16–21.

Árnadíóttir OT-ADL Neurobehavioral Evaluation. See A-One.

Arthritis Hand Function Test

Backman, C., and H. Mackie. 1996. The Arthritis Hand Function Test. *Physical Disabilities Special Interest Section Newsletter* 19(4): 1–2.

Backman, C., S. Cork, and J. Parsons. 1996. Assessment of hand function: The relationship between pegboard dexterity and applied dexterity. *Canadian Journal of Occupational Therapy* 59: 208–213.

Backman, C., and H. Mackie. 1995. Arthritis Hand Function Test: Interrater reliability among self-trained raters. *Arthritis Care and Research* 8(1): 10–15.

Backman, C., H. Mackie, and J. Harris. 1991. Arthritis Hand Function Test: Development of a standardized assessment tool. *Occupational Therapy Journal of Research* 11(4): 245–256.

Reliability and validity of the Arthritis Hand Function Tests in adults with osteoarthritis. *Occupational Therapy Journal of Research* 1997; 17(1): 55–66.

Assessment for Cursive Writing Skills Training

Benbow, M.D. 1996. *Assessment of Cursive Writing Skills Training*. San Antonio, TX: Therapy Skills Builder/The Psychological Corporation. Videotape.

Assessment Instrument for Problem-Focused Coping

Tollen, A., and G. Ahlstrom. 1998. Assessment instrument for problem-focused coping. *Scandinavian Journal of Caring Science* 12: 18–24.

Assessment Log and Developmental Progress Chart for the Carolina Curriculum for Infants and Toddlers with Special Needs (CCITSN)

Johnson-Martin, N.M., K.G. Jens, S.M. Attermeier, and B.J. Hacker, B.J. 1991. Assessment Log and Developmental Progress Chart for the Carolina Curriculum for Infants and Toddlers with Special Needs. In *The Carolina Curriculum for Infants with Special Needs*, 2nd ed., 47–67. Baltimore, MD: Paul H. Brookes. Also published separately.

Assessment Log and Developmental Progress Chart for the Carolina Curriculum for Preschoolers with Special Needs (CCPSN)

Johnson-Martin, N.M., S.M. Attermeier, and B.J. Hacker. 1990. Assessment Log and Developmental Progress Chart for the Carolina Curriculum for Preschoolers with Special Needs. In *The Carolina Curriculum for Preschoolers with Special Needs*, 37–65. Baltimore, MD: Paul H. Brookes. Also published separately.

Assessment of Awareness of Disability

Tham, B., B. Berspang, and A.G. Fisher. 1999. Development of the Assessment of Awareness of Disability. *Scandinavian Journal of Occupational Therapy* 6: 184–190.

Assessment of Communication and Interaction Skills (ACIS).

Forsyth, I., J.S. Lai, and G. Kielhofner. 1999. The Assessment of Communication and Interaction Skills (ACIS): Measurement properties. *British Journal of Occupational Therapy* 62(2): 69–74.

Kielhofner, G. 1995.' *Model of human occupation: Theory and practice,* 2nd ed., 207–209, 232–234, 366. Baltimore, MD: Williams & Wilkins. Sample and additional information.

Mentrup, C., A. Niehaus, and G. Kielhofner. 1999. Applying the model of human occupation in work-focused rehabilitation: A case illustration. *Work: Journal of Prevention, Assessment, and Rehabilitation* 12(1): 61–70.

Salamy, M., S. Simon, and G. Kielhofner. 1989, 1993. Assessment of communication and interacting skills. Model of Human Occupation Clearinghouse, Department of Occupational Therapy (M/C 811). University of Illinois at Chicago, 1919 West Taylor Street, Chicago, IL 60612. Fax: (312) 413-0256. Also available from American Occupational Therapy Association, 4720 Montgomery Lane, Bethesda, MD 20814-3425.

Simon, S. 1989. The development of an assessment for communication and interaction skills. Unpublished master's thesis, University of Illinois at Chicago.

Assessment of Hand Skills in the Primary Child

Benbow, M.D. 1996. *Assessment of hand skills in the primary child.* San Antonio, TX: Therapy Skills Builder/The Psychological Corporation. Videotape.

Assessment of Home Safety of Well Elderly

Buchanan, A. 1986. Assessment of home safety of well elderly. *Gerontology Special Interest Section Newsletter* 9(2): 2–4.

Assessment of Motor and Process Skills (AMPS)

Assessment of Motor and Process Skills. Fort Collins, CO: Three Star Press, 1995.

Baron, K.B. 1994. Clinical interpretation of "The Assessment of Motor and Process Skills of Persons with Psychiatric Disorders." *American Journal of Occupational Therapy* 48(9): 781–782.

Bernspang, B., and A.G. Fisher. 1995. Differences between persons with right and left CVA on the Assessment of Motor and Process Skills. *Archives of Physical Medicine and Rehabilitation* 76(12): 1144–1151.

Bernspang, B., and A.G. Fisher. 1995. Validation of the Assessment of Motor and Process Skills for use in Sweden. *Scandinavian Journal of Occupational Therapy* 2(1): 3–9.

Bryze, K., and A.G. Fisher. 1995. Diane: The use of the Assessment of Motor and Process Skills in treatment planning for an adult with developmental disabilities. In *A model of human occupation: Therapy and application,* 2nd ed., ed. G. Kielhofner, 286–295. Baltimore, MD: Williams & Wilkins.

Culler, K.H. 1993. Assessment of Motor and Processing Skills. In *Willard and Spackman's Occupational Therapy,* 8th ed., eds. Hopkins, H., and H. Smith, 214–215. Philadelphia: J.B. Lippincott. Short Scoring Form.

Dickerson, A.D. 1995. Culture-relevant functional performance assessment of the Hispanic elderly. *Occupational Therapy Journal of Research* 15(1): 50–68.

Dickerson, A.E. 1994. Considering culture in the assessment of elderly persons. *Gerontology Special Interest Section Newsletter* 17(3): 1–2.

Dickerson A.E., and A.G. Fisher. 1993. Age differences in functional performance. *American Journal of Occupational Therapy* 47(8): 686–692.

Doble, E.C., J.D. Fisk, A.G. Fisher, P.G. Ritvo, and T.J. Murray. 1994. Functional competence of community dwelling persons with multiple sclerosis using the Assessment of Motor and Process Skills (AMPS). *Archives of Physical Medicine and Rehabilitation* 75(8): 843–851.

Doble, S. 1991. Test-retest and interrater reliability of a process skills assessment. *Occupational Therapy Journal of Research* 11(1): 8–23.

Duran, L., and S. Park. 1994. An overview of the Assessment of Motor and Process Skills. *Physical Disabilities Special Interest Newsletter* 17(1): 3.

Duran, L.J., and A.G. Fisher. 1996. Male and female performance on the Assessment of Motor and Process Skills. *Archives of Physical Medicine and Rehabilitation* 77(10): 1019–1024.

Fisher, A.G. AMPS Project, Occupational Therapy Building, Colorado State University, Fort Collins, CO 80523.

Fisher, A.G. 1993. The assessment of IADL motor skills: An application of many-faceted Rasch analysis. *American Journal of Occupational Therapy* 47(4): 319–329.

Fisher, A.G. 1994. Functional assessment and occupation: Critical issues for occupational therapy. *New Zealand Journal of Occupational Therapy* 45(2): 13–19.

Fisher, A.G., Y. Liu, C.A. Velozo, and A.L. Pan. 1992. Cross-cultural assessment of process skills. *American Journal of Occupational Therapy* 46(10): 876–885.

Fisher, W.P., and A.G. Fisher. 1993. Applications of Rasch analysis to studies in occupational therapy. *Physical Medicine Rehabilitation Clinics of North America* 4: 551–569.

Goto, S., A.G. Fisher, and W.L. Mayberry. 1996. Assessment of Motor and Process Skills applied cross-culturally to the Japanese. *American Journal of Occupational Therapy* 50(10): 798–806.

Josephsson, S., L. Backman, L. Borell, L. Nygard, and B. Bernspang. 1995. Effectiveness of an intervention to improve occupational performance in dementia. *Occupational Therapy Journal of Research* 15(1): 36–49.

Kielhofner, G. 1995. *A model of human occupation: Theory and practice*, 2nd ed., 233–237, 289–291, 366. Baltimore, MD: Williams & Wilkins. Overview and sample.

Kottorp, A., B. Bernspang, A.G. Fisher, and K. Bryne. 1995. IADL ability measured with the AMPS: Relation to two classification systems of mental retardation. *Scandinavian Journal of Occupational Therapy* 2: 121–128.

Magalhaes, L.C., A.G. Fisher, B. Bernspang, and J.A. Linacre. 1996. Cross-cultural assessment of functional ability. *Occupational Therapy Journal of Research* 16(1): 45–63.

Nygard, L., B. Bernspang, A.G. Fisher, and B. Winblad. 1994. Comparing motor and process ability of persons with suspected dementia in home and clinical settings. *American Journal of Occupational Therapy* 48(8): 689–696.

Pan, A., and A.G. Fisher. 1994. The Assessment of Motor and Process Skills of persons with psychiatric disorders. *American Journal of Occupational Therapy* 48(9): 775–780.

Park, S., A.G. Fisher, and C.A. Velozo. 1994. Using the Assessment of Motor and Process Skills to compare occupational performance between clinic and home settings. *American Journal of Occupational Therapy* 48(8): 697–709.

Puderbaugh, J.K., and A.G. Fisher. 1992. Assessment Motor and Process Skills in normal young children and children with dyspraxia. *Occupational Therapy Journal of Research* 12(4): 195–216.

Robinson, S.E., and A.G. Fisher. 1996. A study to examine the relationship of the Assessment of Motor Processing Skills (AMPS) to other tests of cognition. *British Journal of Occupational Therapy* 59(6): 260–263.

Assessment of Motor and Processing Skills (AMPS), 2nd ed. See also School Assessment of Motor and Process Skills.

Backman, C. 1998. Functional assessment. In *Rheumatologic rehabilitation series: Assessment and management* vol. 1., eds. J. Melvin and G. Jensen, 168–169. Bethesda, MD: American Occupational Therapy Association.

Coulthard-Morris, L., J.S. Burks, and R.M. Herndon. 1998. Assessment of Motor and Process Skills. In *Handbook of neurologic rating scales*, ed. R.M. Herndon, 232, 235–239. New York: Demos Vermande.

Darragh, A.D., P.L. Sample, and A.G. Fisher. 1998. Environment effect of functional task performance in adults with acquired brain injury: Use of the Assessment of Motor and Process Skills. *Archives of Physical Medicine and Rehabilitation* 79(4): 418–423.

Dickerson, A.E., and A.G. Fisher. 1997. The effects of familiarity of task and choice on the functional assessment of young and old adults. *Psychology and Aging* 12: 247–254.

Doble, S.E., J.D. Fisk, N. Lewis, and K. Rockwood. 1999. Test-retest reliability of the Assessment of Motor and Process Skills in elderly adults. *Occupational Therapy Journal of Research* 19(3): 203–215.

Doble, S.E., J.D. Fisk, K.M. MacPherson, A.G. Fisher, and K. Rockwood. 1997. Measuring functional competence in older persons with Alzheimer's disease. *International Psychogeriatrics* 9(1): 25–38.

Duran, L., and A.G. Fisher. 1999. Evaluation and intervention with executive functions impairment. In *Cognitive and perceptual dysfunction: A clinical reasoning approach to evaluation and intervention*, ed. C. Unsworth, 209–255. Philadelphia: F.A. Davis.

Fisher, A.G. 1997. *Assessment of Motor and Process Skills*, 2nd ed. Fort Collins, CO: Three Star Press.

Fisher, A.G. 1997. Multifaceted measurement of daily life task performance: Conceptualizing a test of instrumental ADL and validating the addition of personal ADL tasks. *Physical Medicine and Rehabilitation: State of the Art Reviews* 11(2): 289–303.

Goldman, S.L., and A.G. Fisher. 1997. Cross-cultural validation of the Assessment of Motor and Process Skills (AMPS). *British Journal of Occupational Therapy* 60(2): 77–85.

Goldstein, K., and N. Robins. 1998. Home advantage. *Occupational Therapy Practice* 3(8): 41–42.

Hariz, G.M., A.G. Bergenheim, M.I. Hariz, and M. Lindberg. 1998. Assess of ability/disability in patients treatment with chronic thalamic stimulation for tremor. *Movement Disorders* 13(1):78–83.

Joe, B.E. 1998. OT raises profile at APA Institute. *Occupational Therapy Week* 12(8): 18–19.

Oakley, F., and T. Sunderland. 1997. Assessment of motor and process skills as a measure of IADL functioning in pharmacologic studies of people with Alzheimer's disease: A pilot study. *International Psychogeriatrics* 9(2): 197–206.

Park, S. 1998. Assessment of Motor and Process Skills. In *Stroke rehabilitation: A function-based approach*, eds. G. Gillen and A. Burkhardt, 362–367, 372–383. St. Louis: Mosby.

Robinson, S.E., and A. Lumb. 1997. Use of AMPS to evaluate older adults with mental health problems. *British Journal of Therapy and Rehabilitation* 4: 541–545.

Rogers, J.C., and M.C. Holm. 1998. Assessment of Motor and Process Skills (AMPS). In *Willard and Spackman's Occupational Therapy*, 9th ed., eds. M.E. Neistadt and E.B. Crepeau, 204–205. Philadelphia: J.B. Lippincott.

Stahl, J., R. Shumany, B. Bergstrom, and A.G. Fisher. 1997. On-line performance assessment using rating scales. *Journal of Outcome Measures* 1(3): 173–179.

Unsworth, C. 1999. Assessment of Motor and Process Skills (AMPS). In *Cognitive and perceptual dysfunction: A clinical reasoning approach to evaluation and intervention*, ed. C. Unsworth, 86–87, 89–90. Philadelphia: F.A. Davis.

Assessment of Occupational Functioning (AOF), 1st ed.

Brollier, C. et al. 1988. A content validity study of the Assessment of Occupational Functioning. *Occupational Therapy in Mental Health* 8(4): 29–47.

Brollier, C., and J.H. Watts. 1985. *Assessment of Occupational Functioning*. Unpublished manuscript, Virginia Commonwealth University.

Brollier, C., J.H. Watts, D.F. Bauer, and W. Schmidt. 1988. A concurrent validity study of two occupational therapy evaluation instruments: The AOF and OCAIRS. *Occupational Therapy in Mental Health* 8(4): 49–60.

Watts, J.H., C. Brollier, and W. Schmidt. 1988. Why use standardized patient evaluation? Commentary and suggestions. *Occupational Therapy in Mental Health* 8(4): 89–97. Includes case study.

Watts, J.H., C. Brollier, D.F. Bauer, and W. Schmidt. 1988. A comparison of two evaluation instruments used with psychiatric patients in occupational therapy. *Occupational Therapy in Mental Health* 8(4): 7–27. Sample form included.

Watts, J.H., G. Kielhofner, D.F. Bauer, M.D. Gregory, and D.B. Valentine. 1986. The Assessment of Occupational Functioning: A screening tool for use in long-term care. *American Journal of Occupational Therapy* 40(4): 231–240.

Assessment of Occupational Functioning (AOF), 2nd ed.

Henry, A.D. 1998. Assessment of Occupational Functioning. In *Willard and Spackman's occupational therapy*, 9th ed., ed. M.E. Neistadt and E.B. Crepeau, 163. Philadelphia: J.B. Lippincott.

Kielhofner, G. 1995. *A model of human occupation: Theory and application*, 2nd ed., 221, 233, 237–238. Baltimore, MD: Williams & Wilkins. Overview.

Viik, M.J., J.H. Watts, M.J. Madigan, and D.F. Bauer. 1990. Preliminary validation of the Assessment of Occupational Functioning with an alcoholic population. *Occupational Therapy in Mental Health* 10(2): 19–33.

Watts, J.H., and C. Brollier, ed. 1988. *Instrument development in occupational therapy*, 69–84. New York: Haworth Press. Form included.

Watts, J.H., C. Brollier, D.F. Bauer, and W. Schmidt. 1988. The Assessment of Occupational Functioning: The second revision. *Occupational Therapy in Mental Health* 8(4): 61–88 or the book form, *Instrument development in occupational therapy*, eds. Watts, J.H. and C. Brollier, New York: Haworth Press, 1988.

Watts, J.H., G. Kielhofner, D.F. Bauer, M.D. Gregory and D.B. Valentine. *Assessment of Occupational Functioning*, 2nd ed. Available from Model of Human Occupation Clearinghouse, Department of Occupational Therapy M/C 811, University of Illinois at Chicago, 1919 West Taylor Street, Chicago, IL 60612.

Assessment of Occupational Functioning—Collaborative Version

Watts, J.H., R. Hinson, M.J. Madigan, P.M. McGuigan, and S.M. Newman. 1999. The Assessment of Occupational Functioning—Collaborative Version 193–203. In *Assessments in occupational therapy mental health: An integrative approach*, ed. B.J. Hemphill-Pearson, 193–203. Thorofare, NJ: Slack.

Assessment of Sensorimotor Integration in Pre-School Children

DeGangi, G. 1979. *Assessment of Sensorimotor Integration in Pre-School Children*. Baltimore, MD: John Hopkins University.

DeGangi, G., R.A. Berk, and L.A. Larsen. 1980. The measurement of vestibular-based functions in pre-school children. *American Journal of Occupational Therapy* 34(7): 452–459.

Assessment of Social Interaction

Englund, B., B. Bernspang, and A.G. Fisher. 1995. Development of an instrument for assessment of social interaction skills in occupational therapy. *Scandinavian Journal of Occupational Therapy* 2(1): 17–23.

Asymmetrical Tonic Neck Reflex Rating Scale

Parmenter, C.L. 1983. An asymmetrical tonic neck reflex rating scale. *American Journal of Occupational Therapy* 37(7): 462–465.

Zemke, R. 1985. Application of an ATNR rating scale to normal preschool children. *American Journal of Occupational Therapy* 39(3): 178–180.

ATNR Rating Scale. See Asymmetrical Tonic Neck Reflex Rating Scale.

Australian ADL Index

Spencer, C., M. Clark, and D.S. Smith. 1986. A modification of the Northwick Park ADL Index (the Australian ADL Index). *British Journal of Occupational Therapy* 49(11): 350–353.

Autonomic Nervous System Inventory

Faber, S.D. 1982. Neurorehabilitation evaluation concepts. In *Neurorehabilitation: A multisensory approach*, 109. Philadelphia: Saunders.

Awareness Screen

Abreu, B. 1996. Awareness Screen. In *Occupational therapy: Enabling function and well-being*, 2nd ed., eds. C. Christiansen and C. Baum, 301. Thorofare, NJ: Slack.

Ayres Clinical Observations. See also Clinical Observations Checklist and Guide to Testing Clinical Observation in Kindergartners.

Poulson, A.A., and K.E. Peachey. 1983. Ayres' Clinical Observations: Performance of four- and five-year-old children. *American Journal of Occupational Therapy* 30(1): 15–22.

Ayres Scale of Adaptive Responses

Soper, G., and C.R. Thorley. 1996. Effectiveness of an occupational therapy programme based on sensory integration theory for adults with severe learning disabilities. *British Journal of Occupational Therapy* 59(10): 475–482.

Ayres Space Test

Ayres, A.J. 1962. *Ayres Space Test*. Beverly Hills, CA: Western Psychological Services.

Ayres Space Visualization Test

Zoltan, B. 1996. Visual discrimination skills. In *Vision, perception, and cognition: A manual for the evaluation and treatment of the neurologically impaired adult*, 3rd ed., 102. Thorofare, NJ: Slack.

Azima Battery

Azima, F.J. 1982. The Azima Battery: An overview. In *Evaluative process in psychiatric occupational therapy*, ed. B.J. Hemphill, 57–67, 339–341. Thorofare, NJ: Slack.

Azima, H. 1961. Dynamic occupational therapy. *Diseases of the Nervous System* 22(4): 138–142.

Azima, H., and F.J. Azima. 1959. Outline of a dynamic theory of occupational therapy. *American Journal of Occupational Therapy* 13(5): 215–221.

BH Battery

Hemphill, B.J. 1982. The BH Battery. In *Evaluation in psychiatric occupational therapy*, ed. B.J. Hemphill, 127–138, 355–360. Thorofare, NJ: Slack.

Hemphill, B.J. 1982. *Training manual for the BH Battery*. Thorofare, NJ: Slack.

Hemphill-Pearson, B.J. 1999. How to use the BH Battery. In *Assessments in occupational therapy mental health: An integrative approach*, ed. B.J. Hemphill-Pearson, 139–152. Thorofare, NJ: Slack.

Balcones Sensory Integration Screening, Revised Edition

Jones, C., and M.A. Monkhouse. 1981. *Balcones Sensory Integration Screening*, Rev. ed. Austin, TX: Texas Occupational Therapy Association.

Barth Time Configuration

Barth, T. 1985. *Barth Time Configuration*. New York: Health-Related Consulting Services. 130 West 28th Street, New York, NY 10001.

Barth, T. 1986. A new variation on an old theme: The Barth Time Construction. *Mental Health Special Interest Section Newsletter* 9(1): 4–5.

Barth, J. 1988. Barth Time Construction. In *Mental health assessment in occupational therapy: An integrative approach to the evaluation process*, ed. B.J. Hemphill, 115–129. Thorofare, NJ: Slack.

Basic Living Skills. See Comprehensive Evaluation of Basic Living Skills.

Bay Area Functional Performance Evaluation (BaFPE), 1st ed.

Bloomer, J.S., and S. Williams. 1982. The Bay Area Functional Performance Evaluation. In *The evaluative process in psychiatric occupational therapy*, ed. B.J. Hemphill, 255–308. Thorofare, NJ: Slack.

Bloomer, J.S., S. Williams, and D. Houston. 1980. The Bay Area Functional Performance Evaluation. *Occupational Therapy in Mental Health* 1(2): 41–42.

Brockett, M.M. 1987. Cultural variations in Bay Area Functional Performance Evaluation Scores: Considerations for occupational therapy. *Canadian Journal of Occupational Therapy* 54(4): 195–199.

Williams, S.L., and J. Bloomer. 1978. *Bay Area Functional Performance Evaluation*. Palo Alto, CA: Consulting Psychologists Press.

Bay Area Functional Performance Evaluation (BaFPE), 2nd ed.

Brown, C., K. Harwood, C. Hays, J. Heckman, and J.E. Short. 1993. Effectiveness of cognitive rehabilitation for improving attention in patients with schizophrenia. *Occupational Therapy Journal of Research* 13(2): 71–86.

Denton, P.L. 1987. *Psychiatric occupational therapy: A workbook of practical skills*, 80. Boston: Little, Brown.

Gilliam, A.R., and H.J. Martinson. 1994. Qualitative interpretations of the Bay Area Functional Performance Evaluation in traumatic brain injury. *Physical Disabilities Special Interest Section Newsletter* 17(1): 1–2.

Houston, D., J. Williams, S.L. Bloomer, and W.C. Mann. 1989. The Bay Area Functional Performance Evaluation: Development and standardization. *American Journal of Occupational Therapy* 43(3): 170–183.

Klyczek, J.P. 1999. The Bay Area Functional Performance Evaluation. In *Assessments in occupational therapy mental health: An integrative approach*, ed. B.J. Hemphill-Pearson, 87–107. Thorofare, NJ: Slack.

Klyczek, J.P., and W.C. Mann. 1990. Concurrent validity of a task-oriented component of the Bay Area Functional Performance Evaluation with the American Association on Mental Deficiency Adaptive Behavior Scale. *American Journal of Occupational Therapy* 44(10): 907–912.

Managh, M.F., and J.V. Cook. 1993. The use of standardized assessment in occupational therapy: The BaFPE-R as an example. *American Journal of Occupational Therapy* 47(10): 877–884.

Mann, W.C., and R. Huselid. 1993. An abbreviated task-oriented assessment (Bay Area Functional Performance Evaluation). *American Journal of Occupational Therapy* 47(2): 111–118.

Mann, W.C., and L.S. Russ. 1991. Measuring the functional performance of nursing home patients with the Bay Area Functional Performance Evaluation. *Physical and Occupational Therapy in Geriatrics* 9(3/4): 113–129.

Mann, W.C., J.P. Klyczek, and R.C. Fiedler. 1989. Bay Area Functional Performance Evaluation (BaFPE) standard scores. *Occupational Therapy in Mental Health* 9(3): 1–7.

Margolis, R.L., S.A. Harrison, H.J. Robinson, and G. Jayaram. 1996. Occupational Therapy Task Observation Scale (OTTOS): A rapid method for rating task group function of psychiatric patients. *American Journal of Occupational Therapy* 50(5): 380–385.

Roman, D.D. 1995. Bay Area Functional Performance Evaluation. In *Twelfth mental measurements yearbook*, eds. J.C. Conoley and J.C. Impara, 109–112. Lincoln, NE: Buros Institute of Mental Measurement.

Stanton, E., W.C. Mann, and J.P. Klyczek. 1991. Use of the Bay Area Functional Performance Evaluation with eating-disordered patients. *Occupational Therapy Journal of Research* 11(4): 227–237.

Thibeault, R., and E. Blackner. 1987. Validating a test of functional performance with psychiatric patients. *American Journal of Occupational Therapy* 41(8): 515–521.

Wener-Altman, P., A. Wolfe, and D. Staley. 1991. Utilization of the Bay Area Functional Performance Evaluation with an adolescent psychiatric population. *Canadian Journal of Occupational Therapy* 58(3): 129–136.

Williams, S.L., and J. Bloomer. 1987. *Bay Area Functional Performance Evaluation.* Palo Alto, CA: Consulting Psychologists Press. Also available from Maddak, Inc., 6 Industrial Road, Pequannock, NJ 07440-1993.

Beaded Peg Test

Kellor, M., J. Frost, N. Silberberg, I. Iverson, and R. Cummings. 1971. Hand strength and dexterity. *American Journal of Occupational Therapy* 25(2): 77–83.

Behavior Rating Scale. See MFS-Rehabilitation Rating Scale.

Behavioral Assessment of Oral Functions in Feeding

Ottenbacher, K., V. Grahn, M. Gevelinger, B.S. Dauck, and C. Hassett. 1985. Reliability of the behavioral assessment scale of oral functions in feeding. *American Journal of Occupational Therapy* 39(7): 436–440.

Stratton, M. 1981. Behavioral assessment scale of oral functions in feeding. *American Journal of Occupational Therapy* 35(11): 719–721.

Behavioral Checklist

Soper, G., and C.R. Thorley. 1996. Effectiveness of an occupational therapy programme based on sensory integration theory for adults with severe learning disabilities. *British Journal of Occupational Therapy* 59(10): 475–482.

Body Puzzle

Corbett, A., and S. Shah. 1996. Body scheme disorders following stroke and assessment of occupational therapy. *British Journal of Occupational Therapy* 59(7): 325–329.

Box and Block Test (BBT)

Boissy, P., D. Bourbonnais, M.M. Carlotti, D. Gravel, and B.A. Arsenault. 1999. Maximal grip force in chronic stroke stubjects and its relationship to global upper extremity function. *Clinical Rehabilitation* 13(4): 354–362.

Box and Block Test. Available from Ti-Schu, Inc. P.O. Box 2900, #222, San Antonio, TX 78229-0999; and Sammons Preston, P.O. Box 5071, Bolingbrook, IL 60440-5071.

Desrosiers, J., G. Bravo, R. Hebert, E. Dutil, and L. Mercier. 1994. Validation of the Box and Block Test as a measure of dexterity of elderly people: Reliability, validity, and norms studies. *Archives of Physical Medicine and Rehabilitation* 75(7): 751–755.

Desrosiers, J., R. Hebert, E. Dutil, G. Bravo, and L. Mercier. 1994. Validity of the TEMPA: A measurement instrument for upper extremity performance. *Occupational Therapy Journal of Research* 14(4): 267–281.

Felder, R., K. James, C. Crown, S. Lemon, and M. Reveal. 1994. Dexterity testing as a predictor of oral care ability. *Journal of the American Geriatric Society* 42(10): 1081–1086.

Goodkin, D.E. et al. 1998. Comparing the ability of various compositive outcomes to disciminate treatment effects in MS clinical trails. The Multiple Sclerosis Collaborative Research Group (MSCRG). *Multiple Sclerosis* 4(6): 480–486.

Goodkin, D.E., R.A. Rudick, S. VanderBrug Medendorp, M.M. Daughtry, K.M. Schwetz, J. Fischer, and C. Van Dyke. 1995. Low-dose (7.5 mg) oral methotrexate reduces the rate of progression in chronic progressive multiple sclerosis. *Annuals of Neurology* 37(1):30–40.

Goodkin, D.W., D. Hertsgaard, and J. Seminary. 1988. Upper extremity function in multiple sclerosis: Improving assessment sensitivity with box-and-block and nine-hole peg tests. *Archives of Physical Medicine and Rehabilitation* 69(10): 850–854.

Goodman, G., and S. Bazyk. 1991. The effects of a short thumb opponens splint on hand function in cerebral palsy: A single-subject study. *American Journal of Occupational Therapy* 45(8): 726–731.

Holser, P., and E. Fuchs. 1960. Box and Block Test. In *Primary prevocational evaluation: Occupational therapist's manual for basic skills assessment*, ed. F.S. Cromwell, 29–30. Pasadena, CA: Fair Oaks Printing.

Mathiowetz, V., S. Federman, and D. Wiemer. 1985. Box and Block Test of manual dexterity: Norms for 6–19-year-olds. *Canadian Journal Occupational Therapy* 52(5): 241–245.

Mathiowetz, V., G. Volland, N. Kashman, and K. Weber. 1985. Adult norms for the Box and Block Test of manual dexterity. *American Journal of Occupational Therapy* 39(6): 386–391.

Transon, C.S., C.K. Nitschke, J.J. McPherson, B.J. Spaudling, G.A. Kukamp, L.M. Anderson, and P. Heckt. 1989. Grip strength and dexterity in adults with developmental delays. *Occupational Therapy in Health Care* 6(2/3): 215–226.

Brain Injury Visual Assessment Battery for Adults (biVABA)

Warren, M. 1998. biVABA (Brain Injury Visual Assessment Battery for Adults). visAbilities. Rehab Services, Inc., 12008 West 87th Street, Suite 349, Lenexa, KS 66215, (888) 752-4364.

Brief Activities of Daily Living (BADL)

Tullis, A., and M. Nicol. 1999. A systematic review of the evidence for the value of functional assessment of older people with dementia. *British Journal of Occupational Therapy* 62(12): 554–563.

Turner, A., and G.M. Humphries. 1989. A Brief Activities of Daily Living (BADL) measure to assess dependency of psychogeriatric patients with change of location. *British Journal of Occupational Therapy* 52(9): 339–342.

Build a City

Clark, E.N. Build a city: A projective task concept. In *Assessments in occupational therapy mental health: An integrative approach*, ed. B.J. Hemphill-Pearson, 155–170. Thorofare, NJ: Slack.

Cambridge Apraxia Battery

Fraser, C.M., and A. Turton. 1986. The development of the Cambridge Apraxia Battery. *British Journal of Occupational Therapy* 49(8): 248–252.

Canadian Occupational Performance Measure (COPM), 1st ed.

Lan, M. et al. 1990. The Canadian Occupational Performance Measure: An outcome measure for occupational therapy. *Canadian Journal of Occupational Therapy* 57(2): 82–87.

Law, M., S. Baptiste, M. McColl, A. Opzoomer, H. Polatajko, and N. Pollock. 1987. Canadian Occupational Performance Measure. Canadian Association of Occupational Therapists, 110 Eglinton Avenue West, 3rd Floor, Toronto, Ontario M4R 1A3 Canada.

Pollock, N. 1993. Client-centered assessment. *American Journal of Occupational Therapy* 47(4): 298–301.

Canadian Occupational Performance Measure (COPM), 2nd ed.

Backman, C. 1998. Functional assessment. In *Rheumatologic rehabilitation series: Assessment and management* vol. 1., eds. J. Melvin and G. Jensen, 163–164, 172–175. Bethesda, MD: American Occupational Therapy Association. Case example.

Baptiste, S., and S. Rochon. 1999. Client-centered assessment: The Canadian Occupational Performance Measure. In *Assessments in occupational therapy mental health: An integrative approach*, ed. B.J. Hemphill-Pearson, 41–56. Thorofare, NJ: Slack.

Baptiste, S.E., M. Law, N. Pollock, H. Polatajko, M.A. McColl, and A. Carswell-Opzoomer. 1993. The Canadian Occupational Performance Measure. *WFOT Bulletin* 28(2): 47–51.

Bodiam, C. 1999. The use of the Canadian Occupational Performance Measure for the assessment of outcome on a neurorehabilitation unit. *British Journal of Occupational Therapy* 62(3): 123–126.

Chan, C.C.H., and T.M.C. Lee. 1997. Validity of the Canadian Occupational Performance Measure. *Occupational Therapy International* 4(3): 229–247.

Cresswell, M.K.M. 1998. Focus on research: A study to investigate the utility of the Canadian Occupational Performance Measure as an outcome measure in community mental health occupational therapy. *British Journal of Occupational Therapy* 61(5): 213. Abstract.

Henry, A.D. 1998. Canadian Occupational Performance Measure. In *Willard and Spackman's occupational therapy*, 9th ed., eds. M.E. Neistadt and E.B. Crepeau, 165. Philadelphia: J.B. Lippincott. Overview.

Law, M., S. Baptiste, A. Carswell, M.A. McColl, H. Polatajko, and N. Pollock. 1994. *Canadian Occupational Performance Measure* (COPM), 2nd ed. Canadian Association of Occupational Therapists, Carleton Technology and Training Centre, Suite 3400, 1125 Colonel By Drive, Ottawa, Ontario K1S 5R1, Canada. Also available from the American Occupational Therapy Association, 4720 Montgomery Lane, Bethesda, MD 20814-3425.

Law, M., H. Polatajko, N. Pollock, A. McColl, A. Carswell, and S. Baptiste. 1994. Pilot testing of the Canadian Occupational Performance Measure: Clinical and measurement issues. *Canadian Journal of Occupational Therapy* 61(4): 191–197.

Mew, M.M., and E. Fossey. 1996. Client-centred aspects of clinical reasoning during an initial assessment using the Canadian Occupational Performance Measure. *Australian Occupational Therapy Journal* 43(3/4): 155–166.

Neistadt, M. 1995. Assessing clients' priorities. *Occupational Therapy Practice* 1(1): 1, 37–39.

Neistadt, M. 1995. Methods of assessing clients' priorities: A survey of adult physical dysfunction settings. *American Journal of Occupational Therapy* 49(5): 428–436.

Packer, T.L., and X. Yun. Needs of people with disabilities used to determine clinical education. *International Journal of Rehabilitation Research* 30(3): 303–313.

Park, S. 1998. Canadian Occupational Performance Measure. In *Stroke rehabilitation: A function-based approach*, eds. G. Gillen and A. Burkhardt, 359–360. St. Louis: Mosby.

Pollock, N., M.A. McColl, and A. Carswell. 1999. The Canadian Occupational Performance Measure. In *Client-centred practice in occupational therapy: A guide to implementation*, ed. T. Sumsion, 103–114. Edinburgh, Scotland: Churchill-Livingstone.

Reid, D., P. Rigby, and S. Ryan. 1999. Functional impact of a rigid pelvic stabilizer on children with cerebral palsy who use wheelchairs: Users' and caregivers' perception. *Pediatric Rehabilitation* 3(3): 101–118.

Toomey, M., D. Nicholson, and A. Carswell. 1995. The clinical utility of the Canadian Occupational Performance Measure. *Canadian Journal of Occupational Therapy* 62(5): 242–249.

Trombly, C.A., M. Vining Radomski, and E. Schold Davis. 1998. Achievement of self-identified goals by adults with traumatic brain injury: Phase I. *American Journal of Occupational Therapy* 52(10): 810–818.

Waters, D. 1995. Clinical practice report: Recovering from a depressive episode using the Canadian Occupational Performance measure. *Canadian Journal of Occupational Therapy* 62(5): 278–282.

Yasuda, Y.L. 1996. Functional outcome measure: An application of the Canadian Occupational Performance Measure. *Physical Disabilities Special Interest Section Newsletter* 19(4): 3–4.

Checklist for Personal Care and Hygiene. See Comprehensive Evaluation of Basic Living Skills.

Checklist for Practical Evaluation. See Comprehensive Evaluation of Basic Living Skills.

Chessington Occupational Therapy Neurological Assessment Battery (COTNAB)

Kennedy, A.M., M. Grocott, M.S. Schwartz, H. Modarres, M. Scott, and F. Schon. 1998. Median nerve injury: An underrecognized complication of brachial artery cardiac catheterisation? *Journal of Neurology, Neurosurgery, and Psychiatry* 63(4): 532–546.

Laver, A.J., and S. Huchinson. 1994. The performance and experience of normal elderly people on the Chessington Occupational Therapy Neurological Assessment Battery (COTNAB). *British Journal of Occupational The*rapy 57(4): 137–142.

Stanley, M., J. Buttfield, S. Bowden, and C. Williams. 1995. Chessington Occupational Therapy Neurological Assessment Battery: Comparison of performance of people aged 50–60 years with people aged 66 years and over. *Australian Occupational Therapy Journal* 42(2): 55–65.

Tyerman, R., A. Tyerman, P. Howard, and C. Hadfield. 1986. *Chessington Occupational Therapy Neurological Assessment Battery (COTNAB)*. Nottingham, United Kingdom: Nottingham Rehab Limited. In United States, distributed by North Coast Medical, 187 Stauffer Boulevard, San Jose, CA 95125-1042.

Unsworth, C. 1999. Chessington Occupational Therapy Neurological Assessment Battery (COTNAB). In *Cognitive and perceptual dysfunction: A clinical reasoning approach to evaluation and intervention*, ed. C. Unsworth, 86–87, 93–94. Philadelphia: F.A. Davis.

Children's Handwriting Evaluation Scale (CHES)

Phelps, J., L. Stempel, and G. Speck. 1984. *Children's Handwriting Evaluation Scale*. 6831 St. Andrews, Dallas, TX 75205.

Children's Handwriting Evaluation Scale for Manuscript Writing (CHES-M)

Phelps, J., and L. Stempel. 1987. Children's Handwriting Evaluation Scale for Manuscript Writing. 6831 St. Andrews, Dallas, TX 75205.

Children's Self Assessment of Occupational Functioning

Curtin, C., and K. Baron. 1990. *A Manual for use with the Children's Self-Assessment of Occupational Functioning*. Chicago: University of Illinois. Available from Model of Human Occupation Clearinghouse. Department of Occupational Therapy, (M/C 811): University of Illinois at Chicago, 1919 West Taylor Street, Chicago, IL 60612–7250. (312) 996-6901, 1999.

Henry, A.D. 1998. Self-Assessment of Occupational Functioning. In *Willard and Spackman's occupational therapy*, 9th ed., eds. M.E. Neistadt and E.B. Crepeau, 166. Philadelphia: J.B. Lippincott. Overview.

Kielhofner, G. 1995. *A model of human occupation: Theory and application*, 2nd ed., 218–220, 233, 246–247, 366. Baltimore, MD: Williams & Wilkins. Overview and sample.

Client-Centred Community Occupational Performance Initial Interview (CCOPII), version 2

Orford, J.E. 1996. Community mental health: The development of the CCOPII, a Client-Centred, Occupational Performance Initial Interview. *British Journal of Occupational Therapy* 58(5): 190–196.

Clinical Examination of the Wrist

Skirven, T. 1996. Clinical examination of the wrist. *Journal of Hand Therapy* 9(2): 96–107.

Clinical Observation of Motor and Postural Skills (COMPS)

Wilson, B.N., N. Pollock, B.J. Kaplan, and M. Law. 1994. Clinical Observation of Motor and Postural Skills (COMPS). San Antonio, TX: Therapy Skills Builders/Psychological Corporation.

Clinical Observations Checklist

Soper, G., and C.R. Thorley. 1996. Effectiveness of an occupational therapy programme based on sensory integration theory for adults with severe learning disabilities. *British Journal of Occupational Therapy* 59(10): 475–482.

Cognitive Adaptive Skills Evaluation (CASE)

The Cognitive Adaptive Skills Evaluation. In *Assessments in occupational therapy mental health: An integrative approach*, ed. B.J. Hemphill-Pearson, 279–284. Thorofare, NJ: Slack, 1999.

Masagatani, G.N., C.S. Nielson, and E.R. Ranslow. 1979. Cognitive Adaptive Skills Evaluation. Eastern Kentucky University, Department of Occupational Therapy, Dizney 103, Richmond, KY 40475-3135.

Masagatani, G.N., C.S. Nielson, and E.R. Ranslow. 1980. The Cognitive Adaptive Skills Evaluation. *Occupational Therapy in Mental Health* 1(2): 43–44.

Cognitive Assessment of Minnesota

Rustad, R., T. DeGroot, M. Jungkunz, K. Freeberg, L. Borowick, and A. Wanttie. 1993. *Cognitive Assessment of Minnesota*. San Antonio, TX: Therapy Skills Builders/The Psychological Corporation.

Cognitive Performance Test

Allen, C, K., K. Kehrberg, and T. Burns. 1992. Evaluation instruments—Part III: Cognitive performance test. In *Occupational therapy treatment goals for the physically and cognitively disabled*, eds. C.K. Allen, C.A. Earhart, and T. Blue, 46–50, 69–84. Bethesda, MD: American Occupational Therapy Association.

Burns, T. 1990. The cognitive performance test: A new tool for assessing Alzheimer's disease. *Occupational Therapy Week* 4(51): 11,15.

Burns, T., J.A. Mortimer, and P. Merchak. 1994. Cognitive performance test: A new approach to functional assessment in Alzheimer's Disease. *Journal of Geriatric Psychiatric and Neurology* 7(1): 46–54.

Common Object Test

Smith, B.T., M.J. Mulcahey, and R.R. Betz. 1996. Quantitative comparison of grasp and release abilities with and without functional neuromuscular stimulation in adolescents with tetraplegia. *Paraplegia* 34:16–23.

Stroh, K., C. Van Doren, G. Thorpe, and C. Wijman. 1989. Common object test: A functional assessment for quadriplegic patients using an FNS hand system. *Proceedings of the RESNA 12th Annual Conference*, 387–388. Washington, DC: RESNA.

Community Dependency Index

Eakin, P.A., and H.E. Baird. 1995. The Community Dependency Index: A standardised measure of outcome for community occupational therapy. *British Journal of Occupational Therapy* 58(1): 17–22.

Ward, G., F. Macaulay, C. Jagger, and W. Harper. 1998. Standardised assessment: A comparison of the Community Dependency Index and the Barthel Index with an elderly hip fracture population. *British Journal of Occupational Therapy* 61(3): 121–126.

Comprehensive Assessment Process

Ehrenberg, F. 1982. Comprehensive Assessment Process. In *Evaluation process in psychiatric occupational therapy*, ed. B.J. Hemphill, 155–167, 367–378. Thorofare, NJ: Slack.

Comprehensive Evaluation of Basic Living Skills

Casanova, J.S., and J. Ferber. 1976. Comprehensive Evaluation of Basic Living Skills. *American Journal of Occupational Therapy* 30(2):101–105.

Comprehensive Occupational Therapy Evaluation (COTE)

Brayman, S.J. 1982. The Comprehensive Occupational Therapy Evaluation. In *Evaluative processes in psychiatric occupational therapy*, ed. B.J. Hemphill, 211–226, 381–388. Thorofare, NJ: Slack.

Brayman, S.J., and T. Kirby. 1976. Comprehensive Occupational Therapy Evaluation. *American Journal of Occupational Therapy* 30(2): 94–100.

Denton, P.L. 1987. *Psychiatric occupational therapy: A workbook of practical skills*, 80. Boston: Little, Brown.

Dutton, R. 1995. *Clinical reasoning in physical disabilities*. Complete form appears on page 212 (Part 1: General Behavior; Part II: Interpersonal) and page 233 (Part III: Task Behavior). Excerpts appear on pages 63, 145, and 193. Baltimore, MD: Williams & Wilkins.

Kunz, K.R., and S.J. Brayman. 1999. The Comprehensive Occupational Therapy Evaluation. In *Assessments in occupational therapy mental health: An integrative approach*, ed. B.J. Hemphill-Pearson, 259–274. Thorofare, NJ: Slack.

Contextual Memory Test

Contextual Memory Test. San Antonio, TX: Therapy Skills Builders/The Psychological Corporation, 1993.

So, Y.P., J. Toglia, and M.V. Donohue. 1997. A study of memory functioning in chronic schizophrenic patients. *Occupational Therapy in Mental Health* 13(2): 1–23.

Toglia, J. 1989. Approaches to cognitive assessment of the brain-injured adult: Traditional methods and dynamic investigation. *Occupational Therapy Practice* 1(1): 36–57.

Zoltan, B. 1996. Orientation, attention, and memory. In *Vision, perception, and cognition: A manual for the evaluation and treatment of the neurologically impaired adult*, 3rd ed., 137–138. Thorofare, NJ: Slack.

Creative Clay Test

Clark, E.N., and M.S. Cross. 1982.Creative Clay Test. In *Evaluative process in psychiatric occupational therapy*, ed. B.J. Hemphill, 309–317. Thorofare, NJ: Slack.

Daily Activities Checklist

Available from Catana Brown, Department of Occupational Therapy, School of Allied Health, University of Kansas Medical Center, 3033 Robinson, Kansas City, KS 66160-7802.

Brown, C. 1998. Comparing individuals with and without mental illness using the Daily Activities Checklist. *Occupational Therapy Journal of Research* 18(3): 84–98.

Brown, C., E. Hamera, and C. Long. 1996. The Daily Activities Checklist: A functional assessment for consumers with mental illness living in the community. *Occupational Therapy in Health Care* 10(3): 33–44. Form included.

Daily Living Activities Questionnaire

Oakley, F., T. Sunderland, J. Hill, S. Phillips, R. Makahon, and J. Ebner. 1991. The Daily Living Activities Questionnaire: A function assessment for people with Alzheimer's disease. *Physical and Occupational Therapy in Geriatrics* 10(2): 67–81.

Tullis, A., and M. Nicol. 1999. A systematic review of the evidence for the value of functional assessment of older people with dementia. *British Journal of Occupational Therapy* 62(12): 554–563.

Daily Living Activities Test for the Cerebral Palsied

Connell, K. 1950. An occupational therapist's approach to the vocational problems of the cerebral palsied. *American Journal of Occupational Therapy* 4(5): 214–238.

DeGangi-Berk Test of Sensory Integration

Berk, R.A., and G.A. DeGangi. 1987. *DeGangi-Berk Test of Sensory Integration*. Los Angeles: Western Psychological Services.

Bornstein, R.A. 1989. DeGangi-Berk Test of Sensory Integration. In *The tenth mental measurements yearbook*, ed. J.C. Conoley and J.J. Kramer, 228–229. Lincoln: University of Nebraska Press.

DeGangi, G.A. 1987. DeGangi-Berk Test of Sensory Integration. In *A therapist's guide to pediatric assessment*, eds. L. King-Thomas and B.J. Hacker, 156–163. Boston: Little, Brown.

DeGangi-Berk Test of Sensory Integration (TSI). In *Special educator's complete guide to 109 diagnostic tests*, eds. R. Pierangelo and G. Giuliani, 215. West Nyack, NY: Center for Applied Research in Education. Critique, 1988.

Deuel's Test of Manual Apraxia

Edwards, D.F., C.M. Baum, and R.K. Deuel. 1991. Constructional apraxia in Alzheimer's disease: Contributions to functional loss. *Physical and Occupational Therapy in Geriatrics* 9(3/4): 53–68.

Edwards, D.F. et al. 1991. A quantitative analysis of apraxia in senile dementia of the Alzheimer type: Stage-related differences in prevalence and type. *Dementia* 2(1): 142–149.

Edwards, D.F. et al. 1991. Contact: Dorothy F. Edwards, Washington University, 4567 Scott Avenue, St. Louis, MO 63105.

Developmental and Sensory Processing Questionnaire

Cermak, S.A., and L.A. Daunhauer. 1997. Sensory processing in the postinstitutionalized child. *American Journal of Occupational Therapy* 51(7): 500–507.

Developmental Programming for Infants and Young Children

Dunn, W. 1990. Establishing inter-rater reliability on a criterion-referenced developmental checklist. *Occupational Therapy Journal of Research* 10(6): 377–380.

Diagnostic Occupational Therapy Test Battery

Androes, L.R., E.A. Dreyfus, and M. Bloesch. 1965. *American Journal of Occupational Therapy* 19(2): 53–59.

Diagnostic Test Battery. See Diagnostic Occupational Therapy Test Battery.

Downey Hand Center Hand Sensitivity Test

Available from North Coast Medical, 18305 Sutter Boulevard, Morgan Hill, CA 35037-2845.

Barber, L.M. 1990. Desensitization of the traumatized hand. In *Rehabilitation of the hand*, 3rd ed., ed. J.M. Hunter, 721–730. St. Louis: Mosby.

Wayett-Rendall, J. 1995. Desensitization of the traumatized hand. In *Rehabilitation of the hand*, 4th ed., eds. J.M. Hunter, E.J. Mackin, and A.D. Callahan, 693–700, St. Louis: Mosby.

Yerxa, E.J., L.M. Barber, O. Diaz, W. Black, and S.P. Azen. 1983. Development of a hand sensitivity test for the hypersensitive hand. *American Journal of Occupational Therapy* 37(3): 176–181.

Dynamic Assessment of Categorization. See Toglia Category Assessment Test.

Dynamic Interactional Assessment

Toglia, J.P. 1994. Attention and memory. In *AOTA self-study series: Cognitive rehabilitation.* Bethesda, MD: American Occupational Therapy Association.

Toglia, J.P. 1992. A dynamic interaction approach to cognitive rehabilitation. In *Cognitive rehabilitation: Models for intervention in occupational therapy,* ed. N. Katz. Boston: Andover Medical Publications.

Toglia, J.P. 1989. Approaches to cognitive assessment of the brain-injured adult: Traditional methods and dynamic investigation. *Occupational Therapy Practice* 1(1): 36–57.

Zoltan, B. 1996. Orientation, attention, and memory. In *Vision, perception, and cognition: A manual for the evaluation and treatment of the neurologically impaired adult,* 3rd ed., 129–130. Thorofare, NJ: Slack.

Dynamic Visual Processing Assessment

Katz, N. 1996. Dynamic Visual Processing Assessment. In *Cognitive rehabilitation: Models for intervention in occupational therapy,* ed. N. Katz, 120–122. Boston: Andover Medical Publishers.

Toglia, J.P., and N. Finkelstein. 1991. *Test protocol. The Dynamic Visual Processing Assessment.* New York: New York Hospital Cornell Medical Center.

Dysphagia Evaluation Protocol

Avery-Smith, W., A.B. Rosen, and D.M. Dellarosa. 1996. *Dysphagia Evaluation Protocol.* San Antonio, TX: Therapy Skill Builders/The Psychological Corporation.

Early Coping Inventory

Zeitlin, S., and G.G. Williamson. 1996. In *New visions for the developmental assessment of infants and young children,* eds. S.J. Meisels and E. Fenichel. Washington, DC: Zero to Three: National Center for Infants, Toddlers, and Families.

Zeitlin, S., G.G. Williamson, and W.P. Rosenblatt. 1987. The coping-with-stress model: A counseling approach for families with a handicapped child. *Journal of Counseling and Development* 65, 443–446.

Zeitlin, S., G.G. Williamson, and M. Szczepanski. 1988. *Early Coping Inventory.* Vensenville, IL: Scholastic Testing Service.

Edinburgh Stroke Rehabilitation Study

Smith, M.E. 1979. The Edinburgh stroke rehabilitation study. *British Journal of Occupational Therapy* 42, 139–142.

Edmans ADL Index

Edmans, J.A., and J. Webster. 1997. The Edmans ADL Index: Validity and reliability. *Disability and Rehabilitation* 19(11): 465–476. Form included.

Employers' Perceptions of Occupational Therapy in Community Mental Health. See Semi-Structured Interview.

Environment Assessment Scale

Kannegiester, R.B. 1986. The development of the Environmental Assessment Scale. *Occupational Therapy in Mental Health* 6(3): 67–83.

Environment-Independence Interaction Scale

Teel, C., W. Dunn, S.T. Jackson, and P. Duncan. 1997. The role of the environment in fostering independence: Conceptual and mythological issues in developing an instrument. *Topics in Stroke Rehabilitation* 4(1): 28–40.

Environmental Questionnaire

Dunning, H.D. 1972. Environmental Questionnaire. *American Journal of Occupational Therapy* 26(6): 292–298.

Erhardt Developmental Prehension Assessment

Dunn, W. 1983. Critique of the Erhardt Developmental Prehension Assessment (EDPA). *Physical and Occupational Therapy in Pediatrics* 3(4): 59–68.

Erhardt, R.P. 1979. *Erhardt Developmental Prehension Assessment*. Fargo, ND: Author.

Erhardt, R.P. 1982. *Developmental hand dysfunction*. Laurel, MD: Ramsco.

Erhardt, R.P., P.A. Beatty, and D.M. Hertsgaard. 1981. A developmental prehension assessment for handicapped children. *American Journal of Occupational Therapy* 35(4):237–242.

Erhardt Developmental Prehension Assessment, Revised (EDPA-R)

Block, M.E., and L.K. Bunker. 1995. In *Twelfth mental measurements yearbook*, eds. J.C. Conoley and J.C. Impacta, 363–366. Lincoln, NE: Buros Institute of Mental Measurement. Review.

Erhardt, R.P. 1984. *Erhardt Developmental Prehension Assessment*. San Antonio, TX: Therapy Skills Builders/The Psychological Corporation.

Erhardt, R.P. 1986. *Developmental hand dysfunction*. San Antonio, TX: Therapy Skill Builders/The Psychological Association.

Pollock, N., M. Law, and L. Jones. 1991. The reliability and validity of a revised version of the Erhardt Developmental Prehension Assessment. *Canadian Journal of Occupational Therapy* 58(2): 77–84.

Scheer, C., S. Morris, J. Williams, and J.J. McPherson. 1994. Intrarater and interrater objectivity of the Erhardt Developmental Prehension Assessment among trained and untrained examiners. *Occupational Therapy Journal of Research* 14(1): 53–66.

Erhardt Developmental Vision Assessment (EDVA)

Erhardt, R.P. 1989. *Erhardt Developmental Vision Assessment* (EDVA). Laurel, MD: Ramsco.

Erhardt Developmental Vision Assessment, Revised (EDVA-R)

Erhardt, R.P. 1993. *Developmental visual dysfunction: Models for assessment and management*. San Antonio, TX: Therapy Skill Builders/The Psychological Association.

Erhardt, R.P. 1987. Sequential levels in the visual-motor development of a child with cerebral palsy. *American Journal of Occupational Therapy* 41(1): 43–49.

Erhardt Developmental Vision Assessment. San Antonio, TX: Therapy Skill Builders/The Psychological Association, 1993.

Erickson, D. 1995. *Twelfth mental measurements yearbook*, eds. J.C. Conoley and J.C. Impacta, 366–370. Lincoln, NE: Buros Institute of Mental Measurement. Review.

Evaluating Movement and Posture Disorganization

Magrun, M.W. 1996. *Evaluating movement and posture disorganization*. San Antonio, TX: Therapy Skill Builders. Video also available.

Evaluation of Home Environment

Kiernat, J.M. 1994. Evaluation of home environment. In *AOTA self-study series: Assessing function*, ed. C. Royeen, 8–9. Rockville, MD: American Occupational Therapy Association.

Evaluation of Oral Function in Feeding. See Behavioral Assessment of Oral Functions in Feeding.

Evaluation of Sensory Procession

LaCroix, J., C. Johnson, and L.D. Parham. 1997. The development of a new sensory history: The Evaluation of Sensory Procession. *Sensory Integration Special Interest Section Quarterly* 20(1): 3–4.

Evaluation Techniques for Older Groups

Kaplan, J. 1959. Evaluation techniques for older groups. *American Journal of Occupational Therapy* 8(5): 222–225, 245.

Evaluation Tool of Children's Handwriting (ETCH)

Amundson, S.J. 1995. *Evaluation tool of children's handwriting*. O.T. Kids, 53805 East End Road, Homer, AK 99603.

Diekema, S.M., J. Deitz, and S.J. Amundson. 1998. Test-retest reliability of the Evaluation Tool of Children's Handwriting-Manuscript. *American Journal of Occupational Therapy* 52(4): 248–255.

Schneck, C.M. 1998. Clinical interpretation of "Test-retest reliability of the Evaluation Tool of Children's Handwriting-Manuscript." *American Journal of Occupational Therapy* 52(4): 256–258.

Extended Activities of Daily Living Scale
(Also called the Nottingham Extended Activities of Daily Living Scale)

Chong, D.K. Measurement of instrumental activities of daily living in stroke. *Stroke* 26(6): 1119–1122.

Fairbrother, G., D. Burke, K. Kell, R. Schwartz, and W. Schuld. 1997. Development of the St. George Hospital Memory Disorders Clinic Occupational Therapy Assessment Scale. *International Psychogeriatrics* 9(2): 115–122.

Kelly, S., and E.G. Jessop. 1996. A comparison of measures of disability and health status in people with physical disabilities undergoing vocational rehabilitation. *Journal of Public Health Medicine* 18(2): 169–174.

Lincoln, N.B., and J.R.F. Gladman. 1992. The Extended Activities of Daily Living Scale: A further validation. *Disability and Rehabilitation* 14(1): 41–43.

Lincoln, N.B., J.R.F. Gladman, P. Berman, A. Luther, and K. Challen. 1998. Rehabilitation needs of community stroke patients. *Disability and Rehabilitation* 20(12): 457–463.

Logan, P.A., A. Ahern, J.R.F. Gladman, and N.B. Lincoln. 1997. A randomized controlled trail of enhanced Social Service occupational therapy for stroke patients. *Clinical Rehabilitation* 11(2): 107–113.

Nouri, F.M., and N.B. Lincoln. 1987. An extended activities of daily living scale for stroke patients. *Clinical Rehabilitation* 1(4): 301–305.

Rodgers, H., J. Soutter, W. Kaiser, P. Pearson, R. Dobson, C. Skilbeck, and J. Bond. 1997. Early supported hospital discharge following acute stroke: Pilot study results. *Clinical Rehabilitation* 11(4): 280–287.

Towle, D. 1988. Use of the Extended Activities of Daily Living Scale with depressed stroke patients. *International Disabilities Studies* 10(4): 148–149.

Turner-Stokes, L., and T. Turner-Stokes. 1997. The use of standardized outcome measures in rehabilitation centres in the UK. *Clinical Rehabilitation* 11(4): 306–313.

Family-Centered Interview

Marmer, L. 1995. Miller tool assesses family strengths and risks. *Advance for Occupational Therapists* 13:22, 58.

Miller, L.J. 1995. *The family-centered interview.* Littleton, CO: KID Foundation.

Feeding Interaction Report-Scale and Treatment (FIRST)

Sparling, J.W., and J.C. Rogers. 1985. Feeding assessment: Development of a biopsychosocial instrument. *Occupational Therapy Journal of Research* 5(1): 3–23.

Fidler Battery. See Fidler Diagnostic Battery.

Fidler Diagnostic Battery

Fidler, G.S., and J.W. Fidler. 1963. *Occupational therapy: A communicative process in psychiatry*, 104–107. New York: Macmillan.

Fieldwork Evaluation for the Occupational Therapist (FWE)

American Occupational Therapy Association. 1987. *Fieldwork evaluation for the occupational therapist.* Rockville, MD: Author.

American Occupational Therapy Association. 1994. *Guide to fieldwork education*, 3rd ed. Bethesda, MD: Author.

American Occupational Therapy Association, Commission on Education. 1988. *Guide to fieldwork education*, rev. ed. Rockville, MD: Author.

Austin, J.T. 1995. Fieldwork evaluation for the occupational therapist. In *Twelfth mental measurements yearbook*, eds. J.C. Conoley and J.C. Impacta, 71–75. Lincoln, NE: Buros Institute of Mental Measurement. Review.

Cooper, R.G. 1985. Nationally speaking—The revised fieldwork performance report: Implementation and implications. *American Journal of Occupational Therapy* 39: 77–78.

Cooper, R.G., and P.A. Crist. 1988. Field test analysis of the fieldwork evaluation for the occupational therapist. *Occupational Therapy Journal of Research* 8: 369–379.

Frum, D. 1988. Frequently asked questions about the new fieldwork evaluation (FWE) #2. *Occupational Therapy News* 42(2): 11.

Hickerson Crist, P.A., and R.G. Cooper. 1988. Nationally speaking—Evaluating clinical competence with the new fieldwork evaluation. *American Journal of Occupational Therapy* 42(12): 771–773.

Fieldwork Evaluation for Occupational Therapy Assistant Students

American Occupational Therapy Association. 1983. *Fieldwork evaluation for occupational therapy assistant students.* Rockville, MD: Author.

Fieldwork Performance Report (FWPR)

Crocker, L.M., J.E. Muthard, J.E. Slaymaker, and L. Samson. 1975. A performance rating scale for evaluating clinical competence of occupational therapy students. *American Journal of Occupational Therapy* 29(2): 81–86.

Slaymaker, J.E. 1978. Occupational therapy: Development of a rating scale. In *Evaluating clinical competence in the healthcare professions*, eds. M.K. Morgan and D.M. Irby, 189–197. St. Louis: Mosby.

Slaymaker, J.E., L.M. Crocker, and J.E. Muthard. 1974. *Field work performance report manual.* Rockville, MD: American Occupational Therapy Association.

Finger Posture Imitation Test

Druker, R.H. 1980. *Development of a posture imitation test for children ages nine through eighteen.* Unpublished master's thesis, University of Southern California, Los Angeles.

Fanchiang, S.P., C. Snyder, J. Zobel-Lachiusa, C.B. Loeffler, and M.E. Thompson. 1990. Sensory integrative processing in delinquent-prone and non-delinquent-prone adolescents. *American Journal of Occupational Therapy* 44(7): 630–639.

FirstSTEP: Screening Test for Evaluating Preschoolers

Miller, L.J. 1993. *FirstSTEP: Screening Test for Evaluating Preschoolers.* San Antonio, TX: Psychological Corporation.

Form A and Form B

Perkins, L.M. 1982. Assessment and management of pscyhogeriatric patients (acute admission) at High Royds Hospital. *British Journal of Occupational Therapy* 45(2): 11–13.

Form to Evaluate Work Behaviors

Ayres, A.J. 1954. A form used to evaluate the work behavior of patients. *American Journal of Occupational Therapy* 8(2): 73–74.

Functional Assessment for Juvenile Rheumatoid Arthritis

MacBain, P.K., and R.H. Hill. 1973. A functional assessment for juvenile rheumatoid arthritis. *American Journal of Occupational Therapy* 26(6): 326–330.

Functional Assessment of Repetitive Strain Injuries

Tsang Wai Ping, C.L., S. Chan Fuk Keung, and P. Lui Wan Yee. 1996. Functional assessment of repetitive strain injuries: Two case studies. *Journal of Hand Therapy* 9(4): 394–398.

Functional Assessment Scale (FAS)

Breines, E. 1983. *Functional Assessment Scale.* Test available from Geri-Rehab, Inc., Hibbler Road, Lebanon, NJ 08833.

Breines, E. 1988. The Functional Assessment Scale as an instrument for measuring changes in levels of function of nursing home residents following occupational therapy. *Canadian Journal of Occupational Therapy* 5(3): 135–140.

Functional Behavior Assessment for Children with Sensory Integrative Dysfunction

Cook, D.G. 1991. The assessment process. In *Pediatric occupational therapy: Facilitating effective service provision*, ed. W. Dunn, 45–49. Thorofare, NJ: Slack.

Functional Behavior Profile (FBP)

Baum, C., D.F. Edwards, and N. Morrow-Howell. 1993. Identification and measurement of productive behaviors in senile dementia of the Alzheimer type. *Gerontologist* 33(3): 403–408.

Baum, C., D.F. Edwards, and N. Morrow-Howell. 1993. Test available from Washington University, 4567 Scott Avenue, St. Louis, MO 64105.

Functional Capacities Evaluation. See also Physical Capacities Evaluation.

Smith, S.L., S. Cunningham, and R. Weinberg. 1983. Predicting reemployment of the physically disabled worker. *Occupational Therapy Journal of Research* 3(3): 178–179.

Smith, S.L., S. Cunningham, and R. Weinberg. 1986. The predictive validity of the Functional Capacities Evaluation. *American Journal of Occupational Therapy* 40(8): 564–567.

Functional Cognitive Index

Labi, M.L.C., M. Brentjens, K. Shaffer, C. Weiss, and M.A. Zielezny. 1998. Functional Cognitive Index: A new instrument to assess cognitive disability after traumatic brain injury. *Journal of Neurologic Rehabilitation* 12(2): 45–51.

Functional Needs Assessment Program for Chronic Psychiatric Patients

Dombrowski, L.B. 1990. *Functional Needs Assessment Program for Chronic Psychiatric Patients.* Tucson, AZ: Therapy Skills Builders, San Antonio, TX: The Psychological Corporation/Therapy Skill Builders.

Graham, J.R. 1995. In *Twelfth mental measurements yearbook*, eds. J.C. Conoley and J.C. Impacta, 395–398. Lincoln, NE: Buros Institute of Mental Measurement. Review.

Porter, J., G. Watson, and S. Capra. 1998. Food skills assessment tools for people with a mental illness. *Australian Occupational Therapy Journal* 45(1): 65–71. Review.

Functional Performance Measure

Carswell, A., C. Dulberg, L. Carson, and J. Zgola. 1995. The Functional Performance Measure for persons with Alzheimer's disease: Reliability and validity. *Canadian Journal of Occupational Therapy* 62(2): 62–69.

Tullis, A., and M. Nicol. 1999. A systematic review of the evidence for the value of functional assessment of older people with dementia. *British Journal of Occupational Therapy* 62(12): 554–563.

Functional Spatial Abilities Questionnaire

Liu, L., L. Gautheir, and S. Gauthier. 1996. The Functional Spatial Abilities Questionnaire for use with persons who are in the early stages of Alzheimer disease: Preliminary data on reliability and validity. *Canadian Journal of Occupational Therapy* 63(4): 224–233.

Functional Status Index for Juvenile Rheumatoid Arthritis. See Juvenile Arthritis Self-Report Index.

Functional Test for the Hemiparetic/Paretic Upper Extremity

Daniel, M.S., and L.R. Strickland. 1992. *Occupational therapy protocol management in adult physical dysfunction*, 22–26. Gaithersburg, MD: Aspen Publishers. Form included.

Wilson, D.J. 1984. Assessment of the Hemiparetic Upper Extremity: A functional test. *Occupational Therapy in Health Care* 1(2): 63–69.

Wilson, D.J., L.L. Baker, and J.A. Craddock. 1984. *Functional Test for the Hemiparetic/Paretic Upper Extremity*. Rancho Los Amigos Occupational Therapy Department, Rehabilitation Engineering Center, 7413 Golondrinas Street, Downey, CA 90242; or available from Los Amigos Research and Education Institute, P.O. Box 3500, Downey, CA 90242.

Wilson, D.J., L.L. Baker, and J.A. Craddock. 1984. Functional Test for the Hemiparetic Upper Extremity. *American Journal of Occupational Therapy* 38(3): 159–164.

Woodson, A.M. 1996. Stroke. In *Occupational therapy for physical dysfunction*, 4th ed., ed. C.A. Trombly, 686–687. Baltimore, MD: Williams & Wilkins. Form included.

Georgia Retardation Center Occupational Therapy Service Assessment Instruments

Georgia Retardation Center Occupational Therapy Service Assessment Instruments. In *Occupational therapy for children*, eds. P.N. Clark and A.S. Allen, 524–534. St. Louis: Mosby, 1985.

Goodman Battery

Goodman, M. 1964. Basic instruction for administering Goodman Battery. In *Regional Institute on the Evaluation Process*. Final Report No. RSA-123-T-68. New York: American Occupational Therapy Association.

Goodman, M. 1982. Goodman Battery. In *Evaluation in psychiatric occupational therapy*, ed. B.J. Hemphill, 85–125, 351–354.Thorofare, NJ: Slack.

Grasp and Release Test

Mulcahey, M.J., R.R. Betz, B.T. Smith, and A.A. Weiss. 1999. A prospective evaluation of upper extremity tendon transfers in children with cervical spinal cord injury. *Journal of Pediaric Orthopaedics* 19: 319–328.

Wuolle, K.S., C.L. Van Doren, G.B. Thorpe, M.W. Keith, and P.H. Peckham. 1994. Development of a quantitative hand grasp and release test for patients with tetraplegia using a hand neuroprothesis. *Journal of Hand Surgery* 19A: 209–218.

Gross Motor Management of Severely Multiply Impaired Students

Fraser, B.A., G. Galka, and R.N. Hensinger. 1987. *Gross motor management of severely multiply impaired students*. Baltimore, MD: University Park Press.

Group-Interaction Skills Survey. See also Occupational Therapist's Evaluation of Group Interaction Skills.

Mosey, A.C. 1973. *Activities therapy*, 92–93. New York: Raven Press.

Guide to Testing Clinical Observation in Kindergartners

Degangi, G.A. 1987. Guide to Testing Clinical Observation in Kindergartners. In *A therapist's guide to pediatric assessment*, eds. L. King-Thomas and B.J. Hacker, 168–174. Boston: Little, Brown.

Dunn, W. 1980. *Guide to Testing Clinical Observation in Kindergartners*. Rockville, MD: American Occupational Therapy Association.

Handwriting Speed Test

Wallen, M., and S. Mackay. 1999. Test-retest, interrater, and intrarater reliability, and construct validity of the Handwriting Speed Test in year 3 and year 6 students. *Physical and Occupational Therapy in Pediatrics* 19(1): 29–42.

Wallen, M., B. Bonney, and L. Lennox. 1996. *The Handwriting Speed Test*. Adelaide, Australia: Helios Art and Book Co.

Wallen, M., B. Bonney, and L. Lennox. 1997. Interrater reliability of the Handwriting Speed Test. *Occupational Therapy Journal of Research* 4: 280–287.

Hawaii Early Learning Profile (HELP)

Furuno, S., K.A. O'Reilly, C.M. Hosaka, T.T. Inatsuka, T.A. Allman, and B. Zeisloft. 1979. *Hawaii Early Learning Profile (HELP): Activity Guide*. VORT Corporation, P.O. Box 60880, Palo Alto, CA 94306.

Lang, W.S. 1992. HELP Checklist (Hawaii Early Learning Profile). In *Eleventh mental measurements yearbook*, eds. J.J. Kramer and J.C. Conoley, 373–375. Lincoln: University of Nebraska Press.

Parks, S., S. Furuno, K. O'Reilly, T. Inatsuka, C. Hosaka, and B. Zeisloft-Falbey. 1992. *HELP at Home.* Palo Alto, CA: VORT Corporation.

Helen Hayes Hospital Functional Shopping Skills Checklist

Golisz, K., and J. Venitelli. 1989. *Helen Hayes Hospital Functional Shopping Skills Checklist.* Haverstraw, NY: Helen Hays Hospital.
Toglia, J. 1989. Approaches to cognitive assessment of the brain-injured adult: Traditional methods and dynamic investigation. *Occupational Therapy Practice* 1(1): 36–57.

Hemiplegia Evaluation

Baum, B., M. Levine, M. Logigian, E. Siev, E.H. Silverman, J. Solet, and N. Wall. 1979. *Hemiplegia Evaluation.* Occupational Therapy Department, Massachusetts Rehabilitation Hospital, Boston. Available from Spaulding Rehabilitation Hospital, 125 Nashua Street, Boston, MA 02114.
Cady Fall, C. 1987. Comparing ways of measuring constructional praxis in the well elderly. *American Journal of Occupational Therapy* 41(8): 500–504.

Home Evaluation

Home Evaluation. In *Occupational therapy*, 4th ed., eds. H. Willard and C.S. Spackman, 248–249. Philadelphia: J.B. Lippincott, 1971.
Lefkovitz, R. 1989. Home Evaluation. In *Occupational therapy for physical dysfunction,* 3rd ed., ed. C.A. Trombly, 435–438. Baltimore, MD: Williams & Wilkins.

Home Evaluation Procedure

Fowles, B.H., M.A. Steward, and S.P. Mahan. 1960. Home evaluation procedure. *Physical Therapy Review* 40(10): 741–744.

Home Hazard Assessment Form. See Westmead Home Safety Assessment.

Home Life Survey

Available from Kavanagh, M. 1982. *Home Life Survey.* 106 Senea Rd., Richmond, VA 23226. No published studies.
Home Life Survey. 1989. In *An annotated index of occupational therapy evaluation tools*, ed. I.E. Asher, 23–25. Bethesda, MD: American Association of Occupational Therapy.

Household Activities Performance Test

Rush, H.A., E.L. Kristeller, J.S. Judson, G.M. Hunt, and M.E. Zimmerman. 1955. *A manual for training the disabled homemaker*, 13–15. New York: Institute of Rehabilitation Medicine, New York University Medical Center.
Zimmerman, M.E. 1963. Household Activities Performance Test: Occupational therapy in the ADL program. In *Occupational therapy*, 3rd ed., eds. H. Willard and C.S. Spackman, 349–352. Philadelphia: J.B. Lippincott.

Household Management Screening Assessment

Olin, D. 1985. Assessing and assisting the persons with dementia: An occupational behavior perspective. *Physical and Occupational Therapy in Geriatrics* 3(4): 25–32.

Housing Enabler

Iwarsson, S. 1999. The Housing Enabler: An objective tool for assessing accessibility. *British Journal of Occupational Therapy* 62(11): 491–497.

Iwarsson, S., and A. Isacsson. 1996. Development of a novel instrument for occupational therapy assessment of the physical environment in the home: A methodologic study on the Housing Enabler. *Occupational Therapy Journal of Research* 16(4): 227–244.

Idiosyncratic Activities Configuration

Cynkin, S. 1995. Idiosyncratic activities configuration. *The practice of the future: Putting occupation back into therapy activities*, ed. C.B. Royeen, 41–44. Rockville, MD: American Occupational Therapy Association.

Independent Living Skills Evaluation (ILSE)

Johnson, T.P., B. Johanson-Vinnicombe, and G.W. Merrill. 1980. The Independent Living Skills Evaluation. *Occupational Therapy in Mental Health*, 1(2): 5–18. Form included.

Johnson, T.P., B. Johanson-Vinnicombe, and G.W. Merrill. 1979. *Independent Living Skills Evaluation.* Toni Johnson, Independent Living Project, 291 North Tenth Street, San Jose, CA 95112, (409) 279-1975.

Marks, R. 1980. Validating the ILSE. *Occupational Therapy in Mental Health* 1(2): 19–20.

Trombly, C.A., M. Vining Radomski, and E. Schold Davis. 1998. Achievement of self-identified goals by adults with traumatic brain injury: Phase I. *American Journal of Occupational Therapy* 52(10): 810–818.

Infant/Toddler Symptom Checklist: A Screening Tool for Parents

Degangi, G.A., S. Poisson, S.Z. Sickel, and A.S. Wiener. 1995. *Infant/toddler symptom checklist: A screening tool for parents.* San Antonio, TX: Therapy Skill Builders/The Psychological Corporation.

Inpatient Rehabilitation—Scale of Therapeutic Occupation

Sass, P.L., and D.L. Nelson. 1998. Pilot study of the Inpatient Rehabilitation—Scale of Therapeutic Occupation. *Occupational Therapy International,* 5(1): 66–81. Form included.

Interdependent Activity Scale

Dawson, P.L. 1985. An interdependence activity scale designed for MPD patients. In *Dissociative disorders: Proceedings of the Second International Conference on Multiple Personal/Dissociative States*, ed. B.G. Braum, 66. Chicago: Rush University. Summary.

Dawson, P.L. 1993. Occupational therapy for inpatients and outpatients with multiple personality disorder. In *Expressive and functional therapies in the treatment of multiple personality disorder*, ed. L.W.S. Kluft, 249–250. Springfield, IL: Charles C. Thomas. Form included.

Integrated Motor Activities Scale

Heiniger, M.C., and C.W. Lewis. 1981. Integrated Motor Activities Scale. In *Neurophysiological concepts of human behavior: The tree of learning*, eds. M.C. Heiniger and S.L. Randolph, 284–322. St. Louis: Mosby.

Integrated Motor Activities Screening

Heiniger, M.C. 1990. *Integrated Motor Activities Screening.* Tucson, AZ: Therapy Skill Builders.

Interest Checklist. See also NPI Interest Checklist and Modified Interest Checklist.

Klyczek, J.P., N. Bauer-Yox, and R.C. Fiedler. 1997. The Interest Checklist: A factor analysis. *American Journal of Occupational Therapy* 51(10): 815–823.

Matsasuya. J. 1969. The Interest Checklist. *American Journal of Occupational Therapy* 23(4): 323–328. Form included.

Interview Form for Sheltered Employment, Rehabilitation, and Training Service

Oxley, C. 1992. Devising an assessment package for an employment rehabilitation services. *British Journal of Occupational Therapy* 55(12): 448–452.

Inventory of Occupational Choice Skills

Shannon, P.D. 1974. Occupational choice: Decision-making play. In *Play as exploratory learning: Studies of curiosity behavior*, ed. M. Reilly, 285–314. Beverly Hills, CA: Sage.

Irena Daily Activity Assessment

Dychawy-Rosner, I., and A. Isacsson. 1996. Interrater reliability and construct validity: An investigation of the IDA Assessment. *Scandinavian Journal of Occupational Therapy* 3(1): 3–13.

Jacobs Pre-Vocational Skills Assessment (JPVA), 1st ed.

Jacobs, K. 1985. *Occupational therapy: Work-related programs and assessment*, 17–91. Boston: Little, Brown.

Jacobs Pre-Vocational Skills Assessment (JPVA), 2nd ed.

Jacobs, K. 1991. *Occupational therapy: Work-related programs and assessment*, 61–136. Boston: Little, Brown.

Jamestown Occupational Therapy Assessment

Gangl, M.L. 1987. The effectiveness of an occupational therapy program for chemically dependent adolescents. *Occupational Therapy in Mental Health* 7(2): 67–88.

Joint Protection Knowledge Assessment

Hammon, A., and N. Lincoln. 1999. The Joint Protection Knowledge Assessment (JPKA): Reliability and validity. *British Journal of Occupational Therapy* 62(3): 117–122.

Juvenile Arthritis Functional Status Index (JAFSI)

Wright, F.V., J.L. Kimber, M. Law, C.H. Goldsmith, V. Crombie, and P. Dent. P. 1996. The Juvenile Arthritis Functional Status Index (JASI): A validation study. *Journal of Rheumatology* 23(6):1066–1079.

Juvenile Arthritis Self-Report Index (JASI)

Brown, G.T. 1996. A review of functional assessment measures for pediatric clients with juvenile rheumatoid arthritis. *Occupational Therapy International* 3(4): 284–299.

Wright, F.V., M. Law, V. Crombie, C.H. Goldsmith, and P. Dent. 1994. Development of a self-report functional status index for juvenile rheumatoid arthritis. *Journal of Rheumatology* 21(3): 536–544.

Wright, F.V., J. Longo-Kimber, M. Law, C.J. Goldsmith, and P. Dent. 1992. Validation of a functional status index for juvenile arthritis. *Physiotherapy Canada* 44: S6. Abstract.

Kenny Self-Care Evaluation, 1st ed.

Gresham, G.E., T.F. Phillips, and M.L.C. Labi. 1980. ADL status in stroke: Relative merits of three standard indexes. *Archives of Physical Medicine and Rehabilitation* 61(8): 355–358.

Iverson, I.A. 1973. Kenny Self-Care Evaluation. Kenny Rehabilitation Institute, 1800 Chicago Avenue, Minneapolis, MN 55404.

Labi, M.L., T.F. Phillips, and G.E. Gresham. 1980. Psychosocial disability in physically restored long-term stroke survivors. *Archives of Physical Medicine and Rehabilitation* 61(12): 561–565.

Schoening, H.A., and I.A. Iverson. 1968. Numerical scoring of self-care status: A study the Kenny Self-Care Evaluation. *Archves of Physical Medicine and Rehabilitation* 49(4): 221–229.

Schoening, H.A., L. Anderegg, D. Bergstrom, M. Fonda, N. Steinke, and P. Ulrich. 1965. Numerical scoring of self-care status of patients. *Archives of Physical Medicine and Rehabilitation* 46(10): 689–697.

Kenny Self-Care Evaluation, 2nd ed.

Available from Dr. Herbert A. Schoening, 4828 Pennsylvania Avenue South, Minneapolis, MN 55409.

Dittmar, S.S., and G.E. Gresham. 1997. Kenny Self-Care Evaluation. In *Functional assessment and outcome measures for the rehabilitation health professional*, eds. S.S. Dittmar and G.E. Gresham, 121–123. Gaithersburg, MD: Aspen Publishers.

Gresham, G.E., M.L. Labi, S.S. Dittmar, J.T. Hicks, S.Z. Joyce, and M.A. Stehlik. 1986. The Quadriplegia Index of Function (QIF): Sensitivity and reliability demonstrated in a study of thirty quadriplegia patients. *Paraplegia* 24(1): 38–44.

Wade, D.T. Kenny Self-Care Evaluation. 1992. *Measurement in neurological rehabilitation*, 188–189. New York: Oxford University Press.

KidCOTE

Kunz, K.R., and S.J. Brayman. The Comprehensive Occupational Therapy Evaluation. In *Assessments in occupational therapy mental health: An integrative approach*, ed. B.J. Hemphill-Pearson, 259–274. Thorofare, NJ: Slack.

Kingston Geriatric Cognitive Battery

Hopkins, R.W., P. Dixon-Medora, and L. Krefting. 1993. The Kingston Geriatric Cognitive Battery. *The Occupational Therapy Journal of Research*, 13(4): 241–252.

Kitchen Task Assessment (KTA)

Baum, C., and D. Edwards. 1993. Cognitive performance in senile dementia of the Alzheimer's type: The Kitchen Task Assessment. *American Journal of Occupational Therapy* 47(5): 431–436.

Porter, J., G. Watson, and S. Capra. 1998. Food skills assessment tools for people with a mental illness. *Australian Occupational Therapy Journal* 45(2): 65–71. Review.

Tullis, A., and M. Nicol. 1999. A systematic review of the evidence for the value of functional assessment of older people with dementia. *British Journal of Occupational Therapy* 62(12): 554–563.

Klein-Bell Activities of Daily Living Scale (K-B ADL Scale)

Bolding, D.M., and L.A. Llorens. 1991. The effects of habilitative hospital admission on self-care, self-esteem, and frequency of physical care. *American Journal of Occupational Therapy* 45(9): 796–800.

Chan, C.C.H., and T.M.C. Lee. 1997. Validity of the Canadian Occupational Performance Measure. *Occupational Therapy International* 4(3): 229–247.

Chen Sea, M.J., A. Henderson, and S.A. Cermak. 1993. Patterns of visual spatial inattention and their functional significance in stroke patients. *Archives of Physical Medicine and Rehabilitation* 74(4): 355–360.

Dittmar, S.S., and G.E. Gresham. 1997. Klein-Bell Activities of Daily Living Scale. In *Functional assessment and outcome measures for the rehabilitation health professional*, eds. S.S. Dittmar and G.E. Gresham, 124–134. Gaithersburg, MD: Aspen Publishers.

Elliott, S.J. 1997. Occupational therapy intervention for residents in skilled nursing: A focus on atypical patients. *Occupational Therapy in Health Care* 10(4): 53–74.

Klein, R.M., and B.J. Bell. 1982. Self-care skills: Behavioral measurements with the Klein-Bell ADL scale. *Archives of Physical Medicine and Rehabilitation* 63(7): 335–338.

Klein, R.M., and B.J. Bell. 1998. The Klein-Bell ADL Scale: An important assessment tool for occupational therapists working in gerontology. *Occupational Therapy Practice* 3(2): 37–39. Available from Health Sciences Center for Educational Resources, Distribution Coordinator, T-281 Health Sciences Building, Box 357161, University of Washington, Seattle, WA 98195, (206) 685-1186.

Kratz, G., I. Soderback, S. Guidetti, C. Hultling, T. Rykatkin, and M. Soderstrom. 1997. Wheelchair users' experience of non-adapted and adapted clothes during sailing, quad rugby, or wheel-walking. *Disability and Rehabilitation* 19(1): 26–34.

Larsson, E.L., S. Aaron, P. Ahlinder, and B. Oberg. 1998. Preoperative evaluation of activity and function in patients with paralytic scoliosis. *European Spine Journal* 7(4): 294–301.

Law, M. and P. Usher. 1988. Validation of the Klein-Bell Activities of Daily Living Scale for children. *Canadian Journal of Occupational Therapy* 55(2): 63–68.

Rockwood, K., B. Joyce, and P. Stolee. 1997. Use of goal attainment scaling in measuring clinically important change in cognitive rehabilitation patients. *Journal of Clinical Epidemiology* 50(5): 581–588.

Rogers, J.C., and M.C. Holm. 1998. Klein-Bell Activities of Daily Living Scale (Klein-Bell). In *Willard and Spackman's occupational therapy*, 9th ed., eds. M.E. Neistadt and E.B. Crepeau, 205–206. Philadelphia: J.B. Lippincott.

Shillam, L.L., C. Beeman, and P.M. Loshin. 1983. Effect of occupational therapy intervention on bathing independence of disabled persons. *American Journal of Occupational Therapy* 37(11): 744–748.

Smith, R.O., M.E. Morrow, J.K. Heitman, W.J. Rardin, J.L. Powelson, and T. Von. 1986. The effects of introducing the Klein-Bell ADL Scale in a rehabilitation service. *American Journal of Occupational Therapy* 40(6): 420–424.

Soderback, I., and A. Lassfolk. 1993. The use of four methods of assessing the benefits of electrically adjustable beds in relation to their costs. *International Journal of Technology Assessment in Health Care* 9(4): 573–580.

Spaulding, S.J., E. Strachota, J.J. McPherson, M. Kuphal, and M. Ramponi. 1989. Wrist muscle tone and self-care skill in persons with hemiparesis. *American Journal of Occupational Therapy* 43(1): 11–16.

Titus, M.N.D., N.G. Gall, E.J. Yerxa, T.A. Roberson, and W. Mack. 1991. Correlation of perceptual performance and activities of daily living in stroke patients. *American Journal of Occupational Therapy* 45(5): 410–418.

Unruh, A.M., S. Fairchild, and J. Versnel. 1993. Patients' and therapists' rating of self-care skills in children with spina bifida. *Canadian Journal of Occupational Therapy* 60(3): 145–158.

Knickerbocker Sensorimotor History Questionnaire (KSHQ)

Carasco, R.C. 1990. Reliability of the Knickerbocker Sensorimotor History Questionnaire. *Occupational Therapy Journal of Research* 10(5): 280–282.

Knickerbocker, B. 1983. *A holistic approach to the treatment of learning disorders*, 349–360. Thorofare, NJ: Slack.

Knox Preschool Play Scale. See also Play Scale and Preschool Play Scale.

Knox, S. 1996. Development and current use of the Knox Preschool Play Scale. In *Play: A clinical focus in occupational therapy for children*, eds. D. Parham and L. Fazio, 35–51. St. Louis, MO: Mosby Yearbooks.

Kohlman Evaluation of Living Skills (KELS), 2nd ed.

Kohlman-Thompson, L. 1979. *Interim manual*, 2nd ed. KELS Research, Box 33503, Seattle, WA 98133.

Radonsky, V.E., H. Jackson, S. Barton, K. Fedak, and M. Martin. 1986. Step ahead: Occupational therapy in the community. *Occupational Therapy in Mental Health* 6(2): 79–82.

Kohlman Evaluation of Living Skills (KELS), 3rd ed.

Kohlman-Thompson, L. 1992. *Kohlman Evaluation of Living Skills*. Bethesda, MD: American Occupational Therapy Association.

Rockwood, K., B. Joyce, and P. Stolee. 1997. Use of goal attainment scaling in measuring clinically important change in cognitive rehabilitation patients. *Journal of Clinical Epidemiology* 50(5): 581–588.

Rogers, J.C., and M.C. Holm. 1998. Kohlman Evaluation of Living Skills. In *Willard and Spackman's occupational therapy*, 9th ed., eds. M.E. Neistadt and E.B. Crepeau, 206. Philadelphia: J.B. Lippincott.

Thomson, L.K. 1999. The Kohlman Evaluation of Living Skills. In *Assessments in occupational therapy mental health: An integrative approach*, ed. B.J. Hemphill-Pearson. Thorofare, NJ: Slack.

Large Allen Cognitive Level Screen (LACLS)

Allen, C.K. 1996. *Large Allen Cognitive Level Test*. Sands, P.O. Box 513, Colchester, CT 06414-0513.

Allen, C.K., and T. Blue. 1998. Cognitive disabilities model: How to make clinical judgments. In *Cognition and occupation in rehabilitation: Cognitive models for intervention in occupational therapy*, ed. N. Katz, 225–279. Bethesda, MD: American Occupational Therapy Association.

Allen, C.K., K. Kehrberg, and T. Burns. 1992. Evaluation instruments—Part II: The Large ACL. In *Occupational therapy treatment goals for the physically and cognitively disabled*, eds. C.K. Allen, C.A. Earhart, and T. Blue, 40–45. Bethesda, MD: American Occupational Therapy Association.

Kehrberg, K.L., M.A. Kaskowski, J.A. Mortimer, and T.D. Shoberg. 1992. Validating the use of an enlarged, easier to see Allen Cognitive Level Test in geriatrics, *Physical Occupational Therapy in Geriatrics* 10(3): 1–14.

Roitman, D., and N. Katz. 1996. Predictive validity of the Large Allen Cognitive Levels Test (LACL) using the Allen Diagnostic Module (ADM) in an aged, non-disabled population. *Physical and Occupational Therapy in Geriatrics* 14(4): 43–57.

Leiter International Performance Scale—Revised

Miller L.J., and D.N. McIntosh. 1998. The diagnosis and treatment and etiology of sensory modulation disorder. *Sensory Integration Special Interest Section Quarterly* 21(1): 1–3.

Roid, G.H., and L.J. Miller. 1997. *Leiter International Performance Scale—Revised*. Wood Dale, IL: Stoelting.

Leng Rating Scale. See Rating Scale for Assessing Elderly Patients.

Level of Interest in Particular Activity

Pizzi, M., J. Mulkand, and M.M. Freed. 1991. HIV infection and occupational therapy. In *Rehabilitation for patients with HIV disease*, ed. J. Mulkand, 300–301. New York: McGraw-Hill. Form included.

Scaffa, M. 1981. Temporal adaptation and alcohol. Unpublished master's thesis, Virginia Commonwealth University, Richmond, Virginia. Available from Occupational Therapy Service, National Institutes of Health, Department of Rehabilitation Medicine, Clinical Center, Building 10, Room 6S235, 9000 Rockville Pike, Bethesda, MD 20892.

Life Strengths Interview

Pomeroy, V.M., M.C. Conroy, and P.G. Coleman. 1997. Setting handicap goals with elderly people: A pilot study of the Life Strengths Interview. *Clinical Rehabilitation* 11(2): 156–161.

Life Style Performance Profile

Fidler, G.S. 1982. Life Style Performance Profile. In *Evaluative process in psychiatric occupational therapy*, ed. B.J. Hemphill, 43–53, 329–331. Thorofare, NJ: Slack.

Fidler, G.S. 1996. Life-style performance: From profile to conceptual model. *American Journal of Occupational Therapy* 50(2): 139–147.

Robertson, S., ed. 1988. *A Focus: Skills for assessment and treatment*, 3:35–3:40. Rockville, MD: American Occupational Therapy Association.

Loewenstein Occupational Therapy Cognitive Assessment (LOTCA)

Annes, G., N. Katz, and S.A. Cermak. 1996. Comparison of younger and older health American adults on the Loewenstein Occupational Therapy Cognitive Assessment (LOTCA). *Occupational Therapy International* 3(3): 157–173.

Averbuch, S., and N. Katz. 1991. Age level standards of the Loewenstein Occupational Therapy Cognitive Assessment (LOTCA). *Israeli Journal of Occupational Therapy* 1: E1–E15.

Averbuch, S., and N. Katz. 1988. Assessment of perceptual cognitive performance: comparison of psychiatric and brain injured adult patients. *Occupational Therapy in Mental Health* 8(1): 57–51.

Cermak, S.A., N. Katz, E. McGuire, P. Greenbaum, C. Peralta, and V.M. Flannagan. 1995. Performance of Americans and Israelis with cerebrovascular accident on the Loewenstein Occupational Therapy Cognitive Assessment (LOTCA). *American Journal of Occupational Therapy* 49(6): 500–506.

Cognitive rehabilitation: A retraining model for clients following brain injuries. In *Cognition and occupation in rehabilitation: Cognitive models for intervention in occupational therapy*, ed. N. Katz, 99–123. Bethesda, MD: American Occupational Therapy Association, 1998.

Itzkovich, M., B. Elazar, S. Averbuch, and N. Katz, Loewenstein Rehabilitation Hospital, Israel. 1990. *Loewenstein Occupational Therapy Cognitive Assessment*. Los Angeles: Western Psychological Services, or Maddox, Inc., 6 Industrial Road, Pequannock, NJ 07440.

Katz, N., D. Champagne, and S.A. Cermak. 1997. Comparison of the performance of younger and older adults on three versions of a puzzle reproduction task. *American Journal of Occupational Therapy* 51(7): 562–568.

Katz, N., D. Hefner, and R. Reuben. 1990. Measuring clinical change in cognitive rehabilitation of patients with brain damage: Two cases—traumatic brain injury and cerebral vascular accident. *Occupational Therapy in Health Care* 7(10): 23–43.

Katz, N., M. Itzkovich, S. Averbuch, and G. Elazer. 1989. Loewenstein Occupational Therapy Cognitive Assessment (LOTCA) battery for brain-injured patients: Reliability and validity. *American Journal of Occupational Therapy* 43(3): 184–192.

Najenson, T., L. Rahmarni, B. Elazar, and S. Averbuch. 1984. An elementary cognitive assessment and treatment of the craniocerebrally injured client. In *Behavioral assessment and rehabilitation of the traumatically brain-damaged*, eds. B.A. Edelstein and E.T. Couture. New York: Plenum Press.

Unsworth, C. 1999. Loewenstein Occupational Therapy Cognitive Assessment (LOTCA). In *Cognitive and perceptual dysfunction: A clinical reasoning approach to evaluation and entervention*, ed. C. Unsworth, 86–87, 97. Philadelphia: F.A. Davis.

Uyanik, M., E. Aki, T. Duger, G. Bumin, and H. Kayihan. 1999. Cognition in 4- to 11-year-old children in Turkey. *Pediatric Rehabilitation* 3(3): 119–124.

Zoltan, B. 1996. Apraxia; Visual discrimination skills; Agnosia; Orientation, attention, and memory. In *Vision, perception, and cognition: A manual for the evaluation and treatment of the neurologically impaired adult*, 3rd ed., 57–58, 98, 110–111, 123–124. Thorofare, NJ: Slack.

Loewenstein Occupational Therapy Cognitive Assessment—Geriatric Version (LOTCA-G)

Averbuch, S., and N. Katz. 1998. Cognitive rehabilitation: A retraining model for clients following brain injuries. In *Cognition and occupation in rehabilitation: Cognitive models for intervention in occupational therapy*, ed. N. Katz, 99–123. Bethesda, MD: American Occupational Therapy Association.

Elazar, B., M. Itzkovich, and N. Katz. 1996. *LOTCA-G Manual*. Pequannock, NJ: Maddak.

Katz, N., B. Elazar, and M. Itzkovich. 1995. Construct validity of a geriatric version of the Loewenstein Occupational Therapy Cognitive Assessment (LOTCA) battery. *Physical and Occupational Therapy in Geriatrics* 13(1): 31–46.

Loma Linda University Medical Center (LLUMC) Activity Sort

Available from West Evaluation System Technology, Long Beach, CA: Loma Linda University.

Magazine Picture Collage

Buck, R., and M.A. Provancher. 1972. Magazine Picture Collages as an evaluative technique. *American Journal of Occupational Therapy* 26(1): 36–39.

Lerner, C. 1979. The Magazine Picture Collage: Its clinical use and validity as an assessment device. *American Journal of Occupational Therapy* 33(8): 500–504.

Lerner, C. 1992. The Magazine Picture Collage. In *Evaluative process in psychiatric occupational therapy*, ed. B.J. Hemphill, 139–154, 361–362. Thorofare, NJ: Slack.

Lerner, C., and G. Ross. 1977. The Magazine Picture Collage: Development of an objective scoring system. *American Journal of Occupational Therapy* 31(3): 156–161.

Sturgess, J. 1983. The Magazine Picture Collage: A suitable basis for pre-fieldwork teaching clinic. *Occupational Therapy in Mental Health* 3(1): 43–53.

Maguire Tri-level ADL Assessment

Maguire, G.H. 1985. Activities of daily living. In *Aging: The health care challenge*, ed. C. Lewis, 35–57. Philadelphia: F.A. Davis.

Maguire, G.H. 1990. Activities of daily living. In *Aging: The health care challenge*, 2nd ed., ed. C. Lewis, 47–68. Philadelphia: F.A. Davis.

Maguire, G.H. 1997. Activities of daily living. In *Aging: The health care challenge*, 3rd ed., ed. C. Lewis, 47–78. Philadelphia: F.A. Davis.

Matchstick Designs

Gregory, M.E., and J.A. Aitken. 1971. Assessment of parietal lobe function in hemiplegia. *Occupational Therapy* 34: 9–17.

Siev, E., and B. Freishtat. 1976. *Perceptual dysfunction in the adult stroke patient: A manual for evaluation and treatment*, 62–63. Thorofare, NJ: Charles B. Slack.

Mayers Lifestyle Questionnaire

Mayers, C.A. 1993. A model for community occupational therapy—stage 1. *British Journal of Occupational Therapy* 56(3): 169–172.

Mayers, C.A. 1995. Defining and assessing quality of life. *British Journal of Occupational Therapy* 58(4): 146–150.

Mayers, C.A. 1998. An evaluation of the use of the Mayers Lifestyle Questionnaire. *British Journal of Occupational Therapy* 61(9): 393–398.

Meaningfulness of Activity Scale

Gregory, M.D. 1983. Occupational behavior and life satisfaction among retirees. *American Journal of Occupational Therapy* 37(8): 548–553.
Weeder, T.C. 1986. Comparison of temporal patterns and meaningfulness of the daily activities of schizophrenic and normal adults. *Occupational Therapy in Mental Health* 6(4): 27–48.

Medical Rehabilitation Follow Along (MRFA)

Baker, J.G., C.V. Granger, and R.C. Fiedler. 1997. A brief outpatient functional assessment measure. *American Journal of Physical Medicine and Rehabilitation*, 76(1): 8–13.
Coulthard-Morris, L., J.S. Burks, and R.M. Herndon. 1998. Medical Rehabilitation Follow Along. In *Handbook of neurologic rating scales*, ed. R.M. Herndon, 260, 262. New York: Demos Vermande.

Melbourne Assessment of Unilateral Upper Limb Function

Johnson, L.M., M.J. Randal, D.S. Reddihough, L.E. Oke, T.A. Burt, and T.M. Bach. 1994. Development of a clinical assessment of quality of movement for unilateral upper-limb function. *Developmental Medicine and Child Neurology* 36(11): 965–973. Form included.

MFS-Rehabilitation Rating Scale

Wolff, R.J. 1961. A behavior rating scale. *American Journal of Occupational Therapy* 15(1): 13–16.

Miller Assessment for Preschoolers (MAP)

Aylward, G.P. 1994. Miller Assessment for Preschoolers. *Practitioner's guide to developmental and psychological testing*, 43–45, 50. New York: Plenum Medical Book. Review.
Banus, B. 1983. The Miller Assessment for Preschoolers (MAP): An introduction and review. *American Journal of Occupational Therapy* 37(5): 333–340.
Daniels, L.E. 1990. The Miller Assessment for Preschoolers: Analysis of score patterns for children with developmental delays. *Canadian Journal of Occupational Therapy* 57(4): 205–210.
Daniels, L.E., and S. Bressler. 1990. The Miller Assessment for Preschoolers: Clinical use with children with developmental delays. *American Journal of Occupational Therapy* 44(1): 48–53.
DeGangi, G.A. 1983. A critique of the standardization of the Miller Assessment for Preschoolers. *American Journal of Occupational Therapy* 37(6): 407–411.
Deloria, D.J. 1985. Miller Assessment for Preschoolers. In *Ninth mental measurements yearbook*, ed. J.V. Mitchell, 975–976. Lincoln: University of Nebraska Press.
Fulks, M.A., and S.R. Harris. 1995. Children exposed to drugs in utero: Their scores on the Miller Assessment for Preschoolers. *Canadian Journal of Occupational Therapy* 62(1): 7–15.
Humphry, R., and L. King-Thomas. 1993. A response and some facts about the Miller Assessment for Preschoolers. *Occupational Therapy Journal of Research* 13(1): 34–49.
Kirkpatrick, L.A., and P.G.W. Schouten. 1993. Authors reply to commentaries. *Occupational Therapy Journal of Research* 13(1): 50–61.
Lane, S.J., C. Attanasio, and R. Huselid. 1994. Prediction of preschool sensory and motor performance by 18-month neurologic scores among children born prematurely. *American Journal of Occupational Therapy* 48(5): 391–396.
Lemerand, P.A. 1988. Predictive validity of the Miller Assessment for Preschoolers (MAP). *Sensory Integration News* (Spring): 1–8. Available from Sensory Integration International, 1402 Cravens Avenue, Torrance, CA 90501.

Linder, T. 1983. Miller Assessment for Preschoolers. In *Test critiques*, vol. 1, eds. D.J. Keyser and R.C. Sweetland, 443–454. Austin TX: Pro-Ed.

McEwan, M.H., R.E. Dihoff, and G.M. Brosvic. 1991. Early infant crawling experience is reflected in later motor skill development. *Perceptual and Motor Skills* 72(1): 75–79.

Michael, W.B. 1985. Miller Assessment for Preschoolers. In *Ninth mental measurements yearbook*, ed. J.V. Mitchell, 976–978. Lincoln: University of Nebraska Press.

Miller Assessment for Preschoolers (MAP). 1998. In *Special educator's complete guide to 109 diagnostic tests*, eds. R. Pierangelo and G. Giuliani, 241. West Nyack, NY: Center for Applied Research in Education. Critique.

Miller, L.J. 1982. *Miller Assessment for Preschoolers*. Littleton, CO: Foundation for Knowledge in Development.

Miller, L.J. 1986. The predictive validity of the Miller Assessment for Preschoolers. University of Denver, Denver, CO. Dissertation available from Bell & Howell Information & Learning, 300 North Zeeb Road, Ann Arbor, MI 48106-1346; (800) 521-0600.

Miller, L.J. 1987. Longitudinal validity of the Miller Assessment for Preschoolers: Study I. *Perceptual and Motor Skills* 65(1): 211–217.

Miller, L.J. 1988. Differentiating children with school-related problems after four years using the Miller Assessment for Preschoolers. *Psychology in the Schools* 25(1): 10–15.

Miller, L.J. 1988. Longitudinal validity of the Miller Assessment for Preschoolers: Study II. *Perceptual and Motor Skills* 66(3): 811–814.

Miller, L.J. 1988. *Miller Assessment for Preschoolers*. San Antonio, TX: The Psychological Corporation.

Miller, L.J. 1993. Response to "Questions and concerns about the Miller Assessment for Preschoolers." *Occupational Therapy Journal of Research* 13(1): 29–33.

Miller, L.J. 1998. The Miller Assessment for Preschoolers: Construct validity and clinical use with children with developmental disabilities. *American Journal of Occupational Therapy* 52(10): 857–865.

Miller, L.J., and P.G.W. Schouten. 1988. Age-related effects on the predictive validity of the Miller Assessment for Preschoolers. *Journal of Psychoeducational Assessment* 6(2): 99–106.

Miller, L.J., and T.A. Sprong. 1986. Psychometric and qualitative comparison of four preschool screening instruments. *Journal of Learning Disabilities* 19(8): 480–484.

Miller, L.J., P.A. Lemerand, and S.H. Cohn. 1987. A summary of three predictive studies with the MAP. *Occupational Therapy Journal of Research* 7: 738–781.

Schneider, E., S. Parush, N. Katz, and J.J. Miller. 1995. Performance of Israeli versus U.S. preschool children on the Miller Assessment for Preschoolers. *American Journal of Occupational Therapy* 49(1): 19–23.

Schouten, P.G.W., and L.A. Kirkpatrick. 1993. Questions and concerns about the Miller Assessment for Preschoolers. *Occupational Therapy Journal of Research* 13(1): 7–28.

Stowers, S., and C.J. Huber. 1987. In *A therapist's guide to pediatric assessment*, eds. L. King-Thomas and B.J. Hacker, 69–77. Boston: Little, Brown.

Widerstrom, A.H., L.J. Miller, and R.J. Marzano. 1986. Sex and race differences in the identification of communicative disorders in preschool children as measured by the Miller Assessment for Preschoolers. *Journal of Communication Disorders* 19(8): 219–226.

Miller Infant and Toddler Test

Einarsson-Backes, L.M., and K.B. Stewart. 1992. Infant neuromotor assessments: A review and preview of selected instruments. *American Journal of Occupational Therapy* 46(3): 224–232.

Miller Screening for Preschoolers

Miller, L.J. 1989. Development of the Miller Screening for Preschoolers. *American Journal of Occupational Therapy* 43(9): 596–601.

Milwaukee Evaluation of Daily Living Skills (MEDLS)

Haertlein, C.L. 1999. The Milwaukee Evaluation of Daily Living Skills. In *Assessments in occupational therapy mental health: An integrative approach*, ed. B.J. Hemphill-Pearson, 245–257. Thorofare, NJ: Slack.

Jones, B.N., G. Jayaram, J. Samuels, and H. Robinson. 1998. Relating competency status to functional status at discharge in patients with chronic mental illness. *Journal of the American Academy of Psychiatry and Law* 26(2): 49–55.

Leonardelli, C.A. 1986. The process of developing a quantifiable evaluation of daily living skills in psychiatry. *Occupational Therapy in Mental Health* 6(4): 17–26.

Leonardelli, C.A. 1988. *Milwaukee Evaluation of Daily Living Skills (MEDLS)*. Thorofare, NJ: Slack. Also in B.J. Hemphill, ed. 1988. *Mental health assessment in occupational therapy: An integrative approach to the evaluative process*, 151–162, 256–259. Thorofare, NJ: Slack.

Margolis, R.L., S.A. Harrison, H.J. Robinson, and G. Jayaram, G. 1996. Occupational Therapy Task Observation Scale (OTTOS): A rapid method for rating task group function of psychiatric patients. *American Journal of Occupational Therapy* 50(5): 380–385.

Rockwood, K., B. Joyce, and P. Stolee. 1997. Use of goal attainment scaling in measuring clinically important change in cognitive rehabilitation patients. *Journal of Clinical Epidemiology* 50(5): 581–588.

Rogers, J.C., and M.C. Holm. 1998. Milwaukee Evaluation of Daily Living Skills (MEDLS). In *Willard and Spackman's occupational therapy*, 9th ed., eds. M.E. Neistadt and E.B. Crepeau, 206–207. Philadelphia: J.B. Lippincott.

Minimal Cerebral Dysfunction

Norton, Y. 1972. Minimal cerebral dysfunction. *American Journal of Occupational Therapy* 26(4): 186–199.

Minimal cerebral dysfunction. In *Occupational therapy for children*, 2nd ed., eds. P.N. Pratt and A.S. Allen, 192–197. St. Louis: Mosby, 1989.

Minnesota Follow-up Study Rehabilitation Rating Scale. See MFS-Rehabilitative Rating Scale.

Minnesota Handwriting Test (MHT). See also Interest Checklist and NPI Interest Checklist.

Reisman, J.E. 1990. Poor handwriting: Who is referred? *American Journal of Occupational Therapy* 45(9): 849–852.

Reisman, J.E. 1999. *Minnesota Handwriting Test*. San Antonio, TX: The Psychological Corporation.

Modified Interest Checklist

Ebb, E.W., W. Coster, and L. Duncombe. 1989. Comparison of normal and psychosocially dysfunctional male adolescents. *Occupational Therapy in Mental Health* 9(2): 53–74.

Furst, G., and C. Stabenow. 1995. Choosing and organizing life occupations. In *A model of human occupation: Application and theory,* 2nd ed., ed. G. Kielhofner, 335–336. Baltimore, MD: Williams & Wilkins. Overview and sample.

Kielhofner, G., and A. Neville. 1983. *The Modified Interest Checklist*. Unpublished manuscript. Coordinator, Model of Human Occupation, Department of Occupational Therapy, M/C 811. University of Illinois at Chicago, 1919 West Taylor Street, Chicago, IL 60612.

Modified Interest Checklist. Available from Occupational Therapy Department, Department of Rehabilitation Medicine, National Institutes of Health, Building 10, Room 6S235, Bethesda, MD 20892.

Scaffa, M.E. 1991. Alcoholism: An occupational behvior perspective. *Occupational Therapy in Mental Health* 11(2/3): 99–111.

Modified Need Satisfaction Schedule. See Need Satisfaction of Activity Interview.

Tickle, L.S., and E.J. Yerxa. 1981. Need satisfaction of older persons living in the community and in institutions—Part 1: The environment. *American Journal of Occupational Therapy* 35(10): 644–649.

Montreal Evaluation

Corriveau, H., F. Guarna, E. Dutil, E. Riley, A.B. Arsenault, and G. Brauin. 1988. An evaluation of hemiplegic subjects based on the Bobath approach—Part II: The evaluation protocol. *Scandinavian Journal of Rehabilitation Medicine* 20(1): 5–11.

Moss Kitchen Assessment

Moss Rehabilitation Hospital. 1980. Moss Kitchen Assessment. In *Sample forms for occupational therapy*, eds. C.A. Hays, J. Kassimir, and J. Parking, 82–83. Rockville, MD: American Occupational Therapy Association.

Porter, J., G. Watson, and S. Capra. 1998. Food skills assessment tools for people with a mental illness. *Australian Occupational Therapy Journal* 45(1): 65–71. Review.

Moss Kitchen Assessment—Revised

Harridge, C., and S. Shah. 1995. The Moss Kitchen Assessment Revised. *New Zealand Journal of Occupational Therapy* 64(2): 5–9.

Mother-Infant Play Rating Scale

Humphry, R., and M.H. Rourk. 1991. When an infant has a feeding problem. *Occupational Therapy Journal of Research* 11(2): 106–120.

Mothers Sensory Developmental Expectation Questionnaire

Parush, S., and F. Clark. 1988. The reliability and validity of a Sensory Developmental Expectation Questionnaire for mothers of newborns. *American Journal of Occupational Therapy* 42(1): 11–16.

Motor Development Chart. See Reflex Testing Methods for Evaluating CNS Development.

Motor Development Checklist

Doudlah, A. 1976. A motor development checklist. Central Wisconsin Center for the Developmentally Disabled, 317 Knutson Drive, Madison, WI 53704.

Gevelinger, M., K.J. Ottenbacker, and T. Tiffany. 1988. The reliability of the Motor Development Checklist. *American Journal of Occupational Therapy* 42(2): 81–86.

Motor Observations (MO) with Regards to Sensory Integration

Norwood, K.W. 1999. Reliability of the Motor Observations with Regards to Sensory Integration: A pilot study. *British Journal of Occupational Therapy* 62(2): 80–88.

Motor Performance Checklist (MPC)

Gwynne, K., B. Blick, and L. Hughes. 1996. Use of an occupational therapy Motor Performance Checklist by a school health service: A pilot study. *Journal of Paediatrics and Child Health* 32: 386–390.

Motor-Free Visual Perception Test—Adult Version. See also Motor-Free Visual Perception Test—Vertical.

Bouska, M.J. 1985. Application of the Motor-Free Visual Perception Test. *Physical Disabilities Special Interest Section* 8(1): 6–7.

Bouska, M.J., and E. Kwatney. 1983. *Manual for application of the Motor-Free Visual Perception Test to the Adult Population*, 6th ed. Philadelphia: Temple University, 1983. Unpublished.

Motor-Free Visual Perception Test—Vertical (MVPT-V)

Mercier, L., J. Hebert, R.P. Colarusso, and D.D. Hammill. 1997. Motor-Free Visual Perception Test—Vertical. Los Angeles: Western Psychological Services.

Movement Assessment of Infants

Ashton, B., M.C. Piper, S. Warren, L. Stewin, and P. Byrne. 1991. Influence of medical history on assessment of at-risk infants. *Developmental Medicine and Child Neurology* 33(5): 412–418.

Bayer, D.J., B. Bleichfeld, S.J. Lane, M.A. Volker, B. Alif, and B. Floss. 1996. The relationship between the Movement Assessment of Infants and the Fagan Test of Infant Intelligence in Infants with prenatal cocaine exposure. *Physical and Occupational Therapy in Pediatrics* 16(1/2): 145–153.

Brander, R., J. Kramer, M. Dancsak, M. Marotta, P. Stratford, and G. Chance. 1993. Inter-retest reliability of the Movement Assessment of Infants. *Pediatric Physical Therapy* 5(1): 9–15.

Campbell, S.K. 1982. Movement Assessment of Infants: An evaluation. *Physical and Occupational Therapy in Pediatrics* 1(4): 53–57.

Chandler, L.S., M.S. Andrews, and M.W. Swanson. 1980. Movement Assessment of Infants. P.O. Box 4631, Rolling Bay, WA 98061.

Darrah, J., M.C. Piper, P.J. Byrne, and S. Warren. 1991. The utilization of the Movement Assessment of Infants risk profile with preterm infants. *Physical and Occupational Therapy in Pediatrics* 11(2): 1–12.

Deitz, J.C., T.K. Crowe, and S.R. Harris. 1987. Relationship between infant neuromotor assessment and preschool motor measures. *Physical Therapy* 67(1): 14–17.

Fetters, L., and E.Z. Tronick. 1996. Neuromotor development of cocaine-exposed and control infants from birth through 15 months: Poor and poorer performance. *Pediatrics* 99(5): 938–943.

Haley, S.M., S.R. Harris, W.L. Tada, and M.W. Swanson. 1986. Item reliability of the Movement Assessment of Infants. *Physical and Occupational Therapy in Pediatrics* 6(1): 21–39.

Harris, S.R. 1987. Early detection of cerebral palsy: Sensitivity and specificity to two motor assessment tools. *Journal of Perinatology* 7(1): 11–15.

Harris, S.R. 1987. Early neuromotor predictors of cerebral palsy in low-birthweight infants. *Developmental Medicine and Child Neurology* 29(4): 508–519.

Harris, S.R. 1989. Early diagnosis of spastic diplegia, spastic hemiplegia, and quadriplegia. *American Journal of Diseases of Children* 143(11): 1356–1360. Comments appear in 1990, 144(9): 958–959.

Harris, S.R., and C.B. Heriza. 1987. Measuring infant movement: Clinical and technological assessment techniques. *Physical Therapy* 67(12): 1877–1880.

Harris, S.R., S.M. Haley, W.L. Tada, and M.W. Swanson. 1984. Reliability of observational measures of the Movement Assessment of Infants. *Physical Therapy* 64(4): 471–477.

Harris, S.R., M.W. Swanson, M.S. Andrews, C.J. Sells, N.M. Robinson, F.C. Bennett, and L.S. Chandler. 1984. Predictive validity of the Movement Assessment of Infants. *Journal of Developmental and Behavioral Pediatrics* 5(6): 337–342.

Lydic, J.S., M.A. Short, and D.L. Nelson. 1983. Comparison of two scales for assessing motor development in infants with Down's syndrome. *Occupational Therapy Journal of Research* 3(4): 213–221.

McGrew, L., P.A. Catlin, and J. Bridgford. The Landau reaction in full-term and preterm infants at four months of age. *Developmental Medicine and Child Neurology* 27(2): 161–169.

Piper, M.C., L.E. Pinnell, J. Darrah, P.J. Byrne, and J.M. Watt. 1992. Early developmental screening: Sensitivity and specificity of chronological and adjusted scores. *Journal of Development and Behavioral Pediatrics* 13(2): 95–101.

Schneider, J.W., and I.J. Chasnoff. 1992. Motor assessment of cocaine/polydrug exposed infants at age 4 months. *Neurotoxicolgy and Teratology* 14(2): 97–101.

Schneider, J.W., W. Lee, and I.J. Chasnoff. 1988. Field testing of the Movement Assessment of Infants. *Physical Therapy* 68(3): 321–327.

Swanson, M.W., F.C. Bennett, K.K. Shy, M.E. Whitfield. 1992. Identification of neurodevelopmental abnormality at four and eight months by the movement assessment of infants. *Developmental Medicine and Child Neurology* 34(4): 321–327. Comments appear in 1992, 34(12):1118–1119.

Umphred, D.A. 1995. *Neurological rehabilitation*, 3rd ed., 259–262. St. Louis: Mosby. Form only.

Musculoskeletal Assessment

Clarkson, H.M., and G.B. Gilewich. 1989. *Musculoskeletal assessment joint range of motion and manual muscle strength.* Baltimore, MD: Williams & Wilkins.

National Institutes of Health (NIH) Activity Record (ACTRE) (NIH Activity Record). See also Occupational Questionnaire.

Available from Furst, G, Department of Rehabilitation Medicine, National Institute of Health, Building 10, Room 6S-235, 10 Center Drive, MSC 1604, Bethesda, MD 20892-1604.

Gerber, L. 1992. Scoring methods and application of the Activity Record (ACTRE) for patients with musculoskeletal disorders. *Arthritis Care Research* 5(3): 151–156.

Gerber, L., and G. Furst. 1992. Validation of the NIH Activity Record: A quantitative measure of life activities. *Arthritis Care Research* 5(2): 81–86.

Kielhofner, G. 1995. *A model of human occupation: Theory and application*, 2nd ed., 217–218, 233, 240–241. Baltimore, MD: Williams & Wilkins. Overview.

Pizzi, M., J. Mulkand, and M.M. Freed. 1993. HIV infection and occupational therapy. In *Rehabilitation of patients with HIV disease*, ed. J. Mulkand, 198–199. New York: McGraw-Hill. Form and instructions.

Pollock, N., S. Baptiste, M. Law, M.A. McColl, A. Opzoomer, and H. Polatajko. 1990. Occupational performance measures: A review based on the guidelines for the client-centered practice of occupational therapy. *Canadian Journal of Occupational Therapy* 57(2): 77–81.

Need Satisfaction of Activity Interview (NSAI). See also Modified Need Satisfaction Schedule.

Tickle, L.S., and E.J. Yerxa. 1981. Need satisfaction of older persons living in the community and in institutions—Part 2: Role of activity. *American Journal of Occupational Therapy* 35(10): 650–655.

Nine-Hole Peg Test

Available from North Coast Medical, 18305 Sutter Boulevard, Morgan Hill, CA. 95037; S&S, 75 Mill Street, Colchester, CT 06415; Smith and Nephew, One Quality Drive, Germantown, WI; and Sammons Preston, 4 Sammons Court, Bolingbrook, IL 60440. Note: Each source has produced a different version of the board for this test.

Backman, C., S. Cork, and J. Parsons. 1992. Assessment of hand function: The relationship between pegboard dexterity and applied dexterity. *Canadian Journal of Occupational Therapy* 59(4): 208–213.

Backman, C., H. Mackie, and J. Harris. 1991. Arthritis Hand Function Test: Development of a standardized assessment tool. *Occupational Therapy Journal of Research* 11(4): 245–256.

Bamberger, H.B., P.J. Stern, T.R. Kielhaber, J.J. McDonough, and R.M. Cantor. 1992. Trapeziometacarpal joint arthrodesis: A functional evaluation. *Journal of Hand Surgery* 17A(4): 605–611.

Davis, J., J. Kayser, P. Matline, S. Mower, and P. Tadano. 1999. Nine-hole peg tests: Are they all the same? *Occupational Therapy Practice* 4(4): 59–61.

Erwin, J.H., C. Keller, S. Anderson, and J. Costa. 1991. Hand and wrist strengthening exercises during rehabilitation of a patient with hereditary distal myopathy. *Archives of Physical Medicine and Rehabilitation* 72(9): 701–702.

Felder, R., K. James, C. Brown, D. Lemon, and M. Reveal. 1994. Dexterity testing as a predictor of oral care ability. *Journal of the American Geriatrics Society* 42(10): 1081–1086.

Goodkin, D.E., D. Hertsgaard, and J. Seminary. 1988. Upper extremity function in multiple sclerosis: Improving assessment sensitivity with box-and-block and nine-hole peg tests. *Archives of Physical Medicine and Rehabilitation* 69(10): 850–854.

Goodkin, D.E., R.L. Pierce, and K.E. Wende. 1998. Comparing the ability of various composite outcomes to discriminate treatment effects in MS clinical trials. The Multiple Sclerosis Collaborative Research Group (MSCRG). *Multiple Sclerosis* 4(6):480–486.

Goodkin, D.E., R.A. Rudick, S. Medendorp, M.M. Daughtry, K.M. Schweta, J. Fischer, and C. Van Dyke. 1995. Low-dose (7.5 mg) oral methotrexate reduces the rate of progression in chronic progressive multiple sclerosis. *Annual of Neurology* 37(1): 30–40.

Heald, A., D. Bates, N.E. Carlidge, J.M. French, and S. Miller. 1993. Longitudinal study of central motor conduction time following stroke: Central motor conduction measured within 72 hours after stroke as a predictor of functional outcome at 12 months. *Brain* 116(6): 1371–1385.

Heller, A., D.T. Wade, V.A. Wood, A. Sunderland, R.L. Hewer, and E. Ward. 1987. Arm function after stroke: Measurement and recovery over the first three months. *Journal of Neurology, Neurosurgery and Psychiatry* 50(6): 714–719.

Holmqvist, L.W., L. vonKoch, V. Kostulas, M. Holm, G. Widsell, H. Tegler, K. Johansson, J. Almazan, and J. de Pedro-Cuesta. 1998. A randomized controlled trial of rehabilitation at home after stroke in southwest Stockhom. *Stroke* 29(3): 591–597.

Kellor, M., J. Frost, N. Silberberg, I. Iversen, and R. Cummings. 1971. Hand strength and dexterity: Norms for clinical use. *American Journal of Occupational Therapy* 25(1): 77–83.

Marque, P., A. Felez, M. Peul, J.F. Demonent, B. Guiraud-Chaumeil, C.F. Rogues, and F. Chollet. 1997. Impairment and recovery of left motor function in patients with right hemiplegia. *Journal of Neurology and Neurosurgery, and Psychiatry* 62(1): 77–81.

Mathiowetz, V., K. Weber, N. Kashman, and G. Volland. 1985. Adult norms for the nine-hole peg test of finger dexterity. *Occupational Therapy Journal of Research* 5(1): 25–38.

Meredith, J.M. 1994. Comparison of three myoelectrically controlled prehensors and the voluntary-opening split hook. *American Journal of Occupational Therapy* 48(10): 932–937.

Parker, V.M., D.T. Wade, and R.L. Hewer. 1986. Loss of arm function after stroke: Measurement, frequency, and recovery. *International Rehabilitation Medicine* 8: 69–73.

Rudick, R.A., S.V. Medendorp, M. Namey, S. Boyle, and J. Fischer. 1995. Multiple sclerosis progression in a natural history study: Predictive value of cerebrospinal fluid free kappa light chains. *Multiple Sclerosis* 1(3): 150–155.

Sunderland, A., D. Tinson, L. Bradley, and R.L. Hewer. 1989. Arm function after stroke. An evaluation of grip strength as a measure of recovery and a prognostic indicator. *Journal of Neurology, Neurosurgery and Psychiatry* 52: 1267–1272.

Transon, C.S., C.K. Nitschke, J.J. McPherson, S.J. Spaulding, G.A. Rukamp, L.M. Anderson, and P. Hecht. 1989. Grip strength and dexterity in adults with developmental delays. *Occupational Therapy in Health Care* 6(2/3): 215–226.

Turner-Stokes, L., and T. Turner-Stokes. 1997. The use of standardized outcome measures in rehabilitation centres in the UK. *Clinical Rehabilitation* 11(4): 306–313.

Wade, D.T. 1989. Measuring arm impairment and disability after stroke. *International Disability Studies* 11(2): 89–92.

Wade, O.T. 1992. Nine-hole peg test. In *Measurement in neurological rehabilitation*, 171. Oxford, UK: Oxford Medical Publications.

Yelnik, A., I. Bonan, M. Debray, E. Lo, F. Gelbert, and B. Bussel. 1986. Changes in the execution of a complex manual task after ipsilateral iscemic cerbral hemispheric stroke. *Archives of Phsyical Medicine and Rehabilitation* 77(8): 806–810.

Northwick Park ADL Index

Benjamin, J. 1976. The Northwick Park ADL Index. *British Journal of Occupational Therapy* 39(12): 301–306.

Brockhurst, J., and D. Mclean. 1980. The Undergraduate. Development of an objective activities of daily living assessment scale. *Australian Occupational Therapy Journal* 27(1): 30–34.

Northwick Park ADL Index—Modified. See Australian ADL Index.

Nottingham Extended Activities of Daily Living Scale. See Extended Activities of Daily Living Scale.

Nottingham Leisure Questionnaire

Drummond, A.E.R., and M.F. Walker. 1994. The Nottingham Leisure Questionnaire for stroke patients. *British Journal of Occupational Therapy* 57(11): 414–418.

Nottingham 10-point ADL Scale

Ebrahim, D., F.M. Nouri, and D. Barer. 1985. Measuring disability after a stroke. *Journal of Epidemiology and Community Health* 39: 86–89.

NPI Interest Checklist. See also Interest Checklist by Matsasuya and Modified Interest Checklist by Kielhofner.

Rogers, J.C. 1988. NPI Interest Checklist. In *Mental health assessment in occupational therapy: An integrative approach to the evaluative process*, ed. B.J. Hemphill, 95–114, 254–255. Thorofare, NJ: Slack. Overview and form.

Rogers, J.C., J.M. Weinstein, and J.J. Figone. 1978. The interest checklist: An empirical assessment. *American Journal of Occupational Therapy* 32(10): 628–630.

Object Manipulation Speed Test

King, L.J. 1978. *The Object Manipulation Speed Test*. Phoenix, AZ: Greenroom Publications.

Occupational and Leisure Assessment for Adults with Epilepsy

Day, S. 1984. Occupational therapy assessment and treatment in a hospital setting for patients with epilepsy. *Occupational Therapy in Health Care* 1(2): 53–62.

Occupational Behavior and Life Satisfaction Among Retirees

Gregory, M.D. 1993. Occupational behavior and life satisfaction among retirees. *American Journal of Occupational Therapy* 35(8): 548–553.

Occupational Case Analysis and Interview Rating Scale (OCAIRS)

Brollier, C., J.H. Watts, D. Bauer, and W. Schmidt. 1988. A concurrent validity study of two occupational therapy evaluation instruments: The AOF and OCAIRS. *Occupational Therapy in Mental Health* 8(4): 49–60.

Cubie, S.H., and K. Kaplan. 1982. A case analysis method for the model of human occupation. *American Journal of Occupational Therapy* 36(10): 645–656.

Denton, P.L. 1987. *Psychiatric occupational therapy: A workbook of practical skills*, 73. Boston: Little, Brown.

Haglund, L., and C. Henriksson. 1994. Testing a Swedish version of OCAIRS on two different patients groups. *Scandinavian Journal of Caring Sciences* 8: 223–230.

Haglund, L., L.H. Thorell, and J. Walinder. 1998. Assessment of occupational functioning for screening of patients to occupational therapy in general psychiatric care. *Occupational Therapy Journal of Research* 18(4): 193–206.

Henriksson, C., and L. Haglund. 1993. *Occupational Case Analysis Interview and Rating Scale*: OCAIRS-S, Version 2. (In Swedish). Halsouniversitetet: Linkopings Universitet.

Henry, A.D. 1998. Occupational Case Analysis and Interview Rating Scale. In *Willard and Spackman's occupational therapy*, 9th ed., eds. M.E. Neistadt and E.B. Crepeau, 163. Philadelphia: J.B. Lippincott.

Kaplan, K. 1983. *Objectifying clinical judgement: Content validity and interrater reliability of the Occupational Case Analysis Interview and Rating Scale*. Unpublished master's thesis. Richmond, VA: Virginia Commonwealth University.

Kaplan, K. 1984. Short-term assessment: The need and a response. *Occupational Therapy in Mental Health* 4(3): 29–43.

Kaplan, K.L., and G. Kielhofner. 1985. *Preliminary manual for the Occupational Case Analysis Interview and Rating Scale*. Arlington, VA: Authors.

Kaplan, K., and G. Kielhofner, eds. 1989. *Occupational case analysis and interview rating scale*. Thorofare, NJ: Slack.

Kielhofner, G. 1995. *A model of human occupation*, 2nd ed., 220–221, 233, 241–242, 366. Baltimore, MD: Williams & Wilkins. Summary.

Watts, J.H., C. Brollier, D. Bauer, and W. Schmidt. 1988. A comparison of two evaluation instruments used with psychiatric patients in occupational therapy. *Occupational Therapy in Mental Health* 8(4): 7–27. Sample of form included.

Occupational Functioning Tool. See Assessment of Occupational Functioning.

Occupational History. See also Occupational Role History and Occupational History Questionnaire—Revised.

Moorhead, L. 1967. *The occupational history in occupational therapy*. Unpublished master's thesis. Occupational Therapy Department, University of Southern California, Los Angeles, CA.

Moorhead, L. 1969. Occupational History. *American Journal of Occupational Therapy* 23(4): 329–332.

Occupational History Questionnaire—Revised. See also Occupational History.

Katz, N., N. Giladi, and C. Peretz. 1988. Cross-cultural application of occupational therapy assessments: Human occupation with psychiatric inpatients and controls in Israel. *Occupational Therapy in Mental Health* 8(1): 7–30.

Kielhofner, G., B. Harlan, D. Bauer, and P. Maurer. 1986. The reliability of a historical interview with physically disabled respondents. *American Journal of Occupational Therapy* 40(8): 551–556.

Smith, N.R., G. Kielhofner, and J.H. Watts. 1986. The relationships between volition, activity pattern, and life satisfaction in the elderly. *American Journal of Occupational Therapy* 40(4): 278–283.

Occupational Performance History Interview (OPHI)

Fossey, E. 1996. Using the Occupational Performance History Interview (OPHI): Therapists' reflections. *British Journal of Occupational Therapy* 59(5): 223–228.

Henry, A.D. 1998. Occupational Performance Interview History Interview. In *Willard and Spackman's occupational therapy*, 9th ed., eds. M.E. Neistadt and E.B. Crepeau, 163–164. Philadelphia: J.B. Lippincott. Overview.

Kielhofner, G. 1995. *A model of human occupation: Theory and application*, 2nd ed., 219–222, 233, 242–243, 366. Baltimore, MD: Williams & Wilkins.

Kielhofner, G., and A.D. Henry. 1988. Developmental and investigation of the Occupational Performance History Interview. *American Journal of Occupational Therapy* 42(8): 489–498.

Kielhofner, G., and T. Mallinson. 1995. Gathering narrative data through interviews: Empirical observations and suggested guidelines. *Scandinavian Journal of Occupational Therapy* 2(2): 63–68.

Kielhofner, G., A.D. Henry, D. Walens, and E.S. Rogers. 1991. A generalizability study of the Occupational Performance History Interview. *Occupational Therapy Journal of Research* 11(5): 292–306.

Mallinson, T., G. Kielhofner, and C. Mattingly. 1996. "Like being stuck in flypaper": Metaphor and meaning in a clinical interview. *American Journal of Occupational Therapy* 50: 338–346.

Mallinson, T., L. Mahaffey, and G. Kielhofner. 1998. The Occupational Performance History Interview: Evidence for three underlying constructs of occupational adaptation. *Canadian Journal of Occupational Therapy* 65(4): 219–228.

Neistadt, M.E. 1995. Assessing clients' priorities. *Occupational Therapy Practice* 1(1): 37–39.

Neistadt, M.E. 1995. Methods of assessing clients' priorities: A survey of adult physical dysfunction settings. *American Journal of Occupational Therapy* 49(5): 428–436.

A user's guide to the Occupational Performance History. Bethesda, MD: American Occupational Therapy Association. 1995. Interview.

Occupational Performance History Interview—II (OPHI-II)

Henry, A.D., and T. Mallinson. 1999. The Occupational Performance History Interview. In *Assessments in occupational therapy mental health: An integrative approach*, ed. B.J. Hemphill-Pearson, 59–70. Thorofare, NJ: Slack.

Kielhofner, G., T. Mallinson, E. Crawford, M. Nowak, M. Rigby, A. Henry, and D. Walens. 1998. *A user's manual for the Occupational Performance History Interview, Version 2*. Chicago: Model of Human Occupation Clearinghouse, University of Illinois.

Occupational Questionnaire. See also NIH Activity Record.

Ebb, E.W., W. Coster, and L. Duncombe. 1989. Comparison of normal and psychosocially dysfunctional male adolescents. *Occupational Therapy in Mental Health* 9(2): 53–74.

Folts, D., K. Tigges, and G. Jackson. 1993. Occupational therapy treatment of anorexia nervosa. In *The eating disorders*, eds. A.J. Giannini and A.E. Slaby, 227–242. New York: Springer-Verlag.

Henry, A.D. 1998. Occupational Questionnaire. In *Willard and Spackman's occupational therapy*, 9th ed., eds. M.E. Neistadt and E.B. Crepeau, 166. Philadelphia: J.B. Lippincott. Overview.

Kielhofner, G. 1995. *A model of human occupation: Theory and application*, 2nd ed., 217–219, 233, 241–242, 366. Baltimore, MD: Williams & Wilkins. Overview and sample.

Smith, N.R. 1986. Occupational Questionnaire. Available from Model of Human Occupation Clearinghouse, University of Illinois at Chicago, Department of Occupational Therapy (M/C 811), 1919 West Taylor Street, Chicago, IL 60612-7250.

Smith, N.R., G. Kielhofner, and J. Watts. 1986. The relationships between volition, activity pattern, and life satisfaction in the elderly. *American Journal of Occupational Therapy* 40(4): 278–283.

Occupational Questions

Pizzi, M., J. Mulkand, and M.M Freed. 1991. HIV infection and occupational therapy. In *Rehabilitation for patients with HIV disease*, ed. J. Mulkand, 283–326. New York: McGraw-Hill.

Occupational Role History. See also Occupational History Questionnaire.

Denton, P.L. 1987. *Psychiatric occupational therapy: A workbook of practical skills*, 73. Boston: Little Brown.

Florey, L., and S.M. Michelman. 1982. The Occupational Role History: A screening tool for psychiatric occupational therapy. *American Journal of Occupational Therapy* 36(5): 301–308.

Occupational Therapist's Evaluation of Group Interaction Skills (Includes Self-Evaluation Form for Patients A and B)

Salo-Chydenius, S. 1996. Changing helplessness to coping: An exploratory study of social skills training with individuals with long-term mental illness. *Occupational Therapy International* 3(3): 174–198.

Occupational Therapy Assessment for Older Adults with Depression

Rogers, J.C. 1987. Occupational therapy assessment for older adults with depression: Asking the right questions. *Occupational and Physical Therapy in Geriatrics* 5(1): 13–33.

Occupational Therapy Assessment of Leisure Time (OTALT)

Kratz, G., I. Soderback, S. Guidette, C. Hulting, T. Kykatkin, and M. Soderstrom. 1997. Wheelchair users' experience of non-adapted and adapted clothes during sailing, quad rugby, or wheel-walking. *Disability and Rehabilitation* 19(1): 26–34.

Soderback, I., and C. Hammarlund. 1993. A leisure-time frame of reference based on a literature analysis. *Occupational Therapy in Health Care* 8(4): 105–133.

Occupational Therapy Assessment Protocol

Bridgett, B. 1993. Occupational therapy evaluation for patients with eating disorders. *Occupational Therapy in Mental Health* 12(2): 79–89.

Occupational Therapy Ethics Self-Assessment Index

Coffey, M.S. 1988. Brief or new: Occupational Therapy Ethics Self-Assessment Index. *American Journal of Occupational Therapy* 42(5): 321–323.

Occupational Therapy Evaluation

Wolf, B. Multiple sclerosis. 1981. In *Interdisciplinary rehabilitation of multiple sclerosis and neuromuscular disorders*, eds. F.P. Maloney, J.S. Burks, and S.P. Ringel, 106–109. Philadelphia: J.B. Lippincott.

Occupational Therapy Evaluation for Older Adults

Szekais, B. 1984. Occupational therapy and assessment of the elderly. *British Journal of Occupational Therapy* 47(8): 240–242.

Occupational Therapy Functional Assessment Compilation Tool (OT Fact)

Bhasin, C.A. 1993. OT Fact: Fact or fiction? *Administration and Management Special Interest Newsletter* 9(4): 1–2.

Bhasin, C.A., and G.D. Goodman. 1992. The use of OT Fact categories to analyze activity configurations of individuals with multiple sclerosis. *Occupational Therapy Journal of Research* 12(2): 67–81.

Smith, R.O. 1990. OT Fact. Rockville, MD: American Occupational Therapy Association. Computer software program.

Smith, R.D. 1990. *OT Fact: Administrative and tutorial manual.* Rockville, MD: American Occupational Therapy Association,.

Smith, R.D. 1999. OT Fact applications in mental health. In *Assessments in occupational therapy mental health: An integrative approach*, ed. B.J. Hemphill-Pearson, 289–307. Thorofare, NJ: Slack.

Occupational Therapy Functional Evaluation Rating Scale

Occupational Therapy Functional Rating Scale. In *The evaluative process in psychiatric occupational therapy*, ed. B.J. Hemphill, 389–392. Thorofare, NJ: Slack, 1982.

Occupational Therapy Referral Form and Behavior Checklist

Merryfield, S. 1991. The referral process. In *Pediatric occupational therapy: Facilitating effective service provision*, ed. W. Dunn, 5–6. Thorofare, NJ: Slack.

Occupational Therapy Task Observation Scale (OTTOS)

Margolis, R.L., S.A. Harrison, H.J. Robinson, and G. Jayaram. 1996. Occupational Therapy Task Observation Scale (OTTOS): A rapid method for rating task group function of psychiatric patients. *American Journal of Occupational Therapy* 50(5): 380–385.

Occupational Therapy Trait Rating Scale (OTTRS)

Clark, J.R., B.A. Koch, and R.C. Nichols. 1965. A factor analytically derived scale. *American Journal of Occupational Therapy* 19(1): 14–18.

Odstock Hand Assessment

Roberts, C. 1990. The Odstock Hand Assessment. *British Journal of Occupational Therapy* 52(7): 256–261.

O'Kane Diagnostic Battery

O'Kane, P. 1969. *The development of a projective technique for use in psychiatric occupational therapy*. New York: University of New York at Buffalo.

O'Neill Hand Function Assessment

O'Neill, G. 1995. The development of a standardized assessment of hand function. *British Journal of Occupational Therapy* 58(11): 477–480.

Ontario Society of Occupational Therapists Perceptual Evaluation (OSOT)

Available from Jenkins, P., J. Martin, R. Oxenham, J. Painter, B. Panturescu, M. Smith, and M. Habal, OSOT, Toronto, Canada: Ontario Society of Occupational Therapists.

Ontario Society of Occupational Therapists Perceptual Evaluation (OSOT)—Revised

Arreola, R.A. 1995. OSOT Perceptual Evaluation. In *Twelfth measurements yearbook*, eds. J.C. Conoley and J.C. Impacts, 724–725. Lincoln, NE: Buros Institute of Mental Measurement.

Boys, M., P. Fisher, C. Holzberg, and D.W. Reid. 1988. The OSOT Perceptual Evaluation: A research perspective. *American Journal of Occupational Therapy* 42(2): 92–98.

Fisher, P., M. Boys, and C. Holzberg. 1991. Ontario Society of Occupational Therapists Perceptual Evaluation (OSOT), Nelson Canada, 1120 Birchmount Road, Scarorough, Ontario M1K 5G4 Canada.

Oromotor Feeding Assessment

Johnson, L.M. 1986. Development of an Oromotor Feeding Assessment. *Occupational Therapy Journal of Research* 6(6): 377–379.

Oswestry Low Back Pain Disability Questionnaire

Fairback, J.C.T., J.B. Davies, J. Couper, and J.P. O'Brien. 1980. The Oswestry Low Back Pain Disability Questionnaire. *Physiotherapy* 66: 271–273.

Oxford Head Injury Service

King, N.S., S. Crawford, F.J. Wenden, N.E.G. Moss, and D.T. Wade. 1997. Interventions and service need following mild and moderate head injury: The Oxford Head Injury Service. *Clinical Rehabilitation* 11(1): 13–27.

Parquetry Block Test

Neistadt, M.E. 1989. Normal adult performance on constructional praxis training tasks. *American Journal of Occupational Therapy* 43(7): 448–455.

Neistadt, M.E. 1993. The relationship between constructional and meal preparation skills. *Archives of Physical Medicine and Rehabilitation* 7(2): 144–148.

Neistadt, M.E. 1994. Using research literature to develop a perceptual retraining treatment protocol. *American Journal of Occupational Therapy* 48(1): 62–72.

Participant Satisfaction Questionnaire

Engel, J.M., and M.A. Rapoff. 1990. Biofeedback-assisted relaxation training for adult and pediatric headache disorders. *Occupational Therapy Journal of Research* 10(5): 283–299.

Pediatric Clinical Test of Sensory Interaction for Balance (P-CTSIB)

Dietz, J.C., P.K. Richardson, S.W. Atwater, T.K. Crowe, and M. Odiorne. 1991. Performance of normal children on the Pediatric Clinical Test of Sensory Interaction for Balance. *Occupational Therapy Journal of Research* 11(6): 336–356.

Richardson, P.K., S.W. Atwater, T.K. Crowe, and J.C. Deitz. 1992. Performance of preschoolers on the Pediatric Clinical Test of Sensory Interaction for Balance. *American Journal of Occupational Therapy* 46(9): 793–800.

Pediatric Evaluation of Disability Inventory (PEDI)

Bloom, K.K., and G.B. Nazar. 1994. Functional assessment following selective posterior rhizotomy in spastic cerebral palsy. *Childs Nervous System* 10(2): 84–86.

Coster, W.J., S. Haley, and M.J. Baryza. 1994. Functional performance of young children after traumatic brain injury: A 6-month follow-up study. *The American Journal of Occupational Therapy* 48(3): 211–218.

Dudgeon, B.J., A.K. Libby, J.F. McLaughlin, R.M. Hays, K.F. Bjornson, and T.S. Roberts. 1994. Prospective measurement of functional changes after selective dorsal rhizotomy. *Archives of Physical Medicine and Rehabilitation* 75(1): 46–53.

Feldman, A.B., S.M. Haley, and J. Coryell. 1990. Concurrent and construct validity of the Pediatric Evaluation of Disability Inventory. *Physical Therapy* 70(10): 602–610.

Haley, S.M., W.J. Coster, L. Ludlow, J.T. Haltiwanger, and P.J. Andrellos. 1992. *Pediatric Evaluation of Disability Inventory Manual*. San Antonio, TX: Therapy Skill Builders.

Hinderer, S.R., and S. Gupta. 1996. Review article: Functional outcome measures to assess interventions for spasticity. *Archives of Physical Medicine and Rehabilitation* 77(10): 1083–1089.

Javernick, J.A. 1993. PEDI: Assessing how young children function. *Occupational Therapy Week* 7(7): 8.

Ketclaar, M., A. Vermeer, and P.J. Helders. 1998. Functional motor abilities of children with cerebral palsy: A systematic literature review of assessment measure. *Clinical Rehabilitation* 12(5): 369–380.

Nichols, D.S., and J. Case-Smith. 1996. Reliability and validity of the Pediatric Evaluation of Disability Inventory. *Pediatric Physical Therapy* 8(1): 15–24.

Reid, D.T., K. Boschen, and V. Wright. 1993. Critique of the Pediatric Evaluation of Disability Inventory (PEDI). *Physical and Occupational Therapy in Pediatrics* 13(4): 57–87. Review.

Perceptual Motor Evaluation for Head-Injured and Other Neurologically Impaired Adults

Zoltan, B., J. Jabri, L. Panikoff, and D. Ryckman. 1983. *Perceptual motor evaluation for head-injured and other neurologically impaired adults.* San Jose, CA: Santa Clara Valley Medical Center, Occupational Therapy Department.

Performance Assessment of Self-Care Skills (PASS)—Version 3.1

Holm, M.B., and J.C. Rogers. 1999. Performance Assessment of Self-Care Skills. In *Assessments in occupational therapy mental health: An integrative approach*, ed. B.J. Hemphill-Pearson, 117–124. Thorofare, NJ: Slack.

Rogers, J.C. 1987. *Performance Assessment of Self-Care Skills.* 3811 O'Hara Street, Pittsburgh, PA 15213.

Rogers, J.C., and M.B. Holm. 1998. Performance Assessment of Self-Care Skills, Version 3.1 (PASS). In *Willard and Spackman's occupational therapy*, 9th ed., eds. M.E. Neistadt and E.B. Crepeau, 207. Philadelphia: J.B. Lippincott.

Rogers, J.C., M.B. Holm, G. Goldstein, M. McCue, and P.D. Nussbaum. 1994. Stability and change in functional assessment of patients with geropsychiatric disorders. *American Journal of Occupational Therapy* 48(10): 914–918.

Performance Evaluation of Occupational Therapy Students

Bridle, M.J. 1981. Profile of an occupational therapist revisited. *Canadian Journal of Occupational Therapy* 48: 107–113.

Canadian Association of Occupational Therapists. 1980. *Performance Evaluation of Occupational Therapy Students.* Toronto, Ontario: CAOT Publications ACE.

Ernest, M. 1985. A comprehensive field placement evaluation instrument: History, development, and implications. *Canadian Journal of Occupational Therapy* 52: 25–29.

Ernest, M. 1995. Evaluation of student clinical competence: An objective approach. *South African Journal of Occupational Therapy* 15(1): 5–11.

Ernest, M. 1987. A fieldwork evaluation instrument: PEOTS. *National: The Newsletter of the Canadian Association of Occupational Therapists* 4(4): 19.

Ernest, M. 1988. Occupational therapy practice: Generic or domain specific? *Canadian Journal of Occupational Therapy* 55(5): 249–254.

Ernest, M., and H. Polatajko. 1982. *Performance Evaluation of Occupational Therapy Students.* Unpublished instrument. University of Western Ontario, London, Canada.

Performance evaluation of occupational therapy students: A validity study. *Canadian Journal of Occupational Therapy* 1986; 53: 265–271.

Polatajko, H., L. Lee, and A. Bossers. 1994. Performance Evaluation of Occupational Therapy Students: A reliability study. *Canadian Journal of Occupational Therapy* 61(1): 20–27.

Performance Evaluation of Occupational Therapy Students—Revised

Ernest, M., H. Polatajko, and A. Bossers. 1990. *Performance Evaluation of Occupational Therapy Students*, rev. ed. Unpublished instrument. University of Western Ontario, London, Canada.

Missiuna, C., H. Polatajko, and M. Ernest-Conibear. 1992. Skill acquisition during fieldwork placements in occupational therapy. *Canadian Journal of Occupational Therapy* 59(1): 28–39.

Polatajko, H.J., L.H. Lee, and A.M. Bossers. 1994. Performance Evaluation of Occupational Therapy Students: A reliability study. *Canadian Journal of Occupational Therapy* 61(1): 20–27.

Performance with Parents Scale

Humphry, R., and S. Geissinger. 1992. Self-rating as an evaluation tool following continuing professional education. *Occupational Therapy Journal of Research* 22(2): 111–121.

Person Symbol

King, L.J. 1982. The Person Symbol as an assessment tool. In *The evaluation process in psychiatric occupational therapy*, ed. B.J. Hemphill, 169–194. Thorofare, NJ: Slack.

Physical Capacities Evaluation

Physical Capacities Evaluation. In *Willard and Spackman's occupational therapy*, 6th ed., eds. H.L. Hopkins and H.D. Smith, 168–173. Philadelphia: J.B. Lippincott, 1983. Form.

Reuss, E.E., D.E. Rawe, and A.E. Sundquist. 1958. Development of a physical capacities evaluation. *American Journal of Occupational Therapy* 12(1): 1–8.

Smith, S. 1978. Physical Capacities Evaluation. In *Willard and Spackman's occupational therapy*, 5th ed., eds. H.L. Hopkins and H.D. Smith, 213–218. Philadelphia: J.B. Lippincott. Form.

Smith, S., and P. Baxter-Petralia. 1992. *The Physical Capacities Evaluation: Its use in four models of clinical practice*. Baltimore, MD: Chess Publications.

Physical Capacities Evaluation of Hand Skills (PCE)

Bell, E., D.K. Jurek, and T. Wilson. 1976. Physical Capacities Evaluation of Hand Skills. *American Journal of Occupational Therapy* 30(2): 80–86.

Physiological Monitored Evaluation (PME)

Shanfield, K.C. 1984. Physiological monitoring: Assessment of energy cost. *Occupational Therapy In Health Care* 1(2): 87–97.

Pizzi Assessment of Productive Living for Adults with HIV Infection and AIDS

Pizzi, M. 1991. HIV infection and AIDS. In *Willard and Spackman's occupational therapy*, 8th ed., eds. H.L. Hopkins and H.D. Smith, 716–729. Philadelphia: J.B. Lippincott. Form included.

Play History

Bryze, K. 1996. Narrative contributions to the Play History. In *Play in occupational therapy for children*, eds. L.D. Parham and L.S. Fazio, 23–34. St. Louis: Mosby.

Takata, N. 1967. Development of a conceptual scheme for analysis of play milieu. Unpublished master's thesis. Occupational Therapy Department, University of Southern California, Los Angeles, CA.

Takata, N. 1969. Play History. *American Journal of Occupational Therapy* 23(4): 314–318.

Takata, N. 1974. Play as a prescription. In *Play as exploratory learning*, ed. M. Reilly, 209–246. Beverly Hills, CA: Sage.

Play Scale. See also Knox Preschool Play Scale and Preschool Play Scale.

Knox, S. 1974. A play scale. In *Play as exploratory learning*, ed. M. Reilly, 247–266. Beverly Hills, CA: Sage.

Play Skills Inventory (PSI)

Hurff, J.M. 1974. A play skills inventory. In *Play as exploratory learning*, ed. M. Reilly, 267–284. Beverly Hills, CA: Sage.

Hurff, J.M. 1980. A play skills inventory: A competency monitoring tool for the 10-year-old. *American Journal of Occupational Therapy* 34(10): 651–656.

Posture and Fine Motor Assessment of Infants (PFMAI)

Case-Smith, J. 1989. Reliability and validity of the Posture and Fine Motor Assessment of Infants. *Occupational Therapy Journal of Research* 9(5): 259–272.

Case-Smith, J. 1992. A validity study of the Posture and Fine Motor Assessment of Infants. *American Journal Occupational Therapy* 46(7): 597–605.

Kuhns, G. 1997. Reliability and validity study of the Posture and Fine Motor Assessment of Infants. *Journal of Occupational Therapy Students* (April): 19–22.

Power-Mobility Indoor Driving Assessment (PIDA)

Dawson, D., R. Chan, and E. Kaiserman. 1994. Development of the Power-Mobility Indoor Driving Assessment for residents of long-term care facilities: A preliminary report. *Canadian Journal of Occupational Therapy* 61(5): 269–276. Form included.

Predischarge Assessment Tool

Rudman, D.L., J. Tooke, T.G. Eimantas, M. Hall, and K.B. Maloney. 1998. Preliminary investigation of the content validity and clinical utility of the Predischarge Assessment Tool. *Canadian Journal of Occupational Therapy* 65(1): 3–11.

Pre/Post-Assessment of Work Behaviors

Daughery, P.M., and M.V. Radomski. 1993. *The Cognitive rehabilitation workbook*, 2nd ed., 21–36. Gaithersburg, MD: Aspen Publishers.

Preschool Occupational Therapy Assessment

Miller, H.E. 1996. The reliability and content validity of the preschool occupational therapy assessment. Unpublished master's thesis. Columbus, OH: Ohio State University.

Miller, H.E. 1997. Development of the Preschool Occupational Therapy Assessment. *Physical and Occupational Therapy in Pediatrics* 17(4): 61–63.

Preschool Play Scale (PPS). See also Knox Preschool Play Scale and Play Scale.

Bledsoe, N.P., and J.T. Shepherd. 1982. A study of reliability and validity of a Preschool Play Scale. *American Journal of Occupational Therapy* 36(12): 783–788, 794–795.

Bundy, A.C. 1989. A comparison of the play skills of normal boys and boys with sensory integrative dysfunction. *Occupational Therapy Journal of Research* 9(2): 84–100.

Clifford, J.M., and A.C. Bundy. 1989. Performance in normal boys and boys with sensory integration dysfunction. *Occupational Therapy Journal of Research* 9(4): 202–217.

Couch, K.J. 1996. Annotated bibliography: the use of the Preschool Play Scale in published research. *Physical and Occupational Therapy in Pediatrics* 16(4): 77–84.

Harrison, H., and G. Kielhofner. 1986. Examining reliability and validity of the Preschool Play Scale with handicapped children. *American Journal of Occupational Therapy* 40(3): 167–173.

Morrison, C.D., A.C. Bundy, and A.G. Fisher. 1991. The contribution of motor skills and playfulness to the play performance of preschoolers. *American Journal of Occupational Therapy* 45(8): 687–694.

Restall, G., and J. Magill-Evans. 1994. Play and preschool children with autism. *American Journal of Occupational Therapy* 48(2): 113–120.

Shepherd, J.T., C.B. Brollier, and R.L. Dandrow. 1994. Research report: Play skills of preschool children with speech and language delays. *Physical and Occupational Therapy in Pediatrics* 14(2): 1–20.
Von Zuben, M.V., P.A. Crist, and W. Mayberry. 1991. A pilot study of differences in play behavior between children of low and middle socioeconomic status. *American Journal of Occupational Therapy* 45(2): 113–118.

Pre-Vocational Assessment of Psychiatric Patients. See Pre-Vocational Evaluation of Rehabilitation Potential.

Pre-Vocational Assessment Package

Oxley, C. 1992. Devising an assessment package for an employment rehabilitation service. *British Journal of Occupational Therapy* 55(12): 448–452.

Pre-Vocational Evaluation of Rehabilitation Potential

Ethridge, D.A. 1968. Pre-Vocational Evaluation of Rehabilitation Potential. *American Journal of Occupational Therapy* 22(3): 161–167.

Profile of Occupational Patterns

Royeen, C.B. 1995. The human life cycle: Paradigmatic shifts in occupation. In *The practice of the future: Putting occupation back into therapy* 11, ed. C.B. Royeen, 14–17. Rockville, MD: American Occupational Therapy Association.

Prone Extension Postural Test

Gregory, J., E. Glock, and E.J. Yerxa. 1984. Standardization of the Prone Extension Postural Test on children ages 4 through 8. *American Journal of Occupational Therapy* 38(3): 187–194.

Psychiatric Occupational Therapy Evaluation of Needs and Treatment Instrument

Spermon, D.M., S.M. Wilson, and M.A. Hill. 1991. The development and validation of the Psychiatric Occupational Therapy Evaluation of Needs and Treatment Instrument. *Occupational Therapy in Mental Health* 11(4): 91–110.

Qual-OT

Robnett, R.H., and J.A. Gliner. 1995. Qual-OT: A quality of life assessment tool. *Occupational Therapy Journal of Research* 15(3): 198–214.

Quality of Upper Extremities Skills Test (QUEST)

DeMatteo, C. et al. 1992. *QUEST: Quality of Upper Extremity Skills Test manual.* Hamilton, Ontario: Neurodevelopmental Research Unit, Chedoke Campus, Chedoke-MacMasters Hospital.
DeMatteo, C. et al. 1993. The reliability and validity of the Quality of Upper Extremity Skills Test. *Physical and Occupational Therapy in Pediatrics* 13(2): 1–18.
Hickey, A., and J. Ziviani. 1998. A review of the Quality of Upper Extremities Skills Test (QUEST) for children with cerebral palsy. *Physical and Occupational Therapy in Pediatrics* 18(3/4): 123–135.
Law, M., D. Cadman, P. Rosenbaum, S. Walter, D. Russell, and C. DeMatteo. 1991. Neurodevelopmental therapy and upper-extremity inhibitive casting for children with cerebral palsy. *Developmental Medicine and Child Neurology* 33: 379–387.

Law, M., D. Russell, N. Pollock, S. Walter, and J. King. 1997. A comparison of intensive neurodevelopmental therapy plus casting and a regular occupational therapy program for children with cerebral palsy. *Developmental Medicine and Child Neurology* 39: 644–670.

Quebec User Evaluation of Satisfaction with Assistive Technology (QUEST)

Demers, L., R. Weiss-Lambrou, and B. Ska. 1996. Development of the Quebec User Evaluation of Satisfaction with Assistive Technology (QUEST). *Assistive Technology* 8(1):3–13.

Demers, L., R.D. Wessles, R. Weiss-Lambrou, B. Ska, and L.P. De Witte. 1999. An international content validation of the Quebec User Evaluation of Satisfaction with Assistive Technology (QUEST). *Occupational Therapy International* 6(3):159–175.

Questionnaire on Adolescent Risk-Taking (Computerized)

Black, M.M., J. Gordon, and J.S. Santelli. 1999. Adolescent risk-taking behaviors: Computer-assisted questionnaire. In *Assessments in occupational therapy mental health: An integrative approach*, ed. B.J. Hemphill-Pearson, 309–319. Thorofare, NJ: Slack.

Questionnaire on Leisure

Howard, L. 1996. A comparison of leisure-time activities between able-bodied children and children with physical disabilities. *British Journal of Occupational Therapy* 59(12): 570–574.

Rabideau Kitchen Evaluation—Revised (RKE-R)

Neistadt, M.E. 1992. The Rabideau Kitchen Evaluation—Revised: An assessment of meal preparation skills. *Occupational Therapy Journal of Research* 12(4):242–253.

Neistadt, M.E. 1993. The relationship between constructional and meal preparation skills. *Archives of Physical Medicine and Rehabilitation* 7(2): 144–148.

Neistadt, M.E. 1994. A meal preparation treatment protocol for adults with brain injury. *American Journal of Occupational Therapy* 48(5): 431–438. Form included.

Neistadt, M.E. 1998. Overview of treatment. In *Willard and Spackman's occupational therapy*, 9th ed., eds. M.E. Neistadt and E.B. Crepeau, 315–322. Philadelphia: J.B. Lippincott.

Porter, J., G. Watson, and S. Capra. 1998. Food skills assessment tools for people with a mental illness. *Australian Occupational Therapy Journal* 45(2): 65–71. Review.

Rabideau, G.M. 1986. Two approaches to improving the functional performance of a cognitively impaired head injured adult. Master's thesis. Tufts University, Medford, MA.

Zoltan, B. 1996. Appendix A. Additional current and related evaluations developed by occupational therapists. In *Vision, perception, and cognition: A manual for the evaluation and treatment of the neurologically impaired adult*, 3rd ed., 199–200. Thorofare, NJ: Slack.

Rating Scale for Assessing Elderly Patients

Leng, N.R.C., S.R. Taylor, and O. Hanley. 1988. A Rating Scale for Assessing Elderly People. *British Journal of Occupational Therapy* 51(2): 60–62.

Rating Scale for Use in Horticultural Therapy

Woodward, S., and P. Holden. 1984. A Rating Scale for Use in Horticultural Therapy. *British Journal of Occupational Therapy* 47(7): 211–214.

Reflex Testing Chart. See Reflex Testing Methods for Evaluating CNS Development.

Reflex Testing Methods for Evaluating CNS Development

Fiorentino, M.R. 1973. *Reflex testing methods for evaluating CNS development*. Springfield, IL: Charles C. Thomas.

Fiorentino, M.R. 1978. Motor Development Chart. In *Willard and Spackman's occupational therapy*, 5th ed., eds. H.L. Hopkins and H.D. Smith, 511–512. Philadelphia: J.B. Lippincott.

Fiorentino, M.R. 1978. Reflex Testing Chart. In *Willard and Spackman's occupational therapy*, 5th ed., eds. H.L. Hopkins and H.D. Smith, 510. Philadelphia: J.B. Lippincott.

Rehabilitation Institute of Chicago Functional Assessment Scale

Intagliata, S., and B.E. Sullivan. 1991. Development and implementation of the Rehabilitation Institute of Chicago Functional Assessment Scale. *Occupational Therapy Practice* 2(2): 26–37.

Reintegration to Normal Living Index

Bethoux, F., R. Calmes, and V. Gautheron. 1999. Changes in the quality of life of hemiplegic stroke patients with time: A preliminary report. *American Journal of Physical Medicine and Rehabilitation* 78(1): 19–23.

Bethoux, F., P. Calmels, V. Gautheron, and P. Minaire. 1996. Quality of life of the spouses of stroke patients: A preliminary study. *International Journal of Rehabilitation Research* 19(4): 291–299.

Carter, B.S., C.S. Ogilvy, G.J. Candia, H.D. Rosas, and F. Buonanno. 1997. One-year outcome after decompressive surgery for massive nondominant hemispheric infarction. *Neurosurgery* 40(6): 1168–1175.

Daverat, P., H. Petti, G. Kemoun, J.F. Dartigues, and M. Barat. 1995. The long-term outcome in 149 patients with spinal cord injury. *Paraplegia* 33(11): 665–658.

Edwards, D.F. 1997. Reintegration to Normal Living Index. In *Enabling function and well-being*, 2nd ed, eds. C.H. Christiansen and C.M. Baum, 566–567. Thorofare, NJ: Slack.

Gauthier-Gagnon, C., and M.C. Grise. 1994. Prosthetic profile of the amputee questionnaire: Validity and reliability. *Archives of Physical Medicine and Rehabilitation* 75(12): 1309–1314.

Korner-Bitensky, N., S. Wood-Dauphinee, J. Siemiatycki, S. Shapiro, and R. Becker. 1994. Health-related information postdischarge: Telephone versus face-to-face interviewing. *Archives of Physical Medicine and Rehabilitation* 75(12): 1287–1296.

Pieper, B., C. Mikols, and T.R. Dawson Grant. 1996. Comparing adjustment to an ostomy for three groups. *Journal of Wound, Ostomy, and Continence Nursing* 23(4): 197–204.

Pollock, N., S. Baptiste, M. Law, M.A. McColl, A. Opzoomer, and H. Polatajko. 1990. Occupational performance measures: A review based on the guidelines for the client-centred practice of occupational therapy. *Canadian Journal of Occupational Therapy* 57(2): 77–81.

Trombly, C.A., M. Vining Radomski, and E. Schold Davis. 1998. Achievement of self-identified goals by adults with traumatic brain injury: Phase I. *American Journal of Occupational Therapy* 52(10): 810–818.

Wade, D.T. 1992. Reintegration to Normal Living Index. In *Measurement in Neurological Rehabilitation*, ed. D.T. Wade, 255–256. New York: Oxford University Press.

Wood-Dauphinee, S.L., and J.I. Williams. 1988. Assessment of global function: The reintegration to normal living index. *Archives of Physical and Medical Rehabilitation* 69(8): 583–590.

Riverdale Hospital's Home and Community Skills Assessment

Brown, H. 1988. The standardization of the Riverdale Hospital's Home and Community Skills Assessment. *Canadian Journal of Occupational Therapy* 55(1): 9–14.

Rivermead Activities of Daily Living (ADL) Scale

Lincoln, N.B., and J.A. Edmans. 1990. A revalidation of the Rivermead ADL Scale for elderly patients with stroke. *Age and Aging* 19(1): 19–24.
Wade, D.T. 1992. *Measurement in neurological rehabilitation*, 181–185. New York: Oxford University Press.

Rivermead Perceptual Assessment Battery

Braden, J.P. 1992. Rivermead Perceptual Assessment Battery. *Eleventh mental measurements yearbook*, eds. J.J. Kramer and J.C. Conoley, 773–775. Lincoln, NE: Buros Institute of Mental Measurement. Review.
Cockburn, J., G. Bhavanani, S.E. Whiting, and N. Lincoln. 1982. Normal performance on some test of perception in adults. *British Journal of Occupational Therapy* 45(2): 67–68.
Cramond, H.J., M.S. Clark, and D.S. Smith. 1989. The effect of using the dominant or nondominant hand on performance of the Rivermead Perceptual Assessment Battery. *Clinical Rehabilitation* 3(3): 215–221.
Donnelly, S.M., D. L. Hextell, and S. Matthey. 1998. The Rivermead Perceptual Assessment Battery: Its relationship to selected functional activities. *British Journal of Occupational Therapy* 61(1): 27–32.
Edmans, J.A. 1987. The frequency of perceptual deficits after stroke. *Clinical Rehabilitation* 1(4): 273–281.
Enderby, P., J. Broeckx, W. Hospers, F. Schildermans, and W. Deberdt. 1994. Effect of piracetam on recovery and rehabilitation after stroke: A double-blind, placebo-controlled study. *Clinical Neuropharmacology* 17(4): 320–331.
Friedman, P.J., and L. Leong. 1992. The Rivermead Perceptual Assessment Battery in acute stroke. *British Journal of Occupational Therapy* 55(6): 233–237.
Gibson, L., W.J. MacLennan, C. Gray, and B. Pentland. 1991. Evaluation of a comprehensive assessment battery for stroke patients. *International Journal of Rehabilitation Research* 14(2): 93–100.
Jesshope, H.J., M.S. Clark, and D.S. Smith. 1991. The Rivermead Perceptual Assessment Battery: Its application to stroke patients and relationship with function. *Clinical Rehabilitation* 5(2): 115–122.
Lincoln, N.B., and D. Clarke. 1987. The performance of normal elderly people on the Rivermead Perceptual Assessment Battery. *British Journal of Occupational Therapy* 50(5): 156–157.
Lincoln, N.B., A.E.R. Drummond, J.A. Edmans, D. Yeo, and D. Willis. 1998. The Rey Figure Copy as a screening instrument for perceptual deficits after stroke. *British Journal of Occupational Therapy* 61(1): 33–35.
Matthey, S., S.M. Donnelly, and D.L. Hextell. 1993. The clinical usefulness of the Rivermead Perceptual Assessment Battery: Statistical considerations. *British Journal of Occupational Therapy* 56(10): 365–370.
Unsworth, C. 1999. Rivermead Perceptual Assessment Battery (RPAB). In *Cognitive and perceptual dysfunction: A clinical reasoning approach to evaluation and intervention*, ed. C. Unsworth, 86–87, 94–96. Philadelphia: F.A. Davis.
Wade, D.T. 1992. Rivermead Perceptual Assessment Battery. *Measurement in Neurological Rehabilitation*, 358. New York: Oxford University Press. Form only.
Whiting, S.E., N. Lincoln, G. Bhavanani, and J. Cockburn. 1985. *Rivermead Perceptual Assessment Battery*. Windsor, England: NFER Nelson; or Western Psychological Services, Los Angeles, CA.

Rivermead Perceptual Assessment Battery—Short Version

Lincoln, N.B., and J.A. Edmans. A shortened version of the Rivermead Perceptual Assessment Battery. *Clinical Rehabilitation* 3(3): 199–204.

Robinson Bashall Functional Assessment for Arthritis Patients

McCloy, L., and L. Jongbloed. 1987. Robinson Bashall Functional Assessment for Arthritis Patients: Reliability and validity. *Archives of Physical Medicine and Rehabilitation* 68(8): 486–489.

Robinson, H.S., and D.A. Bashall. 1962. Functional assessment in rheumatoid arthritis. *Canadian Journal of Occupational Therapy* 29: 123–138.

Role Activity Performance Scale (RAPS)

Denton, P.L. 1987. *Psychiatric occupational therapy: A workbook of practical skills*, 73. Boston: Little, Brown.

Folts, D., K. Tigges, and G. Jackson. 1993. Occupational therapy treatment of anorexia nervosa. In *The eating disorders*, eds. A.J. Giannini and A.E. Slaby, 227–242. New York: Springer-Verlag.

Good-Ellis, M.A. 1999. The Role Activity Performance Scale. In *Assessments in occupational therapy mental health: An integrative approach*, ed. B.J. Hemphill-Pearson, 205–226. Thorofare, NJ: Slack.

Good-Ellis, M.A., S.B. Fine, G.L. Haas, J.H. Spencer Jr., and E.D. Glick. 1986. Quantitative role and performance assessment: Implication and application to treatment of major affective disorders. In *Depression: Assessment and treatment update*, ed. American Occupational Therapy Association, 36–48. Rockville, MD: American Occupational Therapy Association.

Good-Ellis, M.A., S.B. Fine, J.H. Spencer, and A. DiVittis. 1985. Developing a Role Activity Performance Scale. *American Journal of Occupational Therapy* 41(4): 232–241.

Henry, A.D. 1998. Role Activity Performance Scale. In *Willard and Spackman's occupational therapy*, 9th ed., eds. M.E. Neistadt and E.B. Crepeau, 164. Philadelphia: J.B. Lippincott. Overview.

Role Change Assessment

Jackoway, I., J. Rogers, and T. Snow. 1987. Role change assessment. *Occupational Therapy in Mental Health* 7(1): 17–37.

Rogers, J.C., and M.B. Holm. 1995. *The Role Change Assessment, version 2.0: An interview tool for evaluating older adults*. Pittsburgh, PA: Unpublished.

Rogers, J.C., and M.B. Holm. 1999. Role Change Assessment: An interview tool for older adults. In *Assessments in occupational therapy mental health: An integrative approach*, ed. B.J. Hemphill-Pearson, 73–82. Thorofare, NJ: Slack.

Role Checklist, 1st ed.

Barris, R., F. Oakley, and G. Kielhofner. 1988. The Role Checklist. In *Mental health assessment in occupational therapy: An integrative approach to the evaluative process*, ed. B.J. Hemphill, 73–91. Thorofare, NJ: Slack.

Oakley, F. 1984. *Role Checklist*. Occupational Therapy Service, National Institutes of Health, Building 10, Room 6S-235, 10 Center Drive MSC 1604, Bethesda, MD 20892-1604.

Oakley, F., G. Kielhofner, R. Barris, and R.K. Reichler. 1986. The Role Checklist: Development and empirical assessment of reliability. *Occupational Therapy Journal of Research* 6(3): 157–169.

Role Checklist, 2nd ed.

Dickerson, A.E. 1999. The Role Checklist. In *Assessments in occupational therapy mental health: An integrative approach*, ed. B.J. Hemphill-Pearson, 175–191. Thorofare, NJ: Slack.

Ebb, E.W., W. Coster, L. Duncombe. 1989. Comparison of normal and psychosocially dysfunctional male adolescents. *Occupational Therapy in Mental Health* 9(2): 53–74.

Hachey, R., J. Jumorty, and C. Mercier. 1995. Methodology for validating the translation of test measurements applied to occupational therapy. *Occupational Therapy International* 2(3): 190–203.

Kielhofner, G. 1995. *A model of human occupation: Theory and application*, 2nd ed., 214–216, 233, 245–246, 366. Baltimore, MD: Williams & Wilkins. Overview.

Mentrup, C., A. Niehaus, and G. Kielhofner. 1999. Applying the model of human occupation in work-focused rehabilitation: A case illustration. *Work: Journal of Prevention, Assessment and Rehabilitation* 12(1): 61–67.

Oakley, F. 1988. *Role Checklist*, 2nd ed. Occupational Therapy Service, National Institutes of Health, Building 10, Room 6S-235, 10 Center Drive MSC 1604, Bethesda, MD 20892-1604.

Pizzi, M., J. Mulkand, and M.M. Freed. 1991. HIV infection and occupational therapy. In *Rehabilitation for patients with HIV disease*, ed. J. Mulkand, 294–295. New York: McGraw-Hill. Form included.

Sepiol, J.M., and J. Froehlich. 1990. Use of the Role Checklist with the patient with multiple personality disorder. *American Journal of Occupational Therapy* 44(11): 1008–1012.

Role Performance Scale. See Role Activity Performance Scale.

Rosenbusch Test of Finger Dexterity

Stein, C., and E. Yerxa. 1989. A test of finger dexterity. *American Journal of Occupational Therapy* 44(6): 499–504.

Routine Task Inventory (RTI-2)

Allen, C.K., K. Kehrberg, and T. Burns. 1992. Evaluation instrument—Part I: Routine Task Inventory. In *Occupational therapy treatment goals for the physically and cognitively disabled*, eds. C.K. Allen, C.A. Earhart, and T. Blue, 34–40, 54–68. Bethesda, MD: American Occupational Therapy Association.

Earhart, C.A., and C.K. Allen. 1988. *Cognitive disabilities: Expanded activity analysis*, 16–33. Pasadena, CA: Author. 3660 Cartwright Street, Pasadena, CA 91107.

Heimann, N., C. Allen, and E. Yerxa. 1989. The Routine Task Inventory: A tool for describing the functional behavior of cognitively disabled. *Occupational Therapy Practice* 1(1): 67–74.

Porter, J., G. Watson, and S. Capra. 1998. Food skills assessment tools for people with a mental illness. *Australian Occupational Therapy Journal* 45(1): 65–71. Review.

Rogers, J.C., and M.C. Holm. 1998. Routine Task Inventory-2 (RTI-2). In *Willard and Spackman's occupational therapy*, 9th ed., eds. M.E. Neistadt and E.B. Crepeau, 207–208. Philadelphia: J.B. Lippincott.

Wilson, D., C.K. Allen, G. McCormack, and G. Burton. 1989. Cognitive disability and routine task behavior in a community-based population with senile dementia. *Occupational Therapy Practice* 1(1): 58–66.

Safety and Functional ADL Evaluation (SAFE)

Available from Virginia Morgan, Director, Occupational Therapy, Spaulding Rehabilitation Hospital, 125 Nashua Street, Boston, MA 02114.

Safety Assessment of Function and the Environment for Rehabilitation (SAFER)

Community Occupational Therapists and Associates. *Safety Assessment of Function and the Environment for Rehabilitation*. 3101 Bathurst Street, Suite 200, Toronto, Ontario, M6A 2A6. Available from the Canadian Association of Occupational Therapy, CTTC Building, Suite 3400, 1125 Colonel by Brive, Ottawa, Ontario, Canada K1S 5R1.

Letts, L., and L. Marshall. 1995. Evaluating the validity and consistency of the SAFER tool. *Physical and Occupational Therapy in Geriatrics* 13(4): 49–60.

Letts, L., L. Marshall, and B. Cawley, B. 1995. Assessing safe function at home: The SAFER tool. *Home and Community Health Special Interest Section Newsletter* 2(1): 1–2.

Letts, L., S. Scott, J. Burtney, L. Marshall, and M. McKean, M. 1998. The reliability and validity of the Safety Assessment of Function and the Environment for Rehabilitation (SAFER) Tool. *British Journal of Occupational Therapy* 61(3): 127–132.

Oliver, R., J. Blathwayt, C. Brackley, and T. Tamaki. 1993. Development of the Safety Assessment of Function and the Environment for Rehabilitation (SAFER) tool. *Canadian Journal of Occupational Therapy* 60(2): 78–82.

Satisfaction with Performance Scaled Questionnaire (SPSQ)

Chan, C.C.H., and T.M.C. Lee. 1997. Validity of the Canadian Occupational Performance Measure. *Occupational Therapy International* 4(3): 229–247.

Pollock, N., S. Baptiste, M. Law, M.A. McColl, A. Opzoomer, and H. Polatajko. 1990. Occupational performance measures: A review based on the guidelines for the client-centered practice of occupational therapy. *Canadian Journal of Occupational Therapy* 57(2): 77–81.

Rogers, J.C., and M.C. Holm. 1998. Satisfaction with Performance Scaled Questionnaire (SPSQ). In *Willard and Spackman's occupational therapy*, 9th ed., eds. M.E. Neistadt and E.B. Crepeau, 207. Philadelphia: J.B. Lippincott.

Yerxa, E.J., S. Burnet-Beaulieu, S. Stocking, and S.P. Azen. 1988. Development of the Satisfaction with Performance Scaled Questionnaire (SPSQ). *American Journal of Occupational Therapy* 42(4): 215–221.

Scale for Rating Functional Demands for Daily Living

MacLean, F.M. 1949. Occupational therapy in the management of poliomyelitis. *American Journal of Occupational Therapy* 3(1): 20–27.

Scale of Children's Readiness in PrinTing (SCRIPT)

Weil, M.J., and S.J.C. Amundson. 1994. Relationship between visuomotor and handwriting skills of children in kindergarten. *American Journal of Occupational Therapy* 48(11): 982–988.

Scanboard Test

Warren, M. 1989. Identification of visual scanning deficits in adults after cerebrovascular accident. *American Journal of Occupational Therapy* 44(5): 391–399.

Zoltan, B. 1996. Visual processing skills. In *Vision, perception, and cognition: A manual for the evaluation and treatment of the neurologically impaired adult*, 3rd ed., 41–42. Thorofare, NJ: Slack.

School Assessment of Motor and Process Skills (School AMPS)

Atchison, B.T., A.G. Fisher, and K. Bryze, K. 1998. Rater reliability and internal scale and person response validity of the School Assessment of Motor and Process Skills. *American Journal of Occupational Therapy* 52(10): 843–850.

Fisher, A.G. 1997. *School AMPS: School version of the Assessment of Motor and Process Skills*. Fort Collins, CO: Three Star Press.

School Function Assessment

Coster, W., T. Deeney, J. Haltiwanger, and S. Haley. 1997. *School Function Assessment*. San Antonio, TX: The Psychological Corporation.

School Questionnaire

King-Thomas, L., and B.J. Hacker. 1987. *A therapist's guide to pediatric assessment*, 337–338. Boston: Little, Brown. Modified from P. Oetter.

Schroeder Block Campbell Adult Psychiatric Sensory Integration Evaluation (SBC)

Evans, J., and A.A. Salim. 1992. A cross-cultural test of the validity of occupational therapy assessments with patients with schizophrenia. *American Journal of Occupational Therapy* 46(8): 685–695.

Schroeder, C.V. and A.K. Herbert. 1981. *Adult psychiatric sensory integration evaluation*, 3rd. ed. Kailua, HI: Schroeder Publishing and Consulting.

Schroeder, C.V., M.P. Block, M.P. Trottier, and M.S. Stoweel. 1978. *Adult psychiatric sensory integration evaluation*, 2nd ed. LaJolla, CA: SBC Research Associates.

Schroeder, C.V. et al. 1982. The adult psychiatric sensory integration evaluation. In *Evaluative process in psychiatric occupational therapy*, ed. B.J. Hemphill, 227–253. Thorofare, NJ: Slack.

Schultz Structured Interview

Schultz, K.S. 1984. The Schultz Structured Interview for assessing upper extremity pain. *Occupational Therapy in Health Care* 1(3): 69–82.

Scorable Self-Care Evaluation

Clark, E.N., and M. Peters. 1984. *Scorable Self-Care Evaluation*. Thorofare, NJ: Slack.

McGeorge, D. 1990. Critique of the Scorable Self-Care Evaluation. *New Zealand Journal of Occupational Therapy* 4(1): 23–26.

Scorable Self-Care Evaluation—Revised

Clark, E.N., and M. Peters. 1993. *Scorable Self-Care Evaluation*, rev. ed. San Antonio, TX: Therapy Skill Builders/The Psychological Corporation.

Screening for Physical and Occupational Therapy Referral (SPOTR)

Woosley, T., D. Sands, and W. Dunlap. 1987. An instrument to screen sensory impaired persons for referral to physical and occupational therapy. *Journal of Rehabilitation* 53(4): 66–69.

Screening Tool for Cumulative Trauma Disorder

Muffly-Elsey, D., and S. Flinn-Wagner. 1987. Proposed screening tool for the detection of cumulative trauma disorders of the upper extremity. *Journal of Hand Surgery* 5(2): 931–935.

Screening Tool for Occupational Therapy Referrals

Johnson, K. 1996. Screening tool for occupational therapy referrals. *Home and Community Health Special Interest Section Newsletter* 3(3): 1.

Self-Assessment of Leisure Interests

Kautzmann, L.N. 1984. Identifying leisure interests: A self-assessment approach for adults with arthritis. *Occupational Therapy in Health Care* 1(2): 45–52.

Self-Assessment of Leisure Interests. 1984. Eastern Kentucky University, Dizney 103, Richmond, KY 40475.

Self Assessment of Occupational Functioning (SAOF)

Self Assessment of Occupational Functioning (SAOF)—Revised. See also Children's Self Assessment of Occupational Functioning.

Baron, K., and C. Curtin. 1990. *A manual for use with the Self Assessment of Occupational Functioning*. Chicago: University of Illinois.

Baron, K., and C. Curtin. 1990. *Self assessment of occupational functioning*. Available from Model of Human Occupation Clearinghouse, Department of Occupational Therapy, (M/C 811), University of Illinois at Chicago, 1919 West Taylor Street, Chicago, IL 60612-7250. (312) 996-6901.

Henry, A.D. 1998. Self Assessment of Occupational Functioning. In *Willard and Spackman's occupational therapy*, 9th ed., eds. M.E. Neistadt and E.B. Crepeau, 166. Philadelphia: J.B. Lippincott. Overview.

Kielhofner, G. 1995. *A model of human occupation: Theory and application*, 2nd ed., 218–220, 233, 246–247, 366. Baltimore, MD: Williams & Wilkins. Overview and sample.

Self-Awareness of Deficits Interview

Fleming, J.M., J. Strong, and R. Ashton. 1996. Self-awareness of deficits in adults with traumatic brain injury: How best to measure? *Brain Injury* 10(1): 1–15. Form included.

Self-Care Ability Scale for the Elderly

Soderhamn, O., A.C. Ek, and I. Porn. 1996. The Self-Care Ability Scale for the Elderly. *Scandinavian Journal of Occupational Therapy* 3(2): 69–78.

Self-Efficacy Scale

Gage, M., S. Noh, H.J. Polatajko, and V. Kaspar. 1994. Self-Efficacy Scale: Measuring perceived self-efficacy in occupational therapy. *American Journal of Occupational Therapy* 48(9): 783–790.

Self-Report Play Skills Questionnaire

Sturgess, J., and J. Ziviani. 1995. Development of a self-report play questionnaire for children aged 5 to 7 years: A preliminary report. *Australian Occupational Therapy Journal* 42, 107–117.

Sturgess, J., and J. Ziviani. 1996. A self-report play skills questionnaire: Technical development. *Australian Occupational Therapy Journal* 43: 142–154.

Semi-Structured Interview

Tryssenaar, J., J. Ball, and K. Klassen. 1997. Employers' perceptions of occupational therapy in community mental health. *Occupational Therapy in Mental Health* 13(3): 63–79.

Sensorimotor History

Ayres, J. 1987. In *A therapist's guide to pediatric assessment*, eds. L. King-Thomas and B.J. Hacker, 335–336. Boston: Little, Brown.

Sensorimotor Integration Test Battery for CVA Clients

Jongbloed, L.E., J.B. Collins, and W. Jones. 1986. A sensorimotor integration test battery for CVA clients: Preliminary evidence of reliability and validity. *Occupational Therapy Journal of Research* 6(3): 132–150.

Ottenbacher, K.J., and D. Goar. 1986. A sensorimotor integration test battery for CVA clients: Preliminary evidence of reliability and validity. *Occupational Therapy Journal of Research* 6(3): 149–156. Commentary.

Sensorimotor Performance Analysis (SPA)

Richter, E.W., and P.E. Montgomery. 1989. *Sensorimotor Performance Analysis*. San Antonio, TX: Therapy Skill Builders/The Psychological Corporation.

Sensory Assessment for Children Battery

Cooper, J., A. Majnemer, B. Rosenblatt, and R. Birnbaum. 1994. Clinical concern: A standardized sensory assessment for children of school age. *Physical and Occupational Therapy in Pediatrics* 13(1): 61–80.

Sensory Integration and Praxis Tests (SIPT)

Ayres, A.J. 1991. *Sensory Integration and Praxis Tests*. Los Angeles: Western Psychological Services.

Ayres, A.J., and D.B. Marr. 1991. *Sensory Integration and Praxis Tests*. In *Sensory integration: Theory and practice*, eds. A.G. Fisher, E.A. Murray, and A.C. Bundy, 203–233. Philadelphia: F.A. Davis.

Cermak, S.A., and E.A. Murray. 1991. The validity of the constructional subtests of the Sensory Integration and Praxis Tests. *American Journal of Occupational Therapy* 45(6): 539–543.

Chu, S. 1996. Evaluation the sensory integrative functions of mainstream schoolchildren with specific developmental disorders. *British Journal of Occupational Therapy* (10): 465–474.

Conoley, J.J., and J.C. Impacta. 1995. *Twelfth mental measurement yearbook,* 944–946. Lincoln, NE: Buros Institute of Mental Measurement. Review.

Kimball, J. 1990. Using the Sensory Integration and Praxis Tests to measure change: A pilot study. *American Journal of Occupational Therapy* 44(7): 603–608.

Mailloux, Z. 1990. An overview of the Sensory Integration and Praxis Tests. *American Journal of Occupational Therapy* 44(7): 589–594.

McAtee, S., and W. Mack. 1990. Relations between design copying and other tests of sensory integrative dysfunction: A pilot study. *American Journal of Occupational Therapy* 44(7): 596–601.

Mulligan, S. 1998. Patterns of sensory integration dysfunction: A confirmatory factor analysis. *American Journal of Occupational Therapy* 52(10): 819–828.

Pierangelo, R., and G. Giuliani. 1998. Sensory Integration and Praxis Test (SIPT). In *Special educator's complete guide to 109 diagnostic tests*, 243–244. West Nyack, NY: Center for Applied Research in Education. Critique.

Stallings-Sahler, S. 1990. Report of an occupational therapy evaluation of sensory integration and praxis. *American Journal of Occupational Therapy* 44(7): 650–653.

Tupper, L.C. 1990. Report of an occupational therapy evaluation using the Sensory Integration and Praxis Tests. *American Journal of Occupational Therapy* 44(7): 647–649.

Sensory Integration Inventory for Individuals with Developmental Disabilities

Reisman, J.E., and B. Hanschu. 1992. *Sensory integration inventory for individuals with developmental disabilities*. San Antonio, TX: Therapy Skill Builders.

Sensory Integration Inventory for Individuals with Developmental Disabilities—Revised

Reisman, J.E., and B. Hanschu. 1996. *Sensory integration inventory for individuals with developmental disabilities*, rev. ed. San Antonio, TX: Therapy Skill Builders/The Psychological Corporation.

Sensory Profile

Bennet, D., and W. Dunn. In press. Comparison of sensory characteristics of children with and without attention deficit hyperactivity disorders. *American Journal of Occupational Therapy*.

Dunn, W. 1994. Performance of typical children on the Sensory Profile: An item analysis. *American Journal of Occupational Therapy* 48(11): 967–974.

Dunn, W. 1997. The Sensory Profile: A discriminating measure of sensory processing in daily life. *Sensory Integration Special Interest Section Quarterly* 20(1): 1–3.

Dunn, W. 1997. The Sensory Profile: The performance of a national sample of children with disabilities. *American Journal of Occupational Therapy* 51(1): 25–34.

Dunn, W., and C. Brown. 1997. Factor analysis on the Sensory Profile from a national sample of children without disabilities. *American Journal of Occupational Therapy* 51(7): 490–495.

Dunn, W., and K. Westman. 1995. *The Sensory Profile*. Kansas City: University of Kansas Medical Center. Unpublished manuscript.

Ermer, J., and W. Dunn. 1998. Sensory Profile: A discriminant analysis of children with and without disabilities. *American Journal of Occupational Therapy* 52(4): 283–290.

Kientz, M.A., and W. Dunn. 1997. A comparison of the performance of children with and without autism on the Sensory Profile. *American Journal of Occupational Therapy* 51(4): 530–537.

Miller L.J., and D.N. McIntosh. 1998. The diagnosis and treatment and etiology of sensory modulation disorder. *Sensory Integration Special Interest Section Quarterly* 21(1): 1–3.

Sensory Rating Scale for Infants and Young Children

Provost, B., and P. Oetter. 1993. The Sensory Rating Scale for Infants and Young Children: Development and reliability. *Physical and Occupational Therapy in Pediatrics* 13(4): 15–35.

Sensory Sensitivity Checklist

Ayres, J.A., and L.S. Tickle. 1980. Hyperresponsivity to touch and vestibular stimuli as a predictor of positive response to sensory integration procedures by autistic children. *American Journal of Occupational Therapy* 34(6): 375–381.

Sensory System Inventory

Farber, S.D. 1982. *Neurorehabilitation: A multisensory approach*, 111–113. Philadelphia: Saunders.

Sequential Occupational Dexterity Assessment (SODA)

O'Connor, D., B. Kortman, A. Smith, M. Ahern, M. Smith, and J. Krishnan. 1999. Correlation between objective and subjective measures of hand function in patients with rheumatoid arthritis. *Journal of Hand Therapy* 12(4): 323–329.

Van Lankveld, W., P. van't Pad Bosch, J. Bakker, S. Terwindt, M. Franssen, and P. van Riel. 1996. Sequential Occupational Dexterity Assessment (SODA): A new test to measure hand disability. *Journal of Hand Therapy* 9(1): 27–32.

Shoemyen Battery

Shoemyen, C. 1970. Occupational therapy orientation and evaluation: A study of procedure and media. *American Journal of Occupational Therapy* 24(4): 276–279.

Shoemyen, C. 1982. Shoemyen Battery. In *Evaluative process in psychiatric occupational therapy*, ed. B.J. Hemphill, 63–83, 343–350. Thorofare, NJ: Slack.

Similarity Scale

Eberhart, K.E., and W. Mayberry. 1994. *Similarity Scale*. Ohio State University Medical Center, 287 Doon Hall, 410 West 10th Avenue, Columbus, OH 43210.

Factors influencing entry-level occupational therapists' attitudes toward persons with disabilities. *American Journal of Occupational Therapy* 1995; 49(7): 629–636.

Sitting Assessment for Children with Neuromotor Dysfunction (SACND)

Reid, D.T. 1996. Sitting Assessment for Children with Neuromotor Dysfunction. San Antonio, TX: Therapy Skill Builders/The Psychological Association.

Smaga and Ross Integrated Battery (SARIB)

Smaga, B., and M. Ross. 1997. Smaga and Ross Integrated Battery. In *Integrative group therapy mobilizing coping abilities with the five-stage group*, ed. M. Ross, 121–166, 179–189. Bethesda, MD: American Occupational Therapy Association.

Smith Hand Function Evaluation

Baron, M., E. Dutil, L. Berkson, P. Lander, and R. Becker. 1987. Hand function in the elderly: Relation to osteoarthritis. *Journal of Rheumatology* 14(4): 815–819.

Smith, H.B. 1973. Smith Hand Function Evaluation. *American Journal Occupational Therapy* 27(5): 244–251.

Smith Physical Capacities Evaluation. See Physical Capacities Evaluation.

Social Support Inventory for Stroke Survivors
McColl, M.A., and J. Friedland. 1989. Development of a multidimensional index for assessing social support in rehabilitation. *Occupational Therapy Journal of Research* 9(4): 218–234.

Solet Test for Apraxia
Available from Jo M. Solet, MOT, OTR, *Solet Test for Apraxia*, 5 Channing Road, Newton Center, MA 02159.
Siev, E., and B. Freishtat. 1976. *Perceptual dysfunction in the adult stroke patient: A manual for evaluation and treatment*, 71–72. Thorofare, NJ: Slack.
Siev, E., B. Freishtat, and B. Zoltan. 1986. *Perceptual dysfunction in the adult stroke patient: A manual for evaluation and treatment*, 2nd ed., 48–49. Thorofare, NJ: Slack.
Zoltan, B. 1996. *Vision, perception, and cognition: A manual for the evaluation and treatment of the neurologically impaired adult*, 3rd ed., 57. Thorofare, NJ: Slack.

Sorting Pictures of Objects
Toglia, J.P. 1989. Approaches to cognitive assessment of the brain-injured adult: Traditional methods and dynamic investigation. *Occupational Therapy Practice* 1(1): 36–57.

Southern California Figure-Ground Visual Perception Test
Ayres, A.J. 1966. *Southern California Figure-Ground Visual Perception Test*. Los Angeles: Western Psychological Services.
Bieliauskas, L.A., B.H. Newberry, and T.J. Gerstenberger. 1988. Young adult norms for the Southern California Figure-Ground Visual Perception Test. *Clinical Neuropsychologist* 2(3): 239–245.
Petersen, P., and R.L. Wikoff. 1983. The performance of adult males on the Southern California Figure-Ground Visual Perception Test. *American Journal of Occupational Therapy* 37(8): 354–360.
Peterson, P., D. Goar, and J. Van Deusen. 1985. Performance of female adults on the Southern California Visual Figure-Ground Perception Test. *American Journal of Occupational Therapy* 39(8): 525–530.
Zoltan, B. 1996. Visual discrimination skills. In *Vision, perception, and cognition: A manual for the evaluation and treatment of the neurologically impaired adult*, 3rd ed., 96–98. Thorofare, NJ: Slack.

Southern California Kinesthesia and Tactile Perception Tests
Ayres, A.J. 1966. *Southern California Kinesthesia and Tactile Perception Tests*. Beverly Hills CA: Western Psychological Services.

Southern California Motor Accuracy Test
Ayres, A.J. 1964. *Southern California Motor Accuracy Test*. Los Angeles: Western Psychological Services.

Southern California Motor Accuracy Test—Revised
Bunker, L.K. 1985. Review of Southern California Motor Accuracy Test—Revised. In *Ninth mental measurements yearbook*, ed. J.V. Mitchell, 1413–1415. Lincoln: University of Nebraska Press.
Hogan, J. 1985. *Southern California Motor Accuracy Test—Revised*. In *Critiques*, vol. 3, eds. D.J. Keyser and R.C. Sweetland, 615–620. Austin, TX: PRO-ED.
Saeki, K., F. Clark, and S.P. Azen. 1985. Performance of Japanese and Japanese-American children on the Motor Accuracy—Revised and design copying tests of the Southern California Sensory Integration Tests. *American Journal of Occupational Therapy* 39(2): 103–109.

Southern California Perceptual-Motor Test

Ayres, A.J. 1968. *Southern California Perceptual-Motor Test.* Los Angeles: Western Psychological Services.

Southern California Postrotary Nystagmus Test

Ayres, A.J. 1975. *Southern California Postrotary Nystagmus Test.* Los Angeles: Western Psychological Services.

DeGangi, G.A. 1987. In *A therapist's guide to pediatric assessments*, eds. L. King-Thomas and B.J. Hacker, 199–205. Boston: Little, Brown.

Deitz, J., C.B. Siegner, and T.K. Crow. 1981. The Southern California Postrotary Nystagmus Test: Test-retest reliability for preschool children. *Occupational Therapy Journal of Research* 1(2): 166–177.

Keating, N.R. 1979. A comparison of duration of nystagmus as measured by the Southern California Postrotary Nystagmus Test and electronystagmography. *American Journal of Occupational Therapy* 33(2): 92–97.

Kimball, J.G. 1981. Normative comparison of the Southern California Postrotary Nystagmus Test: Los Angeles vs. Syracuse data. *American Journal of Occupational Therapy* 35(1): 21–25.

Morrison, D., and J. Sublett. 1983. Reliability of the Southern California Postrotary Nystagmus Test with learning-disabled children. *American Journal of Occupational Therapy* 37(10): 694–698.

Nelson, D.L., N.K. Weidensaul, V.G. Anderson, and L.S. Shih. 1984. The Southern California Postrotary Nystagmus Test and electronystagmography under different conditions of visual input. *American Journal of Occupational Therapy* 38(8): 535–540.

Polatajko, H.J. 1983. The Southern California Postrotary Nystagmus Test: A validity study. *Canadian Journal of Occupational Therapy* 50(4): 119–123.

Punwar, A. 1982. Expanded normative data: Southern California Postrotary Nystagmus Test. *American Journal of Occupational Therapy* 36(3): 183–187.

Rourke, B.P. 1985. Review of Southern California Postrotary Nystagmus. In *Ninth mental measurements yearbook*, ed. J.V. Mitchell, 1416–1417. Lincoln: University of Nebraska Press.

Royeen, C. 1980. Factors affecting test-retest reliability of the Southern California Postrotary Nystagmus Test. *American Journal of Occupational Therapy* 34(1): 37–39.

Royeen, C.B., G. Lesinski, S. Ciani, and D. Schneider. 1981. Relationship of the Southern California Sensory Integrations Tests, the Southern California Postrotary Nystagmus Test, and clinical observations accompanying them to evaluations in otolaryngology, ophthalmology, and audiology: Two descriptive case studies. *American Journal of Occupational Therapy* 35(7): 443–450.

Weiss-Lambrou, R., S. Messier, and U. Maag. 1988. Montreal normative data for the Southern California Postrotary Nystagmus Test. *Canadian Journal of Occupational Therapy* 55(4): 200–205.

Wilson, B.N., B.J. Kaplan, and P.D. Farris. 1992. Test-retest reliability of the Southern California Postrotary Nystagmus Test in children with motor coordination problems. *Occupational Therapy Journal of Research* 12(2): 83–95.

Southern California Sensory Integration Tests

Ayres, A.J. 1980. *Southern California Sensory Integration Tests.* Los Angeles: Western Psychological Services.

Ayres, A.J. 1981. Standard errors of measurement of the SCSIT converted into proportions of a standard deviation and smoothed to best fit. *Center for the Study of Sensory Integrative Dysfunction Newsletter* 9(2): 5.

DeGangi, G.A. 1987. In *A therapist's guide to pediatric assessment*, eds. L. King-Thomas and B.J. Hacker, 206–214. Boston: Little, Brown.

Evans, P.R., and A.S. Peham. 1981. *Testing and measurement in occupational therapy: A review of current practice with special emphasis on the Southern California Sensory Integration Tests*. Monograph No. 15. Minneapolis, MN: University of Minnesota Institute for Research on Learning Disabilities.

Fairgrieve, E.M. 1989. Alternative means of assessment: A comparison of standardised tests identifying minimal cerebral dysfunction. *British Journal of Occupational Therapy* 52(3): 88–92.

Reed, H.B. 1978. Southern California Sensory Integration Tests. In *Eighth mental measurements yearbook*, ed. O.K. Buros, 874–876. Lincoln: University of Nebraska Press.

Royeen, C.B., G. Lesinski, S. Ciani, and D. Schneider. 1981. Relationship of the Southern California Sensory Integration Tests, the Southern California Postrotary Nystagmus Test, and clinical observations accompanying them to evaluations in otolaryngology, ophthalmology, and audiology: Two descriptive case studies. *American Journal of Occupational Therapy* 35(7): 443–450.

Saeki, K., F.A. Clark, and S.P. Azen. 1985. Performance of Japanese and Japanese-American children on the Motor Accuracy-Revised and Design Copying tests of the Southern California Sensory Integration Tests. *American Journal of Occupational Therapy* 39(2): 103–109.

Sattler, J.M. 1982. Southern California Sensory Integration Tests. In *Assessment of children's intelligence and special abilities*, 304–305. Boston: Allyn and Bacon. Review.

Yerxa, E.J. 1982. A response to testing and measurement in occupational therapy: A review of current practice with special emphasis on the Southern California Sensory Integration Tests. *American Journal of Occupational Therapy* 36(6): 399–404.

Spatial, Temporal, and Physical Analysis of Motor Control: A Comprehensive Guide to Reflexes and Reactions

McCormack, D.B., and K.R. Perrin. 1997. *Spatial, temporal, and physical analysis of motor control: A comprehensive guide to reflexes and reactions*. San Antonio, TX: Therapy Skill Builders/The Psychological Corporation.

Special Services Screening Tool

Short, M.A., and G.N. Fincher. 1983. Intercorrelations among three preschool screening instruments. *Occupational Therapy Journal of Research* 3(3): 181–182.

Spinal Function Sort

Matheson, L.M., and M.L. Matheson. *Spinal Function Sort*. Rancho Santa Margarita, CA: Performance Assessment and Capacity Testing.

Matheson, L.N., M.L. Matheson, and J.E. Grant. 1993. Development of a measure of perceived functional ability. *Journal of Occupational Rehabilitation* 3: 15–30.

Matheson, L.N., V. Mooney, J.E. Grant, M. Affleck, H. Hall, T. Melles, R.L. Lichter, and G. McIntosh. 1995. A test to measure lift capacity of physically impaired adults—Part 1: Development and reliability testing. *Spine* 20: 2119–2129.

St. George Hospital Memory Disorders Clinic Occupational Therapy Assessment Scale (OTAS)

Fairbrother, G., D. Burke, K. Kell, R. Schwartz, and W. Schuld. 1997. Development of the St. George Hospital Memory Disorders Clinic Occupational Therapy Assessment Scale. *International Psychogeriatrics* 9(2): 115–122.

St. Mary's CVA Evaluation

Harlowe, D., and Van Deusen, J. 1984. Construct validation of the St. Mary's CVA Evaluation: Perceptual measures. *American Journal of Occupational Therapy* 38(3): 184–186.

Van Deusen, J., and D. Harlowe. 1984. Construct validation or occupational therapy measures used in CVA evaluation: A beginning. *American Journal of Occupational Therapy* 38(2): 101–106.

Van Deusen, J., and D. Harlowe. 1986. Continued construct validation of the St. Mary's CVA Evaluation: Brunnstrom arm and hand stage ratings. *American Journal of Occupational Therapy* 40(8): 561–563.

Van Deusen, J., and D. Harlowe. 1987. Continued construct validation of the St. Mary's CVA Evaluation: Bilateral Awareness Scale. *American Journal of Occupational Therapy* 41(4): 242–245.

Van Deusen, J., L. Shalik, and D. Harlowe. 1990. Construct validation of an acute care occupational therapy cerebral vascular accident assessment tool. *Canadian Journal of Occupational Therapy* 57(3): 155–159.

Standardized Test of Hand Function

Fraser, C., and J. Fusco. 1981. A standardized test of hand function. *British Journal of Occupational Therapy* 44(8): 258–260.

Stereognostic Test

Tyler, N.B. 1972. A stereognostic test for screening tactile sensation. *American Journal of Occupational Therapy* 26(5): 256–260.

Stress Management Questionnaire

Stein, F., and S. Nikolic. 1989. Teaching stress management techniques to a schizophrenic patient. *American Journal of Occupational Therapy* 43(3): 162–169. Form included.

Stein, F., D.E. Bentley, and M. Natz. 1999. Computerized assessment: The Stress Management Questionnaire. In *Assessments in occupational therapy mental health: An integrative approach*, ed. B.J. Hemphill-Pearson, 321–337. Thorofare, NJ: Slack.

Structured Observational Test of Function (SOTOF)

Laver, A.J. 1994. The Structured Observational Test of Function. *Gerontology Special Interest Section Newsletter* 17(1): 1–3.

Laver, A.J. 1995. Structured Observational Test of Function. NFER-NELSON Publishing Company Ltd., Windsor, Berkshire SL4 1DF, England

Laver, A.J., and C. Unsworth. 1999. Evaluation and intervention with simple perceptual impairment (Agnosias). In *Cognitive and perceptual dysfunction: A clinical reasoning approach to evaluation and intervention*, ed. C. Unsworth, 299–356. Philadelphia: F.A. Davis. Form included.

Unsworth, C. 1999. Structured Observational Test of Function (SOTOF). In *Cognitive and perceptual dysfunction: A clinical reasoning approach to evaluation and intervention*, ed. C. Unsworth, 86–89. Philadelphia: F.A. Davis.

Student Role Expectation Inventory

Furgang, N.T., and E.J. Yerxa. 1979. Expectations of teachers for physically handicapped and normal first-grade students. *American Journal of Occupational Therapy* 33(11): 697–704.

Sunnaas Index of ADL

Korpelainen, J.T., E. Niileksela, and V.V. Myllyla. 1997. The Sunnaas Index of Activities of Daily Living: Responsiveness and concurrent validity in stroke. *Scandinavian Journal of Occupational Therapy* 4, 31–36.

Vardeberg, K. 1994. The Sunnaas Index of ADL: Applicable, reliable, and valid? In *Proceedings of the Eleventh International Congress of the World Federation of Occupational Therapists*. London. Abstract.

Vardeberg, K., M. Kolsrud, and T. Laberg. 1991. Sunnaas Index of ADL. *WFOT Bulletin* 24, 30–35.

Tactile Sensitivity Profile

Parush, S., A. Gal, and N. Heimann. 1994. Age-related profiles of tactile sensitivity in normal children ages 1½ and 2½ years old. *Israel Journal of Occupational Therapy* 3(1): E14–E28.

Takata Play History. See Play History.

Teacher Questionnaire on Sensorimotor Behavior (TQSB)

Carrasco, R.C., and C.E. Lee. 1993. Development of a teacher questionnaire on sensorimotor behavior. *Sensory Integration Special Interest Newsletter* 16(3): 5,6. Available from R.C. Carrasco, Medical College of Georgia, EF-102, Augusta, GA 30912.

Telephone Interview Instrument

Lawlor, M.C. 1994. Development of a standardized Telephone Interview Instrument. *Occupational Therapy Journal of Research* 14(1): 39–52.

Tell Us What Your Drawings Say

Sheffer, M., and S. Harlock. 1980. Tell Us What Your Drawings Say. *Occupational Therapy in Mental Health* 1(2): 21–38.

Williams, S.K. Next steps in validation: Comments on "Tell Us What Your Drawings Say." *Occupational Therapy in Mental Health* 1(2): 39–40.

TEMPA

Desrosiers, J., R. Hebert, G. Bravo, and E. Dutil. 1994. Upper extremity performance test for the elderly (TEMPA): Normative data and correlates with sensorimotor parameters. *Archives of Physical Medicine and Rehabilitation* 76(12): 1125–1129.

Desrosiers, J., R. Hebert, E. Dutil, and G. Bravo. 1993. Development and reliability of an upper extremity function test for the elderly: The TEMPA. *Canadian Journal of Occupational Therapy* 60(1): 9–16.

Desrosiers, J., R. Hebert, E. Dutil, and G. Bravo. 1993. *TEMPA administration manual*. Sherbrook, Quebec: Centre de Recherche Gerontlogie et Geriatrie.

Derosiers, J., R. Hebert, E. Dutil, G. Bravo, and L. Mercier. 1994. Validity of the TEMPA: A measurement instrument for upper extremity performance. *Occupational Therapy Journal of Research* 14(4): 267–281.

Temporal Pattern Questionnaire. See also Activity Configuration (Watanabe). (Modification of Watanabe's Activity Configuration and Gregory's Meaningfulness of Activity Scale)

Weeder, T.C. 1986. Comparison of temporal patterns and meaningfulness of daily activities of schizophrenic and normal adults. *Occupational Therapy in Mental Health* 6(4): 27–48.

Test for Apraxia

Longs-Christopher, B. 1993. Life's a maze: Treating patients with apraxia. *Occupational Therapy Forum* 8(8): 4–5, 8–9.

Test of Body Scheme

MacDonald, C.J. 1960. An investigation of body scheme in adults with cerebral vascular accidents. *American Journal of Occupational Therapy* 14(2): 75–79.

Test of Fine Finger Dexterity

Stein, C., and E.J. Yerxa. 1990. Test of Fine Finger Dexterity. *American Journal of Occupational Therapy* 44(6): 499–504.

Test of In-Hand Manipulation Skills

Exner, C.E. 1990. *Test of in-hand manipulation skills.* Occupational Therapy Department, Towson State University, Towson, MD 21204.

Exner, C.E. 1990. The zone of proximal development in in-hand manipulation skills of nondysfunctional 3- and 4-year-old children. *American Journal of Occupational Therapy* 44(10): 884–891.

Test of Infant Motor Performance (TIMP)

Campbell, S.K., E.T. Osten, T.H.A. Kolobe, and A.G. Fisher. 1993. Test of Infant Motor Performance. In *New developments in functional assessment,* eds. C.V. Granger and G.E. Gresham, 541–550. Philadelphia: W.B. Saunders.

Test of Motor and Neurological Functions

DeGangi, G.A., R.A. Berk, and J. Valvano. 1983. Test of Motor and Neurological Functions in high-risk infants: Preliminary findings. *Journal of Developmental and Behavioral Pediatrics* 4(3): 182–189.

Valvano, J., and G.A. DeGangi. 1986. Atypical posture and movement findings in high risk pre-term infants. *Physical and Occupational Therapy in Pediatrics* 6(2): 71–84.

Test of Orientation for Rehabilitation Patients (TORP)

Deitz, J., C. Beeman, and D.W. Thorn. 1993. *Test of Orientation for Rehabilitation Patients.* Tucson, AZ: Therapy Skill Builders. Protocol form.

Deitz, J.C., V.S. Tovar, D.W. Thorn, and C. Beeman. 1990. The Test of Orientation for Rehabilitation Patients: Interrater reliability. *American Journal of Occupational Therapy* 44(9): 784–790.

Zoltan, B. 1996. Orientation, attention, and memory. In *Vision, perception, and cognition: A manual for the evaluation and treatment of the neurologically impaired adult,* 3rd ed., 122. Thorofare, NJ: Slack.

Test of Playfulness (ToP)

Bundy, A. 1993. Test of playfulness. Department of Occupational Therapy, Colorado State University, Room 219, Occupational Therapy Building, Fort Collins, CO 80523.

Parham, L.D. and L. Fazio 1996. *Play in occupational therapy for children,* 52–66. St. Louis: Mosby Yearbook.

Test of Sensory Function in Infants (TSFI)

Albanese, M. 1992. Test of Sensory Functions in Infants. In *Eleventh mental measurements yearbook,* eds. J.J. Kramer and J.C. Conoley, 974–976. Lincoln: University of Nebraska Press.

Benson, A.M., and S.J. Lane. 1994. Intrarater reliability of the Test of Sensory Functions in Infants as used with infants exposed to cocaine in utero. *Occupational Therapy Journal of Research* 14(3): 170–177.

DeGangi, G.A. 1988. *Test of Sensory Function in Infants.* Los Angeles, CA: Western Psychological Services.

DeGangi, G.A., and S.I. Greenspan. 1988. The development of sensory functions in infants. *Physical and Occupational Therapy in Pediatrics* 8(4): 21–33.

DeGangi, G.A., R.A. Berk, and S.I. Greenspan. 1988. The clinical measurement of sensory functioning in infants: A preliminary study. *Physical and Occupational Therapy* 8(2/3): 1–23.

Jirikowic, T.L., J.M. Engel, and J.C. Deitz. 1997. The Test of Sensory Functions in Infants: Test-retest reliability for infants with developmental delays. *American Journal of Occupational Therapy* 51(9): 733–738.

Wiener, A.A., T. Long, G.A. DeGangi, and B. Battaile. 1996. Research report: Sensory processing of infants born prematurely or with regulatory disorders. *Physical and Occupational Therapy in Pediatrics* 16(4): 1–17.

Texture Discrimination and Object Recognition Test

King, P.M. 1997. Sensory function assessment: A pilot comparison study of touch pressure threshold with texture and tactile discrimination. *Journal of Hand Therapy* 10(1): 24–28.

Therapeutic Home Visit Survey

Durham, D.P. 1992. Occupational and physical therapists' perspective of the perceived benefits of a therapeutic home visit program. *Physical and Occupational Therapy in Geriatrics* 10(3): 15–33.

Toddler and Infant Motor Evaluation (TIME)

Miller, L.J., and G.H. Roid. 1994. *Toddler and Infant Motor Evaluation.* San Antonio, TX: Therapy Skill Builders/The Psychological Corporation.

Toglia Category Assessment (TCA) Test

Josman, N. 1994. Toglia Categorization Assessment (TCA) Test: Application in Israel. *Israel Journal of Occupational Therapy* 3(3): E94–E95.

Reliability and validity of the Toglia Category Assessment Test. *Canadian Journal of Occupational Therapy* 1999; 66(1): 33–42.

Toglia, J.P. 1989. Approaches to cognitive assessment of the brain-injured adult: Traditional methods and dynamic investigation. *Occupational Therapy Practice* 1(1): 36–55.

Toglia, J.P. 1992. Dynamic assessment of categorization: The Toglia Category Assessment. In *Cognitive rehabilitation: Models for intervention in occupational therapy,* ed. N. Katz, 118–124. Boston: Andover Medical Publishers.

Toglia, J.P. 1994. *Dynamic Assessment of Categorization: The Toglia Category Assessment.* Maddak, Inc., 6 Industrial Road, Pequanrock, NJ 07440-1993; or AliMed, Inc., 297 High Street, Dedham, MA 02026-9135.

Touch Inventory for Elementary-School-Aged Children (TIE)

Royeen, C.B. 1986. The development of a touch scale for measuring tactile defensiveness in children. *American Journal of Occupational Therapy* 40(6): 414–419.

Royeen, C.B. 1987. Test-retest reliability of a touch scale for tactile defensiveness. *Physical and Occupational Therapy in Pediatrics* 7(3): 45–52.

Royeen, C.B. 1990. Touch Inventory for Elementary School Aged Children. *American Journal of Occupational Therapy* 44(2): 155–159.

Royeen, C.B. 1997. *A research primer in occupational and physical therapy,* 67–72. Bethesda, MD: American Occupational Therapy Association.

Touch Inventory for Preschoolers (TIP)

Royeen, C.B. 1987. Touch Inventory for Preschoolers. *Physical and Occupational Therapy in Pediatrics* 7(1): 29–40.

Tri-Level ADL Assessment. See Maguire Tri-level ADL Assessment.

Tseng Teacher Handwriting Checklist

Tseng, M.H. 1994. Construct validity of the Tseng Teacher Handwriting Checklist. *Occupational Therapy International* 1(2): 90–102.

Tufts Assessment of Motor Performance

Gans, B.M., S.M. Haley, S.C. Hallenborg, N. Mann, C.A. Inacio, and R.M. Faas. 1988. Description and interobserver reliability of the Tufts Assessment of Motor Performance. *American Journal of Physical Medicine and Rehabilitation* 67(5): 202–210.

Haley, S.M., and L.H. Ludlow. 1992. Applicability of hierarchical scales of the Tufts Assessment of Motor Performance for school-aged children and adults with disabilities. *Physical Therapy* 72(3): 191–206.

Haley, S.M., L.H. Ludlow, B.M. Gans, R.M. Faas, and C.A. Inacio. 1991. Tufts Assessment of Motor Performance: An empirical approach to identifying motor performance categories. *Archives of Physical Medicine and Rehabilitation* 72(5): 359–366.

Upper Extremity Fitness for Duty Evaluation (UEFFDE)

King, J.W. 1993. Upper Extremity Fitness for Duty Evaluation. *Journal of Hand Therapy* 6(1): 57–58. Abstract.

Vancouver Burn Scar Assessment

deLinde, L.G. and W.K. Miles. 1995. Remodeling of scar tissue in the burned hand. In *Rehabilitation of the hand: Surgery and therapy*, eds. J.M. Hunter, E.J. Mackin, and A.D. Callahan, 1281–1282. St. Louis: Mosby.

Sullivan, T., J. Smith, J. Kermode, E. McIver, and D.J. Courtemanche. 1990. Rating the burn scar. *Journal of Burn Care and Rehabilitation* 11(3): 256–260.

Visual Neglect and Extinction Test

Anton, H.A., C. Hershler, and P. Lloyd. 1988. Visual neglect and extinction: A new test. *Archives of Physical Medicine and Rehabilitation* 69(12): 1013–1016.

Visual Response Evaluation

Davis, A.L. 1991. The Visual Response Evaluation: A pilot study of an evaluation tool for assessing visual responses in low-level brain-injured patients. *Brain Injury* 5(3): 315–320.

Volitional Questionnaire

Chern, J.S., G. Kielhofner, C.G. de las Heras, and L.C. Magelhaes. 1996. The volitional questionnaire: Pschyometric developments and practical use. *American Journal of Occupational Therapy* 50(7): 516–525.

De las Heras, C.G. 1988; 1993. *Volitional Questionnaire*. Available from Model of Human Occupation Clearinghouse, University of Illinois at Chicago, Department of Occupational Therapy, M/C 811, 1919 West Taylor Street, Chicago, IL 60612-7250; also available from American Occupational Therapy Association, 4720 Montgomery Lane, Bethesda, MD 20814-3425.

De las Heras, C.G. 1993. Validity and reliability of the Volitional Questionnaire. Unpublished master's thesis, Tufts University, Boston, MA.

Kielhofner, G. 1995. *A model of human occupation: Theory and Application*, 2nd ed., 209, 211–213, 247–249. Baltimore, MD: Williams & Wilkins. Questions, sample, and scoring.

Vulpe Assessment Battery

Jain, M., D. Turner, and T. Worrell. 1994. The Vulpe Assessment Battery and the Peabody Developmental Motor Scales: A preliminary study of concurrent validity between gross motor sections. *Physical and Occupational Therapy in Pediatrics* 14(1): 23–33.

Stowers, S., and C.J. Huber. 1987. Vulpe Assessment Battery. In *A therapist's guide to pediatric assessment*, eds. L. King-Thomas and B.J. Hacker, 122–129: Boston: Little, Brown.

Venn, J. 1987. Vulpe Assessment Battery. In *Test critiques*, vol. 4, eds. D. Keyser and R. Sweetland, 622–627. Austin TX: PRO-ED.

Vulpe, S. 1969. *Home care and management of the mentally retarded child and the assessment battery.* Downsview, Ontario, Canada. NIMR Publications.

Vulpe Assessment Battery—Revised (VAB-R)

Vulpe, S. 1994. *Vulpe Assessment Battery—Revised.* East Aurora, NY: Slosson Educational Publications.

WeeFIM—Functional Independence Measure for Children

Braun, S.L., and C.V. Granger. 1991. A practical approach to functional assessment in pediatrics. *Occupational Therapy Practice* 2(2): 46–51.

Braun, S.L., M.E. Msall, and C.V. Granger. 1991. *Manual for the Functional Independence Measure for Children (WeeFIM).* Buffalo, NY: Center for Functional Assessment Research, Uniform Data System for Medical Rehabilitation, State University of New York.

Dittman, S.S., G.E. Gresham, and C.V. Granger. 1997. *Functional assessment and outcome measures for the rehabilitation health profession,* 190–195. Gaithersburg, MD: Aspen Publishers.

Msall, M.E., S.L. Braun, and C.V. Granger. 1990. Use of the Functional Independence Measure for Children (WeeFIM): An interdisciplinary training tape. *Developmental Medicine and Child Neurology* 32(Suppl. 62): 46. Abstract.

Msall, M.E., K.M. DiGaudio, and L.C. Duffy. 1993. Use of functional assessment in children with disabilities. *Physical Medicine and Rehabilitation Clinics of North America* (3): 517–527.

Msall, M.E., K.M. DiGaudio, L.C. Duffy, S. LaForest, S. Braun, and C.V. Granger. 1994. WeeFIM normal sample of an instrument for tracking functional independence in children. *Clinical Pediatrics* 33(7): 421–430.

Msall, M.E., S. Mallen, B.T. Rogers, N. Catanzaro, and L.C. Duffy. 1991. Pilot use of a functional status measure at age 4-5 years in extremely premature infants after surfactant. *Developmental Medicine and Child Neurology* 33(Suppl. 64): 15–16.

Sperle, P.A., K.J. Ottenbacker, S.L. Braun, S.J. Lane, and S. Nochajski. 1997. Equivalence reliability of the Functional Independence Measure for Children (WeeFIM) administration methods. *American Journal of Occupational Therapy* 51(1): 35–41.

Westmead Home Safety Assessment

Clemson, L. 1997. *Home fall hazards and the Westmead Home Safety Assessment.* West Brunswick, Australia: Coordinates Publications.

Clemson, L., and M.H. Fitzgerald. 1998. Understanding assessment concepts with the occupational therapy context. *Occupational Therapy International* 5(1): 18–34.

Clemson, L., M.H. Fitzgerald, and R. Heard. 1999. Content validity of an assessment tool to identify home fall hazards: The Westmead Home Safety Assessment. *British Journal of Occupational Therapy* 62(4): 171–179.

Clemson, L., M.H. Fitzgerald, R. Heard, and R.G. Cumming. 1997. Types of hazards in the homes of elderly people. *Occupational Therapy Journal of Research* 17(3): 200–213.

Clemson, L., M.H. Fitzgerald, R. Heard, and R.G. Cumming. 1999. Inter-rater reliability of a home fall hazards assessment tool. *Occupational Therapy Journal of Research* 19(2): 83–100.

Clemson, L., M. Roland, and R.G. Cumming. 1992. Occupational therapy assessment of potential hazards in the homes of elderly people: An interrater reliability study. *Australian Occupational Therapy Journal* 39(3): 23–26.

Wheel Diagram

Bell, C.H., and P.L. Ingeman. 1983. A strategy for assessing occupational behavior. *Occupational Therapy in Mental Health* 3(2): 23–34.

Bell, C.H., M.M. Kavanaugh, K.C. Ridout, and F.E. Gainer. 1986. A strategy for assessing occupational behavior—Part II: An inter-rater reliability study. *Occupational Therapy in Mental Health* 6(3): 1–16.

Work Assessment Questions

Backman, C. 1998. Functional assessment. In *Rheumatologic rehabilitation series: Assessment and management* vol. 1., eds. J.L. Melvin and G. Jensen, 192–194. Bethesda, MD: American Occupational Therapy Association. Form included.

Melvin, J.L. 1989. Evaluation of activities of daily living at home, work, and leisure. In *Rheumatic disease in the adult and child: Occupational therapy and rehabilitation*, 3rd ed., ed. J.L. Melvin, 359–361. Philadelphia: F.A. Davis.

Work Box

Black, M.K., C.E. Nelson, P.A. Maurer, and D.F. Bauer. 1993. Test-retest reliability of the Work Box. *Work: A Journal of Prevention, Assessment, and Rehabilitation* 3(4): 26–34.

Speller, L., J.A. Trollinger, P.A. Maurer, C.E. Nelson, and D.F. Bauer. 1997. Comparison of the test-retest reliability of the Work Box using three administrative methods. *American Journal of Occupational Therapy* 51(7): 516–522.

Work Environment Impact Scale (WEIS)

Corner, R.A., G. Kielhofner, and F.L. Lin. 1997. Construct validity of a Work Environment Impact Scale. *Work: A Journal of Prevention, Assessment, and Rehabilitation* 9(1): 21–34.

Corner, R.A., G. Kielhofner, and F.L. Lin. 1997. *Work Environment Impact Scale*. Available from Model of Human Occupational Clearinghouse, University of Illinois at Chicago, Department of Occupational Therapy (M/C 811), College of Associated Health Professions, 1919 West Taylor Street, Chicago, IL 60612-7250; also available from American Occupational Therapy Association, 4720 Montgomery Lane, Bethesda, MD 20814-3425.

Kielhofner, G., J.S. Lai, L. Olson, L. Haglund, E. Ekbadh, and M. Hedlund. 1999. Psychometric properties of the work environment impact scale: A cross-cultural study. *Work: A Journal of Prevention, Assessment, and Rehabilitation* 12(1): 71–77.

Work Performance Inventory

Allen, C.K. 1985. *Occupational therapy for psychiatric diseases: Measurement and management of cognitive disabilities.* Boston: Little, Brown.

Worker Role Interview (WRI)

Baron, K.B., and M.J. Littleton. 1999. The model of human occupation: A return to work case study. *Work: Journal of Prevention, Assessment, and Rehabilitation* 12(1): 37–46.

Biernacki, S. 1993. Reliability of the Worker Role Interview. *American Journal of Occupational Therapy* 47(9): 797–803.

Fisher, G.S. 1999. Administration and application of the Worker Role Interview: Looking beyond functional capacity. *Work: Journal of Prevention, Assessment, and Rehabilitation* 12(1): 25–36.

Henry, A.D. 1998. Worker Role Interview. In *Willard and Spackman's occupational therapy*, 9th ed., eds. M.E. Neistadt and E.B. Crepeau, 164–165. Philadelphia: J.B. Lippincott. Overview.

Kielhofner, G. 1995. *A model of human occupation: Theory and application*, 2nd ed., 222–225, 233, 249–250, 366. Baltimore, MD: Williams & Wilkins. Overview.

Velozo, C., G. Kielhofner, and G. Fisher. 1992. *Worker Role Interview*. Available from Model of Human Occupational Clearinghouse, University of Illinois at Chicago, Department of Occupational Therapy (M/C 811), College of Associated Health Professions, 1919 West Taylor Street, Chicago, IL; also available from the American Occupational Therapy Association, 4720 Montgomery Lane, Bethesda, MD 20814-3425.

Working with Young Children and Their Families

Humphry, R., and S. Geissinger. 1992. Self-rating as an evaluation tool following continuing professional education. *Occupational Therapy Journal of Research* 12(2): 111–121.

Appendix D

References for Evaluation Procedures

COORDINATION (SEE MOTOR CONTROL AND MOTOR BEHAVIOR)

ENDURANCE

Trombly, C.A. 1996. Evaluation of motor performance-endurance. In *Occupational therapy for physical dysfunction*, 4th ed., ed. C.A. Trombly, 152–154. Baltimore, MD: Williams & Wilkins.

GRIP STRENGTH

Flood-Joy, M., and V. Mathiowetz. 1987. Grip-strength measurement: A comparison of three Jamar dynamometers. *Occupational Therapy Journal of Research* 7(4):235–243.

Mathiowetz, V. 1990. Effects of three trials on grip and pinch strength measurements. *Journal of Hand Therapy* 3(4):195–198.

Mathiowetz, V. 1990. Grip and pinch strength measurements. In *Muscle strength testing: Instrumented and non-instrumented systems*, ed. L.R. Amundsen, 163–177. New York: Churchill Livingstone.

Mathiowetz, V., et al. 1985. Grip and pinch strength: Normative data for adults. *Archives of Physical Medicine and Rehabilitation* 66:69–72.

Mathiowetz, V., C. Rennells, and L. Donahoe. 1985. Effect of elbow position on grip and key pinch strength. *Journal of Hand Surgery* 10A:694–697.

Mathiowetz, V. et al. 1984. Reliability and validity of hand strength evaluations. *Journal of Hand Surgery* 9A:222–226.

Mathiowetz, V., D.M. Wiemer, and S.M. Federman. 1986. Grip and pinch strength: Norms for 6- to 19-year-olds. *American Journal of Occupational Therapy* 40(10):705–711.

Trombly, C.A. 1996. Evaluation of biomechanical and physiological aspects of motor performance— Measurement of grasp and pinch. In *Occupational therapy for physical dysfunction*, 4th ed., ed. C.A. Trombly, 150–152. Baltimore, MD: Williams & Wilkins.

Woody, R., and V. Mathiowetz. 1988. Effect of forearm position on pinch strength measurements. *Journal of Hand Surgery* 1(3):123–126.

MOTOR CONTROL AND MOTOR BEHAVIOR

Mathiowetz, V., and J. Bass-Haugen. 1996. Evaluation of motor behavior: Traditional and contemporary views. In *Occupational therapy for physical dysfunction*, 4th ed., ed. C.A. Trombly, 157–185. Baltimore, MD: Williams & Wilkins.

Solomon, J.W. 1998. Evaluation of motor control. In *Physical dysfunction practice skills for the occupational therapy assistant*, ed. M.B. Early, 114–127. St. Louis: Mosby.

Undzis, M.F., B. Zoltan, and L.W. Pedretti. 1996. Evalution of motor control. In *Occupational therapy: Practice skills for physical dysfunction*, 4th ed., ed. L.W. Pedretti, 151–164. St. Louis: Mosby.

MUSCLE STRENGTH

Kendal, F.P., and E.K. McCreary. 1983. *Muscles: Testing and function*, 3rd ed. Baltimore, MD: Williams & Wilkins (not occupational therapists).

Pedretti, L.W. 1996. Evaluation of muscle strength. In *Occupational therapy: Practice skills for physical dysfunction*, 4th ed., ed. L.W. Pedretti, 109–149. St. Louis: Mosby.

Pedretti, L.W., and M.K. Davis. 1998. Evaluation of muscle strength. In *Physical dysfunction practice skills for the occupational therapy assistant*, ed. M.B. Early, 93–113. St. Louis: Mosby.

Trombly, C.A. 1996. Evaluation of biomechanical and physiological aspects of motor performance— Muscle strength. In *Occupational therapy for physical dysfunction*, 4th ed., ed. C.A. Trombly, 107– 150. Baltimore, MD: Williams & Wilkins.

MUSCLE TONE (SEE MOTOR CONTROL AND MOTOR BEHAVIOR)

PERCEPTUAL AND PERCEPTUAL MOTOR DEFICITS

Abreu, B. 1994. Perceptual and motor skills: Assessment and intervention strategies. In *AOTA self-study series: Cognitive rehabilitation, 8*, ed. C.B. Royeen, 1–48. Bethesda, MD: American Occupational Therapy Association.

Pedretti, L.W., B. Zoltan, and C.J. Wheatley. 1996. Evaluation and treatment of perceptual and perceptual motor deficits. In *Occupational therapy: Practice skills for physical dysfunction*, 4th ed., ed. L.W. Pedretti, 231–239. St. Louis: Mosby.

Pedretti, L.W., B. Zoltan, and C.J. Wheatley. 1998. Evaluation of perceptual and perceptual motor deficits. In *Physical dysfunction practice skills for the occupational therapy assistant*, ed. M.B. Early, 141–144. St. Louis: Mosby.

Quintana, L.A. 1996. Evaluation of perception and cognition. In *Occupational therapy for physical dysfunction*, 4th ed., ed. C.A. Trombly, 201–224. Baltimore, MD: Williams & Wilkins.

RANGE OF MOTION

American Academy of Orthopaedic Surgeons. 1965. *Joint motion: Method of measuring and recording*. Chicago: The Academy. Standard reference.

Pedretti, L.W. 1996. Evaluation of joint range of motion. In *Occupational therapy: Practice skills for physical dysfunction*, 4th ed., ed. L.W. Pedretti, 79–107. St. Louis: Mosby.

Pedretti, L.W., and M.K. Davis. 1998. Evaluation of joint range of motion. In *Physical dysfunction practice skills for the occupational therapy assistant*, ed. M.B. Early, 75–92. St. Louis: Mosby.

Trombly, C.A. 1996. Evaluation of biomechanical and physiological aspects of motor performance— Range of motion. In *Occupational therapy for physical dysfunction*, 4th ed., ed. C.A. Trombly, 73–106. Baltimore, MD: Williams & Wilkins.

REFLEXES AND REACTIONS

Fiorentino, M.R. 1973. *Reflex testing methods for evaluating CNS development*. Springfield, IL: Charles C. Thomas.

SENSATION

Bentzel, K. 1996. Evaluation of sensation. In *Occupational therapy for physical dysfunction*, 4th ed., ed. C.A. Trombly, 187–200. Baltimore, MD: Williams & Wilkins.

Pedretti, L.W. 1990. Evaluation of sensation and treatment of sensory dysfunction. In *Occupational therapy: Practice skills in physical dysfunction*, 3rd ed., eds. L.W. Pedretti and B. Zoltan, 177–193. St. Louis: Mosby.

Pedretti, L.W. 1998. Evaluation of sensation. In *Physical dysfunction practice skills for the occupational therapy assistant*, ed. M.B. Early, 129–140. St. Louis: Mosby.

Appendix E

References to Models in Occupational Therapy

ABREU'S QUADRAPHONIC APPROACH

Abreu, B.C. 1992. The quadraphonic approach: Management of cognitive-perceptual and postural control dysfunction. *Occupational Therapy Practice* 3(4):12–29.

Abreu, B.C. 1994. Perceptual motor skills. In *AOTA self-study series: Cognitive rehabilitation, 8*, ed. C.B. Royeen, 1–48. Rockville, MD: American Occupational Therapy Association.

Abreu, B.C. 1995. The effect of environmental regulations on postural control after stroke. *American Journal of Occupational Therapy* 49:517–525.

Abreu, B.C. 1998. The quadraphonic approach: Holistic rehabilitation for brain injury. In *Cognition and occupational rehabilitation: Cognitive models for intervention in occupational therapy*, ed. N. Katz, 51–97. Bethesda, MD: American Occupational Therapy Association.

Abreu, B.C., and J. Hinojosa. 1992. Process approach for cognitive-perceptual and postural control dysfunction for adults with brain injury. In *Cognitive rehabilitation: Models for intervention in occupational therapy*, ed. N. Katz, 167–194. Stoneham, MA: Butterworth-Heinemann.

Abreu, B.C., M. Duval, D. Gerber, et al. 1994. Occupational performance and the functional approach. In *AOTA self study series: Cognitive rehabilitation, 9*, ed. C.B. Royeen, 1–44. Rockville, MD: American Occupational Therapy Association.

Abreu, B., and J.P. Toglia. 1987. Cognitive rehabilitation: A model for occupational therapy. *American Journal of Occupational Therapy* 41:439–448.

Abreu, B.C. and P. Price-Lackey. 1994. Documentation and additional consideration. In *AOTA self-study series: Cognitive rehabilitation, 12*, ed. C.B. Royeen, 1–44. Rockville, MD: American Occupational Therapy Association.

Abreu, B.C., G. Seale, J. Podlesak, et al. 1996. Development of critical paths for postacute brain injury rehabilitation: Lesson learned. *American Journal of Occupational Therapy* 50:417–427.

Duchek, J.M., and B.C. Abreu. 1996. Meeting the challenges of cognitive disabilities. In *Occupational therapy: Enabling function and well-being*, eds. C. Christiansen and B. Baum, 288–311. Thorofare, NJ: Slack.

Farber, S.D., and B.C. Abreu. 1994. Understanding the brain and learning theories related to cognitive function and rehabilitation. *AOTA self-study series: Cognitive rehabilitation, 2*, ed. C.B. Royeen, 1–28. Rockville, MD: American Occupational Therapy Association.

ALLEN'S MODEL OF COGNITIVE DISABILITIES

Allen, C.K. 1982. Independence through activity: The practice of occupational therapy. *American Journal of Occupational Therapy* 36:731–739.

Allen, C.K. 1985. *Occupational therapy for psychiatric diseases: Measurement and management of cognitive disabilities.* Boston: Little, Brown.

Allen, C.K. 1987. Activity: Occupational therapy's treatment method. *American Journal of Occupational Therapy* 41:563–575.

Allen, C.K. 1988. Cognitive disabilities. In *Mental health focus skills for assessment and treatment,* ed. S.E. Robertson, 3–32. Rockville, MD: American Occupational Therapy Association.

Allen, C.K. 1988. Occupational therapy: Functional assessment of the severity of mental disorders. *Hospital and Community Psychiatry* 39(2):140–142.

Allen, C.K. 1988. Preface. The development of standardized clinical evaluations in mental health. *Occupational Therapy in Mental Health* 8:(1).

Allen, C.K. 1989. Psychiatry. In *Physical and occupational therapy: Drug implications for practice,* ed. T. Malone, 207–228. Philadelphia: J.B. Lippincott Co.

Allen, C.K. 1989. Treatment plans in cognitive rehabilitation. *Occupational Therapy Practice* 1(1): 1–8.

Allen, C.K. 1991. Cognitive disability and reimbursement for rehabilitation and psychiatry. *Journal of Insurance Medicine* 23:145–147.

Allen, C.K. 1992. Cognitive disabilities. In *Cognitive rehabilitation: Models for intervention in occupational therapy,* ed. N. Katz, 1–21. Boston: Andover Medical Publishers.

Allen, C.K. 1994. Creating a need-satisfying, safe environment: Management and maintenance approaches. In *AOTA self-study series: Cognitive rehabilitation, 11,* ed. C.B. Royeen, 1–36. Rockville, MD: American Occupational Therapy Association.

Allen, C.K. 1996. *Allen Cognitive Level Test manual.* Colchester, CT: S & S Worldwide.

Allen, C.K., and R.E. Allen. 1987. Cognitive disabilities: Measuring the social consequences of mental disorders. *Journal of Clinical Psychiatry* 48:185–191.

Allen, C.K., and T. Blue. 1996. Cognitive disabilities model: How to make clinical judgment. In *Cognition and occupation in rehabilitation: Cognitive models for intervention in occupational therapy,* ed. N. Katz, 225–279. Bethesda, MD: American Occupational Therapy Association.

Allen, C.K., C.A. Earhart, and T. Blue. 1992. *Occupational therapy treatment goals for the physically and cognitively disabled.* Bethesda, MD: American Occupational Therapy Association.

Allen, C.K., C.A. Earhart, and T. Blue. 1993. *Allen Diagnostic Model manual.* Colchester, CT: S & S Worldwide.

Allen, C.K., C.A. Earhart, and T. Blue. 1996. *Understanding the models of performance.* Ormond Beach, FL: Allen Conferences.

Allen, C.K., M. Foto, T. Moon-Sperling, et al. 1989. A medical review approach to Medicare outpatient documents. *American Journal of Occupational Therapy* 43:793–800.

Allen, C.K., J. Goldberg, and J. Tryssenaar. 1995. Treating attentional impairment. *Canadian Journal of Occupational Therapy* 62(1):49–51.

AYRES' MODEL OF SENSORY INTEGRATION

Ayres, A.J. 1954. Ontogenetic principles in the development of arm and hand functions. *American Journal of Occupational Therapy* 3:95–99.

Ayres, A.J. 1955. Proprioceptive facilitation elicited through the upper extremities. Part I: Background. *American Journal of Occupational Therapy* 9(1):1–9,50.

Ayres, A.J. 1955. Proprioceptive facilitation elicited through the upper extremities. Part II: Application. *American Journal of Occupational Therapy* 9(2):57–58,76–77.

Ayres, A.J. 1955. Proprioceptive facilitation elicited through the upper extremities. Part III: Specific application of occupational therapy. *American Journal of Occupational Therapy* 9(3):121–126,143.

Ayres, A.J. 1958. The visual-motor function. *American Journal of Occupational Therapy* 12(3):130–138,155–156.

Ayres, A.J. 1960. Occupational therapy for motor disorders resulting from impairment of the central nervous system. *Rehabilitation Literature* 21:302–310.

Ayres, A.J. 1961. Development of the body scheme in children. *American Journal of Occupational Therapy* 15(3):99–102,128.

Ayres, A.J. 1961. The role of gross motor activities in the training of children with visual motor retardation. *Journal of the American Optometric Association* 33:121–125.

Ayres, A.J. 1962. *Ayres Space Test*. Los Angeles: Western Psychological Services.

Ayres, A.J. 1962. Methods of evaluating perceptual-motor dysfunction. In *Proceedings of the World Federation of Occupational Therapy*, 113–117. Philadelphia: University of Pennsylvania.

Ayres, A.J. 1962. Perception of space of adult hemiplegic patients. *Archives of Physical Medicine and Rehabilitation* 43:552–555.

Ayres, A.J. 1963. Integration of information. In *Approaches to the treatment of patients with neuromuscular dysfunction, study course VI*, ed. C. Sattely, 49–57. Third International Congress of the World Federation of Occupational Therapy. Dubuque, IA: William C. Brown.

Ayres, A.J. 1963. Occupational therapy directed toward neuromuscular integration. In *Occupational therapy*, 3rd ed., eds. H.S. Willard and C.S. Spackman, 358–466. Philadelphia: J.B. Lippincott Co.

Ayres, A.J. 1963. Perceptual-motor training for children. In *Approaches to the treatment of patients with neuromuscular dysfunction, study course VI*, ed. C. Sattely, 17–22. Third International Congress of the World Federation of Occupational Therapy. Dubuque, IA: William C. Brown.

Ayres, A.J. 1963. The development of perceptual-motor abilities: A theoretical basis for treatment of dysfunction. *American Journal of Occupational Therapy* 17(6):221–225.

Ayres, A.J. 1964. *Perceptual-motor dysfunction in children*. Cincinnati: Greater Cincinnati District of the Ohio Occupational Therapy Association.

Ayres, A.J. 1964. Perspectives on neurological bases of reading. *Claremont Reading Conference* 28:113–118.

Ayres, A.J. 1964. *Southern California Motor-Accuracy Test*. Los Angeles: Western Psychological Services.

Ayres, A.J. 1964. Tactile functions: Their relation to hyperactive and perceptual motor behavior. *American Journal of Occupational Therapy* 18(1):6–11.

Ayres, A.J. 1965. A factor analytic study. *Perceptual and Motor Skills* 20:335–368.

Ayres, A.J. 1965. A method of measurement of degree of sensorimotor integration. *Archives of Physical Medicine and Rehabilitation* 46:433–435.

Ayres, A.J. 1966. Interrelations among perceptual-motor abilities in a group of normal children. *American Journal of Occupational Therapy* 20:288–292.

Ayres, A.J. 1966. Interrelationships among perceptual-motor functions in children. *American Journal of Occupational Therapy* 20:68–71.

Ayres, A.J. 1966. Interrelation of perceptual function and treatment. *Physical Therapy* 46(7):741–744.

Ayres, A.J. 1966. *Southern California Figure Ground Visual Perception Tests*. Los Angeles: Western Psychological Services.

Ayres, A.J. 1966. *Southern California Kinesthesia and Tactile Perception Tests*. Los Angeles: Western Psychological Services.

Ayres, A.J. 1967. Remedial procedures based on neurobehavioral constructs. In *Proceedings of the 1967 International Convocation on Children and Young Adults with Learning Disabilities*. Pittsburgh.

Ayres, A.J. 1968. *Effect of sensorimotor activity on perception and learning in the neurologically handicapped child (Project No. H-126)*. Los Angeles: University of Southern California (ERIC Document No. ED033757).

Ayres, A.J. 1968. Reading—A product of sensory integrative process. In *Perception and reading*, ed. H.K. Smith, 77–82. Newark, DE: International Reading Association.

Ayres, A.J. 1968. Reading—A product of sensory integrative process. In *The Development of sensory integrative theory and practice*, ed. A. Henderson, 167–175. Dubuque, IA: Kendall/Hunt Publishing.

Ayres, A.J. 1968. Sensory integrative processes and neuropsychological learning disabilities. In *Learning disabilities*, vol. III. Seattle, WA: Special Child Publication.

Ayres, A.J. 1968. *Southern California Perceptual-Motor Tests*. Los Angeles: Western Psychological Services.

Ayres, A.J. 1969. Deficits in sensory integration in educationally handicapped children. *Journal of Learning Disabilities* 2:160–168.

Ayres AJ. 1969. Relation between Gesell developmental quotients and later perceptual-motor performance. *American Journal of Occupational Therapy* 23:11–17.

Ayres, A.J. 1971. Characteristics of types of sensory integrative dysfunction. *American Journal of Occupational Therapy* 25(7):329–334.

Ayres, A.J. 1972. Basic concepts of occupational therapy for children with perceptual-motor dysfunction. In *Proceedings of the Twelfth World Congress of Rehabilitation International*. Sydney, Australia.

Ayres, A.J. 1972. Improving academic scores through sensory integration. *Journal of Learning Disabilities* 5:338–343.

Ayres, A.J. 1972. *Sensory integration and learning disorders*. Los Angeles: Western Psychological Services.

Ayres, A.J. 1972. Sensory integrative processes: Implications for the deaf-blind from research with learning disabled children. In *Proceedings of the National Symposium for Deaf-Blind*, ed. W.A. Blea, 81–89. Pacific Grove, CA: Asilomar.

Ayres, A.J. 1972. *Southern California Sensory Integration Tests*. Los Angeles: Western Psychological Services.

Ayres, A.J. 1972. Types of sensory integrative dysfunction among disabled learners. *American Journal of Occupational Therapy* 26(1):13–18.

Ayres, A.J. 1973. An interpretation of the role of the brain stem in intersensory integration. In *The body senses and perceptual deficit*, eds. A. Henderson and J. Coryell, 81–89. Rockville, MD: U.S. Department of Health, Education and Welfare.

Ayres, A.J. 1973. The influence of the vestibular system on the auditory and visual systems. In *New techniques for work with deaf-blind children*, eds. J.L. Horsley and W.J. Smith, 1–13. Denver, CO: Mountain Plains Regional Center.

Ayres, A.J. 1975. Sensorimotor foundations of academic ability. In *Perceptual and learning disabilities in children: Research and theory*, vol. 2, eds. W.M. Cruickshank and D.P. Hallahan, 301–358. Syracuse, NY: Syracuse University Press.

Ayres, A.J. 1975. *Southern California Postrotary Nystagmus Test*. Los Angeles: Western Psychological Services.

Ayres, A.J. 1976. *The effect of sensory integrative therapy on learning disabled children*. Los Angeles: University of Southern California.

Ayres, A.J. 1976. *Interpreting the Southern California Sensory Integration Tests*. Los Angeles: Western Psychological Services.

Ayres, A.J. 1977. Cluster analyses of measures of sensory integration. *American Journal of Occupational Therapy* 31(6):362–366.

Ayres, A.J. 1977. Dichotic listening performance in learning disabled children. *American Journal of Occupational Therapy* 31(7):441–446.

Ayres, A.J. 1977. Effects of sensory integrative therapy on the coordination of children with choreoathetoid movements. *American Journal of Occupational Therapy* 31(5):291–293.

Ayres, A.J. 1978. Learning disabilities and the vestibular system. *Journal of Learning Disabilities* 11:18–29.

Ayres, A.J. 1980. *Sensory integration and the child*. Los Angeles: Western Psychological Services.

Ayres, A.J. 1980. *Southern California Motor Accuracy Test, Revised*. Los Angeles: Western Psychological Services.

Ayres, A.J. 1980. *Southern California Sensory Integration Tests, Revised.* Los Angeles: Western Psychological Services.

Ayres, A.J. 1985. *Developmental dyspraxia and adult-onset apraxia.* Torrance, CA: Sensory Integration International.

Ayres, A.J. 1988. *Sensory Integration and Praxis Tests.* Los Angeles: Western Psychological Services.

Ayres, A.J., and Z.K. Mailloux. 1981. Influence of sensory integration procedures on language development. *American Journal of Occupational Therapy* 35(6):383–390.

Ayres, A.J., and Z.K. Mailloux. 1983. Possible pubertal effect on therapeutic gains in an autistic girl. *American Journal of Occupational Therapy* 37(8):535–540.

Ayres, A.J., and D.B. Marr. 1991. Sensory Integration and Praxis Tests. In *Sensory integration theory and practice*, eds. A.G. Fisher, E.A. Murray, and A.C. Bundy, 203–229. Philadelphia: F.A. Davis.

Ayres, A.J., and W. Reid. 1966. The self-drawing as an expression of perceptual-motor dysfunction. *Cortex* 2:254–265.

Ayres, A.J., and L.S. Tickle. 1980. Hyper-responsivity to touch and vestibular stimuli as a predictor of positive response to sensory integration procedures by autistic children. *American Journal of Occupational Therapy* 34(6):375–381.

Ayres, A.J., Z.K. Mailloux, and S. McAtee. 1985. An update of the Sensory Integration and Praxis Tests. *Sensory Integration Special Interest Section Newsletter* 8(3):1, 3–4.

Ayres, A.J., Z.K. Mailloux, and C.L. Wendler. 1987. Developmental dyspraxia. Is it a unitary function? *Occupational Therapy Journal of Research* 7(2):93–110.

BIOMECHANICAL MODEL

Colangelo, C.A. 1999. Biomechanical frame of reference. In *Frame of reference for pediatric occupational therapy*, 2nd ed., eds. P. Kramer and J. Hinojosa, 257–322. Baltimore: Lippincott, Williams & Wilkins.

Dutton, R. 1995. Biomechanical frame of reference. In *Clinical reasoning in physical disabilities*, ed. R. Dutton, 29–78. Baltimore: Williams & Wilkins.

Dutton, R. 1998. Biomechanical frame of reference. In *Willard and Spackman's occupational therapy*, 9th ed., eds. M.E. Neistadt and E.B. Crepeau, 540–542. Philadelphia: J.B. Lippincott.

Trombly, C.A. 1996. Evaluation of biomechanical and physiological aspects of motor performance. In *Occupational therapy for physical dysfunction*, 4th ed., ed. C.A. Trombly, 73–156. Baltimore: Williams & Wilkins.

BOBATH'S MODEL OF NEURODEVELOPMENT THERAPY

Bobath, B. 1948. For the physiotherapist: A new treatment of lesions of the upper motor neurone. *British Journal of Physical Medicine* 11:26–29.

Bobath, B. 1948. The importance of the reduction of muscle tone and the control of mass reflex action in the treatment of spasticity. *Occupational Therapy and Rehabilitation* 27:371–383.

Bobath, B. 1953. Control of postures and movements in the treatment of cerebral palsy. *Physiotherapy* 39:99–104.

Bobath, B. 1954. A study of abnormal postural reflex activity in patients with lesions of the central nervous system. *Physiotherapy* 40(9):259–267;40(10):295–300; 40(11):326; 40(12):295–300; 40(12):368; 41(1):146.

Bobath, B. 1955. The treatment of motor disorders of pyramidal and extra-pyramidal origin by reflex inhibition and by facilitation of movements. *Physiotherapy* 41(5):146–153.

Bobath, B. 1959. Observations on adult hemiplegia and suggestions for treatment. *Physiotherapy* 45(12):279–289.

Bobath, B. 1960. Observations on adult hemiplegia and suggestions for treatment. *Physiotherapy* 46(1):5–15.

Bobath, B. 1963. Treatment principles and planning in cerebral palsy. *Physiotherapy* 49(4):122–124.

Bobath, B. 1963. A neuro-developmental treatment of cerebral palsy. *Physiotherapy* 49(8):242–244.

Bobath, B. 1967. The very early treatment of cerebral palsy. *Developmental Medicine and Child Neurology* 9(4):373–390.

Bobath, B. 1967. The neuro-developmental treatment of cerebral palsy. *Journal of the American Physical Therapy Association* 47(11):1039–1041.

Bobath, B. 1969. The treatment of neuromuscular disorders by improving patterns of coordination. *Physiotherapy* 55(1):18–22.

Bobath, B. 1970. *Adult hemiplegia: Evaluation and treatment.* London, England: William Heinemann Medical Books.

Bobath, B. 1971. *Abnormal postural reflex activity caused by brain lesion,* 2nd ed. London, England: William Heinemann Medical Books.

Bobath, B. 1977. Treatment of adult hemiplegia. *Physiotherapy* 63:310–313.

Bobath, B. 1985. *Abnormal postural reflex activity caused by brain lesions,* 3rd ed. Gaithersburg, MD: Aspen Publishers.

Bobath, B. 1990. *Adult hemiplegia: evaluation and treatment,* 3rd ed. London, England: Heinemann Medical Books.

Bobath, K. 1959. The neuropathology of cerebral palsy and its importance in treatment and diagnosis. *Cerebral Palsy Bulletin* 1(8):13–33.

Bobath, K. 1959. The effect of treatment by reflex-inhibition and facilitation of movement in cerebral palsy. *Folia Psychiatric Neurologica et Neurochirurgica Neelandica* 62(5):448–457.

Bobath, K. 1960. The nature of the paresis in cerebral palsy. In *Child neurology and cerebral palsy,* 88–93. Oxford, England: Spastic Society Study Group.

Bobath, K. 1962. The prevention of mental retardation in patients with cerebral palsy. *Acta Paedopsychiatrica* 30:141–154.

Bobath, K. 1966. *The motor deficits in patients with cerebral palsy.* Clinics in Development Medicine, no. 23. London, England: Heinemann Medical Books.

Bobath, K. 1969. *The motor deficit in patients with cerebral palsy.* Clinics in Development Medicine, no. 23. London, England: The Spastic Society and William Heinemann Medical Books.

Bobath, K. 1971. The problem of spasticity in the treatment of patients with lesions of the upper motor neuron. In *Proceedings of the Sixth International Congress of the World Federation for Physical Therapists,* 456–464. Amsterdam: Assen van Gorcus.

Bobath, K. 1971. The normal postural reflex mechanism and its deviation in children with cerebral palsy. *Physiotherapy* 57:515–525.

Bobath, K. 1980. *A neurophysiological basis for the treatment of cerebral palsy.* Clinics in Development Medicine, no. 75. London, England: The Spastic Society and William Heinemann Medical Books.

Bobath, B., and K. Bobath. 1975. *Motor development in the different types of cerebral palsy.* London, England: William Heinemann Medical Books.

Bobath, B., and K. Bobath. 1984. The neurodevelopmental treatment. In *Management of the motor disorders of children with cerebral palsy,* ed. D. Scrutton, 6–18. Philadelphia: J.B. Lippincott.

Bobath, K., and B. Bobath. 1950. Spastic paralysis: Treatment of by the use of reflex inhibition. *British Journal of Physical Medicine* 13(6):121–127.

Bobath, K., and B. Bobath. 1952. A treatment of cerebral palsy: Based on the analysis of the patient's motor behaviour. *British Journal of Physical Medicine* 15:107–117.

Bobath, K., and B. Bobath. 1954. Treatment of cerebral palsy by the inhibition of abnormal reflex action. *British Orthopedic Journal* 11:88–98.

Bobath, K., and B. Bobath. 1955. Tonic reflexes and righting reflexes in the diagnosis and assessment of cerebral palsy. *Cerebral Palsy Review* 16(5):4–10.

Bobath, K., and B. Bobath. 1956. The diagnosis of cerebral palsy in infancy. *Archives of Diseases and Childhood* 31:408–414.

Bobath, K., and B. Bobath. 1956. Control of motor function in the treatment of cerebral palsy. *Australian Journal of Physiotherapy* 2(2):75–85.

Bobath, K, and B. Bobath. 1957. Control of motor function in the treatment of cerebral palsy. *Physiotherapy* 43(10):295–303.

Bobath, K., and B. Bobath. 1962. An analysis of the development of standing and walking patterns in patients with cerebral palsy. *Physiotherapy* 48(6):144–153.

Bobath, K., and B. Bobath. 1964. The facilitation of normal postural reactions and movements in the treatment of cerebral palsy. *Physiotherapy* 50(8):246–262.

Bobath, K., and B. Bobath. 1972. Diagnosis and assessment of cerebral palsy. Part 1. In *Physical therapy services in the developmental disabilities*, eds. P. Pearson and C. Williams, 31–113. Springfield, IL: Charles C. Thomas.

Bobath, K., and B. Bobath. 1972. The neurodevelopmental approach to treatment. Part 2. In *Physical therapy services in the developmental disabilities*, eds. P. Pearson and C. Williams, 114–185. Springfield, IL: Charles C. Thomas.

Bobath, K., and B. Bobath. 1974. The importance of memory traces of motor efferent discharges for learning skilled movement. *Developmental Medicine and Child Neurology* 16:837–838.

Bobath, B., and E. Cotton. 1965. A patient with residual hemiplegia: And his response to treatment. *Journal of the American Physical Therapy Association* 45:849–864.

Bobath, B., and N. Finnie. 1958. Re-education of movement patterns for everyday life in the treatment of cerebral palsy. *Occupational Therapy* 21(6):23–30.

BRUNNSTROM'S MODEL OF RECOVERY FROM HEMIPLEGIA

Brunnstrom, S. 1956. Associated reactions of the upper extremity in adult patients with hemiplegia. *Physical Therapy Review* 36:225–236.

Brunnstrom, S. 1961. Motor behavior in adult hemiplegic patients. *American Journal of Occupational Therapy* 15:6–12.

Brunnstrom, S. 1964. Recording gait patterns of adult hemiplegic patients. *Journal of the American Physical Therapy Association* 44(1):11–18.

Brunnstrom, S. 1964. Training the adult hemiplegic patient: Orientation of techniques to patient's motor behavior. In *Approach to the treatment of patients with neuromuscular dysfunction*, ed. C. Sattely, 44–48. Dubuque, IA: William C. Brown.

Brunnstrom, S. 1965. Walking preparation for adult patients with hemiplegia. *Journal of the American Physical Therapy Association* 45(1):17–29.

Brunnstrom, S. 1966. Motor testing procedures in hemiplegia based on recovery stages. *Journal of the American Physical Therapy Association* 46(4):357–375.

Brunnstrom, S. 1970. *Movement therapy in hemiplegia*. New York: Harper & Row.

COGNITIVE DISABILITIES

David, S.K., and W.T. Riley. 1990. The relationship of the Allen Cognitive Level Test to cognitive ability and psychopathology. *American Journal of Occupational Therapy* 44(6):493–498.

Heinmann, N.E., C.K. Allen, and E.J. Yerxa. 1989. The Routine Task Inventory: A tool for describing the functional behavior of the cognitively disabled. *Occupational Therapy Practice* 1:67–74.

Josman, N., and N. Katz. 1991. Problem-solving version of the Allen Cognitive Level (ACL) Test. *American Journal of Occupational Therapy* 45:331–338.

Katz, N., N. Josman, and N. Steinmetz. 1988. Relationship between cognitive disability theory and the model of human occupation in the assessment of psychiatric and nonpsychiatric adolescents. *Occupational Therapy in Mental Health* 8:31–43.

Kehrberg, K.L., M.A. Kuskowski, J.A. Mortimer, and T.D. Shoberg. 1992. Validating the use of an enlarged, easier-to-see Allen Cognitive Level Test in geriatrics. *Physical and Occupational Therapy in Geriatrics* 10(3):1–14.

Kiernan, K., and A. Stoudemire. 1989. Occupational therapy program development for medical-psychiatry units: A cognitive model. *General Hospital Psychiatry* 11:109–118.

Levy, L.L. 1986. A practical guide to the care of the Alzheimer's disease victim: The cognitive disability perspective. *Topics in Geriatric Rehabilitation* 1(2):16–26.

Levy, L.L. 1986. Coping with confusion: The cognitive disability perspective. *Gerontology Special Interest Section Newsletter* 9(3):1–3.

Levy, L.L. 1989. Activity adaptation in rehabilitation of the physically and cognitively disabled aged. *Topics in Geriatric Rehabilitation* 4(4):53–66.

Levy, L.L. 1998. The cognitive disabilities model in rehabilitation of older adults with dementia. In *Cognition and occupational rehabilitation: Cognitive models for intervention in occupational therapy*, ed. N. Katz, 195–221. Bethesda, MD: American Occupational Therapy Association.

Maddox, M.K., and T. Burns. 1997. Positive approaches to dementia care in the home. *Geriatrics* 52(Suppl.2):254–258.

Mayer, M.A. 1988. Analysis of information processing and cognitive disability therapy. *American Journal of Occupational* Therapy 42(3):176–183.

Wilson, D.S., C.K. Allen, G. McCormack, et al. 1989. Cognitive disability and routine task behaviors in a community based population with senile dementia. *Occupational Therapy Practice* 1:58–66.

DUNN ECOLOGY OF HUMAN PERFORMANCE

Dunn, W., C. Brown, L. McClain, and K. Westman. 1994. The ecology of human performance: A contextual perspective on human occupation. In *AOTA self-study series: The practice of the future: Putting occupation back into therapy, 1*, ed. C.B. Royeen, 1–56. Rockville, MD: American Occupational Therapy Association.

Dunn, W., C. Brown, and A. McGuigan. 1994. The ecology of human performance: A framework for considering the effect of context. *American Journal of Occupational Therapy* 48:595–607.

Dunn, W., L.H. McClain, C. Brown, and M.J. Youngstrom. 1998. The ecology of human performance. In *Willard and Spackman's occupational therapy*, 9th ed., eds. M.E. Neistadt and E.B. Crepeau, 521–524. Philadelphia: J.B. Lippincott.

DYNAMIC INTERACTIONAL MODEL/MULTICONTEXT MODEL

Josman, N. 1998. The dynamic interactional model in schizophrenia. In *A dynamic interactional model to cognitive rehabilitation*, ed. N. Katz, 151–164. Bethesda, MD: American Occupational Therapy Association.

KIELHOFNER'S MODEL OF HUMAN OCCUPATION

Barris, R., and G. Kielhofner. 1985. Generating and using knowledge in occupational therapy: Implication for professional education. *Occupational Therapy Journal of Research* 5(2):113–124.

Barris, R., and G. Kielhofner. 1986. Beliefs, perspectives, and activities of psychosocial occupational therapy educators. *American Journal of Occupational Therapy* 40(8):535–541.

Barris, R., G. Kielhofner, and D. Bauer. 1985. Educational experience and changes in learning and value preferences. *Occupational Therapy Journal of Research* 5(4):243–256.

Barris, R., G. Kielhofner, and D. Bauer. 1985. Learning preferences, values and student satisfaction. Occupational therapy students and physical therapy students. *Journal of Allied Health* 14(1):13–23.

Barris, R., G. Kielhofner, R. Burch-Martin, et al. 1986. Occupational function and dysfunction in three groups of adolescents. *Occupational Therapy Journal of Research* 6(5):301–317.

Barris, R., G. Kielhofner, R.E. Levine, et al. 1985. Occupation as interaction with the environment. In *A model of human occupation: Theory and application*, ed. G. Kielhofner, 42–62. Baltimore: Williams & Wilkins.

Barris, R., G. Kielhofner, and J. Watts. 1983. *Psychosocial occupational therapy: Practice in a pluralistic arena*. Laurel, MD: RAM Associates.

Barris, R., G. Kielhofner, and J. Watts. 1988. *Occupational therapy in psychosocial practice*. Thorofare, NJ: Slack.

Borell, L., P. Sandman, and G. Kielhofner. 1991. Clinical decision making in Alzheimer's disease. *Occupational Therapy in Mental Health* 11:111–124.

Duellman, M.K., R. Barris, and G. Kielhofner. 1986. Organized activity and the adaptive status of nursing home residents. *American Journal of Occupational Therapy* 40(9):618–622.

Fisher, A.G., G. Kielhofner, and C. Davis. 1989. Research values of occupational and physical therapists. *Journal of Allied Health* 18(2):143–155.

Harrison, H., and G. Kielhofner. 1986. Examining reliability and validity of the Preschool Play Scale with handicapped children. *American Journal of Occupational Therapy* 40(3):167–173.

Kielhofner, G. 1977. Temporal adaptation: A conceptual framework for occupational therapy. *American Journal of Occupational Therapy* 31(4):235–242.

Kielhofner, G. 1978. General systems theory. *American Journal of Occupational Therapy* 32(10):637–645.

Kielhofner, G. 1979. The temporal dimension in the lives of retarded adults: A problem of interaction and intervention. *American Journal of Occupational Therapy* 33(3):161–168.

Kielhofner, G. 1980. A model of human occupation. Part 2. Ontogenesis from the perspective of temporal adaptation. *American Journal of Occupational Therapy* 34(10):657–663.

Kielhofner, G. 1980. A model of human occupation. Part 3. Benign and vicious cycles. *American Journal of Occupational Therapy* 34(11):731–737.

Kielhofner, G. 1982. A heritage of activity: Development of theory. *American Journal of Occupational Therapy* 35(11):723–812.

Kielhofner, G., ed. 1983. *Health through occupation: Theory and practice in occupational therapy*. Philadelphia: F.A. Davis.

Kielhofner, G. 1984. An overview of research on the model of human occupation. *Canadian Journal of Occupational Therapy* 51(2):59–67.

Kielhofner, G., ed. 1985. *A model of human occupation: Theory and application*. Baltimore: Williams & Wilkins.

Kielhofner, G. 1985. The demise of diffidence: An agenda for occupational therapy. *Canadian Journal of Occupational Therapy* 52(4):165–171.

Kielhofner, G. 1986. A review of research on the model of human occupation. Part 1. *Canadian Journal of Occupational Therapy* 53(2):69–74.

Kielhofner, G. 1986. A review of research on the model of human occupation. Part 2. *Canadian Journal of Occupational Therapy* 53(3):129–134.

Kielhofner, G., and L. Barrett. 1998. The model of human occupation. In *Willard and Spackman's occupational therapy*, 9th ed., eds. M.E. Neistadt and E.B. Crepeau, 527–529. Philadelphia: J.B. Lippincott.

Kielhofner, G., and R. Barris. 1984. Collecting data on play: a critique of available methods. *Occupational Therapy Journal of Research* 4(3):150–180.

Kielhofner, G., and R. Barris. 1984. Mental health occupational therapy: Trends in literature and practice. *Occupational Therapy in Mental Health* 4(4):35–50.

Kielhofner, G., and R. Barris. 1986. Organization of knowledge in occupational therapy: A proposal and a survey of the literature. *Occupational Therapy Journal of Research* 6(2):67–84.

Kielhofner, G., and M. Brinson. 1989. Development and evaluation of an aftercare program for young chronic psychiatrically disabled adults. *Occupational Therapy in Mental Health* 9(2):1–25.

Kielhofner, G., and J.P. Burke. 1977. Occupational therapy after 60 years: an account of changing identity and knowledge. *American Journal of Occupational Therapy* 31(10): 676–689.

Kielhofner, G., and J.P. Burke. 1980. A model of human occupation. Part 1. Conceptual framework and content. *American Journal of Occupational Therapy* 34(9):572–581.

Kielhofner, G., and A.D. Henry. 1988. Development and investigation of the Occupational Performance History Interview. *American Journal of Occupational Therapy* 42(8):489–498.

Kielhofner, G., and S. Miyake. 1981. The therapeutic use of games with mentally retarded adults. *American Journal of Occupational Therapy* 35(6):375–382.

Kielhofner, G., and G. Nelson. 1983. A study of patient motivation and cooperation/participation in occupational therapy. *Occupational Therapy Journal of Research* 3(1):35–46.

Kielhofner, G., and M. Nicol. 1989. The model of human occupation: A developing conceptual tool for clinicians. *British Journal of Occupational Therapy* 52(6):210–214.

Kielhofner, G., and N. Takata. 1980. A study of mentally retarded persons: Applied research in occupational therapy. *American Journal of Occupational Therapy* 34(4):252–258.

Kielhofner, G., R. Barris, D. Bauer, et al. 1983. A comparison of play behavior in nonhospitalized and hospitalized children. *American Journal of Occupational Therapy* 37(5):304–312.

Kielhofner, G., R. Barris, and J.H. Watts. 1982. Habits and habit dysfunction: A clinical perspective for psychosocial occupational therapy. *Occupational Therapy in Mental Health* 2(1):1–21.

Kielhofner, G., J.P. Burke, and C.H. Igi. 1980. A model of human occupation. Part 4. Assessment and intervention. *American Journal of Occupational Therapy* 34(12):777–788.

Kielhofner, G., B. Harlan, D. Bauer, et al. 1986. The reliability of a historical interview with physically disabled respondents. *American Journal of Occupational Therapy* 40(8):551–556.

Lederer, J.M., G. Kielhofner, and J.H. Watts. 1985. Values, personal causation and skills of delinquents and nondelinquents. *Occupational Therapy in Mental Health* 5(2):59–77.

Neville, A., A. Kreisberg, and G. Kielhofner. 1985. Temporal dysfunction in schizophrenia. *Occupational Therapy in Mental Health* 5(1):1–19.

Oakley, F., G. Kielhofner, and R. Barris. 1985. An occupational therapy approach to assessing psychiatric patients' adaptive functioning. *American Journal of Occupational Therapy* 39(3):147–154.

Oakley, F., G. Kielhofner, R. Barris, et al. 1986. The Role Checklist: Development and empirical assessment of reliability. *Occupational Therapy Journal of Research* 6(3):157–170.

Smith, N.R., G. Kielhofner, and J.H. Watts. 1986. The relationships between volition, activity pattern, and life satisfaction in the elderly. *American Journal of Occupational Therapy* 40(4):278–283.

Smyntek, L., R. Barris, and G. Kielhofner. 1985. The model of human occupation applied to psychosocially functional and dysfunctional adolescents. *Occupational Therapy in Mental Health* 5(1):21–39.

Watts, J.H., G. Kielhofner, D.F. Bauer, et al. 1986. The assessment of occupational functioning: A screening tool for use in long-term care. *American Journal of Occupational Therapy* 40(4):231–240.

LAW'S CLIENT-CENTERED MODEL (OR THE PERSON-ENVIRONMENT-OCCUPATION MODEL OR THE CANADIAN MODEL)

Law, M. 1991. Muriel Driver memorial lecture: The environment: A focus for occupational therapy. *Canadian Journal of Occupational Therapy* 58:171–180.

Law, M. 1993. Evaluating activities of daily living: Directions for the future. *Canadian Journal of Occupational Therapy* 47:233–237.

Law, M., ed. 1998. *Client-centered occupational therapy*. Thorofare, NJ: Slack.

Law, M., S. Baptiste, A. Carswell, et al. 1994. Canadian occupational performance measure manual, 2nd ed. Toronto, Ontario, Canada: CAOT Publications ACE.

Law, M., S. Baptiste, and J. Mills. 1995. Client-centred practice: What does it mean and does it make a difference? *Canadian Journal of Occupational Therapy* 62:250–257.

Law, M., B. Cooper, D. Stewart, et al. 1994. Person-environment relations. *Work* 4:228–238.

Law, M., B. Cooper, S. Strong, et al. 1996. The person-environment-occupation model: A transactive approach to occupational performance. *Canadian Journal of Occupational Therapy* 63(1):9–23.

Law, M., B. Cooper, S. Strong, et al. 1996. Theoretical contexts for the practice of occupational therapy. In *Occupational therapy: Enabling function and well-being*, eds. C. Christensen and C. Baum, 72–102. Thorofare, NJ: Slack.

Law, M., H. Polatajko, S. Baptiste, et al. 1997. Core concepts in occupational therapy. In *Enabling occupation: An occupational therapy perspective*, 29–56. Ottawa, Ontario, Canada: Canadian Association of Occupational Therapists.

Law, M., S. Steinwender, and L. LeClair. 1998. Occupation, health and well-being: A review of research evidence. *Canadian Journal of Occupational Therapy* 65:81–91.

Letts, L., M. Law, P. Rigby, et al. 1994. Person-environment assessments in occupational therapy. *American Journal of Occupational Therapy* 48:608–618.

Sumsion, T. 1993. Client-centred practice: The true impact. *Canadian Journal of Occupational Therapy* 60(1):6–8.

Sumsion, T. 1997. Environmental challenges and opportunities of client-centred practice. *British Journal of Occupational Therapy* 60(2):53–56.

Sumsion, T., ed. 1999. *Client-centred practice in occupational therapy: A guide to implementation.* Edinburgh, Scotland: Churchill Livingstone.

MATHIOWETZ AND BASS-HAUGEN'S MOTOR CONTROL MODEL

Bass-Haugen, J., and V. Mathiowetz. 1996. Contemporary task-oriented approach. In *Occupational therapy for physical dysfunction*, 4th ed., ed. C.A. Trombly, 510–528. Baltimore: Williams & Wilkins.

Mathiowetz, V., and J. Bass-Haugen. 1994. Motor behavior research: Implications for therapeutic approaches to central nervous system dysfunction. *American Journal of Occupational Therapy* 48:733–745.

MODEL OF HUMAN OCCUPATION (MOHO)

Baron, K.B. 1987. The model of human occupation: A newspaper treatment group for adolescents with a diagnosis of conduct disorder. *Occupational Therapy in Mental Health* 7(2):89–104.

Baron, K.B. 1991. The use of play in child psychiatry: Reframing the therapeutic environment. *Occupational Therapy in Mental Health* 11:37–56.

Barris, R. 1986. Occupational dysfunction and eating disorders: Theory and approach to treatment. *Occupational Therapy in Mental Health* 6(1):27–45.

Barris, R., V. Dickie, and K.B. Baron. 1988. A comparison of psychiatric patients and normal subjects based on the model of human occupation. *Occupational Therapy Journal of Research* 8(1):3–23.

Blakeney, A.B. 1985. Adolescent development: An application to the model of human occupation. In *Occupational therapy and adolescents with disability*, ed. F.S. Cromwell, 19–40. New York: Haworth Press.

Burrows, E. 1989. Clinical practice: An approach to the assessment of clinical competencies. *British Journal of Occupational Therapy* 52(6):222–226.

Burton, J.E. 1989. The model of human occupation and occupational therapy practice with elderly patients: I. Characteristics of aging. *British Journal of Occupational Therapy* 52(6):215–218.

Burton, J.E. 1989. The model of human occupation and occupational therapy practice with elderly patients: II. Application. *British Journal of Occupational Therapy* 52(6):219–221.

Cubie, S.H., and K. Kaplan. 1982. A case analysis for the model of human occupation. *American Journal of Occupational Therapy* 36(10):645–656.

Curtin, C. 1991. Psychosocial intervention with an adolescent with diabetes using the model of human occupation. *Occupational Therapy in Mental Health* 11:23–36.

DeForest, D., J.H. Watts, M.J. Madigan. 1991. Resonation in the model of human occupation: A pilot study. *Occupational Therapy in Mental Health* 11:57–71.

DePoy, E., and J.P. Burke. 1992. Viewing cognition through the lens of the model of human occupation. In *Cognitive rehabilitation: Models for intervention in occupational therapy*, ed. N. Katz, 240–257. Boston: Andover Medical Publishers.

Ebb, E.W., W. Coster, and L. Duncombe. 1989. Comparison of normal and psychosocially dysfunctional male adolescents. *Occupational Therapy in Mental Health* 9(2):53–74.

Elliott, M.S., and R. Barris. 1987. Occupational role performance and life satisfaction in elderly persons. *Occupational Therapy Journal of Research* 7(4):215–224.

Gerardi, S.M. 1996. The management of battle-fatigue solders: an occupational therapy model. *Military Medicine* 161:483–488.

Gusich, R.L. 1984. Occupational therapy for chronic pain: A clinical application of the model of human occupation. *Occupational Therapy in Mental Health* 4(3):59–73.

Gusich, R.L. 1991. Basava day clinic: The model of human occupation as applied human occupation. *Occupational Therapy in Mental Health* 11:113–134.

Josephsson, S., L. Backman, L. Borell, et al. 1995. Effectiveness of an intervention to improve occupational performance in dementia. *Occupational Therapy Journal of Research* 15(1):36–49.

Kaplan, K. 1984. Short-term assessment: The need and a response. *Occupational Therapy in Mental Health* 4(3):29–45.

Kaplan, K.L. 1986. The directive group: Short-term treatment for psychiatric patients with a minimal level of functioning. *American Journal of Occupational Therapy* 40(7):474–481.

Katz, N., N. Giladei, and C. Peretz. 1988. Cross-cultural application of occupational therapy assessment: Human occupation with psychiatric inpatients and controls in Israel. *Occupational Therapy in Mental Health* 8(1):7–30.

Katz, N., N. Josman, N. Steinmetz. 1988. Relationship between cognitive disability theory and the model of human occupation in the assessment of psychiatric and nonpsychiatric adolescents. *Occupational Therapy in Mental Health* 8(1):31–43.

Khoo, S.W., and R.M. Renwick. 1989. A model of human occupational perspective on the mental health of immigrant women in Canada. *Occupational Therapy in Mental Health* 9(3):31–49.

Levine, R.E. 1984. The cultural aspects of home care delivery. *American Journal of Occupational Therapy* 38(11):734–738.

Morgan, D., and L. Jongbloed. 1990. Factors influencing leisure activities following a stroke: An exploratory study. *Canadian Journal of Occupational Therapy* 57(4):223–229.

Oakley, F. 1987. Clinical application of the model of human occupation in dementia of the Alzheimer's type. *Occupational Therapy in Mental Health* 7(4):37–50.

Olin, D.W. 1984. Assessing and assisting the persons with dementia: An occupational behavior perspective. *Physical and Occupational Therapy in Geriatrics* 3(4):25–32.

Pizzi, M. 1990. The model of human occupation and adults with HIV infection and AIDS. *American Journal of Occupational Therapy* 44(3):257–264.

Rust, K., R. Barris, and F.H. Hooper. 1987. Use of the model of human occupation to predict women's exercise behavior. *Occupational Therapy Journal of Research* 7(1):23–35.

Salz, C. 1983. A theoretical approach to the treatment of work difficulties in borderline personalities. *Occupational Therapy in Mental Health* 3(3):33–46.

Sholle-Martin, S. 1987. Application of the model of human occupation: Assessment in child and adolescent psychiatry. *Occupational Therapy in Mental Health* 7(2):3–22.

Wieringa, N., and M. McColl. 1987. Implications of the model of human occupation for the intervention with Native Canadians. *Occupational Therapy in Health Care* 4(1):73–91.

MOTOR CONTROL MODEL

Giuffrida, C.G. 1998. Motor control theories and models: Emerging occupational performance treatment principles and assumptions. In *Willard and Spackman's occupational therapy*, 9th ed., eds. M.E. Neistadt and E.B Crepeau, 421–428. Philadelphia: Lippincott-Raven Publishers.

NEURODEVELOPMENTAL THERAPY MODEL

Adler, L.J. 1983. Neurodevelopmental treatment perspective of disorders in sensory integration. *Sensory Integration Special Interest Section Newsletter* 6(4):1–3.

Arsenault, A.B. 1988. An evaluation of the hemiplegic subject based on the Bobath approach: A validation study. Part 3. *Scandinavian Journal of Rehabilitation Medicine* 20(1):13–16.

Basmajian, J.V., et al. 1987. Stroke treatment: Comparison of integrated behavioral-physical therapy vs. traditional physical therapy programs. *Archives of Physical Medicine and Rehabilitation* 68(5, part 1):267–272.

Bay, J.B. 1991. Positioning for head control to access an augmentative communication machine. *American Journal of Occupational Therapy* 45:544–549.

Bertoti, D.B. 1986. Effect of short leg casting on ambulation in children with cerebral palsy. *Physical Therapy* 66(1):1522–1529.

Blanche, E.I., and M. Hallway. 1998. Historical perspective: Neurodevelopmental treatment in occupational therapy. *Developmental Disabilities Special Interest Section Quarterly* 21(3):1–3.

Blanche, E.I., T.M. Botticelli, and M.K. Hallway. 1995. *Combining neurodevelopmental treatment and sensory integration principles: An approach to pediatric therapy.* Tucson, AZ: Therapy Skill Builders.

Boehme, R. 1983. Self-care assessment and treatment from an NDT perspective. *Developmental Disabilities Special Interest Section Newsletter* 6(4):1,3.

Campbell, P.H., and B. Steart. 1986. Measuring changes in movement skills with infants and young children with handicaps. *Journal of the Association of Severely Handicapped* 11(3):153–161.

Carlson, P. 1975. Comparison of two occupational therapy approaches for treating the young cerebral palsied child. *American Journal of Occupational Therapy* 29:267–271.

Chakerian, D.L., and M.A. Larson. 1993. Effects of upper-extremity weight-bearing on hand-opening and prehension patterns in children with cerebral palsy. *Developmental Medicine and Child Neurology* 35:216–229.

Colan, B.J. 1996. Helping children grow: Therapists cite effectiveness of NDT. *Advance for Occupational Therapists* 12(27):16.

Corriveau, H., et al. 1988. An evaluation of the hemiplegic subject based on the Bobath approach: The evaluation protocol. Part 2. *Scandinavian Journal of Rehabilitation Medicine* 20(1):5–11.

Davis, J.Z. 1990. Neurodevelopmental treatment. In *Occupational therapy: Practice skills in physical dysfunction,* 3rd ed., eds. L.W. Pedretti and B. Zoltan, 351–362. St. Louis: Mosby.

DeGangi, G.A. 1994. Examining the efficacy of short-term NDT intervention using a case study design: Part 1. *Physical and Occupational Therapy in Pediatrics* 14(1):71–87.

DeGangi, G.A. 1994. Examining the efficacy of short term NDT intervention using a case study design: Part 2. *Physical and Occupational Therapy in Pediatrics* 14(2):21–61.

DeGangi, G.A., L. Hurley, and T.R. Linscheid. 1983. Toward a methodology of the short-term effects of neurodevelopmental treatment. *American Journal of Occupational Therapy* 37(7):479–484.

Dickstein, R., et al. 1986. Stroke rehabilitation. Three exercise therapy approaches. *Physical Therapy* 66(8):1233–1238.

Dutton, R. 1995. Neurodevelopmental frame of reference. In *Clinical reasoning in physical disabilities,* ed. R. Dutton, 79–162. Baltimore: Williams & Wilkins.

Edwards, S.J., and H.K. Yuen. 1991. An intervention program for a fraternal twin with Down syndrome. *American Journal of Occupational Therapy* 45(4):374–375.

Fetters, L., and J. Sluzik. 1996. The effects of neurodevelopmental treatment versus practice on the reaching of children with spastic cerebral palsy. *Physical Therapy* 76:346–358.

Goodman, M. 1985. Effect of early neurodevelopmental therapy in normal and at-risk survivors of neonatal intensive care. *Lancet* 2:1327–1330.

Guarna, R. 1988. An evaluation of the hemiplegic subject based on the Bobath approach: The model. Part 1. *Scandinavian Journal of Rehabilitation Medicine* 20(1):1–4.

Harris, S.R. 1981. Effects of neurodevelopmental therapy on motor performance of infants with Down's syndrome. *Developmental Medicine and Child Neurology* 23:477–483.

Herndon, W.A., et al. 1987. Effects of neurodevelopmental treatment on movement patterns of children with cerebral palsy. *Journal of Pediatric Orthopedics* (4):395–400.

Iammatteo, P.A., C. Trombly, and L. Luecke. 1990. The effect of mouth closure on drooling and speech. *American Journal of Occupational Therapy* 44:686–691.

Kinghorn, J., and G. Roberts 1996. The effective of an inhibitive weight-bearing splint on tone and function: A single-case study. *American Journal of Occupational Therapy* 50:807–815.

Kong, E. 1966. Very early treatment of cerebral palsy. *Developmental Medicine and Child Neurology* 8:198–202.

Laskas, C.A., S.L. Mullen, D.L. Nelson, et al. 1985. Enhancement of two motor functions of the lower extremity in a child with spastic quadriplegia. *Physical Therapy* 65(1):11–16.

Lilly, L.A., and N.J. Powell. 1990. Measuring the effectiveness of neurodevelopmental treatment on the daily living skills of two children with cerebral palsy. *American Journal of Occupational Therapy* 44:139–145.

Logigian, M.K., M.A. Samuels, J. Falconer, et al. 1983. Clinical exercise trial for stroke patients. *Archives of Physical Medicine and Rehabilitation* 64(8):364–367.

McPherson, J.J., R. Schild, S.J. Spauling, et al. 1991. Analysis of upper extremity movement in four sitting positions: A comparison of persons with and without cerebral palsy. *American Journal of Occupational Therapy* 34:123–129.

Morrison, D., and J. Sublett. 1986. The effects of sensory integration therapy on nystagmus duration, equilibrium reactions and visual-motor integration in reading retarded children. *Child: Care, Health and Development* 12(2):99–110.

Mulder, T., W. Hulstign, and J. van der Meer. 1986. EMG feedback and the restoration of motor control. A controlled group study of 12 hemiparetic patients. *American Journal of Physical Medicine* 65(4):173–188.

Ottenbacher, K.J. 1986. Quantitative analysis of the effectiveness of pediatric therapy. Emphasis on the neurodevelopmental treatment approach. *Physical Therapy* 66(7):1095–1101.

Parette, H.P., Jr., L.F. Holder, and J.D. Sears. 1984. Correlates of therapeutic progress by infants with cerebral palsy and motor delay. *Perceptual and Motor Skills* 58(11):159–163.

Piper, M.C., et al. 1986. Early physical therapy effects on the high-risk infants: A randomized controlled trial. *Pediatrics* 78:216–224.

Ryerson, S., and K. Levit. 1997. *Functional movement reeducation*. New York: Churchill-Livingstone.

Sadsad, C. 1998. Research articles pertaining to the efficacy of neurodevelopmental treatment. *Developmental Disabilities Special Interest Section Quarterly* 21(4):1–2

Scherzer, A., V. Mike, and J. Ilson. 1976. Physical therapy as a determinant of change in the cerebral palsied infant. *Pediatrics* 58:47–52.

Smith, M.M. 1983. Applying the neurodevelopmental treatment approach to OT. *Developmental Disabilities Special Interest Section Newsletter* 6(4):1–2.

Stahl, C. 1998. NTD: Which way should you go? Fifty-plus years and still going strong. *Advance for Occupational Therapists* 14(24):27–28.

Sussman, M.D. 1983. Casting as an adjunct to neurodevelopmental therapy for cerebral palsy. *Developmental Medicine and Child Neurology* 25(6):804–805.

Watt, J., et al. 1986. A prospective study of inhibitive casting as an adjunct to physiotherapy for cerebral-palsied children. *Developmental Medicine and Child Neurology* 28(4):480–488.

Wright, T., and J. Nicholson. 1973. Physiotherapy for the spastic child: An evaluation. *Developmental Medicine and Child Neurology* 15:146–163.

NEUROFUNCTIONAL APPROACH

Giles, G.M. 1989. Demonstrating the effectiveness of occupational therapy after severe brain trauma. *American Journal of Occupational Therapy* 43:613–615.

Giles, G.M. 1998. A neurofunctional approach to rehabilitation following severe brain injury. In *Cognition and occupation in rehabilitation: Cognitive models for intervention in occupational therapy*, ed. N. Katz, 125–147. Bethesda, MD: American Occupational Therapy Association.

OCCUPATIONAL ADAPTATION

Ford, K. 1995. Occupational adaptation in home health: An occupational therapist's viewpoint. *Home and Community Health Special Interest Section Newsletter* 2:3–4.

Garrett, S., and J.K. Schkade. 1995. The occupational adaptation model of professional development as applied to level II fieldwork in occupational therapy. *American Journal of Occupational Therapy* 49:119–126.

Pasek, P.B., and J.K. Schkade. 1996. Effects of a skiing experience on adolescents with limb deficiencies: An occupational adaptation perspective. *American Journal of Occupational Therapy* 50(1):24–31.

OCCUPATIONAL BEHAVIOR

Barrett, L., and G. Kielhofner. 1998. An overview of occupational behavior. In *Willard and Spackman's occupational therapy*, 9th ed., eds. M.E. Neistadt and E.B. Crepeau, 525–527. Philadelphia: Lippincott-Raven Publishers.

Black, M.M. 1976. The occupational career. *American Journal of Occupational Therapy* 30:225–228.

Borys, S.S. 1974. Implications of interest theory. *American Journal of Occupational Therapy* 30:225–228.

Burke, J.P. 1977. A clinical perspective on motivation: Pawn versus origin. *American Journal of Occupational Therapy* 31:254–258.

Dunning, H. 1972. Environmental occupational therapy. *American Journal of Occupational Therapy* 26:292–298.

Florey, L. 1969. Intrinsic motivation: The dynamics of occupational therapy theory. *American Journal of Occupational Therapy* 23(4):319–322.

Matsutsuyu, J. 1971. Occupational behavior—A perspective on work and play. *American Journal of Occupational Therapy* 25:291–292.

Primeau, L.A., and J.M. Ferguson. 1999. Occupational frame of reference. In *Frames of reference for pediatric occupational therapy*, 2nd ed., eds. P. Kramer and J. Hinojosa, 469–516. Baltimore: Lippincott, Williams & Wilkins.

Shannon, P. 1972. Work-play theory and the occupational therapy process. *American Journal of Occupational Therapy* 26(4):169–172.

Shannon, P. 1977. The derailment of occupational therapy. *American Journal of Occupational Therapy* 31(4):229–234.

OCCUPATIONAL SCIENCE

Clark, F. 1993. Occupation embedded in a real life: Interweaving occupational science and occupational therapy. *American Journal of Occupational Therapy* 47:1067–1078.

Clark, F., and E.A. Larson. 1993. Developing an academic discipline. The science of occupation. In *Willard and Spackman's occupational therapy*, 8th ed., eds. H. Hopkins and H.D. Smith, 44–57. Philadelphia: J.B. Lippincott.

Clark, F.A., D. Parham, M.E. Carlson, et al. 1991. Occupational science: Academic innovation in the service of occupational therapy's future. *American Journal of Occupational Therapy* 45:300–310.

Clark, F., W. Wood, and E.A. Larson. 1998. Occupational science: Occupational therapy legacy for the 21st century. In *Willard and Spackman's occupational therapy*, 9th ed., eds. M.E. Neistadt and E.B. Crepeau, 13–21. Philadelphia: J.B. Lippincott.

Yerxa, E.J., F. Clark, G. Frank, et al. 1989. An introduction to occupational science: A foundation for occupational therapy in the 21st century. *Occupational Therapy in Health Care* 6:1–17.

RECOVERY FROM HEMIPLEGIA MODEL

Hughes, E. 1972. Bobath and Brunnstrom: Comparison of two methods of treatment of a left hemiplegia. *Physiotherapy Canada* 24(5):262–266.

Pedretti, L.W. 1990. Movement therapy: The Brunnstrom approach to treatment of hemiplegia. In *Occupational therapy: Practice skills in physical dysfunction*, 3rd ed., eds. L.W. Pedretti and B. Zoltan, 334–350. St. Louis: Mosby.

Perry, C. 1967. Principles and techniques of the Brunnstrom approach to the treatment of hemiplegia. *American Journal of Physical Medicine* 46:789–797.

Reynolds, G.G., K.C. Archibald, S. Brunnstrom, et al. 1958. Preliminary report on neuromuscular function testing of the upper extremity in adult hemiplegic patients. *Archives of Physical Medicine and Rehabilitation* 39(5):303–310.

Shah, S.K. 1984. Reliability of the original Brunnstrom recovery scale following hemiplegia. *Australian Occupational Therapy Journal* 31(4):144–151.

Shah, S.K. 1986. Stroke rehabilitation outcome based on Brunnstrom recovery stages. *Occupational Therapy Journal of Research* 6:365–376.

REED AND SANDERSON'S PERSONAL ADAPTATION MODEL

Reed, K.L. 1984. A proposed model: Adaptation through occupation. In *Models of practice in occupational therapy*, 491–513. Baltimore: Williams & Wilkins.

Reed, K.L., and S.R. Sanderson. 1980. Towards a theory of occupational therapy. In *Concepts of occupational therapy*, 225–231. Baltimore: Williams & Wilkins.

Reed, K.L., and S.R. Sanderson. 1983. Toward a theoretical model of occupational therapy. In *Concepts of occupational therapy*, 2nd ed., 74–80. Baltimore: Williams & Wilkins.

Reed, K.L., and S.R. Sanderson. 1992. Toward a theoretical model of occupational therapy. In *Concepts of occupational therapy*, 3rd ed., 87–93. Baltimore: Williams & Wilkins.

REILLY'S OCCUPATIONAL BEHAVIOR MODEL

Reilly, M. 1962. Occupational therapy can be one of the great ideas of 20th century medicine. *American Journal of Occupational Therapy* 16(1):1–9.

Reilly, M. 1969. The educational process. *American Journal of Occupational Therapy* 23:299–307.

Reilly, M. 1974. An explanation of play. In *Play as exploratory learning: Studies of curiosity behavior*, 117–149. Beverly Hills, CA: Sage.

ROOD'S SENSORIMOTOR APPROACH

Goff, B. 1972. The application of recent advances in neurophysiology to Miss M. Rood's concept of neuromuscular facilitation. *Physiotherapy* 58(12):409–415.

McCormack, G.L. 1996. The Rood approach to treatment of neuromuscular dysfunction. In *Occupational therapy: Practice skills for physical dysfunction*, ed. L.W. Pedretti, 377–400. St. Louis: Mosby.

Rood, M. 1952. Occupational therapy in the treatment of cerebral palsy. *Physical Therapy Review* 32(2):76–82.

Rood, M. 1954. Neurophysiological reactions as a basis for physical therapy. *Physical Therapy Review* 34(9):444–449.

Rood, M. 1956. Neurophysiological mechanisms utilized in the treatment of neuromuscular dysfunction. *American Journal of Occupational Therapy* 10(4, part II):220–224.

Rood, M. 1958. Every one counts. *American Journal of Occupational Therapy* 12(6):326–329.

Rood, M. 1959. Use of reflexes as an aid in occupational therapy. In *Occupational therapy as a link in rehabilitation. Proceedings of the Second International Congress of the World Federation of Occupational Therapists*, 166–176. Copenhagen: Clemenstrykkeriet Arbus.

Rood, M. 1963. The use of sensory receptors to activate, facilitate, and inhibit motor responses, autonomic and somatic, in developmental sequence. In *Approaches to the treatment of patients with neuromuscular dysfunction, study course VI*, ed. C. Satterly, 26–37. Third International Congress of the World Federation of Occupational Therapy. Dubuque, IA: William C. Brown.

Rood, M. 1969. Proprioceptive neuromuscular facilitation and demonstration. *South Africa Cerebral Palsy Journal* 13(3):12–15.

Rood, M. 1976. Neurodevelopmental theory and application. *In Feeding the handicapped child. Proceedings of the Conference for University Affiliated Programs*, eds. E. McKibbin and H. Cloud, 36–65. Birmingham, AL: Center for Development and Learning Disorders, University of Alabama in Birmingham.

Stockmeyer, S.A. 1967. An interpretation of the approach of Rood to the treatment of neuromuscular dysfunction. *American Journal of Physical Medicine* 46(1):900–955.

Trombly, C.A. 1996. Rood approach. In *Occupational therapy for physical dysfunction*, 4th ed., ed. C.A. Trombly, 437–445. Baltimore: Williams & Wilkins.

ROSS AND BURDICK'S SENSORY INTEGRATION MODEL

Robichaud, L., R. Hebért, and J. Desrosiers. 1994. Efficacy of a sensory integration program on behaviors of inpatients with dementia. *American Journal of Occupational Therapy* 48(4):355–360.

Ross, M., and D. Burdick. 1981. *Sensory integration: A training manual for therapists and teachers for regressed, psychiatric and geriatric patient groups*. Thorofare, NJ: Slack.

SCHKADE AND SCHULTZ'S OCCUPATIONAL ADAPTATION MODEL

Schkade, J.K., and S. Schultz. 1992. Occupational adaptation: Toward a holistic approach for contemporary practice. Part 1. *American Journal of Occupational Therapy* 46:829–837.

Schkade, J.K., and S. Schultz. 1993. Occupational adaptation—An integrative frame of reference. In *Willard and Spackman's occupational therapy*, 8th ed., eds. H. Hopkins and H. Smith. Philadelphia: J.B. Lippincott.

Schkade, J.K., and S. Schultz. 1998. Occupational adaptation: An integrative frame of reference. In *Willard and Spackman's occupational therapy*, 9th ed., eds. M.E. Neistadt and E.B. Crepeau, 529–531. Philadelphia: J.B. Lippincott.

Schultz, S., and J.K. Schkade. 1992. Occupational adaptation: Toward a holistic approach to contemporary practice. Part 2. *American Journal of Occupational Therapy* 46:917–926.

Schultz, S., and J.K. Schkade. 1994. Home healthcare: A window of opportunity to synthesize practice. *Home & Community Health Special Interest Section Newsletter* 1:1–4.

Schultz, S., and J. Schkade. 1996. Adaptation. In *Occupational therapy: Enabling function and well-being*, eds. C. Christiansen and C. Baum, 458–481. Thorofare, NJ: Slack.

SENSORY DIET

Wilbarger, P. 1995. The sensory diet: Activity programs based on sensory processing theory. *Sensory Integration Special Interest Section Newsletter* 18(2):1–4.

Wilbarger, P. and J. Wilbarger. 1992. *Sensory defensiveness in children aged 2–12: An intervention guide for parents and other caretakers.* Santa Barbara, CA: Avanti Educational Programs.

SENSORY INTEGRATION

Arendt, R.E., W.E. MacLean Jr., and A.A. Baumeister. 1988. Critique of sensory integration therapy and its application in mental retardation. *American Journal of Mental Retardation* 92(5):401–409.

Atwood, R.M., and S.A. Cermak. 1986. Crossing the midline as a function of distance from midline. *American Journal of Occupational Therapy* 40(10):685–690.

Babayov, D., H. Omer, and J. Menczel. 1985. Sensorimotor integration therapy for hip fracture and CVA patients. *Canadian Journal of Occupational Therapy* 52(3):133–137.

Blanche, E.I., T.M. Botticelli, and M.K. Hallway. 1995. *Combining neuro-developmental treatment and sensory integration principles: An approach to pediatric therapy.* Tucson, AZ: Therapy Skill Builders.

Bochner, S. 1978. Ayres, sensory integration and learning disorders: Question of theory and practice. *American Journal of Mental Retardation* 5:41–45.

Bochner, S. 1980. Sensory integration therapy and learning disabilities: A critique. *Australian Occupational Therapy Journal* 27:125–138.

Bright, T., K. Bittick, and B. Fleeman. 1981. Reduction of SIB using sensory integrative techniques. *American Journal of Occupational Therapy* 35:167–172.

Carte, E., D. Morrison, J. Sublett, et al. 1984. Sensory integration theory: A trial of a specific neurodevelopmental therapy for the remediation of learning disabilities. *Journal of Developmental and Behavioral Pediatrics* 5(4):189–194.

Cermak, S.A. 1991. Somatodyspraxia. In *Sensory integration theory and practice*, eds. A.G. Fisher, E.A. Murray, A.C. Bundy, 137–165. Philadelphia: F.A. Davis.

Cermak, S.A., E.A. Ward, and L.M. Ward. 1986. The relationship between articulation disorders and motor coordination in children. *American Journal of Occupational Therapy* 40(8):546–550.

Chappiro, C. 1985. Australian Association of Occupational Therapists position paper on sensory integration. *Australian Occupational Therapy Journal* 32:23–26.

Chee, F.K.W., J.R. Kreutzberg, and D.L. Clark. 1978. Semicircular canal stimulation in cerebral palsied children. *Physical Therapy* 58:1071–1075.

Clark, E., A. Mailloux, and D. Parham. 1985. Sensory integration and children with learning disabilities. In *Occupational therapy for children*, eds. P.N. Clark and A.S. Allen, 359–405. St. Louis: Mosby.

Committee on Children with Disabilities. 1985. School aged children with motor disabilities. *Pediatrics* 76:648–649.

Cummins, R.A. 1991. Sensory integration and learning disabilities: Ayres' factor analyses reappraised. *Journal of Learning Disabilities* 24(3):160–168.

Densem, J.F., et al. 1989. Effectiveness of a sensory integrative therapy program for children with perceptual-motor deficits. *Journal of Learning Disabilities* 22(4):221–229.

Dilts, C.V., C.A. Morris, and C.O. Leonard. 1990. Hypothesis for development of a behavioral phenotype in Williams Syndrome. *American Journal of Medical Genetics Supplement* 6:126–131.

Doyle, B.A., and D.C. Higginson. 1984. Relationships among self-concept and school achievement, maternal self-esteem and sensory integration abilities for learning disabled children, ages 7 to 12 years. *Perceptual and Motor Skills* 58(1):177–178.

Dura, J.R., J.A. Mulick, and D. Hammer. 1988. Rapid clinical evaluation of sensory therapy for self-injurious behavior. *Mental Retardation* 26(2):83–87.

Evan, P.R., and M.A. Peham. 1981. *Testing and measurements in occupational therapy: A review of current practice with special emphasis on the Southern California Sensory Integration Tests.* Minneapolis: University of Minnesota.

Fisher, A.G. 1991. Vestibular-proprioceptive processing and bilateral integration and sequencing deficits. In *Sensory integration theory and practice*, eds. A.G. Fisher, E.A. Murray, and A.C. Bundy, 71–107. Philadelphia: F.A. Davis.

Fisher, A.G., and W. Dunn. 1983. Tactile defensiveness: Historical perspectives, new research. A theory grows. *Sensory Integration Special Interest Section Newsletter* 6(3):1–2.

Fisher, A.G., and E.A. Murray. 1991. Introduction to sensory integration theory. In *Sensory integration theory and practice*, eds. A.G. Fisher, E.A. Murray, and A.C. Bundy, 3–26. Philadelphia: F.A. Davis.

Fisher, A.G., E.A. Murray, and A.C. Bundy. 1991. *Sensory Integration Theory and Practice*. Philadelphia: F.A. Davis.

Harten, G., U. Stephani, G. Henze, et al. 1984. Slight impairment of psychomotor skills in children after treatment of acute lymphoblastic leukemia. *European Journal of Pediatrics* 142(3):189–197.

Hixson, V.J., and A.W. Mathews. 1984. Sensory integration and chronic schizophrenia: Past, present and future. *Canadian Journal of Occupational Therapy* 51(1):19–24.

James, M.R. 1984. Sensory integration: A theory for therapy and research. *Journal of Music Therapy* 21(2):79–88.

Jaroma, M., P. Danner, and E. Koiveuniemi. 1984. Sensory integrative therapy and speech therapy for improving the perceptual motor skills and speech articulation of a dyspractic boy. *Folia Phoniatrica* 36(6):261–266.

Jenkins, J.R., R. Fewell, and S.R. Harris. 1983. Comparison of sensory integrative therapy and motor programming. *American Journal of Mental Deficiency* 88(2):221–224.

Kantner, R., et al. 1976. Effects of vestibular stimulation on nystagmus response and motor performance in the developmentally delayed infant. *Physical Therapy* 56:414–421.

Kavale, K., and P.D. Mattson. 1983. One jumped off the balance beam: Meta-analysis of perceptual motor training. *Journal of Learning Disabilities* 16(3):165–173.

Kimball, J.G. 1986. Prediction of methylphenidate (Ritalin) responsiveness through sensory integrative testing. *American Journal of Occupational Therapy* 40(4):241–248.

Kimball, J.G. 1988. Hypothesis for prediction of stimulant drug effectiveness utilizing sensory integrative diagnostic methods. *Journal of the American Osteopathic Association* 88(6):757–762.

Knox, S., W. Mack, and Z. Mailloux. 1988. *Interpreting the Sensory Integration and Praxis Tests*. Los Angeles: Sensory Integration International.

Koomar, J.A., and A.C. Bundy. 1991. The art and science of creating direct intervention from theory. In *Sensory integration theory and practice*, eds. A.G. Fisher, E.A. Murray, and A.C. Bundy, 251–314. Philadelphia: F.A. Davis.

Kuharski, T., et al. 1985. Effects of vestibular stimulation on sitting behaviours among preschoolers with service handicaps. *Journal of the Association of Persons with Severe Handicaps* 10:137–145

Larson, K.A. 1982. The sensory history of developmentally delayed children with and without sensory defensiveness. *American Journal of Occupational Therapy* 36:590–596.

Lever, R.J. 1981. An open letter to an occupational therapist. *Journal of Learning Disabilities* 14:3–4.

Montgomery, P., and E. Richter. 1977. Effect of sensory integrative therapy on the neuromotor development of retarded children. *Physical Therapy* 57:799–806.

Morrison, D., and J. Sublett. 1986. The effects of sensory integration therapy on nystagmus duration equilibrium reactions and visual-motor integration in reading retarded children. *Child: Care, Health and Development* 12(2):99–110.

Ottenbacher, K. 1982. Patterns of postrotary nystagmus in three learning-disabled children. *American Journal of Occupational Therapy* 36(10):657–663.

Ottenbacher, K. 1982. Sensory integration therapy: Affect or effect. *American Journal of Occupational Therapy* 36(9):571–578.

Ottenbacher, K. 1983. Developmental implications of clinically applied vestibular stimulation. *Physical Therapy* 63(3):338–342.

Ottenbacher, K.J., and P. Pedersen. 1983. The efficacy of vestibular stimulation as a form of specific sensory enrichment. *Clinical Pediatrics* 23(8):428–433.

Ottenbacher, K.J., and P. Pederson. 1985. A meta-analysis of applied vestibular stimulation research. *Physical and Occupational Therapy in Pediatrics* 5:119–134.

Ottenbacher, K., and M.A. Short. 1985. Sensory integrative dysfunction in children: A review of theory and treatment. *Advances in Developmental and Behavioral Pediatrics* 6:287–329.

Ottenbacher, K., M.A. Short, and P.J. Watson. 1981. The effects of a classically applied program of vestibular stimulation on the neuromotor performance of children with severe developmental disability. *Physical and Occupational Therapy in Pediatrics* 1:1–11.

Ottenbacher, K.J., et al. 1987. The effectiveness of tactile stimulation as a form of early intervention: A quantitative evaluation. *Journal of Developmental and Behavioral Pediatrics* 8(2):68–76.

Parmenter, C.L. 1983. An asymmetrical tonic neck reflex rating scale. *American Journal of Occupational Therapy* 37(7):462–465.

Parush, S., and F. Clark. 1988. The reliability and validity of a sensory developmental expectation questionnaire for mothers of newborns. *American Journal of Occupational Therapy* 42(1):11–16.

Peterson, P., and R.L. Wikoff. 1983. The performance of adult males on the Southern California Figure-Ground Visual Perception Test. *American Journal of Occupational Therapy* 37(8):554–560.

Polatajko, H.J. 1985. A critical look at vestibular dysfunction in learning-disabled children. *Developmental Medicine and Child Neurology* 27:283–292.

Posthuma, B.W. 1983. Sensory integration: Fact or fad. *American Journal of Occupational Therapy* 37:343–345.

Pothier, P.C., and K. Cheek. 1984. Current practices in sensory motor programming with developmentally delayed infants and young children. *Child: Care, Health and Development* 10:341–348.

Potter, C.N., and L.N. Silverman. 1984. Characteristics of vestibular function and static balance skills in deaf children. *Physical Therapy* 64(7):1071–1075.

Royeen, C.B., and J.C. Fortune. 1990. TIE: Touch inventory for elementary school aged children. *American Journal of Occupational Therapy* 44:165–170.

Royeen, C.B., and S.J. Lane. 1991. Tactile processing and sensory defensiveness. In *Sensory integration theory and practice*, eds. A.G. Fisher, E.A. Murray, and A.C. Bundy, 108–133. Philadelphia: F.A. Davis.

Saeki, K., F.A. Clark, and S.P. Azen. 1985. Performance of Japanese and Japanese-American children on the Motor Accuracy-Revised and Design Copying Tests of the Southern California Sensory Integration Tests. *American Journal of Occupational Therapy* 39(2):103–109.

Sellick, K.J., and T. Over. 1980. Effects of vestibular stimulation on motor development of cerebral palsied children. *Developmental Medicine and Child Neurology* 22:476–483.

Shaffer, R. 1984. Sensory integration therapy with learning disabled children: A critical review. *Canadian Journal of Occupational Therapy* 51(2):73–77.

Shaffer, R. 1990. Play behavior and occupational therapy. *American Journal of Occupational Therapy* 44(1):68–75.

Short, M.A., P.J. Watson, K. Ottenbacher, et al. 1983. Vestibular-proprioceptive functions in 4 year olds: Normative and regressive analyses. *American Journal of Occupational Therapy* 37(2):102–109.

Sieben, R.I. 1977. Controversial medical treatments of learning disabilities. *Academic Therapy* 13:133–147.

Smith, C.M., S.A. Cermak, and D.L. Nelson. 1984. Sequential versus simultaneous graphesthesia tasks in 6- and 10-year-old children. *American Journal of Occupational Therapy* 38(6):377–381.

Stepp-Gilbert, E. 1988. Sensory integration: A reason for infant enrichment. *Issues in Comprehensive Pediatric Nursing* 11(5–6):319–331.

Stepp-Gilbert, E. 1988. Sensory integration dysfunction. *Issues in Comprehensive Pediatric Nursing* 11(5–6):313–318.

Storey, K., et al. 1984. Reducing the self-stimulatory behavior of a profoundly retarded female through sensory awareness training. *American Journal of Occupational Therapy* 38:510–516.

Tickle-Degnen, L. 1988. Perspectives on the status of sensory integration theory. *American Journal of Occupational Therapy* 42(7):427–433.

Walker, K.F. 1991. Sensory integrative therapy in a limited space. An adaptation of the Ayres Clinic design. *Sensory Integration Special Interest Section Newsletter* 14(3):1–2,4.

Werry, J.S., R. Scaletti, and F. Mills. 1990. Sensory integration and teacher-judged learning problems: A controlled intervention trial. *Journal of Paediatrics and Child Health* 26(1):31–35.

White, M. 1979. A first-grade intervention program for children at risk for reading failure. *Journal of Learning Disabilities* 12(4):231–237.

Wilbarger, P., and J.L. Wilbarger. 1990. *Defensiveness in children: An intervention guide for parents and other caregivers.* Hugo, MN: PDP Products.

Wilson, B.N., and C.A. Trombly. 1984. Proximal and distal function in children with and without sensory integrative dysfunction: An E.M.G. study. *Canadian Journal of Occupational Therapy* 51(1):11–17.

Yack, E. 1989. Sensory integration: A survey of its use in the clinical setting. *Canadian Journal of Occupational Therapy* 56(5):229–235.

Ziviani, J., A Poulsen, and A. O'Brien. 1982. Correlation of the Bruninks-Oseretsky Test of Motor Proficiency with the Southern California Sensory Integration Tests. *American Journal of Occupational Therapy* 36(8):519–523.

Also see all articles in the *American Journal of Occupational Therapy* 44(7):610–657, 1990.

TOGLIA'S MULTICONTEXTUAL MODEL AND DYNAMIC INTERACTIONAL APPROACH

Abreu, B., and J.P. Toglia. 1987. Cognitive rehabilitation: A model for occupational therapy. *American Journal of Occupational Therapy* 41:439–448.

Golisz, K.M., and J.P. Toglia. 1998. Occupational therapy evaluation: Evaluation of perception and cognition. In *Willard and Spackman's occupational therapy*, 9th ed., eds. M.E. Neistadt and E.B. Crepeau, 260–281. Philadelphia: J.B. Lippincott.

Toglia, J.P. 1989. Approaches to cognitive assessment of the brain injured adult: Traditional methods and dynamic investigation. *Occupational Therapy Practice* 1:36–57.

Toglia, J.P. 1989. Visual perception of objects: An approach to assessment and intervention. *American Journal of Occupational Therapy* 43(9):587–595.

Toglia, J.P. 1991. Generalization of treatment: A multicontext approach to cognitive perceptual impairment in adults with brain injury. *American Journal of Occupational Therapy* 45:505–516.

Toglia, J.P. 1991. Unilateral visual inattention: Multidimensional components. *Occupational Therapy Practice* 3(1):18–34.

Toglia, J.P. 1992. A dynamic interactional approach to cognitive rehabilitation. In *Cognitive rehabilitation: Models for interaction in occupational therapy*, ed. N. Katz, 104–143. Boston: Andover Medical Publishers.

Toglia, J.P. 1993. Attention and memory. In *AOTA self-study series: Cognitive rehabilitation,* ed. C.B. Royeen, 1–72. Rockville, MD: American Occupational Therapy Association.

Toglia, J.P. 1993. *The Contextual Memory Test.* Tucson, AZ: Psychological Corporation/Therapy Skills Builders.

Toglia, J.P. 1994. *Toglia Category Assessment* (TCA). Paquannock, NJ: Maddak.

Toglia, J.P. 1998. A dynamic interactional model to cognitive rehabilitation. In *A dynamic interactional model to cognitive rehabilitation*, ed. N. Katz, 5–50. Bethesda, MD: American Occupational Therapy Association.

Toglia, J.P. 1998. Cognitive-perceptual retraining and rehabilitation. In *Willard and Spackman's occupational therapy*, 9th ed., eds. M.E. Neistadt and E.B. Crepeau, 428–450. Philadelphia: J.B. Lippincott.

Toglia, J.P., and K. Golisz. 1990. *Cognitive rehabilitation: Group games and activities.* Tucson, AZ: Therapy Skill Builders.

VISUAL INFORMATION ANALYSIS (VISION THERAPY)

Downing-Baum, S., and D. Marino. 1996. Case studies show success in OT-OD treatment plans. *Advance for Occupational Therapists* 12(44):18,46.

Scheiman, M. 1997. *Understanding and managing vision deficits: A guide for occupational therapists.* Thorofare, NJ: Slack.

Todd, V.P. 1999. Visual information analysis: Frames of reference for visual perception. In *Frames of reference for pediatric occupational therapy*, eds. P. Kramer and J. Hinojosa, 205–256. Philadelphia: Lippincott, Williams & Wilkins.

Warren, M. 1990. Identification of visual scanning deficits in adults after cerebrovascular accident. *American Journal of Occupational Therapy* 44:391–399.

Warren, M. 1993. A hierarchical model for evaluation and treatment of visual perceptual dysfunction in adult acquired brain injury. Parts 1 and 2. *American Journal of Occupational Therapy* 47:42–66.

Warren, M. 1994. Visual-spatial skills: Assessment and intervention strategies. In *AOTA self-study series: Cognitive rehabilitation, 7*, ed. C.B. Royeen, 1–76. Rockville, MD: American Occupational Therapy Association.

Warren, M. 1995. Providing low vision rehabilitation services with occupational therapy and ophthalmology: A program description. *American Journal of Occupational Therapy* 49:877–883.

Warren, M. 1996. Evaluation and treatment of visual deficits. In *Occupational therapy: Practice skills for physical dysfunction*, ed. L.W. Pedretti, 193–212. St. Louis: Mosby.

WILLIAMSON'S COPING FRAME OF REFERENCE

Williamson, G.G. 1987. *Children with spinal bifida: Early intervention and preschool programming.* Baltimore: Paul H. Brookes Publishing.

Williamson, G.G., and M. Szczepanski. 1999. Coping frame of reference. In *Frames of reference for pediatric occupational therapy*, 2nd ed., eds. P. Kramer and J. Hinojosa, 431–468. Philadelphia: Lippincott, Williams & Wilkins.

Williamson, G.G., S. Zeitlin, and M. Szczepanski. 1989. Coping behavior: Implications for disabled infants and toddlers. *Infant Mental Health Journal* 10:3–13.

Zeitlin, S., and G.G. Williamson. 1988. Developing family resources for adaptive coping. *Journal of the Division for Early Childhood* 12:137–146.

Zeitlin, S., and G.G. Williamson. 1990. Coping characteristics of disabled and nondisabled young children. *American Journal of Orthopsychiatry* 60:404–411.

Zeitlin, S., and G.G. Williamson. 1994. *Coping in young children: Early intervention practices to enhance adaptive behavior and resilience.* Baltimore: Paul H. Brookes Publishing.

Zeitlin, S., G.G. Williamson, and W.P. Rosenblatt. 1987. The coping with stress model: A counseling approach for families with a handicapped child. *Journal of Counseling and Development* 65:443–446.

Zeitlin, S., G.G. Williamson, and M. Szczepanski. 1988. *Early coping inventory.* Bensenville, IL: Scholastic Testing Service.

Appendix F

Disorders with One Major Reference or No Major Reference

Note: The following disorders each have one major reference that may be useful to the practitioner but does not provide sufficient information for a unit in the regular text.

ACALCULIA

Zoltan, B. 1996. Acalculia. In *Vision, perception and cognition: A manual for the evaluation and treatment of the neurologically impaired adult*, ed. B. Zoltan, 177–184. Thorofare, NJ: Slack.

BENIGN CONGENITAL HYPOTONIA

Parush, S., A. Tenenbaum, E. Tekuzener, et al. 1998. Developmental correlates of school-age children with a history of benign congenital hypotonia. *Developmental Medicine and Child Neurology* 40:448–452.

BLINDNESS IN ADULTS

Yuen, H.K. 1993. Improved productivity through purposeful use of additional template for a woman with cortical blindness. *American Journal of Occupational Therapy* 47(2):105–110.

BLOOD VESSEL REPAIR

Theisen, L. 1997. Upper extremity vessel repair. In *Hand rehabilitation: A practical guide*, 2d ed., eds. G.L. Clark, E.F.S. Wilgis, B. Aiello, et al., 43–46. New York: Churchill Livingstone.

CARDIAC CONDITIONS IN CHILDREN

Balouf, O. 1993. Cardiopulmonary dysfuntion in children. In *Willard and Spackman's occupational therapy*, 8th ed., eds. H.L.Hopkins and H.D. Smith, 615–616. Philadelphia: J.B. Lippincott.

CENTRAL CORD INJURY

Fowler, S.B., and H. Hardaway. 1996. Collaborative efforts in achieving patient outcomes in central cord injury syndrome in the acute care setting. *SCI Nursing* 12(4):121–123.

CONGENITAL DISORDERS OF THE UPPER EXTERMITY

Fuller, M. 1999. Treatment of congenital differences of the upper extremity: Therapist's commentary. *Journal of Hand Therapy* 12(2):174–177.

ENCEPHALITIS

Katzmann, S., and C. Mix. 1994. Improving functional independence in a patient with encephalitis through behavior modification shaping techniques. *American Journal of Occupational Therapy* 48(3):259–262.

EOSINOPHILIC FACIITIS

O'Laughlin, T.J., R.R Klima, and D.E. Kenney. 1994. Rehabilitation of eosinophilic faciitis: A case report. *American Journal of Physical Medicine and Rehabilitation* 73:286–292.

FICTITIOUS DISORDERS

Barnitt, R.E. 1996. Fictitious disorders in occupational therapy: Sad cases or incorrigible rogues. *British Journal of Occupational Therapy* 59(2):50–55.

MALARIA

Stock, C., and D.M. Joss. 1998. Malaria. *Work: A Journal of Prevention, Assessment & Rehabilitation* 10:85–99.

OSTEOGENESIS IMPERFECTA

Beeler, L.M., and M. Hallway. 1992. Case report: Pediatric osteogensis imperfecta. *REHAB Management* 5(4):147–149.

Francesco, G. 1992. The unknown script of a mysterious people: An occupational therapy consultation for a child with osteogenesis imperfecta. *World Federation of Occupational Therapists Bulletin* 26:60–63.

Hardwick, K., L. Feichtinger, and D. Wiederhold. 1997. Daniel's story. *TeamRehab Report* 8(7):34–36, 38.

RADIAL CLUB HAND

Kennedy, S.M. 1996. Neoprene wrist brace for correction of radial club hand in children. *Journal of Hand Therapy* 9(4):387–390.

SHOULDER DISORDERS

Sagerman, S.D., and K.L. Truppa. 1998. Diagnosis and managment of occupational disorders of the shoulder. In *Occupational hand and upper extremity injuries and diseases*, 2nd ed., ed. M.L. Kasdan, 277–285. Philadelphia: Handley & Belfus.

SPINAL FUSION

Budge G. 1997. An evaluation of the occupational therapy for spinal fusion hip spica patients. *British Journal of Occupational Therapy* 60(9):365–369.

SUICIDE

Marmer, L. 1997. How skill building can help prevent suicide. *Advance for Occupational Therapists* 13(39):15, 46.

TORTURE

Kerr, T. 1998. Coming out of the shadows: Torture treatment. *Advance for Occupational Therapy Practitioners* 14(49):18–19, 42.

TRANSPLANTATION

Ma, H.S., T.A. El-Gammal, and F.C. Wei. 1996. Current concepts of toe-to-hand transfer: Surgery and rehabilitation. *Journal of Hand Therapy* 9(1):41–46.

ULNAR NEUROPATHY

Blackmore, S.M., and R.N. Hotchkiss. 1995. Therapist's management of ulnar neuropathy at the elbow. In *Rehabiltation of the hand*, 4th ed., eds. J.M. Hunter, E.J. Mackin, and A.D. Callahan, 665–678. St. Louis: Mosby.

WILLIAMS SYNDROME

Joe, B.E. 1994. Williams syndrome. *OT Week* 8(45):18–19.

Appendix G

Resource Bibliography on Media, Modalities, and Techniques

ACCESSIBILITY—BARRIER-FREE DESIGN (see also Home Modification and Accessibility)

Christenson, M.A. 1999. Embracing universal design. *OT Practice* 4(9):12–15.

Figoni, S.F., L. McClain, A.A. Bell, et al. 1998. Accessibility of physical fitness facilities in the Kansas City metropolitan area. *Topics in Spinal Cord Injury Rehabilitation* 3(3):66–78.

Hadly, M. 1997. Making learning accessible. *Advance for Occupational Therapy Practitioners* 13(9):17. Also in *Advance for Directors in Rehabilitation* 1996;5(9):24,26.

Meade, K.M. 1995. Breaking down barriers: Bringing patients home to accessible housing. *Advance for Directors in Rehabilitation* 4(5):15–17.

Spokojny, J.D. 1994. Barrier-free design. *Rehab Management* 7(6):122–123.

ACTIVITIES OF DAILY LIVING (ADL)

Daly, M.P., and J.H.Fouche. 1997. *Critical thinking for activities of daily living and communication.* San Antonio, TX: Communication Skills Builders.

Foti, D., and L.W. Pedretti. 1998. Activities of daily living. In *Physical dysfunction: Practice skills for the occupational therapy assistant,* ed. M.B. Early, 237–275. St. Louis: Mosby.

McCarthy, K. 1993. *Activities of daily living: A manual of group activities and written exercises.* Framingham, MA: Therapro.

ALTERNATIVE MEDICINE

Gosman-Hedstrom, G., L. Claesson, U. Klingenstierna, et al. 1998. Effects of acupuncture treatment on daily life activities and quality of life: A controlled, prospective, and randomized study of acute stroke patients. *Stroke* 29:2100–2108.

Huelskamp, S. 1998. Magnet therapy: What's the attraction? *Advance for Occupational Therapy Practitioners* 14(42):42–43.

O'Reilly, A. 1998. Alternative medicine: The controversial cure. *Advance for Occupational Therapy Practitioners* 14(23):26–29.
O'Reilly, A. 1998. Alternative medicine: The controversial cure. *Advance for Occupational Therapy Practitioners* 14(24):34–35,66.
Stahl, C. 1996. Movement by pattern. *Advance for Occupational Therapy Practitioners* 12(10):13.

ANIMAL-ASSISTED THERAPY (see also Pet Therapy)

Amabile, M.J., K. Howe, and L.L. Knis. 1997. Creature comforts: How animals aid therapy. *Advance for Occupational Therapy Practitioners* 13(24):14–15.
Bernard, S. 1995. *Animal assisted therapy: A guide for health care professionals and volunteers.* Whitehouse, TX: Therapet[P.O. Box 1696, Whitehouse, TX 75791].
Darrah, J.P. 1996. A pilot survey of animal-facilitated therapy in southern California and South Dakota nursing homes. *Occupational Therapy International* 3(2):105–121.
Diffendal, J. 1998. Nature *and* nurture: When animals go to school. *Advance for Occupational Therapy Practitioners* 34(39):34,38.
Gross, K., 1997. They talk with the animals. *Advance for Occupational Therapy Practitioners* 13(49):6–8.
Marmer, L. 1997. A llama at school: It makes the children laugh and play. *Advance for Occupational Therapy Practitioners* 13(40):14,50.

AQUATIC THERAPY

Adams, R.C. 1995. Combining aquatic and land therapy offers patients the best of both worlds. *Advance for Occupational Therapy Practitioners* 11(37):19,21.
Feeney, T. 1995. Some aquatic maintenance puts new life into elderly. *Advance for Occupational Therapy Practitioners* 11(37):18.
Garret, G. 1994. A stroke of genius. *Rehab Management* 7(3):56–60.
Garrett, G. 1995. Making a big splash with small pools. *Advance for Directors in Rehabilitation* 5(8):63–64.
Garrett, G. 1995. Occupational therapy's perspective. *Rehab Management* 8(3):47,49.
Garrett, G. 1997. Coordinating the planning of your water clinic. *Advance for Occupational Therapy Practitioners* 13(19):12.
Garrett, G. 1997. Designing and constructing water clinics. *Advance for Directors in Rehabilitation* 6(5):43–44.
Glassman, S. 1998. The benefit of buoyancy: Where TBI rehab gets all wet. *Advance for Occupational Therapy Practitioners* 14(24):29–30.
Jamison, L., and D. Ogden. 1994. *Aquatic therapy using PNF patterns.* Tucson, AZ: Therapy Skill Builders.
Jamison, L., and D. Ogden. 1996. Strong strokes: Water ideal for patients with neurological disorders. *Advance for Directors in Rehabilitation* 5(10):53–61.
Johnson, C., and L. Haskell. 1996. Making temperatures 'just right' for therapy goals. *Advance for Directors in Rehabilitation* 5(4):57–59.
Kearney, C., and K. Britsch. 1998. When to use—and not use—aquatic therapy. *Advance for Occupational Therapy Practitioners* 14(50):8,23.
Kerr, T. 1996. Aquatic therapy network to ask for AOTA statement. *Advance for Occupational Therapists,* 12(44):15–46.
Kerr, T. 1997. 'Everybody into the pool!' The debate over aquatic therapy. *Advance for Occupational Therapy Practitioners* 13(2):14–15,46.

Pantanella, T. 1997. How water really works in therapy. *Advance for Occupational Therapy Practitioners* 13(28):17.

Rohland, P. 1996. Small pools, big business. *Advance for Occupational Therapy Practitioners* 12(44):14.

Salzman, A.P. 1998. Digging in? STOP!: Here are a few questions to answer before starting construction on a new therapy pool. *Advance for Occupational Therapy Practitioners* 14(1):23–25.

Vogle, L.K., D.M. Morris, and B.G. Denton. 1998. An aquatic program for adults with cerebral palsy living in group homes. *Physical Therapy Case Reports* 1(5):250–259.

Westerfield, V. 1998. New people in the pool: What aquatics can do for your DD clients. *Advance for Occupational Therapy Practitioners* 14(1):20–22.

ART AND CRAFTS

Breines, E.B. 1995. *Occupational therapy: Activities from clay to computers: Theory and practice.* Philadelphia: F.A. Davis.

Breines, E. 1997. Paint can be all-purpose medium in the OT clinic. *Advance for Occupational Therapy Practitioners* 13(24):5.

Diffendal, J. 1998. How to go back to the future with therapeutic activities. *Advance for Occupational Therapy Practitioners* 14(50):19–21.

Drake, M. 1992. *Crafts in therapy and rehabilitation.* Thorofare, NJ: Slack.

Fidler, G.S. 1981. From crafts to competence. *American Journal of Occupational Therapy* 35(9):567–573.

Johnson, C., K. Lobdell, J. Nesbitt, et al. 1996. *Therapeutic crafts: A practical approach.* Thorofare, NJ: Slack.

Kerr, A. 1998. Have some problem patients? Try tanning their hides. *Advance for Occupational Therapy Practitioners* 14(1):27–28.

Stahl, C. 1998. VSA recaptures the 'Very Special Arts' of therapy. *Advance for Occupational Therapy Practitioners* 14(35):22–23.

ASSISTIVE TECHNOLOGY

Angelo, J. 1997. *Assistive technology for rehabilitation therapists.* Philadelphia: F.A. Davis.

Bain, B.K. 1998. Assistive technology. In *Stroke rehabilitation: A function based approach*, eds. G. Gillen and A. Burkhardt, 465–478. St. Louis: Mosby.

Bain, B.K., and D. Leger. 1997. *Assistive technology: An interdisciplinary approach.* New York: Churchill Livingstone.

Bell, P., and J. Hinojosa. 1995. Perception of the impact of assistive devices on daily life of three individuals with quadriplegia. *Assistive Technology* 7(2):87–94.

Burstein, A.R., M.L. Wright-Drechsel, and A. Wood. 1998. Promoting function in daily living skills. In *Caring for children with cerebral palsy: A team approach*, eds. J.P. Dormans and L. Pellegrino, 371–389. Baltimore: Paul H. Brookes Publishing.

Cook, A.M., and S.M. Hussey. 1995. *Assistive technologies: Principles and practice.* St. Louis: Mosby.

Cook, A.M., and S.M. Hussey. 1998. Electronic assistive technologies. In *Physical dysfunction: Practice skills for the occupational therapy assistant*, ed. M.B. Early, 325–338. St. Louis: Mosby.

Demers, L., R. Weiss-Lambrou, and B. Ska. 1996. Development of the Quebec user evaluation of satisfaction with assistive technology (QUEST). *Assistive Technology* 8(1):3–12.

Fahlgren, K.J. 1993. Use of assistive devices by persons with quadriplegia: A literature review. *Journal of Occupational Therapy Students* 7(1):55–62.

Flippo, K.F., K.J. Inge, and J.M. Barcus. 1995. *Assistive technology: A resource for school, work, and community.* Baltimore: Paul H. Brookes Publishing.

Frantz, G.C., M.A. Christenson, and A. Lindquist. 1998. *Assistive products: An illustrated guide to terminology.* Bethesda, MD: American Occupational Therapy Association.

Freire, E.K., and B.E. Donleavy. 1995. Maximizing potential in young lives with assistive devices. *Advance for Directors in Rehabilitation* 4(3):21–2.

Gitlin, L., and R. Schemm. 1993. Adaptive device use by older adults with mixed disabilities. *Archives of Physical Medicine and Rehabilitation* 74(2):149–152.

Gitlin, L, and R. Schemm. 1996. Maximizing assistive device use among older adults. *TeamRehab Report* 7(4):25–26, 28.

Hammel, J. 1996. What's the outcome? Multiple variables complicate the measurement of assistive technology outcomes. *Rehab Management* 9(2):97–99.

Hammel, J., and J. Angelo. 1996. Technology competencies for occupational therapy practitioners. *Assistive Technology* 8(1):34–42.

Iskowitz, M. 1998. Matchmaking in AT. *Advance for Occupational Therapy Practitioners* 14(14):34.

Luebben, A.J. 1995. Keeping up with assistive technology. *Rehab Management* 8(1):128–129.

Lusa, H.Y., and K.F. Ortmann. 1996. Adaptive equipment and assistive devices. In *Rehabilitation of persons with rheumatoid arthritis*, ed. R.W. Chang, 173–190. Gaithersburg, MD: Aspen Publishers

MacNeil, V. 1998. 'Electronic aids to daily living': A change for the better. *TeamRehab Report* 9(11):53–56.

Mann, W.C., and J.P. Lane. 1995. *Assistive technology for persons with disabilities.* Rockville, MD: American Occupational Therapy Association.

Mann, W.C., and M. Tomita. 1998. Perspectives on assistive devices among elderly persons with disabilities. *Technology and Disability* 9(3):119–148.

Mann, W.C., D. Hurren, B. Charvat, et al. 1996. Changes over one year in assistive device use and home modifications by home-based older persons with Alzheimer's disease. *Topics in Geriatric Rehabilitation* 12(2):9–16.

Mann, W.C., D. Hurren, B. Charvat, et al. 1997. The use of phones by elders with disabilities: Problems, intervention, costs. *Assistive Technology* 8(1):23–33.

Mann, W.C., D. Hurren, and M. Tomita. 1993. Comparison of assistive device use and needs of home-based older persons with different impairments. *American Journal of Occupational Therapy* 47(11):980–987.

Mann, W.C., D. Hurren, M. Tomita, et al. 1995. Assistive devices for home-based older stroke survivors. *Topics in Geriatric Rehabilitation* 10(3):75–86.

Nochajski, S.M., M.R. Tomita, and W.C. Mann. 1996. The use and satisfaction with assistive devices by older persons with cognitive impairments: A pilot intervention study. *Topics in Geriatric Rehabilitation* 12(2):40–53.

Rosenblatt, R.L. 1994. A communication system established for a C-5 quadriplegic and his hearing impaired parents. *Proceedings of the Rehabilitation Engineering Society of North America (RESNA '94)*, 86–88.

Schmeler, M. 1998. 10 tips on documenting the need for assistive technology. *TeamRehab Report* 9(8):16–17.

Shafer, D. 1995. Exploring solutions for vocational re-entry with assistive technology. *Advance for Directors in Rehabilitation* 4(9):59–62.

Shafer, D., and J. Hammel. 1994. A comparison of computer access devices for persons with high level spinal cord injuries. *Proceedings of the Rehabilitation Engineers Society of North America (RESNA '94)*, 394–396.

Stern, P., and E. Trefler. 1997. An interdisciplinary problem-based learning project for assistive technology education. *Assistive Technology* 9(2):152–157.

Struck, M. 1997. How AT coincides with occupation. *Advance for Occupational Therapy Practitioners* 13(41):4.

Struck, M. 1997. Technology to extend independence. *Advance for Occupational Therapy Practitioners* 13(49):6.

Tomita, M.R., W.C. Mann, L.F. Fraas, et al. 1997. Racial differences of frail elders in assistive technology. *Assistive Technology* 9(2):140–151.

CAREGIVING/CARE PROVIDERS

Baum, C.M. 1996. Women as care providers and care receivers: Effective strategies. In *Women with physical disabilities: Achieving and maintaining health and well-being*, eds. D.M. Krotoski, M.A. Nosek, and M.A. Turk, 243–258. Baltimore: Paul H. Brookes Publishing.

Broone, A., and B.J. Rodrigues. 1998. Working with families and caregivers of elders. In *Occupational therapy with elders: Strategies for the COTA*, eds. H. Lohman, R.L. Padilla, and S. Byers-Connon, 121–128, St. Louis: Mosby.

Corradetti, E.V., and G.A. Hills. 1998. Assessing and supporting caregivers of the elderly. *Topics in Geriatric Rehabilitation* 14(1):12–35.

Grott, G. 1998. The caregiving therapist. *Advance for Occupational Therapy Practitioners* 14(11):19.

Hills, G.A. 1998. Caregivers of the elderly: Hidden patients and health team members. *Topics in Geratic Rehabilitation* 14(1)1–11.

Jeng-Ru, L., G.A. Hills, S. Kaplan, et al. 1998. Burden among caregivers of stroke patients in Taiwan. *Topics in Geriatric Rehabilitation* 14(1):74–81.

CASTING (see Serial and Plaster Casting)

CLOTHING ADAPTATIONS

Kratz, G., I. Soderback, S. Guidetti, et al. 1997. Wheelchair users' experience of non-adapted and adapted clothes during sailing, quad rugby or wheel-walking. *Disability and Rehabilitation* 19(1):26–34.

COGNITIVE RETRAINING OR COGNITIVE REHABILITATION

Allen, C.K., T. Blue, and C.A. Earhart. 1995. *Understanding cognitive performance modes*. Ormond Beach, FL: Allen Conferences.

Annoni, J.M., D.G. Jenkins, and J. Williams. 1995. Four case reports illustrating the contribution of intensive cognitive rehabilitation in patients neuropsychologically handicapped as a result of brain damage. *Disability and Rehabilitation* 17(8):449–455.

Katz, N., and N. Hada. 1995. Cognitive rehabilitation: Occupational therapy models for intervention in psychiatry. *Psychosocial Rehabilitation Journal* 19(2):29–36.

COMMUNICATION AIDS

Havard, A. 1998. Up to speed: Dale Stone finds new opportunities through improved mobility and communication. *TeamRehab Report* 9(7):42–44,46.

COMPUTERS

Anson, DK. 1997. *Alternative computer access: A guide to selection*. Philadelphia: F.A. Davis.

Breines, EB. 1995. *Occupational therapy: Activities from clay to computers: Theory and practice*. Philadelphia: F.A. Davis.

Herman, G., and T. Nakashima. Mouse breakout: Relations of mouse switch functions. *Rehabilitation Engineering Society of North America (RESNA '94)*, 409–410.

Nichols, C. 1998. Windows to accessibility: Enabling people with disabilities to access computers. *Advance for Occupational Therapy Practitioners* 14(43):28–30.

Struck, M. 1996. Augmentative communication and computer access. In *Occupational Therapy for Children*, 3rd ed., eds. J. Case-Smith, A.S. Allen, and P.N. Pratt, 545–561. St. Louis: Mosby.

Struck, M. 1997. Keyboarding: It's a skill workers need. *Advance for Occupational Therapy Practitioners* 13(10):4.

Yeomans, J. 1998. Conversations with a computer. *Advance for Occupational Therapy Practitioners* 14(2):30–31.

CRANIOSACRAL THERAPY

Joyce, P., and C. Clark. 1996. The use of craniosacral therapy to treat gastroesophageal reflux in infants. *Infants and Young Children* 9(2):51–58.

Rosenbaum, P.L., and M. Law. 1996. Craniosacral therapy and gastroesophageal reflux: A commentary. *Infants and Young Children* 9(2):69–74.

DRIVER EVALUATION AND TRAINING

Blanc, C. 1997. On the way to work. *TeamRehab Report* 8(12):20–22.

Blanc, C., and J.T. Hunt. 1994. Getting in gear. *TeamRehab Report* 5(8):33–34,36,38–39.

Garber, S.L., and P. Lathem. 1995. Adaptive driving: Mobility and community integration for person with spinal cord injury. *Topics in Spinal Cord Injury Rehabilitation* 1(1):59–65.

Jacobs, K. 1994. OTs in the driver's seat. *Rehab Management* 7(2):126–127.

Johnson, M. 1997. Driver evaluation—it's your choice. *Accent on Living* 42(1):82–83.

Kalina, T. 1997. The road ahead. *TeamRehab Report* 8(7):25–26,28,30,32.

Lillie, S.M. 1998. Driving with a physical dysfunction. In *Physical dysfunction: practice skills for the occupational therapy assistant*, ed. M.B. Early, 312–318. St. Louis: Mosby.

Pierce, S. 1995. Getting a green light for starting a driving program. *Advance for Directors of Rehabilitation* 4(9):52–54,56.

Pierce, S.L. 1998. Driving. In *Stroke rehabilitation: A function-based approach*, eds. G. Gillen, and A. Burhardt, 385–406. St. Louis: Mosby.

Stadwick, K.L. 1998. Back in the driver's seat with General Motors. *Advance for Directors in Rehabilitation* 7(9):75.

Varnell, M.A. 1998. Keeping seniors behind the wheel. *Advance for Occupational Therapy Practitioners* 14(42:34–35.

DYSPHASIA

Avery-Smith, W. 1996. Eating dysfunction (position paper). *American Journal of Occupational Therapy* 50(10):846–847. Also in Eating dysfunction position paper. 1998. *Reference Manual of the Official Documents of the American Occupational Therapy Association*, 7th ed., 197–199. Bethesda, MD: American Occupational Therapy Association.

Avery-Smith, W. 1998. An occupational therapist-coordinated dysphagia program. *OT Practice* 3(10):20–23.

Avery-Smith, W., and D.M. Dellarosa. 1994. Approaches to treating dysphagia in patients with brain injury. *American Journal of Occupational Therapy* 48(3):235–239. (Literature review)

Fucile, S., P.M. Wright, I. Chan, et al. 1998. Function oral-motor skills: Do they change with age? *Dysphagia.* 13:195–201.
Lambert, H.C., and E.G. Gisel. 1996. The assessment of oral, pharyngeal, and esophageal dysphagia in elderly persons. *Physical and Occupational Therapy in Geriatrics* 14(4):1–25. (Literature review)
Morawski, D. 1994. Dysphagia: Its psychological impact. *Physical Disabilities Special Interest Section Newsletter* 17(2):1–2.
Morawski, D., and T. Davis. 1998. Dysphagia and other eating and nutritional concerns with elders. In *Occupational therapy with elders: Strategies for the COTA*, eds. H. Lohman, R.L. Padilla, and S. Byers-Connon, 202–212. St. Louis: Mosby.
Nelson, K.L. 1996. Dysphagia: Evaluation and treatment. In *Occupational therapy: Practice skills for physical dysfunction*, 4th ed., ed. L.W. Pedretti, 165–192. St. Louis: Mosby.
Nelson, K.L. 1998. Treatment of dysphagia. In *Physical dysfunction: practice skills for the occupational therapy assistant*, ed. M.B. Early, 298–311. St. Louis: Mosby.
Noll, S.F., C.E. Bender, and M.C. Nelson. 1996. Rehabilitation of patients with swallowing disorders. In *Physical Medicine and Rehabilitation*, ed. R.L. Braddom, 533–554. Philadelphia: W.B. Saunders.
O'Sullivan, N., ed. 1995. *Dysphagia care: Team approach with acute and long-term patients*, 2nd ed. Los Angeles: Cottage Square.
Skvaria, A.M., and R.A. Schroeder-Lopez. 1998. Dysphagia management. In *Stroke rehabilitation: A function-based approach*, eds. G. Gillen and A. Burhardt, 407–422. St. Louis: Mosby.
Stinnett, K.A., and E.C. Adams. 1995. The institutionalized frail older person and the dining experience. *Topics in Geriatric Rehabilitation* 11(2):26–34.
Williams-Santa, K. 1994. The dysphagia program of the National Rehabilitation Hospital. *Physical Disabilities Special Interest Section Newsletter* 17(2):5–8.

EARLY INTERVENTION

Brown, S.E, and J.L. Valluzzi. 1995. Do not resuscitate orders in early intervention settings: Who should make the decision? *Infants and Young Children* 7(3):13–27.
Feinberg, E.A., B. Hanft, and N. Marvin. 1996. Program evaluation and strategic planning in early intervention: General principles and a case example. *Infants and Young Children* 8(4):41–48.
Hanft, B.E. 1997. Toward the development of a framework for determining the frequency and intensity of early intervention services. *Infants and Young Children* 10(1):27–37.
Jackson, L. 1998. Who's paying for therapy in early intervention? *Infants and Young Children* 11(2):65–72.
Johnson, D.E., and K. Dole. 1999. International adoptions: Implications for early intervention. *Infants and Young Children* 11(4):34–45.
Rush, D.D., M. Shelden, L. Stanfill. 1995. Facing the challenges: Implementing a statewide system of inservice training in early intervention. *Infants and Young Children* 7(4):55–61.
Schultz-Krohn, W. 1997. Early intervention: Meeting the unique needs of parent-child interaction. *Infants and Young Children* 10(1):47–60.
Vergara, E. 1993. *Foundations for practice in the neonatal intensive care unit and early intervention: A self-guided practice manual*, vol. 1. Rockville, MD: American Occupational Therapy Association.
Vergara, E. 1993. *Foundations for practice in the neonatal intensive care unit and early intervention: A self-guided practice manual*, vol. 2. Rockville, MD: American Occupational Therapy Association.

EDEMA CONTROL

Burkhard, A. 1998. Edema control. In *Stroke rehabilitation: A function-based approach*, eds. G. Gillen and A. Burkhard, 152–160. St. Louis: Mosby.

ENERGY CONSERVATION

Kerr, T. 1997. One video is worth more than 1,000 words. *Advance for Occupational Therapy Practitioners* 13(22):13,46.

Packer, T.L., N. Brink, and A. Sauriol. 1995. *Managing fatigue: A six-week course for energy conservation.* Tucson, AZ: Therapy Skill Builders.

ENVIRONMENT CONTROL TECHNOLOGY

Bartholomew, E., and M. Deatherage. 1995. Making the right choice. *TeamRehab Report* 6(5):32–36.

Dickey, R. 1996. Assessment for selection of environmental control. *TeamRehab Report* 7(7):23–26.

Graf, M., E. Severe, and A. Holle. 1997. Environmental control unit: Considerations for the person with high-level tetraplegia. *Topics in Spinal Cord Injury Rehabilitation* 2(3):30–40.

Kangas, K.M. 1995. Staying in control: ECUs offer level of independence. *Advance for Directors in Rehabilitation* 4(10):65–67.

Lange, M. 1995. 1995. Selecting an ECU. *TeamRehab Report* 6(11):43–45.

Lange, M. 1997. What's new and different in environmental control systems. *TeamRehab Report* 8(9):19–23.

Marmer, L. 1997. Electronics that make life easier. *Advance for Occupational Therapy Practitioners* 13(4):14–15,50.

Marmer, L. 1997. This old house: Home improvement was never like this! *Advance for Occupational Therapy Practitioners* 13(6):14–15.

Rizzo, C., and A. Koontz. 1998. Control his environment: Phil Macri's environmental control system helps him reach out from his home office. *TeamRehab Report* 9(3):26–28,30.

ERGONOMICS

Bodenhamer, A. 1993. Ergonomics. In *Rehabilitation of the spine: Science and practice*, eds. S.H. Hochschuler, H.B. Cotler, and R.D. Guyer, 699–702. St. Louis: Mosby.

Glassman, S. 1997. Same old grind: An ergonomic evaluation can help prevent overuse syndromes for developing or continuing. *Advance for Occupational Therapy Practitioners* 13(49):22–23.

Hedman, G., and T. Nakashima. 1994. Modification of industrial hose nozzle and work area for worker with arthritis. *Proceedings of the Rehabilitation Engineering Society of North America (RESNA '94)*, 487–489.

Isernhagen, S.J. 1998. Ergonomics at work: Six keys combine science and art to make you more ergonomically effective, and your clients injury-free. *Advance for Occupational Therapy Practitioners* 14(36):36–37.

Jacobs, K. 1994. Job analysis. *Rehab Management* 7(3):113–114.

Jacobs, K. 1995. Ergonomic certification update. *Rehab Management* 8(1):125–126.

Jacobs, K. 1995. Ergonomic protection standard. *Rehab Management* 8(4):149–153.

Jacobs, K., and C.M. Bettencourt. 1995. *Ergonomics for therapists.* Boston: Butterworth-Heinemann.

Rice, V.J. 1997. Rehabilitation ergonomics: a client-centered ecological approach. *Work* 9:191–194.

Rice, V.J. 1998. *Ergonomics in health care and rehabilitation.* Boston: Butterworth-Heinemann.

Werrell, M. 1997. Eight ways to a healthier workplace: Proper ergonomics can result in fewer injuries to workers. *Advance for Occupational Therapy Practitioners* 13(47):32–34.

FEEDING/SWALLOWING AND ORAL MOTOR DEVELOPMENT—CHILD

Case-Smith, J., and R. Humphry. 1996. Feeding: An oral motor skill. In *Occupational therapy for children,* 3rd ed., eds. J. Case-Smith, A.S. Allen, and P.N. Pratt, 430–460. St. Louis: Mosby.

Geyer, L.A., and J.S. McGowan. 1995. Positioning infants and children for videofluoroscopic swallowing function studies. *Infants and Young Children* 8(2):58–64.

Gisel, E.G. 1996. Oral-motor skills following sensorimotor therapy in two groups of moderately dysphagic children with cerebral palsy: Aspiration vs. nonaspiration. *Dysphagia* 11:59–71.

Gisel, E.G. 1998. Effect of oral appliance (ISMAR) therapy in children with cerebral paralyzed moderate dysphagia. *AACPDM Abstracts*, 8. [Published with *Developmental Medicine and Child Neurology*]

Iskowitz, M. 1998. Pediatrics and DD: Airway issues and dysphagia. *Advance for Occupational Therapy Practitioners* 14(23):18, 66.

Joe, B.E. 1996. Swallowing problems call for gentle touch. *OT Week* 10(30):14–16.

Kazman, W. 1997. What OT has taught me about myself. *Advance for Occupational Therapy Practitioners* 13(14):12.

Tapper, B.E. 1995. Hard to swallow. *OT Week* 9(1):16–17.

Yossem, F. 1998. *Clinical management of feeding disorders: Case studies.* Boston: Butterworth-Heinemann.

FEEDING/SWALLOWING PROBLEMS—ADULT (see Dysphasia)

FUNCTIONAL SKILLS

Wamboldt, J.J. 1996. *Functional skills program for the neurologically impaired client.* Tucson, AZ: Therapy Skills Builders.

GROUP TECHNIQUES

Byers-Connon, S., and S. Hoff. 1998. Group treatment with elders. In *Occupational therapy with elders: Strategies for the COTA*, eds. H. Lohman, R.L. Padilla, and S. Byers-Connon, 137–144. St. Louis: Mosby

Ross, M. 1997. *Integrative group therapy: Mobilizing coping abilities with the five-stage group.* Bethesda, MD: American Occupational Therapy Association.

HAND FUNCTIONS—ADULT

Bergmann, K.P. 1990. Incidence of atypical pencil grasps among nondysfunctional adults. *American Journal of Occupational Therapy* 44(8):736–740.

Desrosiers, J. et al. 1993. Development and reliability of an upper extremity function test for the elderly: The TEMPA. *Canadian Journal of Occupational Therapy* 60(1):9–16.

Marmer, L. 1998. OTs put FUN in FUNctional rehab: The upper limb exerciser 'takes hold' in U.S. *Advance for Occupational Therapy Practitioners* 14(19):29–30,32.

Thompson, S.T., and M.A. Wehbe. 1995. Extensor physiology in the hand and wrist. *Hand Clinics* 11(3):367–371.

HAND FUNCTIONS—CHILD

Boehme, R. 1993. Developing hand function. In *Therapeutic exercise in developmental disabilities*, 2nd ed., eds. B.H. Connolly and P.C. Montgomery, 155–166. Hixson, TN: Chattanooga Group, Inc. [P.O. Box 489, 4717 Adams Road, Hixson, TN 37343].

Case-Smith, J. 1995. Grasp, release, and bimanual skills in the first two years of life. In *Hand function in the child: Foundations for remediation*, eds. A. Henderson and C. Pehoski, 113–135. St. Louis: Mosby.

Case-Smith, J. and C. Pehoski. 1992. *Development of hand skills in the child.* Rockville, MD: American Occupational Therapy Association.

Erhardt, R.P. 1997. Hand development: Answers to some common questions. *Advance for Occupational Therapy Practitioners* 13(23):12.

Erhardt, R.P. 1997. The prehension/vision connection: Implications for skill development. *Advance for Occupational Therapy Practitioners* 13(25):12.

Erhardt, R.P. 1997. Early hand development: What children need for future adult performance. *Advance for Occupational Therapy Practitioners* 13(27):12–13.

Exner, C.E. 1996. Development of hand skills. In *Occupational therapy for children,* 3rd ed., eds. J. Case-Smith, A.S. Allen, and P.N. Pratt, 268–306. St. Louis: Mosby.

Pehoski, C. 1995. Cortical control of skilled movements of the hand. In *Hand function in the child: Foundations for remediation,* eds. A. Henderson and C. Pehoski, 2–15. St. Louis: Mosby.

Pehoski, C. 1995. Objective manipulation in infants and children. In *Hand function in the child: Foundations for remediation,* eds. A. Henderson and C. Pehoski, 236–253. St. Louis: Mosby.

Rosblad, B. 1995. Reaching and eye-hand coordination. In *Hand function in the child: Foundations for remediation,* eds. A. Henderson and C. Pehoski, 81–92. St. Louis: Mosby.

Shaperman, J., and M. LeBlanc. 1995. Prehensor grip for children: A survey of the literature. *JPO: Journal of Prosthetics and Orthotics* 7(2):61–64.

Stilwell, J.M., and S.A. Cermak. 1995. Perceptual functions of the hand. In *Hand function in the child: Foundations for remediation,* eds. A. Henderson and C. Pehoski, 55–80. St. Louis: Mosby.

HANDEDNESS

Marmer, L. 1997. Climbing to maturity hand over hand. *Advance for Occupational Therapy Practitioners* 13(20):13,19.

Murray, E.A. 1995. Hand preference and its development. In *Hand function in the child: Foundations for remediation,* eds. A. Henderson and C. Pehoski, 154–163. St. Louis: Mosby.

HANDWRITING

Amundson, S.J. 1998. *TRICS for written communication: Techniques for rebuilding and improving children's school skills.* Homer, AL: O.T. KIDS.

Amundson, S.J., and M. Weil. 1996. Prewriting and handwriting skills. In *Occupational therapy for children,* 3rd ed., eds. J. Case-Smith, A.S. Allen, and P.N. Pratt, 524–544. St. Louis: Mosby.

Benbow, M. 1995. Principles and practices in teaching handwriting. In *Hand function in the child: Foundations for remediation,* eds. A. Henderson and C. Pehoski, 255–281. St. Louis: Mosby.

Ziviani, J. 1995. The development of graphomotor skills. In *Hand function in the child: Foundations for remediation,* eds. A. Henderson and C. Pehoski, 184–193. St. Louis: Mosby.

HIPPOTHERAPY (see Therapeutic Horse Riding and Hippotherapy)

HOME MANAGEMENT

Law, M. 1998. Home management. In *Introduction to disability,* eds. M.A. McColl and J.E. Bickenbach, 91–98. Philadelphia: W.B. Saunders.

HOME MODIFICATION AND ACCESSIBILITY

Bulger-Tsapos, D. 1996. Kitchen accessibility: Recipes for success. *Advance for Directors in Rehabilitation* 5(7):17,19,22.

Burgess, L. 1999. Home modification: Bridging the gap between inpatient and community practice. *OT Practice* 4(6):38–42.

Fieman, R., and S. Rogers. 1995. An accessible habitat. *TeamRehab Report* 6(10):14–17.

Gitlin, L.N., and M.A.Corcoran. 1996. Managing dementia at home: the role of home environment modifications. *Topics in Geriatric Rehabilitation* 12(2):28–39.

Kalupa, K.J., S. Apte-Kakade, and S.V. Fisher. 1994. Assistive devices and environmental modifications. In *Rehabilitation of the aging and elderly patient*, eds. G. Felsenthal, S.J. Garrison, and F.U. Steinberg, 449–465. Baltimore: Williams & Wilkins.

Mann, W.C., D. Hurren, B. Charvat, et al. 1996. Changes over one year in assistive device use and home modifications by home-based older persons with Alzheimer's disease. *Topics in Geriatric Rehabilitation.* 12(2):9–16.

Salerno, C.A. 1998. Home evaluation and modification. In *Stroke rehabilitation: A function-based approach*, eds. G. Gillen and A. Burhardt, 452–464. St. Louis: Mosby.

Shamberg, S., and A. Shamberg. 1996. Building an accessible home from the ground up. *TeamRehab Report* 7(4):16–17,20–22.

Tempio, S. 1995. Right at home: Effective home accessibility recommendations require a comprehensive evaluation of the client, his or her lifestyle and environment. *TeamRehab Report* 6(3):14–16.

HOME SAFETY AND ACCIDENT PREVENTION

Salerno, C.A. 1998. Home assessments and safety modifications. In *Stroke rehabilitation: A function-based approach*, eds. G. Gillen and A. Burhardt, 543–553. St. Louis: Mosby.

McLean, D., and S. Lord. 1996. Falling in older people at home: Transfer limitations and environmental risk factors. *Australian Occupational Therapy Journal* 43(1):13–18.

HORTICULTURE/GARDENING

Carlson, J. 1998. The PLANT, the whole PLANT, nothing but the PLANT. *Advance for Occupational Therapy Practitioners.* 34(43):26–27,36.

INDEPENDENT LIVING

McGeorge, D.W.F., C.R. Clark, and R.E.A. Goble. 1993. St. Loye's independent living centre: An analysis of assessment. *Disability and Rehabilitation* 15(3):136–142.

Shepherd, J., S.A. Procter, and I.L. Coley. 1996. Self-care and adaptations for independent living. In *Occupational therapy for children,* 3rd ed., eds. J. Case-Smith, A.S. Allen, and P.N. Pratt, 461–503. St. Louis: Mosby.

Stahl, C. 1998. Spaulding's therapeutic overnight stay. *Advance for Occupational Therapy Practitioners* 14(11):31–32.

INDUSTRIAL REHABILITATION

Breske, S. 1997. Getting a grip: Hand issues in industrial rehab. *Advance for Occupational Therapy Practitioners* 13(20):16–17.

Keegan, D.M., and L.F. Murphy. 1997. Industrial rehabilitation services. In *Hand rehabilitation: A practical guide*, 2nd ed., eds. G.L. Clark, E.F.S. Wilgis, B. Aiello, et al., 315–420. New York: Churchill Livingstone.

Lawn, G. 1996. OT/PT: Finding a place in industrial medicine. *Advance for Physical Therapists* (July 15):6–7.

Marmer, L. 1996. Offering 'alternatives' in industrial medicine. *Advance for Occupational Therapists* 7(6):8–9.

Melnik, M.S. 1993. Industrial back school. In *Rehabilitation of the spine: Science and practice*, eds. S.H. Hochschuler, H.B. Cotler, and R.D. Gyer, 703–709. St. Louis: Mosby.

Stahl, C. 1997. On-site industrial rehabilitation: Reduces worker's comp costs, boosts moral. *Advance for Occupational Therapy Practitioners* 13(17):12–13.

JOB MODIFICATION

Volz, D. 1998. Low-cost solutions to common job problems. *Advance for Occupational Therapy Practitioners* 14(27):18.

JOINT PROTECTION

Hammond, A. 1994. Joint protection behavior in patients with rheumatoid arthritis following an education program: A pilot study. *Arthritis Care and Research* 7(1):5–9.

LEISURE/RECREATION SKILLS

Dress, L. 1997. Kid zone: A fitness park on a rehab hospital's campus benefits people in both the hospital and the community. *Advance for Occupational Therapy Practitioners* 13(49):32–34.

Glantz, C.H., and N. Richman. 1996. Evaluation and intervention for leisure activities. In *ROTE: The role of occupational therapy with the elderly,* 2nd ed., eds. K.O. Larson, R.G. Stevents-Ratchford, L. Pedretti, et al., 729–742. Bethesda, MD: American Occupational Therapy Association.

McCree, S.T. 1993. *Leisure and play in therapy: Theory, goals, and activities.* Tucson, AZ: Therapy Skill Builders.

Ravetz, C. 1995. Leisure. In *Occupational therapy in short-term psychiatry,* 3rd ed., ed. M. Willson, 195–216. New York: Churchill Livingstone.

Stangler, K. 1997. Adapted equipment for recreation. *Advance for Occupational Therapy Practitioners* 13(46):25–26.

Whyte, N.C., and D.A. Supon. 1998. Leisure: Methods to improve skills. In *Stroke rehabilitation: A function-based approach*, eds. G. Gillen and A. Burhardt, 496–507. St. Louis: Mosby.

LIFE SKILLS

Gadberry, L., and T. Frauenheim-Finke. 1996. *Motivating life skill modules for individuals with spinal cord injury.* Bethesda, MD: American Occupational Therapy Association.

Precin, P. 1999. *Living skills recovery workbook.* Boston: Butterworth-Heinemann.

MEDICATIONS

Flynn, B., and B.M. Coppard. 1998. Use of medications by elders. In *Occupational therapy with elders: Strategies for the COTA*, eds. H. Lohman, R.L. Padilla, and S. Byers-Connon, 145–154. St. Louis: Mosby.

MOBILE ARM SUPPORTS (BALL-BEARING FOREARM ORTHOSES OR BALANCED FOREARM ORTHOSES)

Adler, C., and L.W. Pedretti. 1998. Balanced forearm orthosis and suspension sling. In *Physical dysfunction: Practice skills for the occupational therapy assistant*, ed. M.B. Early, 319–324. St. Louis: Mosby.

MOBILITY (see also Positioning, Seating, and Wheelchairs and Accessories)

Adler, C., M. Tipton-Burton, and R.M. Lehman. 1998. Wheelchairs and wheelchair mobility, functional mobility and transfer training, and ambulation aids. In *Physical dysfunction: Practice skills for the occupational therapy assistant*, ed. M.B. Early, 276–296. St. Louis: Mosby.

Casey, P., and M. Smith. 1995. U-step helps patients walk. *Advance for Directors in Rehabilitation* 4(10):80.

Copperman, L., C. Harley, P. Scharf, et al. 1994. Fatigue and mobility. *Journal of Neurologic Rehabilitation* 8(3):131–136.

de Mello, M.A.F., and W.C. Mann. 1995. The use of mobility related devices by older individuals with developmental disabilities living in community residences. *Technology and Disability* 4(4):275–285.

Galyen, K., S.H. Okada, and P.J. Lavoot. 1998. Considerations of mobility. In *Occupational therapy with elders: Strategies for the COTA*, eds. H. Lohman, R.L. Padilla, and S. Byers-Connon, 155–173, St. Louis: Mosby.

Havard, A. 1998. Up to speed: Dale Stone finds new opportunities through improved mobility and communication. *TeamRehab Report* 9(7):42–44,46.

Kane, L.A., and K.A. Buckley. 1998. Functional mobility. In *Stroke rehabilitation: A function-based approach*, eds. G. Gillen and A. Burhardt, 205–242. St. Louis: Mosby.

LePostelec, M. 1998. Upward mobility: The benefits of standing chairs. *Advance for Occupational Therapy Practitioners* 14(19):31–32.

Mann, W.C., S.M. Nochajski, S.H. Sprigle, et al. 1995. Custom device development and professional training in developmental disabilities. *Technology and Disability* 4(4):295–329.

Marmer, L. 1996. Putting the power in powered mobility. *Advance for Directors in Rehabilitation* 5(9):11–12,15.

Murphy, J. 1995. Scooters aren't just for kids anymore. *Advance for Occupational Therapy Practitioners* 11(8):16.

Pohland, P. 1997. Limiting time in 'walkers' may avoid back pain later in life. *Advance for Occupational Therapy Practitioners* 13(46):35–36.

Tanquay, S., and M. Wayland. 1998. Power chairs and scooters. *Exceptional Parent* 28(9):62,64–65.

Taylor, S.J. 1995. Powered mobility evaluation and technology. *Topics in Spinal Cord Injury Rehabilitation* 1(1):23–36.

Taylor, S.J, and D. Kreutz. 1994. Manual or powered mobility. *Advance for Directors in Rehabilitation* 3(10):23–29.

Trefler, E., D.A. Hobson, S.J. Taylor, et al. 1993. *Seating and mobility for persons with physical disabilities.* Tucson, AZ: Therapy Skill Builders.

Vander Schaaf, P. 1995. Cody goes mobile. *TeamRehab Report* 7(4):36–39.

Wright-Ott, C., and S. Egilson. 1996. Mobility. In *Occupational therapy for children,* 3rd ed., eds. J. Case-Smith, A.S. Allen, P.N. Pratt, 562–580. St. Louis: Mosby.

MUSIC ACTIVITIES

Walters, S.L., and P. Seretny. 1997. A therapeutic duet: OTs and MTs pair up to restore function. *Advance for Directors in Rehabilitation* 6(9):29–30.

ONE-HANDED TECHNIQUES

Herrington, M., and A.J. Luebben. 1994. The gripper: A one-handed cattle castrator. *Rehabilitation Engineering Society of North America (RESNA '94)*, 433–435.

Mayer, T. 1996. *One-handed in a two-handed world: Your personal guide to managing single-handedly.* Boston: Prince-Gallison Press.

Sullivan, J.W., R.A. Ryan. 1998. Activities of daily living adaptations: Managing the environment with one-handed techniques. In *Stroke rehabilitation: A function-based approach*, eds. G. Gillen and A. Burhardt, 479–495. St. Louis: Mosby.

ORTHOSES (Other Than Splints)

Kerrick, R.C., and C. French. 1993. Torticollis: A head and neck immobilizer. *American Journal of Occupational Therapy* 47(1):79–80.

Kirshblum, S., C. O'Connor, B.T. Benevento, et al. 1998. Spinal and upper extremity orthotics. In *Rehabilitation medicine: Principles and practice*, 3rd ed., ed. J.A. DeLisa, 635–650. Philadelphia: Lippincott-Raven Publishers.

Kjeken, I., G. Moller, and T.K. Kvien. 1995. Use of commercially produced elastic wrist orthoses in chronic arthritis: A controlled study. *Arthritis Care and Research* 8(2):108–113.

Lohman, M., and H. Goldstein. 1993. Alternative strategies in tone-reducing AFO design. *Journal of Prosthetics and Orthotics* 5(1):21–24.

Osterioh, T.C. 1994. Fabricating TLSOs can be quick and easy. *Advance for Directors of Rehabilitation* 3(9):58.

Ridgway, C.L., and G.D. Warden. 1995. Evaluation of vertical mouth stretching orthosis: Two case reports. *Journal of Burn Care and Rehabilitation* 16(1):74–78.

Stern, E.B., S.R. Ytterberg, L.M. Larson, et al. 1997. Commercial wrist extensor orthoses: A descriptive study of use and preference in patients with rheumatoid arthritis. *Arthritis Care and Research* 10(1):27–35.

PET THERAPY (see also Animal-Assisted Therapy)

Bernard, S. 1995. Rehab is going to the dogs. *Advance for Occupational Therapy Practitioners* 11(14):17.

Breines, E. 1996. Are pets the therapy tool your practice is missing? *Advance for Occupational Therapy Practitioners* 12(7):5.

Copley-Nigro, J. 1995. A friend indeed. *Advance for Occupational Therapy Practitioners* 11(43):19.

Copley-Nigro, J. 1997. How to use pets in home care: Animals deliver therapy with unconditional love. *Advance for Occupational Therapy Practitioners* 14(28):35–36.

Fick, K.M. 1993. The influence of an animal on social interactions of nursing home residents in a group setting. *American Journal of Occupational Therapy* 47(6):529–534.

Zisselman, M.N., B.W. Rovner, Y. Shmuely, et al. 1996. A pet therapy intervention with geriatric psychiatry inpatients. *American Journal of Occupational Therapy* 50(1):47–51.

PHYSICAL AGENT MODALITIES

Colan, B.J. 1995. The other side of FES: Strengthening the arms. *Advance for Occupational Therapy Practitioners* 11(43):9.

Diffendal, J. 1998. FES to walk again. *Advance for Occupational Therapy Practitioners* 14(31):24–27,66.

Johnson, C., and L. Haskell. 1996. Making temperatures 'just right' for therapy goals. *Advance for Directors in Rehabilitation* 5(4):57–59.

Kohlmeyer, K.M., J.P. Hill, G.M. Yarkony, et al. 1996. Electrical stimulation and biofeedback effect on recovery of tenodesis grasp: A controlled study. *Archives of Physical Medicine and Rehabilitation* 77(7):702–706.

Smith, B.T., R.R. Betz, M.J. Mulcahey, et al. 1994. Reliability of percutaneous intramuscular electrodes for upper extremity functional neuromuscular stimulation in adolescents with C5 tetraplegia. *Archives of Physical Medicine and Rehabilitation* 75(9):939–945.

PLAY

Morrison, C.D., P. Metzger, and P.N. Pratt. 1996. Play. In *Occupational therapy for children,* 3rd ed., eds. J. Case-Smith, A.S. Allen, and P.N. Pratt, 504–523. St. Louis: Mosby.

Parham, L.D., and L.S. Fazio. 1997. *Play in occupational therapy for children.* St. Louis: Mosby.

POSITIONING (see also Mobility, Seating, and Wheelchairs and Accessories)

Doherty, J., and M. Robdau. 1998. Static/dynamic head control: It is possible? *TeamRehab Report* 9(8):18–20.

Trefler, E., and J. Angeo. 1997. Comparison of anterior trunk supports for children with cerebral palsy. *Assistive Technology* 9(1):15–21.

Weiler, J. 1998. Positioning for pennies: You can cut costs with cardboard, creativity. *Advance for Occupational Therapy Practitioners* 14(29):29–30.

POSTURAL CONTROL

Nichols, D.S. 1996. The development of postural control. In *Occupational therapy for children,* 3rd ed., eds. J. Case-Smith, A.S. Allen, and P.N. Pratt, 247–267. St. Louis: Mosby.

POWERED MOBILITY (see Mobility)

PRESSURE GARMENTS

Pratt, J., G. West. 1995. *Pressure garments: A manual on their design and fabrication.* Oxford: England: Butterworth-Heinemann.

RELAXATION TECHNIQUES

Cooper, J., ed. 1997. *Occupational therapy in oncology and palliative care.* Appendices 8–12, Relaxation, 247–262. San Diego: Singular Press.

Keable, D. 1997. Active relaxation techniques. In *The management of anxiety: A guide for therapists*, ed. D. Keable, 103–108. New York: Churchill Livingstone.

Keable, D. 1997. Mental relaxation techniques. In *The management of anxiety: A guide for therapists*, ed. D. Keable, 83–86. New York: Churchill Livingstone.

Keable, D. 1997. Physiological relaxation techniques. In *The management of anxiety: A guide for therapists*, ed. D. Keable, 77–81. New York: Churchill Livingstone.

SAFETY AND ACCIDENT/INJURY PREVENTION

Clemson, L., R.G. Cumming, and M. Roland. 1996. Case-control study of hazards in the home and risk of falls and hip fractures. *Age and Aging* 25:97–101.

Ehrlich, P., and C. Piersol. 1997. Keeping your clients safe and independent at home. *Advance for Occupational Therapy Practitioners* 13(38):16.

Kerr, T. 1997. Helmets protect infants' head shapes. *Advance for Occupational Therapy Practitioners* 13(14):13,66.

King, P.M. 1995. The psychosocial work environment: Implications for workplace safety and health. *Professional Safety* 40(3):36–39.

Marmer, L. 1997. Keeping older adults 'safe and sound' in the community. *Advance for Occupational Therapy Practitioners* 13(9):20.
Nieman, D., and M. Silver. 1997. Safe homes for people with Alzheimer's. *Advance for Occupational Therapy Practitioners* 13(42):21.
Valluzzi, J. 1995. Safety issues in community-based settings for children who are medically fragile: Program planning for natural disasters. *Infants and Young Children* 7(4):62–76.

SEATING (see also Mobility, Positioning, and Wheelchairs and Accessories)

Barkley, R., and J. Root. 1996. Improved seating and head position: It's never too late. *TeamRehab Report* 9(7):28–30.
Boeker, C., and S. Edwards. 1995. Seating solutions: Choosing the appropriate cushion. *Advance for Directions in Rehabilitation* 4(3):9–11.
Colman, M. 1995. Assessing and meeting seating and positioning needs. *Advance for Direction in Rehabilitation* 4(10):37–38,41.
Freney, D. 1995. Pediatric seating and positioning. *Rehab Management* 8(4):155–156,159.
Freney, D. 1997. Pediatric seating and mobility: The challenges of changing children. *Rehab Management* 10(4):38,40, 42.
Freney, D., K. Denning-Goldner, and M. Peterson. 1995. The stroller option. *TeamRehab Report* 6(3):26–28,30.
Johann, C.M. 1998. Seating and wheeled mobility prescription. In *Stroke rehabilitation: A function-based approach*, eds. G. Gillen and A. Burhardt, 437–451. St. Louis: Mosby.
Kreutz, D., S.J. Taylor, and D.F. Apple. 1995. A wheelchair seating challenge. *Topics in Spinal Cord Injury Rehabilitation* 1(1):37–41.
Lachman, S.M., E. Greenfield, and A. Wrench. 1993. Assessment of need for special seating and/or electronic control systems for wheelchairs among people with severe physical disabilities. *Clinical Rehabilitation* 7:151–156.
Lange, M.L., C. McDonald, and J. Marcoux. 1995. A custom fit. *TeamRehab Report* 6(1):22–26.
Lemaire, E.D., D. Upton, J. Paialung, et al. 1996. Clinical analysis of a CAD/CAM system for custom seating: A comparison with hand-sculpting methods. *Journal of Rehabilitation Research and Development* 33(3):311–320.
Reid, D.T. 1995. The effects of the saddle seat on seated postural control and upper extremity movement in children with cerebral palsy. *Developmental Medicine and Child Neurology* 38(9):805–815.
Schoger, S. 1996. Years of effort pay off: Bringing up Debra. *TeamRehab Report* 7(3):18–22.
Shasin, C.A. 1995. Understanding MS. *TeamRehab Report* 6(8):20–23.
Sommerfreund, J., and M. Masse. 1995. Combining tilt and recline. *TeamRehab Report* 6(10):18–20.
Stinnett, K.A. 1995. Issues in geriatric settings: Health, comfortable seating. *Advance for Directors in Rehabilitation* 4(6):22–23,26.
Stinnett, K.A. 1998. Developing a seating/positioning system. *Advance for Occupational Therapy Practitioners* 14(2):27–28.
Taylor, S.J., and D. Kreutz. 1996. Using a clinical framework for seating evaluation. *Advance/Rehabilitation* 5(5):11–12,14.
Trefler, E. 1993. Selecting a seating system. *Exceptional Parent* 23(5):42,44.
Trefler, E. 1995. Proper seating and positioning. *Exceptional Parent* 25(2):38–39.
Trefler, E., D.A. Hobson, S.J. Taylor, et al. 1993. *Seating and mobility for persons with physical disabilities*. Tucson, AZ: Therapy Skill Builders.
Wagner, D., M. Fox, and E. Ellis. 1994. Developing a successful interdisciplinary seating program. *Ostomy/Wound Management* 40(1):32–34,36–38,40–41.

SELF-CARE

Christiansen, C.H., and K.J. Ottenbacher. 1998. Evaluation and management of daily self-care requirements. In *Rehabilitation medicine: Principles and practice*, 3rd ed., ed. J.A. DeLisa, 137–166. Philadelphia: Lippincott-Raven Publishers.

Henderson, A. 1995. Self-care and hand skill. In *Hand function in the child: Foundations for remediation*, eds. A. Henderson and C. Pehoski, 164–183. St. Louis: Mosby.

Shepherd, J., S.A. Procter, and I.L. Coley. 1996. Self-care and adaptations for independent living. In *Occupational therapy for children,* 3rd ed., eds. J. Case-Smith, A.S. Allen, and P.N. Pratt, 461–503. St. Louis: Mosby.

SELF-HELP DEVICES

MacCormac, B. 1996. Transfer handle offers independence. *Advance for Directors in Rehabilitation* 5(1):19.

SELF-REGULATION

Williams, M.S., and S. Shellenberger. 1996. *"How does your engine run?": A leader's guide to the Alert Program for Self-Regulation.* Albuquerque, NM: TherapyWorks, Inc. [4901 Butte Place N.W., Albuquerque, NM 87120].

SENSORIMOTOR DEVELOPMENT

DeGangi, G.A. 1994. *Documenting sensorimotor progress: A pediatric therapist's guide.* Tucson, AZ: Therapy Skill Builders.

Eliasson, A.C. 1995. Sensorimotor integration of normal and impaired development of precision movement of the hand. In *Hand function in the child: Foundations for remediation*, eds. A. Henderson and C. Pehoski, 40–54. St. Louis: Mosby.

Haldy, M. 1998. Making learning accessible. *Advance for Occupational Therapy Practitioners* 14(13):23–34.

Haldy, M., and L. Haack. 1995. *Making it easy: Sensorimotor activities at home and school.* Tucson, AZ: Therapy Skill Builders.

Sheda, C.H., and P.R. Ralston. 1997. *Sensorimotor processing activity plans.* San Antonio, TX: Therapy Skill Builders.

SENSORY INTEGRATION/DYSFUNCTION

Anderson, E., and P. Emmons. 1996. *Unlocking the mysteries of sensory dysfunction: A resource for anyone who works with, or lives with, a child with sensory issues.* Arlington, TX: Future Horizons.

Anzalone, M.E. 1993. Sensory contributions to action: A sensory integrative approach. *Zero to Three* 14(2):17–20.

Downing-Baum, S., and D. Maino. 1996. Case studies show success in OT-OD treatment plans. *Advance for Occupational Therapy Practitioners* 12(44):18,46.

Inamura, K.N. 1998. *SI for early intervention: A team approach.* San Antonio: Therapy Skill Builders.

Kadrmas, C.J. 1993. Is sensory integration therapy an effective treatment for children with learning disabilities? *Journal of Occupational Therapy Students* 7(2):15–22.

Kaplan, B.J, H.J. Polatajko, B.N. Wilson, et al. 1993. Reexamination of sensory integration treatment: A combination of two efficacy studies. *Journal of Learning Disabilities* 26(5):342–347.

Kranowitz, C.S. 1998. *The out-of-sync child: Recognizing and coping with sensory integration dysfunction*. New York: Skylight Press.

Mora, J., and N. Kashman. 1998. 'Teaming' model provides holistic approach to autism treatment. *Advance for Occupational Therapy Practitioners* 14(17):27–29.

Motola, B. 1996. A case report: How SI increased the independence of a teen with DD. *Advance for Occupational Therapy Practitioners* 12(2):14.

Motola, B. 1996. Using the SI inventory for individuals with developmental disabilities. *Advance for Occupational Therapy Practitioners* 12(9):16–17.

Parham, L.D., and Z. Mailloux. 1996. Sensory integration. In *Occupational therapy for children,* 3rd ed., eds. J. Case-Smith, A.S. Allen, and P.N. Pratt, 307–356. St. Louis: Mosby.

Tupper, L.C., and K.E.K. Miesner. 1995. *School hardening: Sensory integration strategies for class and home*. Tucson, AZ: Therapy Skill Builders.

White, C. 1996. My trial by fire with sensory defensiveness. *Advance for Occupational Therapy Practitioners* 12(30):10.

Williamson, G.G. 1997. Sensory integration: A key component of evaluation and treatment of young children with difficulties in relating and communicating. *Zero to Three* 17(5):29–36.

SENSORY RETRAINING

Pedretti, L.W. 1998. Treatment of sensory dysfunction. In *Physical dysfunction: Practice skills for the occupational therapy assistant*, ed. M.B. Early, 389–392. St. Louis: Mosby.

SERIAL AND PLASTER CASTING

Copley, J., and K. Kuipers. 1999. *Management of upper limb hypertonicity*. San Antonio, TX: Therapy Skill Builders. (Chapter 11).

Joachim-Grizzaffi, L. 1998. Casting applications. In *Stroke rehabilitation: A function-based approach*, eds. G. Gillen and A. Burhardt, 185–204. St. Louis: Mosby.

Kelly, LB. 1996. *Upper extremity casting: A practical guide*. Tucson, AZ: Therapy Skill Builders.

Staley, M., and M. Serghious. 1998. Casting guidelines, tips, and techniques: Proceedings from the 1997 American Burn Association PT/OT casting workshop. *Journal of Burn Care & Rehabilitation* 19(3):254–260.

SEXUALITY FOR PERSONS WITH HANDICAPS/DISABILITIES

Burton, G.U. 1998. Sexuality: An activity of daily living. In *Physical dysfunction practice skills for the occupational therapy assistant*, ed. M.B. Early, 185–199. St. Louis: Mosby.

Farman, J., and J.D. Friedman. 1998. Sexual function and intimacy. In *Stroke rehabilitation: A function-based approach*, eds. G. Gillen and A. Burhardt, 423–436. St. Louis: Mosby.

Guest, K.L., and B.K. Miller. 1997. The development of the Survey of Attitudes toward the Sexuality of Adults and Disabilities (SASAD). *Topics in Geriatric Rehabilitation* 12(4):61–71.

Lohman, H. 1998. Addressing sexuality of elders. In *Occupational therapy with elders: Strategies for the COTA*, eds. H. Lohman, R.L. Padilla, and S. Byers-Connon, 129–136, St. Louis: Mosby.

Miller, P.A., and N.C. Couloumbis. 1996. Sexual expression in later life. In *ROTE: The role of occupational therapy with the elderly,* 2nd ed., eds. K.O. Larson, R.G. Stevents-Ratchford, L. Pedretti, et al., 679–689. Bethesda, MD: American Occupational Therapy Association.

SPIRITUALITY AND SPIRITUALISM

Christiansen, C. 1997. Acknowledging a spiritual dimension in occupational therapy practice. *American Journal of Occupational Therapy* 51(3):169–172.

Collins, M. 1998. Occupational therapy and spirituality: Reflecting on quality of experience in therapeutic interventions. *British Journal of Occupational Therapy* 61(6):280–283.

Desai, F.A. 1997. The force that underlies the power of occupation. *Advance for Occupational Therapy Practitioners* 13(42):13,58.

Desai, F.A. 1997. The real meaning of 'spirituality' in OT. *Advance for Occupational Therapy Practitioners* 13(41):13.

Egan, M., and M. Delaat. 1994. Considering spirituality in occupational therapy practice. *Canadian Journal of Occupational Therapy* 61(2):95–101.

Egan, M., and M. Delaat. 1997. The implicit spirituality of occupational therapy practice. *Canadian Journal of Occupational Therapy* 64(3):115–121.

Enquist, D., M. Short De Graft, J. Gliner, et al. 1997. Occupational therapists' beliefs and practices with regard to spirituality and therapy. *American Journal of Occupational Therapy* 51(3):173–180.

Howard, B., and J. Howard. 1997. Occupation as spiritual activity. *American Journal of Occupational Therapy* 51(3):181–185.

McLean, V. 1997. Learning to live is learning awareness. *Advance for Occupational Therapy Practitioners* 13(47):7.

Spencer, J., H. Davidson, and V. White. 1997. Help clients develop hopes for the future. *American Journal of Occupational Therapy* 51(3):191–198.

Stahl, C. 1997. The unity of mind and spirit. *Advance for Occupational Therapy Practitioners* 13(50):18–20.

Wolensky, J. 1997. Spreading light through body, mind, spirit. *Advance for Directors in Rehabilitation* 6(3):82

SPLINTS, SPLINT MAKING—CHILD

Copley, J., and K. Kuipers. 1999. *Management of upper limb hypertonicity*. San Antonio: Therapy Skill Builders. (Chapters 9 and 10).

Duvall-Riley, B. 1998. Big goals for little hands: Mixing kids and splints. *Advance for Occupational Therapy Practitioners* 14(16):28–29.

Hogan, L., and T. Uditsky. 1998. *Pediatric splinting: Selection, fabrication, and clinical application of upper extremity splints*. San Antonio, TX: Therapy Skill Builders.

Kerr, T. 1997. Splints and kids: You can make it work. *Advance for Occupational Therapist* 13(7):14–15.

Thompson, E., and A.B. Tobin. 1997. The modified MacKinnon: A low temperature approach to ped splinting. *Advance for Occupational Therapy Practitioners* 13(48):32–33.

SPLINTS, SPLINT MAKING—ADULT

Berger, S., and L.W. Pedretti. 1998. Hand splinting. In *Physical dysfunction: Practice skills for the occupational therapy assistant*, ed. M.B. Early, 339–356. St. Louis: Mosby.

Bledsoe, S. 1994. To fabricate or not to fabricate: Splinting options. *Advance for Directors in Rehabilitation* 3(9):51–52,54,56.

Colditz, J.C. 1995. Anatomic considerations for splinting the thumb. In *Rehabilitation of the hand*, 4th ed., eds. J.M. Hunter, E.J. Mackin, A.D. Callahan, 1161–1172. St. Louis: Mosby.

Coppard, B.M., and H. Lohman. 1996. *Introduction to splinting: A critical-thinking and problem solving approach*. St. Louis: Mosby.

Curtin, M. 1994. Development of a tetraplegic hand assessment and splinting protocol. *Paraplegia* 32(3):159–169.

Ensor, C. 1996. Splint sense: Pre-fabricated UE choices. *Advance for Directors in Rehabilitation* 5(8):65–67.

Jensen C., and G. Rayan. 1996. Buddy strapping of mismatched fingers: The offset buddy strap. *Journal of Hand Surgery* 21:317–318.

Milazzo, S., G. Gillen. 1998. Splinting applications. In *Stroke rehabilitation: A function-based approach*, eds. G. Gillen and A. Burhardt, 161–184. St. Louis: Mosby.

Pearson, L. 1995. Hands on. *TeamRehab Report* 6(4):21–23, 27.

Thompson, T., and M. Malloy. 1997. The computer access splint. *Advance for Occupational Therapy Practitioners* 13(48):30.

Wilson, G. 1997. Custom neoprene supports for UE disorders. *Advance for Occupational Therapy Practitioners* 13(48):31,33.

Wilton, J.C. 1997. *Hand splinting: Principles of design and fabrication*. London: W.B. Saunders Company.

SPORTS

Kerr, T. 1997. Handling the hopes of young disabled drivers. *Advance for Occupational Therapy Practitioners* 13(25):17,50.

STRESS MANAGEMENT

Keable, D. 1995. Managing stress. In *Occupational therapy in short-term psychiatry*, ed. M. Wilson, 149–172. Edinburgh, Scotland: Churchill Livingstone.

Kerr, T. 1997. Home for the holidays. *Advance for Occupational Therapy Practitioners* 13(49):18–20.

SUPPORT AND SURVIVOR'S GROUPS

Tomlinson, J.L. 1998. Helping the family support the patient. In *Stroke rehabilitation: A function-based approach*, eds. G. Gillen and A. Burhardt, 512–518. St. Louis: Mosby.

THERAPEUTIC HORSE RIDING AND HIPPOTHERAPY

MacKinnon, J.R., S. Noh, J. Lariviere, et al. 1995. A study of therapeutic effects of horseback riding for children with cerebral palsy. *Physical and Occupational Therapy in Pediatrics* 15(1):17–34.

Pfaff , K. 1993. Creature comforts. *TeamRehab Report* 4(4):18–20,22,24,26.

Stancliff, B.L. 1996. Careers: do what you love, the career will follow: OTs recognize animals in therapy. *OT Practice* 1(2):12–13.

TOYS

Kerr, T. 1998. The OT art of making toys accessible. *Advance for Occupational Therapy Practitioners* 14(47):18–19.

Tobias, M.V., and I.M. Goldkopf. 1995. Toys and games: Their role in hand development. In *Hand function in the child: Foundations for remediation*, eds. A. Henderson and C. Pehoski, 223–254. St. Louis: Mosby.

URINARY INCONTINENCE

Collins, L.F. 1998. Using biofeedback to treat incontinence. *OT Practice* 3(5):30–31.

Gitlin, L.N., and M. Corcoran. 1993. Expanding caregiver ability to use environmental solutions for problems of bathing and incontinence. *Technology and Disability* 2(1):12–21.
Joe, B.E. 1998. Urinary incontinence. *OT Week* 12(14):13.
Meissner, D. 1996. Stopping incontinence. *OT Week* 10(36):116–117.
Sahoo, K. 1998. Treating urinary incontinence in the geriatric population. *Advance for Occupational Therapy Practitioners* 14(34):34–35.
Reichenback, V. 1998. From secrecy to self-esteem: Addressing incontinence can restore dignity and independence to clients. *OT Practice* 3(5):26–29, 32.
Reichenback, V.R. 1998. Incontinence. *Gerontology Special Interest Section Quarterly* 21(1):1–3.
Toto, P. 1997. Occupational therapy for functional incontinence. *Advance for Occupational Therapy Practitioners* 13(45):10.

VIRTUAL REALITY

Cohen, B. 1996. Down-to-earth applications of virtual reality. *Advance for Occupational Therapy Practitioners* 12(6):16.
Cunningham, D. 1998. In Alabama, OT is a virtual reality. *Advance for Occupational Therapy Practitioners* 14(17):19.

WELLNESS PROGRAMS

Berg J. 1997. A wellness model for cancer recover. *OT Week* June 5:16–17.
Mandel, D.R., M.H. Jackson, R. Zemke, et al. 1999. *Lifestyle redesign: Implementing the well elderly program*. Bethesda, MD: American Occupational Therapy Association.
Swarbrick, P. 1997. Wellness model for clients. *Mental Health Special Interest Section Quarterly* 20(1):1–4.

WHEELCHAIRS AND ACCESSORIES (see also Mobility, Positioning, and Seating)

Adler, C., M. Tipton-Burton, and R.M. Lehman. 1998. Wheelchairs and wheelchair mobility, functional mobility and transfer training, and ambulation aids. In *Physical dysfunction: practice skills for the occupational therapy assistant*, ed. M.B. Early, 276–296. St. Louis: Mosby.
Brienza, D.M., and J. Angelo. 1996. A force feedback joystick and control algorithm for wheelchair obstacle avoidance. *Disability and Rehabilitation* 19(3):123–129.
Brienza, D., J. Angelo, and K. Henry. 1995. Consumer participation in identifying research and development priorities for power wheelchair input devices and controllers. *Assistive Technology* 7(1):55–62.
Currie, D.M., K. Hardwick, R.A. Marburger. 1998. Wheelchair prescription and adaptive seating. In *Rehabilitation medicine: principles and practice*, 3rd ed., ed. J.A. DeLisa, 789–828. Philadelphia: Lippincott-Raven Publishers.
Edwards, S., and W.D. Hammon. 1997. Choosing the right recline chair. *Advance for Directors in Rehabilitation* 6(2):10–11.
Garber, S., and T. Krouskop. 1997. Technical advances in wheelchairs and seating systems. *Physical Medicine and Rehabilitation: State of the Art Reviews* 11(1):93–106.
Kirby, R.L., B.D. Ashton, S.A. Ackroyd-Stolarz, et al. 1996. Adding loads to occupied wheelchairs: Effect on static rear and forward stability. *Archives of Physical Medicine and Rehabilitation* 77(2):183–186.

Kirby, R.L., F.A.V. Thoren, B.D. Ashton, et al. 1994. Wheelchair stability and maneuver ability: Effect of varying the horizontal and vertical position of a rear anti-tip device. *Archives of Physical Medicine and Rehabilitation* 75(5):525–534.

Lange, M., and M. Racicot. 1997. A comparison of wheelchair mounting systems. *TeamRehab Report* 8(6):14–15, 16.

Lynch, S.M., and S.L. Edwards. 1995. Meeting the challenge. *TeamRehab Report* 6(8):24–28.

Perks, B.A., R. Mackintosh, C.P.U. Stewart, et al. 1994. A survey of marginal wheelchair users. *Journal of Rehabilitation Research and Development* 31(4):297–302.

Perr, A., and K. Barnicle. 1993. Van lifts: The ups and downs and ins and outs. *TeamRehab Report* 4(4):49–53.

Petty, L., and S.S. Laurence. 1995. Pediatric power. *TeamRehab Report* 6(5):41–42, 44.

Rovig, S., and A. Hasdai. 1997. Randy moves on. *TeamRehab Report* 8(3):14–16,18

Rushmore, H., and E. Trefler. 1997. In focus. *TeamRehab Report* 8(6):41–43.

Saur, T. 1996. Jamie's dream machine. *TeamRehab Report* 7(8):38–41.

Stinnett, K.A. 1997. Geriatric seating and positioning within a wheeled mobility frame of reference in the long-term care setting. *Topics in Geriatric Rehabilitation* 13(2):75–84.

Thacker, J.G., S.H. Sprigle, and B.O. Morris. 1994. *Understanding the technology when selecting wheelchairs.* Arlington, VA: RESNA Press.

WORK HARDENING

Carranza, C.B. 1996. Work hardening. In *Rehabilitation of the spine: Science and practice*, eds. S.H. Hochschuler, H.B. Cotler, and R.D. Guyer, 741–746. St. Louis: Mosby.

Ziller, J., G. Sturm, and C.W. Cruse CW. 1993. Patients with burns are successful in work hardening programs. *Journal of Burn Care and Rehabilitation* 14(2, Part 1):189–196.

WORK-RELATED PROGRAMS

Holmes, D., and S.D. Lopez. 1998. How early is early? Onsite early return-to-work programs cut losses and costs. *Rehab Management* 11(2):28–33,35.

Howe, M.C. 1994. Work, productivity, and worth in old age. In *The clinical care of the aged person: An interdisciplinary perspective*, ed. D.G. Satin, 294–310. New York: Oxford University Press.

Kornblau, B.L. 1994. Occupational therapist's role in vocational evaluation. *Vocational Evaluation and Work Adjustment Bulletin* 27(4):154–159.

Index